FACIAL TRAUMA SURGERY

From Primary Repair
to Reconstruction

FACIAL TRAUMA SURGERY

From Primary Repair to Reconstruction

Amir H. Dorafshar MD, FACS, FAAP

John W. Curtin, MD Chair of Plastic and Reconstructive Surgery
Professor of Surgery and Neurological Surgery
Division of Plastic and Reconstructive Surgery
Rush University Medical Center
Chicago, IL, USA

Adjunct Professor
Department of Plastic and Reconstructive Surgery
Johns Hopkins University School of Medicine
Baltimore, MD, USA

Eduardo D. Rodriguez MD, DDS

Helen L. Kimmel Professor of Reconstructive Plastic Surgery
Hansjörg Wyss Department of Plastic Surgery
NYU Langone Medical Center
New York University
New York, NY, USA

Paul N. Manson MD

Distinguished Service Professor
Department of Plastic, Reconstructive and Maxillofacial Surgery
Johns Hopkins University School of Medicine
Professor of Surgery
R Adams Cowley Shock Trauma Center
University of Maryland School of Medicine
Baltimore, MD, USA

For additional online content visit ExpertConsult.com

ELSEVIER

Edinburgh   London   New York   Oxford   Philadelphia   St Louis   Sydney   2020

ISBN: 978-0-323-49755-8
E-ISBN: 978-0-323-50960-2

Content Strategist: Belinda Kuhn
Content Development Specialist: Sharon Nash
Project Manager: Anne Collett
Design: Ryan Cook
Illustration Manager: Amy Faith Heyden
Illustrator: MPS North America LLC
Marketing Manager: Claire McKenzie

Printed in China

Last digit is the print number: 9   8   7   6   5   4   3   2   1

Working together
to grow libraries in
developing countries

www.elsevier.com • www.bookaid.org

VIDEO CONTENTS

CONTENTS

Additional evidence-based content can be found online at expert consult.com

vii

"PRECISION MEDICINE" AND FACIAL INJURIES, 2018

In the past 30 years, much progress has occurred in the treatment of facial injuries with regard to classification, treatment options, timing, and technique of reductions of both the bone and soft tissue. Treatment planning options are numerous, and patient-specific implants and computerized plans are used more frequently. Facial injuries now benefit from refined classifications, which incorporate outcome data, which then cycle refinement of the classification and treatment options, producing a recurring cycle of continuous treatment improvements.

Since all disease occurs in patterns, recognition of the patterns of facial injuries allows the use of specific algorithms for management of the various categories, which include minimal, intermediate, and severe injuries to each anatomical portion of the facial skeleton. The recurring process of diagnosis, treatment, and outcome analysis yields progressive changes and improvements to both the taxonomy and thereby the future treatment algorithms, perpetuating the recurring cycle of improvement.[1,2]

Practically, division of the face by functional parts creates an anatomical treatment algorithm organized on "CT-based fracture classification"[3] determined by (1) anatomical area of the face and (2) the energy or "comminution and displacement" of the particular anatomical part injured.

The papers cited[3–8] propose a comprehensive treatment organization for both the bone and soft tissue. Functionally, there are four areas of the facial skeleton:

(I) Frontal bone (supraorbital and frontal sinus areas)
(II) Upper midface (zygomas and nasoethmoid)
(III) Lower midface and occlusion
(IV) Mandible (horizontal and vertical sections)

These papers[1–15] cover exposure, reduction, and fixation for each degree of bone injury (low energy – mild; middle energy – moderate; high energy – severe) in each anatomical area (zygoma, horizontal mandible, nasoethmoid, etc.), and then deal with how to improve the quality of the soft tissue in terms of the original injury, timing of fracture repair, and repair and replacement of soft tissue onto the anatomically restored facial skeleton.

Within each of the four areas, each section may be classified as minimally, moderately or severely displaced, and therefore treated with (a) no or (b) minimal open reduction, (c) a standard open reduction, or (d) an extended open reduction. The latter is reserved for the most comminuted and displaced fractures requiring multiple and complete exposures for alignment and fixation at all buttress articulations of a particular anatomical area.

For the zygomatic portion of a panfacial fracture, it could be so minimally displaced that no reduction would be necessary. More frequently, the standard minimally displaced zygoma (incomplete or "greensticked" at the zygomaticofrontal suture) could be approached by inferior alone approaches at the zygomatic buttress and inferior orbital rim. For the standard displacement, a more complete set of anterior incisions, the "anterior alone" approaches of the lower midface gingival buccal sulcus and upper/lower eyelid incisions, allows complete exposure and fixation of all anterior zygoma buttress articulations. The severely comminuted zygoma would require the anterior complete exposure plus the zygomatic arch (anterior and posterior exposures) via a coronal incision for reduction and fixation at each zygomatic buttress and within the orbit laterally and inferiorly.

Similarly, for the nasoethmoid area,[5] the simplest fractures would be undisplaced or "greensticked" at the articulation with the internal angular process of the frontal bone, and therefore would, like the "greensticked" zygoma, be amenable to inferior alone approaches where the infraorbital rim and pyriform aperture fractures are aligned and stabilized through only a gingival buccal sulcus incision, perhaps supplementing it with the eyelid for the next degree of severity. With increasing displacement and comminution of the nasoethmoidal orbital area, the lower eyelid and coronal approaches would have to be added to permit more complete exposure and perhaps also provide for detachment and reattachment of the medial canthal ligament in extreme cases.

The approaches and degree of fracture displacements would be summed over all the anatomical areas of fracture in the patient, permitting a comprehensive treatment plan for all areas to be developed for what is necessary in each area, and then an order of treatment is developed for the entire case, linking and sequencing the anatomical areas by a plan which combines segmental reductions. In this way, the treatment is the least (but still maximally effective) for each anatomical area according to the procedures necessary for each component of the fracture. Such approaches were first described in an article about "CT-based fracture treatment".[3]

Generally, my preference, if no neurosurgical urgency is present, is to begin with stabilization of the occlusion by reduction of the split palate and mandible alveolar fractures, and then to address the vertical and horizontal mandible. Or if one needs to begin in the frontal bone because of simultaneous brain injury, the frontal bone is reduced after defunctionalizing the frontal sinus; perhaps first using wires for temporary positioning, and then proceeding to rigid fixation after the multiple areas of reduction required are confirmed as accurate. Then, the upper midface could be reduced and stabilized, then completing the reduction of the lower face, then linking the upper and lower face at the Le Fort I level.

Several comments about the soft tissue bear repeating:

1. Every facial fracture has an injury to the soft tissue, and it may be minimal, moderate or severe. How the soft tissue responds (and therefore the ultimate quality and the position of the soft tissue) depends on when and what you do to the bone, and whether or not the soft tissue can respond by healing and remodeling over a precisely reconstructed bony facial skeleton. The early bone reduction and the repair of the incisions and refixation of the soft tissue to a reduced skeleton become the method of "treatment" of the soft tissue, the "soft tissue reduction".

2. Timing and facial fracture management: Since the soft tissue has an initial injury, it makes good sense to confine the incisions and dissection and repair to this initial injury period, rather than to create a second soft tissue injury with the definitive reduction in the vulnerable period of soft tissue healing 1–2 weeks after the initial soft tissue trauma.

   While many isolated, simple fractures may be operated on at any time after the injury with little compromise in the ultimate soft tissue quality, true high-energy facial injuries begin to develop soft tissue scar and contracture immediately from the time of the initial injury, and the soft tissue becomes stiffened, thicker, discolored, and less pliable with each day of initial healing.

   Soft tissue contracture and stiffness develop in the shape of the underlying displaced bone fracture. Making reduction incisions and dissecting in the "vulnerable period" 1–3 weeks after the initial injury creates a second set of soft tissue injuries from the surgery, further damaging the soft tissue, whereas confining the incisions to the initial injury period isolates the two soft tissue injuries to a single reaction where the soft tissue reacts to a single insult, yielding the best result one could achieve in terms of soft tissue quality and position.

3. Dehiscence and displacement of soft tissue: The layered closure of incisions prevents soft tissue dehiscence. Reattaching the repaired soft tissue to the facial skeleton places the soft tissue correctly over the reconstructed and realigned facial skeleton, allowing the soft tissue to heal in the correct position and with the correct contour. The shape and position of the bone are the pattern for the remodeling and repair by internal scar of the soft tissue injury. In some cases, such as the nasoethmoidal orbital area, placing soft tissue bolsters over the soft tissue pressing it against the maxilla and the lateral nose keeps the tissue aligned to the repaired facial skeleton over the complex contours and angles of the central upper midface area, prevents hematoma (minimizing excess fibrosis and thickness of soft tissue), and keeps the soft tissue stretched to length over the entire curving surface of the anatomically reduced bone.

These several considerations create a comprehensive plan for treatment of any facial injury, both for the bone and for the soft tissue. Of course, immediate bone grafting and microvascular flap transfer may be added where necessary to replace critical missing areas of the facial skeleton and soft tissue. Mismatched cutaneous soft tissue islands from microvascular transfer may be removed secondarily by serial excision or standard facial cutaneous flap reconstruction, covering the mismatched soft tissue added with a contoured area of soft tissue with matching cutaneous color.

So read on, enjoy, and benefit from the mastery of experienced practitioners who are ready to assist you with these difficult problems.

Paul N. Manson MD
Distinguished Service Professor of Plastic Surgery
Johns Hopkins School of Medicine
Professor of Surgery, The University of Maryland
R Adams Cowley Shock Trauma Unit

REFERENCES

1. Manson P, Clark N, Robertson B, et al. Subunit principles in midface fractures: the importance of sagittal buttresses, soft tissue reductions and sequencing treatment of segmental fractures. *Plast Reconstr Surg.* 1999;103:1287–1306.

2. Manson P, Markowitz B, Mirvis S, et al. Toward CT-based facial fracture treatment. *Plast Reconstr Surg.* 1990;85:202–212.

3. Markowitz B, Manson P, Sargent L, et al. Management of the medial canthal tendon in nasoethmoid orbital fractures: The importance of the central fragment in treatment and classification. *Plast Reconstr Surg.* 1991;87:843–853.

4. Crawley W, Clark N, Azman P, Manson P. The edentulous Le Fort fracture. *J Craniofacial Surg.* 1997;8:298–308.

5. Hendrickson M, Clark N, Manson P. Sagittal fractures of the maxilla: classification and treatment. *Plast Reconstr Surg.* 1998;101:319–332.

6. Rodriguez ED, Stanwix MG, Nam AJ, et al. Twenty-six-year experience treating frontal sinus fractures: a novel algorithm based on anatomical fracture pattern and failure of conventional techniques. *Plast Reconstr Surg.* 2008;122(6):1850–1866.

7. Manson PN, Stanwix M, Yaremchuk M, et al. Frontobasilar fractures: anatomy, classification and clinical significance. *Plast Reconstr Surg.* 2009;124:2096–2106.

8. Manson P, Iliff N. Management of blowout fractures of the orbital floor: early repair of selected injuries. *Surv Ophthalmol.* 1991;35:280–291.

9. Lee R, Gamble B, Manson P. Facial lacerations: patterns, associated injuries and the McFontz classification system. *Plast Reconstr Surg.* 1995;99:1544–1554.

10. Lee RH, Gamble B, Manson P, et al. Patterns of facial lacerations from blunt trauma. *Plast Reconstr Surg.* 1997;99:1544–1554.

11. Clark N, Birely B, Manson PN, et al. High-energy ballistic and avulsive facial injuries: classification, patterns, and an algorithm for primary reconstruction. *Plast Reconstr Surg.* 1996;98:583–601.

12. Robertson B, Manson P. The importance of serial debridement and "a second look" procedures in high-energy ballistic and avulsive facial injuries. *Oper Tech Plast Reconstr Surg.* 1998;5(3):236–246.

13. Rodriguez E, Martin M, Bluebond-Langner R, et al. Microsurgical reconstruction of post-traumatic high-energy maxillary defects: establishing the effectiveness of early reconstruction. *Plast Reconstr Surg.* 2007;120(7):103S–117S.

14. Rodriguez E, Bluebond-Langner R, Park J, et al. Preservation of contour in periorbital & midfacial craniofacial microsurgery: reconstruction of the soft tissue elements and skeletal buttresses. *Plast Reconstr Surg.* 2008;121(5):1738–1747.

15. Fisher M, Dorafshar A, Bojovic B, et al. The evolution of critical concepts in aesthetic craniofacial microsurgical reconstruction. *Plast Reconstr Surg.* 2012;130(2):389–398.

PREFACE

"If I have seen further it is by standing on the shoulders of Giants."
Isaac Newton, 1675

The idea for the genesis of this textbook originated from being invited to co-author a book chapter on facial trauma with Drs. Eduardo Rodriguez and Paul Manson in the fourth edition of Neligan's *Plastic Surgery* textbook. In helping to co-author this book chapter I realized that to provide a comprehensive text on the subject area in the limited number of words was impossible; we therefore decided to expand the book chapter into a textbook. The textbook initially set out to cover primary traumatic repair, but as we conceived the book chapters, we thought that no textbook on facial trauma surgery would be complete without describing delayed posttraumatic reconstruction.

This textbook has been based on the principles and concepts of craniofacial surgery for the care of patients with facial traumatic injuries that were originally described and taught by Dr. Paul Manson, and later expanded upon by Dr. Eduardo Rodriguez to include microsurgical applications to craniofacial reconstruction over the last 40 years at the R Adams Cowley Shock Trauma Center at the University of Maryland Medical Center. I have also tried to add my own perspective and insights, which I have gained over the last decade treating patients with traumatic facial injuries at the R Adams Cowley Shock Trauma Center and at the Johns Hopkins Hospital.

We decided to ask internationally recognized authors across the disciplines of Plastic and Reconstructive Surgery, Oral & Maxillofacial Surgery, Otolaryngology and Facial Plastic Surgery, Oculoplastic Surgery and Neurological Surgery to contribute their perspectives in their respective expert areas in the treatment of patients with craniofacial traumatic injuries. Each book chapter has a concluding "Expert Commentary" by Dr. Paul Manson offering his viewpoint on the subject. Several book chapters also include evidence-based summaries in areas of controversy and video attachments to supplement and clarify surgical technique. We have also included chapters on virtual surgical planning, 3D printing, intraoperative surgical navigation, and the roles of microsurgery and facial transplantation in the treatment of facial traumatic injuries to provide an advanced and modern approach.

This book is focused towards the young reconstructive surgeon or surgical trainee wishing to understand basic principles and concepts of primary traumatic facial injury repair and secondary facial reconstruction. It is designed to be of value to all the subspecialties of reconstructive surgery and we hope to improve the delivery of traumatic facial injury care to patient populations not only in the United States but around the world.

Amir H. Dorafshar MD, FACS, FAAP
John W. Curtin, MD Chair of Plastic and Reconstructive Surgery
Professor of Surgery and Neurological Surgery
Division of Plastic and Reconstructive Surgery
Rush University Medical Center, Chicago, IL, USA
Adjunct Professor
Department of Plastic and Reconstructive Surgery
Johns Hopkins University School of Medicine
Baltimore, MD, USA

LIST OF CONTRIBUTORS

Bizhan Aarabi MD, FRCSC
Professor
Department of Neurosurgery
University of Maryland Medical Center and
    R Adams Cowley Shock Trauma Center
Baltimore, MD, USA

**Zahid Afzal BDS, MBChB, MPhil
    (OMFS), MFDS RCS(Eng)**
Resident
Department of Oral and Maxillofacial
    Surgery
University of Maryland
Baltimore, MD, USA

Majd Al Mardini DDS, MBA, FRCD(C)
Director of Ocular and Maxillofacial
    Prosthetics Unit
Department of Dentistry and Maxillofacial
    Prosthetics
University Health Network, Princess
    Margaret Cancer Center
Toronto, ON, Canada

Brian Alpert DDS, FACD, FICD, FACS
Professor of Oral and Maxillofacial Surgery
University of Louisville School of Dentistry;
Chief, Oral and Maxillofacial Surgery and
    Dentistry
University of Louisville Hospital
Louisville, KY, USA

Oleh Antonyshyn MD, FRCSC
Associate Professor
Department of Plastic and Reconstructive
    Surgery
University of Toronto
Toronto, ON, Canada

Krystal Archer-Arroyo MD
Assistant Professor
Department of Radiology and Nuclear
    Medicine
University of Maryland School of Medicine
Baltimore, MD, USA

Said C Azoury MD
Resident Physician
Division of Plastic Surgery
Department of Surgery University of
    Pennsylvania Health System
Philadelphia, PA, USA

Craig Birgfeld MD, FACS
Associate Professor
Department of Surgery, Division of Plastic
    Surgery
University of Washington
Seattle, WA USA

Kofi D.O. Boahene MD
Associate Professor
Department of Otolaryngology – Head and
    Neck Surgery
Johns Hopkins University School of
    Medicine
Baltimore, MD, USA

Colin M. Brady MD
Craniofacial Fellow
Division of Plastic and Maxillofacial Surgery
Department of Surgery
University of Southern California
Los Angeles, CA, USA

Steven R. Buchman MD
M. Haskell Newman Professor in Plastic
    Surgery
Professor of Neurosurgery, University of
    Michigan Medical School;
Chief, Pediatric Plastic Surgery, CS Mott
    Children's Hospital;
Director, Craniofacial Anomalies Program,
    University of Michigan Medical Center
University of Michigan Medical Center
Ann Arbor, MI, USA

Patrick Byrne MD, MBA
Professor and Director
Division of Facial Plastic and Reconstructive
    Surgery
Department of Otolaryngology – Head and
    Neck Surgery
Johns Hopkins School of Medicine
Baltimore, MD, USA

Daniel Cantu DDS
Philip J. Boyne and Peter Geistlich Research
    Fellow
Department of Oral and Maxillofacial
    Surgery
Loma Linda University
Loma Linda, CA, USA

John P. Carey MD
Professor and Division Chief for Otology,
    Neurotology and Skull Base Surgery
Department of Otolaryngology – Head and
    Neck Surgery
Johns Hopkins University School of
    Medicine
Baltimore, MD, USA

**Edward H. Davidson MD, MA (Cantab),
    MBBS**
Assistant Professor
Department of Plastic Surgery and
    Reconstructive Surgery
Montefiore Medical Center
Albert Einstein College of Medicine
Bronx, NY, USA

Kristopher M. Day MD
Plastic Surgery Resident
Department of Plastic Surgery
University of Tennessee Chattanooga
Chattanooga, TN, USA

A. Lee Dellon MD, PhD
Professor of Plastic Surgery and Professor of
    Neurosurgery
Johns Hopkins University
Baltimore, MD, USA

Sarah W. DeParis MD
Oculoplastic Surgeon
Department of Ophthalmology
The Permanente Medical Group
San Rafael, CA, USA

J. Rodrigo Diaz-Siso MD
Postdoctoral Research Fellow
Hansjörg Wyss Department of Plastic
    Surgery
New York University Langone Medical
    Center
New York, NY, USA

Amir H. Dorafshar, MD, FACS, FAAP
John W. Curtin, MD Chair of Plastic and
    Reconstructive Surgery
Professor of Surgery and Neurological
    Surgery
Division of Plastic and Reconstructive Surgery
Rush University Medical Center
Chicago, IL, USA
Adjunct Professor
Department of Plastic and Reconstructive
    Surgery
Johns Hopkins University School of Medicine
Baltimore, MD, USA

Edward Ellis III, DDS, MS
Professor and Chair
Department of Oral and Maxillofacial
    Surgery
University of Texas Health Science Center at
    San Antonio
San Antonio, TX, USA

Jeffrey Fialkov MD, MSc FRCSC
Associate Professor
Department of Plastic and Reconstructive
    Surgery
University of Toronto
Toronto, ON, Canada

Robert L. Flint DMD, MD
Assistant Professor of Oral and Maxillofacial
    Surgery
University of Louisville School of Dentistry
Louisville, KY, USA

**Christopher R. Forrest MD, MSc,
    FRCSC, FACS**
Chief, Plastic and Reconstructive Surgery,
    Medical Director
The Centre for Craniofacial Care and
    Research
The Hospital for Sick Children
Toronto, ON, Canada;
Chair/Professor
Division of Plastic and Reconstructive
    Surgery
University of Toronto
Department of Surgery
Toronto, ON, Canada

Nils-Claudius Gellrich MD, DDS
Professor and Chair
Department of Oral and Maxillofacial
    Surgery
Hannover Medical School
Hannover, Germany

Dane J. Genther MD
Professional Staff
Division of Facial Plastic and Reconstructive
    Surgery
Department of Otolaryngology – Head and
    Neck Surgery
Head and Neck Institute
Cleveland Clinic
Cleveland, OH, USA

Jesse A. Goldstein MD
Assistant Professor of Pediatric Plastic
    Surgery
Department of Plastic Surgery
Children's Hospital of Pittsburgh
University of Pittsburgh Medical Center
Pittsburgh, PA, USA

Chad R. Gordon DO, FACS
Director, Neuroplastic and Reconstructive
    Surgery
Fellowship Director, Neuroplastic &
    Reconstructive Surgery (Plastic Surgery)
Co-Director, Multidisciplinary Adult
    Cranioplasty Center
Associate Professor of Plastic Surgery and
    Neurosurgery
Department of Plastic and Reconstructive
    Surgery
Johns Hopkins University School of
    Medicine

Michael Grant MD, PhD, FACS
Professor and Chief
Trauma Plastics
R Adams Cowley Shock Trauma Center
University of Maryland School of Medicine
Baltimore, MD, USA

Joseph S. Gruss MD
Professor
Division of Plastic Surgery
Seattle Children's Hospital
University of Washington
Seattle, WA, USA

Corbett A. Haas DDS MD
Resident in Oral and Maxillofacial Surgery
Department of Oral and Maxillofacial
    Surgery
Harvard School of Dental Medicine/
    Harvard Medical School
Massachusetts General Hospital
Boston, MA, USA

Alan S. Herford DDS, MD, FACS
Professor and Chair
Department of Oral and Maxillofacial
    Surgery
Loma Linda University
Loma Linda, CA, USA

Larry H. Hollier MD, FACS, FAAP
Surgeon in Chief
Texas Children's Hospital
S. Baron Hardy Endowed Chair
Professor of Plastic Surgery, Orthopedic
    Surgery, and Pediatrics
Chief of Plastic Surgery
Baylor College of Medicine
Houston, TX, USA

Richard A. Hopper MD
Professor
Division of Plastic Surgery
Seattle Children's Hospital
University of Washington
Seattle, WA, USA

Matthew G. Huddle MD
Resident Physician
Department of Otolaryngology – Head and
    Neck Surgery
Johns Hopkins School of Medicine
Baltimore, MD, USA

Lewis C. Jones DMD, MD
Adjunct
Assistant Professor of Oral and Maxillofacial
    Surgery
University of Louisville School of Dentistry
Louisville, KY, USA

Bartlomiej Kachniarz MD, MBA
Resident Physician
Plastic and Reconstructive Surgery
Johns Hopkins University School of
    Medicine
Baltimore, MD, USA

Leslie Kim MD, MPH
Assistant Professor and Director
Division of Facial Plastic and Reconstructive
    Surgery
Department of Otolaryngology – Head and
    Neck Surgery
The Ohio State University School of
    Medicine
Columbus, OH, USA

George M. Kushner DMD, MD, FACS
Professor of Oral and Maxillofacial Surgery
    and Residency Program Director
University of Louisville School of Dentistry
Louisville, KY, USA

Matthew E. Lawler DMD MD
Resident in Oral and Maxillofacial Surgery
Department of Oral and Maxillofacial
    Surgery
Harvard School of Dental Medicine/
    Harvard Medical School
Massachusetts General Hospital
Boston, MA, USA

Andrew Lee MD
Resident Physician
Division of Otology, Neurotology and Skull
    Base Surgery
Department of Otolaryngology – Head and
    Neck Surgery
Johns Hopkins University School of
    Medicine
Baltimore, MD, USA

Jeffrey Lee MD
Craniofacial Reconstructive and Aesthetic
 Surgery Fellow
Division of Plastic and Reconstructive
 Surgery
Massachusetts General Hospital
Boston, MA, USA

Jonathan Y. Lee MD, MPH
Craniofacial and Pediatric Plastic Surgery
 Fellow
Department of Plastic Surgery
Children's Hospital of Pittsburgh
University of Pittsburgh Medical Center
Pittsburgh, PA, USA

Fan Liang MD
Assistant Professor
Trauma Plastics
R Adams Cowley Shock Trauma Center
University of Maryland School of Medicine
Baltimore, MD, USA

Joseph Lopez MD, MBA
Resident
Department of Plastic and Reconstructive
 Surgery
Johns Hopkins Medical Institution
Baltimore, MD, USA

Joseph E. Losee MD
Ross H. Musgrave Professor of Pediatric
 Plastic Surgery
Department of Plastic Surgery
Children's Hospital of Pittsburgh
University of Pittsburgh Medical Center
Pittsburgh, PA, USA

Matthew R. Louis MD
Resident
Department of Plastic and Reconstructive
 Surgery
Johns Hopkins Hospital
Baltimore, MD

**Alexandra Macmillan MA (Cantab.),
 MBBS**
Research Fellow
Department of Plastic and Reconstructive
 Surgery
Johns Hopkins Medical Institution
Baltimore, MD, USA

Paul N. Manson MD
Distinguished Service Professor
Department of Plastic, Reconstructive and
 Maxillofacial Surgery
Johns Hopkins University School of
 Medicine;
Professor of Surgery
R Adams Cowley Shock Trauma Center
University of Maryland School of Medicine
Baltimore, MD, USA

Meagan Miller DDS
Resident
Department of Oral and Maxillofacial
 Surgery
Loma Linda University
Loma Linda, CA, USA

Shannath L. Merbs MD, PhD, FACS
Professor
Departments of Ophthalmology and
 Oncology
Johns Hopkins University School of
 Medicine
Baltimore, MD, USA

Stuart E. Mirvis MD, FACR
Retired Professor, Department of Radiology
 and Nuclear Medicine
University of Maryland School of Medicine
Baltimore, MD, USA

Corey M. Mossop MD
Interim Chief – Neurosurgery Service and
 Instructor
Department of Surgery
Tripler Army Medical Center and the
 Uniformed Services University of the
 Health Sciences
Honolulu, HI and Bethesda, MD, USA

Gerhard S. Mundinger MD
Assistant Professor, Plastic and
 Reconstructive Surgery
Assistant Professor, Department of Cell
 Biology and Anatomy
Craniofacial Center Director
Director of Pediatric Plastic Surgery
Children's Hospital of New Orleans
Louisiana State University Health Sciences
 Center
New Orleans, LA, USA

Arthur J. Nam MD, MS
Assistant Professor
Division of Plastic, Reconstructive and
 Maxillofacial Surgery
R Adams Cowley Shock Trauma Center
University of Maryland School of Medicine
Baltimore, MD, USA

Lauren T. Odono DDS
Oral Maxillofacial Surgery Resident
Division of Plastic and Maxillofacial Surgery
Department of Surgery
University of Southern California
Los Angeles, CA, USA

Devin O'Brien-Coon MD, MSE
Assistant Professor
Department of Plastic and Reconstructive
 Surgery
Johns Hopkins University School of
 Medicine
Baltimore, MD, USA

Ira D. Papel MD
Professor
Division of Facial Plastic and Reconstructive
 Surgery
Department of Otolaryngology – Head and
 Neck Surgery
Johns Hopkins University School of
 Medicine
Facial Plastic Surgicenter
Baltimore, MD, USA

Zachary S. Peacock DMD, MD, FACS
Assistant Professor
Department of Oral and Maxillofacial
 Surgery
Harvard School of Dental Medicine/
 Harvard Medical School
Massachusetts General Hospital
Boston, MA, USA

Daniel Perez DDS
Associate Professor
Department of Oral and Maxillofacial
 Surgery
University of Texas Health Science Center at
 San Antonio
San Antonio, TX, USA

Christian Petropolis MD, FRCSC
Assistant Professor
Department of Plastic and Reconstructive
 Surgery
University of Manitoba
Winnipeg, MB, Canada

David B. Powers MD, DMD, FACS, FRCS (Ed)
Associate Professor of Surgery
Director, Duke Craniomaxillofacial Trauma
    Program
Duke University Medical Center
Durham, NC, USA

Andrew M. Read-Fuller MD, DDS
Clinical Assistant Professor, Oral and
    Maxillofacial Surgery
Texas A&M University College of Dentistry
    and Baylor University Medical Center
Dallas, TX, USA

Richard J. Redett MD
Professor
Department of Plastic and Reconstructive
    Surgery
Johns Hopkins University School of
    Medicine
Baltimore, MD, USA

Likith V. Reddy MD, DDS, FACS
Clinical Professor and Program Director
Department of Oral and Maxillofacial
    Surgery
Texas A&M University College of Dentistry
    and Baylor University Medical Center;
Clinical Professor, Surgery
Texas A&M University College of Medicine
Dallas, TX, USA

Sashank Reddy MD, PhD
Resident
Department of Plastic and Reconstructive
    Surgery
Johns Hopkins Medical Institution
Baltimore, MD, USA

Douglas D. Reh MD
Associate Professor, Otolaryngology – Head
    and Neck Surgery
Department of Otolaryngology – Head and
    Neck Surgery
Johns Hopkins University School of
    Medicine
Baltimore, MD, USA

Isabel Robinson BA
Medical Student
Hansjörg Wyss Department of Plastic
    Surgery
New York University Langone Medical
    Center
New York, NY, USA

Eduardo D. Rodriguez MD, DDS
Helen L. Kimmel Professor of
    Reconstructive Plastic Surgery
Hansjörg Wyss Department of Plastic
    Surgery
New York University Langone Medical
    Center
New York, NY, USA

Christopher R. Roxbury MD
Resident
Department of Otolaryngology – Head and
    Neck Surgery
Johns Hopkins University School of
    Medicine
Baltimore, MD, USA

Shai M. Rozen MD, FACS
Professor of Plastic and Reconstructive
    Surgery
Director of Microsurgery
Director of The Facial Palsy Program
Director of Clinical Research
Department of Plastic and Reconstructive
    Surgery
UT Southwestern Medical Center
Dallas, TX, USA

Larry Sargent MD, FACS, FAAP
Board-Certified Plastic and Craniofacial
    Surgeon
Sargent Plastic Surgery
Salt Lake City, UT, USA

Tatyana A. Shamliyan MD, MS
Senior Director
Evidence-Based Medicine Quality Assurance
Elsevier Inc.
Philadelphia, PA, USA

David A. Shaye MD
Instructor
Department of Otolaryngology
Harvard Medical School
Massachusetts Eye & Ear
Boston, MA, USA

Ghassan G. Sinada DDS, MBA
Director, Oral Oncology and Maxillofacial
    Prosthodontics
Milton J. Dance Jr. Head and Neck Cancer
    Center
Greater Baltimore Medical Center
Baltimore, MD, USA

Ryan M. Smith MD
Assistant Professor, Facial Plastic Surgery
    and Reconstruction
Department of Otorhinolaryngology – Head
    and Neck Surgery
Rush University Medical Center
Chicago, IL, USA

Mark W. Stalder MD
Assistant Professor of Clinical Surgery
Division of Plastic and Reconstructive
    Surgery
Louisiana State University Health Sciences
    Center
New Orleans, LA, USA

E. Bradley Strong MD
Professor
Department of Otolaryngology
University of California at Davis
Sacramento, CA, USA

Marcelo Suzuki DDS
Associate Professor
Assistant Division Head, Undergraduate
    Prosthodontics
Department of Prosthodontics
Tufts University School of Dental Medicine
Boston, MA, USA

Jeffrey G. Trost Jr. MD
Resident
Division of Plastic and Reconstructive
    Surgery
Baylor College of Medicine
Houston, TX, USA

Anthony P. Tufaro DDS, MD, FACS
Professor of Surgery, Plastic Surgery &
    Surgical Oncology
Department of Surgery
University of Oklahoma Health Science
    Center
Oklahoma City, OK, USA

Mark Urata, MD, DDS, FACS, FAAP
Audrey Skirball Kenis Endowed Chair and
    Chief
Division of Plastic and Reconstructive
    Surgery
Chair, Keck School of Medicine of USC
Division of Oral and Maxillofacial Surgery
Ostrow School of Dentistry of USC
Los Angeles, CA, USA

Christian J. Vercler MD, MA, FACS, FAAP
Associate Professor
Section of Plastic Surgery
Department of Surgery
University of Michigan Medical Center
Ann Arbor, MI, USA

Gary Warburton DDS, MD, FDSRCS, FACS
Associate Professor
Program Director & Division Chief Oral & Maxillofacial Surgery
University of Maryland
Baltimore, MD, USA

Heather M. Weinreich, MD MPH
Assistant Professor
Department of Otolaryngology – Head and Neck Surgery
University of Illinois
Chicago, IL, USA

Tyler Wildey MD, DDS
Past Resident, Oral and Maxillofacial Surgery
Texas A&M University College of Dentistry and Baylor University Medical Center
Dallas, TX, USA

S. Anthony Wolfe MD
Chief, Division of Plastic Surgery
Miami Children's Health System
Miami, FL, USA

Bradford A. Woodworth MD
James J. Hicks Professor of Otolaryngology
Department of Otolaryngology – Head and Neck Surgery
University of Alabama at Birmingham
Birmingham, AL, USA

Robin Yang DDS, MD
Chief Resident
Department of Plastic and Reconstructive Surgery
Johns Hopkins University
Baltimore, MD, USA

Michael J. Yaremchuk MD
Clinical Professor of Surgery, Harvard Medical School
Chief of Craniofacial Surgery, Massachusetts General Hospital
Boston, MA, USA

Elizabeth Zellner MD
Craniofacial Fellow
The Centre for Craniofacial Care and Research
Division of Plastic and Reconstructive Surgery
The Hospital for Sick Children
Toronto, ON, Canada

Rüdiger M. Zimmerer MD, DDS
Assistant Professor and Consultant
Department of Oral and Maxillofacial Surgery
Hannover Medical School
Hannover, Germany

ACKNOWLEDGMENTS

While there are too many people to name individually in this acknowledgment section, I would like to mention the enormous gratitude I have for the author contributors to this book who have come together from various subspecialties to give their unique perspectives on facial trauma surgery for this multidisciplinary comprehensive textbook. I greatly appreciate the sacrifice of their time taken away from their families, friends and practices to make this book a reality. Shianne Pietrowksi, my administrative assistant, who helped with the formatting and re-typing of several book chapters, deserves special recognition for her humor and determination to help me get through the multiple revisions of each chapter. The team at Elsevier, particularly Sharon, Belinda, Elaine and Tatyana, whom I have worked with individually and collectively through various phases of the book, have been excellent throughout. Lastly, I would like to thank my close family and friends for your patience with me for the many nights and weekends that I have not been present or with you. Your encouragement and support have been instrumental in my determination to complete this book.

Amir H. Dorafshar
January 2019

First and foremost, I would like to thank God for providing me the opportunity to share the knowledge of my fellow authors with you. Next, to my parents who sacrificed their lives for me to succeed; to my mentors who helped inspire me; to my trainees who have made me a better teacher; and to my patients who have taught me humility.

Assessment of the Patient With Traumatic Facial Injury

Arthur J. Nam, Edward H. Davidson, Paul N. Manson

BACKGROUND

Incidence of Facial Trauma in the United States and Worldwide

The spectrum of facial trauma includes soft tissue and bone, and ranges from the simple to the complex. Epidemiology varies with local and global demographic factors and reflects a complex interplay of influences, including those related to the environment, economics, age, gender, and mechanism of injury. Any understanding of the incidence of facial trauma is further confounded by the presumptive underreporting and treatment of minor injuries. As a result, the plethora of data is often conflicting. Nonetheless, the incidence of facial fractures presenting to the emergency room is approximately 500,000 per year in the United States, with nasal fractures likely the most common, followed by mandible fractures.[1] These commonly occur in males more than females, are most frequent in the second and third decades of life, and are most frequently the result of altercations, assaults, falls, work or home accidents, and motor vehicle or motorcycle collisions (MVCs). While many studies cite mandible fractures as being more common than nasal fractures, this has been attributed to a sampling bias favoring inpatient admissions or requirement for in-hospital treatment rather than capturing all emergency room presentations. Several older studies show higher rates of injury from MVCs, prior to the mandatory implementation of airbags and restraining devices.[2] Despite this, MVCs remain the most important cause of facial trauma all over the world. Global trends also reflect an increase in the male/female injury ratio in countries where the social custom is for women to be more confined to the home.[3] Associated soft tissue trauma is the most common concomitant injury, occurring in approximately 30% of facial fractures. Concomitant fractures of the skull, upper limbs, and associated areas are estimated to occur in around 25% of facial fractures; these include intracranial injuries in 12%–45.5%, and associated cervical spine injury with facial injury in up to 9.7%.[1,4] One must therefore always exclude brain and cervical spine injuries in the patient with facial injuries as trauma is often a geographic injury to the head and neck. Missed injuries of the spine, extremities, and pelvis are also frequent (10%) and are easily missed.

Patterns of Facial Trauma and Causes

Patterns of facial injuries may be subdivided into soft tissue, bony skeleton, and/or dentoalveolar trauma. Descriptions can also be made based on location in facial thirds: the upper third (including the frontal bone, frontal sinuses, and orbital roofs), middle third (including the orbit, nose, malar region, and maxilla), and lower third (including the mandible and its dentition) (Fig. 1.1.1). Blunt trauma can result in relatively predictable fracture patterns due to the presence of facial buttresses and resultant functional skeletal units (Fig. 1.1.2).[5] Injury to the upper third may reveal frontal sinus fractures, which require the determination of whether injury affects the inner table, outer table, or both, degree of displacement, and the presence of nasofrontal outflow tract obstruction.[6] Midface fracture patterns may include the characteristic Le Fort fracture patterns, but are more frequently asymmetric and more extensive on the side of the force application, or orbito-zygomaticomaxillary complex (OZMC), orbital, nasal and naso-orbito-ethmoid (NOE) fractures in isolation or in combination. Lower third facial fractures, i.e., those of the mandible, also demonstrate reproducible patterns. The most prevalent site of mandibular fracture reported in the literature is variable, though mandibular angle and condyle are the most frequently cited.[7] Based on the mandibular "ring" concept, mandibular fractures have conventionally been thought to involve at least two sites, however, unifocal mandibular fractures commonly occur. Common multifocal patterns include mandibular body and contralateral angle/ramus/condyle, angle and contralateral parasymphysis, symphysis/parasymphysis, and bilateral condyle. True panfacial fractures involve all thirds of the face simultaneously and are less involved on the contralateral side, both in terms of fracture extent and comminution.[8] These fracture patterns differ depending on mechanism, with most panfacial fractures usually resulting from MVCs and, less commonly, from gunshot wounds (GSWs). Sports injuries typically are isolated to the mandible or upper midface, and assaults are predictive of isolated mandible, midface or zygoma fractures. MVCs and GSWs each predict a higher severity of injury than assaults, falls, or sports injuries.[9,10]

Patterns of facial trauma in the pediatric population differ from those in adults. Facial fractures are relatively less common in children due to parental supervision as well as intrinsic anatomical factors such as larger fat pads, decreased pneumatization of sinuses, increased skeletal flexibility secondary to more malleable bone stock, and compliant sutures. The large cranium partially shields the rest of the face from injury. Atypical craniofacial fracture patterns precede the Le Fort patterns seen in adulthood and as an incompletely pneumatized frontal sinus transmits energy directly from the site of impact to the supraorbital foramen and then to the orbit, superior NOE and anterior maxillary wall or zygoma.[11,12] Younger patients are at higher risk of dentoalveolar trauma, including crown fractures (the most common injury), luxations, avulsions, subluxations, root fractures, and intrusions, with approximately one-third occurring in those younger than 10 years of age. These most often result from activities of daily living, play, MVCs, and sports.[13]

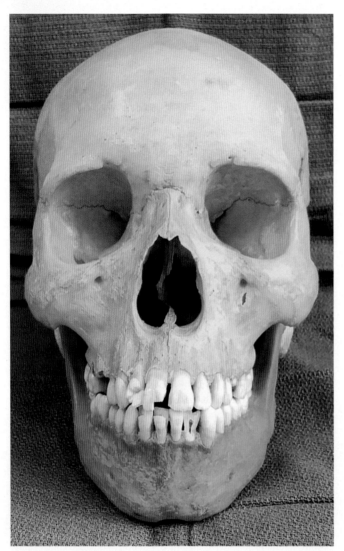

Fig. 1.1.1 Facial skeleton in thirds: upper (*yellow*), middle (*blue*), lower (*pink*).

The relative incidence of fracture patterns is debated; mandible fractures are often cited as the most common pediatric facial fracture, accounting for 20%–50% of all pediatric facial fractures.[14–17] Anatomical distribution varies with age; isolated condylar fracture incidence decreases, while body and angle fractures increase.[18] Others have reported that nasal fractures comprise up to 50% of pediatric facial fractures, but usually escape hospital registries.[14,19] Nasal and maxillary fractures were the most common osseous injuries among infants in the US National Trauma Databank, while mandible fractures were more common in older teenagers, with mandible fractures being the overall most common facial fracture.[20] Nasal fractures are likely often underreported, with many treated as an outpatient or not treated and thus not reported.[21] One review found 54% of fractures to occur in the skull, one-third in the upper and middle thirds of the face, and the remainder in the lower third.[22] Another group stratified patients by dental maturity – primary, mixed, and permanent dentition – and concluded orbital fracture was the most common fracture type for all age groups combined. This group showed activities of daily living as the most common cause of injury in 0- to 5-year-olds, MVCs, sports, and play in ages 6–11, and violence, sports, and MVCs as the most common causes of injury in 12- to 18-year-olds.[23]

Similarly, fracture patterns, demographics, and mechanisms of injury differ significantly between geriatric and nongeriatric adult craniofacial trauma patients. Falls are more frequent causes of fractures in geriatric patients whereas assaults, MVCs, and pedestrians struck were significantly more frequent causes in the nongeriatric adult population. Mandible fractures and panfacial fractures are more common in the nongeriatric population while higher incidences of orbital floor, maxillary, and condylar fractures are more common in geriatric patients and are dependent on geriatric age status, rather than mechanism of injury alone.[24,25] The most common cause of soft tissue injury has been shown to be falls and therefore older people seem excessively prone to this injury.

Penetrating soft tissue trauma, including that resulting from bites, stab wounds, gunshot, and other ballistic injuries, can result in injury configurations and fracture patterns that fall outside the usual predictable blunt trauma patterns. Distribution of soft tissue injury is frequently concentrated in a "T-shaped" area that includes the forehead, nose, lips, and chin as well as commonly affecting the lateral brows, malar eminences, forehead, and occiput.[26] Patterns may be described by facial

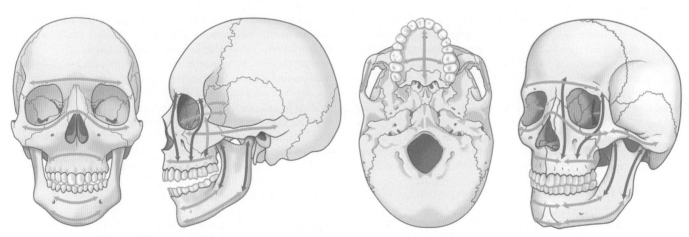

Fig. 1.1.2 Transverse (*blue*), vertical (*red*), and sagittal (*green*) buttresses of the facial skeleton. (From Prein J, Ehrenfeld M, Manson PN, editors. Principles of internal fixation of the craniomaxillofacial skeleton: trauma and orthognathic surgery. AO Foundation, Thieme; 2012, Fig. 1.3.1-5, p.24.)

aesthetic units[27] or in reference to bony landmarks. Depth and structures suspected to be injured are also important considerations, especially the globe, eyelids, canthi, lacrimal system, lips, nose, facial nerve, and parotid duct. Ballistic injuries including GSWs are further uniquely characterized by blast vasospasm.[28] These may be further complicated by a combination of blunt, penetrating, and burn injuries.[29]

These patterns of injury and interplay with epidemiology, mechanism, and patient demographics emphasize the importance of a meticulous history and a sequential and directed physical examination as central to the evaluation of a patient with facial trauma. This process collects information that predicts the injury pattern, which is further documented by examination and radiographs to serve as a basis for diagnosis and management.

SURGICAL ANATOMY

Facial Soft Tissue Anatomy

Knowledge of the functional anatomy of the face is fundamental to the understanding of facial trauma management. Important soft tissue considerations are the exact locations of the unique structures of the face and their relations to aesthetic units, layers of the face, and surface landmarks of deep structures such as the lacrimal system, Stenson's duct, and neurovascular networks, including facial nerve "danger zones"[30] (Fig. 1.1.3). The eyelids, nose, ears, and lips are unique structures of the face. A detailed description of their component tissues is beyond the scope of this chapter but an appreciation of this detailed anatomy is vital for reapproximation, repair, and reconstruction following injury and is found in individual sections dealing with regional areas. Similarly,

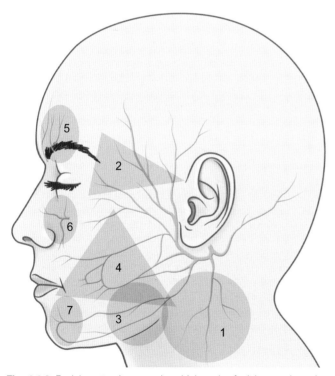

Fig. 1.1.3 Facial anatomic zones in which major facial nerve branches are susceptible to injury. Zone 1 – great auricular nerve; Zone 2 – temporal branch of VII; Zone 3 – marginal mandibular branch of VII; Zone 4 – zygomatic and buccal branches of VII; Zone 5 – supraorbital and supratrochlear nerves of V_1; Zone 6 – infraorbital nerve of V_2; Zone 7 – mental nerve of V_3. (Modified from Holzman NL, Doherty ST, Seckel BR. Facial nerve danger zones, Fig. 7-1. Plastic Surgery Key. https://plasticsurgerykey.com/facial-nerve-danger-zones/.)

aesthetic facial subunits and the lines of skin tension (Langer's lines) can help guide soft tissue repair strategy. The tenet from tumor surgery that loss of more than 50% of a subunit requires consideration of excision of the remainder of that subunit and reconstruction of it as a whole should be considered, but may not be as valid in youth or in cutaneous facial injury. The soft tissue planes of the face from superficial to deep are skin, subcutaneous fat, superficial musculoaponeurotic system (SMAS), containing mimetic muscles, deep fascia and fat compartments, and periosteum. The lacrimal system is the apparatus that produces tears and manages their transfer and drainage; it extends from the lacrimal gland in the lateral upper eyelid, over the corneal surface to the lacrimal canaliculi, through the lacrimal sac and the nasolacrimal duct to the inferior meatus of the nose. Injuries in the region of the eyelids, medial canthus, and upper lateral posterior nasal region should raise suspicion of potential injury to these structures. Stenson's duct is the conduit for saliva from the parotid gland to the mouth, emerging at a papilla adjacent to the second maxillary molar. An evaluation of Stenson's duct integrity is important in deep lacerations of the central cheek (especially those that occur near a reference line from the tragus to the lateral oral commissure). Sialocele, fistulae, and infection follow duct or gland injury. The trigeminal nerve branches that supply sensory innervation to the face may be injured as they exit bony foramina approximately in line with the mid-pupil, the supraorbital foramen/notch, infraorbital foramen, and mental foramen for the three principal sensory branches of V_1, V_2, and V_3 respectively. The blood supply to the face is exceedingly robust and focal injury of single vessels rarely results in clinically significant tissue ischemia in otherwise virgin tissue due to efficient and profuse collateral supply. Injury to the facial artery and its branches such as the labial arteries of the lips, the superficial temporal artery, angular vessels and its other branches can cause significant bleeding and, if untreated, near exsanguination. Identification of foci of blood loss, along with ability to control epistaxis, are essential for control of bleeding from facial injuries as discussed further below. Facial nerve deficit can be one of the most devastating ramifications of an injury to the face. While the facial nerve can be injured anywhere along its course, there are "danger zones" where it is particularly vulnerable to injury; the temporal branch along Pitanguy's line (from 0.5 cm below the tragus to 1.5 cm above the lateral eyebrow), the zygomatic and buccal branches around Zuker's point (halfway point along a reference line from the helical root to the oral commissure),[31] and the marginal mandibular branch overlying the inferior mandibular body border. Nerve injuries medial to the lateral canthus are less clinically significant due to arborization of the nerve, but any cut nerve seen should be repaired. For those more proximal branches, operative exploration and repair within 72 hours optimizes recovery of motor function.

Facial Skeletal Anatomy

The structural support of the facial skeleton may be organized by the description of the facial buttresses. Nasofrontal/nasomaxillary, zygomatic, and pterygomaxillary buttresses are the major structures of vertical support of the maxilla; mandibular, maxillary–palatal, zygomatic, and frontal buttress are responsible for anteroposterior projection; and the orbital buttress has both vertical and horizontal components (see Fig. 1.1.2). These are the supporting pillars of the facial skeleton; alignment and stabilization following injury literally provides the bony foundation for the restoration of facial form and support.[5]

Adult and Primary Dentition and Nomenclature

Assessment of dental trauma requires fluent knowledge of the nomenclature of dentition, both adult (permanent) and primary (deciduous) teeth. There are 20 primary teeth denoted by letters A to T proceeding from upper right second molar (A), to upper left second molar (J),

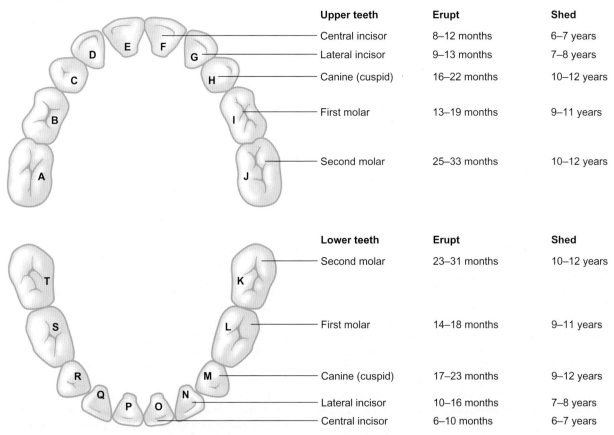

Upper teeth	Erupt	Shed
Central incisor	8–12 months	6–7 years
Lateral incisor	9–13 months	7–8 years
Canine (cuspid)	16–22 months	10–12 years
First molar	13–19 months	9–11 years
Second molar	25–33 months	10–12 years

Lower teeth	Erupt	Shed
Second molar	23–31 months	10–12 years
First molar	14–18 months	9–11 years
Canine (cuspid)	17–23 months	9–12 years
Lateral incisor	10–16 months	7–8 years
Central incisor	6–10 months	6–7 years

Fig. 1.1.4 Primary teeth nomenclature and eruption chart.

then lower left second molar (K) to lower right second molar (T) (Fig. 1.1.4). Similarly, permanent teeth are denoted by numbers 1–32 from upper right third molar (1) to upper left third molar (16) and then lower left third molar (17) to lower right third molar (32) (Fig. 1.1.5). The mandibular first molar is the first permanent tooth to erupt, typically at 6 years, followed by incisors at age 6–9, then canines between 9 and 12 years, first premolars at 10–11, second premolars at 11–12, second molars at 11–13, and finally third molars around 17–21 years of age. There is specific anatomical terminology for orientation when referencing teeth, namely mesial (towards midline) and distal (away from midline) in reference to the dental arch, as well as lingual (towards tongue)/palatal (towards palate) versus buccal (towards cheek), labial (toward the lip) (Fig. 1.1.6).

The practical application of the anatomy of the soft tissue, osseous, and dentoalveolar structures enables accurate diagnosis and nomenclature of facial injury, forms the basis for surgical exposure of the craniofacial skeleton, and as such is the cornerstone of fracture management. Incisions and exposures must be designed to respect aesthetic units, navigating the various layers of the face without injury to vital structures, preserving nerves and vessels to expose underlying fractures and skeletal buttresses.

CLASSIFICATION

There is no widely adopted classification of facial trauma that encompasses all of the soft tissue, dentoalveolar, and bony injuries. Rather, certain injury patterns do have well described and accepted classification systems, such as Le Fort fractures, NOE fractures, and dentoalveolar fractures, and each will be discussed below. Facial injuries are usually classified descriptively and largely by pattern. Soft tissue injuries may

be classified by descriptions of their mechanism (sharp, crush, ballistic, blunt, burn), laceration and/or avulsion, location, orientation (vertical, transverse, oblique), and depth. In general, fractures can be classified by pattern: location, displacement, comminution, and whether they are open/closed to the skin. Most commonly, facial fractures are classified as being upper, middle or lower third (i.e., mandible) fractures or a combination; a true "panfacial" fracture has components involving upper, middle, and lower thirds simultaneously.

The Le Fort classification is a widely adopted and historical description of midface fracture patterns and fracture line locations in the maxilla with strong historical roots to original French cadaver experiments.[32,33] The hallmark of Le Fort fractures is traumatic *pterygomaxillary separation*, which signifies fractures of the pterygoid plates. Le Fort Type I fractures involve the lateral and medial walls of the maxillary sinus, propagating posteriorly above the alveolar process from the pyriform aperture (Fig. 1.1.7). Le Fort Type II fractures extend through the inferior orbital rim and orbital floor and the maxillary sinuses, and across the nose either high or low, forming a pyramidal shape of varying heights (Fig. 1.1.8). Le Fort Type III fractures extend horizontally from the nasofrontal suture to the frontozygomatic suture, through the orbits, and transect the zygomatic arches (Fig. 1.1.9). Le Fort I, II, and III fractures are conceptualized as a "floating palate," "floating maxilla," and "craniofacial dysfunction," respectively.[34,35] Most Le Fort fractures are usually bilateral, but asymmetric due to the asymmetric forces creating the fracture. It is thus common to have a higher-level fracture (i.e., Le Fort III) on the side of force application, and a lower-level fracture (i.e., Le Fort II) on the contralateral side. Lesser Le Fort segments usually exist within the overall Le Fort fracture pattern, reflecting comminution. Accurate bilateral description of the fracture pattern is critical for planning of the open reduction. The fracture pattern is defined by stating

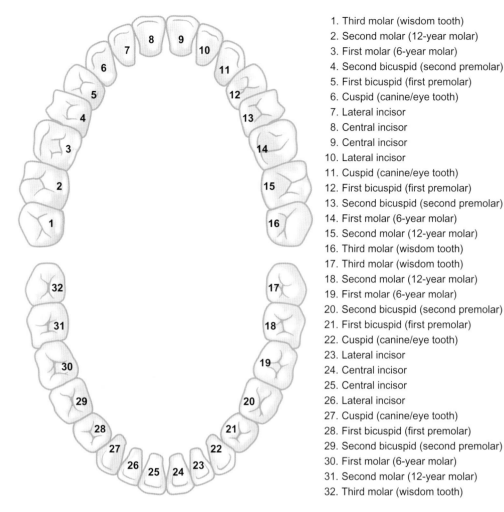

1. Third molar (wisdom tooth)
2. Second molar (12-year molar)
3. First molar (6-year molar)
4. Second bicuspid (second premolar)
5. First bicuspid (first premolar)
6. Cuspid (canine/eye tooth)
7. Lateral incisor
8. Central incisor
9. Central incisor
10. Lateral incisor
11. Cuspid (canine/eye tooth)
12. First bicuspid (first premolar)
13. Second bicuspid (second premolar)
14. First molar (6-year molar)
15. Second molar (12-year molar)
16. Third molar (wisdom tooth)
17. Third molar (wisdom tooth)
18. Second molar (12-year molar)
19. First molar (6-year molar)
20. Second bicuspid (second premolar)
21. First bicuspid (first premolar)
22. Cuspid (canine/eye tooth)
23. Lateral incisor
24. Central incisor
25. Central incisor
26. Lateral incisor
27. Cuspid (canine/eye tooth)
28. First bicuspid (first premolar)
29. Second bicuspid (second premolar)
30. First molar (6-year molar)
31. Second molar (12-year molar)
32. Third molar (wisdom tooth)

Fig. 1.1.5 Permanent (adult) teeth chart.

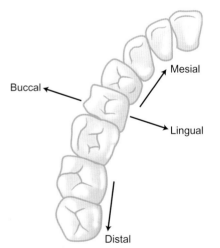

Fig. 1.1.6 Orientation terminology in reference to the dental arch.

the highest level of Le Fort fracture on each side up to (and including) the frontal bone and the nature of the fragment that includes the maxillary dentition (i.e., dentoalveolar fracture, split palate).[36] The Le Fort fracture pattern is thus precisely defined and guides the surgeon where open reduction should be performed.

Markowitz and colleagues classified NOE fractures based on comminution and its impact on the medial canthal tendon-bearing bone fragment ("central fragment" of the NOE fracture)[37] (Fig. 1.1.10). Type I fractures are characterized by a single noncomminuted "central" fragment without medial canthal tendon detachment/avulsion. The simplest fractures are "greensticked," or incomplete superiorly and displaced inferiorly, at the inferior orbital rim and pyriform aperture. Complete Type I fractures have a complete fracture at all buttresses including the nasofrontal suture. Type II fractures are characterized by a comminuted central fragment without medial canthal tendon disruption, and no fractures extending underneath the insertion of the medial canthal ligament. Type III fractures are characterized by a severely comminuted central fragment with fractures extending under the medial canthal tendon insertion and avulsion of the medial canthal ligament. Type I require open reduction internal fixation (ORIF) with junctional miniplates, Types II and III also require transnasal wiring and peripheral miniplate fixation.

Dentoalveolar injuries can be classified as tooth fractures, injuries of the periodontal apparatus, and/or injuries to supporting bone tissues.[38] There are numerous classification systems, such as that by Andreasen[39] and Garcia-Godoy.[40] Most are based on the World Health Organization Classification (I = Fracture of enamel of tooth, II = Fracture of crown without pulpal involvement, III = Fracture of crown with pulpal involvement, IV = Fracture of root of tooth, V = Fracture of crown and root

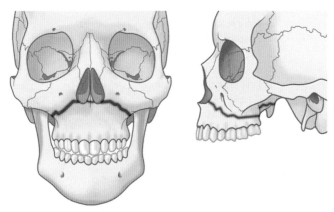

Fig. 1.1.7 Le Fort I fracture is located transversally above the dental apices and separates the dentoalveolar process, the hard palate, and the pterygoid processes, resulting in "floating palate." (From Prein J, Ehrenfeld M, Manson PN, editors. Principles of internal fixation of the craniomaxillofacial skeleton: trauma and orthognathic surgery. AO Foundation, Thieme; 2012, Fig. 3.1-1a–b, p.183.)

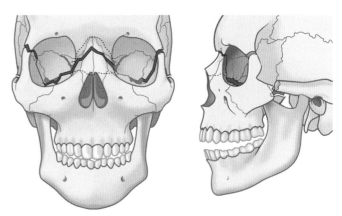

Fig. 1.1.9 Le Fort III fracture extends horizontally from the nasofrontal suture to the frontozygomatic suture and zygomatic arches, resulting in "craniofacial dissociation." (From Prein J, Ehrenfeld M, Manson PN, editors. Principles of internal fixation of the craniomaxillofacial skeleton: trauma and orthognathic surgery. AO Foundation, Thieme; 2012, Fig. 3.2-3a–b, p.194.)

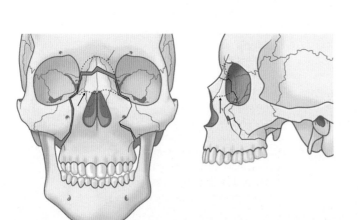

Fig. 1.1.8 Le Fort II fracture forms a pyramidal shape, resulting in "floating maxilla." There may be high and low variations as it crosses the nasal bridge: high at frontal bone (*blue arrow*), and low under the nasal bone (*black arrow*). (From Prein J, Ehrenfeld M, Manson PN, editors. Principles of internal fixation of the craniomaxillofacial skeleton: trauma and orthognathic surgery. AO Foundation, Thieme; 2012, Fig. 3.2-2a–b, p.194.)

of tooth, VI = Fracture of tooth unspecified, VII = Luxation of tooth, VIII = Intrusion or extrusion of tooth, IX = Avulsion of tooth, X = Other injuries, including laceration of oral soft tissues).[41]

CLINICAL PRESENTATION

The spectrum of facial trauma encompasses the superficial skin laceration to the panfacial fracture with overlying composite soft tissue injury, and everything in between. Strategies of evaluation should therefore obviously be tailored to the severity of the clinical presentation, but must always be thorough and complete. ATLS guidelines should always be adhered to for evaluation of airway, bleeding, and circulation. Screening for life-threatening injuries, bleeding, brain injury, and cervical spine assessment should precede facial trauma evaluation. Assuming the airway is patent, the patient is breathing adequately, and is hemodynamically stable, it is then prudent not to delay assessment of the face for soft tissue and bone injuries. Indeed, facial injuries may threaten

the airway and may be the source of massive bleeding, demanding emergent evaluation/control of hemorrhage in such cases. Finally, a directed, complete history and physical examination of the face is performed.

History

Pertinent information from the patient's clinical history includes mechanism of injury (blunt, sharp, dog bite, assault, MVC, etc.), previous injuries/trauma to the face, comorbidities, medications (especially anticoagulants and antiplatelet medications), and allergies.

Physical Examination

There is no universal convention for the sequencing of a thorough facial examination but the examination should progress in an orderly fashion and be complete; one may elect to work cephalad to caudad or vice-versa. Once the sequential examination is complete, second examinations are conducted in each anatomical area. One must be systematic, and complete; with experience, the entire exam is completed first and then a specific detailed exam can be more targeted toward focal, obvious injuries. For example, working from cephalad to caudad, one may proceed through inspection, palpation, and special tests as follows. Inspect for ecchymosis/edema/hematoma/lacerations throughout (including scalp, ears, and under the chin), pupillary reaction to light, and assessment of visual acuity/double vision; globe position (hypoglobus/enophthalmos/exophthalmos) and globe rupture, subconjunctival hemorrhage, chemosis (swelling of the conjunctiva), hyphema (blood in the anterior chamber, as sign of globe injury) (Fig. 1.1.11), telecanthus, rounding of eyelid commissure; note asymmetries, deviations (e.g. of the nose), and drainage. A cranial nerve exam can then be performed (typically olfactory examination of CN I is deferred) but testing of extraocular movements, pupil response, and visual acuity, assessment for diplopia and inspection of globe are mandatory in any periorbital trauma or generalized injury (a detailed discussion of the eye examination is presented later in this chapter). Examination of sensation in the three principal distributions of CN V should be performed in the frontal, maxillary, and mandibular regions. CN VII facial motor function can then be assessed with instruction to "raise eyebrows, squeeze eyes closed, puff out cheeks, smile and show teeth." A crude hearing (VIII) and balance assessment can be performed by basic questioning. Gag reflex can be assessed (IX) and instruction to "shrug" shoulders (XI), turning

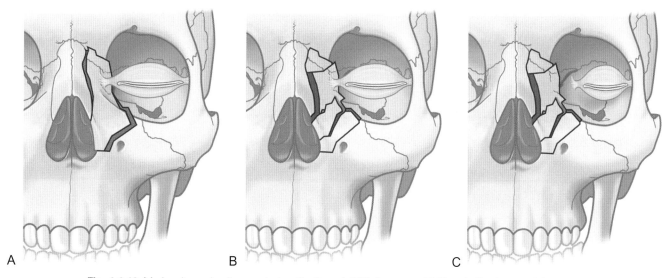

Fig. 1.1.10 Markowitz and colleagues' classification of NOE fractures. (A) Type I: Single central fragment bearing the medial canthal ligament. (B) Type II: Comminuted central fragment with medial canthal ligament attached to a bone fragment. (C) Type III: Comminuted central fragment with detached medial canthal ligament. (From Prein J, Ehrenfeld M, Manson PN, editors. Principles of internal fixation of the craniomaxillofacial skeleton: trauma and orthognathic surgery. AO Foundation, Thieme; 2012, Fig. 3.5-3a–c, p.236.)

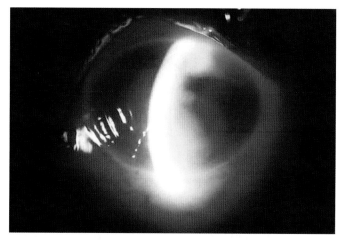

Fig. 1.1.11 Slit-lamp photograph of eye demonstrating total hyphema.

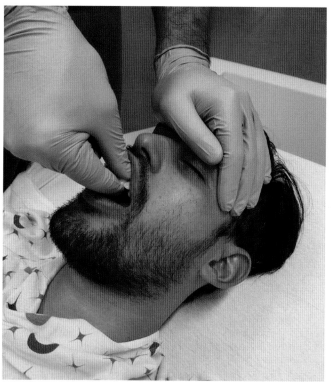

Fig. 1.1.12 Assessment for maxillary mobility while stabilizing the head.

of the head from side to side, and protrusive movement of the tongue (XII) completes the cranial nerve examination. Sequential palpation of all bony surfaces is performed; first the scalp, for hematoma/depression/skull fractures, then the frontal process of the zygoma, lateral and medial orbital rims, nasal bones, body of zygoma for tenderness and step-offs (bilateral examination helps identify differences), and zygomatic arches. The nose is examined for deviation, crepitus, lacerations, and contour. Flattening of the nasal bridge and an upturned nasal tip indicate frontal impact nasal or nasoethmoid fractures. Assessment for any maxillary mobility can be performed to detect movement of the maxillary dental arch while stabilizing the head with the second hand (Fig. 1.1.12). A test for lateral mobility of the dentition reflects split palate or palato-alveolar fractures. Intraoral exam should include inspection for ecchymosis, lacerations, edema, state of dentition, fractured, missing teeth or bleeding gums (including counting of teeth), presence of any malocclusion or trismus, and a bimanual mandible exam to test stability (Fig. 1.1.13). The mandible should be ranged and the temporal mandibular joints assessed for stability and tenderness.

For any nasal injury, intranasal examination should be performed with a nasal speculum to detect intranasal lacerations or septal hematoma. Clear nasal or bloody but watery drainage should create suspicion for CSF leak, which can be tested by beta-2 transferrin assay or with the "halo" or "ring" test (created by collecting a drop of the draining fluid on tissue paper – CSF moves further from the center than blood by capillary action) creating a "double ring" sign of clear fluid surrounding an inner blood ring. Similarly, for ear trauma/bleeding otoscopy

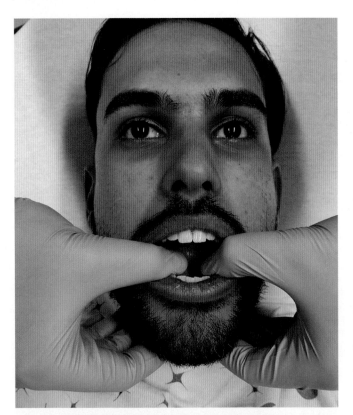

Fig. 1.1.13 Bimanual examination of mandible.

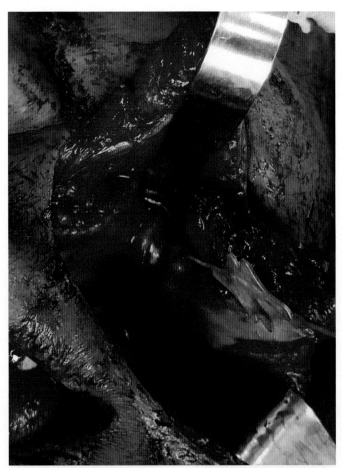

Fig. 1.1.14 Cannulating the Stenson's duct with lacrimal probe. The transection of the duct is clear with the probe visible within the intraoral laceration. The duct was repaired with 8-0 nylon interrupted sutures under loupe magnification.

is indicated to examine for hemotympanum (which may be indicative of ear canal lacerations from temporomandibular joint, mandibular condyle or skull base trauma) and otorrhea. Battle's sign is a hematoma of the mastoid from a basal skull fracture.

For suspected injury to Stenson's duct, the duct can be cannulated with a size 22 plastic angiocath sleeve and flushed (Fig. 1.1.14). One technique for this is to dilate the papilla of the duct on the buccal mucosa at the level of the second maxillary molar with a lacrimal dilator then probe (Fig. 1.1.14), with serial dilation as necessary, until an angiocath sleeve can be passed to cannulate the duct. Once passed, the cannulated duct can be irrigated with normal saline, and any drainage of fluid from the facial laceration indicates a duct injury. Most commonly, duct transection is accompanied by buccal branch facial nerve palsy.

For any periorbital or orbital trauma, examination of the eye should be more extensive than that previously described as part of the cranial nerve screening examination. Any telecanthus or rounding of eyelid commissure indicates canthal detachment which can be confirmed by the eyelid traction test, which assesses the status of the medial canthal tendon's attachment to the bone. Grasping the eyelid and pulling it displays abnormal canthal mobility in canthal avulsion. A bimanual examination can move the "central fragment" of an NOE fracture between a clamp placed under the canthus intranasally (not the nasal bone) and a palpating finger placed directly over the canthus externally (Fig. 1.1.15). Testing of visual acuity (Snellen® pocket card), diplopia, pupillary light reflex, and any limitation of extraocular movements may be supplemented with forced duction testing (Fig. 1.1.16). Presence of Marcus Gunn pupil or relative afferent pupillary defect (RAPD) (Fig. 1.1.17) may be suggestive of injury to the optic nerve or retina, and ophthalmological consultation should be obtained. In a RAPD, a patient's affected eye has decreased pupillary response to light, and will dilate when a

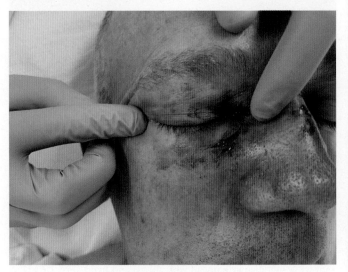

Fig. 1.1.15 Lid retraction test

bright light is swung from the unaffected eye to the affected eye. The affected eye may sense the light and produce pupillary sphincter constriction to some degree, albeit reduced. In suspected nasolacrimal duct injury, Jones testing is performed. For the Jones I test, a drop of fluorescein is placed on the conjunctiva and if detected in the nose within

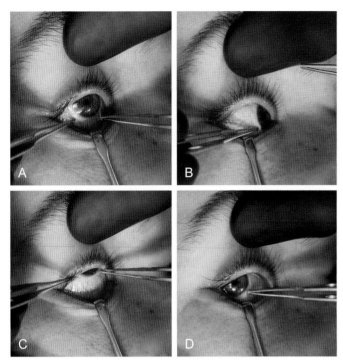

Fig. 1.1.16 Forced duction test of the right globe. (A) Bulbar conjunctiva is grasped with a toothed pick-up and forced (B) medially, (C) superiorly, and (D) laterally.

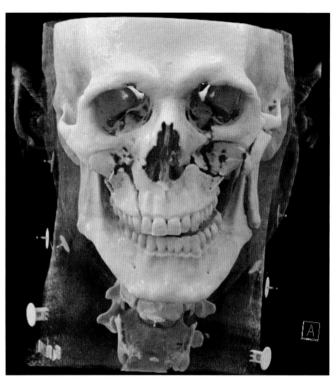

Fig. 1.1.18 Three-dimensional CT reconstruction of facial bones with multilevel fractures.

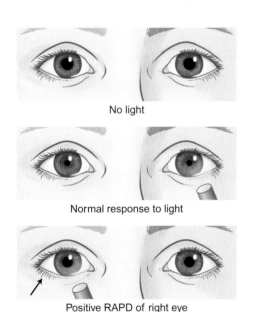

No light

Normal response to light

Positive RAPD of right eye

Fig. 1.1.17 Marcus Gunn or relative afferent pupillary defect (RAPD).

5 minutes, the test is said to be positive and indicative of a patent duct. A Jones II test follows a negative Jones I test. Remaining excess fluorescein is irrigated with saline and if detected in the nose Jones II test is positive and there is a functional/partial obstruction; if no saline appears in the nose there is complete obstruction. Partial stenosis of the canaliculi can respond to prolonged intubation/stenting of the lacrimal drainage system, otherwise dacrocystorhinostomy (DCR) is necessary. In the context of orbital and periorbital trauma, consultation to ophthalmology can be considered for suspected globe injury, optic nerve

dysfunction (normal globe with absent vision, direct optic nerve injury or indirect optic nerve injury, e.g. deceleration injuries), compartment syndrome (the orbit feels firm, visual loss, decreased extra-ocular motility, proptosis from hemorrhage/edema, guitar pick sign on CT scan, in which the back of the globe is no longer round), or for a confirmatory preoperative visual evaluation/test.

RADIOLOGICAL EVALUATION

The initial diagnostic imaging of choice for evaluating facial injuries is computed tomography (CT). In addition, many patients have concomitant head injuries requiring head and brain CT scan, which can be obtained at the same time as the CT of facial bones. Plain facial radiographs provide little information and are not worthwhile. CT scans in several planes and with 3-dimensional reconstructions provide precise anatomic identification and quantification of facial fractures which can be viewed in axial, coronal, and sagittal 2-dimensional images. Three-dimensional reconstruction of facial bones augments the information obtained, but does not replace 2-dimensional images. 3D images provide spatial relationships which aid in planning complex repairs (Fig. 1.1.18). Panoramic radiographs (orthopantomograms) are occasionally necessary and show the entire mandible, including the condyles, dentoalveolar bone, dentition, and the location/path of the inferior alveolar nerves (Fig. 1.1.19). The benefits of panoramic radiographs include ease of obtaining in dental offices and they are less expensive than the CT images, however, 2D representation of a 3D object will carry inherent limitations in accurately portraying the displacement, extent, and angulation of the fractures. They also have the disadvantage of blurring the symphysis and they require a standing patient for the study. For these reasons, CT is the imaging modality of choice by most practitioners for evaluating facial trauma patients.

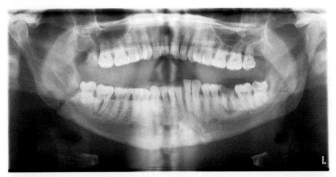

Fig. 1.1.19 Panoramic radiograph of right angle and left parasymphyseal fractures. Dentoalveolar diseases involving the right second molar and left first molar are visualized.

SURGICAL TREATMENTS

Initial Considerations

Evaluation of facial injury is followed with synchronous initiation of treatment to control bleeding as well as presurgical interventions that may include wiring of teeth or fractures, application of arch bars, manual reduction of grossly displaced fractures, and cleansing/irrigation of wounds, removal of gross contamination, and initiation of tetanus protection, antibiotic, and analgesic therapy. Repair of soft tissue injuries may commence at any time.

Substantial bleeding can occur from soft tissue injuries, especially scalp lacerations and injuries to superficial temporal and facial arteries. Large bleeding scalp lacerations typically require debridement and closure with combinations of sutures possibly over a drain to limit blood loss and fluid accumulation. Suture ligation of vessels and laceration closure both achieve control of bleeding vessels. Facial nerve branches should be avoided in clamps and ligatures. A low threshold for formal intraoperative exploration of these injuries best prevents low-quality wound repairs and recurrent wound problems, including hematomas, and best ensures meticulous hemostasis and ideal tissue approximation. Sharp but minimal debridement of irregular lacerations at the marginal zone of contusion ensures healthy, surgically created wound edges for optimal healing. Problem areas for debridement include the eyelids, lips, distal nose, nostril rims, ear, and eyebrow.

Midface fractures can result in significant epistaxis requiring hemostatic control by anterior–posterior nasal packing (usually posteriorly with nasal balloons/Foley catheters) and anteriorly (with nasal packing). Open fractures causing hemorrhage can also be covered with sterile dressings after cleansing; debridement dressings can be impregnated with hemostatic adjuncts but are of secondary importance to definitive control. Definitive treatment of bleeding may benefit from operative intervention or interventional radiology-guided embolization. Manually repositioning grossly displaced fractures and application of maxillary reduction/rest with intermaxillary fixation (IMF) can also help with bleeding. Patients transferred to the radiology suite must be monitored, observed, and properly resuscitated and stabilized prior to transfer out of the trauma bay.

It is also appropriate in the emergency room setting to close lacerations (after adequate debridement and irrigation). Debridement must be complete but purposefully conservative. Heavily contaminated wounds and those with significant tissue loss will likely warrant formal operating room management. All foreign material, road tattoo, and particles must be removed completely. Secondary procedures to remove foreign material are largely ineffective. Septal and auricular hematomas should be promptly incised, drained, and dressed with an intranasal Doyle

splint or soft lubricated compression dressings, as failure to recognize and manage these results in septal necrosis and perforations, and skin and/or cartilage necrosis or "cauliflower ear."

Patients With Concomitant Neurological, Cardiopulmonary, or Extremity Trauma

Facial injuries do not necessarily occur in isolation, and practitioners should be cognizant of issues regarding management of patients with simultaneous neurological, cardiopulmonary or extremity trauma. Although there are injuries that require immediate operative intervention, such as entrapped muscle in orbital fractures and blindness, in the absence of active bleeding from major named vessels in the face, most facial trauma is not a life-threatening situation; however, the benefits of definitive prompt management of facial injuries have been underemphasized in the literature.

Partially avulsed or flail segments of fractured facial bones should be stabilized in the ER by replacement into proper position, perhaps wired, and then definitively managed in the operating room. A dental "bridle wire" for mandible fractures may be used in the emergency room for initial control of positioning flail mandibular fragments. Maxillomandibular fixation using intermaxillary fixation screws or arch bars can be placed for temporary stabilization of mandible or palate fractures at the bedside, or at the time of treatment of other injuries such as craniotomy or repair of open lower extremity/pelvic fractures. The possibilities for treatment of facial injuries in the operating room while other definitive or life-saving treatments are occurring have also been understated in the literature. Consideration should be given to tetanus vaccination, initiation of antibiotics, especially for soft tissue wounds caused by burns or bites and fractures violating sinuses and the dentition.

All facial interventions as outlined above should be performed in compliance with general trauma guidelines and in the context of working together as a multidisciplinary team with other trauma care subspecialists and healthcare providers achieving communication and consensus for optimal management of each individual patient's care needs.

Various Surgical Exposures of Craniofacial Skeleton
Exposure of Upper Third and Upper Midface (Frontal Sinus, Le Fort II and III)

The coronal incision allows the wide exposure necessary to access the frontal bone, upper NOE, medial/superior/lateral orbital walls, zygoma, the zygomatic arch and temporomandibular joint. The coronal incision location can be adjusted based on the hairline pattern (possibly using a zig-zag in the hair for camouflage), and inferior/lateral extension will be necessary to expose the zygomatic arch/temporal mandibular joint areas (Fig. 1.1.20). The coronal incision may be extended retroauricularly as well as preauricularly. The infraorbital rim and orbital floor can be accessed through local incisions via subciliary, midtarsal, or transconjunctival approaches with or without lateral canthotomy (Fig. 1.1.21). The extent and pattern of the fracture, lid anatomy/laxity, and presence of concomitant lacerations will influence the choice of eyelid incision. Exposure of the upper lateral orbital rim (i.e., zygomaticofrontal suture area) can be achieved through local incisions such as the lateral portion of the upper blepharoplasty incision (1–2 cm only), or the transconjunctival incision with lateral cantholysis and superior dissection (Fig. 1.1.22). Considerable postoperative swelling accompanies the latter approach.

Exposure of Lower Midface (Le Fort I and Palate)

The standard approach for exposure of the maxilla is the intraoral vestibular incision around the maxillary arch 8–10 mm away from the

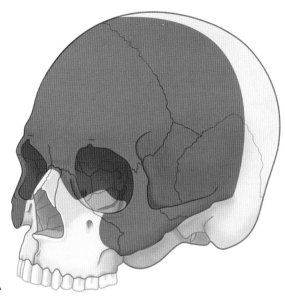

Fig. 1.1.20(A) Coronal approach: wide area of exposure (pink) is possible through coronal incision. (From Prein J, Ehrenfeld M, Manson PN, editors. Principles of internal fixation of the craniomaxillofacial skeleton: trauma and orthognathic surgery. AO Foundation, Thieme; 2012, Fig. 3.4-4, p.227.)

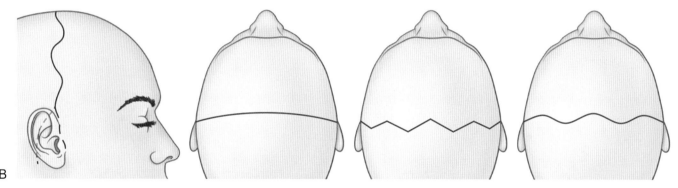

Fig. 1.1.20(B) Coronal approach: various modifications of coronal incision. (From Prein J, Ehrenfeld M, Manson PN, editors. Principles of internal fixation of the craniomaxillofacial skeleton: trauma and orthognathic surgery. AO Foundation, Thieme; 2012, Fig. 3.2-5b–c, p.196.)

attached gingival mucosa (Fig. 1.1.23), leaving a myomucosal cuff for multilayered suture-layered closure. The central area over the incisors frequently may be preserved, which assists alignment and closure. Layered closure of the muscle and mucosa is recommended and sutures besides chromic have more secure staying power and may have to be removed in the postoperative period.

Exposure of Lower Face (Mandible)

Typically, intraoral incisions are used for exposure of symphysis, parasymphysis, body and angle of the mandible. However, under certain circumstances transcutaneous incisions will allow improved exposure for complicated fracture reduction and fixation. Extraoral incisions are preferred for comminuted fractures. The intraoral vestibular incision is typically located on the mobile mucosa 8–10 mm from the attached gingival mucosa (Fig. 1.1.24). Again, this provides a healthy myomucosal cuff for incision closure at the end of the procedure. Layered muscle repair of the mentalis/buccinators incisions for intraoral closure is essential, and if omitted can result in lip or cheek ectropion. Transcutaneous incisions may be considered if there are existing facial lacerations in proximity to the fractures, or when significant comminution or loss of bone are present requiring access to the inferior border of the mandible for placement of a load-bearing reconstruction plate (Fig. 1.1.25A). Cephalad retraction of the facial vessels (which often need to be ligated) protects the marginal branch of the facial nerve (Fig. 1.1.25B). Transcutaneous approaches offer the best exposure to the condyle and ascending ramus (i.e., posterior mandible); although intraoral ramal incisions are preferred by some but are generally acknowledged to be more challenging (Fig. 1.1.26).

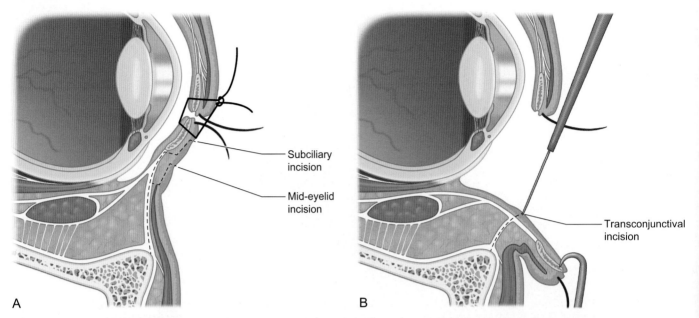

A

B

Fig. 1.1.21 Approaches to infraorbital rim and floor. (A) Subciliary and mid-eyelid incisions. (B) Transconjunctival incision. (From Prein J, Ehrenfeld M, Manson PN, editors. Principles of internal fixation of the craniomaxillofacial skeleton: trauma and orthognathic surgery. AO Foundation, Thieme; 2012, Fig. 3.2-8a–b, p.198.)

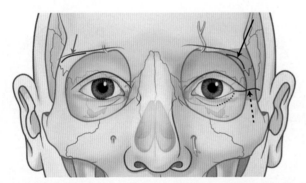

Fig. 1.1.22 Local exposure of the zygomaticofrontal suture area (*shaded pink*). Upper blepharoplasty (*solid black arrow*) and lateral brow (*blue arrow*) incisions, and transconjunctival incision with lateral canthotomy (*dotted black arrow*). (From Prein J, Ehrenfeld M, Manson PN, editors. Principles of internal fixation of the craniomaxillofacial skeleton: trauma and orthognathic surgery. AO Foundation, Thieme; 2012, Fig. 3.2-7a, p.197.)

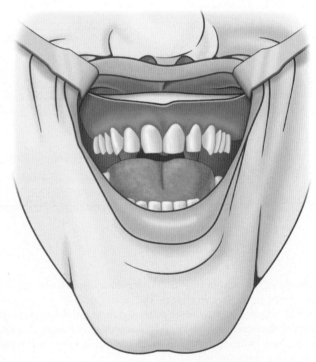

Fig. 1.1.23 Upper intraoral vestibular incision for exposure of maxilla. (From Prein J, Ehrenfeld M, Manson PN, editors. Principles of internal fixation of the craniomaxillofacial skeleton: trauma and orthognathic surgery. AO Foundation, Thieme; 2012, Fig. 3.1-4, p.186.)

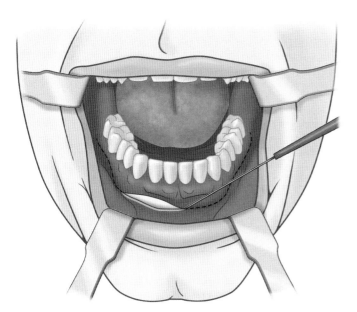

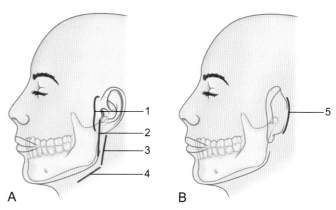

Fig. 1.1.26 (A–B) Transcutaneous approaches to the posterior mandible: 1 = preauricular approach, 2 = transparotid approach, 3 = retromandibular approach, 4 = submandibular approach, 5 = retroauricular approach. (From Prein J, Ehrenfeld M, Manson PN, editors. Principles of internal fixation of the craniomaxillofacial skeleton: trauma and orthognathic surgery. AO Foundation, Thieme; 2012, Fig. 2.3-6a–b, p.163.)

Fig. 1.1.24 Lower intraoral vestibular incision for exposure of mandible. (From Prein J, Ehrenfeld M, Manson PN, editors. Principles of internal fixation of the craniomaxillofacial skeleton: trauma and orthognathic surgery. AO Foundation, Thieme; 2012, Fig. 2.1-4, p.138.)

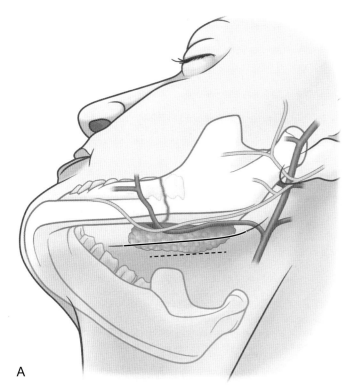

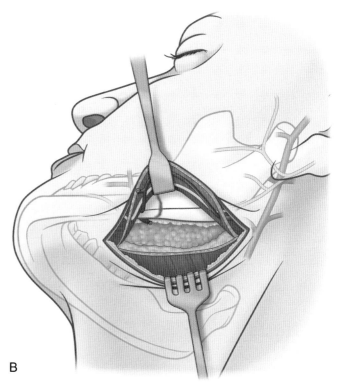

Fig. 1.1.25(A) Transcutaneous (submandibular) incision to approach the body of mandible. Skin incision (*solid line*) is usually made 2 cm below the inferior border of the mandible, followed by dissection through platysma, superficial cervical fascia and deep cervical fascia. (From Prein J, Ehrenfeld M, Manson PN, editors. Principles of internal fixation of the craniomaxillofacial skeleton: trauma and orthognathic surgery. AO Foundation, Thieme; 2012, Fig. 2.2-4a, p.151.)

Fig. 1.1.25(B) The facial vessels often need to be ligated, and its cephalad retraction protects the marginal mandibular branch of the facial nerve. (From Prein J, Ehrenfeld M, Manson PN, editors. Principles of internal fixation of the craniomaxillofacial skeleton: trauma and orthognathic surgery. AO Foundation, Thieme; 2012, Fig. 2.2-4b, p.151.)

EXPERT COMMENTARY

One of the wonderful things about the evaluation of patients with facial injuries is that the physical examination is still valuable and important in making a diagnosis and in determining the treatment. Indeed, I often challenge the residents to make all the diagnoses from the initial physical examination, and then confirm their findings on the CT scan, and then go back to the patient and see what findings were underestimated or overlooked.

In this way, one refines and improves one's perception, and many times there are few facts that elude the careful, organized physical examination. In the older text books [1–4] this was all they had except for plain X-rays, and so the clinicians of that era were extraordinarily good diagnosticians, and were alert to the subtle signs of the obscure injury, and by necessity had expert knowledge of dental anatomy. All of these things can be learned with careful study – for instance, the best way to learn dental anatomy is to review a text, then to take impressions and make models on every patient with a fracture involving the occlusion, counting the teeth to determine any that are missing. Many patients have had orthodontia or previous dental extractions, and teeth may be missing; there may be old dental records and models available, and old photographs brought by the family may suggest previous skeletal differences, or asymmetries of appearance that cannot be overcome or corrected by open reductions that try to achieve symmetry. Only this repetitive combination of physical examination/CT training, constantly looking at both data sets, can teach the practitioner the detailed knowledge that serves to make one become expert in physical diagnosis and initial patient diagnosis and management. Postoperative CT training and critical review of patient results, interviewing patients to see what they think, will do wonders for your expertise. Good discussion with the patient may well be one of the most useful teaching exercises.

Stability of the patient is paramount to determine and continuously access, and one must always consider the facial injury a geographic injury to the head and neck region, ruling out brain and cervical spine injury routinely. Lacerations and bruises are symptoms of underlying bony or organ injury until proven otherwise. Training in examination of the eye and its adnexae must be mastered, and again confirming and augmenting the findings of the ophthalmic consultant will improve the perception of the non-ophthalmologist, and improve the determination and monitoring of the physiological events following orbital surgery.

References

1. Rowe NL, Killey HC. *Fractures of the Facial Skeleton.* 2nd ed. London: E&S Livingstone; 1968.
2. Kazanjian VH, Converse JC. *Kazanjian and Converse's Surgical Treatment of Facial Injuries.* 3rd ed. Baltimore, MD: Williams & Wilkins; 1974.
3. Dingman R, Natvig P. *Surgery of Facial Fractures.* Philadelphia: WB Saunders; 1964.
4. Irby WB. *Facial Trauma and Concomitant Problems – Evaluation and Treatment.* St. Louis: C.V. Mosby Co.; 1974.

 Evidence-based medicine (EBM) content available in Appendix 1 (online only)

REFERENCES

1. Allareddy V, Allareddy V, Nalliah RP. Epidemiology of facial fracture injuries. *J Oral Maxillofac Surg.* 2011;69(10):2613–2618.
2. VandeGriend ZP, Hashemi A, Shkoukani M. Changing trends in adult facial trauma epidemiology. *J Craniofac Surg.* 2015;26(1):108–112.
3. Boffano P, Kommers SC, Karagozoglu KH, Forouzanfar T. Aetiology of maxillofacial fractures: a review of published studies during the last 30 years. *Br J Oral Maxillofac Surg* [Internet]. 2014;52(10):901–906. Available from: http://www.sciencedirect.com/science/article/pii/S0266435614005531.
4. Mithani SK, St.-Hilaire H, Brooke BS, et al. Predictable patterns of intracranial and cervical spine injury in craniomaxillofacial trauma: analysis of 4786 patients. *Plast Reconstr Surg* [Internet]. 2009;123(4):1293–1301. Available from: http://content.wkhealth.com/linkback/openurl?sid=WKPTLP:landingpage&an=00006534-200904000-00016.
5. Manson PN, Hoopes J, Su CT. Structural pillars of the facial skeleton: an approach to the management of Le Fort fractures. *Plast Reconstr Surg.* 1980;66(1):54–62.
6. Rodriguez ED, Stanwix MG, Nam AJ, et al. Twenty-six-year experience treating frontal sinus fractures: a novel algorithm based on anatomical fracture pattern and failure of conventional techniques. *Plast Reconstr Surg.* 2008;122(6):1850–1866.
7. Buch K, Mottalib A, Nadgir RN, et al. Unifocal versus multifocal mandibular fractures and injury location. *Emerg Radiol.* 2016;23(2):161–167.
8. Manson P, Clark N, Robertson B, et al. Subunit principles in midface fractures: the importance of sagittal buttresses, soft-tissue reductions, and sequencing treatment of segmental fractures. *Plast Reconstr Surg.* 1999;103(4):1287–1306.
9. Breeze J, Tong D, Gibbons A. Contemporary management of maxillofacial ballistic trauma. *Br J Oral Maxillofac Surg* [Internet]. 2017;55(7):661–665. Available from: http://dx.doi.org/10.1016/j.bjoms.2017.05.001.
10. Stefanopoulos PK, Soupiou OT, Pazarakiotis VC, Filippakis K. Wound ballistics of firearm-related injuries – Part 2: Mechanisms of skeletal injury and characteristics of maxillofacial ballistic trauma. *Int J Oral Maxillofac Surg* [Internet]. 2015;44(1):67–78. Available from: http://dx.doi.org/10.1016/j.ijom.2014.07.012.
11. Moore M, David D, Cooter R. Oblique craniofacial fractures in children. *J Craniofac Surg.* 1990;1(1):4–7.
12. MacMillan A, Lopez J, Faateh M, et al. How do Le-Fort type fractures present in a pediatric cohort? *J Oral Maxillofac Surg.* 2017;In press.
13. Kraft A, Abermann E, Stigler R, et al. Craniomaxillofacial trauma: synopsis of 14,654 cases with 35,129 injuries in 15 years. *Craniomaxillofac Trauma Reconstr* [Internet]. 2012;5(1):41–50. Available from: http://www.pubmedcentral.nih.gov/articlerender.fcgi?artid=3348752&tool=pmcentrez&rendertype=abstract.
14. Kaban L, Mulliken J, Murray J. Facial fractures in children: an analysis of 122 fractures in 109 patients. *Plast Reconstr Surg.* 1977;59(1):15–20.
15. Thaller S, Huang V. Midfacial fractures in the pediatric population. *Ann Plast Surg.* 1992;29(4):348–352.
16. Reedy B, Bartlett S. Pediatric facial fractures. In: Bentz M, ed. *Pediatric Plastic Surgery.* Stamford: Appleton & Lange; 1998:463–486.
17. McCoy F, Chandler R, Crow M. Facial fractures in children. *Plast Reconstr Surg.* 1966;37(3):209–215.
18. Smartt JM, Low DW, Bartlett SP. The pediatric mandible: II. Management of traumatic injury or fracture. *Plast Reconstr Surg.* 2005;116(2):28e–41e.
19. Zimmermann CE, Troulis MJ, Kaban LB. Pediatric facial fractures: recent advances in prevention, diagnosis and management. *Int J Oral Maxillofac Surg* [Internet]. 2006;35(1):2–13. Available from: http://www.ncbi.nlm.nih.gov/pubmed/16425444.
20. Imahara SD, Hopper RA, Wang J, et al. Patterns and outcomes of pediatric facial fractures in the United States: a survey of the National Trauma Data Bank. *J Am Coll Surg* [Internet]. 2008;207(5):710–716. Available from: http://www.ncbi.nlm.nih.gov/pubmed/18954784.
21. Cole P, Kaufman Y, Hollier LH Jr. Managing the pediatric facial fracture. *Craniomaxillofac Trauma Reconstr* [Internet]. 2009;2(2):77–83. Available from: http://www.ncbi.nlm.nih.gov/pubmed/22110800%5Cnhttp://www.pubmedcentral.nih.gov/articlerender.fcgi?artid=PMC3052668.
22. Eggensperger Wymann NM, Hölzle A, Zachariou Z, Iizuka T. Pediatric craniofacial trauma. *J Oral Maxillofac Surg.* 2008;66(1):58–64.
23. Grunwaldt L, Smith DM, Zuckerbraun NS, et al. Pediatric facial fractures: demographics, injury patterns, and associated injuries in 772 consecutive patients. *Plast Reconstr Surg* [Internet]. 2011;128(6):1263–1271. Available from: http://www.ncbi.nlm.nih.gov/pubmed/21829142.
24. Mundinger G, Bellamy J, Miller D, et al. Defining population-specific craniofacial fracture patterns and resource use in geriatric patients: a comparative study of blunt craniofacial fractures in geriatric versus nongeriatric adult patients. *Plast Reconstr Surg.* 2016;137(2):386e–393e.

25. Zelken JA, Khalifian S, Mundinger GS, et al. Defining predictable patterns of craniomaxillofacial injury in the elderly: analysis of 1,047 patients. *J Oral Maxillofac Surg* [Internet]. 2014;72(2):352–361. Available from: http://dx.doi.org/10.1016/j.joms.2013.08.015.

26. Hussain K, Wijetunge DB, Grubnic S, Jackson IT. A comprehensive analysis of craniofacial trauma [Internet]. *J Trauma Injury Infect Crit Care*. 1994;34:34–47.

27. Gonzalez-Ulloa M. Regional aesthetic units of the face. *Plast Reconstr Surg*. 1987;79(3):489–490.

28. Foisie P. Traumatic arterial vasospasm. *N Engl J Med*. 1947;237(9):295–302.

29. Kaufman Y, Cole P, Hollier L. Facial gunshot wounds: trends in management. *Craniomaxillofac Trauma Reconstr*. 2009;2(2):85–90.

30. Seckel B. *Facial Danger Zones: Avoiding Nerve Injury in Facial Plastic Surgery*. 2nd ed. New York: Thieme Medical Publishers, Inc.; 2010:1–52.

31. Dorafshar AH, Borsuk DE, Bojovic B, et al. Surface anatomy of the middle division of the facial nerve: Zuker's point. *Plast Reconstr Surg* [Internet]. 2013;131(2):253–257. Available from: http://www.ncbi.nlm.nih.gov/pubmed/23357986.

32. Tessier P. The classic reprint. Experimental study of fractures of the upper jaw. I and II. René Le Fort, MD. *Plast Reconstr Surg*. 1972;50(5):497–506.

33. Tessier P. The classic reprint: experimental study of fractures of the upper jaw. 3. René Le Fort, M.D., Lille, France. *Plast Reconstr Surg*. 1972;50(6):600–607.

34. Daffner R. Imaging of facial trauma. *Curr Probl Diagn Radiol*. 1997;26(4):153–184.

35. Salvolini U. Traumatic injuries: imaging of facial injuries. *Eur Radiol*. 2002;1253–1261.

36. Manson PN. Some thoughts on the classification and treatment of Le Fort fractures. *Ann Plast Surg*. 1986;17(5):356–363.

37. Markowitz BL, Manson PN, Sargent L, et al. Management of the medial canthal tendon in nasoethmoid orbital fractures: the importance of the central fragment in classification and treatment. [Internet]. *Plast Reconstr Surg*. 1991;87:843–853. Available from: http://www.ncbi.nlm.nih.gov/pubmed/2017492.

38. Bastone EB, Freer TJ, McNamara JR. Epidemiology of dental trauma: a review of the literature. *Aust Dent J*. 2000;45(1):2–9.

39. Andreasen J. *Traumatic Injuries of the Teeth*. 2nd ed. Copenhagen: Munksgaard; 1981:19–24.

40. Garcia-Godoy F. A classification for traumatic injuries to primary and permanent teeth. *J Pedod*. 1981;5:295–297.

41. World Health Organization. *Application of the International Classification of Diseases to dentistry and stomatology (ICD-DA)*. Geneva: World Health Organization; 1978:88–89.

Radiological Evaluation of the Craniofacial Skeleton

Krystal Archer-Arroyo, Stuart E. Mirvis

BACKGROUND

It was the discovery of X-rays by Wilhelm Roentgen in 1895 that allowed visualization of the internal structures of the body for the first time in history. In 1972, an electrical engineer, Godfrey Hounsfield, advanced the use of X-rays with the invention of computed tomography, allowing the complete visualization of the internal solid organs, soft tissues, and bones of the body using image reconstruction mathematics. A new imaging modality, magnetic resonance imaging, shortly followed in 1973. This modality using a magnetic field and mathematical analysis of the signals for image reconstruction, allowed unprecedented evaluation of the internal architecture of the soft tissues, such as the globe of the eye and individual muscle groups. Now all of these modalities are used in the emergent, surgical, and clinical setting to evaluate both the osseous and soft tissue components of the craniofacial region in its entirety.

SURGICAL ANATOMY

The surgical anatomy is shown in Figs. 1.2.1–1.2.10:
- Plain radiography: Figs. 1.2.1–1.2.2
- Computed tomography (CT): Figs. 1.2.3–1.2.7
- Magnetic resonance imaging (MRI): Figs. 1.2.9–1.2.10

RADIOLOGICAL EVALUATION

Radiography

Radiographs of the skull at various angles allow visualization of the major osseous structures of the face and mandible. Plain radiographs are named based on the projection of the X-ray beam.[1] The most common radiographs of the face in the trauma setting include: standard occipitomental (30 degrees OM or Waters view), posteroanterior (PA skull or Towne view), reverse Towne's and the true lateral skull (Fig. 1.2.1). The submentovertex view, which requires hyperextension of the neck, is not obtained given the risk of a concomitant cervical spine injury seen in 2.2% of patients with maxillofacial fractures.[2] Each projection of the face best demonstrates certain osseous features of the craniofacial skeleton (Table 1.2.1). However, overlapping osseous structures limit evaluation of the entire craniofacial skeleton, especially the midface, sinuses, and skull base. Moreover, the patient must be able to cooperate with positioning to obtain the various projections. This is impossible with patients suffering from traumatic brain injuries associated with craniofacial fractures.

Panoramic Radiography

The panoramic radiograph (orthopantomogram or panorex) displays the entire maxillomandibular region on a single image (Fig. 1.2.2A).

The term panoramic radiography is derived from panorama, "an unobstructed view of a region in every direction."[3] There are two different ways of obtaining panoramic views, which are defined by the location of the radiation source: intraoral or extraoral.

The intraoral technique requires a small X-ray tube be placed in the patient's mouth where radiation is directed through the jaws to expose a film placed just outside of the targeted facial anatomy. The first patient undergoing this procedure was reported by a German inventor, Horst Berger.[3] The extraoral technique, which is the most popular method in use today, employs an extraoral source of radiation that rotates around the patient. To create a panoramic view, objects in front or behind the focal trough are blurred, leaving a sharp image of the entire mandible in one 2-dimensional plane facilitating the diagnosis of mandible fractures and dentoalveolar trauma (Fig. 1.2.2B).

Panoramic radiographs are fast and convenient with minimal training needed for the operating technician. Moreover, panoramic radiography provides the lowest radiation dose with broad coverage of maxillomandibular bones and teeth. This imaging modality is most advantageous for stable patients who cannot tolerate intraoral procedures or examination. The limitations of the radiographs include unequal magnification across the image, making linear measurements

TABLE 1.2.1	Craniofacial Radiographs			
	Waters (30 degrees OM)	Towne's (AP Skull)	Reverse Towne's	True Lateral Skull
Cranium		X		X
Midface fractures				
Le Fort I	X			
Le Fort II	X			
Le Fort III	X			
Paranasal sinuses				
Frontal sinus		X		X
Sphenoid sinus				X
Maxillary sinus				X
Mandible			X	
Mandibular condyle			X	
Coronoid process	X			

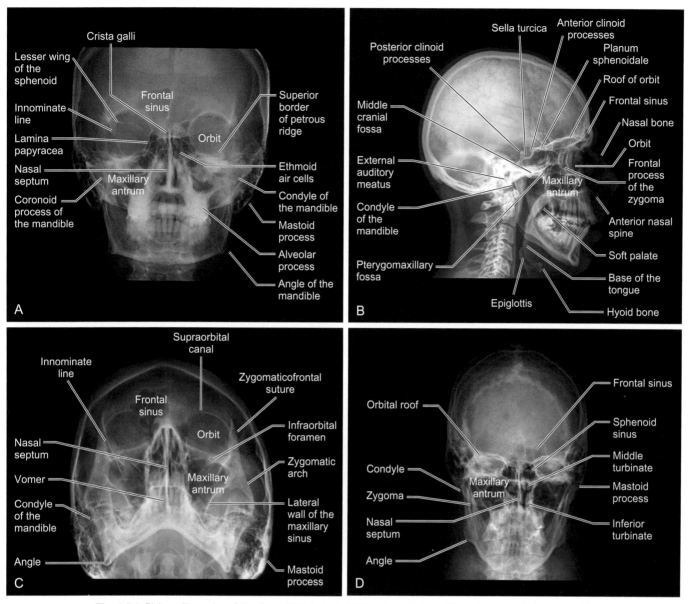

Fig. 1.2.1 Plain radiographs of the face: (A) PA view, (B) true lateral view, (C) occipitomental view, and (D) reverse Towne's view.

unreliable, as well as difficulty imaging both sides of the mandible when the patient has severe maxillomandibular discrepancies causing malocclusion.[4] The tomographic technique of the exam also creates artifacts, including double images of the hyoid bone, cervical spine, and epiglottis. Ghost artifacts, which are higher than the true anatomic location on the opposite side of the image, are created by the upward inclination of the X-ray beam.[4] These artifacts, in addition to the superimposition of overlying structures, limit the complete evaluation of the maxillomandibular structures, especially the mandibular condyle and coronoid process which overlap the mastoid prominence and midface, respectively.

Computed Tomography (CT)

In computed tomography, an X-ray tube rotates around the patient emitting a fan-shaped beam of X-rays that are detected by a row of detectors on the opposite side. Initially, the X-ray tube and detector rotated synchronously around the patient for one cycle then the table would move a small increment (i.e., 5 mm) for the next scan or slice image. This was known as the "step and shoot" method or so-called incremental scanners.[4] In 1989, CT scanners acquired image data in a helical fashion where the X-ray tube and detectors continuously revolve around the patient while the table advances the patient through the gantry. This overlapping image data results in higher spatial resolution, improved multiplanar reconstructions, faster scanning and reduction in radiation dose. Multidetector CT scanners were introduced in 1998 beginning with a 4-detector row CT scanner and progressing to the current state-of-the art CT scanners with up to 320-detector rows allowing for multiple slices to be captured quickly and simultaneously, reducing exposure time and motion artifact. This also results in improved resolution and quality of the axial, reformatted, and 3-dimensional images of the face. Current technology allows data obtained via CT to be transmitted to the operating room for computer-assisted surgery, including

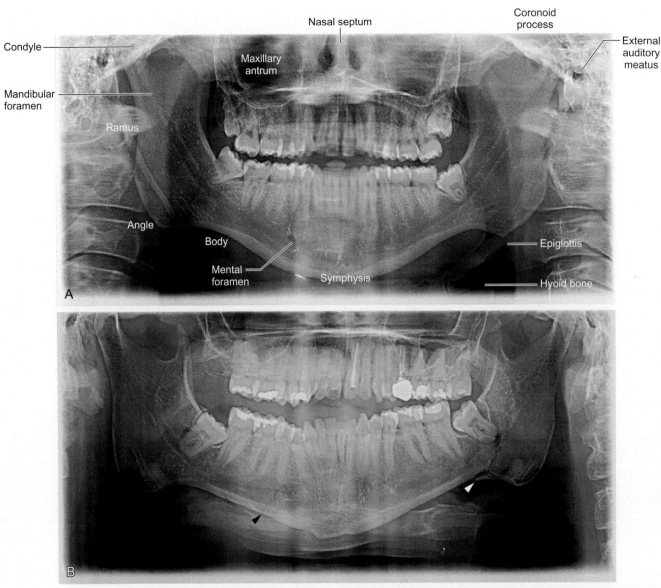

Fig. 1.2.2 (A) Normal panoramic radiograph of the mandible. (B) Panoramic radiograph of the mandible demonstrates bilateral mandible fractures. There is a nondisplaced fracture through the anterior body of the right mandible (*black arrowhead*) and a displaced, comminuted fracture through the angle of the left mandible (*white arrowhead*) extending to the root of a partially erupted molar tooth.

presurgical planning and intraoperative navigation during the repair of craniomaxillofacial injuries.

In comparison to plain radiographs of the face, CT eliminates the superimposition of structures and provides high-resolution contrast of the osseous structures and soft tissues that can be viewed simultaneously in three orthogonal planes as well as 3D (Figs. 1.2.3–1.2.7). This allows for complete evaluation of the face, skull base, cranium, and brain. In a large study, it was reported that the most common fractures were to the midface (71.5%) with supraorbital and frontobasal skull fractures present in 4.2% of the cases.[5] CT is superior to plain radiographs when assessing the mandible, especially nondisplaced symphyseal fractures, given the overlapping spine on the AP Towne's view.[6] CT has a higher accuracy, sensitivity, and specificity (90%, 90%, 87%, respectively) for condylar fractures when compared to panoramic radiographs

(73%, 70%, 77%, respectively).[7] CT has also been shown to detect additional fractures not seen on plain or panoramic radiographs, often leading to a change in operative management.[8] In the setting of penetrating trauma, multidetector CT is the best imaging modality to assess the trajectory of the missile and injury to the adjacent soft tissues and vascular structures (Fig. 1.2.8).[9]

Magnetic Resonance Imaging (MRI)

The first MR image was described by Paul Lauterbur in 1973.[1] By the early 1980s, MRI was available for clinical use. The patient is placed into a magnetic field that causes the spin of the hydrogen atoms within the soft tissues to align with the magnetic field. The scanner then directs a radiofrequency (RF) pulse into the patient that redirects the spin of the hydrogen atoms. When the RF pulse is turned off, as the spin of

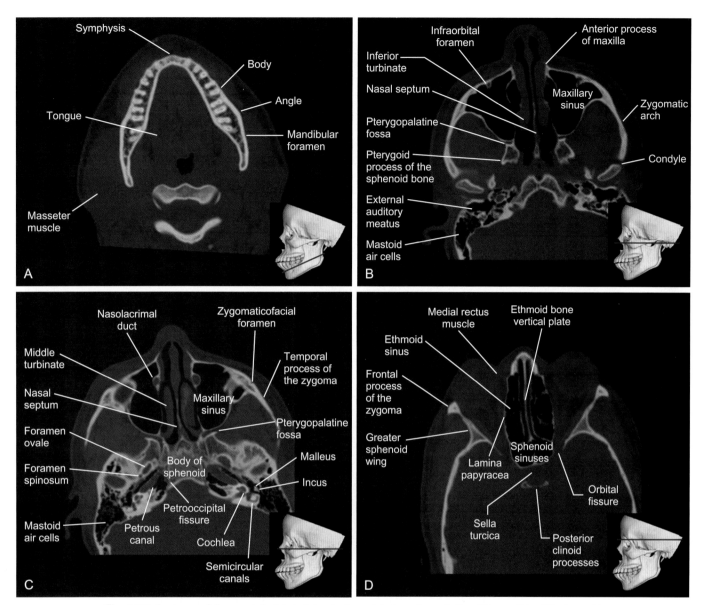

Fig. 1.2.3 Anatomy of the craniofacial skeleton in the axial plane through the: (A) mandible, (B) pterygoid plates, (C) skull base, and (D) orbits.

the hydrogen atoms returns to that of the external magnetic field, a signal is released and detected by a coil in the scanner which is used to create the MR image.

Advantages of MRI include noninvasive imaging without ionizing radiation, and soft tissue resolution in multiple planes that is superior to computed tomography (Figs. 1.2.9 and 1.2.10). In the setting of craniomaxillofacial trauma, MRI can be used to evaluate the optic nerve for traumatic optic neuropathy (TON) (Fig. 1.2.11), as well as herniation of orbital contents into the adjacent maxillary sinus or traumatic encephaloceles. A study by Freund[10] et al. demonstrated that MRI showed the inferior rectus muscle to be herniated through the orbital floor fractures twice as often as when compared to the evaluation of the orbital contents using CT. Although MRI is suboptimal in assessing cortical bone given the paucity of hydrogen atoms, it can depict bone marrow edema associated with chronic complications of trauma such as mandibular osteomyelitis, ischemic necrosis of the condylar head,

and traumatic damage to the articular disc.[6] The disadvantages of MRI include high cost, long scan times, metallic hardware that can obscure adjacent structures, and other relative contraindications to MRI.

Radiation Dose

In the United States, it is estimated that each person is exposed to 3 milliSieverts (mSv) of radiation from background sources such as radon gas and cosmic radiation from airplane flights at high altitudes.[11] In diagnostic radiology, this is the reference to which the radiation patients receive during imaging is compared (Table 1.2.2). Plain radiographs, which can be used in the initial evaluation of craniofacial trauma, are the lowest in radiation dose. Although higher in radiation in comparison to plain radiographs, computed tomography has become the standard modality in imaging facial trauma given it allows rapid assessment of the entire craniofacial skeleton.[12] The dose of radiation from CT varies with the number of channels as well as the number

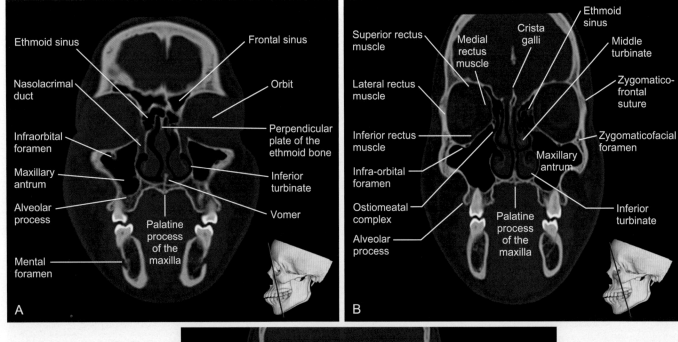

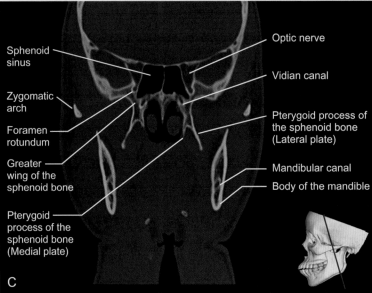

Fig. 1.2.4 Anatomy of the craniofacial skeleton in the coronal plane through the: (A) anterior, (B) middle, and (C) posterior nasal cavity.

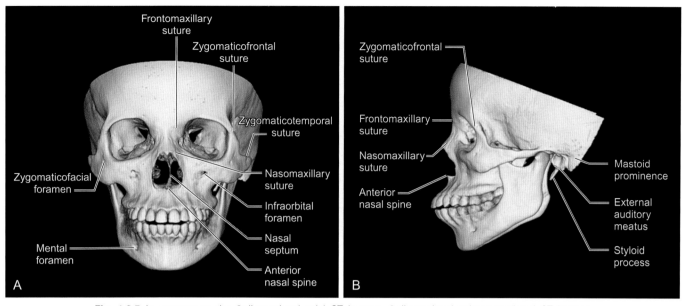

Fig. 1.2.5 In contrast to the 2-dimensional axial CT images, 3-dimensional volume-rendered CT images demonstrate the entire craniofacial skeleton in one image. (A) Frontal view of the face. (B) Lateral view of the face.

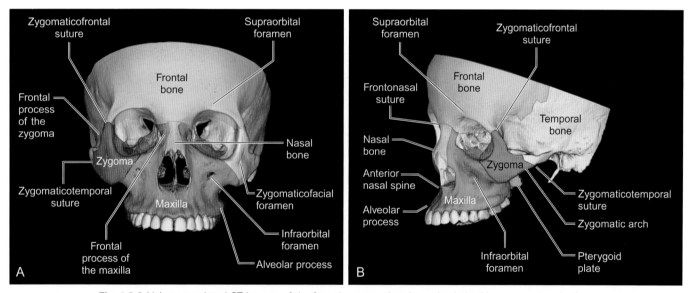

Fig. 1.2.6 Volume-rendered CT images of the face demonstrating the main skeletal bones creating the face and orbits. (A) Frontal view of the face. (B) Oblique view of the face.

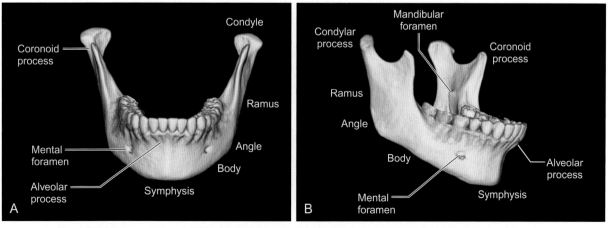

Fig. 1.2.7 Volume-rendered CT images of the mandible illustrating normal anatomy. (A) Frontal view of the mandible. (B) Oblique view of the mandible.

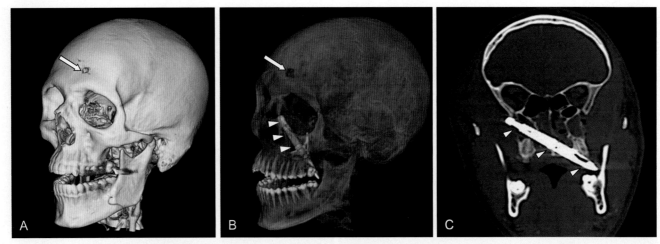

Fig. 1.2.8 CT images of a 25-year-old male after a suicide attempt. (A) Volume-rendered CT image of the craniofacial skeleton demonstrates a circular defect in the frontal bone superior to the left orbit (*white arrow*). (B) Shaded volume-rendered CT image of the craniofacial skeleton reveals the tip of a crossbow arrow extending through the midface (*white arrowheads*) in addition to the circular skull fracture created by another arrow (*white arrow*). (C) Coronal CT image of the midface shows the obliquely oriented crossbow arrow extending through the right maxillary sinus, inferior nasal cavity, and hard palate with tip in the left masticator space.

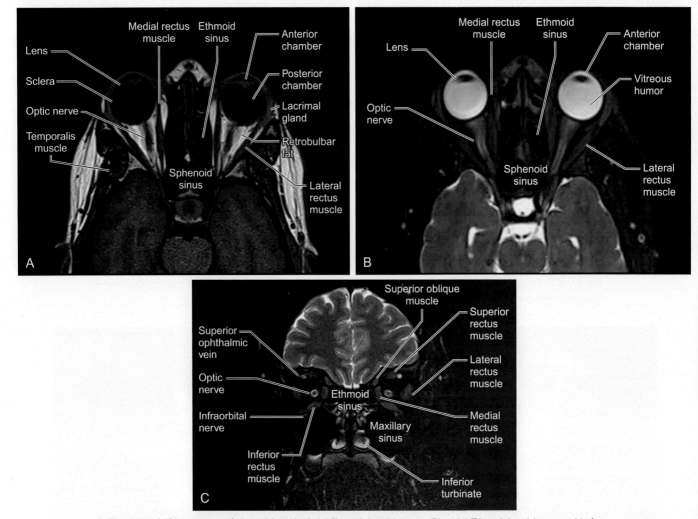

Fig. 1.2.9 MRI anatomy of the orbits. (A) Axial T1-weighted image. (B) Axial T2-weighted image with fat saturation. (C) Coronal T2-weighted image with fat saturation.

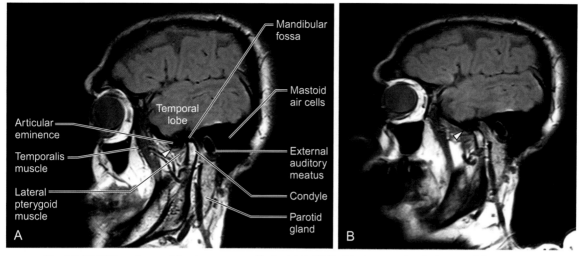

Fig. 1.2.10 MRI anatomy of the temporomandibular joint. (A) Sagitttal proton density image of the temporo-mandibular joint with the mouth closed. (B) Sagitttal proton density image of the temporomandibular joint with the mouth open shows the mandibular condyle articulating with the articular disc (*white arrowhead*). (Courtesy Dr. Frank Berkowitz.)

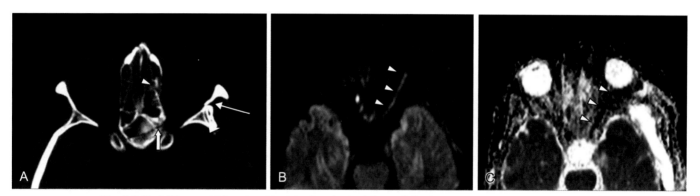

Fig. 1.2.11 A 34-year-old female with vision loss in the left eye following a high-speed motor vehicle collision. (A) Axial CT image through the face demonstrates a fracture in the anterior cranial fossa extending to the apex of the left orbit (*thick white arrow*) as well as fractures in the lamina papyracea (*white arrowhead*) and sphenozygomatic suture (*thin white arrow*). (B) Axial diffusion-weighted image from a subsequent MRI demonstrates restricted diffusion in the left optic nerve (*white arrowheads*). (C) Apparent diffusion coefficient map image with low signal intensity throughout the left optic nerve (*white arrowheads*) consistent with acute ischemia related to traumatic optic neuropathy.

of X-ray tubes in use (Table 1.2.2). Dual energy CT (DECT) may use two X-ray tubes at different kilovoltages (kV), i.e., Tube A at 90 kV and Tube B at 150 kV, allowing low-dose imaging with image optimization using iterative reconstruction. In comparison to the multidetector CT (MDCT) scanners, DECT scanners can help reduce the radiation dose by almost 50%.

CLASSIFICATION

Computed tomography (CT) is the best imaging modality to classify and characterize injuries to the craniofacial skeleton. Please see Video 1.2.1, "Systematic method for reading a craniofacial CT scan," to review a real-time systematic approach to interpreting a CT of the face.

POSTOPERATIVE IMAGING

There is no indication for the use of plain radiographs following open reduction and internal fixation (ORIF).[13] There is a consensus in the literature that after the direct visualization and fixation of the facial

TABLE 1.2.2 Radiation Dose of Craniofacial Imaging

Exam	Effective Dose (mSv)
Panoramic radiograph[a]	0.01
Face radiographs (3 views)	0.05
Chest radiograph[a]	0.1
DECT of the face[b]	0.73
MDCT of the face – 64 channel[c]	1.5
MDCT of the face – 256 channel[c]	1.8
Annual background exposure	3.0

[a]http://www.dentalbuzz.com/wp-content/uploads/2010/08/dental-radiation-doses.pdf.
[b]SOMATOM Force, Siemens Healthcare, Forchheim, Germany.
[c]Brilliance, Philips Medical Systems, Cleveland, OH.
DECT = dual energy computed tomography; MDCT = multidetector computed tomography.

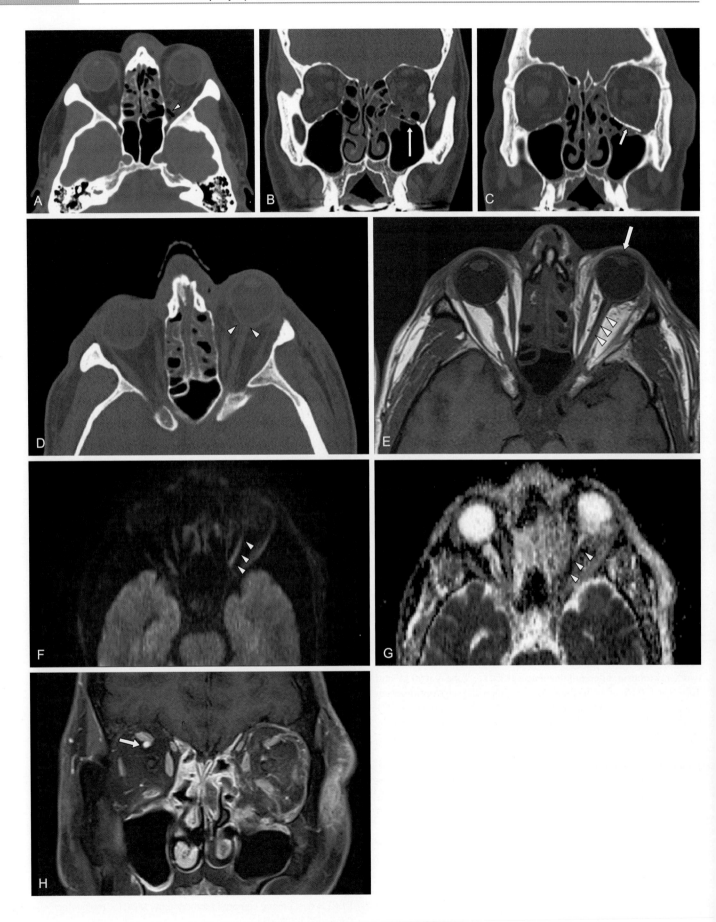

Fig. 1.2.12 A 56-year-old male presented to the hospital after a 12-foot fall from a ladder with complaints of diplopia and pain with upward gaze. Unenhanced CT images of the face (A–B) show mild proptosis of the left globe with retrobulbar gas (*white arrowhead*) and hematoma related to a displaced orbital floor fracture (*white arrow*). Herniation of the intraconal fat and inferior rectus muscle were reduced and the orbital floor repaired with titanium mesh (C). Shortly after the intraoperative repair and imaging, the patient developed near complete vision loss. The titanium mesh was emergently removed and repeat imaging (D) demonstrates marked increase in proptosis with straightening of the optic nerve and tenting at its insertion (*white arrowheads*). The patient underwent an emergent lateral cantholysis and canthotomy. Subsequent T1-weighted imaging demonstrates straightening of the optic nerve (*white arrowheads*) with asymmetric narrowing of the anterior chamber of the left eye (E) consistent with increased intraocular pressure. Diffusion-weighted imaging (F) shows restricted diffusion as well as decreased signal intensity on the apparent diffusion coefficient map (G) consistent with acute ischemia. A coronal T1-weighted image post gadolinium administration (H) only shows a normal enhancing right superior ophthalmic vein (*white arrow*) with loss of flow in the left superior ophthalmic vein consistent with orbital apex syndrome.

fractures, radiographs do not show any postoperative complications or abnormalities. Complications (i.e., malocclusion) are most likely to occur in the subacute or remote postoperative period.

CT is often completed immediately after ORIF to assess and confirm the alignment of the osseous fragments and hardware. This is most helpful in the evaluation of orbital floor repairs to ensure the complete reduction of the herniated orbital contents and ensure the allopathic mesh is not entrapping or impinging retrobulbar structures, such as the rectus muscles or optic nerve. CT is also used to rapidly assess acute postoperative complications causing vision loss, such as retrobulbar hematoma. Furthermore, CT is the modality of choice in imaging the craniofacial skeleton in the subacute and remote postoperative period with the use of intravenous contrast when evaluating soft tissue infection or vascular complications, i.e., carotid-cavernous fistula.

MRI is useful in the evaluation of injury to the optic nerve, which may result from direct trauma or shearing injury at the juncture of the intraorbital and intracanalicular segments resulting in disruption of its vascular supply.[14] The incidence of blindness following reduction of facial fractures is known to be about 0.2%.[15] Traumatic optic neuropathy (TON) has been seen after orbital surgery, Le Fort I osteotomies, and maxillofacial fracture fixation.[14] Just like an ischemic stroke within the brain, ischemic change within the optic nerve will demonstrate increased signal intensity on diffusion weighted (DWI) imaging and decreased signal intensity on the apparent diffusion coefficient (ADC) map (Fig. 1.2.11). MR angiography (MRA) and the administration of intravenous gadolinium can also be used to evaluate the etiology of vision loss such as thrombosis of the superior ophthalmic vein or compromised perfusion due to orbital compartment syndrome (Fig. 1.2.12).

ACUTE AND LONG-TERM COMPLICATIONS

While plain radiographs may be used in a community setting to initially evaluate craniofacial trauma, CT is the modality of choice given the detail it provides in assessing overlapping osseous structures, especially those of the orbit. It has been reported that approximately 5% of adults with head trauma have occult orbital floor fractures with approximately half of them requiring surgical intervention.[12] Entrapment occurs in 12% of cases of orbital floor fractures presenting with decreased ocular motility.[12] Retrobulbar hematoma and edema can also reduce ocular motility mimicking entrapment.[16] The classic appearance of the inferior rectus muscle completely entrapped within the maxillary sinus is most commonly seen in the pediatric population.[16] The plasticity

of the bone allows the free edge of the orbital fragment to snap back into place. In adults, entrapment most commonly involves the inferior rectus muscle as well as the medial, lateral, and superior recti with decreasing frequency.[16] The inferior rectus muscle is most commonly entrapped within the mid to posterior orbit (Fig. 1.2.13). Alteration in the course of the inferior rectus muscle and particularly its shape, changing from ovoid to circular, are additional CT or MR signs of herniation resulting from displacement of the orbital floor and tearing of the fascial investment of the muscle.[17] Entrapment may also result from a bone spicule piercing the muscle body and impeding its movement (Fig. 1.2.14). Diplopia is a typical sign of entrapment, but can also result from injury to cranial nerves innervating extraocular muscles (EOMs), altered angle of the muscle's action, mass effect from adjacent intraorbital hematoma or herniation, direct contusion or shearing of EOMs.[18]

Orbital emphysema can occur as a result of orbital wall fractures; most often from an isolated medial wall fracture or in combination with the orbital floor in 82% of cases (Fig. 1.2.15).[19,20] Rarely, air from a paranasal sinus may track into the orbit in a one-way mechanism producing tension orbital emphysema. Air may also track from the mediastinum superiorly into the face and hence the orbit. Tension orbital emphysema presents with proptosis, and without orbital decompression, progresses to visual loss potentially leading to blindness.[21,22] Sudden increases of intraorbital pressure may also result from sneezing or nose-blowing if there is a traumatic tract from a paranasal sinus into the orbit. Urgent orbital decompression is needed to manage this complication.[20,22] Rarely, intraorbital air under pressure can also track through mucoperiosteal tears related to orbital fractures through the various compartments of the face and neck, i.e., retropharyngeal, pretracheal, etc., into the mediastinum.[20]

Enophthalmos results from an increase in orbital volume, typically resulting from outward displacement of one or usually more orbital walls allowing the globe to settle into the expanded orbital capacity. Concurrent intraorbital edema and/or retrobulbar hematoma can mask the appearance of enophthalmos initially.

Portions of the orbital walls are involved in most major fracture patterns including the naso-orbital-ethmoid (medial orbit), Le Fort II (medial orbital floor), and III (medial, lateral walls, and floor), and zygomaticomaxillary complex (lateral orbit). Orbital roof fractures can be minimally displaced but fragments can "blow-in" or be inferiorly displaced into the orbit with high potential for orbital hematoma, globe damage and herniation of contused brain into the orbit (Fig. 1.2.16). Roof fragments can also "blow-up" into the anterior cranial fossa

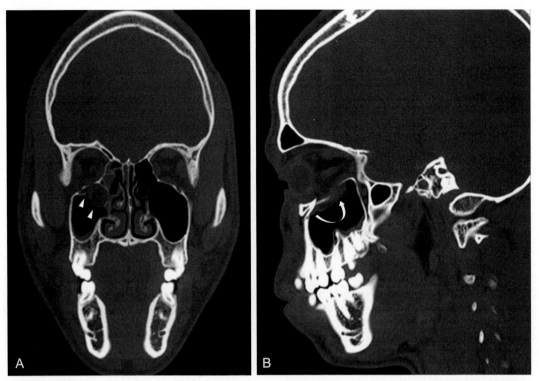

Fig. 1.2.13 A 17-year-old male presents with complaints of right eye pain, diplopia, and vertical gaze after being punched in the face. Coronal CT of the face (A) demonstrates a narrow osseous defect in the right orbital floor with herniation of orbital fat and the inferior rectus muscle (*white arrowheads*) into the maxillary sinus. Sagittal CT of the face (B) shows the herniated inferior rectus muscle (*curved arrow*) entrapped between the fragments of the right orbital floor.

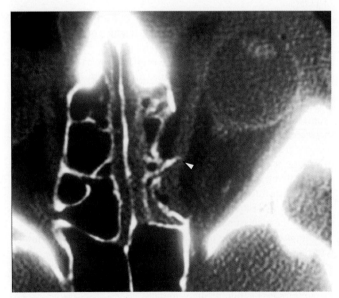

Fig. 1.2.14 Medial rectus muscle impaled. Axial CT image shows a spicule of bone from the ethmoid air cells embedded in the medial rectus muscle (*arrowhead*) preventing normal motion and leading to diplopia.

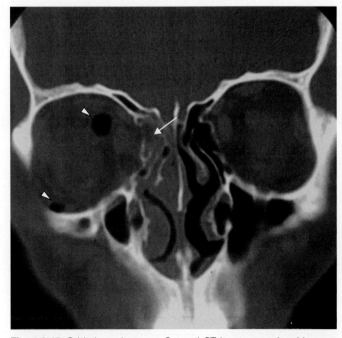

Fig. 1.2.15 Orbital emphysema. Coronal CT image reveals a blow-out fracture of the medial right orbital wall (*arrow*). Two dots of air are present within the orbit, one intraconal (*top arrowhead*) and one extraconal (*bottom arrowhead*). Orbital emphysema most commonly arises from the ethmoid sinus since air from the maxillary sinus is blocked by herniating tissue.

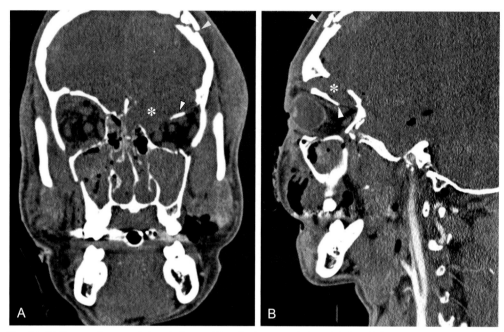

Fig. 1.2.16 Traumatic encephalocele from a blow-in fracture of the orbital roof. Coronal (A) and sagittal (B) views of a CT-angiogram of the face show comminuted and inferiorly displaced left orbital roof fragments (*arrowheads*). The parenchyma of the left frontal lobe (*asterisk*) herniates inferiorly into the superior orbit. The left globe is compressed by the herniating tissue and bone fragments with mild proptosis. This injury typically lacerates the dura, as well as contusing the brain, requiring repair by a neurosurgeon.

producing frontal lobe injury. Both injuries can lead to leakage of cerebrospinal fluid (CSF) into the orbit and potential spread of infection via sinus–cerebral communication.[23,24] MRI is recommended to fully assess injured intra- and periorbital soft tissue, particularly when involving the cerebral tissue.

Superior Ophthalmic Fissure/Orbital Apex Syndrome

Another complication of orbital trauma includes the optic nerve and innervation of the extraocular muscles. The nerves supplying the extraocular muscles (cranial nerves III and IV and the ophthalmic divisions of cranial nerves V and VI) traverse the superior ophthalmic fissure and can be injured when deep facial fractures traverse the region or by hematomas compressing the adjacent nerves (Fig. 1.2.17). This syndrome includes ptosis, fixed dilated pupil, ophthalmoplegia, and paresthesia in the distribution of the supratrochlear, supraorbital, and inferior orbital nerve.[20,22]

Acute Traumatic Cataract

After penetrating or blunt eye trauma, acute traumatic cataracts may develop. Traumatic cataracts occur in 24% of patients with globe contusions.[25] The presence of facial soft tissue swelling, opacified anterior chamber, or other complications can preclude direct examination of the lens. In patients with orbital injury, the CT attenuation of the patient's cataractous lens is markedly lower than in the contralateral lens (mean density difference, 30 H, $P < .0001$) (Fig. 1.2.18).[25] This decreased attenuation corresponds to acute cataract formation with increased fluid within the lens.[25] This low CT attenuation results from osmotic hydration with laceration of the lens capsule and failure of the sodium–potassium ion pump causing increased permeability and swelling of intra- and extracellular components of the lens.[25] Patients with normal attenuation values of the lens in the traumatized globe (as compared with the contralateral lens) do not have acute traumatic cataract or will develop a cataract within a 1-year follow-up period.[25]

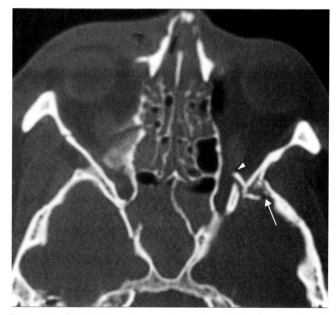

Fig. 1.2.17 Ophthalmic fissure syndrome. Axial CT in 47-year-old male injured in a fall demonstrates a comminuted fracture of the greater curvature of the left sphenoid (*arrow*) with a bone fragment impinging on the optic nerve (*arrowhead*) Fracture plane traverses the superior ophthalmic fissure with injury to cranial nerves supplying extraocular muscles.

Traumatic Optic Neuropathy

Traumatic optic neuropathy (TON) occurs in 2.5% of patients with midface fractures and 0.5%–5% of patients sustaining closed head injury.[26] TON results from direct and indirect injuries, with direct injuries occurring from penetrating objects such as knives or projectiles and bone fragments. Indirect injury results from contusion-induced necrosis from adjacent fractures in the canal region transmitting energy to the fixed optic nerve.[26] Craniofacial fractures occur in 75% of patients with TON, varying from isolated orbital wall fractures to more complex Le Fort and zygomaticomaxillary patterns. MRI of acute optic neuropathy shows increased signal on diffusion-weighted sequences and decreased apparent diffusion coefficient (diminished diffusion) predominantly involving the posterior optic nerve. While this MRI finding is 100% specific, it is only 28% sensitive (Fig. 1.2.11).[26]

Nasolacrimal System

Injury to the lacrimal drainage system (canaliculi, duct, and fossa) usually results from naso-orbital-ethmoid (NOE) fracture patterns, including the medial orbit and lateral nose (Fig. 1.2.19).[4] Nasolacrimal duct injuries are seen in about 10% of NOE fractures with displacement of the nasolacrimal buttress, bone fragments in the sac or duct, or avulsion of the lacrimal crest, and duct compression greater than 50%.[27] Injury to the nasolacrimal duct is associated with telecanthus in about 50% of NOE injuries.[27] Dacrocystitis and epiphora are the most common

clinical complications.[28] Other facial fractures occur in 83% of patients and 54% have concurrent intracranial injury.[29,30]

MANDIBLE

Mandibular factures are the second most common facial fractures after the nasal bones. CT is the most valuable tool to assess the extent of injury and assist in the surgical approach to fixation.[30–33] CT is helpful in evaluating patients presenting with trismus, which may result from restriction of the mandibular opening secondary to impaction of the coronoid process against a depressed zygomatic fracture (Fig. 1.2.20). Additional major acute and subacute complications of mandibular injuries include infection with altered bone density such as sclerosis, destructive or resorption changes, sequestration, nonunion, abscess or fixation plate exposure. Paresthesia may occur from pre- or postoperative

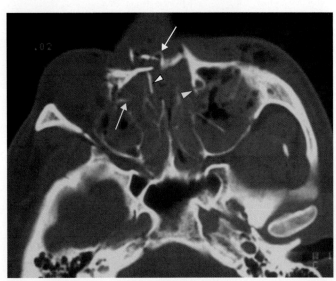

Fig. 1.2.19 Adult male patient with naso-orbital-ethmoid (NOE) and displaced nasolacrimal duct fractures. Axial CT demonstrates high energy comminuted NOE. The left lacrimal duct is in near anatomic position traversed by a fracture plane (*yellow arrowhead*). The right duct is fractured and markedly posteriorly displaced (*yellow arrow*). Multiple additional nasal (*white arrow*) and nasal septal (*white arrowhead*) fractures are present. Patient had bilateral epiphora.

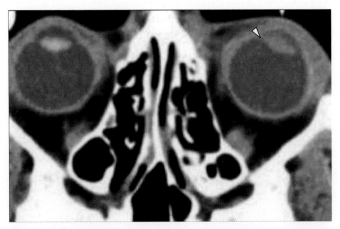

Fig. 1.2.18 Traumatic cataract. Axial CT of the orbits shows lower attenuation of left lens (*arrowhead*). Blunt trauma to the globe may disrupt the lens capsule, which may lead to edema within the lens that may eventually result in the development of a cataract.

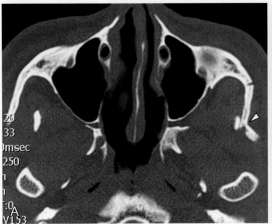
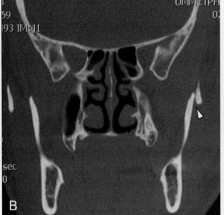
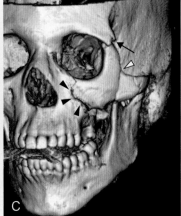

Fig. 1.2.20 Depressed zygomaticomaxillary complex (ZMC) with trismus. Axial (A) and coronal (B) images show the depressed mid-zygomatic arch fragments impacted on the coronoid process impairing motion of the mandible (*white arrowheads*). The patient has a ZMC fracture involving the anterior maxillary wall (*black arrowheads*), zygomatic arch (*white arrowhead*), and frontozygomatic suture (*black arrow*).

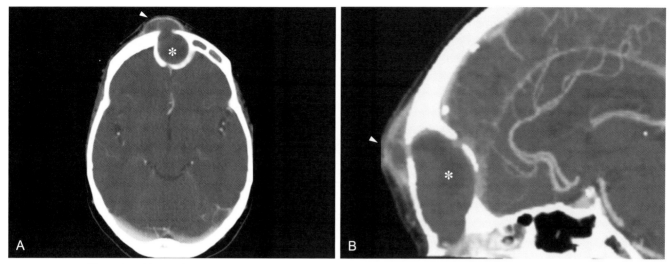

Fig. 1.2.21 Traumatic mucopyocele (*asterisk*) secondary to occluded nasofrontal ducts after trauma and continuing mucous secretions from retained mucosa in sinus.

nerve injury. Postoperative complications include malocclusion, failure of surgical fixation, and residual deformity.[30] Factors that are associated with an increase in major complications include mandibular angle and parasymphyseal fractures, with up to a 30% complication rate, removal of a tooth along the fracture line, interpersonal violence as an etiology, readmission or return to surgery, patient noncompliance and unexpected postoperative hospital stay.[31–33]

Frontal Sinus Injury

Frontal sinus fractures make up approximately 5%–15% of cranio-maxillofacial fractures and are usually associated with NOE fracture patterns.[34] This high-energy injury is commonly associated with other facial fractures, and can lead to significant complications such as meningitis, encephalitis, intracranial abscesses, osteomyelitis, and mucoceles (Fig. 1.2.21).

Vascular Injury

As mentioned before, CT is the preferred imaging modality in the setting of blunt and penetrating trauma within the craniofacial region not only for osseous injury, but also the soft tissues. In the setting of blunt trauma, displaced and depressed fracture fragments may lacerate branches of the external carotid artery resulting in injuries requiring emergent endovascular intervention. Vascular injuries in the setting of penetrating trauma include direct injury from laceration or indirect injury from shock wave formation and temporary cavitation from gunshot wounds.[35,36] Multidetector computed tomography angiography (MDCTA) accurately demonstrates the vascular injuries associated with projectile and non-projectile penetrating trauma of the neck, including: pseudoaneurysm, arteriovenous fistula, intimal injury with flap formation, active bleeding or dissection with partial or complete occlusion of the artery (Fig. 1.2.22). Metallic streak artifact from ballistic fragments may limit the evaluation of the adjacent vascular structures necessitating a conventional angiogram of both the internal and external carotid arteries.

MRI is contraindicated in the presence of nonferromagnetic metal or shrapnel. Moreover, MRI is often not a viable option given the prolonged amount of time required to image patients who may be hemodynamically unstable. The use of vascular ultrasound is also limited by lack of access from the overlying osseous structures of the midface and mandible as well as the numerous branches of the external carotid artery.

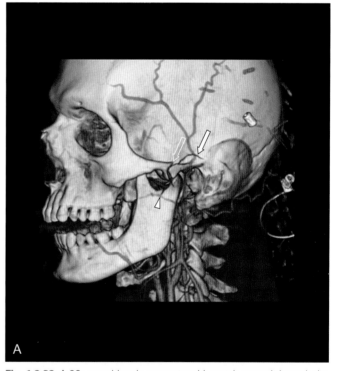

Fig. 1.2.22 A 26-year-old male presents with a stab wound through the left posterior aspect of the face. 3-D reconstruction of the face (A) shows mildly displaced fractures through the squama of the temporal bone (*white arrow*), zygomatic arch (*open white arrow*) and mandibular notch (*white arrowhead*). An unenhanced image of the face (B) demonstrates hemorrhage within the soft tissues of the parotid (*white arrowheads*) and parapharyngeal spaces (*white arrow*). CT angiogram of the neck (C) demonstrates a bilobed vascular abnormality in the left masticator space (*small white arrowhead*). A coronal maximum intensity projection image (D) shows a pseudoaneurysm (*yellow arrow*) arising from the left internal maxillary artery with venous drainage into the left external jugular vein consistent with an arteriovenous fistula (*white arrowheads*).

Continued

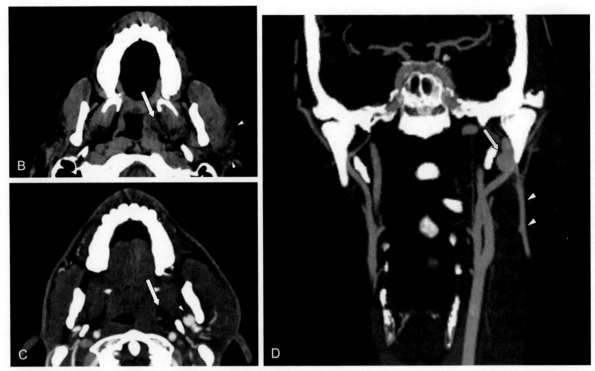

Fig. 1.2.22 cont'd

EXPERT COMMENTARY

'T.E.A.M.' we say, in the words of Brad Robertson, who ran the Shock Trauma Plastic Surgery Unit at the University of Maryland in Baltimore, Maryland for years. It means "together, we achieve more." Nowhere is this more helpful than in the combination of multiple specialists to solve challenging problems like medical issues, infectious disease, and imaging. While the dedicated maxillofacial physician can become an expert in imaging interpretation, knowledge and accuracy is facilitated by discussing images with colleagues: neurosurgeons, general surgical colleagues, and most essentially, radiologists. Neuro-ophthalmologists and sinus endoscopists are also essential for coordinated learning of the facial structures which allows the maxillofacial surgeon to sharpen his skills in the interpretation of the occasional, subtle problems encountered.

Mirvis, over 30+ years, has accumulated perhaps the most sophisticated radiological experience in facial trauma, with the world-class Shock Trauma Unit presenting a vast volume of injuries for learning. I learned early the value of a number of educational experiences: (1) a daily conference with the radiologists about our patients and their radiographs, which proved invaluable for us both, and especially the residents; (2) the value of postoperative critical imaging interpretation, as a training tool for residents and faculty to improve their reductions and the perception of disease. The value of postoperative imaging was taught to me by an orthopedist, Andy Burgess, who (when I finished a zygoma and was in the hall outside the operating room) was in the same hall, awaiting the technician taking an intraoperative film of an open tibia fracture. "Why would you want to image the reduction of a fracture you are treating open?" I asked. Andy appeared shortly in the recovery room with the film, which he was anxious to show me and which showed an error in fixation placement. I then ordered a postoperative CT on the patient with the zygoma I had just finished, and it showed a slight malreduction; the incident which became indelibly etched in my memory as a step-check in the confirmation postoperatively for open reduction. Postoperative imaging has become the single most helpful tool in helping me achieve more accurate reductions, and I remember the mistakes I have made, and check intraoperatively to assess whether the error has been avoided. And thanks

to our German colleagues [1], the advent of intraoperative imaging has further improved operative results. Michael Grant tells me that the rate of revision following an intraoperative CT scan is 20%–30%, avoiding a return to the operative room [2].

All of these steps [3–10] help achieve better results: interpretation, conference learning, intraoperative and postoperative assessment. The best results are achieved by using all three methods of radiological evaluation.

References

1. Gellrich NC, Schramm A, Hammer B, et al. Computer-assisted secondary reconstruction of unilateral posttraumatic orbital deformity. *Plast Reconstr Surg.* 2002;110(6): 1417–1429.
2. Personal communication with Dr. Michael Grant.
3. Van Hout WM, Van Camm EM, Muradin MS, et al. Intraoperative imaging for the repair of zygomaticomaxillary complex fractures: a comprehensive review of the literature. *J Craniomaxillofac Surg.* 2014;42(8):1918–1923.
4. Zimmerer RM, Ellis E, Aniceto GS, et al. A prospective multicentre study to compare the precision of posttraumatic internal orbital reconstruction with standard preformed and individualized orbital implants. *J Craniomaxillofac Surg.* 2016;44(9): 1485–1497.
5. Zhang Y, He Y, Zhang ZY, et al. Evaluation of the application of computer-aided shape-adapted fabricated titanium mesh for mirroring–reconstructing orbital walls in cases of late post-traumatic enophthalmos. *J Oral Maxillofac Surg.* 2010;68(9):2070–2075.
6. Rana M, Chul CHK, Wagner M, et al. Increasing the accuracy of orbital reconstruction with selective laser-melted patient-specific implants combined with intraoperative navigation. *J Oral Maxillofac Surg.* 2015;73(6):1113–1118.
7. Schmelzeisen R, Gellrich NC, Schoen R, et al. Navigation-aided reconstruction of medial orbital wall and floor contour in cranio-maxillofacial reconstruction. *Injury.* 2004;35(10): 955–962.
8. Kim JS, Lee BW, Scawn RL, et al. Secondary orbital reconstruction in patients with prior orbital fracture repair. *Ophthalmic Plast Reconstr Surg.* 2016;32(6):445–447.
9. Yung HN, Byun JY, Hyung-Jin K, et al. Prognostic CT findings of diplopia after surgical repair of pure orbital blowout fracture. *J Craniomaxillofac Surg.* 2016;44: 1479–1484.
10. Thai KN, Hummel RP, Kitzmiller WJ, et al. The role of computed tomographic screening in the management of facial trauma. *J Trauma.* 1997;43:214–217.

REFERENCES

1. Whaites E. *Essentials of Dental Radiography and Radiology*. Edinburgh: Churchill Livingstone; 2007.
2. Mukherjee S, Abhinav K, Revington P. A review of cervical spine injury associated with maxillofacial trauma at a UK tertiary referral centre. *Ann R Coll Surg Engl*. 2015;97(1):66–72.
3. Langland OE, ed. History of panoramic radiography. In: *Panoramic Radiology*. Philadelphia: Lea & Febiger; 1989.
4. White SC, Pharoah MJ, eds. Intraoral projections. In: *Oral Radiology: Principles and Interpretation*. St. Louis, MO: Elsevier; 2014.
5. Gassner R, Tuli T, Hächl O, et al. Cranio-maxillofacial trauma: a 10 year review of 9543 cases with 21,067 injuries. *J Craniomaxillofac Surg*. 2003;31:51–61.
6. Schuknecht B, Graetz K. Radiologic assessment of maxillofacial, mandibular, and skull base trauma. *Eur Radiol*. 2005;15(3):560–568.
7. Chacon GE, Dawson KH, Myall RW, et al. A comparative study of 2 imaging techniques for the diagnosis of condylar fractures in children. *J Oral Maxillofac Surg*. 2003;61:668–673.
8. Wilson IF, Lokeh A, Benjamin CI, et al. Prospective comparison of panoramic tomography (zonography) and helical computed tomography in the diagnosis and operative management of mandibular fractures. *Plast Reconstr Surg*. 2001;107:1369–1375.
9. Mahoney PF. *Imaging triage for ballistic trauma. Ballistic Trauma: A Practical Guide*. London: Springer; 2005:470–471.
10. Freund M, Hähnel S, Sartor K. The value of magnetic resonance imaging in the diagnosis of orbital floor fractures. *Eur Radiol*. 2002;12:1127–1133.
11. http://www.dentalbuzz.com/wp-content/uploads/2010/08/dental-radiation-doses.pdf.
12. Exadaktylos AK, Sclabas GM, Smolka K, et al. The value of computed tomographic scanning in the diagnosis and management of orbital fractures associated with head trauma: a prospective, consecutive study at a level I trauma center. *J Trauma*. 2005;58(2):336–341.
13. Jain MK, Alexander M. The need of postoperative radiographs in maxillofacial fractures – a prospective multicentric study. *Br J Oral Maxillofac Surg*. 2009;47(7):525–529.
14. Kumaran AM, Sundar G, Chye LT. Traumatic optic neuropathy: a review. *Craniomaxillofac Trauma Reconstr*. 2015;8(1):31–41.
15. Girotto JA, Gamble WB, Robertson B, et al. Blindness after reduction of facial fractures. *Plast Reconstr Surg*. 1998;102(6):1821–1834, Review.
16. Roth FS, Koshy JC, Goldberg JS, Soparkar CNS. Pearls of orbital trauma management. *Semin Plast Surg*. 2010;24(4):398–410.
17. Hopper RA, Salemy S, Sze RW. Diagnosis of midface fractures with CT: what the surgeon needs to know. *Radiographics*. 2006;26(3):783–793.
18. Sari A, Adiguzel U, Ismi T. An unexpected outcome of blunt ocular trauma: rupture of three muscles. *Strabismus*. 2009;17(3):95–97.
19. Moon H, Kim Y, Wi JM, Chi M. Morphological characteristics and clinical manifestations of orbital emphysema caused by isolated medial orbital wall fractures. *Eye (Lond)*. 2016;30(4):582–587.
20. van Issum C, Courvoisier DS, Scolozzi P. Posttraumatic orbital emphysema: incidence, topographic classification and possible pathophysiologic mechanisms. A retrospective study of 137 patients. *Oral Surg Oral Med Oral Parhol Oral Radiol*. 2013;115(6):7373–7742.
21. Oura H, Hirose M, Ishiki M. Diplopia and blepharoptosis associated with orbital emphysema following thoracotomy with lung cancer; report of a case. *Kyobu Geka*. 2004;57(6):501–504.
22. Tomasetti P, Jacbosen C, Gander T, Zemann W. Emergency decompression of tension retrobulbar emphysema secondary to orbital floor fracture. *J Surg Case Rep*. 2013;2013(3):rjt011.
23. Borumandi F. Traumatic orbital CSF leak. *BMJ Case Rep*. 2013;doi:10.1136/bcr-2013-202216.
24. Righi S, Boffano P, Gugliemlmi V, et al. Diagnosis and imaging of orbital roof fractures: a review of the current literature. *Oral Maxillofac Surg*. 2015;19(1):1–4.
25. Boorstein JM, Titelbaum DS, Patel Y, et al. CT diagnosis of unsuspected traumatic cataracts in patients with complicated eye injuries: significance of attenuation value of the lens. *AJR Am J Roentgenol Radiother*. 1995;164(1):181–184.
26. Bodanapally UK, Shanmuganathan K, Shin RK, et al. Hyperintense optic nerve due to diffusion restriction: diffusion-weighted imaging in traumatic optic neuropathy. *AJNR Am J Neuroradiol*. 2015;36:1536–1541.
27. Garg RK, Hartman MJ, Lucarelli MJ, et al. Nasolacrimal system fractures: a description of radiologic findings and associated outcomes. *Ann Plast Surg*. 2015;75(4):407–413.
28. Ramkumar VA, Agarkar S, Mukherjee B. Nasolacrimal duct obstruction: does it really increase the risk of amblyopia in children? *Indian J Ophthalmol*. 2016;64(7):496–499.
29. Becelli R, Renzi G, Mannino G, et al. Posttraumatic obstruction of lacrimal pathways: a retrospective analysis of 58 consecutive naso-orbitoethmoid fractures. *J Craniofac Surg*. 2004;15(1):29–33.
30. McRae M, Momeni R, Naravan D. Frontal sinus fractures: a review of trends, diagnosis, treatment, and outcomes at a level 1 trauma center in Connecticut. *Conn Med*. 2008;72(3):133–138.
31. Dreizin D, Nam AJ, Tirada N, et al. Multidetector CT of mandibular fractures, reductions, and complications: a clinically relevant primer for the radiologist. *Radiographics*. 2016;36(5):1539–1564.
32. Christensen BJ, Mercante DE, Neary JP, King BJ. Risk factors for severe complications of operative mandibular fractures. *J Oral Maxillofac Surg*. 2016;75(4):787.e1–787.e8.
33. Munante-Cardenas JL, Fachina Nunes PH, Passeri LA. Etiology, treatment, and complications of mandibular fractions. *J Craniofac Surg*. 2015;26(3):611–615.
34. Rosado P, de Vicente JC, Villalain L, et al. Posttraumatic frontal mucocele. *J Craniofac Surg*. 2011;22(4):1537–1539.
35. Bush K, Huikeshoven M, Wong N. Nasofrontal outflow tract visibility in computed tomography imaging of frontal sinus fractures. *Craniomaxillofac Trauma Reconstr*. 2014;7(2):167–168.
36. Offiah C, Hall E. Imaging assessment of penetrating injury of the neck and face. *Insights Imaging*. 2012;3(5):419–431.

Intraoperative Imaging and Postoperative Quality Control

Rüdiger M. Zimmerer, Nils-Claudius Gellrich

BACKGROUND

The idea behind intraoperative imaging is to avoid postoperative imaging and secondary revision procedures by allowing the intraoperative confirmation and adjustment of fracture reduction and hardware placement as necessary. This should save time, resources, reduce the number of operations, and improve results. Different imaging modalities are available intraoperatively, including magnetic resonance imaging (MRI), computed tomography (CT), ultrasound (US), and cone beam computed tomography (CBCT).[1,2] Today, intraoperative imaging using CBCT mainly refers to so-called 3D C- and O-arms. The terms "C-arm" and "O-arm" originate from the shape of the device (Fig. 1.3.1). Basically, intraoperative imaging can be performed using either portable or static devices. C- and O-arms are available as mobile and static devices. CT and MRI scanners are usually static devices and might be integrated into hybrid operation theaters.

The usage of intraoperative C-arms or image intensifiers began in the 1960s.[2,3] Contrary to craniomaxillofacial surgery, intraoperative imaging has been performed for more than half a century in orthopedic surgery. Today, orthopedic surgery without intraoperative imaging is unimaginable. This is based on the fact that initially only 2-dimensional (2D) images could be obtained which were not suitable to display the complex 3-dimensional (3D) anatomy of the facial skeleton, particularly of the orbit. Plain radiographs of the skull, for example, panoramic, Waters view, submentovertex (jug-handle view), or lateral radiographs, are difficult to interpret because of the effects of superimposition. In midface fractures, orbital wall involvement cannot be ruled out using conventional 2D imaging. Furthermore, the resolution of those images, particularly concerning orbital walls, is inadequate for accurate diagnosis. Thus, 2D and 3D imaging should be used for diagnosis and treatment planning of craniomaxillofacial fractures, particularly of the orbit.[4,5] Today, multislice computed tomography (MSCT) and cone beam computed tomography (CBCT) are the imaging modalities of choice for diagnosing midface fractures.[4,6,7] Both techniques were found to be suitable for imaging midface fractures in all 3 dimensions and to help assess whether orbital reconstruction is required.

The transfer of the postoperative radiological examination into the operation theater has not only offered the chance of immediate revisional surgery but has also substituted conventional radiographs with a 3D data set. Thus, CT and CBCT should not only be used for diagnosis and treatment planning in craniomaxillofacial trauma but also for postoperative quality control.[8] In most institutions postoperative CT or CBCT scans are used. Not until motorized cone beam systems with 3D CT-like image data sets were introduced, was intraoperative imaging attractive to craniomaxillofacial surgery.[2]

Intraoperative Cone Beam Computed Tomography

Three-dimensional C-arm devices that are also referred to as angiographic image intensifiers were initially used in cardiac and vascular surgery. Meanwhile, they have increasingly been used since the end of the 1990s.[2,3,9] These advances have also enabled the use of such 3D C-arms for intraoperatively displaying the facial skeleton. Thus, this technology has increasingly been used over the last decade in oral and maxillofacial surgery.[2,10–12] As mentioned above, C-arms are portable or can be fixed or mounted to the ceiling, to the ground, or even to robotic arms.

The principle behind this technique is a cone-shaped X-ray bundle. The conical shape of the beam distinguishes this technique from helical or spiral CT, which used a fan-shaped beam. The X-ray source and the detector (image intensifier or flat panel detector) rotated around a field of interest of the patient. By rotating the beam around a fixed point (isocenter) in the object of interest and acquiring projections from many different angles, a typically cylindrical 3D volume can be reconstructed. Although a 360 degree rotation is used in general, some devices have implemented a 180 degree or slightly greater rotation arc, which suffices for image reconstruction and leads to significant radiation reduction. Conventional intraoperative 3D C-arm devices consist of an isocentric C-arm and the motorized devices allow rotations of 190 degrees around the patient.[2] As a result of the acquisition of 2D projections throughout this rotation, only a single rotation 360 degrees or less is needed to acquire a full (3D) data set.

The images received by the detector are then compiled into volumetric data (primary reconstruction). This can then be visualized as 2D multiplanar reformatted slices or in three dimensions by using surface reconstruction or volume rendering. Typically, a few hundreds of projections are collected. The 2D attenuation profiles obtained from all angles are then reconstructed into a 3D matrix, containing volume elements (voxels), each having a certain grey value which represents the average density within this volume element. As examples, a few devices that are frequently used in craniomaxillofacial surgery are described in Table 1.3.1.[2]

Today, intraoperative 3D C-arms should be connectable to devices that allow for intraoperative real-time navigation.[2,8,13] In addition, DICOM-Data generated by the 3D C-arm can be fused with the preoperatively created virtual planning so that an immediate intraoperative superimposition of planning and result are possible in the operating room.

Indications for Intraoperative CBCT

Basically, the indications are more or less the same as compared to conventional postoperative CBCT or CT. The major advantage of intraoperative imaging can be seen in procedures in which intraoperative verification of the surgical result is crucial and would lead to secondary corrections. According to recent literature, the major indication for intraoperative CBCT is craniomaxillofacial trauma, particularly fractures of the zygomaticomaxillary complex (ZMC), including posttraumatic orbital deformities.[10,11] However, multiple different indications have been described in the literature. Intraoperative CBCT has also been

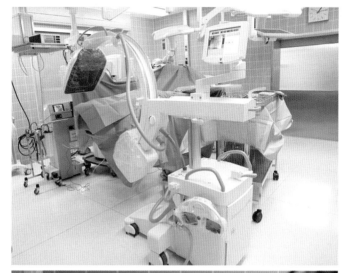

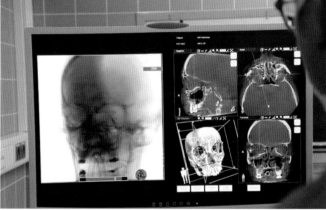

Fig. 1.3.1 Portable intraoperative 3D imaging device. C-arm in an intraoperative setting (Ziehm Vision RFD, Ziehm Imaging, Nürnberg, Germany). The device can be covered with sterile drapes. Using an integrated laser the device can be adjusted according to the patient and the area of interest. Intraoperatively, some C-arms can be linked with intraoperative navigation devices. Intraoperatively, the result of reconstruction or reduction can be analyzed immediately on a separate screen.

used in orthognathic surgery, in maxillary and mandibular reconstructions with bone grafts. In gunshot injuries it was shown to be useful in the detection and removal of metallic foreign bodies. Intraoperative imaging using a 3D C-arm was used during mandibular fracture repair, particularly of the condylar process and the condylar head. In those cases the postreduction result of the fragments or the position of the condylar head in the glenoid fossa are crucial. Three-dimensional intraoperative imaging using a C-arm device was also described as a practical device in evaluation and verification following bone grafting procedures, including sinus floor augmentation. Furthermore, CBCT data generated by intraoperative mobile systems were shown to be sufficient for the planning of dental implant position.[23] As mentioned above, intraoperative imaging can also be used in combination with intraoperative real-time navigation. Finally, preoperative CT or MRI in infants often requires general anesthesia. In children with preoperatively proven indications for surgical treatment, preoperative imaging under general anesthesia was substituted by intraoperative CBCT scans.

In summary, hard tissues can be displayed sufficiently using intraoperative 3D C-arm devices. The integration of flat panel detectors in advanced mobile CBCT systems will overcome the current disadvantages, such as limited data volume and insufficient soft tissue visualization.

However, one disadvantage is the fact that the field of view cannot be altered in this system, resulting in imaging of areas that are not of primary interest.

Intraoperative CT and MRI

CT and MRI scanners are usually static devices and are mainly part of so-called hybrid operation theaters. Meanwhile, CT scans have emerged as standard imaging modalities in the diagnosis and treatment of craniomaxillofacial trauma and reconstruction, particularly of the orbit.[5,10,14,15] Multislice systems with secondary coronal reconstructions have superseded primary coronal scans. However, the installation of an intraoperative fan beam CT scanner in a hybrid operation theater is associated with enormous costs and requires a complex infrastructure. However, the high resolution of intraoperative CT scans and the size of the scanning volume can be considered a major advantage, particularly in panfacial fractures.[16] So far, CT is superior to all other imaging modalities in craniomaxillofacial trauma. Particularly, the fine anatomy of the orbit can be displayed most suitably using CT. Its disadvantages include high doses of radiation emitted, the high procurement costs and, as with magnetic resonance imaging, the imperative need for the presence of a radiologist with basic knowledge in craniomaxillofacial surgery, surgical demands, and sterility.[2] This final disadvantage may result in intraoperative delays as well. Therefore, intraoperative CT is so far not recommended as a routine intraoperative imaging modality in craniomaxillofacial surgery.

In addition, intraoperative MRI is also not in routine use in craniomaxillofacial surgery. This is due to the fact that bony structures and inserted radiopaque implants are not displayed sufficiently. Further disadvantages include the extended scanning time, the complex intraoperative handling, and the need for a radiologist to be present.[2]

Intraoperative Real-Time Navigation

The use of intraoperative real-time navigation has been increasingly described in the field of craniomaxillofacial surgery.[6,7,17–20] Today, this technique is routinely used in many institutions. The major advantage of intraoperative infrared-based navigation includes its radiation-free application in the operating room. In addition, multiple instruments including drills and burrs can be registered and tracked that allow their intraoperative real-time navigation.[21] According to virtually determined trajectories, position, orientation, and path of movement of the instrument can be controlled in real time using an autopilot function (Figs. 1.3.2 and 1.3.3). However, a preoperative CT or CBCT data set is always required for the determination of registration markers.[22] The fact that this technique is based on a preoperative scan means that topographic changes during surgery result in discrepancies between the preoperative image data and the surgical site.[23,24]

There are various markers that can be used for registration, including anatomical landmarks, dental-based navigation splints with radiopaque markers (screws), or previously inserted navigation screws.[22] Anatomical landmarks for registration can be defined using the initial CT or CBCT scan. However, an additional CT or CBCT scan is required in case navigation splints or navigation screws are used (Fig. 1.3.3B). Meanwhile, frameless registration can be realized in the craniomaxillofacial region using a laser surface scanning system in order to avoid radiation exposure.[23] Computer-assisted preoperative planning is required to virtually reduce fractures or reconstruct defects by mirroring.[25] Intraoperatively, the patient's position and anatomy need to be registered to the preoperative CT or CBCT data set using a "skull reference base" that needs to be fixed to the patient's skull. Thereby, the patient's position during the procedure can be tracked. Intraoperatively, the quality of fracture reduction as well as the planned position and shape of an implant can be checked in real-time sensing. It could be shown that

TABLE 1.3.1   Selection of Different Intraoperative 3D C-arms

Company	Product Name	Intended Use	H × W × D of C-arm frame, cm (in.)	Image Intensifier, cm (in.)	Image Matrix Size	Generator	Navigation Aids	Differences From Competition
Ziehm Imaging	Vision RFD 3D	Fluoroscopy, interventional radiology	30 (12) FD: 159 × 80 × 188 (62.6 × 31.5 × 74); 20 (8) FD:160.3 × 80 × 189.4 (63.1 × 31.5 × 74.6)	Flat-panel detector 30 (12)/flat-panel detector 20 (8)	1024 × 1024	25 kW	Roadmapping; interface to image-guided surgery 2D	20 kW powerful monoblock generator; SmartVascular; up to three synchronized touchscreen user-interfaces; large flat-panel; advanced active cooling for nearly unlimited X-ray time; SmartArchive; SmartDose
Siemens Healthcare	Arcadis Orbic 3D	Surgical fluoroscopic imaging	215 × 80 × 180 (84 × 31 × 71)	23 (9)	1024 × 1024	2.3 kW	Yes	3D visualization and navigation
Philips Healthcare	Veradius Neo	Interventional procedure visualization	169 × 81 × 73 (66 × 32 × 29)	Flat detector 26 (10)	1280 × 1024	15 kW	Digital navigation link, landmarking, pixel shift, roadmapping, SmartMask, trace mode	Optimized C-Arm geometry; new distortion-free Trixell FD with 103 dB dynamic range; 15 kW generator; cardiovascular packages; 12-in. stand monitor for operator

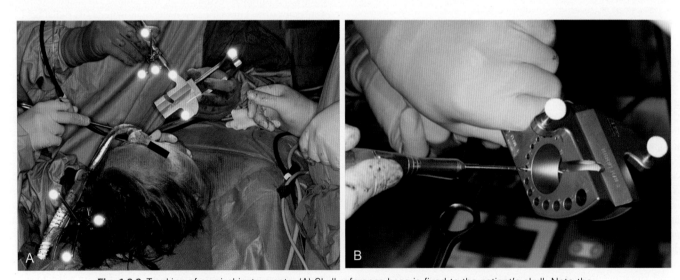

Fig. 1.3.2 Tracking of surgical instruments. (A) Skull reference base is fixed to the patient's skull. Note the Brainlab ready-to-use adapter for instrument tracking with the Brainlab calibration matrix in the back (Kolibri™, Brainlab, Feldkirchen, Germany). With the Brainlab instrument calibration matrix any instrument geometry, including diameter and vector, can be included and tracked in real-time sensing. (B) Close-up of the adapter for instrument tracking (diameter and length). All instruments used for navigation were provided by Brainlab (Feldkirchen, Germany).

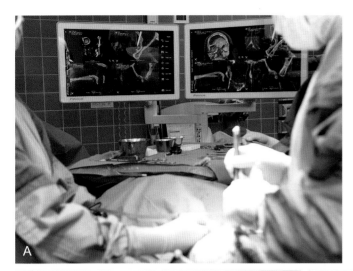

Fig. 1.3.3 Intraoperative real-time navigation using trajectories and instrument tracking (Kolibri™, Brainlab, Feldkirchen, Germany). (A) Intraoperative setting with the Brainlab Curve system (Curve™, Brainlab, Feldkirchen, Germany). (B) Virtual plan of a functionalized, customized orbital implant (IPS Orbit, KLS Martin, Tuttlingen, Germany) in the right orbit. (*Left*) Two trajectories (*blue*) in the oblique sagittal plane (*) and the transition zone (#) between medial orbital wall and orbital floor. Screws for intraoperative registration included in a navigational splint. (*Right*) Intraoperative autopilot function.

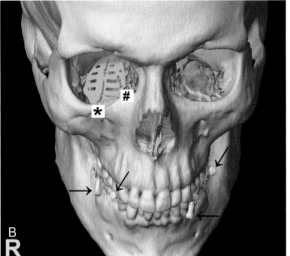

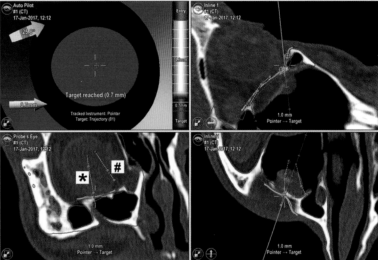

intraoperative infrared-based navigation significantly improves the precision of orbital reconstruction using different titanium implants.[6,20] The use of navigation also had a significant effect on the precision of the orbital volume reconstruction.[6]

Recently, intraoperative imaging has opened up new perspectives in the field of intraoperative navigation. The renewal of intraoperative 3D imaging in maxillofacial surgery was mainly driven by the disadvantage of intraoperative navigation systems being based on preoperatively acquired imaging data that increasingly differ from the surgical site with ongoing surgery.[24] Today, 3D C-arm devices generate DICOM data sets that are usable for intraoperative navigation. However, contrary to real-time navigation that is planned and registered on preoperative CT or CBCT data sets, fluoroscopic images (2D/3D) are used for the combination of intraoperative imaging and intraoperative navigation as originally described and used in spinal surgery.[26] Meanwhile, the intraoperative acquisition of 3D fluoroscopic data sets for real-time navigation in craniomaxillofacial surgery has already been introduced.[10] Finally, it could also be shown that 3D fluoroscopic data sets revealed an accuracy for navigation comparable to CT.[13] Unfortunately, fusion of 3D fluoroscopy data with other 3D modalities could not be clinically realized up to today. But regarding high-contrast structures, an intraoperative updating by 3D fluoroscopy seems possible in the near future.[23]

SURGICAL ANATOMY IN 3D IMAGING

As previously mentioned, 2D images are not suitable to display the complex 3D anatomy of the facial skeleton, particularly in complex post-traumatic and congenital deformities, contour-relevant reconstructions, skull base surgery, and orbital deformities.[5,10] Thus, high-resolution 3D imaging is recommended in the diagnosis as well as in the postoperative or intraoperative quality control of those cases.[5] Distinct anatomical regions in the facial skeleton require distinct pre- and postoperative images, or if available, intraoperative imaging in order to be able to reconstruct complex anatomical regions. Those regions particularly include midface (zygomaticomaxillary region) and orbit, skull base, and the frontobasal region, as well as the condylar processes. Today, the indication for surgery should depend on the results of the diagnostic 3D imaging rather than 2D radiographs.[5] Thus, the detailed anatomical information provided by 3D imaging allows craniomaxillofacial surgery to meet the requirements of a true-to-original reconstruction.

Goals of Reconstruction

The goals of reconstruction in the craniomaxillofacial region are:
  To get things …
  • Right, that were right (e.g. primary trauma)
  • Better, that had been made wrong (e.g. secondary trauma)

- Adequate, that were never right (e.g. congenital)
- More adequate after tissue loss (e.g. postablative)

In order to achieve a true-to-original reconstruction, the anatomical features discussed below have to be taken into consideration.[5,6,27–29]

Radiological key elements exist that should be analyzed in the preoperative 3D trauma scan first and, in case of reconstruction, again in the post- or intraoperative 3D imaging. The advances of high-resolution 3D imaging and computer-assisted surgery have given new insights into the details of orbital anatomy and have transformed the basic understanding of internal surface contours in relation to volume, ocular globe position, and binocular function.[6] In general, the contralateral unaffected side should always be analyzed and provide a template.

Radiological Key Elements in Orbital Reconstruction

- Shape of the orbital walls, e.g. "lazy-S shape" of the orbital floor
- Volume of the orbit
- Posteromedial bulge
- The posterior ledge
- The nasolacrimal canal
- The inferomedial orbital buttress (transition zone between medial orbital wall and floor)

A common clinical observation is the loss of support in the posteromedial portion of the orbital floor, so that the profile of the posterior orbital floor changes from convex to concave.[28,30] After trauma, the shape of the orbital wall changes from a complex undulating cone to a sphere, where all the subtle curves of the internal orbit are lost.[28,31] It is the inferior displacement of the posterior orbital floor that results in deviation of the globe.[6,7] An increase of orbital volume correlates with enophthalmos.[28,32,33] Dystopia of the ocular globe including enophthalmos and hypoglobus and diplopia might result from inadequate diagnosis and treatment of posttraumatic orbital deformities in terms of a true-to-original reconstruction of orbital volume, internal orbital buttresses, posteromedial bulge, and the lazy-S-shape of the floor.[6,7,34] In summary, both the preoperative diagnostic imaging and the intra- or postoperative imaging should provide reliable information about the key elements of orbital anatomy for adequate diagnosis and treatment. CT or CBCT (pre-, intra-, or postoperative) are recommended for the diagnosis, treatment, and postoperative quality control in orbital traumatology and reconstruction[4,6] (Fig. 1.3.4).

Radiological Key Elements for the Orbitozygomaticomaxillary (OZMC) Complex

In the radiological assessment of ZMC fractures it is crucial to analyze the midfacial buttresses and the vertical, transverse, and sagittal dimensions of the facial skeleton.
- Axial, coronal, and sagittal projection of the zygoma
- Bilateral shape of the zygomatic arch starting from the zygomatic process of the temporal bone (sagittal and transverse dimensions of the facial skeleton)
- Dorsolateral wall of the maxillary sinus (first signs of ZMC fracture)
- Sutures:
  - zygomaticofrontal suture
  - infraorbital rim
  - zygomaticomaxillary buttress
  - zygomatic arch
  - zygomaticosphenoid sutures

In more comminuted OZMC fractures, the junction between the orbital process of the zygoma and the greater wing of sphenoid facilitates correction of rotational alignment of the zygoma. This suture is a broad surface, the alignment of which may be used to help ascertain that the zygoma has been repositioned correctly. In more complex cases the anterior lip of the greater wing of the sphenoid is disrupted, and one has to be sure that the lateral orbit, zygoma, and greater wing of the sphenoid junction are entirely in a straight line with the intact greater wing of the sphenoid (Fig. 1.3.4).

Radiological Key Elements for Mandible and Condylar Processes

The indications for condylar process fracture treatment are still discussed controversially, even among expert surgeons. At this point in time, consensus about treatment of all fractures has not been reached. In many cases, clinical examination and conventional radiographs (panoramic and Waters view) are sufficient to basically diagnose fractures of the mandible and the condylar processes. However, 3D imaging (CT and CBCT) might help to decide whether surgery is indicated or not, particularly in cases with involvement of the condylar region. Using 3D imaging, the following fracture parameters have to be considered in order to choose the best therapeutic option for the patient (Fig. 1.3.5):
- Transversal width of the mandible
- Bilateral vertical ramus height
- Direction of condylar head luxation
- Fragmentation pattern (comminuted, simple) and length and architecture of the comminuted segments
- Association with other mandibular injuries and other facial bone injuries (such as palate and maxilla)
- Injuries of the mandibular fossa

Important clinical parameters including dental occlusion, status of dentition, association with systemic injuries, and the condition of the patient (comorbidity factors) must be taken into consideration as well.

RADIOLOGICAL EVALUATION

The radiological evaluation of a posttraumatic orbital defect is shown in Fig. 1.3.6 and Video 1.3.1. After assessment and analysis of the fracture pattern, the defect size was measured in order to plan an adequate reconstruction. In the axial view the defect of the medial orbital wall starting from the posteromedial bulge can be seen. In the coronal view the width of the defect is measured as well as the dislocation of the orbital floor into the maxillary sinus. Compared to the contralateral side, the fracture includes the transition zone between medial orbital wall and floor. This can clearly be seen by comparing the angles in the transition zone. In the sagittal view the length of the defect and the dislocation of the orbital floor into the maxillary sinus can be measured. The defect includes the posterior ledge and the lazy-S shape of the orbital floor is no longer present (see Fig. 1.3.4 and Surgical anatomy in 3D imaging, above). For didactic reasons, the case demonstrated here will be shown again after reconstruction using intraoperative imaging and intraoperative real-time navigation in the following section (see Fig. 1.3.7 and Video 1.3.4).

SURGICAL TECHNIQUES

After orbital reconstruction was indicated based on clinical and radiological findings (Video 1.3.1), the patient was treated with a patient-specific orbital implant (IPS Orbit, KLS Martin, Tuttlingen, Germany). Following preparation of a transconjunctival, retroseptal approach, the patient-specific orbital implant was inserted using intraoperative real-time navigation (Brainlab Curve, Brainlab, Feldkirchen, Germany). Navigation was used to verify the correct implant position in the orbital cavity according to the preoperative virtual plan (Video 1.3.2). In order to facilitate the intraoperative navigation, the virtual model

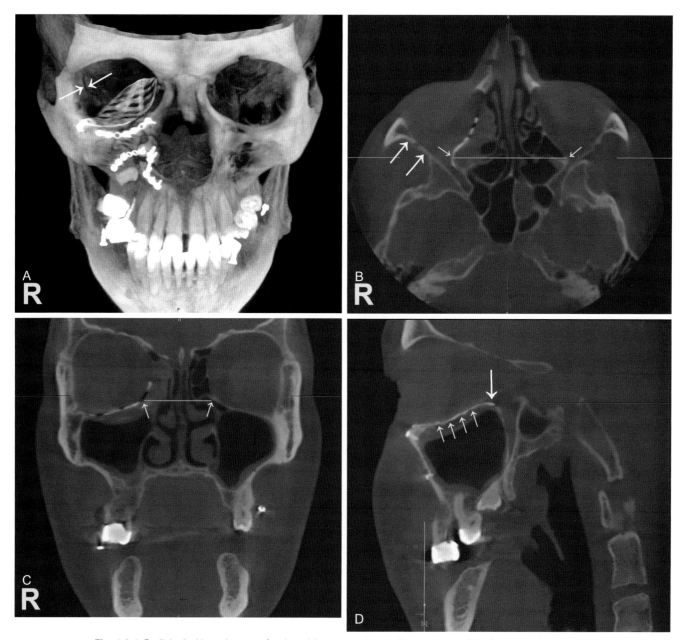

Fig. 1.3.4 Radiological key elements for the orbitozygomaticomaxillary complex (OZMC) in a postreconstruction 3D CBCT. (A) Fluoroscopic image. Reduction of an OZMC fracture and reconstruction of the orbital floor with a patient-specific orbital implant (IPS Orbit, KLS Martin, Tuttlingen, Germany). The junction between the orbital process of the zygoma and the greater wing of sphenoid facilitates correction of rotational alignment of the zygoma (*white arrows*). (B) Axial view. Reduction of the zygomatico-sphenoid suture (*white arrows*) and reconstruction of the posteromedial bulge (*yellow arrows*) compared to the contralateral side (*horizontal line*). (C) Coronal view. Reconstruction of the transition zone between medial orbital wall and orbital floor (*yellow arrows*) compared to the contralateral side (*horizontal line*). (D) Oblique sagittal view. Reconstruction of the orbital floor using a functionalized customized titanium orbital implant (IPS Orbit, KLS Martin, Tuttlingen Germany). Note the lazy-S shape of the orbital floor (*yellow arrows*). The implant lies on the posterior ledge (*white arrow*).

of the patient-specific implant was imported into the planning platform as an STL-file (stereolithographic) prior to surgery. In this case, the patient-specific orbital implant was equipped with two tracks that provide guidance for correct insertion of the implant and allow for intraoperative navigation (Video 1.3.2, Fig. 1.3.3, and see Surgical anatomy in 3D imaging, above). Following implant insertion using intraoperative navigation, intraoperative 3D imaging was performed using a mobile 3D C-arm (Ziehm Vision RFD, Ziehm Imaging, Nürnberg, Germany) (Video 1.3.3). After data acquisition, the generated DICOM data were imported into the navigation and planning platform to fuse preoperative virtual planning and the intraoperative CBCT whilst the patient is still under general anesthesia (Fig. 1.3.7, Video 1.3.4). If the reconstruction is in line with a preoperative virtual plan, the patient can be closed-up and surgery is finished. In case of implant malposition or inadequate

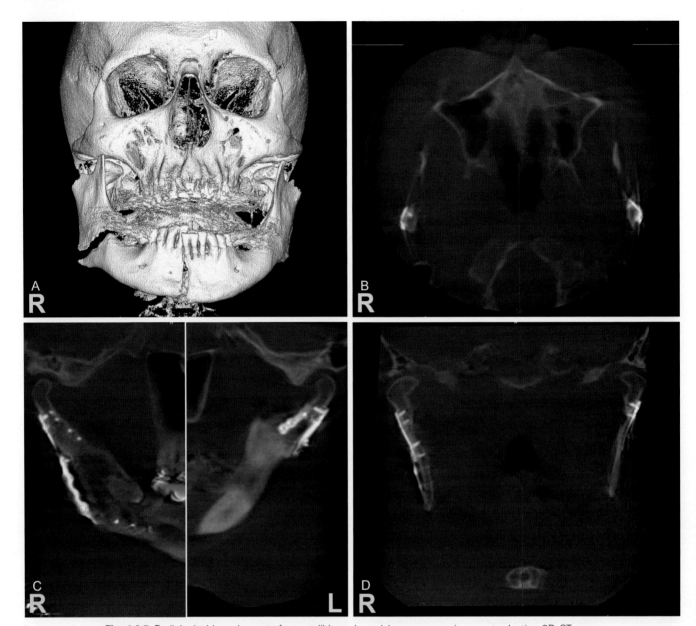

Fig. 1.3.5 Radiological key elements for mandible and condylar processes in a postreduction 3D CT scan. Following preoperative 3D imaging the fracture pattern was evaluated showing a multiple fractured mandible including a bilateral condylar neck fracture with medial dislocation, reduction of the vertical height and luxation out of the glenoid fossa. Due to the complex fracture pattern, reduction and fixation were performed via extraoral approaches. The postreduction imaging showed an adequate reduction, fixation, and position of the fragments and the condyles. (A) 3D reconstruction shows bilateral condylar neck fracture with medial displacement, fracture of the mandibular body (median) and the right mandibular angle. Note the changes in the transversal width of the mandible and the shortening of the vertical height. (B) Axial view. Reconstruction of the transversal mandibular width. (C) Oblique sagittal views. Reduction of the condylar processes back into the glenoid fossa in sagittal dimensions. (D) Coronal view. Reconstruction of the vertical mandibular height. Reduction of the condylar processes back into the glenoid fossa in transversal dimensions.

fracture reduction, immediate corrective surgery can be performed (Fig. 1.3.8).

POSTOPERATIVE COURSE

In general, intra- and postoperative 3D imaging (CT or CBCT) as recommended by the authors must only be implemented if therapeutic consequences would arise from the results of the scan. Depending on the experience of the surgeon and the anatomical region treated, there might be no need for intra- or postoperative 3D imaging in craniomaxillofacial trauma. In this context, simple mandibular and zygomaticomaxillary fractures should be mentioned. However, in displaced zygomaticomaxillary fractures and posttraumatic orbital deformities reconstructed with radiopaque (metallic) orbital implants, intra- and postoperative imaging facilitates the evaluation of fracture reduction and implant placement. Inadequately reconstructed posttraumatic orbital deformities (in terms of volume and shape or severely displaced [orbital] implants) can be diagnosed and revised immediately (see Fig. 1.3.8).

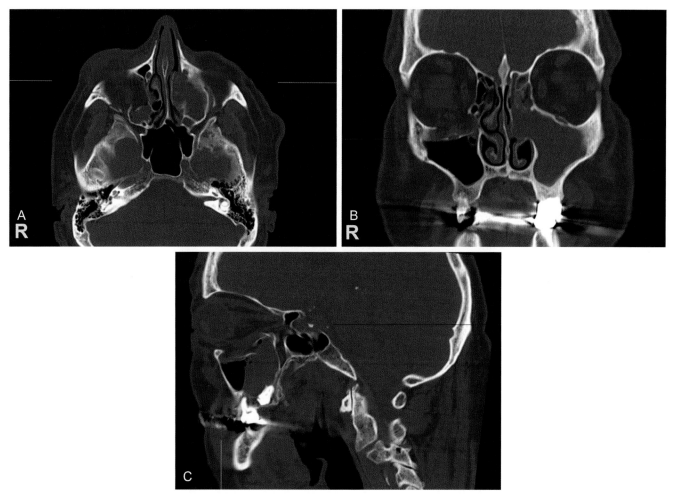

Fig. 1.3.6 Radiological evaluation of a posttraumatic orbital deformity. (A) Axial view. Defect of the medial orbital wall starting from the posteromedial bulge. (B) Coronal view. Defect in the orbital floor and fracture of the transition zone between medial orbital wall and orbital floor. (C) Oblique sagittal view. The length of the defect of the orbital floor which includes the posterior ledge. Note the loss of the lazy-S shape of the orbital floor. For distinct radiological evaluation refer to Video 1.3.1.

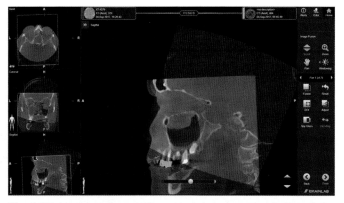

Fig. 1.3.7 Intraoperative quality control. Intraoperative fusion of the intraoperative 3D CBCT data with the preoperative virtual plan (Brainlab Curve, Brainlab, Feldkirchen, Germany). The preoperative CT scan (*yellow*) was fused with the intraoperative CBCT (*blue*). *Pink line* represents the virtual model of the patient-specific orbital implant (IPS Orbit, KLS Martin, Tuttlingen Germany). Slightly above this line, the orbital implant can be seen. For distinct radiological evaluation refer to Video 1.3.4.

Otherwise, severe late complications, including dystopia of the optical globe deformity and diplopia, might develop that are challenging to correct secondarily. As stated by Paul Manson: "You'll never get a second chance at primary treatment." However, if intraoperative or secondary interventions are not intended by the surgeon in the first place, intra- or postoperative imaging should not be performed. In recent literature it could be shown that intraoperative imaging has led to immediate consequences in 26% of the cases enrolled in this study. In those cases, fracture reduction turned out to be insufficient and was further optimized. In the same study, intraoperative CBCT was used to diagnose incorrectly positioned titanium orbital implants that were used for the reconstruction of posttraumatic orbital deformities. In addition, intraoperative CBCT allows for the detection of foreign bodies and bony fragments. In the majority of cases intraoperative imaging using 3D C-arms is suitable and sufficient to evaluate fracture reduction and implant placement.[2,10] Generally, additional postoperative CT or CBCT scans are not indicated and should not be routinely performed automatically. Only in cases of severe intra- or postoperative complications additional imaging (CT, CBCT, or even MRI) might be indicated depending on the condition. In summary, intraoperative imaging provides a number of advantages over posttherapeutic imaging in the management of facial fractures.

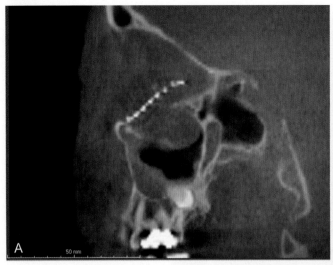
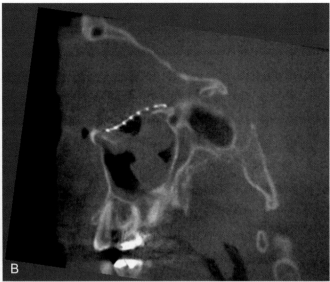

Fig. 1.3.8 Corrective surgery. (A) Oblique sagittal view. Displaced and malpositioned orbital titanium mesh in the intraoperative CBCT scan. The titanium mesh does not lie on the posterior ledge. (B) Oblique sagittal view after immediate revision and repositioning of the titanium mesh in the intraoperative CBCT scan. Adequate position and shape of the orbital titanium mesh.

ACUTE COMPLICATIONS

Intraoperative imaging does influence the initial set-up time and the length of the procedure. The set-up time depends on several factors including training status of the personnel, imaging modality (intra-operative CT, CBCT, or MRI), and the kind of device (mobile, static, or mounted to a robotic arm). For a well-trained team, including surgeons, nurses, and anesthesiologists, the additional set-up time for a mobile 3D C-arm ranges between 5 and 10 minutes. In addition, the length of the procedure is also influenced and again depends on the training status of the team and their experience. According to recent literature, the mean additional time for an experienced team ranges again between 5 and 10 minutes for the intraoperative scanning procedure. In terms of intraoperative CT, it could be shown that at the end of the learning curve, intraoperative CT examination was reported to necessitate an extra time of about 20 minutes.[10,35]

However, compared to the additional time and resources required if a secondary intervention would be indicated after a postoperative scan, the extra time for intraoperative imaging can almost be negated.

LONG-TERM COMPLICATIONS

Long-term complications of intra- or postoperative imaging might only exist in terms of radiation dose emitted to the patient. However, compared to a postoperative helical CT scan, intraoperative imaging using a 3D C-arm was shown to emit lower doses of radiation.[36] In the majority of cases intraoperative imaging is suitable and sufficient to evaluate fracture reduction and implant placement.[2,10] Generally, additional postoperative CT or CBCT scans are not indicated and should not be performed automatically. In cases of severe intra- or postoperative complications additional imaging (CT, CBCT, or even MRI) might be indicated depending on the condition. However, imaging must only be performed if therapeutic consequences arise from the results of the scan.

To the knowledge of the authors, the benefits of intra- and postoperative imaging outweigh the risks of additional radiation exposure. Particularly, in cases of orbital trauma, severely displaced zygomaticomaxillary fractures, frontobasal and skull base fractures, and condylar fractures intraoperative imaging is particularly useful because the number of secondary interventions can significantly be reduced. The complications resulting from not performing intra- or postoperative imaging depend on the anatomical region treated. In general, if any contour-relevant implant was placed its position and shape should be evaluated intra- or postoperatively using 3D imaging, preferably CBCT in order to keep the emitted dose of radiation to a minimum. The dose of radiation emitted depends on the device used. More precisely, on its tube power, image repetition frequency, and fluoroscopy time. Although no comparative studies have been conducted, the applied radiation dose per C-arm rotation can be assumed to be less than for a comparable conventional CT of the facial skeleton.[36] This assumption is derived from the fact that the underlying technology is CBCT which is known for emitting a radiation dose in comparable facial skeleton scans that is below that of CT.[37]

THE NEED FOR QUALITY CONTROL

Quality control is defined as a process to ensure that outcomes are predictable. A predictable outcome requires a pretherapeutic treatment plan that should rely on constant, unchanging fundamentals and facts (imaging) that has been proven to be relevant (CT/CBCT). But most importantly, the posttherapeutic result must be evaluated in relation to the pretherapeutic treatment plan in order to assess whether the plan has been accomplished. Otherwise, inaccurate and deficient planning and implementation will not be uncovered which leads to the absence of individual and general improvement. As mentioned above, diagnoses and treatment planning in craniomaxillofacial trauma should rely on multislice CT scan or CBCT. To finally assess quality control, multiple tools are available, including intra- and postoperative imaging which allow comparison of the results achieved with the pretherapeutic plan. Today, postoperative results in craniofacial trauma should be evaluated using 3D imaging.[5] If available, intra- or postoperative CBCT or CT can be used, assuming a suitable 3D volume and an adequate resolution of the devices that avoids additional postoperative imaging. Intraoperatively, the acquired CBCT data can directly be fused with preoperative virtual treatment plan to verify the quality of reduction or reconstruction (see Fig. 1.3.7). If an inadequate result can be assessed using intraoperative imaging, an immediate revision could be performed while the patient is still under general anesthesia.

In cases where neither an intra- nor a postoperative CBCT is available, a postoperative thin-slice CT scan should be the imaging modality of choice in traumatology.[4] As an additional radiation-free tool, intraoperative real-time navigation can be used as described earlier this chapter.

DICOM Data and Quality Control

If carried out correctly by the radiologist according to the surgeon's needs (Table 1.3.2), and the raw digital imaging and communication data (DICOM) are provided, the preoperative trauma CT scan can be used for preoperative diagnostics, preoperative virtual planning, the production of patient-specific implants or biomodels of the patient, and intraoperative navigation. Today, there is no need for printed-out

X-rays, radiographic films, reformatted, or reconstructed image sets from the radiologist in coronal and sagittal views or 3D reconstructions. However, the surgeon should be provided with the raw DICOM data of the axial scan. Using DICOM data implies, however, a technically skilled and trained surgeon and an imaging platform (DICOM viewer) that allows the individual adjustment of virtual planes and not only the predetermined axial, coronal, and sagittal views as delivered by the radiologist or available in the picture archiving and communication system (PACS) of the corresponding hospital. In this context, two imaging platforms have been proven and tested by the authors in their daily clinical routine, including CoDiagnostiX® (Version 9.7.1, Dental Wings GmbH, Chemnitz, Germany) and Visage® (Visage 7®, Visage Imaging, Pro Medicus Limited, Richmond, Australia). Frequently, image data sets from radiologists or colleagues are exported together with an integrated viewer in a different format but not the DICOM format. This makes it sometimes impossible to work with the provided data (Fig. 1.3.9C). It has to be mentioned that any radiological device is capable

TABLE 1.3.2 Recommendations for CT Scans in Craniomaxillofacial Surgery		
Preferred Scanning Parameters		**Patient Positioning**
Scan spacing	Less than 1.25 mm (equal to slice thickness)	Occlusal plane should be parallel to the gantry
Slice thickness	Less than 1.25 mm (equal to scan spacing)	
Field of view	25.0 cm	
Algorithm: (examples)	GE: Standard (not bone or detail) Siemens: H30s Toshiba: FC20 Philips: B	
Gantry tilt	0 degree	
Archive media	CD or DVD	
File type	DICOM (uncompressed)	
Series	Original/Primary/Axial (No recon, reformat or postprocess data)	

It is recommended to use a 3D scanning routine that provides high-resolution images as comparable to image-guided surgery, stereotactic planning, or other 3D applications. Scans should be acquired at a high spatial resolution. Series should be acquired with thin, contiguous image slices (equivalent thickness and spacing of 1.25 mm or less) and as small a field of view (FOV) as possible while still including the patient's external contour. Scan at least 2 cm above and below the area of interest. For cranial defects, the entire defect plus 2 cm above and below the defect should be scanned. In severe craniomaxillofacial trauma (panfacial fractures) a full head scan (hyoid – vertex) should be performed. Images should be provided in the original scanning plane. If software postprocessing is performed to reorient or reformat the scan volume, then a series of thin slice images in the original acquisition plane *must* be included. Do *not* use a gantry tilt during image acquisition. Images acquired with gantry tilt and then postprocessed to reorient images (i.e., "take out" tilt) are not acceptable. Please ensure that scans are free from motion artifact. The patient must remain completely still through the entire scan. If patient motion occurs, the scan must be restarted. Image distortion from patient motion can severely compromise the accuracy of a model, particularly if patient-specific implants are planned.

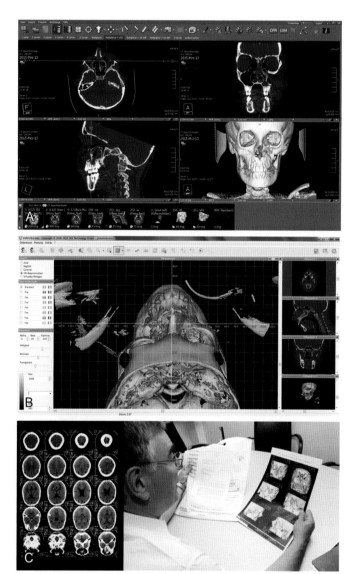

Fig. 1.3.9 Selection of different DICOM viewers. (A) Visage® (Visage 7 ®, Visage Imaging, Pro Medicus Limited, Richmond, Australia). (B) VoXim® (IVS Technology GmbH i. L., Version 6.5.1.1, Dental Wings GmbH, Chemnitz, Germany). (C) Example of print-out radiographs that are not suitable for detailed deformity analysis.

of generating and exporting DICOM data and any medical specialist should use only the DICOM format if medical images are transferred. In cases of further surgical procedures, follow-up 3D data will be available even in pathologies that would not have justified a CT or CBCT scan. In general, the acquired DICOM data can be imported in a variety of software tools, including platforms for virtual planning of patient-specific implants and intraoperative navigation. Due to the rapid progress and technical innovations in medical imaging and computer-assisted surgery, nowadays surgeons must be able to completely manage and utilize, and interpret, DICOM data independently from radiologists.

EXPERT COMMENTARY

"Why do you do this?" I asked Nils when I studied his work on intraoperative imaging.

"Because I don't want to spend 30 years learning the difficult aspects of orbital reconstruction, like you," he replied.

His brilliant intraoperative analyses were initiated by information from postoperative films which predicted the need for intraoperative monitoring of reduction accuracy. Today, plans made preoperatively, models, splints, and reduction templates all help the practitioner deal with challenging cases with unprecedented accuracy, reproducibility, and time saving for operative procedures.

Younger surgeons particularly benefit from these teaching and planning guides, which also improve the accuracy of older individuals like myself. Their use is becoming routine for complex procedures, and particularly where the demands of the procedure require a degree of perfection otherwise not attainable. In this chapter you can begin your study with a master teacher and planner, who will introduce you to this rapidly expanding field, which you will want to employ.

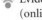 Evidence-based medicine (EBM) content available in Appendix 1 (online only)

REFERENCES

1. McCann PJ, Brocklebank LM, Ayoub AF. Assessment of zygomatico-orbital complex fractures using ultrasonography. *Br J Oral Maxillofac Surg.* 2000;38(5):525–529.
2. Wilde F, Schramm A. Intraoperative imaging in orbital and midface reconstruction. *Facial Plast Surg.* 2014;30(5):545–553.
3. Gebhard F, Riepl C, Richter P. The hybrid operating room: home of high-end intraoperative imaging. *Unfallchirurg.* 2012;115(2):107–120, [in German].
4. Wilde F, Lorenz K, Ebner AK, et al. Intraoperative imaging with a 3D C-arm system after zygomatico-orbital complex fracture reduction. *J Oral Maxillofac Surg.* 2013;71(5):894–910.
5. Manson PN, Markowitz B, Mirvis S, et al. Toward CT-based facial fracture treatment. *Plast Reconstr Surg.* 1990;85(2):202–212, discussion 213–214.
6. Zimmerer RM, Ellis E 3rd, Aniceto GS, et al. A prospective multicenter study to compare the precision of posttraumatic internal orbital reconstruction with standard preformed and individualized orbital implants. *J Craniomaxillofac Surg.* 2016;44(9):1485–1497.
7. Zimmerer RM, Gellrich NC, von Bülow S, et al. Is there more to the clinical outcome in posttraumatic reconstruction of the inferior and medial orbital walls than accuracy of implant placement and implant surface contouring? A prospective multicenter study to identify predictors of clinical outcome. *J Craniomaxillofac Surg.* 2018;46(4):578–587.
8. Heiland M, Schulze D, Rother U, et al. Postoperative imaging of zygomaticomaxillary complex fractures using digital volume tomography. *J Oral Maxillofac Surg.* 2004;62(11):1387–1391.
9. Rock C, Linsenmaier U, Brandl R. Introduction of a new mobile C-arm/CT combination equipment (ISO-C-3D). Initial results of 3-D sectional imaging. *Unfallchirurg.* 2001;104(9):827–833, [in German].
10. Heiland M, Schulze D, Blake E, et al. Intraoperative imaging of zygomaticomaxillary complex fractures using a 3D C-arm system. *Int J Oral Maxillofac Surg.* 2005;34(4):369–375.
11. Pohlenz P, Blessmann M, Blake F, et al. Clinical indications and perspectives for intraoperative cone-beam computed tomography in oral and maxillofacial surgery. *Oral Surg Oral Med Oral Pathol Oral Radiol Endodontol.* 2007;103(3):412–417.
12. Heiland M, Schulze D, Adam G, et al. 3D-imaging of the facial skeleton with an isocentric mobile C-arm system (Siremobil Iso-C3D). *Dentomaxillofac Radiol.* 2003;32(1):21–25.
13. Euler E, Heining S, Riquarts C, et al. C-arm-based three-dimensional navigation: a preliminary feasibility study. *Comput Aided Surg.* 2003;8(1):35–41.
14. Gilbard SM, Mafee MF, Lagouros PA, et al. Orbital blowout fractures the prognostic significance of computed tomography. *Ophthalmology.* 1985;92(11):1523–1528.
15. Ploder O, Plug C, Vorachek M, et al. Evaluation of computer-based area and volume measurement from coronal computed tomography scans in isolated blowout fractures of the orbital floor. *J Oral Maxillofac Surg.* 2002;60(11):1267–1272.
16. Singh M, Ricci JA, Caterson EJ. Use of intraoperative computed tomography for revisional procedures in patients with complex maxillofacial trauma. *Plast Reconstr Surg Global Open.* 2015;3(7):e463.
17. Schramm A, Gellrich NC, Schmelzeisen R. *Navigational Surgery of the Facial Skeleton.* Berlin: Springer; 2007.
18. Gellrich NC, Schramm A, Hammer B, et al. Computer-assisted secondary reconstruction of unilateral posttraumatic orbital deformity. *Plast Reconstr Surg.* 2002;110(6):1417–1429.
19. Schramm A, Suarez-Cunqueiro MM, Barth EL, et al. Computer-assisted navigation in craniomaxillofacial tumors. *J Craniofac Surg.* 2008;19(4):1067–1074.
20. Rana M, Chui CH, Wagner M, et al. Increasing the accuracy of orbital reconstruction with selective laser-melted patient-specific implants combined with intraoperative navigation. *J Oral Maxillofac Surg.* 2015;73(6):1113–1118.
21. Schmelzeisen R, Gellrich NC, Schramm A, et al. Navigation-guided resection of temporomandibular joint ankylosis promotes safety in skull base surgery. *J Oral Maxillofac Surg.* 2002;60(11):1275–1283.
22. Essig H, Rana M, Kokemueller H, et al. Referencing of markerless CT data sets with cone beam subvolume including registration markers to ease computer-assisted surgery – a clinical and technical research. *Int J Med Robotics Computer Assist Surg.* 2013;9(3):e39–e45.
23. Heiland M, Pohlenz P, Blessmann M, et al. Navigated implantation after microsurgical bone transfer using intraoperatively acquired cone-beam computed tomography data sets. *Int J Oral Maxillofac Surg.* 2008;37(1):70–75.
24. Heiland M, Habermann CR, Schmelzle R. Indications and limitations of intraoperative navigation in maxillofacial surgery. *J Oral Maxillofac Surg.* 2004;62(9):1059–1063.
25. Hohlweg-Majert B, Schon R, Schelzeisen R, et al. Navigational maxillofacial surgery using virtual models. *World J Surg.* 2005;29(12):1530–1538.
26. Foley KT, Simon DA, Rampersaud YR. Virtual fluoroscopy: computer-assisted fluoroscopic navigation. *Spine.* 2001;26(4):347–351.
27. Cornelius C-P, Mayer P, Ehrenfeld M, et al. The orbits – anatomical features in view of innovative surgical methods. *Facial Plast Surg.* 2014;30(05):487–508.
28. Metzger MC, Schön R. Tetzlaf R. Topographical CT-data analysis of the human orbital floor. *Int J Oral Maxillofac Surg.* 2007;36(1):45–53.
29. Ellis IIIE, El-Attar A, Moos KF. An analysis of 2,067 cases of zygomatico-orbital fracture. *J Oral Maxillofac Surg.* 1985;43(6):417–428.
30. Ramieri G, Spada MC, Bianchi SD, et al. Dimensions and volumes of the orbit and orbital fat in posttraumatic enophthalmos. *Dentomaxillofac Radiol.* 2000;29(5):302–311.

31. Manson PN. The orbit after Converse: seeing what is not there. *J Craniofac Surg.* 2004;15(3):363–367.

32. Manson PN, Clifford CM, Su CT, et al. Mechanisms of global support and posttraumatic enophthalmos: I. The anatomy of the ligament sling and its relation to intramuscular cone orbital fat. *Plast Reconstr Surg.* 1986;77(2):193–202.

33. Manson PN, Grivas A, Rosenbaum A, et al. Studies on enophthalmos: II. The measurement of orbital injuries and their treatment by quantitative computed tomography. *Plast Reconstr Surg.* 1986;77(2):203–214.

34. Raskin EM, Millman AL, Lubkin V, et al. Prediction of late enophthalmos by volumetric analysis of orbital fractures. *Ophthal Plast Reconstr Surg.* 1998;14(1):19–26.

35. Hoelzle F, Klein M, Schwerdiner O, et al. Intraoperative computed tomography with the mobile CT Tomoscan M during surgical treatment of orbital fractures. *Int J Oral Maxillofac Surg.* 2001;30(1):26–31.

36. Schulze D, Heiland M, Thurmann H, et al. Radiation exposure during midfacial imaging using 4- and 16-slice computed tomography, cone beam computed tomography systems and conventional radiography. *Dentomaxillofac Radiol.* 2004;33(2):83–86.

37. Cohnen M, Kemper J, Möbes O, et al. Radiation dose in dental radiology. *Eur Radiol.* 2002;12(3):634–637.

1.4

Primary Repair of Soft Tissue Injury and Soft Tissue Defects

Christian Petropolis, Oleh Antonyshyn

BACKGROUND

Reconstruction of soft tissue craniofacial trauma represents a challenging and common problem. The soft tissue structures of the head and neck contain complex 3-dimensional geometry spanning across multiple subunits and structures. Each anatomic region requires careful attention in its repair to meet exacting aesthetic and functional demands. No other region of the body is as scrutinized during social interaction as the face, where even minute deformity is readily detectable at conversational distance.

Craniofacial trauma is common at all ages, accounting for upwards of 7% of patients presenting to adult emergency rooms. Cases of isolated soft tissue craniofacial trauma greatly outnumber cases involving bony injury.[1] Most injuries occur on the forward most projecting surfaces of the head, including the forehead, nose, lips, and chin. Injury types vary from contusions, lacerations to areas of skin, and soft tissue loss. Full-thickness lacerations are most commonly seen and are often small.[2] Left-sided injuries predominate when the cause is an altercation.[1,2]

The etiology and rates of injury vary significantly with age, sex, and occupation of the patient.[1–3] In children less than 15 years old the most common cause of injury is falls, with a peak incidence between 1 and 6 years of age. Males are more likely to sustain injury compared to females in this age group.[2,3] In adults 15–50 years of age, interpersonal violence with assault becomes the most common cause of trauma. Other common causes include motor vehicle collisions (MVCs), sports injuries, and occupational injuries. In this age group males were far more likely than females to present with craniofacial trauma. Over the age of 50 falls again become the main cause of injury, followed by assaults and MVCs.

SURGICAL ANATOMY

The surface topography of the face, represented by complex 3-dimensional variations in the size, position, proportions, and shape of facial surface contours, defines and characterizes facial appearance. Reconstruction relies on an understanding of subunit classification systems, which serve to describe the extent of injury, and guide surgical management (Fig. 1.4.1).[4–7] Although many of these classifications were originally developed for extirpative and congenital defects, they are also applicable to the posttraumatic deformity.

The nasal subunit classification, originally developed by Burget and Menick, is particularly well utilized clinically. It divides the nose into tip, soft triangles, alae, sidewalls, dorsal subunits (Fig. 1.4.2).[5] The underlying principle of nasal subunit reconstruction dictates that defects greater then 50% of a given subunit are best treated with excision of the remaining tissue and reconstruction of the entire subunit. This ensures that subunits or defined surfaces are reconstructed with similar homogenous tissues, while scars are hidden along boundaries or junctions of anatomical units.

Similar to the nose, it is helpful to think of reconstruction of the perioral region based on aesthetic subunits and anatomic layers (Fig. 1.4.1).[8] Although excision of the remaining subunit can minimize visibility of scars, compromise is often required. This is especially true in traumatic injuries where aggressive use of flaps may not always be an option due to the zone of injury and questionable tissue viability. It is important to understand the cross-sectional anatomy of the lips and the relationship of the orbicularis muscle, white roll, and location of the labial arteries, which run just deep to the muscle at the wet dry vermillion junction.

The case illustrated in Fig. 1.4.3 demonstrates the utility of the subunit principle. Initially the remaining lip is significantly splayed, making it difficult to assess the true defect. Repositioning the lateral lip segments to their natural position allows for proper assessment of the remaining subunits. A lip switch flap was chosen to reconstruct the lip defect and nasal sill. Note that the flap design maintains the integrity of the labiomental crease and leaves the chin intact. A full-thickness graft provides coverage for the columella and a composite graft from the right ear is used for the alar defect.

Knowledge of surface anatomy plays an important role in diagnosing damage to vital structures such as the facial nerve, trigeminal nerve, and Stenson's (parotid) duct. This is demonstrated by the patient in Fig. 1.4.4, who sustained a full-thickness laceration across the cheek with exposure of the mandible. The relative positions of the facial nerve branches and parotid duct are depicted. The frontal branch of the facial nerve has multiple branches that cross the central third to half of the zygomatic arch.[9] Cephalad to the zygomatic arch these branches run in a plane just deep to the temporoparietal fascia.[10] At the level of the zygomatic arch the temporal branch is found in a deeper plane directly adjacent to the periosteum.[11] The zygomatic and buccal branches of the facial nerve exit the parotid and run in a plane deep to both the SMAS (superficial musculoaponeurotic) and parotid masseteric fascia. They then travel through the buccal space and go on to innervate the facial musculature on their undersurface. Significant arborization occurs between the terminal zygomatic and buccal branches, and because of this spontaneous recovery from injury is commonly seen.[10] Exploration and attempted repair of these branches medial to the lateral canthus is not recommended due to their small size and chance for spontaneous recovery.[12] The marginal mandibular branch of the facial nerve has been extensively studied and most often its course remains above the inferior border of the mandible. However, the nerve can travel from 1–3 cm below the inferior edge in some individuals, specifically in the region between the mandibular angle and the point the nerve crosses superficial to the facial vessels. After exiting the caudal parotid the nerve travels in a plane deep to the parotid masseteric fascia, crosses superficial to the facial vessels and then pierces the deep cervical fascia to innervate the lower lip depressors and mentalis.[10,11]

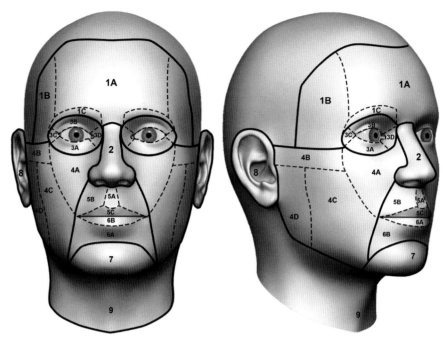

Fig. 1.4.1 The topographic subunits of the face. 1, forehead unit (1A, central; 1B lateral; 1C eyebrow); 2, nasal unit; 3, eyelid unit (3A, lower lid; 3B, upper lid; 3C, lateral canthus; 3D, medial canthus); 4, cheek unit (4A, medial; 4B, zygoma; 4C, lateral; 4D, buccal); 5, upper lip unit (5A, philtrum; 5B, lateral; 5C, mucosa); 6, lower lip unit (6A, central; 6B, mucosa); 7, mental unit; 8, auricular unit; 9, neck unit. (Courtesy Christian Petropolis.)

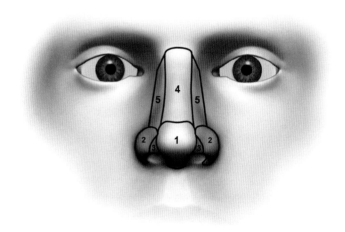

Fig. 1.4.2 The topographic subunits of the nose. 1, tip; 2, alar lobules; 3, soft triangles; 4, dorsum; 5, sidewalls. (Courtesy Christian Petropolis.)

The parotid duct exits the anterior edge of the parotid gland roughly at the level of the tragus and initially runs on the anterior surface of the masseter muscle. At the anterior edge of the masseter it passes through the buccal fat pad and pierces the buccinator muscle to emerge into the oral cavity adjacent to the 2nd maxillary molar. It is approximately 7 cm in length. The superficial landmark for the path of the duct is a line drawn between the tragus and the midline of the lip (Fig. 1.4.4). Any laceration deep to the SMAS in this region should prompt further investigation into parotid duct integrity.[12]

CLINICAL PRESENTATION

The initial presentation of patients with soft tissue facial trauma will vary significantly depending on mechanism and extent of injury. The Advanced Trauma Life Support (ATLS) protocol should be used to efficiently evaluate and stabilize all major trauma patients. Thorough history should first be obtained, including details relating to timing, mechanism, location of incident, and the degree of contamination. Any dangerous mechanisms of injury such as fall from elevation (3 feet, 5 stairs), high speed MVC, rollover or ejection should prompt further evaluation for possible brain and C-spine injury.[13,14] The mechanism also provides useful information on the zone of injury and risk to underlying structures. For example, even small sharp lacerations may penetrate deeply and injure vital structures, and when found in critical areas must raise suspicion. In the case of ballistic trauma, information should be obtained on the gun as well as the projectile characteristics (velocity, shape, and mass) and the firing range.[15]

In the case of an animal bite, attention should be paid to whether the attack was provoked or unprovoked, the immunization status of the animal, and if the animal has been detained, monitoring for developing signs of rabies.[16] Due to the widely varying incidence and risk of rabies from animal bites, any concern in this regard should prompt a consult to the infectious disease service or public health medical officer.

Classifying traumatic wounds as either clean or dirty helps to determine need for prophylactic antibiotics and tetanus treatment. Clean traumatic wounds or lacerations are those without evidence of macroscopic contamination or signs of infection and do not require prophylactic antibiotic treatment. This is especially true in craniofacial trauma where the soft tissues are highly vascularized. Dirty traumatic wounds include those with macroscopic contamination, with devitalized tissue, caused by animal bites, or occurring in a contaminated environment. Prophylactic antibiotics should be used in most dirty wounds.

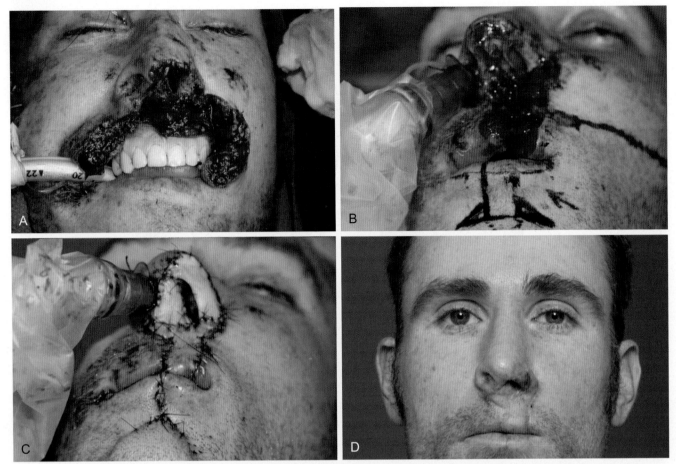

Fig. 1.4.3 (A) Traumatic avulsion of the upper lip and nose resulting from a dog bite. (B) True defect after repositioning of the residual subunits with planned lip switch flap. (C) Immediate postoperative picture with lip switch flap reconstruction of the lower lip and nasal sill, full-thickness skin graft of the columella and helical rim composite graft to the alar rim. (D) Early postoperative result following division of the lip switch flap.

Tetanus immunization status should be assessed in every patient as all wounds are potentially at risk. If vaccination history is unknown, less than three doses have been received or it has been more than 10 years since the last dose of tetanus vaccine, a booster should be given. If the wound is not considered clean, then tetanus immunoglobulin should also be given to these nonimmune patients.[17]

Physical exam should be approached in a systematic way, from the top of the head down. Each site should be assessed for possible embedded foreign body, glass or particulate matter. The scalp is a common location of missed lacerations due to the obstruction of hair. Palpation over the entire scalp should be performed, examining for obvious lacerations or areas of dry blood and matted hair. Scalp lacerations have significant risk of prolonged bleeding due to the rich vascular supply and the lack of retraction due to the galea aponeurosis. Untreated scalp lacerations are a known cause of hemorrhagic shock and can be fatal.[18]

Examination of the periorbital region should focus on each structural region to avoid missing subtle injuries. Depth of laceration and involvement of the lid margin should be noted. Orbital fat observed in the wound is a sign of violation of the orbital septum and possible injury to underlying structures such as the globe and levator palpebrae superioris. If there is injury to one or more of the lids then associated injury to the globe must also be ruled out with suspected injury prompting an immediate consultation with ophthalmology. Assessment of the lacrimal system, levator palpebrae function, and medial and lateral

canthal tendon integrity should also be assessed. Testing the integrity of the lacrimal system in traumatic injuries is usually done simply by probing of the lacrimal system and examining for defects. In children, lacrimal probing is usually not tolerated without sedation and so a Jones 1 test with fluorescein placed into the conjunctival fornices can be performed. If fluorescein is detected under the inferior nasal meatus, the drainage system is likely intact.[19]

Exam of the traumatized nose must include inspection of both the external and internal structures. Integrity of the external skin, the cartilaginous and bony supporting structures, and the internal lining must be examined. Specific care should be taken to rule out a septal hematoma due to the devastating consequences of septal necrosis and secondary nasal collapse. This can occur after even minor trauma, especially in children where the softer cartilage is more easily deformed.[20] Damage to the septal cartilage can occur within 24 hours and necrosis between 72–96 hours if not treated. On intranasal examination, a septal hematoma will appear as a bulging, boggy, ecchymotic mass often causing obstruction bilaterally, as seen in Fig. 1.4.5.[21]

Examination of the ears should assess both the anterior and posterior surface for lacerations and signs of hematoma. Auricular hematoma seen in blunt trauma carries the risk of developing cauliflower ear if not identified and treated.[22] Lacerations should be assessed for involvement of the underlying cartilage framework. If there is extension into the external auditory meatus, as seen in Fig. 1.4.6, otoscopy should be performed

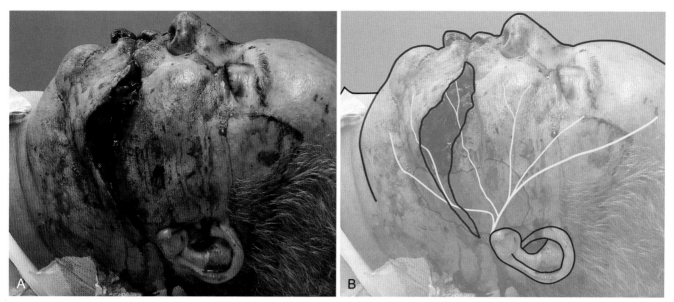

Fig. 1.4.4 (A) Full-thickness laceration with exposure of the mandible secondary to motor vehicle trauma. (B) Relative positions of the facial nerve (*yellow*), parotid duct (*blue*), and parotid gland (*orange*).

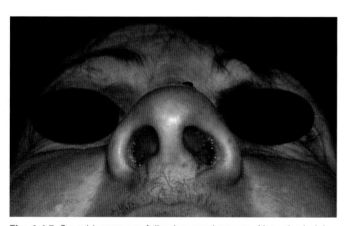

Fig. 1.4.5 Septal hematoma following nasal trauma. Note the bulging ecchymotic mucosa causing bilateral nasal obstruction.

to rule out damage to middle ear structures. Penetrating or ballistic injuries in this area can also cause damage to the facial nerve trunk, and its intratemporal course, therefore its integrity must be assessed.

Lacerations and injury to the lips should be evaluated for the extent of tissue loss and which subunits are affected. Intraoral examination should follow to assess for through-and-through lacerations, and associated injury to the buccal mucosa or tongue.

Lacerations overlying the path of the facial nerve (described previously) require careful examination to rule out damage to one or more of its branches. The location of the laceration is important clinically because damage to buccal or zygomatic branches medial to the lateral canthus are generally not repaired due to the small size and high rate of crossover between the facial nerve branches, leading to spontaneous recovery.[12] Each facial nerve innervated muscle should be tested and compared to the uninjured side if possible. Any weakness should be documented with a systematic top-down approach. If nerve laceration is suspected on examination, early operative exploration is indicated. Early recognition is essential as locating the distal cut ends of the nerve is much easier within the first 2–6 days following injury before the distal nerve undergoes Wallerian degeneration and can no longer be

stimulated.[23] Sensation in all distributions of the trigeminal nerve should also be assessed and documented during the initial examinations.

The course of the parotid duct follows a line from the tragus to the upper lip cupid's bow, with the duct entering the oral cavity adjacent to the maxillary second molar. Exploration should be performed to determine the extent and location of damage to the duct and gland. Cannulation of the duct intraorally with a lacrimal probe or angiocath (angiocath can be left *in situ* to stent the subsequent repair) can be helpful in diagnosing an injury on exam.

Penetrating neck injuries (PNI) are potentially life-threatening secondary to hypovolemic shock and airway loss. Hard clinical signs of major vascular injury include severe active bleeding, rapidly expanding hematoma, hypovolemic shock not responsive to fluid resuscitation, and diminished radial pulse.[24] In the case of a hemodynamically unstable patient, resuscitation following the ATLS protocol and emergent surgical exploration should be carried out. Some centers will attempt Foley catheter balloon tamponade before operative exploration, and if successful, follow with angiography.[25] In the case of a hemodynamically stable patient with PNI, monitoring for at least 24 hours and possible CT angiography should be carried out.

RADIOLOGICAL EVALUATION

Radiological investigation in facial trauma usually focuses on the underlying bony skeleton with high-resolution CT being the primary modality. Soft tissue structures can also be assessed on these scans, revealing depth of injury, involved structures, the presence of radiopaque foreign bodies or hematoma. If an infused scan is performed, the presence of active extravasation can also be assessed. In the case of soft tissue injuries with secondary infection and abscess, CT provides useful information of size and location which can guide surgical management.

CT imaging may not be sufficient if there is concern for retained foreign body with low radio density such as wood or plastic. MRI can detect these materials, however access to this modality is often limited.[26] Ultrasound is readily available and it has increasingly been used in the detection of radiolucent materials.[26,27] Most often, detailed physical examination and exploration of the wound with magnification are all that is required.[28]

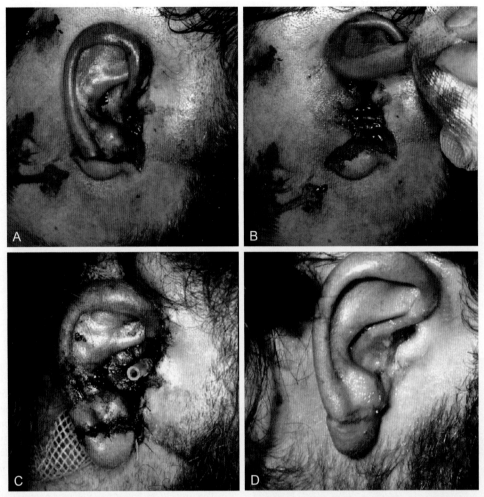

Fig. 1.4.6 (A–B) Near total avulsion of the ear. (C) Repair including stenting of the external auditory meatus and bolster dressing in the conchal bowl. (D) Early result showing maintenance of all subunits. The patient eventually required only minor revisions.

Sialography can be used in the diagnosis of parotid duct injuries, however it is rarely performed as most injuries are readily diagnosed on examination and exploration. If a duct injury is suspected in a small but penetrating injury, sialography may be useful in avoiding an operative exploration that would put adjacent facial nerve branches at risk.[29]

CLASSIFICATION OF SOFT TISSUE INJURIES

Contusion and Hematoma

Blunt soft tissue injuries can result in diffuse damage to the subcutaneous tissues without overt damage to the skin. This mechanism can result in fat necrosis with eventual depression and contour irregularity. Contusions resulting in significant hematoma can exaggerate this effect due to the elevated pressure placed on the soft tissues. Hematomas are best drained immediately before they coagulate, otherwise a small stab incision or delayed drainage will be required.

Abrasive Injuries

Abrasive wounds are diffuse injuries caused by motion across an irregular surface. Typically, these are superficial injuries without exposure of the underlying subcutaneous tissue. Depending on the mechanism and abrasive surface there could be significant embedded dirt, foreign body, and loose devitalized skin which should be removed with scrubbing

and debridement. This should be performed before healing of the tissue entraps the particles leading to traumatic tattooing. The Versajet hydrosurgery system has been successfully used for this purpose, and may facilitate the process by providing a finely tunable debridement.[30] Healing of partial-thickness wounds of this type will occur within 2 weeks with proper wound care, including gentle cleansing and light, greasy dressings. Deep partial-thickness wounds need careful consideration of their healing potential as prolonged healing will greatly increase the risk of scarring. If healing is not expected to occur within 3 weeks, consideration should be given to definitive debridement and grafting.

Lacerations

Lacerations can range from simple clean-line cuts caused by sharp mechanisms, to stellate bursts from blunt force or ballistic mechanisms, causing tearing of skin. The trauma mechanism will affect the zone of injury, with blunt or tearing forces resulting in diffuse damage to the skin and soft tissues with the possibility of an underlying hematoma. Although clearly devitalized tissue should be removed, the generous blood supply to facial soft tissues allows for conservative debridement. All irreplaceable tissues, such as those of the lip, should be given a chance to declare themselves as they may survive on even small vascular pedicles. When tissues have undergone diffuse damage, and viability is questionable, the objective should be to close the wound in as simple a manner as possible to avoid additional stress on the tissues. To achieve this the smallest number of sutures possible should be used and tissue rearrangement should be avoided during the initial closure.

In simple lacerations without diffuse damage, revision of the wound edges during the initial closure can be considered to potentially avoid the need for secondary revision. This is applicable in hyper-beveled lacerations that would result in overriding edges, or lacerations with ragged edges or multiple parallel cuts. Trapdoor scars occur in curvilinear and U-shaped lacerations and result in raised areas secondary to circumferential contraction. Immediate or early Z-plasty to break up the contracting forces can be considered.

Avulsive Injuries

Partial soft tissue avulsions of facial tissues have the advantage of the generous blood supply of the head and neck region. Avulsed tissue maintained on small pedicles can survive, however closure must not impair tissue vascularity. The treatment of venous congestion in partial avulsion injuries with medicinal leeches has been shown to be effective. Brisk arterial inflow into the part should be confirmed prior to leeching. If arterial inflow is compromised, arterial microvascular repair should be considered.[31]

Avulsive injuries that result in exposure of critical structures require immediate resurfacing with vascularized tissues. Reasonable options include local flaps, galea frontalis flap, or temporalis muscle flap.

The patient in Fig. 1.4.7 presented as a cyclist involved in an MVC. He sustained a Manson Type II naso-orbito-ethmoid fracture, nasal bone fracture, and avulsive injury resulting in a glabellar defect. Coverage of the bony structures and fixation hardware was achieved using a galeal frontalis flap pedicled on the right supratrochlear vessels with application of a full-thickness skin graft.

Fig. 1.4.8 demonstrates a devastating injury resulting from a high-velocity projectile penetrating through a windshield. The patient sustained a ruptured globe and compound panfacial fractures with disruption and exposure of the left anterior cranial base. Following skeletal fixation, the patient required soft tissue coverage of the left orbit and anterior cranial base. Reconstruction was completed with orbital exenteration and temporalis muscle transposition.

Complete avulsions of head and neck tissues should be considered for microvascular replantation. Numerous successful replantations have been reported, including small partial ear avulsions, composite lip and nose and large full-scalp and forehead segments.[32–34] Anastomosis of

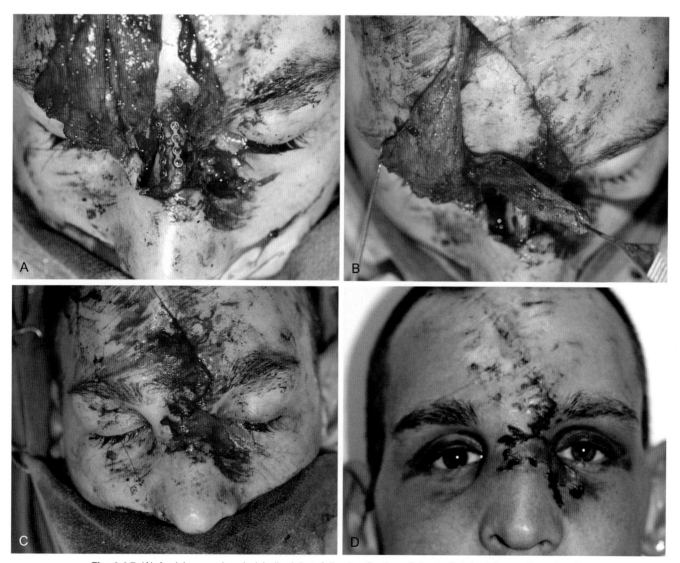

Fig. 1.4.7 (A) Avulsive nasal and glabellar injury following fixation of the underlying Manson Type II NOE fracture. (B–C) Galeal frontalis flap pedicled on the right supratrochlear vessels. Full-thickness skin graft was then applied to the flap. (D) Early postoperative result.

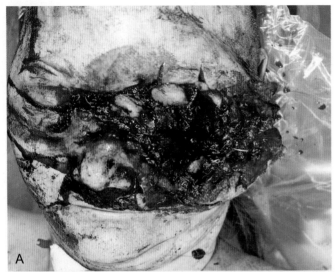

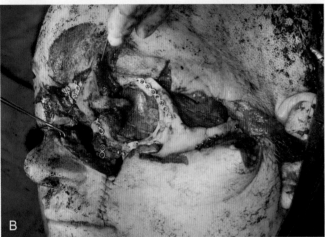

Fig. 1.4.8 Devastating injury resulting from a high-velocity projectile penetrating through a windshield. The patient sustained a ruptured globe, compound panfacial fractures with disruption and exposure of the left anterior cranial base. Following skeletal fixation, the patient required soft tissue coverage of the left orbit and anterior cranial base. Reconstruction was completed with orbital exenteration and temporalis muscle transposition.

even a single artery can supply a segment larger than the scalp, and it is often the venous drainage which is the limiting factor in survival of these parts.[34] Small parts may not have a vein sufficient for anastomosis and therefore must rely on either medicinal leeches or bleeding encouraged by dermabrasion and the application of heparin-soaked pledgets. If relying on these methods to salvage a larger avulsed segment, numerous blood transfusions should be anticipated until new venous ingrowth occurs after several days.[32]

SURGICAL TECHNIQUES

Preamble

Surgical repair of facial soft tissue injuries requires care and attention to obtain optimal results. Initial irrigation and debridement of tissues is required, however debridement of irreplaceable tissues such as the lip, eyelid, nose tip, nostril rims, helix and anthelix of the ear should be avoided if possible. Even when badly damaged, the patient's own tissue will often have a superior appearance compared to a part

reconstructed with flaps. Thorough irrigation and removal of dirt, debris, and other foreign material should precede closure of tissues. Closure technique and suture material will vary based on injury location and type, however there are some generalizable principles. Lacerations located in visible areas should be closed with 6-0 nonresorbable sutures removed in 5–7 days to minimize the risk of permanent stitch marks. To facilitate closure with fine stitches, and to allow early removal, tension must be adequately offloaded using buried dermal sutures. Repair of underlying muscle and fascial structures will also offload tension from the overlying skin. In certain cases deep structures can be resuspended to periosteum to restore proper contour and facilitate closure of the overlying skin. For example, closing a defect at the junction of the lower eyelid and cheek would lead to excess pull on the lower lid, potentially causing an ectropion. By suspending the lower flap of the defect to the periosteum of the maxilla, the downward force is eliminated and the skin can be closed without tension.

Scalp, Forehead, and Brow

The methods used for repair of scalp defects encompass the entire reconstructive ladder. The choice of reconstruction will depend on defect size, which layers are involved, and the defect location. Although small defects can be closed primarily, the convex shape of the skull and tightly adherent galea aponeurotica make even simple defects difficult to close.[35]

Direct closure is usually possible in simple lacerations and small defects of the scalp. If significant bleeding is encountered it will typically be from vessels running just superficial to the galea. Aggressive use of cautery should be avoided in hair-bearing areas to avoid damage to hair follicles. Closure should be done in layers with absorbable sutures placed in the galea taking up most of the tension. Skin stitches or staples can also be used for the superficial skin closure, however staples should be avoided in non-hair-bearing areas or areas with excess tension. To reduce tension, the defect can be undermined circumferentially in the bloodless subgaleal plane.

Under circumstances where the scalp avulsion is very extensive, revascularization may be indicated. In the attached example depicted in Fig. 1.4.9, near total avulsion of the scalp was associated with diminished perfusion of the forehead. Anastomosis of the superficial temporal artery ensured vascularization and improved healing of the flap, although partial-thickness necrosis of the leading edge of the avulsion flap resulted in scarring and alopecia.

Skin grafting is a simple technique which can quickly close large scalp defects. It requires a clean, well-vascularized bed for success, and therefore in the setting of trauma is usually performed after a delay to allow full declaration of the tissues. There are several concerns in the use of grafts, including alopecia, color mismatch, and contour irregularity. However, its simplicity makes grafting a viable temporizing measure which can later be revised secondarily if required, usually with expansion of the remaining scalp.

Pedicled flap closure of scalp defects is a common technique with a multitude of described options, including rotation, transposition, and advancement flaps. Indications for flap closure include coverage of exposed calvarium and hardware, or to avoid the cosmetic aspects of skin grafting. Consideration should be given to the zone of injury surrounding the defect, and if there is any doubt over the tissue viability, reconstruction should be delayed if possible. Flaps should be planned with extra redundancy to compensate for the unyielding galea. For larger defects multiple flaps should be planned to facilitate closure in the event the first flap is insufficient. The base of the flap should ideally be located in an area of laxity off of the scalp to allow for a back cut and greater advancement. Scoring of the galea perpendicular to the direction of desired advancement will allow for a small gain in length. Care must be taken not to disrupt the vascular supply which will be

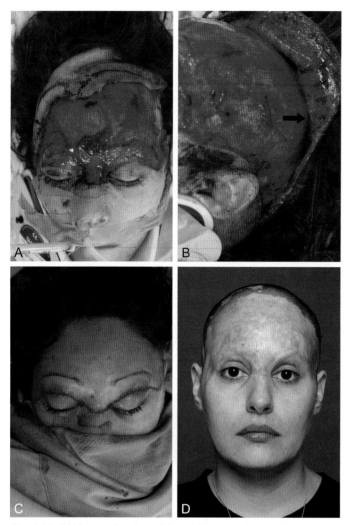

Fig. 1.4.9 (A) Near-total scalp avulsion with poor perfusion. (B) Superficial temporal artery was located and microvascular repair carried out. (C) Immediate postoperative result. (D) Despite revascularization, the patient experienced partial-thickness necrosis with scarring and alopecia.

directly superficial to the galea. Distortion of the anterior hairline should be avoided whenever possible.

If regional tissues are insufficient to reconstruct a scalp defect, free tissue transfer can supply enough tissue to resurface the entire scalp.[36] The most commonly used flaps for this purpose are the latissimus dorsi and the anterolateral thigh (ALT) flap, with the preference being center-dependent.[36,37] Supporters of the latissimus dorsi favor its large size and ability to be raised as a chimeric flap supplying large amounts of tissue, including muscle bone and multiple skin paddles. Atrophy of the muscle over time is a known issue that may result in dehiscence and exposure of vital structures or hardware requiring reoperation. The ALT flap has the advantage of being raised in the supine position, allowing for a two-team approach. It also provides significant tissue as well as the possibility for chimeric muscle flaps. Flap thickness may be an issue in obese individuals requiring multiple debulking procedures to achieve appropriate contour. The superficial temporal vessels are usually used as recipients, with the facial vessels being an alternative option.

Repair of simple lacerations through the eyebrow requires careful alignment to prevent step deformity or distortion in the hair follicle direction. If a partial eyebrow defect is present there are several described

flaps to aid in closure, including rotation flaps, V–Y island advancement flaps, and A–T closure.[38] If the entire eyebrow is lost, reconstruction with scalp hair based on the temporoparietal fascia can be used.[39] Alternatively the defect can be closed and reconstructed secondarily with a composite graft or with hair transplantation techniques.[40]

Eyelid and Lacrimal System

Simple cutaneous eyelid lacerations not involving the lid margins can be closed primarily using the principles previously described for other facial lacerations. Full-thickness lacerations require close attention to ensure proper alignment of the lid margin, underlying tarsal plate, and skin. Anatomic landmarks such as the grey line and lash line should be first approximated with a 6-0 permanent stitch, leaving the tails long so they can be later tied down away from the margin. With the lid margin approximated, the tarsal plate can then be repaired with absorbable suture, ensuring to orientate the knot towards the superficial surface. It is critical that no suture material protrude through the conjunctiva towards the globe due to the risk of corneal irritation. The lid margin should have no notching and if present could be a sign of excessive tension, incorrect suture placement or failure to adequately repair the tarsoligamentous sling. The skin is then closed as usual while also ensuring to capture the long tails of the margin sutures, pulling them away from the globe.[41]

The patent in Fig. 1.4.10 sustained full-thickness lacerations of both the upper and lower lids extending into the brow, cheek, and lip. His levator palpabrae superioris was identified in the wound and repaired to the tarsal plate. Supratrochlear, supraorbital nerves and infraorbital nerves were each identified and found to be grossly intact. Accurate repair of the lids was then carried out as described above.

Lacerations involving the canaliculus require repair within 3–5 days for optimal outcome. Although repair of monocanalicular injuries, especially the upper canaliculus, has been debated, most authors agree that repair of monocanalicular injuries is the best way to avoid post-traumatic epiphora.[41–43] Repair over a silicone stent is the most common method of repair. The stent prevents stenosis as well as provides medial traction to offload tension on the lid repair. Identification of the medial end of the cut end can be difficult and it is helpful to reduce the soft tissue swelling with a short delay for head elevation and cool compresses. If the medial end cannot be identified, air can be passed through an intact canaliculus while placing pressure on the lacrimal sac. Once identified the stent is passed through the medial cut end of the canaliculus into the nose where the metal probe is retrieved under the inferior turbinate. Repair can then proceed with 6-0 polyglactin suture used for the medial canthal tendon and soft tissues and 7-0 placed for the canaliculus. The sutures should be tied only after they are all placed to facilitate an accurate repair. The silicone stent is then secured in the nose and left in place for 3–6 months.[41]

Repair of medial and lateral canthal injuries is required to prevent a canthal dystopia. The mechanism of injury is typically direct laceration or avulsion and may be associated with an underlying bony injury. Any injury to the medial canthus should prompt investigation into the integrity of the closely associated canalicular system. For lacerations, if direct repair is possible this can be performed as described above with 6-0 polyglactin suture. If complete disinsertion from the bone occurs, repair can be facilitated using bone anchors or drill holes. Our preference for lateral canthal tendon reinsertion is with drill holes placed in the lateral orbital rim using stainless steel suture. For medal canthal reinsertion the choice between bone anchors or transnasal wires depends on the quality of bone and available surgical access. Proper reinsertion must ensure the vector of pull accurately conforms the lids to the globe. Comparison to the contralateral side should ensure symmetric intercanthal distance and palpebral aperture width. Defects of the

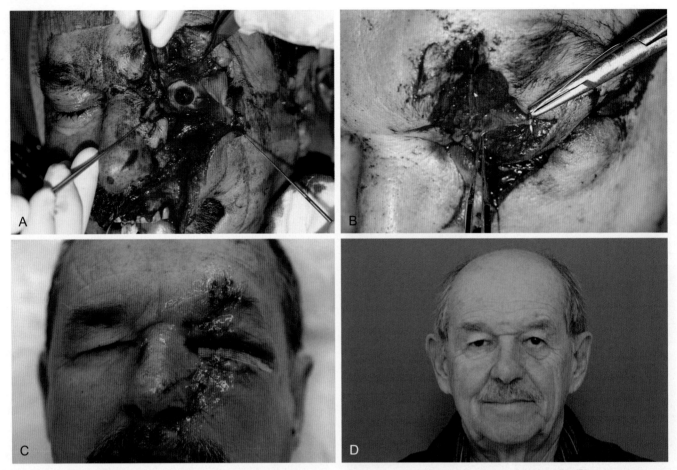

Fig. 1.4.10 (A) Chainsaw injury resulting in laceration to brow, upper and lower lids, cheek and upper lip. (B) The cut and retracted levator palpabrae superioris was identified and repaired. (C) Immediate postoperative result. (D) Long-term result.

canthal tendon can be reconstructed using a strip of periosteum raised as a flap.

If there is an associated bony defect to the canthal insertion, as seen in Fig. 1.4.11, reconstruction with stable bone is required. This is typically done with a rigidly fixated bone graft. Accurate contouring and placement of the graft is required to appropriately set the intercanthal distance. The medial canthal tendon is then anchored to the bone graft using one of the methods previously discussed.

If a defect is present in either the upper or lower lid there are several local and regional flap options available for reconstruction. Defects less than one-third of the lid can often be closed primarily, especially in the elderly with more laxity of the lids. If direct closure is not possible, lateral canthotomy can provide additional mobility to the lateral lid segment. If additional tissue is required, laterally based flaps such as the Tenzel or Mustarde, can be employed. Wide shallow defects of the lower lid can be reconstructed with the Hughes tarsoconjunctival flap.

Nasal Reconstruction

Initial management of traumatic nasal wounds should include irrigation and careful debridement. All deficits in cutaneous coverage, nasal lining, and support should be documented. Simple cutaneous lacerations can be closed as previously described. Involvement of the cartilage and lining requires additional care with three-layered closure. Chromic 5-0 stitches should be used to close the mucosa followed by 5-0 or 6-0 polypropylene or PDS on a taper needle to repair the cartilage. Cartilage

stitches should be placed such that the knots are buried and not palpable. Repair of the alar rim should be properly everted to prevent a secondary notch deformity.

If a septal hematoma is identified, drainage should be performed with an incision through the mucosa, followed by thorough irrigation to remove all clot. To prevent reaccumulation, a combination of nasal packing and septal quilting stitches should be used. If packing is placed, prophylactic antibiotics should be given until the packing is removed. Close follow-up is required to ensure no reaccumulation or continued bleeding occurs.

The timing of definitive reconstruction for traumatic nasal defects requires careful consideration. In severe injuries local and regional reconstructive options may be involved in the zone of injury. It is also ideal if the viability of tissues is fully declared prior to definitive reconstruction. If the viability of the tissues is questionable, loose closure should be performed with delayed definitive reconstruction. If there is exposure of the bony or cartilaginous framework, gel dressings can be applied to prevent desiccation.

To be successful in nasal reconstruction, a surgeon must address defects in lining, cartilaginous support, and cutaneous cover. Cutaneous reconstruction without adequate support will contract and distort. Cartilaginous reconstruction without adequate lining and cover will become exposed and resorb.[44] The avulsive injury displayed in Fig. 1.4.12 has a relatively simple cutaneous component, however without meticulous closure of the nasal lining defect and repair of the cartilage framework, the final outcome will be unsatisfactory.

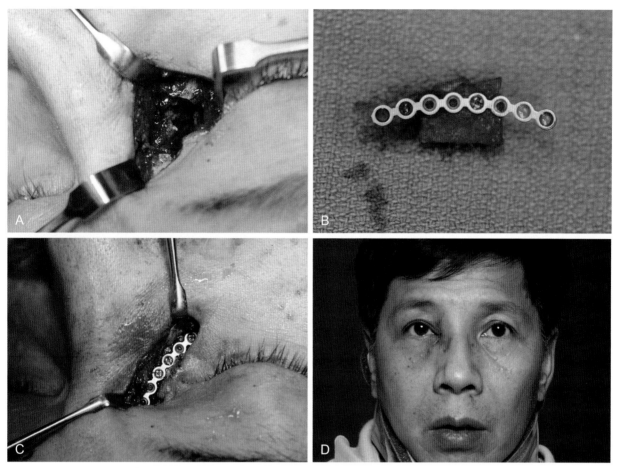

Fig. 1.4.11 (A) Small caliber gunshot wound to medial orbit resulting in bone loss and a Manson Type III NOE fracture. (B–C) Iliac crest bone graft, cut, contoured, and fitted to a plate which reconstructs the bony defect in the medial orbit. The medial canthal tendon is then anchored to the bone graft. (D) Early postoperative result.

There are several options for reconstruction of the lining, including local tissue rearrangements, mucosal advancement flaps, nasolabial flaps, and septal hinge flaps, which may also provide cartilage if required. Large lining defects may require reconstruction with a forehead flap or free tissue transfer.[45] With an intact lining restored cartilaginous reconstruction follows, with repair or replacement of cartilage structures. If grafting is required cartilage can be obtained from a variety of sources, such as an intact septum, ear, rib or allograft depending on the structural and size requirements. As previously described, the nasal subunit principle can help guide the cutaneous reconstruction. Scars are camouflaged when placed at the junction of the subunits and contraction around the base of the reconstructed subunit can accentuate the convex shape of the tip and ala. Each subunit should be accurately mapped and a template of the defect created. Small defects that do not encroach on the alar rim can be reconstructed with local flaps such as the Marchac or bilobe flap. Larger defects or those involving the alar rim usually require tissue brought in from a non-nasal source such as a forehead or nasolabial flap.

Ear Reconstruction

The skin of the ear is tightly adherent to the underlying cartilage framework, and because of this, lacerations of the skin will usually also involve the cartilage. Laceration repair should begin with alignment of the disrupted anatomic landmarks such as the helix, anti-helix, and other cartilage prominences. Buried sutures, usually 5-0 polyglactin, can be placed into the perichondrium if intact. If placing sutures into the cartilage, care must be taken as it is quite fragile, especially in older patients. Cutaneous stitches can then be placed on the anterior and posterior surface. To prevent notching of the helical rim and lobule, everting stitches should be used. Immediate use of Z-plasty can also prevent this notching. If the injury has a component of skin degloving from the cartilage a bolster dressing should be applied to prevent collection.

A near-total ear avulsion is displayed in Fig. 1.4.6. Management begins with irrigation of tissues and minimal debridement, preserving critical areas of anatomy if possible. Tissue viability and vascular perfusion are confirmed. Cases of vascular insufficiency are difficult to manage, however arterial inflow can be reestablished with microvascular techniques. Venous drainage is usually managed with leeching or dermabrasion and heparin pledgets until vascular ingrowth occurs.[46] In this case perfusion was adequate and closure was achieved along with stenting of the external auditory meatus. Despite marginal necrosis all anatomic structures are preserved, allowing for a simplified secondary correction.

Patients presenting with auricular hematoma require drainage to prevent secondary calcification and cauliflower deformity. A small incision should be made in an inconspicuous location to facilitate drainage. A conforming bolster dressing should then be sewn into place with through-and-through ear stitches. This can be removed in several days once the risk of reaccumulation has passed.

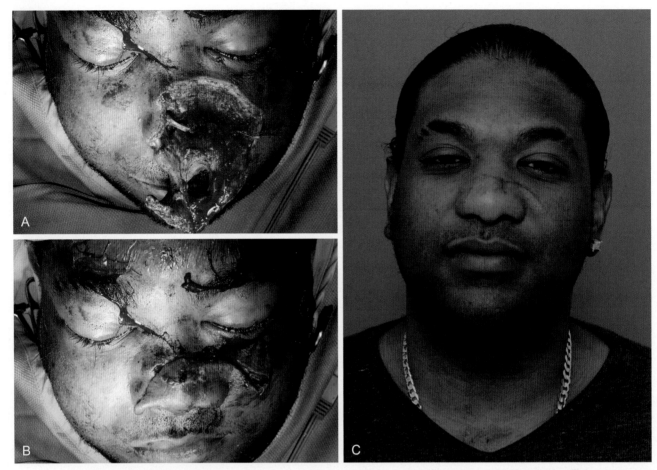

Fig. 1.4.12 (A–B) Complex nasal laceration with disruption of the cartilage framework and nasal lining. (C) Late postoperative result following meticulous closure of the lining, reestablishment of the cartilage framework, and skin closure.

Small defects of the helical rim can be closed by completing a wedge excision. Larger marginal defects can be reconstructed with a chondrocutaneous Antia Buch flap. These flaps allow advancement of the helical rim based on a posterior auricular skin pedicle and are useful for both middle and upper third defects. Mastoid skin flaps can also be used to reconstruct helical defects of the middle third as a two-stage procedure and have been described by multiple authors.[47] Upper third defects can be covered with superiorly-based preauricular or postauricular skin flaps.

Nonmarginal cutaneous defects can be treated with either full- or split-thickness skin grafting. If perichondrium is not present for grafting, the underlying cartilage can be excised and the graft placed on the underlying soft tissue. Defects involving the external auditory meatus can result in secondary contraction and obstruction. Consideration should be given to postoperative stenting of the meatus to prevent this complication.

Lips

The lips are complex functional and aesthetic structures required for communication, oral competence, and social interaction. Full-thickness lip lacerations will often appear to have a significant defect due to splaying of tissues resulting from the pull of the orbicularis muscle. A quick assessment of laxity in the splayed lip segments can determine if there is a true deficiency present. When repairing a lip laceration the white roll and red line of the vermillion margin should be identified and marked prior to injection of local anesthetic. Mental or infraorbital nerve blocks can be used to avoid direct injection into the lips and the resulting distortion of soft tissues. Loop magnification and adequate lighting are beneficial for accurate repair. Full-thickness lip lacerations require repair of the mucosa, orbicularis oris muscle and skin. Repair should begin with 4-0 polyglactin sutures placed into the orbicularis oris muscle, ensuring accurate repair without bunching of the muscle as this will result in an animation deformity. 6-0 polypropylene sutures are then placed directly above and below the white roll prior to closure of the remaining skin. The mucosa is then closed with 5-0 chromic gut suture.

Defects of the lips are best repaired with local tissue as it is extremely difficult to match the color and texture of the vermillion, or the structure of the white roll using distant tissues. For vermillion-only defects, grafting to lip has been described from donor sites including tongue, upper lip and labia minora.[48,49] More commonly sliding mucosa or vermillion advancement flaps are employed. Use of the facial artery myomucosal flap has also been described for this purpose. Small defects involving the white roll can be reconstructed by completing a wedge excision and repairing the defect as described above. Full-thickness defects up to one-quarter of the upper lip or one-third of the lower lip can be closed directly with good aesthetic and functional result as long as the commissure is intact. Upper and lower lip defects involving the commissure can be reconstructed using the Estlander flap.

Larger upper lip defects not involving the commissure can be reconstructed with several options, each with advantages and disadvantages. Three examples are the Abbe lip switch flap, Bernard-Burrow advancement of the intact upper lip or reverse Karapanzic advancement of the lower lip. The Abbe flap is most likely to maintain the proper anatomic relationships of the philtrum and commissure, but requires two stages and relies on spontaneous neurotization for sensation and orbicularis function. The Bernard-Burrow and Karapanzic both provide innervated lip and orbicularis in one stage, but result in distortion of the philtrum and commissure respectively. Another option for upper lip reconstruction is lateral lip advancement using peri-alar crescentic excisions. This can be combined with an Abbe flap to reconstruct defects up to three-quarters of the upper lip (see Fig. 1.4.3).

Upper and lower lip defects greater than 80% of the total lip present a significant challenge. In the past, regional flap reconstruction was used in these cases with microstomia being a common complication.[50] With the advent of free tissue transfer tissue quantity is no longer an issue, however function still suffered as these reconstructions were static and insensate. With advances in technique, sensate and dynamic free tissue transfers are now possible. The most common microsurgical lower lip reconstruction employs a folded free radial forearm flap with palmaris longus tendon. To create a dynamic reconstruction, the tendon is weaved into the remaining orbicularis oris as well the musculature of the modiolus bilaterally. The lateral antebrachial cutaneous nerve of the arm can be anastomosed to a mental nerve stump.[51] Aesthetics remain a concern in these free tissue transfers as they do not recreate the vermillion or white roll. Vermillion tattooing, contouring with liposuction and fat injection as well as mucosal and tongue flaps have been attempted to correct this deficiency.[50,52]

Parotid Gland, Stenson's Duct, Facial Nerve

Lacerations over the cheek require thorough exploration to ensure integrity of the facial nerve and Stenson's duct. Lacerations that do not violate the SMAS can be irrigated and closed. Small skin defects can usually be closed primarily with limited superficial undermining. Larger cutaneous defects may require local or regional flap coverage, however if the zone of injury is extensive it is prudent to temporize a wound with a skin graft and perform a secondary revision. Free tissue transfer may be required for definitive closure if there is exposed bone and vital structures, or through-and-through cheek defects. Fasciocutaneous flaps are usually employed for this purpose, with the ALT flap being our preference due to its large size, long pedicle, and ability to be raised supine for a two-team approach. The ALT flap can also be folded or raised with multiple skin paddles if combined external and intraoral coverage is required.

Intraoperative assessment of Stenson's duct can be done by cannulation of the duct with a lacrimal probe or by injection of dilute methylene blue solution with a small cannula. Identification of the proximal duct can be difficult in avulsion or irregular injuries. In these cases the parotid gland can be milked while looking for the flow of saliva in the proximal duct. Treatments for duct lacerations can be divided into primary repair, diversion of flow with creation of a salivary fistula or salivary gland suppression.[53,54] The preferred treatment is anastomosis when possible. Dissection of the proximal and distal ends of the duct should be done with magnification to prevent injury to nearby buccal facial nerve branches. Repair with 8-0 nylon suture over a silicone stent or angiocath prevents secondary stenosis. The stent is then secured to the buccal mucosa and left in place for 2 weeks.[53,54]

If repair to the distal duct is not possible, salivary flow should be diverted into the oral cavity. The intact proximal duct can be brought through and sutured to the oral mucosa using 8-0 nylon suture. If the proximal duct is damaged and diversion not possible, ligation of the duct is performed. Initial swelling and discomfort is to be expected, with gland atrophy occurring with time. Compression dressings and medical treatment with antisialogogues can be used in the interim while awaiting gland atrophy.[54] Botulinum toxin has been used successfully to suppress parotid function by blocking acetocholine release.[55]

Facial nerve injuries should be explored within 2–6 days so that distal nerve endings can still be identified with nerve stimulation.[56] There may be multiple cut branches in close proximity and care must be taken to ensure that proximal and distal cut ends are matched appropriately. Repair should be completed with a 9-0 nylon suture without tension using an operative microscope. If a nerve gap exists, an autologous interposition nerve graft should be used to facilitate repair. Fig. 1.4.13 demonstrates the repair of a small distal temporal branch following an avulsion injury.

Tongue

Traumatic injuries to the tongue rarely require more then direct closure or healing by secondary intention. The functioned capabilities of the tongue are maintained as long as at least 50% of it remains. Significant injury to the tongue and oral cavity should raise concern for possible airway obstruction due to swelling. Defects greater than 50% are best reconstructed with free tissue transfer. The free radial forearm flap allows for a thin pliable reconstruction when greater than 33% of the tongue remains and mobility of the residual tongue is maintained.[57] In

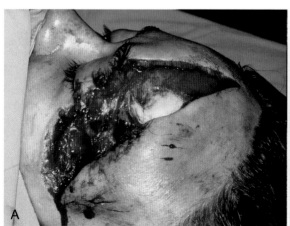
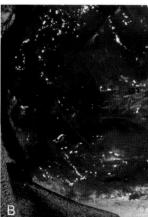
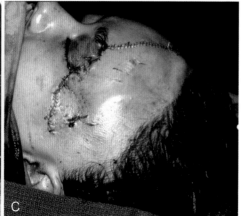

Fig. 1.4.13 (A) Avulsion injury resulting in transaction of the temporal branch of the facial nerve and loss of the lateral brow. (B) Nerve following microsurgical repair. (C) Completed repair.

the case of total or near total loss of the tongue the larger ALT or rectus abdominis flap are able to provide bulk for obturation. This allows for functional swallowing despite their lack of mobility.[58,59] To ensure proper egress of saliva the reconstructed tongue base must not obstruct the pharynx.

EXPERT COMMENTARY

Most facial injury chapters do not emphasize how very important soft tissue management is to the final outcome and appearance of the patient.

Indeed, definitive soft tissue management, cleaning, and debridement of lacerations, excising where possible that millimeter or two of contused edge of lacerations, draining hematomas, and cleaning soft tissue will provide superior results when administered at the time of primary repair. Indeed, late soft tissue management can never replace immediate definitive management in terms of treatment outcomes. Too often I have seen patients late who could have been better managed initially in the acute setting, but the delayed setting often is complicated by risks and issues that are not as easily dealt with.

Indeed, just as facial fractures have patterns, soft tissue injuries have patterns, and their patterns are reproducible and knowing them and scrupulously caring for these injuries will pay rich rewards in the final appearance of the patient. Indeed, the acute management setting often presents unequalled opportunities for proper definitive management which cannot be recaptured in the late setting.

The advantage of judicious debridement and resection of 2 mm of the edge of the laceration can contribute to good results, as can trimming of contused, partially devitalized tissue. Uneven tissue lacerations can frequently be improved where debridement can be tolerated, avoiding debridement/resection in the eyelid, distal nose, and perhaps vermillion border. The advantage of definitive, more aggressive treatment of the surfaces of the wound and the wound edge have been underemphasized in the literature.

Do *not* debride eyebrows, the nasal alae, eyelids, lips, and nostril rim, and be careful with ears.

The patterns of soft tissue injuries and my management recommendations are resources you may consider [1–7].

References

1. Manson P. Reconstruction of traumatic cutaneous facial defects. *Operat Tech Plast Reconstr Surg.* 1998;5(4):368–379.
2. Manson PN. Facial injuries. In: McCarthy J, ed. *Plastic Surgery.* Vol. 2. Philadelphia: W.B. Saunders; 1998:867–1142.
3. Lee RH, Gamble B, Manson P, Mayer M. Patterns of facial lacerations from blunt trauma. *Plast Reconstr Surg.* 1997;99:1544–1554.
4. Robertson B, Manson P. The importance of serial debridement and "A second look" procedures in high-energy ballistic and avulsive facial injuries. *Operat Tech Plast Reconstr Surg.* 1998;5(3):236–246.
5. Robertson B, Manson P. High-energy ballistic and avulsive injuries: a management protocol for the next millennium. *Surg Clin North Am.* 1999;79:1489–1503.
6. Lee R, Gamble B, Robertson B, Manson P. The MC FONTZL classification of facial soft tissue injuries to the face. *Plast Reconstr Surg.* 1999;103:1150–1158.
7. Lee RH, Robertson B, Gamble WB, Manson P. Blunt trauma craniofacial injuries: a comprehensive analysis. *J Craniomaxillofac Trauma.* 2000;6(2):7–16.

REFERENCES

1. Ong TK, Dudley M. Craniofacial trauma presenting at an adult accident and emergency department with an emphasis on soft tissue injuries. *Injury.* 1999;30(5):357–363.
2. Hussain K, Wijetunge DB, Grubnic S, Jackson IT. A comprehensive analysis of craniofacial trauma. *J Trauma.* 1994;36(1):34–47.
3. Mitchener TA, Canham-Chervak M. Oral-maxillofacial injury surveillance in the Department of Defense, 1996-2005. *Am J Prev Med.* 2010;38(1 suppl):S86–S93.
4. Gonzalez-Ulloa M, Castillo A, Stevens E, et al. Preliminary study of the total restoration of the facial skin. *Plast Reconstr Surg.* 1954;13(3):151–161.
5. Burget GC, Menick FJ. The subunit principle in nasal reconstruction. *Plast Reconstr Surg.* 1985;76(2):239–247.
6. Fattahi T. An overview of facial aesthetic units. *J Oral Maxillofac Surg.* 2003;61:1207–1211.
7. Spinelli HM, Jelks GW. Periocular reconstruction: a systematic approach. *Plast Reconstr Surg.* 1993;91:1017–1024.
8. Iwahira Y, Maruyama Y, Yoshitake M. A miniunit approach to lip reconstruction. *Plast Reconstr Surg.* 1994;93(6):1282–1285.
9. Roostaeian J, Rohrich RJ, Stuzin JM. Anatomical considerations to prevent facial nerve injury. *Plast Reconstr Surg.* 2015;135(5):1318–1327.
10. Stuzin JM, Wagstrom L, Kawamoto HK, et al. Anatomy of the frontal branch of the facial nerve: the significance of the temporal fat pad. *Plast Reconstr Surg.* 1989;83:265–271.
11. Owsley JQ, Agarwal CA. Safely navigating around the facial nerve in three dimensions. *Clin Plast Surg.* 2008;35:469–477.
12. Van Sickels JE, Alexander JM. Parotid duct injuries. *Oral Surg Oral Med Oral Pathol.* 1981;52(4):364–367.
13. Stiell IG, Wells GA, Vandemheen K, et al. The Canadian CT Head Rule for patients with minor head injury. *Lancet.* 2001;357(9266):1391–1396.
14. Stiell IG, Wells GA, Vandemheen KL, et al. The Canadian C-spine rule for radiography in alert and stable trauma patients. *JAMA.* 2001;286(15):1841–1848.
15. Powers DB, Delo RI. Characteristics of ballistic and blast injuries. *Atlas Oral Maxillofac Surg Clin North Am.* 2013;21:15–24.
16. Willoughby RE. Rabies: rare human infection – common questions. *Infect Dis Clin North Am.* 2015;29:637–650.
17. Hamborsky J, Kroger A, Wolfe S. *Epidemiology and Prevention of Vaccine-Preventable Diseases.* 13th ed. Public Health Foundation; 2015.
18. Hamilton JR, Sunter JP, Cooper PN. Fatal hemorrhage from simple lacerations of the scalp. *Forensic Sci Med Pathol.* 2005;1:26772.
19. Guzek JP, Ching AS, Hoang TA, et al. Clinical and radiologic lacrimal testing in patients with epiphora. *Ophthalmology.* 1997;104(11):1875–1881.
20. Wright RJ, Murakami CS, Ambro BT. Pediatric nasal injuries and management. *Facial Plast Surg.* 2011;27(5):483–490.
21. Sanyaolu LN, Farmer SE, Cuddihy PJ. Nasal septal haematoma. *BMJ.* 2014;349:g6075.
22. Stuteville OH, Janda C, Pandya NJ. Treating the injured ear to prevent a "cauliflower ear." *Plast Reconstr Surg.* 1969;44(3):310–312.
23. Bendet E, Vajtai I, Maranta CE, et al. Rate and extent of early axonal degeneration of the human facial nerve. *Ann Otol Rhinol Laryngol.* 1998;107(1):1–5.
24. Harris R, Olding C, Lacey C, et al. Changing incidence and management of penetrating neck injuries in the South East London trauma centre. *Ann R Coll Surg Engl.* 2012;94(4):240–244.
25. Petrone P, Verde JM, Asensio JA. Management of penetrating neck injuries. *Br J Surg.* 2012;99(suppl 1):149–154.
26. Blankenship RB, Baker T. Imaging modalities in wounds and superficial skin infections. *Emerg Med Clin North Am.* 2007;25:223–234.
27. Turkcuer I, Atilla R, Topacoglu H, et al. Do we really need plain and soft-tissue radiographies to detect radiolucent foreign bodies in the ED? *Am J Emerg Med.* 2006;24(7):763–768.
28. Hart RG, Hall J. The value of loupe magnification: an underused tool in emergency medicine. *Am J Emerg Med.* 2007;25:704–707.
29. Abdel-Wahed N, Amer ME, Abo-Taleb NS. Assessment of the role of cone beam computed sialography in diagnosing salivary gland lesions. *Imaging Sci Dent.* 2013;43(1):17–23.
30. Vrints I, Den Hondt M, Van Brussel M, et al. Immediate debridement of road crash injuries with Versajet® hydrosurgery: traumatic tattoo prevention? *Aesthetic Plast Surg.* 2014;38(2):467–470.
31. Frodel JL, Barth P, Wagner J. Salvage of partial soft tissue avulsions with medicinal leeches. *Otolaryngol Head Neck Surg.* 2004;131(6):934–939.
32. Larsson J, Klasson S, Arnljots B. Successful nose replantation using leeches for venous draining. *Facial Plast Surg.* 2016;32(04):469–470.
33. Baptista RR, Barreiro GC, Alonso N. Pediatric lip replantation: a case of supermicrosurgical venous anastomosis. *J Reconstr Microsurg.* 2015;31(02):154–156.

34. Plant MA, Fialkov J. Total scalp avulsion with microvascular reanastomosis: a case report and literature review. *Can J Plast Surg.* 2010;18(3):112–115.

35. Desai SC, Sand JP, Sharon JD, et al. Scalp reconstruction an algorithmic approach and systematic review. *JAMA Facial Plast Surg.* 2015;17(1):56–66.

36. Herrera F, Buntic R, Brooks D, et al. Microvascular approach to scalp replantation and reconstruction: a thirty-six-year experience. *Microsurgery.* 2012;32(8):591–597.

37. Sosin M, De la Cruz C, Bojovic B, et al. Microsurgical reconstruction of complex scalp defects: an appraisal of flap selection and the timing of complications. *J Craniofac Surg.* 2015;26(4):1186–1191.

38. Silapunt S, Goldberg LH, Peterson SR, et al. Eyebrow reconstruction: options for reconstruction of cutaneous defects of the eyebrow. *Dermatol Surg.* 2004;30(4 Pt 1):530–535.

39. Motomura H, Muraoka M, Nose K. Eyebrow reconstruction with intermediate hair from the hairline of the forehead on the pedicled temporoparietal fascial flap. *Ann Plast Surg.* 2003;51(3):314–318.

40. Pensler JM, Dillon B, Parry SW. Reconstruction of the eyebrow in the pediatric burn patient. *Plast Reconstr Surg.* 1985;76(3):434–440.

41. Chang EL, Rubin PA. Management of complex eyelid lacerations. *Int Ophthalmol Clin.* 2002;42(3):187–201.

42. Kalin-Hajdu E, Cadet N, Boulos PR. Controversies of the lacrimal system. *Surv Ophthalmol.* 2016;61(3):309–313.

43. Murchison AP, Bilyk JR. Canalicular laceration repair: an analysis of variables affecting success. *Ophthal Plast Reconstr Surg.* 2014;30(5):410–414.

44. Austin GK, Shockley WW. Reconstruction of nasal defects: contemporary approaches. *Curr Opin Otolaryngol Head Neck Surg.* 2016;24(5):453–460.

45. Haack S, Fischer H, Gubisch W. Lining in nasal reconstruction. *Facial Plast Surg.* 2014;30(03):287–299.

46. Jung SN, Yoon S, Kwon H, et al. Successful replantation of an amputated earlobe by microvascular anastomosis. *J Craniofac Surg.* 2009;20(3):822–824.

47. Shonka DC, Park SS. Ear defects. *Facial Plast Surg Clin North Am.* 2009;17(3):429–443.

48. Kroll SS, Weber RS, Goldberg DP, et al. The vermilion-sharing graft for repairing a vermilionectomy defect. *Plast Reconstr Surg.* 1996;98(5):876–879.

49. Ahuja RB. Vermilion reconstruction with labia minora graft. *Plast Reconstr Surg.* 1993;92(7):1418–1419.

50. Baumann D, Robb G. Lip reconstruction. *Semin Plast Surg.* 2008;22(4):269–280.

51. Ozdemir R, Ortak T, Koçer U, et al. Total lower lip reconstruction using sensate composite radial forearm flap. *J Craniofac Surg.* 2003;14(3):393–405.

52. Serletti JM, Tavin E, Moran S, et al. Total lower lip reconstruction with a sensate composite radial forearm–palmaris longus free flap and a tongue flap. *Plast Reconstr Surg.* 1997;99(2):559–561.

53. Van Sickels JE. Management of parotid gland and duct injuries. *Oral Maxillofac Surg Clin North Am.* 2009;21(2):243–246.

54. Steinberg MJ, Herréra AF. Management of parotid duct injuries. *Oral Surg Oral Med Oral Pathol Oral Radiol Endod.* 2005;99(2):136–141.

55. Ellies M, Gottstein U, Rohrbach-Volland S, et al. Reduction of salivary flow with botulinum toxin: extended report on 33 patients with drooling, salivary fistulas, and sialadenitis. *Laryngoscope.* 2004;114(10):1856–1860.

56. Bendet E, Vajtai I, Maranta C, et al. Rate and extent of early axonal degeneration of the human facial nerve. *Ann Otol Rhinol Laryngol.* 1998;107(1):1–5.

57. Engel H, Huang JJ, Lin CY, et al. A strategic approach for tongue reconstruction to achieve predictable and improved functional and aesthetic outcomes. *Plast Reconstr Surg.* 2010;126(6):1967–1977.

58. Hurvitz KA, Kobayashi M, Evans GR. Current options in head and neck reconstruction. *Plast Reconstr Surg.* 2006;118(5):122e–133e.

59. Lyos AT, Evans GR, Perez D, et al. Tongue reconstruction: outcomes with the rectus abdominis flap. *Plast Reconstr Surg.* 1999;103:442–447.

Traumatic Facial Nerve Injury

Shai M. Rozen

INTRODUCTION

The field of facial paralysis provides the reconstructive surgeon an incredible opportunity to help patients with what is undoubtedly a devastating injury. The field intricately involves restoration of function, form, and even emotion, demanding that the surgeon use a wide spectrum of surgical tools and principles, including microsurgery, peripheral nerve surgery, and aesthetic facial surgery with the goal of restoring the patient's appearance, as feasibly as possible, to normalcy. Although traumatic facial palsy may differ in etiology and mechanism from other facial palsies, the reconstructive principles, philosophy, approach, and techniques remain quite similar. Hopefully this chapter will provide the reader a thinking process and technical tools to achieve optimal outcomes.

EPIDEMIOLOGY AND ETIOLOGY

Each year approximately 20 of 100,000 people are diagnosed with facial palsy.[1] Among more than 40 different etiologies, the most common include facial palsy of unknown etiology (Bell's palsy), infections, trauma, and iatrogenic facial nerve injury during extirpative surgery. The exact incidence of traumatic facial palsy is not as clear, but is approximated at 16%.[2] Although intraoperative facial nerve injury, whether inadvertent or during cosmetic or extirpative surgery, may not be considered as trauma in the classic sense, this chapter discusses these types of injuries due to similarities in clinical presentation, diagnoses, and management principles.

SURGICAL ANATOMY

The facial nerve is a mixed nerve that carries fibers from and into three distinct nuclei in the midbrain.[3-5] The motor nucleus originates fibers that innervate the mimetic musculature, the superior salivatory nucleus sends preganglionic parasympathetic fibers to the lacrimal, sublingual, and submandibular glands, and the solitary tract nucleus receives sensory fibers from the external auditory canal and taste fibers from the anterior two-thirds of the tongue. Upper motor neurons from the cerebrum converge via the corticobulbar tract into the facial motor nucleus in the pons. The forehead is innervated by fibers from both cortices while the lower two-thirds of the face is innervated from the contralateral side. As the fibers converge in the brain stem to synapse in the facial nerve motor nucleus, the remainder of the nerve, the lower motor neuron, innervates the entire ipsilateral hemiface. From the brain stem, the facial nerve enters the petrous portion of the temporal bone at the internal auditory meatus, coursing through the bone until it exits through the styloid–mastoid foramen. This is the longest and narrowest course of a nerve within a bone in the body, making it susceptible to compression (Fig. 1.5.1). Along its intratemporal portion, the facial nerve gives off several branches, including parasympathetic fibers innervating the lacrimal gland via the greater petrosal nerve and more distally the sublingual and submandibular glands via the chorda tympani, motor fibers innervating the stapedius muscle, and taste fibers innervating the anterior two-thirds of the tongue.

Although variations exist in the extracranial facial nerve anatomy, once the facial nerve exits the stylomastoid foramen, it sends a small sensory branch to the posterior wall of the external auditory canal and tympanic membrane, followed by the postauricular nerve that innervates the posterior auricular and occipitalis muscles, and two small branches innervating the stylohyoid and posterior belly of the digastric muscles. It courses 1–2 cm and at the pes anserinus divides into two major trunks: the superior temporofacial trunk and the inferior cervicofacial trunk. The first divides into the temporal (frontal) branch with minimal arborizations and the zygomatic and buccal branches that have significantly more arborizations creating an intertwining network of nerves in the midface. The cervical trunk divides into the mandibular branch and the cervical branch with minimal arborizations between them. The frontal branch innervates the frontalis muscles and is responsible for brow elevation, anterior and superior auricular muscles, corrugator and procerus muscles, and contributions to the orbicularis oculi muscle. The zygomatic and buccal branches innervate the mimetic muscles of the midface, including the orbicularis oculi, levators of the lip, buccinator and rizorius muscles, and the orbicularis oris muscle, and depressors of the lip. The cervical trunk innervates the mentalis muscle via the marginal mandibular nerve and the platysma via the cervical division. A full review of the facial nerve anatomy and its branches may be found in any anatomy atlas[4] (Table 1.5.1).

Based on the anatomic level of facial nerve injury, different deficits will occur. Unilateral upper motor neuron injuries will cause injuries to the contralateral lower two-thirds of the face sparing the forehead, while injuries distal to the facial nerve nucleus will affect both the upper and lower parts of the ipsilateral face. More proximal injuries may involve the lacrimal gland via the greater petrosal nerve, the auditory apparatus via the stapedial nerve, and taste via the chorda tympani and lingual nerve, in addition to motor deficits. More distal injuries may spare the former and create purer motor deficits and small sensory deficits. Knowledge of this anatomy is consequential in both the diagnosis and localization of the facial nerve injury as well as the treatment plan.[5]

HISTORY AND PHYSICAL EXAM

A thorough history and physical examination is critical in the evaluation and treatment plan. Establishing the duration, mechanism, and pretraumatic facial nerve function, especially in older patients, is pertinent. Age, comorbidities, and previous surgical history will also partially dictate the type of future intervention.

In multitrauma cases, initial assessment must include a full trauma evaluation for other injuries. Low Glasgow Coma Scores suggest traumatic brain injuries and possible skull base fractures affecting the facial

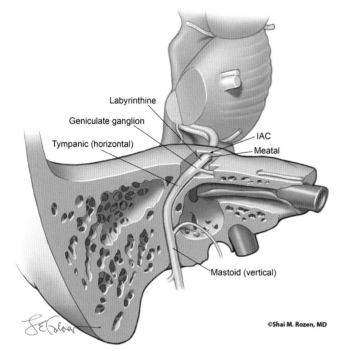

Fig. 1.5.1 Intratemporal course of the facial nerve. IAC = internal auditory canal. (Courtesy Shai M. Rozen. Copyright Shai M. Rozen.)

nerve. External auditory canal otoscopic examination can reveal a step deformity or laceration. If hemotympanum or tympanic membrane perforation with blood or CSF is seen, longitudinal fracture of the temporal bone should be suspected. Conductive hearing loss is also generally associated to longitudinal temporal fractures while sensorineural loss is most commonly associated to transverse fractures. Regional facial examination for resting tone and voluntary activity is necessary. Thorough mimetic muscle assessment from forehead to neck is crucial. Whether an intracranial or extracranial nerve injury is suspected, any facial motion suggests a contusion rather than laceration and implies continuity of nerve and excellent prognosis. In midface penetrating injuries, parotid duct injuries must be excluded. Additionally, remaining cranial nerves must be evaluated for both injury and their potential as donor nerves for reanimation.

Clinical presentation may suggest the level of facial nerve injury. Injuries proximal to the midbrain nuclei, termed upper motor neuron injuries, will spare the forehead due to the bilateral contributions of the cerebral hemispheres yet produce contralateral lower two-third paralysis. In the trauma setting these injuries usually result in death or preclude rehabilitation, but patients must be assessed individually. Injuries inclusive and distal to the midbrain nuclei will result in complete ipsilateral facial paralysis. The more proximal the injury, the more fiber types are included, and symptoms will include decreased lacrimation, hyperacousis, changes in taste, sensory, and motor deficits. The more distal the injury, the resultant injury is more localized. Hence complete knowledge of facial nerve anatomy is paramount in the diagnosis of facial nerve trauma. Midface lacerations involving proximal buccal and zygomatic nerve injuries will mostly cause midface paralysis unless they are isolated to single branches, in which cases the injury may be unnoticeable due to arborization between the branches. In this setting, concomitant parotid duct injury should be ruled out.

TABLE 1.5.1 Mimetic Muscle Innervation by Facial Nerve Branch

Branch of CN VII	Muscle	Action
Posterior auricular	Posterior auricular	Pulls ear up and backwards
	Occipitofrontalis, occipital belly	Moves scalp backward
Temporal	Anterior auricular	Pulls ear up and forwards
	Superior auricular	Raises ear
	Occipitofrontalis, frontal belly	Wrinkles forehead and raises eyebrow
	Corrugator supercilii	Pulls eyebrow medially and down
	Procerus	Pulls medial angle of eyebrow down producing transverse wrinkles over bridge of nose
Temporal and zygomatic	Orbicularis oculi	Closes eyelids gently (palpebral part) or forcefully (orbital part) and contracts skin around eye
Zygomatic and buccal	Zygomaticus major	Pulls corners of mouth up and lateral
Buccal	Zygomaticus minor	Elevates upper lip
	Levator labii superioris	Elevates upper lip (helps form nasolabial furrow)
	Levator labii superioris alaeque nasi	Elevates medial nasolabial fold and nasal ala (opens nostril)
	Risorius	Pulls corner of mouth lateral (aids smile)
	Buccinator	Pulls corner of mouth backward and compresses cheek against teeth
	Levator anguli oris	Raises angles of mouth upward (helps form nasolabial furrow)
	Orbicularis oris	Closes and protrudes lips
	Nasalis, alar part	Flares nostrils by pulling cartilage down and laterally
	Nasalis, transverse part	Compresses nostrils
Buccal and marginal mandibular	Depressor anguli oris	Pulls corner of mouth down and lateral
	Depressor labii inferioris	Pulls lower lip down and lateral
Marginal mandibular	Mentalis	Pulls skin of chin upward
Cervical	Platysma	Pulls down corners of mouth

Special attention needs to be given to patients suffering from high-energy injuries involving blast or high velocity projectiles or patients with multilevel injuries as seen in animal bites. These patients usually present with facial nerve injuries at several levels, coinciding with soft tissue trauma including muscle, skin, mucosa and bone.

Ancillary Testing
CT Scans

Temporal bone fractures are a product of high-energy blunt trauma commonly resulting in fracture, hemorrhage, nerve trauma, vascular damage, with disruption of the middle or inner ear structures, classically classified into longitudinal, transverse, or oblique fractures. Longitudinal fractures often result from lateral to medial forces extending through the facial nerve canal, possibly causing intraneural hemorrhage, transection, or bone compression. They can disrupt the ossicular chain, resulting in conductive hearing loss. Transverse fractures often result from anterior posterior forces with a fracture line often traversing the vestibulocochlear apparatus causing sensorineural hearing loss and equilibrium disorders. Transverse fractures more commonly injure the facial nerve due to proximity to the nerve's labyrinthine segment. Oblique, also termed mixed, fractures include both longitudinal and transverse components. Additional classifications are based on degree of involvement of the petrous portion of the temporal bone, or the otic capsule.[6] Temporal bone computed tomography (CT) scans should be performed in thin-section 1 mm cuts to avoid interpreting normal suture lines as fractures.

MRI

Magnetic resonance imaging (MRI) has lower sensitivity and specificity in depicting temporal bone fractures compared to CT scans. It may demonstrate fluid in the middle ear and mastoid air cells as a high signal on T2-weighted images or suggest hemorrhage, revealed by a bright signal in the labyrinth or middle ear. Recent MR neurography has some promise in depicting intratemporal facial nerve injury.

ENoG

Electroneurography is an objective test that measures evoked compound muscle action potentials using skin electrodes. Nerve injury is expressed as percentage of function relative to the healthy contralateral side. It is preferable to perform ENoG only after 3 days, when Wallerian degeneration is completed otherwise there is a risk for a false negative since conduction will still occur. Conversely, ENoG is of little value if performed after 21 days since interpretation is unreliable. Optimally it should be performed at 3 days followed every 3–5 days to demonstrate a trend. Some surgeons use a decrease of 90% on the injured side as an indication for temporal bone decompression, although this remains controversial.

EMG

Electromyography measures voluntary mimetic muscle response with needle electrodes detecting action potentials during muscle contraction. Denervated muscles display fibrillation potentials while muscle that are reinnervating demonstrate polyphasic potentials. Electrical silence indicates severe muscle atrophy and degradation of motor end plates. EMG is best performed at least 10–14 days after injury to allow Wallerian degeneration to set in. The value of the EMG in the acute facial nerve injury period is unclear but may have some value in the subacute period, up to 12–18 months, possibly helping decide between nerve transfers relying on salvageability of the patient's native mimetic muscles versus using a new muscle for reanimation. A more detailed discussion will follow.

LOCATION, MECHANISM, AND DURATION OF INJURY – EFFECTS ON MANAGEMENT STRATEGIES

The evaluation of a new patient with facial palsy must include the three crucial factors in future treatment decisions: location, mechanism, and perhaps most important, the duration of paralysis. Location can be grouped into intracranial or extracranial, mechanism into blunt or penetrating, and duration into acute, subacute, and chronic.

Location and Mechanism of Injury
Intracranial Facial Nerve Injuries

Most intracranial nerve injuries occur secondary to blunt trauma. Penetrating injuries are usually associated to gunshot wounds and are frequently lethal. The mechanism is usually either complete transection of the nerve or irreversible compression injury due to collapse of the osseous canal within the petrous portion of the temporal bone. The zone of injury is usually beyond the area of transection and difficult to assess (Fig. 1.5.2).

Blunt injuries resulting in temporal bone fractures are often encountered in motor vehicle accidents, altercations, or falls from heights. Approximately 7%–10% of temporal bone fractures result in facial nerve injury. Temporal bone fractures have several classifications. Fracture line orientation relative to the petrous bone defines fractures as longitudinal (70%–80%), transverse (10%–20%), and oblique (10%). Facial paralysis occurs most commonly in transverse fractures (50%) but may also occur in longitudinal fractures (25%).[7] More modern CT-based classifications assess whether fractures are otic capsule sparing or violating, the latter being twice as likely to cause facial paralysis.[8,9] Four types of facial nerve trauma have been found in temporal bone fractures. In 76% of longitudinal fractures either bony impingement or intraneural hematoma was found, and in 15% the nerve was transected. In the remainder of patients, no visible pathology was found other than neural edema. In transverse fractures, 92% were transected and 8% had impingement[10] (Fig. 1.5.3). Similar to penetrating intracranial facial nerve injuries, surviving patients are initially often in critical condition and the facial paralysis is often unnoticed.

Extracranial Facial Nerve Injuries

Extracranial penetrating trauma may include either low-energy penetrating objects, higher-energy projectiles or blasts, or a combination of sharp, crush, and avulsion injuries.

Low-energy penetrating trauma, commonly secondary to sharp objects as knives or broken glass, usually results in localized cuts through the facial nerve branches resulting in paralysis of one or more of the facial nerve branches. These injuries are mostly clean, associated with minimal nerve gaps, and frequently result in well-aligned proximal and distal nerve endings. These injuries may span proximally from the styloid foramen to the small distal branches just proximal to the mimetic muscles. Proximal injuries at the level of the pes anserinus result in complete unilateral facial paralysis while more distal injuries may result in more regional palsies or none. Injuries at nearly any level of the frontal or marginal mandibular branches will result in complete paralysis of the forehead or depressors of the lip due to the lack of arborization with synergistic nerve branches, while injury to the zygomatic or buccal branches is more forgiving due to increased branch arborization.

Combined sharp, crush, or avulsion injuries, as often seen in animal bites, high-energy projectiles, or blasts, are usually characterized by contaminated, multilevel traumatic injury that may involve multilevel facial nerve injury, often creating long nerve gaps with or without muscle injury or overlying tissue deficiencies. Blunt injury to the extracranial

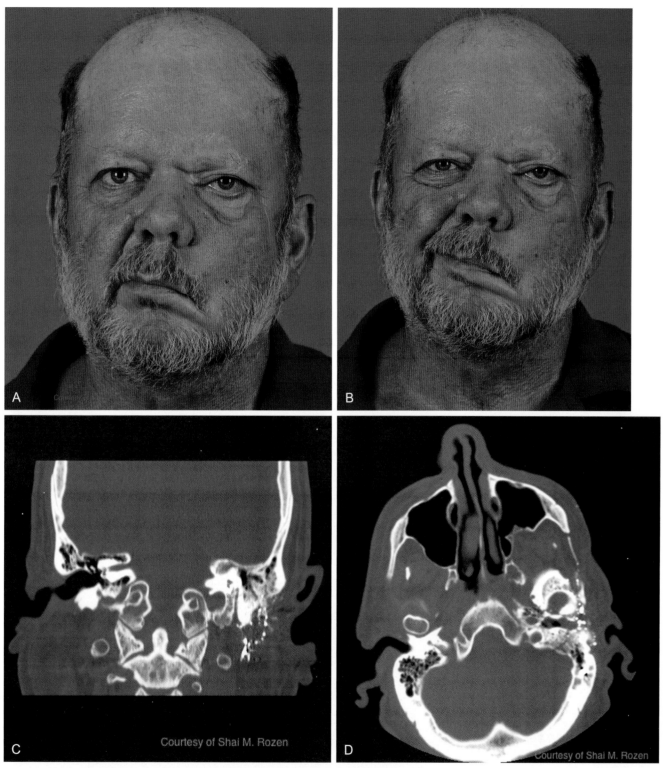

Fig. 1.5.2 A 61-year-old male 10 months after gunshot injury obliterating the left zygomatic arch and temporal bone, presenting with complete left facial palsy. (A) Repose. (B) Animation. (C) Coronal CT scan. (D) Axial CT scan. (Courtesy Shai M. Rozen. Copyright Shai M. Rozen.)

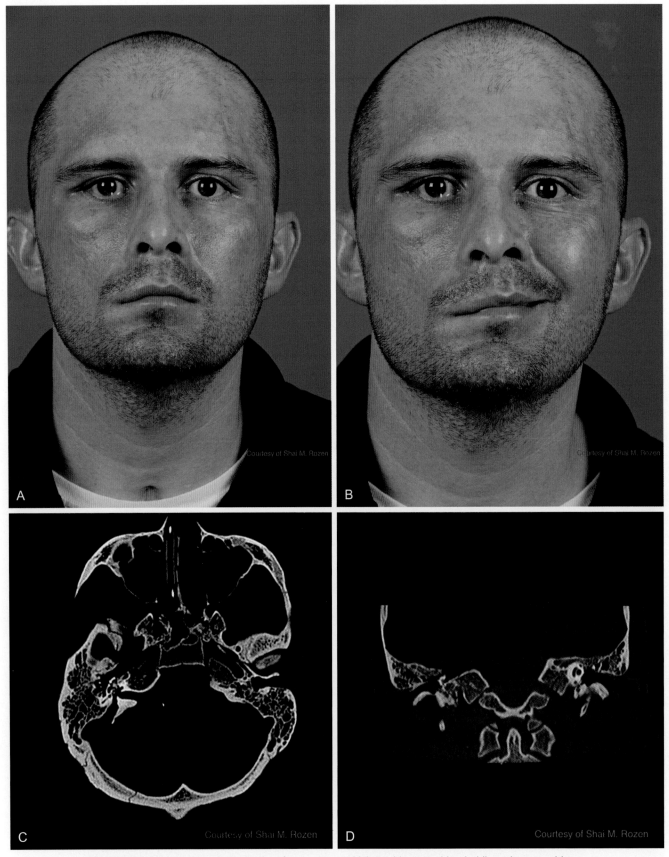

Fig. 1.5.3 A 36-year-old-male 8 months after a motor vehicle accident resulting in bilateral temporal bone fracture – right transverse fracture resulting in near-complete paralysis and left oblique fracture resulting in near-complete recovery. (A) Repose. (B) Animation. (C–D) Axial and coronal CT scan revealing bilateral temporal bone fractures – right transverse otic violating and left otic sparing. (Courtesy Shai M. Rozen. Copyright Shai M. Rozen.)

portion of the face is a rare cause of facial paralysis, and will usually result in temporary neuropraxia and complete recovery.

Muscle Injury

Although not a common cause of facial paralysis, muscle injury may have similar effects and clinical presentation as nerve injuries, especially in the setting of acute trauma, in which both muscle and nerve may be contused. Over time, when the nerve recovers the muscle injury usually becomes more apparent since motion is seen in the proximal innervated muscle but animation is inhibited because the distal muscle is detached and will not produce the intended motion at the muscle insertion. These injuries usually result in more focal akinesia compared with proximal nerve injuries (Fig. 1.5.4).

Duration of Paralysis, Pre-Injury Function, and Choice of Surgical Techniques

The most important variable when evaluating facial palsy patients is the duration of paralysis and degree of function prior to injury. As opposed to patients whose facial palsy is due to neoplasms, infections, or Bell's palsy, in whom palsy duration is not always clear, most facial nerve trauma patients have no history of prior paralysis, are frequently younger, and palsy duration is directly traced to the time of injury. Duration may be divided into three quite indistinct periods: acute (0–72 hours), subacute (up to 6–12 months), and longstanding facial paralysis (beyond 12–18 months). Differentiation should be more physiological than chronological. Distinction between acute and subacute facial paralysis is somewhat artificial since management may be similar and depends more on the type of injury rather than duration of paralysis, but common to both is the potential to salvage the patient's mimetic muscles, as opposed to longstanding facial paralysis, when a new neuromuscular unit must be introduced as part of the treatment strategy due to mimetic muscle denervation atrophy.

Acute Facial Paralysis

Historically, acute facial palsy may be defined as a period between the time of trauma up to 72 hours, after which Wallerian degeneration begins and stimulation of the distal nerve branches is not feasible. This is likely the period in which treating the paralysis with either direct

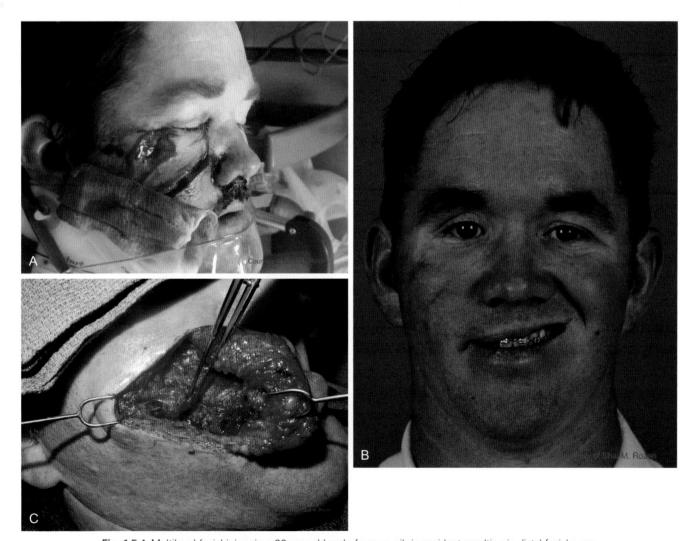

Fig. 1.5.4 Multilevel facial injury in a 26-year-old male from an oil rig accident resulting in distal facial nerve contusion and mimetic muscle lacerations. (A) Preoperative injury at presentation to an outside institution. (B) Preoperative photo 12 months after injury and prior to muscle repair. (C) Intraoperative photo revealing lacerated distal zygomatic and levator muscle of the lip before repair – pickup holding cut muscle plexus.

Continued

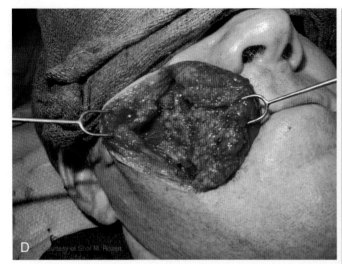

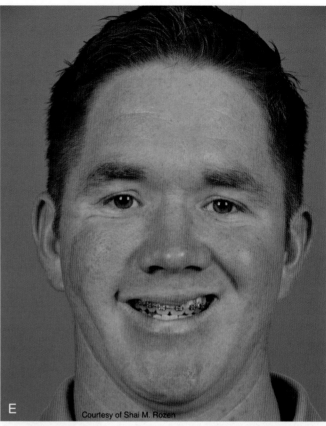

Fig. 1.5.4, cont'd (D) After repair. (E) Postoperative photo 9 months after repair. (Courtesy Shai M. Rozen. Copyright Shai M. Rozen.)

nerve repair, nerve grafting, or nerve transfer will yield the best results although results may vary with each of these techniques depending on the mechanism and location of facial nerve injury.

Acute Intracranial Facial Nerve Injuries

Decompression. The use of steroids in these cases has not been demonstrated to confer the benefit it has in the setting of Bell's palsy, therefore the benefits versus risks of infection should be weighed. There is scant high-level evidence as to whether acute intracranial facial nerve decompression helps prevent facial paresis,[11,12] and only few reports support this approach and are mainly retrospective, lack controls, and suffer from small patient numbers.[13,14] The main difficulty in achieving high-level evidence is the difficulty in comparing a control group whose natural history is often favorable, to an intervention group, proving the latter fare better. Additionally, these injuries are frequently in the setting of traumatic brain injuries with most patients intubated and either intentionally sedated or in comatose conditions, rendering early clinical assessment of facial nerve function difficult. If examination is possible, sensorineural hearing loss bears a poorer prognosis than conductive hearing loss and partial facial palsy is highly predictive of full recovery versus poorer prognosis with complete palsy. Overall, many of these patients recover facial nerve function without intervention.

ENoG, if performed within 14 days of injury and demonstrating more than 95% degeneration compared to the normal side, has been suggested by some authors as a criterion for surgery, but no strong supportive data exists. In most cases, especially when several weeks have passed since the trauma, treatment is directed more by a combination of high-resolution CT scans and EMGs demonstrating fibrillation

potentials,[13,15] and is often based on the surgeon's personal opinion and experience with intracranial decompression. Technical details of intracranial nerve decompression are beyond the scope of this text and are more relevant for the neuro-otologist than the plastic and reconstructive surgeon, but close collaboration is paramount.

Primary nerve repair. In the setting of trauma, primary neuroraphy would be a rare scenario, since most injuries would necessitate nerve grafting due to some degree of zone of injury to the nerve and the inability to mobilize the nerve sufficiently and perform a tension-free coaptation.

Nerve grafting. In cases of intracranial trauma with laceration and discontinuity of the facial nerve, acute nerve grafting may be considered. The literature is scant and the situation is further complicated by the difficulty in assessing the zone of nerve injury. If the injury is close to the brain stem, a proximal nerve may not be available for coaptation, rendering grafting impossible. If a nerve graft is optional, suturing may be difficult and using fibrin glue may be preferable, although there is no evidence of superiority of one technique over another. Additionally, current literature on immediate intracranial nerve grafting in the setting of tumor resection demonstrates poor functional results, albeit restoration of some facial tone, especially in the perioral, periorbital, and buccinator muscle areas,[16] but the trauma setting provides even less optimal conditions for immediate nerve grafting.

Acute Extracranial Facial Nerve Injuries

Primary repair. Primary neuroraphy is always the treatment of choice if feasible and provides the best results.[17–19] The advantages of repair at this stage are twofold. Distal branches are still stimulable prior to onset of Wallerian degeneration and identification of branches is easier in the unscarred environment. Two conditions must be met for primary neurorraphy to result in successful outcomes. The first is that both proximal and distal nerve endings must exist. The second is that direct nerve coaptation must be absent of tension. Any tension on repair will uniformly result in scarring and inhibit axonal regeneration through the coaptation.[17] Prior to induction, communicating with the anesthesiologist to avoid the use of paralytics is important and local injection should include only epinephrine for hemostasis. Depending on the location of injury, exploration may be performed via the wound edges or a preauricular incision. A nerve stimulator with several options of amperage and frequency enabling repetitive stimulation and tetany is necessary for accurate facial nerve branch mapping. Ragged nerve edges may be trimmed with a fresh blade while cutting on a sterile wooden tongue blade. Repair of midface branches, including the zygomatic and buccal branches, results in better function than repairs of the marginal mandibular and temporal branches, although repair of the latter is recommended in the acute setting.

Nerve grafting. Where a nerve gap exists despite mobilization of the nerve endings, the second-best option is nerve grafting the gap.[20] The options for nerve grafting are abundant. Where only one branch needs repair, the great auricular nerve may be used since it is usually within the same operative field, but more commonly several branches may need repair, in which case a sural nerve would provide more graft material. The advantage of the latter is that one nerve may be either cut into several longitudinal nerve segments or if size mismatch exists, i.e. the sural nerve is too large, the sural nerve can usually be safely neurolyzed along its fascicles for relatively long distances, providing several fascicles of decreased diameter for better size match. Additional potential donor nerves are the medial or lateral antebrachial cutaneous nerves.

Whether direct nerve repair or nerve grafting is performed, coaptation is usually performed with either 9-0 or 10-0 nylon under microscopy. Prior to coaptation, the nerve endings may be cleared from any surrounding connective tissue to alleviate identification of the epineurium and prevent any redundant tissue disrupting the coaptation. The key is to approximate the nerve ending via epineural sutures, minimizing fascicular injury and avoiding tension. If a fascicle has "escaped" between the nerve endings, it may either be gently pushed back or shortened and reinserted into the coaptation. Some authors use fibrin sealants to minimize the need for sutures in coaptation, but the potential exists that glue may infiltrate the interface and inhibit axonal growth.

In cases where a proximal nerve is not found or is too close to the styloid foramen, unroofing the mastoid portion of the nerve is warranted to enable nerve grafting. If a proximal nerve is not found, then nerve transfers are justified, enabling the use of native mimetic muscles. In younger patients (under 60), concomitant cross facial nerve grafting can be performed, with future planning to perform selective end-to-end coaptation once axons have reached the contralateral side or performing end-to-side coaptations in the primary surgery. In rare cases when a distal branch is not found, but a proximal branch is available, the latter may be used to innervate a functional muscle transplant.

Nerve transfers. Although acute nerve transfers in the trauma setting are uncommon, they may be used concomitantly in cases where planned extirpation of the facial nerve is performed and nerve grafting is unlikely to yield optimal results or is not feasible. Nerve transfers are used much more frequently in the subacute phase and are detailed below (Fig. 1.5.5).

Subacute Facial Paralysis

Subacute facial paralysis includes a period in which the native mimetic muscles have the potential to be salvaged and can produce significant function if they are reinnervated. The exact duration of this period is somewhat vague and far from consensus, but some authors would consider this a year. In our experience, some recovery can be established even after a year of denervation, but the best results are seen with earlier reinnervation at around 6 months after injury, in concordance with a few other studies on the subject.[21–23] Reinnervation may be attempted via direct nerve coaptation, nerve grafting or nerve transfers depending on the clinical scenario.

Intracranial Subacute Facial Nerve Injuries

Nerve decompression. Although there is weak evidence suggesting possible benefits of delayed intracranial nerve decompression in patients with severe Bell's palsy,[24] literature is scant to support delayed intracranial facial nerve decompression for an established facial paralysis.[12,25]

Nerve grafting. Attempts at resecting the presumed intratemporal nerve segment with subsequent nerve grafting can be considered and necessitate an experienced skull base surgeon, but supporting evidence does not exist. Current literature discusses intracranial nerve grafting in the acute setting of tumor resection, demonstrating poor functional outcomes yet providing some facial tone.[16] Delayed intracranial grafting carries a poor prognosis since it may require both longer grafts due to scarring and prolonged regeneration time necessary to reach the neuromuscular junction, possibly rendering the mimetic muscles nonsalvageable.

Nerve transfers. A more feasible treatment option in the subacute phase of intracranial injuries, granted that distal facial nerve branches exist, is nerve transfers with or without concomitant cross facial nerve grafting, also known as the baby-sitter procedure.[23,26] The premise for this approach is the potential for mimetic muscle renervation using the extracranial facial nerve as a conduit for axonal growth while the source of the new innervation is from an ipsilateral nonfacial nerve. The most common donor nerves are the masseter nerve, the spinal accessory nerve, and the hemihypoglossal nerve, which has fallen out of favor as it yields lesser results and higher complication rates. In younger patients, up to the sixth decade in life, additional cross facial nerve grafts may be considered, potentially bringing in contralateral facial nerve axons, in theory increasing spontaneity. This is still somewhat of a controversial subject, since the contribution of the cross facial axons compared to those of the ipsilateral nerve transfer axons is not entirely defined. Although the longest duration of paralysis in which effective nerve transfers can be performed is unclear, there is growing consensus that better results are seen when performed within the first 6 months.[22] The additional pertinent operative decision is the anatomic location within the facial nerve into which the nerve transfer is performed. The more proximal the coaptation, the more mimetic muscle will be reinnervated at the price of increased synkinesis, albeit not significant in the author's opinion. The more distal the transfer is performed, the less mimetic muscles are salvaged, but theoretically synkinesis decreases (Fig. 1.5.6).

Extracranial Subacute Facial Nerve Injuries

Many patients who are seen in facial palsy centers at this stage have been previously operated at other institutions and are referred for evaluation because of failure to recover. The question as to when to intervene is perhaps one of the most difficult the surgeon must answer, but as a general guideline, if patients fail to demonstrate any motion at 6 months, regardless of EMG findings, surgical intervention is highly recommended to avoid losing a chance to salvage native mimetic muscles. If some degree of motion is seen, frequent follow-up is necessary to assess if a functional plateau is reached and whether function is satisfactory or

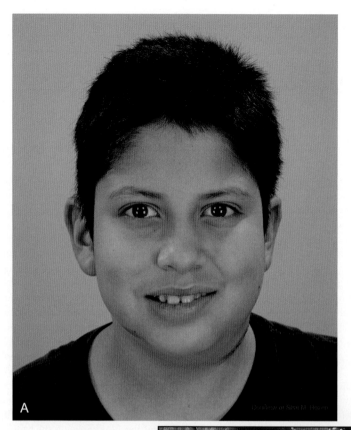

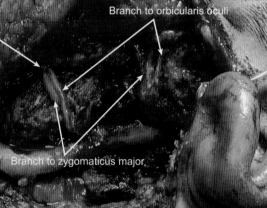

CFNG x 2
1. From OO
2. From ZM

Branch to orbicularis oculi

Branch to zygomaticus major

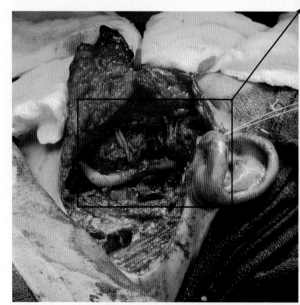

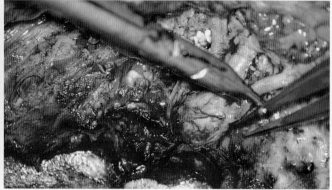

B   Courtesy of Shai M. Rozen

Fig. 1.5.5 A 10-year-old boy who had undergone a masseter to facial nerve transfer with concomitant two cross facial nerve grafts (CFNG) during an extra and distal mastoid intracranial nerve resection for tumor. (A) Before surgery. (B) Intraoperative photo demonstrating a V to VII nerve transfer with two CFNGs.

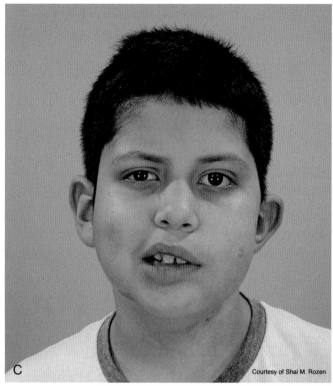
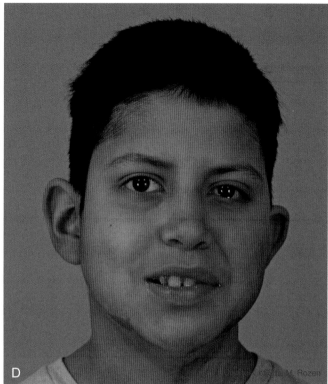

Courtesy of Shai M. Rozen

Fig. 1.5.5, cont'd Postoperative photos at 7 weeks (C) and 13 weeks (D) after surgery. (Courtesy Shai M. Rozen. Copyright Shai M. Rozen.)

may be improved. In these situations, every effort should be made to obtain previous operative notes (Fig. 1.5.7).

Direct repair. If both proximal and distal nerve ending of the injured facial nerve can be retrieved and a tension-free coaptation is possible, it should be attempted. Realistically, the chances of having only a minimal nerve gap after exploration within scar tissue are low and most often a nerve graft is necessary.

Nerve grafting. In theory, ipsilateral nerve grafting may be performed in a delayed fashion if salvage of the mimetic muscles is deemed possible. The main problems that may be encountered in this setting are identification of the proximal and distal nerve endings beyond the scar and zone of injury. Additional considerations are salvageability of mimetic muscles based on the duration of the palsy, nerve gap length, and injury distance from muscle. Nerve grafting from the contralateral side should only be attempted if combined with concomitant ipsilateral nerve transfers. Alone, they do not consistently provide sufficient axonal load and power, and by the time they provide limited axons, irreversible mimetic muscle atrophy will have occurred.

Nerve transfers. Considerations for nerve transfers in the setting of subacute extracranial nerve injuries are like those of intracranial injuries and are detailed above. The additional factor to be weighed is the existence of intact distal nerve branches. When the injury is solely intracranial, the extracranial facial nerve is nearly always intact, but in cases of extensive extracranial nerve injuries, the surgeon must absolutely verify the continuity of facial nerve branches from the site of nerve transfer to the neuromuscular junction, otherwise regenerating axons will fail to reach the targeted muscle.

Acute and Subacute Intracranial and Extracranial Facial Nerve Injuries Without Existing Distal Facial Nerve Branches

These scenarios are not common but should be treated similarly to longstanding facial palsy patients since regenerating axons will not reach the mimetic muscles. Although some literature exists as to techniques of direct muscle neurotization,[27] meaning directly inserting a nerve graft into the paralyzed muscle, the few results that have been reported did not demonstrate strong motion and are unpredictable. In these cases, a functional muscle transplant may be innervated from an ipsilateral or contralateral facial nerve source or ipsilateral nonfacial nerve source. Considerations as to source of innervation are detailed in the following sections on treatment of longstanding facial paralysis.

Longstanding Facial Paralysis

Longstanding facial paralysis is usually considered a period of between 12–18 months of palsy duration, when reinnervation of the mimetic musculature is less likely to produce effective motion due to denervation atrophy. If incomplete denervation is present, successful attempts at renervation or functional upgrading after longer than a year remains a disputed subject, with some success reported even several years after injury, but pervasive literature is scant.[28] When denervation is complete, the approaches to longstanding facial paralysis vary, but common to all techniques is introduction of a new vascularized neuromuscular unit, either via a free functional muscle transfer or local muscle advancements. The optimal goal in any facial palsy patient is to obtain symmetry in repose and animation, as well as synchronicity and spontaneity during animation. Depending on the clinical scenario and age of the patient, these goals are sometimes obtainable but it must be recognized that in certain subpopulations including older patients, patients with comorbidities, heavy-set faces, or patient preference, the ideal is not always achievable nor necessarily optimal. Often, achieving excellent results in some of the noted goals is preferable than achieving sub-par results in all the goals. In other words, some patients may have better overall results by obtaining good excursion with decreased chance of spontaneity rather than little function with spontaneity or no function at all. Also, it is important to recognize that patients will often need several

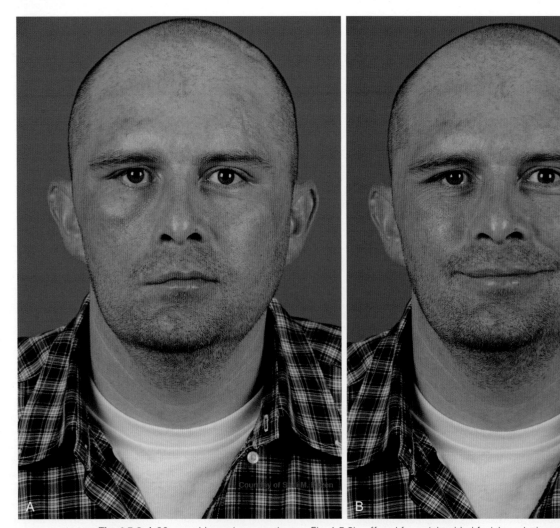

Fig. 1.5.6 A 36-year-old man (same patient as Fig. 1.5.3) suffered from right-sided facial paralysis secondary to skull base trauma. Five and a half months after selective V to VII nerve transfer in addition to two CFNGs, each coapted end to side to the respective facial nerve branches to the orbicularis oculi and zygomaticus major muscles. (A) Repose. (B) Animation. (Courtesy Shai M. Rozen. Copyright Shai M. Rozen.)

ancillary procedures, including treatment of additional facial subunits affected by the paralysis to optimize the results.

Free Functional Muscle Transplants

When performing free functional muscle transplant two choices exist: a choice of donor nerve and a choice of muscle.

Choosing a donor nerve is perhaps more important than choosing a muscle. The only nerve that reliably provides spontaneity is the facial nerve, either via a cross facial nerve graft from the contralateral facial nerve or less frequently from the ipsilateral side if a proximal facial nerve stump exists (Fig. 1.5.8). The latter is not an option when the facial nerve injury is proximal, as in intracranial injuries. The cross facial nerve graft is usually used as the first step of a two-step reconstruction, followed by a functional muscle transplant. Although spontaneity is expected, muscle excursion is often weaker compared to an ipsilateral nonfacial nerve and likely less reliable in older patients.[29,30]

Nonfacial nerve input, providing less of a chance for spontaneity, may include an ipsilateral nerve to masseter,[31–33] spinal accessory nerve,[34–35] or less commonly used today, a hemi-hypoglossal nerve.[36,37] The most frequent nonfacial nerve used today is the anterior branch of the masseter nerve,[38,39] which may be used in one-stage procedures, and provides

strong excursion but is less reliable in providing spontaneity and associated with secondary involuntary motion.[40]

A donor muscle should answer several criteria: sufficient muscle excursion, anatomical consistency allowing easy dissection, minimal function loss, and negligible donor site morbidity. Several muscles have been described in the treatment of longstanding facial palsy. Today, the most commonly used muscle is the gracilis muscle, as has been initially described by Harii[41] and the partial gracilis muscle described originally by Manktelow and Zuker.[42] The gracilis muscle has appropriate excursion, is easily dissected by a second team concomitantly with the facial dissection, has minimal donor site morbidity, and a sufficient vascular and nerve pedicle length, allowing proper vector positioning of the muscle. Videos of surgical techniques are provided and referred to later in the chapter.

Two-Stage Reanimation

First stage – facial nerve donor selection. The first step in a two-step reconstruction is deciding on the donor nerve – the facial nerve or a nonfacial nerve. The facial nerve can be used in two situations. The more common is using the contralateral normal facial nerve as a first stage cross facial nerve graft (CFNG). The less common scenario,

3 Month after injury and repair.

Courtesy of Shai M. Rozen

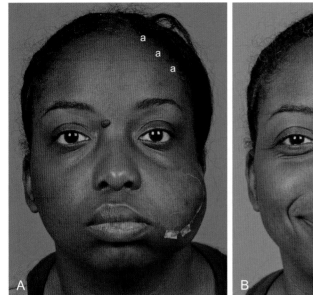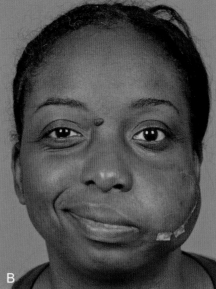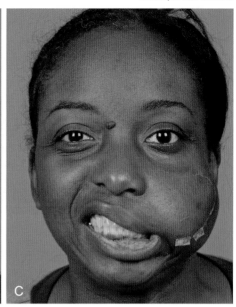

15 Month after injury and repair.

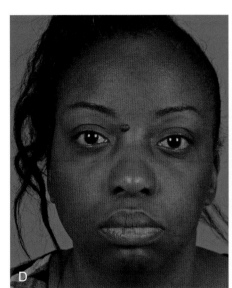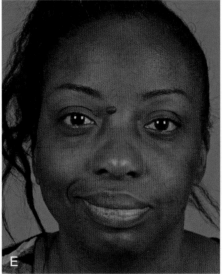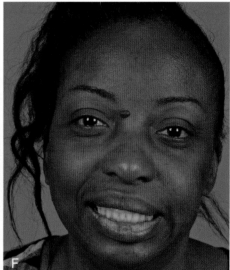

Fig. 1.5.7 A 42-year-old woman with knife laceration of the left cheek who presented without any motion 3 months after primary repair at an outside institution. At 6 months she started showing very minute motion of her left face, encouraging her to wait without surgical intervention. (A–C) Three months after repair. (D–F) Fifteen months after repair. (Courtesy Shai M. Rozen. Copyright Shai M. Rozen.)

is the use of a proximal facial nerve stump, if it exists, to innervate the transplanted muscle.

When using a CFNG, several key principles exist. The first is selecting the facial donor branch that provides the facial movement the CFNG is targeting. For example, smile or eye closure. Most commonly the CFNG aims to reconstitute the smile but often an additional nerve graft may be used for other purposes, as in eye closure. Once the facial nerve branches are mapped for their exact function via nerve stimulation, it is imperative that at least two branches perform the same function thereby avoiding paralysis when one is cut. It is extremely rare that a redundant branch is not identified. If that occurs, avoiding cutting the branch is likely a safer approach. There is an increasing amount of evidence that larger axonal loads are key to improved function of the

muscle transplant.[43,44] For that reason, a 5–10 mm retrograde parotid dissection is advisable, verifying redundancy and accuracy of action is maintained. Additionally, larger diameter nerves correlate to larger axonal loads.[45] Hence choosing the larger branches is recommended. This is even more important in older ages, since a correlation between axonal counts and age has been demonstrated.[46]

Once the facial nerve donor branch is selected, the harvested sural nerve is crossed from the healthy side to the paralyzed side of the face, and coapted to the healthy selected facial nerve branch. Coaptation is performed in the regular manner under a microscope and the distal edge is either secured over the contralateral canine tooth as a short nerve graft,[47] or the contralateral preauricular area as a long graft (Video 1.5.1).

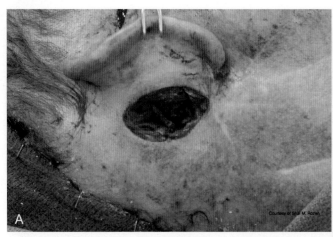
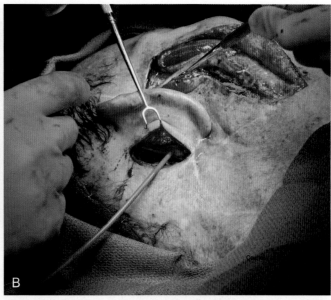

Fig. 1.5.8 A gracilis functional free flap is coapted to the intramastoid facial nerve stump. (A) Mastoid portion of the facial nerve exposed. (B) Obturator nerve from gracilis muscle transferred to intracranial proximal facial nerve. (Courtesy Shai M. Rozen. Copyright Shai M. Rozen.)

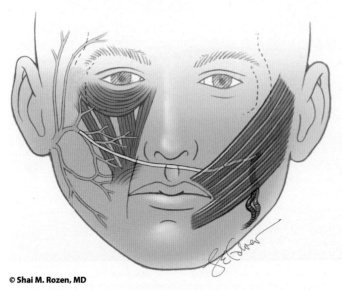

© Shai M. Rozen, MD

Fig. 1.5.9 Depiction of a two-stage procedure. (Courtesy of Shai M. Rozen. Copyright Shai M. Rozen.)

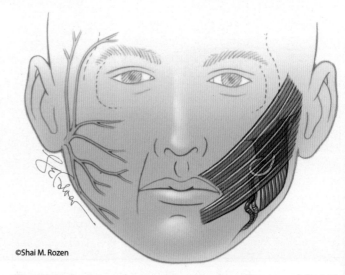

©Shai M. Rozen

Fig. 1.5.10 Depiction of a one-stage procedure. (Courtesy of Shai M. Rozen. Copyright Shai M. Rozen.)

Second stage – functional muscle transplant. In the two-stage approach a waiting period between 6–12 months is usually necessary for axonal growth through the nerve graft, depending on the length of the nerve graft. Clinically, axonal growth is monitored by a Tinel sign. Now the second stage muscle transfer is planned. Several muscles have been described and may be used.[48–51] Most commonly, a partial gracilis muscle is used, but latissimus dorsi, serratus anterior, and pectoralis minor muscles have all been described (Fig. 1.5.9). In common to all these muscles – they are transferred as a neurovascular-functional muscle unit. Insetting the muscle in the correct vector and tension is the most important portion of the surgery, notwithstanding a viable and neurotized muscle. Partial gracilis muscle harvest and inset can be viewed in Video 1.5.2.

One-Stage Reanimation With Functional Muscle Transplant Coapted to the Masseter Nerve

The technical principles of one-stage reanimation are similar to the second stage muscle transplant of a two-stage reanimation aside from innervation by the masseter or other nonfacial donor nerve (Fig. 1.5.10). In the trauma setting, several situations exist when a donor facial nerve is not feasible or desired. These may include rare cases of bilateral facial palsy in severe trauma cases, older patients in which a CFNG often yields poor excursion, obese patients with heavy-set faces, or simply patients who prefer not waiting a prolonged period that is necessary in a two-stage procedure. Several techniques have been described for localizing the masseter nerve but our preference is basing the dissection on anatomical landmarks just superior to the mandibular notch[38,39,52] (Fig. 1.5.11).

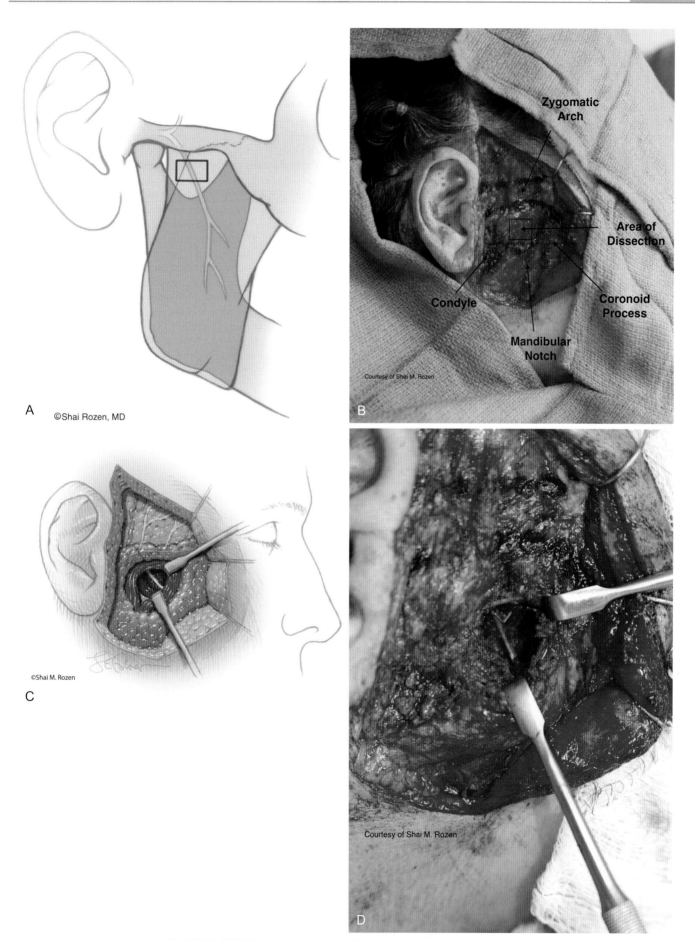

A ©Shai Rozen, MD

B
Zygomatic Arch
Area of Dissection
Coronoid Process
Condyle
Mandibular Notch
Courtesy of Shai M. Rozen

C ©Shai M. Rozen

D Courtesy of Shai M. Rozen

Fig. 1.5.11 (A–D) Anatomical landmarks for dissection of the masseter nerve.

Conceptually, the main difference between one-stage reanimation with a nonfacial nerve, as in the case of a masseter nerve, versus a two-stage reanimation using the facial nerve, is the spontaneity provided by the latter. This apparently should serve as a decisive argument in favor of a two-stage procedure, since an effortless, spontaneous, and emotional smile is the ultimate goal. The problem with this supposition is that the two-stage procedure is less consistent with its results, which may range from a perfectly symmetric, synchronous, and spontaneous smile, through more commonly observed weaker excursions due to lack of sufficient axonal loads, to near lack of motion, likely seen in older patients.[29,53] In addition, a two-stage procedure may take 18 months until effective motion is seen, versus 4–6 months in one-stage functional muscle transplants, and 3–6 weeks in cases of temporalis lengthening myoplasties. Generally, younger patients fare better than older with two-stage procedures that necessitate a long nerve graft with the resultant decreased axonal loads (Fig. 1.5.12).

Postoperative Care

In all scenarios of the different extracranial reconstructions, postoperative instructions tend to be similar and include avoiding laying on the repaired side, avoiding situations that may risk hitting the face on the repaired side, avoiding bending down or participating in activities that risk elevated blood pressure, controlling hypertension, and a soft diet for 3 weeks. Once motion is observed, all patients are referred to a specialized facial nerve physical therapist to begin exercises both in front of the mirror and increasingly in a social setting. In cases in which a nonfacial nerve is used the emphasis is on coordination and synchronization of the smile as well as practicing an emotional smile.

Lengthening Temporalis Myoplasty (LTM)

Local muscle flaps have been described for decades, including variations of masseteric muscle advancement and temporalis muscle slings. The more common local muscle transfer used today, reliably providing good results, is the temporalis muscle lengthening myoplasty, also known as the Labbe procedure, named after Daniel Labbe, who popularized the technique in 1997.[54–57] Although some authors contend that spontaneity does not occur, results have demonstrated that in many cases patients have undergone cortical adaptation and display spontaneity.[58] Potential advantages include shorter surgeries, quick recovery to motion, and no need for microsurgery expertise. Also, the ability to transpose the temporalis muscle insertion in a deep plane through Bichet's fat pad avoids cheek deformation and bulkiness, as occasionally seen with free muscle transfers. LTM may likely provide better symmetry in repose, possibly due to the tendinous portion of the muscle. For the same reason, LTM likely provides weaker excursion than a functional muscle transplant, its use is possibly limited in severely scarred or previously radiated tissue, and may cause a slight temporal hollowing. Several excellent technical papers including videography exist describing the LTM technique in detail.[54,57,59]

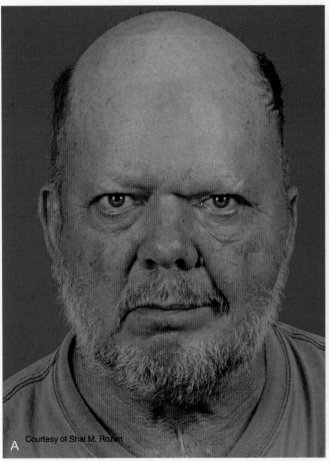
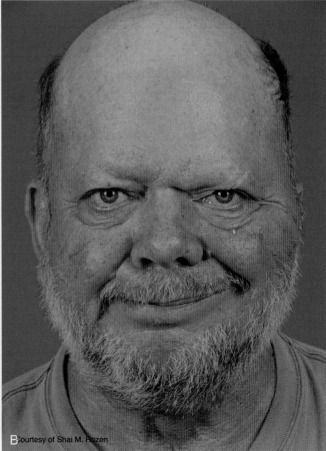

Courtesy of Shai M. Rozen

Fig. 1.5.12 A 61-year-old male (same patient as Fig. 1.5.2) after gunshot to the left face obliterating the left zygomatic arch and temporal bone. (A) Repose and (B) animation 11 months after free functional gracilis muscle transplant to masseter nerve. (Courtesy Shai M. Rozen. Copyright Shai M. Rozen.)

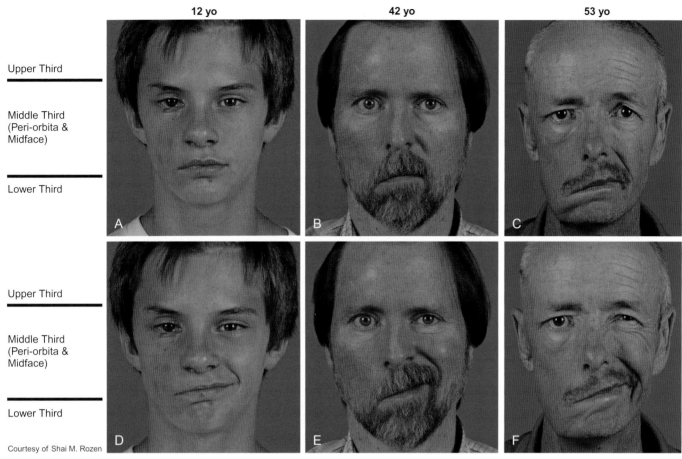

| 12 yo | 42 yo | 53 yo |

Upper Third

Middle Third
(Peri-orbita &
Midface)

Lower Third

Upper Third

Middle Third
(Peri-orbita &
Midface)

Lower Third

Courtesy of Shai M. Rozen

Fig. 1.5.13 Increased asymmetry in repose with increasing age in upper, mid- and lower face – note descent of brow, midface, lower eyelid, and oral commissure with increasing age. (Courtesy Shai M. Rozen. Copyright Shai M. Rozen.)

Static and Other Ancillary Procedures

Although static procedures do not provide motion, they constitute essential tools in the treatment of facial paralysis, providing both protective and improved aesthetic outcomes. These procedures may be performed prior, during, and after dynamic procedures and are part of the necessary surgical toolbox in the treatment of facial palsy. Many of these procedures are not necessary in younger populations that have good skin tone, but become more essential for older patients with decreased tone and soft tissue descent (Fig. 1.5.13).

ADDITIONAL PROCEDURES

Protection of the Eye

When a new patient with facial palsy is seen, the priority is protection of the eye. Most patients with complete palsy will suffer from a combination of paralytic lagophthalmos and an inferiorly displaced lower lid, rendering the eye susceptible to exposure keratitis, ulceration, scarring, and subsequent blindness. This is even worsened with proximal injuries when tear production is decreased due to disruption of parasympathetic fibers into the lacrimal gland. Therefore, most older patients will need surgery for paralytic lagophthalmos and lower eyelid support, regardless of whether reinnervation of the orbicularis oculi is planned.

Treatment of Upper Eyelid Paralytic Lagophthalmos

Several options exist for treatment of upper eyelid paralytic lagophthalmos including springs,[60–62] temporalis slings,[63,64] and the most commonly used technique of upper eyelid weight.[65–67] Traditionally, the weight, made of either gold or platinum, is inserted deep to the pretarsal orbicularis oculi muscle. This location is advantageous from an inferior vector displacement perspective but has several major disadvantages, including visibility, entropion, high risk of extrusion and infection. For these reasons, another approach was developed to insert the weight in a postseptal position.[68] This allows placement of the weight on the levator aponeurosis, covered by the postseptal fat and septum, followed by the overlaying orbicularis oculi muscle and skin. Because of the more posterior positioning, the weight is generally 0.2–0.4 g heavier than that measured in clinic, which is taped on the pretarsal skin during examination and weight assessment. The advantages of this technique are a nearly invisible weight, decreased risk of extrusion, and avoidance of entropion. Full technical details are available in the literature.[68]

Treatment of Lower Eyelid Inferior Malposition

Young patients in their first decade of life and teens very frequently have excellent skin tone and often will not need lower eyelid surgery, but as patients age, midface descent as well as lower eyelid malposition increases.

In younger patients, who do not have horizontal lid laxity, a canthoplasty is the preferred procedure. In older patients with horizontal lid laxity, a tarsal strip will address both the inferior malposition and the laxity. It is rare that a permanent tarsorraphy is necessary but a temporary one is often used at the end of the tarsal strip for temporary support. For technical details on canthoplasty and tarsal strip the reader is referred to several sources of excellent reading materials.[69,70]

© Stefania Tuinder
Artist: Greet Mommen

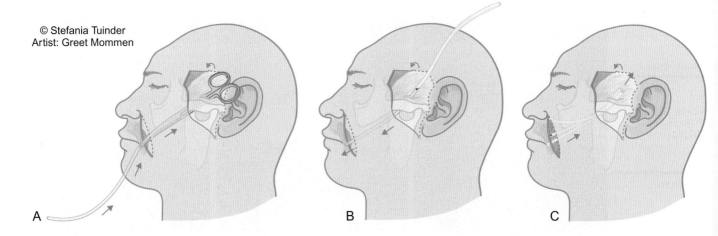

A   B   C

Fig. 1.5.14 Multiple fascia lata strips for midface support. (Copyright Stefania Tuinder.)

Treatment of Brow Ptosis

Similar to the lower eyelid, brow ptosis does not pose a problem in young patients, but increases with age and may affect line of vision. As opposed to traditional aesthetic techniques that tend to elevate the brow from a distance to hide scars, patients with paralytic brow ptosis need a significantly stronger and longer-lasting elevation which is only achieved with different variations of direct brow lifts.[70–72] In elderly patients with significant skin ptosis, direct skin excisions immediately above the brow line prove to be the most effective. An incision with very small zig-zags tends to hide the scar extremely well and is nearly unnoticeable. In younger patients with less skin laxity and ptosis another option is brow elevation via four separate small incisions just above the brow line in which the deep dermis on the brow side is secured to the periosteum in a higher position with nonabsorbable sutures. The incisions are well hidden and long-term elevation is achieved. Dynamic reanimation of the long-term paralyzed forehead with functional muscle has not become a common treatment option but in the subacute period nerve transfers may be considered.[73]

Treatment of Midface and Commissure Ptosis

The use of static midface procedures can range from rhytidectomies to insertion of tendons or fascial strips to support the midface. These procedures may be used alone, as in the case of high-risk patients, or in tandem with dynamic procedures.

Rhytidectomy

A rhytidectomy may help in achieving symmetry but is usually not performed at the time of dynamic reanimation. It is more commonly used on the contralateral healthy side, since the reconstructed side is usually volume repleted with a muscle flap and often looks younger and fuller. In cases of patients who are not good candidates for longer surgeries rhytidectomies can be used in conjunction with static slings.

Static Midface Slings

Several options for static slings exist, including palmaris tendon, fascia lata slings, dermal substitutes, or artificial meshes.[74–76] Typically, these techniques suffer from gradual weakening and elongation over time. In our opinion dermal substitutes do not provide lasting results and the use of artificial materials is highly discouraged due to excess scarring, increased chances for infections, and contour deformity.

The most commonly used material is tensor fascial lata, providing sufficient autologous material and the ability to use it in several strips.

Commonly in the past, one wide strip was used to provide elevation to the upper lip and commissure, but splitting the fascia into three to four strips enables providing differential tension of the lower lip, commissure, mid upper lip, and nasal alar root. The strips are passed via Bichet's fat pad under the zygomatic arch and secured into the temporalis fascia with permanent sutures[77] (Figs. 1.5.14 and 1.5.15).

Treatment of Lower Lip Depressor Asymmetry

Dynamic and static procedures of the paralyzed lip are not mainstream treatment options, although several options have been described but not uniformly reproduced.[78,79] Current mainstay of treatment consists of weakening the contralateral lip. The best initial option is weakening the contralateral depressors with botulinum toxin injections. This is a temporary solution that necessitates repetition if the patient desires, or it may serve as a demonstration for the patient of the potential end results of neurectomy and partial depressor myectomy for a more definitive solution.

Botulinum Toxin Injection

The use of botulinum toxin has two main roles in the treatment of facial paralysis. The first is in patients who need or want to weaken the nonparalyzed side. The most common muscles for weakening are the depressor anguli oris of the normal side. Weakening the midface or forehead on the normal side has its inherent risks, namely excessive weakening which may cause midface or brow ptosis. The second is in patients that have partially recovered and developed synkinesis. Although surgical procedures have been suggested and have merit in the treatment of severe synkinesis, further discussion is beyond the scope of this text. Most patients may effectively be treated with repeated botulinum injections. The most common and significant is oral-ocular synkinesis, which may be temporized with injections into the lower preseptal and orbital parts of the orbicularis oculi muscle. Conservative doses should be used in new patients (12.5 units) to assess the effect yet avoid ectropion.[80]

Supplementary Procedures to Achieve Aesthetic Outcomes

Beyond the procedures mentioned above that may be useful in achieving improved aesthetic outcomes, any additional procedures in the armamentarium of the reconstructive surgeon can and should be used to achieve aesthetic excellence. These may include brow lifts, blepharoplasties, fat grafting, correction of previous surgical mishaps often

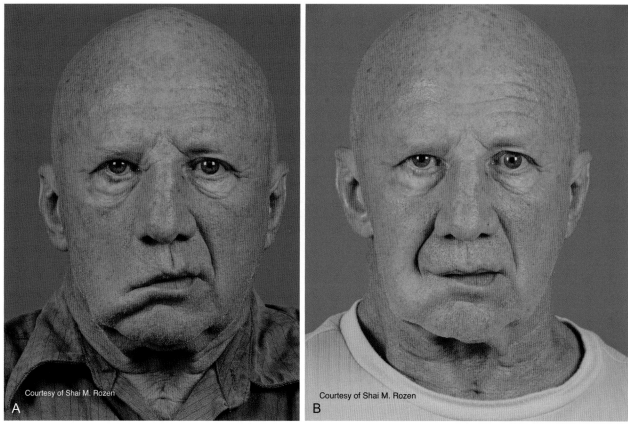

Courtesy of Shai M. Rozen

A

Courtesy of Shai M. Rozen

B

Fig. 1.5.15 A 66-year-old patient after tensor fascia lata strips. (A) Preoperative. (B) Four months postoperative. (Courtesy Shai M. Rozen. Copyright Shai M. Rozen.)

referred to facial palsy centers, as in cases of deforming tarsorraphies, effacement of supratarsal folds, or excess scarring from previously used foreign materials. The final desired result should be achieved with any surgical technique the surgeon may offer to optimally approach a normal appearance.

COMPLICATIONS
Acute Complications
Hematoma
Hematomas usually occur in the first 24 hours after surgery. The most common presentation is swelling in the side of dissection. Risk factors include history of high blood pressure or acute bouts of hypertension often associated with an unsmooth extubation. Treatment involves immediate incision and drainage of the hematoma. Occurrence of hematoma formation can be decreased by blood pressure control, deep extubation, and avoiding any medications that may increase bleeding.

Acute Vascular Compromise
Acute vascular compromise will usually result in flap failure. Several authors do not monitor functional muscle flaps with the belief that the muscle would not be salvageable but monitoring may be performed with frequent Doppler checks over the muscle for the first 24–48 hours. During extubation, the surgeon must stay in the room and assure the safe transport of the patient from the operating to recovery bed and ensure no pressure is inadvertently applied to the surgical area.

Infection
Infections may be either local due to suture abscess or panfacial with significant risk to the flap. The former usually does not occur acutely

but rather after several weeks or even months and is more typical if using a braided permanent suture to secure a functional muscle flap. The latter may occur within the first several days to weeks and is most commonly caused by insertion sutures that inadvertently penetrated the oral mucosa. Since the facial planes have recently been dissected, these infections commonly spread into the entire hemiface and require surgical drainage and intravenous antibiotics and may result in flap loss if not drained in time. Aside from incision and drainage, the culprit sutures must be removed and the mucosa reclosed.

Excessive Botulinum Toxin Injection
Excessive botulinum injection into the periorbital region in patients who have synkinesis may create ectropion and difficulty in shutting the eye, and in extreme cases may weaken the midface. This must be discussed with the patients prior to injection and if this occurs, the patient should be reassured that function will return within 3 months. In cases of ectropion the physician must verify that the eye remains protected.

Long-Term Complications
Failure of Functional Muscle Flaps
On average, functional muscle flaps demonstrate motion in 4–6 months after neurotization. Although in some patients it may take longer, this is a time to discuss with patients the potential of flap failure and possible reexploration and the need to repeat the surgery depending on the findings. If the muscle flap has vascular compromise, some type of reanimation procedure should be considered. If the muscle has bleeding when cut, consideration should be given to adding or converting neurotization of the muscle with a masseter nerve if a two-stage procedure was previously performed. If previous neurotization was performed with a masseteric nerve then using a new muscle should be considered,

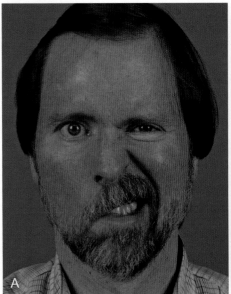
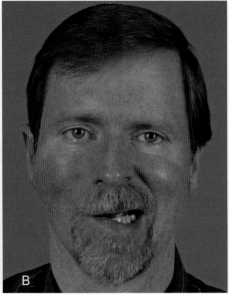
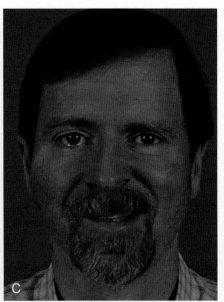

Pre OP

12 months after Gracilis to V

15 months after Gracilis to V
3 months after advancement

Courtesy of Shai M. Rozen

Fig. 1.5.16 A 44-year-old male underwent reanimation with functional muscle transplant with dehiscence of insertion 12 months after surgery. (A) Preoperative. (B) Twelve months postoperative, with dehiscence of muscle insertion. (C) Fifteen months after initial surgery and 3 months after re-advancement of muscle. (Courtesy Shai M. Rozen. Copyright Shai M. Rozen.)

since reexploration of the masseter nerve is difficult in the previously scarred area and can likely be successfully tried only once, in which case a new muscle would likely have the best chance of success.

Dehiscence of Insertion

Perhaps one of the most critical portions of any dynamic reanimation procedure is the placement of the muscle insertion. Successful dynamic reanimation is judged not only by establishing motion, but as importantly, by an aesthetic result. If the distance between the insertion of the muscle to the oral commissure is too long the nasolabial fold is lateralized and the philtral to commissure distance is elongated, resulting in a very unaesthetic result. These scenarios are difficult to manage, and necessitate readvancement of the muscle into the proper insertion (Fig. 1.5.16).

Excessive Muscle Bulk

Excessive muscle bulk can occur after implantation of the functional muscle flap. Although all free functional muscle flaps undergo significant atrophy, once motion begins, some of the bulk returns. The surgeon can decrease this occurrence by harvesting a smaller flap if possible and sometimes debulking it on its superficial aspect. If excess bulkiness persists, debulking is generally performed one year after the muscle transplant, based on surgeon's preference and experience.

Suture Abscess

Suture abscess and penetration through the skin can occur over time, and is more typical of permanent braided sutures at either the insertion or origin of the muscles. Since exposure often usually occurs months after the procedure, the exposed sutures can safely be removed.

CONCLUSION

The treatment of facial paralysis is a fascinating field allowing the reconstructive surgeon to help patients with devastating injuries by utilizing all reconstructive and aesthetic principles and surgical tools to restore form and function. Both patients and surgeons need to understand that achieving optimal results necessitates a staged approach, a journey, requiring several surgeries, and it is often the small subsequent surgeries that yield the highest impact in final surgeon and patient satisfaction.

EXPERT COMMENTARY

Great progress has been made in the last 30 years in the area of facial palsy, facial nerve repair, and techniques for facial rehabilitation following nerve injury. Remotely (30 years ago), facial nerve injuries were simply neglected, accepted as sequelae to the accident. Now, great progress has been made in diagnosis, primary repair, rehabilitation, and in reconstructive surgical procedures for the patient with nerve deficits. Rosen, as a current expert in facial nerve injuries and rehabilitation, summarizes all the nuances in diagnosis and treatment that have greatly improved the management of these injuries. Facial nerve injuries should now be precisely diagnosed, treated/repaired where possible, and rehabilitated with a variety of techniques and procedures available to the well informed. This chapter serves to summarize what is possible, and where to find more extensive information.

REFERENCES

1. Jackson CG, von Doersten PG. The facial nerve. Current trends in diagnosis, treatment, and rehabilitation. *Med Clin North Am.* 1999;83(1):179–195, x.
2. May M. Trauma to the facial nerve. *Otolaryngol Clin North Am.* 1983;16(3):661–670.
3. Wilson-Pauwels L, Akesson EJ, Stewart PA. *cranial Nerves: Anatomy and Clinical Comments.* St. Louis, MO: C.V. Mosby; 1988:xiii.
4. Moore KL, Agur AMR, Dalley AF. *Essential Clinical Anatomy.* 4th ed. Baltimore, MD: Lippincott Williams & Wilkins; 2011:xxviii.
5. Monkhouse WS. The anatomy of the facial nerve. *Ear Nose Throat J.* 1990;69(10):677–683, 686–687.

6. Ishman SL, Friedland DR. Temporal bone fractures: traditional classification and clinical relevance. *Laryngoscope.* 2004;114(10):1734–1741.

7. Gurdjian ES, Lissner HR. Deformation of the skull in head injury; a study with the stresscoat technique. *Surg Gynecol Obstet.* 1945;81:679–687.

8. Dahiya R, Keller JD, Litofsky NS, et al. Temporal bone fractures: otic capsule sparing versus otic capsule violating clinical and radiographic considerations. *J Trauma.* 1999;47(6):1079–1083.

9. Brodie HA, Thompson TC. Management of complications from 820 temporal bone fractures. *Am J Otol.* 1997;18(2):188–197.

10. Chang CY, Cass SP. Management of facial nerve injury due to temporal bone trauma. *Am J Otol.* 1999;20(1):96–114.

11. Nash JJ, Friedland DR, Boorsma KJ, Rhee JS. Management and outcomes of facial paralysis from intratemporal blunt trauma: a systematic review. *Laryngoscope.* 2010;120(7):1397–1404.

12. Darrouzet V, Duclos JY, Liguoro D, et al. Management of facial paralysis resulting from temporal bone fractures: our experience in 115 cases. *Otolaryngol Head Neck Surg.* 2001;125(1):77–84.

13. Ulug T, Arif Ulubil S. Management of facial paralysis in temporal bone fractures: a prospective study analyzing 11 operated fractures. *Am J Otolaryngol.* 2005;26(4):230–238.

14. Liu Y, Han J, Zhou X, et al. Surgical management of facial paralysis resulting from temporal bone fractures. *Acta Otolaryngol.* 2014;134(6):656–660.

15. Bodenez C, Darrouzet V, Rouanet-Larriviere M, et al. Facial paralysis after temporal bone trauma]. *Ann Otolaryngol Chir Cervicofac.* 2006;123(1):9–16.

16. Rozen SM, Harrison BL, Isaacson B, et al. Intracranial facial nerve grafting in the setting of skull base tumors: global and regional facial function analysis and possible implications for facial reanimation surgery. *Plast Reconstr Surg.* 2016;137(1):267–278.

17. Millesi H. Microsurgery of peripheral nerves. *Hand.* 1973;5(2):157–160.

18. Siemionow M, Brzezicki G. Chapter 8: Current techniques and concepts in peripheral nerve repair. *Int Rev Neurobiol.* 2009;87:141–172.

19. Sunderland S. *Nerve injuries and Their Repair : A Critical Appraisal.* Edinburgh: Churchill Livingstone; 1991:x.

20. Millesi H. The nerve gap. Theory and clinical practice. *Hand Clin.* 1986;2(4):651–663.

21. Terzis JK, Konofaos P. Nerve transfers in facial palsy. *Facial Plast Surg.* 2008;24(2):177–193.

22. Terzis JK, Konofaos P. Experience with 60 adult patients with facial paralysis secondary to tumor extirpation. *Plast Reconstr Surg.* 2012;130(1):51e–66e.

23. Mersa B, Tiangco DA, Terzis JK. Efficacy of the "baby-sitter" procedure after prolonged denervation. *J Reconstr Microsurg.* 2000;16(1):27–35.

24. Kim SH, Jung J, Lee JH, et al. Delayed facial nerve decompression for Bell's palsy. *Eur Arch Otorhinolaryngol.* 2016;273(7):1755–1760.

25. Quaranta A, Campobasso G, Piazza F, et al. Facial nerve paralysis in temporal bone fractures: outcomes after late decompression surgery. *Acta Otolaryngol.* 2001;121(5):652–655.

26. Kalantarian B, Rice DC, Tiangco DA, Terzis JK. Gains and losses of the XII–VII component of the "baby-sitter" procedure: a morphometric analysis. *J Reconstr Microsurg.* 1998;14(7):459–471.

27. Terzis JK, Karypidis D. Outcomes of direct muscle neurotization in pediatric patients with facial paralysis. *Plast Reconstr Surg.* 2009;124(5):1486–1498.

28. Frey M, Giovanoli P, Michaelidou M. Functional upgrading of partially recovered facial palsy by cross-face nerve grafting with distal end-to-side neurorrhaphy. *Plast Reconstr Surg.* 2006;117(2):597–608.

29. Hontanilla B, Marre D, Cabello A. Facial reanimation with gracilis muscle transfer neurotized to cross-facial nerve graft versus masseteric nerve: a comparative study using the FACIAL CLIMA evaluating system. *Plast Reconstr Surg.* 2013;131(6):1241–1252.

30. Bae YC, Zuker RM, Manktelow RT, Wade S. A comparison of commissure excursion following gracilis muscle transplantation for facial paralysis using a cross-face nerve graft versus the motor nerve to the masseter nerve. *Plast Reconstr Surg.* 2006;117(7):2407–2413.

31. Klebuc MJ. Facial reanimation using the masseter-to-facial nerve transfer. *Plast Reconstr Surg.* 2011;127(5):1909–1915.

32. Hontanilla B, Marre D, Cabello A. Masseteric nerve for reanimation of the smile in short-term facial paralysis. *Br J Oral Maxillofac Surg.* 2014;52(2):118–123.

33. Hontanilla B, Marre D. Masseteric-facial nerve transposition for reanimation of the smile in incomplete facial paralysis. *Br J Oral Maxillofac Surg.* 2015;53(10):943–948.

34. Lu JC, Chuang DC. One-stage reconstruction for bilateral Mobius syndrome: simultaneous use of bilateral spinal accessory nerves to innervate 2 free muscles for facial reanimation. *Ann Plast Surg.* 2013;70(2):180–186.

35. Placheta E, Tinhofer I, Schmid M, et al. The spinal accessory nerve for functional muscle innervation in facial reanimation surgery: an anatomical and histomorphometric study. *Ann Plast Surg.* 2016;77(6):640–644.

36. Darrouzet V, Dutkiewicz J, Chambrin A, et al. [Hypoglosso-facial anastomosis: results and technical development towards end-to-side anastomosis with rerouting of the intra-temporal facial nerve (modified May technique)]. *Rev Laryngol Otol Rhinol (Bord).* 1997;118(3):203–210.

37. Pellat JL, Bonnefille E, Zanaret M, Cannoni M. [Hypoglossal-facial anastomosis. A report of 60 cases]. *Ann Chir Plast Esthet.* 1997;42(1):37–43.

38. Cheng A, Audolfsson T, Rodriguez-Lorenzo A, et al. A reliable anatomic approach for identification of the masseteric nerve. *J Plast Reconstr Aesthet Surg.* 2013;66(10):1438–1440.

39. Borschel GH, Kawamura DH, Kasukurthi R, et al. The motor nerve to the masseter muscle: an anatomic and histomorphometric study to facilitate its use in facial reanimation. *J Plast Reconstr Aesthet Surg.* 2012;65(3):363–366.

40. Rozen S, Harrison B. Involuntary movement during mastication in patients with long-term facial paralysis reanimated with a partial gracilis free neuromuscular flap innervated by the masseteric nerve. *Plast Reconstr Surg.* 2013;132(1):110e–116e.

41. Harii K, Ohmori K, Torii S. Free gracilis muscle transplantation, with microneurovascular anastomoses for the treatment of facial paralysis. A preliminary report. *Plast Reconstr Surg.* 1976;57(2):133–143.

42. Manktelow RT, Zuker RM. Muscle transplantation by fascicular territory. *Plast Reconstr Surg.* 1984;73(5):751–757.

43. Snyder-Warwick AK, Fattah AY, Zive L, et al. The degree of facial movement following microvascular muscle transfer in pediatric facial reanimation depends on donor motor nerve axonal density. *Plast Reconstr Surg.* 2015;135(2):370e–381e.

44. Terzis JK, Wang W, Zhao Y. Effect of axonal load on the functional and aesthetic outcomes of the cross-facial nerve graft procedure for facial reanimation. *Plast Reconstr Surg.* 2009;124(5):1499–1512.

45. Hembd A, Nagarkar PA, Saba S, et al. Facial nerve axonal analysis and anatomical localization in donor nerve: optimizing axonal load for cross-facial nerve grafting in facial reanimation. *Plast Reconstr Surg.* 2017;139(1):177–183.

46. Hembd AN, Perez J, Gassman A, et al. Correlation between facial nerve axonal load and age and its relevance to facial reanimation. *Plast Reconstr Surg.* 2017;in press.

47. Manktelow RTZ, Zuker RM. Cross-facial nerve graft – the long and short graft: The first stage for microneurovascular muscle transfer. *Oper Tech Plast Reconstr Surg.* 1999;6(3):174–179.

48. Zuker RM, Goldberg CS, Manktelow RT. Facial animation in children with Mobius syndrome after segmental gracilis muscle transplant. *Plast Reconstr Surg.* 2000;106(1):1–8, discussion 9.

49. Ueda K, Harii K, Asato H, Yamada A. Neurovascular free muscle transfer combined with cross-face nerve grafting for the treatment of facial paralysis in children. *Plast Reconstr Surg.* 1998;101(7):1765–1773.

50. Ueda K, Harii K, Yamada A. Free neurovascular muscle transplantation for the treatment of facial paralysis using the hypoglossal nerve as a recipient motor source. *Plast Reconstr Surg.* 1994;94(6):808–817.

51. Takushima A, Harii K, Asato H, et al. Neurovascular free-muscle transfer for the treatment of established facial paralysis following ablative surgery in the parotid region. *Plast Reconstr Surg.* 2004;113(6):1563–1572.

52. Fisher MD, Zhang Y, Erdmann D, Marcus J. Dissection of the masseter branch of the trigeminal nerve for facial reanimation. *Plast Reconstr Surg.* 2013;131(5):1065–1067.

53. Manktelow RT, Tomat LR, Zuker RM, Chang M. Smile reconstruction in adults with free muscle transfer innervated by the masseter motor nerve: effectiveness and cerebral adaptation. *Plast Reconstr Surg.* 2006;118(4):885–899.

54. Labbe D. [Lengthening of temporalis myoplasty and reanimation of lips. Technical notes]. *Ann Chir Plast Esthet.* 1997;42(1):44–47.

55. Benateau H, Labbe D, Elissalde JM, Salame E. [Anatomical study of the temporalis tendon. Value in temporalis lengthening myoplasty]. *Ann Chir Plast Esthet.* 2001;46(6):611–616.

56. Har-Shai Y, Metanes I, Badarny S, et al. Lengthening temporalis myoplasty for facial palsy reanimation. *Isr Med Assoc J.* 2007;9(2):123–124.

57. Labbe D, Huault M. Lengthening temporalis myoplasty and lip reanimation. *Plast Reconstr Surg.* 2000;105(4):1289–1297, discussion 98.

58. Garmi R, Labbe D, Coskun O, et al. Lengthening temporalis myoplasty and brain plasticity: a functional magnetic resonance imaging study. *Ann Chir Plast Esthet.* 2013;58(4):271–276.

59. Aljudaibi N, Bennis Y, Duquennoy-Martinot V, et al. Lengthening temporalis myoplasty: virtual animation-assisted technical video. *Plast Reconstr Surg.* 2016;138(3):506e–509e.

60. Terzis JK, Kyere SA. Experience with the gold weight and palpebral spring in the management of paralytic lagophthalmos. *Plast Reconstr Surg.* 2008;121(3):806–815.

61. Demirci H, Frueh BR. Palpebral spring in the management of lagophthalmos and exposure keratopathy secondary to facial nerve palsy. *Ophthal Plast Reconstr Surg.* 2009;25(4):270–275.

62. Chan RC, Chan JY. Application of palpebral spring in Asian patients with paralytic lagophthalmos. *Ophthal Plast Reconstr Surg.* 2017;33(4):300–303.

63. Zhang GC, Zheng TS. [Correction of lagophthalmos in leprosy by transfer of a temporalis muscle bundle and fascial sling – report of 26 cases]. *Zhonghua Zheng Xing Shao Shang Wai Ke Za Zhi.* 1987;3(1):14–15, 77.

64. Gupta RC, Kushwaha RN, Budhiraja I, et al. Modified silicone sling assisted temporalis muscle transfer in the management of lagophthalmos. *Indian J Ophthalmol.* 2014;62(2):176–179.

65. Townsend DJ. Eyelid reanimation for the treatment of paralytic lagophthalmos: historical perspectives and current applications of the gold weight implant. *Ophthal Plast Reconstr Surg.* 1992;8(3):196–201.

66. Gladstone GJ, Nesi FA. Management of paralytic lagophthalmos with a modified gold-weight implantation technique. *Ophthal Plast Reconstr Surg.* 1996;12(1):38–44.

67. Lavy JA, East CA, Bamber A, Andrews PJ. Gold weight implants in the management of lagophthalmos in facial palsy. *Clin Otolaryngol Allied Sci.* 2004;29(3):279–283.

68. Rozen S, Lehrman C. Upper eyelid postseptal weight placement for treatment of paralytic lagophthalmos. *Plast Reconstr Surg.* 2013;131(6):1253–1265.

69. Anderson RL, Gordy DD. The tarsal strip procedure. *Arch Ophthalmol.* 1979;97(11):2192–2196.

70. Fagien S. *Putterman's Cosmetic Occuloplastic Surgery.* 4th ed. Amsterdam: Elsevier; 2008.

71. Leatherbarrow B. *Oculoplastic Surgery.* 2nd ed. New York: Informa; 2011.

72. Meltzer NE, Byrne PJ. Management of the brow in facial paralysis. *Facial Plast Surg.* 2008;24(2):216–219.

73. Dauwe PB, Hembd A, De La Concha-Blankenagel E, et al. The deep temporal nerve transfer: an anatomical feasibility study and implications for upper facial reanimation. *Plast Reconstr Surg.* 2016;138(3):498e–505e.

74. Lemound J, Stoetzer M, Kokemuller H, et al. Modified technique for rehabilitation of facial paralysis using autogenous fascia lata grafts. *J Oral Maxillofac Surg.* 2015;73(1):176–183.

75. Graillon N, Colson T, Bardot J. [Rehabilitation of facial paralysis using autogenous fascia lata graft. Stable results over time]. *Ann Chir Plast Esthet.* 2015;60(5):442–447.

76. Liu YM, Sherris DA. Static procedures for the management of the midface and lower face. *Facial Plast Surg.* 2008;24(2):211–215.

77. Puddu GS, Tuinder S, Lataster A, Santoro A. A new way to insert fascia lata in static suspensions for facial palsy. 2013 International Facial Nerve Symposium; June 28–July 2, 2013; Boston, MA.

78. Terzis JK, Tzafetta K. Outcomes of mini-hypoglossal nerve transfer and direct muscle neurotization for restoration of lower lip function in facial palsy. *Plast Reconstr Surg.* 2009;124(6):1891–1904.

79. Watanabe Y, Sasaki R, Agawa K, Akizuki T. Bidirectional/double fascia grafting for simple and semi-dynamic reconstruction of lower lip deformity in facial paralysis. *J Plast Reconstr Aesthet Surg.* 2015;68(3):321–328.

80. Bennis Y, Duquennoy-Martinot V, Guerreschi P. Epidemiologic overview of synkinesis in 353 patients with longstanding facial paralysis under treatment with botulinum toxin for 11 years. *Plast Reconstr Surg.* 2016;138(2):376e–378e.

Diagnosis and Multimodality Management of Skull Base Fractures and Cerebrospinal Fluid Leaks

Corey M. Mossop, Bizhan Aarabi

BACKGROUND

History

The description, diagnosis, and management of skull base cerebrospinal fluid (CSF) leaks has a long, controversial history dating back to the first report of this entity in the 17th century by Bidloo.[1,2] In his report, the Dutch surgeon described a case of profuse posttraumatic CSF rhinorrhea that resulted in the death of his patient 7 months later from meningitis. Then, in the late 1800s, Chiari was the first to document the link between CSF rhinorrhea and traumatic injuries to the paranasal sinuses with concomitant pneumocephalus.[3] These early cases highlighted the end result modern practitioners aim to prevent and the impetus behind the increasingly sophisticated methods and techniques used to treat this condition.

The early 1900s saw further classification of skull base CSF leaks and the first descriptions of the surgical repair of dural defects causing these leaks. Using his experience with both closed and penetrating brain injuries, Hugh Cairns in a 1937 paper classified CSF rhinorrhea into four categories that are still applicable today (see Table 1.6.1).[4] In addition, Walter Dandy visualized and repaired a dural tear at the base of the skull with tensor fascia lata in the same time frame.[5,6]

Military conflicts since World War I have revealed CSF leaks to be harbingers of significant morbidity and mortality. In the Iran–Iraq War, CSF leaks were an independent variable contributing to deep central nervous system (CNS) infections in military missile head wounds in a regression model.[7] Additionally, as modern protective gear and helmets have improved, the incidence of individuals' sustaining penetrating injuries to the skull base via transfrontal, transorbital, and transfacial routes have only increased.[8] Finally, the high energy imparted by modern penetrating and nonpenetrating blast injuries creates closed head and paranasal sinus injuries classically associated with CSF rhinorrhea and otorrhea in the civilian population.

Demographics and Associated Injuries

In the general population, head trauma is the major cause of morbidity and mortality between the ages of 1 and 44, with approximately 50,000 Americans dying annually from traumatic brain injury (TBI).[9] Among those sustaining closed head injuries (CHI), 10%–20% have a basilar skull fracture and 1%–3% have CSF leaks.[10,11] Additionally, approximately 1.7% of individuals with blunt mechanism facial fractures will sustain basilar skull fractures and 9.7% will have cervical spine fractures.[12] Among those experiencing CSF leaks, over 80% present with CSF rhinorrhea and the other 20% with otorrhea.[13,14] Also, between 20% and 50% of patients with CSF leaks will develop CNS infections if left

untreated with no resolution of their leak.[1,15,16] Of note, for those sustaining basilar skull fractures, a CSF leak does not have to be present for meningitis to occur and said event can be quite remote from its antecedent trauma.[17,18]

SURGICAL ANATOMY

The anterior skull base is formed by the confluence of the frontal, ethmoid, and sphenoid bones with their corresponding paranasal sinuses being the most common sources of CSF rhinorrhea given their intimate relationship with the basal dura of the frontal lobes (see Fig. 1.6.1).

Positioned at the apex of the nasal cavity, the frontal sinus derives from the extension of the frontal recess into the frontal bones. The sinus begins to pneumatize at 2 years of age and is usually apparent radiographically beginning at 6 years of age, reaching an average volume of approximately 3.5 cm^3.[19] Its mucosal drainage via the nasofrontal outflow tract into the semilunar hiatus is critically important in the clinical decision making regarding fractures of this complex.[20]

Typically present at birth, the ethmoid sinuses reach their average volume of approximately 4.5 cm^3 by 16 years of age and are classically divided into anterior, middle, and posterior divisions.[19] Pneumatization of the sphenoid sinus is usually apparent by 1 year of age and reaches its average full volume of 3.5 cm^3 by the age of 15, with a growth spurt occurring between 6 and 10 years of age.[19]

CLINICAL PRESENTATION

History, Clinical, and Laboratory Assessment

One must consider several important historical findings in those with skull base fractures and concomitant CSF leaks. In addition to the timing and mechanism of injury, one should also note any reports of loss of consciousness, seizure activity, or periods of hypoxia or hypotension as these can independently affect prognosis and subsequent decision making. While severe craniomaxillofacial trauma can be dramatic at first glance, one should always remember the basic tenets of trauma care and resuscitation. ATLS guidelines and protocol should be followed on presentation and no further neurosurgical treatment planning should commence until it is certain that the patient is stable from a cardiopulmonary standpoint. During this time, one may perform a neurological examination (to attain a Glasgow Coma Score [GCS]) prior to intubation (if possible) and stop any arterial hemorrhage from scalp or facial wounds by simple closure with staples or sutures. In addition to standard trauma protocols utilizing the placement of rigid cervical collars and universal spine precautions, those in which there

TABLE 1.6.1 Cairns' Classification of CSF Rhinorrhea

1. Those that occur in the acute stage of a head injury
2. Those that occur as a delayed complication of a head injury
3. Those produced during operation on the cranium or the accessory sinuses
4. Cases of spontaneous CSF rhinorrhea

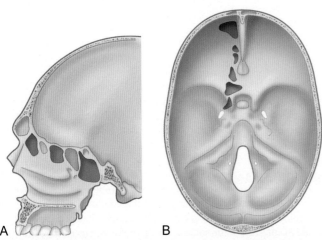

Fig. 1.6.1 Lateral (A) and basal (B) views of the skull illustrating the anatomy of the paranasal air sinuses. (Reproduced with permission from Aarabi B, O'Malley BW, Martin JE, Eisenberg HM. Surgical management of cerebrospinal fluid leaks. In: Sekhar LN, Fessler RG, editors. Atlas of neurosurgical techniques: Brain. New York: Thieme; 2006; p.927–938. Figure 80-1, p.928.)

is a significant concern for cervical spine injury should undergo a full American Spinal Injury Association (ASIA) exam to fully describe and characterize the completeness and neurological level of any potential spinal cord injury. Finally, all cooperative patients should undergo cranial nerve testing to rule out an orbital apex syndrome or optic nerve injury.

The clinical and physical signs of those with skull base CSF leaks typically mimic those with all basilar skull fractures (mastoid ecchymosis [Battle's sign], periorbital ecchymosis [raccoon eyes], etc.). When found clinically and/or radiographically, one should have a high index of suspicion for CSF leakage and perform a detailed physical examination as such. Aside from the obvious signs of CSF rhino/otorrhea, one should attempt to examine the posterior oropharynx for the "glistening" sight of CSF drainage. In addition, CSF accumulation behind the tympanic membrane should be examined for using an otoscope. In the obtunded or sedated patient, endoscopy may be utilized to examine the paranasal sinuses, skull base, posterior oropharynx, and Eustachian tube in a more detailed manner for CSF drainage. Additionally, examination of the orbit may reveal CSF leakage or a pulsatile globe due to an orbital roof fracture that may have a corresponding dural tear. In awake patients, additional symptoms such as positional headaches, the sensation of postnasal drip, a "salty" taste in the back of the mouth, or a feeling of fluid/fullness in the ear should be identified.

For cases in which the clinical diagnosis of CSF rhino or otorrhea is uncertain, certain laboratory findings can assist in confirming what may be a presumptive diagnosis. Glucose and protein levels have been

used in the past, utilizing normative values to help establish whether the fluid in question is in fact CSF. One should use caution with this method alone though, as these values can vary in the presence of infection/meningitis and in those with diabetes, which can affect the interpretation of results. Beta-2 transferrin (beta-2 trf), the desialated isoform of transferrin, is only present in CSF and has a sensitivity and specificity of 84% and 100% (respectively) in the diagnosis of CSF leakage.[21] However, most assays require between 2 mL and 5 mL of fluid for successful analysis, which may be problematic for those with low-flow/volume or intermittent CSF leakage (which account for the majority of cases with clinical/diagnostic uncertainty).[21] Additionally, the laboratory assay for beta-2 transferrin is not readily available at all hospital/clinical laboratories and as such may take several days to weeks to process at outside facilities. As a result, laboratory analysis of fluid concerning for CSF leakage serves a limited role and should be used as only one of the factors that seasoned clinicians use in diagnosis.

RADIOLOGICAL EVALUATION

Computed Tomography (CT)

In modern practice, fine-cut (less than 1 mm) CT scans of the face, sinuses, and head in the axial, sagittal, and coronal planes are the best way to examine for the skull base and sinus fractures typically associated with CSF leakage and pneumocephalus.[22] With regards to the frontal sinus, the status of both the anterior and posterior walls in addition to the patency of the nasofrontal ducts should be assessed. Given the multiplicity and thin bony architecture of the ethmoid sinuses, fractures can often be difficult to detect. However, the presence of ethmoid opacification on CT, air cells appearing to communicate with the intracranial compartment, or frank pneumocephalus are harbingers of injury to this complex.

Basilar skull injuries affecting the middle cranial fossa typically result in either longitudinal or transverse fracture patterns of the petrous pyramid. Of note, longitudinal fractures are more likely to result in CSF otorrhea given their tendency to involve the posterior portion of the external auditory canal and the tegmen tympani.[9,23] One should also examine for any involvement of the carotid canal, facial canal, cochlea, and semicircular canals in these particular fractures.

The injection of intrathecal contrast in conjunction with CT imaging as specified above is another method to more precisely localize the potential site(s) of CSF leakage. Additionally, the use of intrathecal fluorescein can be of great assistance in localizing the site of CSF leak either pre- or intraoperatively utilizing endoscopic assistance.

Magnetic Resonance Imaging (MRI)

For cases in which clinical uncertainty exists regarding actual CSF leakage or where further anatomic clarification of potential leak sites would be beneficial further imaging studies may be indicated on a case-by-case basis. Multiplanar fine-cut T2-weighted MR imaging can reveal CSF accumulation into particular paranasal sinuses and even the site of potential dural tears or pseudo-meningoceles (see Fig. 1.6.2).[9,24–29] This information can be invaluable for clinical decision making and planning the surgical approach (open vs. endoscopic) one takes for a particular case.

Nuclear Medicine (NM) Studies

When the clinical signs, symptoms, and imaging work-up to date are equivocal for the absence or presence of a skull base CSF leak, nuclear medicine studies can assist in basic diagnosis. By performing an intrathecal injection of metrizamide with nasal pledgets placed beforehand, technicians can then examine for the presence (or absence) of the tracer

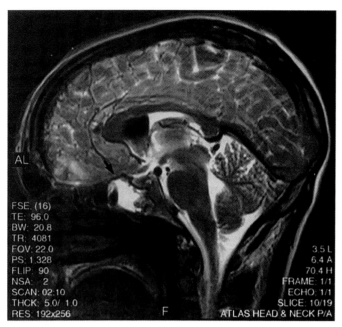

Fig. 1.6.2 MRI appearance of skull base CSF leaks. Sagittal T2-weighted MRI illustrating CSF accumulation into the sphenoid sinus. (Reproduced with permission from Aarabi B, O'Malley BW, Martin JE, Eisenberg HM. Surgical management of cerebrospinal fluid leaks. In: Sekhar LN, Fessler RG, editors. Atlas of neurosurgical techniques: Brain. New York: Thieme; 2006; p.927–938. Figure 80-4, p.929.)

at various intervals (usually up to 24 hours) after the injection.[30–34] This modality is typically reserved more for an absolute determination of CSF leakage when other modalities have failed to yield adequate diagnostic information.

CONSIDERATIONS IN THE INITIAL MANAGEMENT OF SKULL BASE CSF LEAKS

Timeframe and Mechanism of Injury

When considering the aggressiveness, modality, and timing of treatment with regards to traumatic skull base CSF leaks, one must take into account the timeframe and underlying mechanism of CSF liquorrhea. The shearing forces typically associated with the acceleration/deceleration mechanisms of closed head injuries usually create linear/simple defects in the paranasal sinuses and surrounding dura. Early CSF leaks associated with these injuries may be more likely to heal with conservative or nonoperative management as presented further in this chapter. It is also important to remember that skull base CSF leaks may present in a delayed manner (more than one week post-injury) as brain parenchymal and sinus mucosal swelling abates after an initial injury.[35]

Medical Stabilization and Management of Concomitant Intracranial Injuries

Once initial cardiopulmonary stabilization and resuscitation has occurred and diagnostic imaging has been obtained, life-threatening intracranial injuries such as acute subdural or epidural hematomas should be searched for. Additionally, the presence of traumatic subarachnoid blood, parenchymal contusions, or diffuse cerebral edema resulting in cisternal effacement should be noted as these may affect the timing and modality of subsequent CSF leak treatment. If any of the above are present, they should be treated appropriately and the patient started on 7 days of antiepileptic medications.

If a patient has an acute cranial neurosurgical emergency with a concomitant skull base CSF leak, it is at the provider's discretion as to whether the two conditions can be managed in a single operative procedure. In an ideal setting this would always be the case, however it is rarely so. Regardless, surgeons should always consider the possibility of future approaches in those at risk of skull base CSF leaks and design their incisions such that they do not preclude adequate access to the paranasal sinuses or sufficient autograft (split-thickness calvarium, pericranium, or temporalis fascia/muscle) for skull base/dural repair if needed at a later point.

Intracranial Pressure Monitoring and CSF Diversion

Of those with acute posttraumatic skull base CSF leaks, approximately 52% will cease spontaneously with a short period (5 days) of observation.[36] For those with persistent skull base CSF leaks after observation or acute high volume leaks in the setting of severe paranasal sinus and skull base trauma, a principle tenet of management is that of CSF diversion. This period of drainage allows for maximal scar tissue to form at the site(s) of dural lacerations to lessen the chance of recurrence. One case series of 24 patients with anterior fossa skull base CSF leaks found that a period (5–7 days) of CSF diversion halted 70% of such leaks.[37]

CSF diversion can occur by multiple means to include ventricular drainage, lumbar drainage, or serial lumbar punctures. For those with intracranial injuries and neurological exams (Glasgow Coma Scale [GCS] <8) in which intracranial pressure monitoring would be useful, the placement of an intraventricular catheter (IVC) would serve to measure and treat intracranial pressure elevations and divert CSF from sites of skull base dural tears.[38]

For those cases in which intracranial pressure monitoring is not indicated, the authors prefer lumbar drainage as the first choice for CSF diversion in skull base CSF leaks. Less ideally, serial lumbar punctures are an option for those with limited resources or supplies.

Nonoperative Management of CSF Leaks and Potential Controversies

As mentioned previously, approximately 52% of skull base CSF leaks will halt spontaneously within 5 days of their onset.[36] As such, observation of those with relatively simple, linear, noncomminuted, and nondepressed skull base/paranasal sinus fractures with a concomitant CSF leak may be observed closely for a short period of time. At the senior author's institution, standard protocol consists of head elevation to greater than 30 degrees at all times, CSF diversion of some form in all patients, and fluid restriction.[9] In addition, supplemental oxygen administration via face mask or nasal cannula is strictly avoided (if needed, a face tent may be used) and nose-blowing (as well as the use of straws for drinking) is prohibited. No prophylactic antibiotics are administered.

With regards to the use of prophylactic antibiotics for those with skull base CSF leaks, a Cochrane review published in 2011 using five randomized controlled trials (RCTs) and 17 non-RCTs found no evidence to support the use of prophylactic antibiotics for those will skull base CSF leaks.[39] As a result, this practice, once controversial, has been steadily on the decline.[40] In fact, only 14% of respondents of a 2014 survey indicated they administer prophylactic antibiotics. Most clinicians cited concerns over inducing bacterial resistance or altering nasopharyngeal flora to more invasive organisms.[41]

However, it is widely known that safe and effective vaccines exist against the three most common pathogens of bacterial meningitis (*Streptococcus pneumoniae*, *Neisseria meningitides*, *Haemophilus influenzae*) with primary and secondary antibody responses taking between 5 and 10 days and 21 days, respectively. Given the lifelong immunity imparted by these vaccinations, some individuals and societies are beginning to recommend administration to all patients with confirmed skull base CSF leaks.[41] At current writing though, more study is needed to examine the effect this intervention may have on those who do and do not develop bacterial meningitis after sustaining a skull base CSF leak.

The use of acetazolamide to decrease CSF production in those with skull base or paranasal sinus injuries has been advocated by some given its ability to decrease CSF production by up to 48%. However, a recent RCT found no significant effect on the duration of CSF leakage in those administered acetazolamide compared to the control group and a significantly higher incidence of medical complications (metabolic acidosis and hypokalemia) in the experimental group.[42]

Surgical Indications and Timing

Penetrating head injuries, in particular those associated with high-velocity projectiles (such as military-grade weaponry) create complex sinus, skull base, and dural injuries that if associated with high-volume CSF leakage are less likely to respond to nonoperative management and CSF diversion. As such, early (within 24–48 hours of presentation) operative coordination and planning may be warranted to prevent subsequent infectious sequelae.

For those with blunt mechanism injuries and persistent CSF rhino- or otorrhea failing to resolve after 5–7 days of observation and subsequent CSF diversion, operative intervention is warranted and planning should proceed as presented below.[1,13,15,35,43–46] Additionally, in those whose leaks halt with nonoperative management, one must be vigilant for the possibility of recurrence in both the short and long term.[35] As such, clinical follow-up should be ensured and patients and their families should be counseled thoroughly about the signs and symptoms of CSF leaks and meningitis.

SURGICAL TECHNIQUES

Preoperative Considerations
Choice of Approach and Patient/Family Counseling
Numerous factors must be considered when determining the best approach for handling a particular skull base CSF leak. The first and foremost includes the comfort level and resources available to a surgeon at the time of presentation. For those with access to a capable neurosurgical endoscopic skull base or otolaryngologic rhinology program, transnasal endoscopic approaches may be more feasible and avoid the traditional risks assumed by a transcranial approach. In addition, endoscopic approaches are ideal for midline frontal, ethmoid, and/or sphenoid defects requiring repair. However, for larger skull base/dural defects associated with penetrating injuries needing more autogenous materials for coverage or repair a transcranial approach may be more advantageous. In addition to the usual risks attendant to any craniotomy, the patient and their family should be specifically counseled as to the high risk of postoperative anosmia for anterior fossa CSF leaks given the need to elevate the olfactory bulbs for adequate visualization of the leak site(s).

Dural Reconstruction Methods/Materials/Adjuncts

In order to attain optimal outcomes, one must be aware of and consider the full spectrum of autogenous and allogenic resources available for skull base reconstruction and the repair/buttressing of dural defects.

Autogenous materials should be given first priority in every case given they pose little to no long-term infectious risk. For a transcranial approach, the availability of split-thickness calvarium for reconstructing osseous defects in addition to pericranium and temporalis muscle/fascia for the repair and buttressing of dural defects are ideal resources. In penetrating head injuries where the pericranium or temporalis muscle/

fascia may be damaged or inadequate, one may consider tensor fascia lata harvesting as an autogenous substitute. Also, abdominal fat is a readily available and easily harvested material for obliterating intracranial dead space from both a transcranial or endoscopic perspective. However, it should be noted that nonvascularized abdominal fat may lead to necrosis and infection and as such has become less commonly used as a method to obliterate intracranial dead space. Finally, for those with large osseous defects, a large concomitant intracranial dead space, or concern over a poorly vascularized pericranial flap, the possibility of de-epitelized or muscle-based free tissue transfer from other regions of the body are increasingly feasible options. While beyond the scope of this text, radial forearm, rectus abdominis, latissimus dorsi, and anterolateral thigh/vastus lateralis free flaps have all been described for the coverage of complex skull base defects but obviously require the assistance of a skilled microsurgeon for harvesting and implantation.[8,14,47–54]

From a transnasal endoscopic route, autogenous reconstructive materials are available but more limited in the pure quantity one can harvest. For the coverage of skull base/paranasal sinus defects, the most common local pedicled flaps used are the middle turbinate and nasal septal flaps.[55,56] In addition, regional extranasal pedicled flaps that are then rotated into the nasal cavity have been described (palatal, pericranial, facial buccinators, and temporoparietal fascia) but add extra time and dissection to any case.[19,53,57–70] These techniques require otolaryngological or neurosurgical endoscopic support and as such may not be available at all medical centers.

Allogenic materials, in an ideal setting, should serve as reinforcement to a water-tight autogenous dural/skull base repair. Several different materials are used in this regard starting with synthetic dural substitutes such as DuraGen (Integra Lifescience Corporation, Plainsboro, New Jersey) and Alloderm (Lifecell Corporation, Branchburg, New Jersey). Commonly used dural/fibrin sealants include DuraSeal (Confluent Surgical, Inc., Waltham, Massachusetts) and Tisseel (Baxter Healthcare Corp., Deerfield, IL).[71,72] These products are readily available and remain an important component of the surgeon's armamentarium as buttresses to autogenous repair.

Intraoperative Adjuncts

In order to precisely localize the site(s) of CSF leakage intraoperatively, some use the intrathecal injection of fluorescein under endoscopic visualization (with a white or blue light filter in addition to a blocking filter to adequately visualize the injected fluorescein). Most protocols use 0.2–0.5 mg of 5% fluorescein mixed with 10 mL of aspirated CSF via lumbar puncture/catheter injected over several minutes approximately 1 hour before visualization is needed followed by a 5 mL flush of CSF.[9]

Surgical Technique(s)

Given that endoscopic skull base and middle cranial fossa approaches are typically within the realm of otolaryngologists and/or skull base neurosurgeons, these topics will not be covered in this text.

On arrival in the operating room, the patient is given appropriate perioperative antibiotics and antiepileptic medications (if not already started preoperatively). A lumbar drain or ventriculostomy is inserted if not already present as it will lessen the amount of frontal or temporal lobe retraction needed intraoperatively, allow for the injection of intrathecal fluorescein, and be a source of postoperative CSF diversion to protect the surgical repair(s) performed. Finally, in the case of patients with known intracranial swelling or injuries, one may give mannitol, furosemide, or hypertonic saline (to maintain the serum sodium in the high normal range [140–145 mEq/L]). These hyperosmolar measures will all serve to further lessen the amount of brain retraction needed during these often challenging cases. In addition, one should always be sure to have sterile access to other regions of the body possibly needed for tissue harvesting (tensor fascia lata, etc.) during the course of the case.

Regardless of whether one decides to use a unilateral or bifrontal approach for the repair of anterior skull base CSF leaks, the objectives of exposure remain the same: to have the inferior border of the craniotomy parallel the floor of the anterior fossa, to have enough exposure to perform a dural repair as far posterior as the tuberculum sellae, to harvest sufficient pericranium to cover the floor of the anterior fossa, and to preserve the supraorbital (V_1) and supratrochlear (V_1) nerves, and the temporal branch of the facial nerve (VII).[9]

The patient is positioned in the usual fashion, either on a horseshoe headrest or with three-point skull fixation and the head elevated above the level of the heart for improved venous drainage. A curvilinear or traditional coronal incision is fashioned depending on the planned approach. The incision is taken through the level of the galea aponeurotica after the injection of local anesthetic, thus preserving the pericranium and temporalis fascia. Upon reaching the temporal fat pad, the dissection is converted to an interfascial approach to remain deep to this structure and protecting the temporal branch of the facial nerve in the process. Once the supraorbital bar is reached, pericranium harvesting is performed and reflected forward, preserving its vascular supply. Another option is to enter the subperiosteal plane and at the level of the temporalis stay superficial to the deep layer of the temporalis fascia. If the pericranial flap is needed it can be dissected free from the underside of the scalp flap at that time. The advantage of this route (while being more technically challenging) is that it preserves the pericranial layer should it not be needed. Proceeding towards the orbital rims in a subperiosteal fashion, the supraorbital nerves are identified and freed from their osseous foramen (if present) with a small osteotome. The scalp and pericranial flaps are then protected with moist gauze and held in place with self-retaining retractors.

Fig. 1.6.3 illustrates suggested craniotomy outlines for both unilateral and bifrontal approaches. After completing a bifrontal craniotomy that is parallel with the floor of the anterior skull base, dissection may proceed in either an extra- or intradural fashion to expose any dural defects responsible for CSF leakage. For an intradural approach, the dura is opened on either side of the superior sagittal sinus, ligated using silk sutures, and subsequently divided near the crista galli (see

Fig. 1.6.4). Aside from the elderly, in whom the dura is usually very thin and adherent to the skull base, the exposure usually proceeds in an extradural manner. Self-retaining retractors are then placed on either side of the dural defect to optimize visualization and one's working corridor.

The dura is then repaired in a watertight manner using various combinations of the materials and methods mentioned above (see Fig. 1.6.4) and sealed using fibrin glue. At this juncture, large osseous defects can be repaired using split-thickness calvarial autograft. The frontal sinus is then cranialized if entered during the course of surgery or known to be injured from the time of initial injury. The posterior wall is removed and the mucosal lining of the sinus is ablated with curettes, drills, and electrocautery. The nasofrontal duct is then obliterated with some combination of bone graft, temporalis muscle/fascia, and again sealed with fibrin glue. Finally, the vascularized pericranial flap is placed over the floor of the anterior fossa and the bone flap is then fastened into position being careful to ensure the pericranial flap is not strangulated of its blood supply.

Postoperative Course

CSF diversion is continued via intermittent hourly lumbar drainage for approximately 3–5 days postoperatively. Antibiotic coverage beyond the 24-hour perioperative window is at the discretion of the treating physician. The author's preferred regimen consists of 1 gram of intravenous cefazolin until the lumbar drain is removed.

EARLY AND DELAYED COMPLICATIONS

As mentioned above, between 20% and 50% of patients with persistent CSF leaks will develop CNS infections.[1,15,16] For those whose leaks halt with nonoperative management, one must be vigilant for the possibility of recurrence in both the short and long term.[35] As such, clinical follow-up should be ensured and patients and their families should be counseled thoroughly about the signs and symptoms of CSF leaks and meningitis that can occur in up to 16% of individuals at an average of 6.5 years post-injury with previously resolved CSF leaks.[73]

For those requiring surgical management of a skull base CSF leak, postoperative infectious complications can still develop in a significant percentage of patients depending on the mechanism of injury. In the senior author's wartime experience with penetrating head injuries

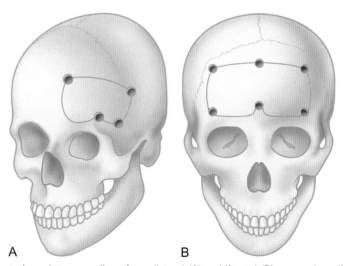

Fig. 1.6.3 Suggested craniotomy outlines for unilateral (A) or bifrontal (B) approaches. (Reproduced with permission from Aarabi B, O'Malley BW, Martin JE, Eisenberg HM. Surgical management of cerebrospinal fluid leaks. In: Sekhar LN, Fessler RG, editors. Atlas of neurosurgical techniques: Brain. New York: Thieme; 2006; p.927–938. Figure 80-5, p.930.)

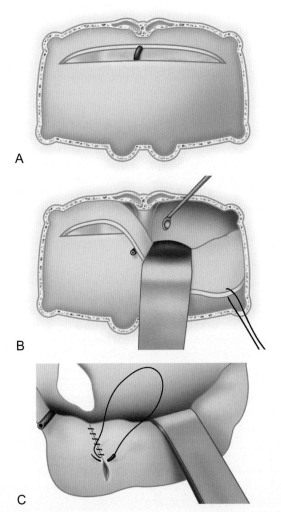

A

B

C

Fig. 1.6.4 Surgical technique for extradural skull base CSF leak repair. After completing a bifrontal craniotomy, the dura is opened on either side of the superior sagittal sinus (SSS) which is then suture ligated (A) in order to release CSF and facilitate safe dural/brain retraction. Self-retaining retractors are then placed in order to visualize both the skull base (B) and dural (C) defects which are repaired as mentioned in the text. (Reproduced with permission from Aarabi B, O'Malley BW, Martin JE, Eisenberg HM. Surgical management of cerebrospinal fluid leaks. In: Sekhar LN, Fessler RG, editors. Atlas of neurosurgical techniques: Brain. New York: Thieme; 2006; p.927–938. Figure 80-6, p.931.)

associated with CSF fistulas, infectious complications developed in 12 of 33 (36%) patients.[7] Of note, Gram-negative organisms such as *Klebsiella pneumoniae* were the most frequent offending organism(s).

For those with blunt mechanism civilian CSF leaks treated appropriately the rate of infectious complications ranges from zero to 21%.[73] The most common infectious scenario is that of meningitis, which can be managed with antibiotic therapy. However, intracranial abscesses, empyemas, or osteomyelitis mandate urgent surgical re-exploration, evacuation of infectious fluid collections, and debridement/removal of any nonviable calvarial bone followed by prolonged antibiotic therapy.

CASE EXAMPLE

See Fig. 1.6.5 for a representative case example.

CONCLUSIONS

The diagnosis and management of skull base fractures and CSF leaks can be complex and requires multidisciplinary consultation and cooperation. Simple, linear, nondisplaced skull base fractures with CSF leakage are more likely to halt with conservative management and can be appropriately managed in this fashion. For those CSF leaks persisting beyond 5 days, or more acute scenarios with large, displaced osseous skull base defects, operative intervention is warranted. Consultation with a specialist familiar with nasal endoscopy and skull base repair should be sought in all such cases to assess the appropriateness for an endoscopic solution to avoid the risks attendant to a transcranial approach. Transcranial approaches currently remain an important part of the treatment armamentarium but will hopefully decline as the experience and familiarity with endoscopic techniques grow.

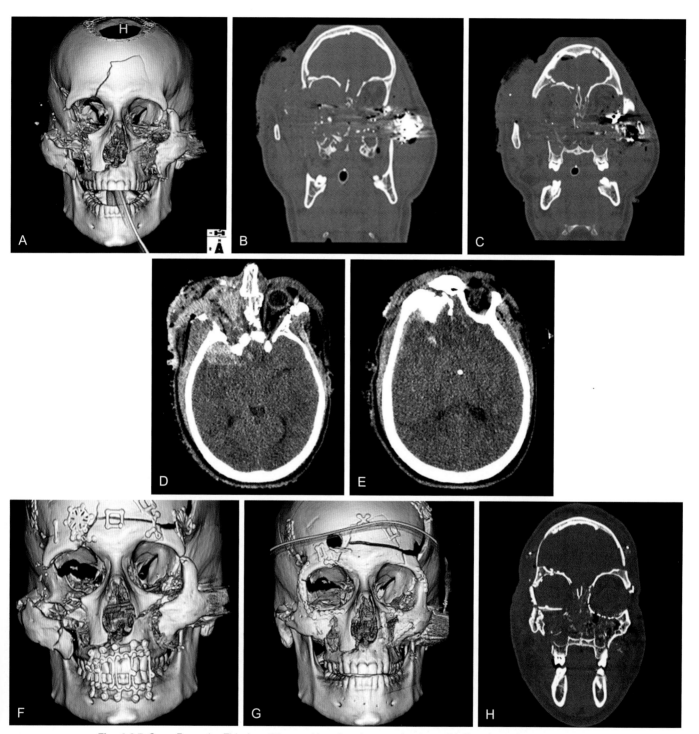

Fig. 1.6.5 Case Example. This is a 24-year-old male who sustained a self-inflicted gunshot wound with resultant severe disruption of his right supraorbital rim, orbital roof, and bilateral orbitozygomaticomaxillary complexes (A–C). On presentation, a high-flow CSF leak was noted through his traumatically enucleated right orbit in association with a right anterior temporal epidural hematoma and bifrontal subarachnoid/subdural hemorrhages/contusions (D–E). Given the high-energy, penetrating mechanism of injury with a high-flow CSF leak he was taken to the operating room the following morning (after a ventriculostomy was placed the evening prior for intracranial pressure monitoring and CSF diversion) for a bifrontal craniotomy, split-thickness calvarial bone harvesting/banking (for later use in facial reconstruction), and dural repair. The supraorbital rim was reconstructed and a 3 × 3 cm basal frontal dural defect was noted over the right orbital roof that was repaired extradurally in a watertight manner using Alloderm (Lifecell Corporation, Branchburg, New Jersey) followed by placement of the pericranial graft. After stabilization of his neurological injuries he was later placed into maxillomandibular fixation (MMF) on hospital day (HD) 5 to maintain his occlusal relationship (F). His facial fractures were definitively fixated on HD 12 (after his ventriculostomy was successfully weaned and discontinued) via coronal, transconjunctival, and intraoral approaches (G). Of final note, the patient lacked a true frontal sinus and as such did not require a cranialization procedure and the split-thickness calvarial bone harvested from the initial skull base repair was used to reconstruct the patient's right lateral orbital rim and orbital floor (H).

REFERENCES

1. Lewin W. Cerebrospinal fluid rhinorrhea in nonmissile head injuries. *Clin Neurosurg.* 1966;12:237–252.
2. Thompson St C. *The Cerebrospinal Fluid: Its Spontaneous Escape From the Nose.* London: Cassell; 1889.
3. Chiari H. Uebereinen Fall, von Luflonsammlong in Der Ventrikeln des Menschlichen Gehoins. *Ztsch Heirk.* 1884;5:383–384.
4. Cairns H. Injuries of the frontal and ethmoidal sinuses with special reference to cerebrospinal rhinorrhoea and aerocele. *J Laryngol.* 1937;52:589–623.
5. Dandy WE. Pneumocephalus (intracranial pneumatocele or aerocedle). *Arch Surg.* 1926;12:949–982.
6. Dandy WE. Treatment of rhinorrhea and otorrhea. *Arch Surg.* 1944;49:75–85.
7. Aarabi B, Taghipour M, Alibaii E, Kamgarpour A. Central nervous system infections after military missile head wounds. *Neurosurgery.* 1998;42:500–507.
8. Kumar A, Tantawi D, Armonda R, Valerio I. Advanced cranial reconstruction using intracranial free flaps and cranial bone grafts: an algorithmic approach developed from the modern battlefield. *Plast Reconstr Surg.* 2012;130(5):1101–1109.
9. Aarabi B, O'Malley BW, Martin JE, Eisenberg HM. Surgical management of cerebrospinal fluid leaks. In: Sekhar LN, Fessler RG, eds. *Atlas of Neurosurgical Techniques: Brain.* New York: Thieme; 2006:927–938.
10. Aarabi B, Leibrock LG. Neurosurgical approaches to cerebrospinal fluid rhinorrhea. *Ear Nose Throat J.* 1992;71:300–305.
11. Coleman CC. Fracture of the skull involving the paranasal sinuses and mastoids. *JAMA.* 1947;109:1613–1616.
12. Mithani SK, St-Hilaire H, Brooke BS, et al. Predictable patterns of intracranial and cervical spine injury in craniomaxillofacial trauma: analysis of 4786 patients. *Plast Reconstr Surg.* 2009;123(4):1293–1301.
13. Jamieson KG, Yelland JDN. Surgical repair of the anterior fossa because of rhinorrhea, aerocele, or meningitis. *J Neurosurg.* 1973;39:328–331.
14. Leech PJ, Paterson A. Conservative and operative management for cerebrospinal-fluid leakage after closed head injury. *Lancet.* 1973;1:1013–1016.
15. Calvert CA, Cairns H. Discussion on injuries of the frontal and ethmoidal sinuses. *Proc R Soc Med.* 1942;35:805–810.
16. Teachenor FR. Intracranial complications of fracture of skull involving frontal sinus. *JAMA.* 1927;88:987–989.
17. Adson AW, Uihlein A. Repair of defects in ethmoid and frontal sinuses resulting in cerebrospinal rhinorrhea. *Arch Surg.* 1949;58:623–634.
18. Davis EDD. Discussion on injuries of the frontal and ethmoidal sinuses. *Laryngology.* 1942;805:13–18.
19. Park I, Song J, Lee H, et al. Volumetric study in the development of paranasal sinuses by CT imaging in Asian: a pilot study. *Int J Pediatr Otorhinolaryngol.* 2010;74:1347–1350.
20. Rodriguez E, Stanwix M, Manson P, et al. Twenty-six-year experience treating frontal sinus fractures: a novel algorithm based on anatomical fracture pattern and failure of conventional techniques. *Plast Reconstr Surg.* 2008;122(6):1850–1866.
21. Risch L, Lisec I, Jutzi M, et al. Rapid, accurate and noninvasive detection of cerebrospinal fluid leakage using combined determination of beta-trace protein in secretion and serum. *Clin Chim Acta.* 2005;351:169–176.
22. Stone JA, Castillo M, Neelon B, Mukherji SK. Evaluation of CSF leaks: high-resolution CT compared with contrast-enhanced CT and radionuclide cisternography. *AJNR Am J Neuroradiol.* 1999;20:706–712.
23. Applebaum EL, Chow JM. Cerebrospinal fluid leaks. In: Cummings CW, Fredrickson JM, Harker LA, et al, eds. *Paranasal Sinuses, Otolaryngology Head and Neck Surgery.* Vol. 2. 3rd ed. St. Louis: Mosby; 1998:1189–1197.
24. Eljamel MS, Pidgeon CN, Toland J, et al. MRI cisternography, and localization of CSF fistulae. *Br J Neurosurg.* 1994;8:433–437.
25. Gupta V, Goyal M, Mishra N, et al. MR evaluation of CSF fistulae. *Acta Radiol.* 1997;38:603–609.
26. Levy LM, Gulya AJ, Davis SW, et al. Flow-sensitive magnetic resonance imaging ion the evaluation of cerebrospinal fluid leaks. *Am J Otol.* 1995;16:591–596.
27. Sillers MJ, Morgan CE, Gammal EL. Magnetic resonance cisternography and thin coronal computerized tomography in the evaluation of cerebrospinal fluid rhinorrhea. *Am J Rhinol.* 1997;11:387–392.
28. Stafford Johnson DBS, Brennan P, Toland J, O'Dwyer AJ. Magnetic resonance imaging in the evaluation of cerebrospinal fluid fistulae. *Clin Radiol.* 1996;51:837–841.
29. Zeng Q, Xiong L, Jinkins JR, et al. Intrathecal gadolinium-enhanced MR myelography and cisternography: a pilot study in human patients. *AJR Am J Roentgenol.* 1999;173:1109–1115.
30. Ahmadi J, Weiss MH, Segall HD, et al. Evaluation of cerebrospinal fluid rhinorrhea by metrizamide computed tomography cisternography. *Neurosurgery.* 1985;16:54–60.
31. Ashburn WL, Harbert JC, Briner WH, et al. Cerebrospinal fluid rhinorrhea studied with the gamma scintillation camera. *J Nucl Med.* 1968;9:523–529.
32. DiChiro G, Ommaya AK, Ashburn WL, et al. Isotope cisternography in the diagnosis and follow-up of cerebrospinal fluid rhinorrheas. *J Neurosurg.* 1968;28:522–529.
33. Drayer BP, Wilkins RH, Boehnke M, et al. Cerebrospinal fluid rhinorrhea demonstrated by metrizamide CT cisternography. *AJR Am J Roentgenol.* 1977;129:149–151.
34. Manelfe C, Guiraud B, Tremoulet M. Diagnosis of CSF rhinorrhea by computerized cisternography using metrizamide. *Lancet.* 1977;2:1073.
35. Russell T, Cummins BH. Cerebrospinal fluid rhinorrhea 34 years after trauma: a case report and review of the literature. *Neurosurgery.* 1984;15:705–706.
36. Scholsem M, Scholtes F, Collignon F, et al. Surgical management of anterior cranial base fractures with cerebrospinal fluid fistulae: a single–institution experience. *Neurosurgery.* 2008;62:463–471.
37. Yilmazlar S, Arslan E, Kocaeli H, et al. Cerebrospinal fluid leakage complicating skull base fractures: analysis of 81 cases. *Neurosurg Rev.* 2006;29(1):64–71.
38. Ziu M, Savage JG, Jimenez DF. Diagnosis and treatment of cerebrospinal fluid rhinorrhea following accidental traumatic anterior skull base fractures. *Neurosurg Focus.* 2012;32:E3.
39. Ratilal BO, Costa J, Sampaio C, Pappamikail L. Antibiotic prophylaxis for preventing meningitis in patients with basilar skull fractures. *Cochrane Database Syst Rev.* 2011;(8):CD004884.
40. Klastersky J, Sadeghi M, Brihaye J. Antimicrobial prophylaxis in patients with rhinorrhea or otorrhea: a double-blind study. *Surg Neurol.* 1976;6:111–114.
41. Rimmer J, Belk C, Lund V, et al. Immunisations and antibiotics in patients with anterior skull base cerebrospinal fluid leaks. *J Laryngol Otol.* 2014;128(7):626–629.
42. Gosal J, Gurmey T, Kursa G, et al. Is acetazolamide really useful in the management of traumatic cerebrospinal fluid rhinorrhea? *Neurol India.* 2015;63(2):197–201.
43. Gil Z, Abergel A, Leider–Trejo L, et al. A comprehensive algorithm for anterior skull base reconstruction after oncological resections. *Skull Base.* 2007;17:25–37.
44. Prosser JD, Vender JR, Solares CA. Traumatic cerebrospinal fluid leaks. *Otolaryngol Clin North Am.* 2011;44(4):857–873, vii.
45. Ray BS, Bergland RM. Cerebrospinal fluid fistula: clinical aspects, techniques of localization and methods of closure. *J Neurosurg.* 1967;30:399–405.
46. Rocchi G, Caroli E, Belli E, et al. Severe craniofacial fractures with frontobasal involvement and cerebrospinal fluid fistula: indications for surgical repair. *Surg Neurol.* 2005;63:559–563.
47. Costa H, Baptista A, Vaz R, et al. The galea frontalis myofascial flap in anterior fossa CSF leaks. *Br J Plast Surg.* 1993;46:503–507.
48. Friedman JA, Ebersold MJ, Quast LM. Persistent posttraumatic cerebrospinal fluid leakage. *Neurosurg Focus.* 2000;9:1–5.
49. Inman J, Ducic Y. Craniomaxillofacial trauma: intracranial free tissue transfer for massive cerebrospinal fluid leaks of the anterior cranial fossa. *J Oral Maxillofac Surg.* 2012;70:1114–1118.

50. Lesavoy MA, Lee GK, Fan K, Dickinson B. Split, temporalis muscle flap for repair of recalcitrant cerebrospinal fluid leaks of the anterior cranial fossa. *J Craniofac Surg.* 2012;23:539–542.

51. Luu Q, Farwell D. Microvascular free flap reconstruction of anterior skull base defects. *Oper Tech Otolayngol Head Neck Surg.* 2010;21:91–95.

52. Reinard K, Basheer A, Jones L, et al. Surgical technique for repair of complex anterior skull base defects. *Surg Neurol Int.* 2015;6(1):99–103.

53. Reyes C, Mason E, Solares C. Panorama of reconstruction of skull base defects: from traditional open to endonasal endoscopic approaches, from free grafts to microvascular flaps. *Int Arch Otorhinolaryngol.* 2014;18:S179–S185.

54. Thakker J, Fernandes R. Surgical oncology and reconstruction: evaluation of reconstructive techniques for anterior and middle skull base defects following tumor ablation. *J Oral Maxillofac Surg.* 2014;72:198–204.

55. Weisman RA. Septal chondromucosal flap with preservation of septal integrity. *Laryngoscope.* 1989;99:267–271.

56. Yessenow RS, McCabe BF. The osteo-mucoperiosteal flap in repair of cerebrospinal fluid rhinorrhea: a 20-year experience. *Otolaryngol Head Neck Surg.* 1989;101:555–558.

57. Amedee RG, Mann WJ, Gilsbach J. Microscopic endonasal surgery for repair of CSF leaks. *Am J Rhinol.* 1993;7:1–4.

58. Anand VK, Murali RK, Glasgold MJ. Surgical decisions in the management of cerebrospinal fluid rhinorrhea. *Rhinology.* 1995;33:212–218.

59. Dodson EE, Gross CW, Swerdloff JL, et al. Transnasal endoscopic repair of cerebrospinal fluid rhinorrhea and skull base defects: a review of twenty-nine cases. *Otolaryngol Head Neck Surg.* 1994;111:600–605.

60. Friedman M, Venkatesan TK, Caldarelli DD. Composite mucochondral flap for repair of cerebrospinal fluid leaks. *Head Neck.* 1995;17:414–418.

61. Hadad G, Rivera-Serrano CM, Bassagaisteguy LH, et al. Anterior pedicle lateral nasal wall flap: a novel technique for the reconstruction of anterior skull base defects. *Laryngoscope.* 2011;121(8):1606–1610.

62. Hosemann W, Goede U, Sauer M. Wound healing of mucosal autografts for frontal cerebrospinal fluid leaks – clinical and experimental investigations. *Rhinology.* 1999;37(3):108–112.

63. Marshall AH, Jones NS, Robertson IJA. An algorithm for the management of CSF rhinorrhea illustrated by 36 cases. *Rhinology.* 1999;37:182–185.

64. Mattox DE, Kennedy DW. Endoscopic management of cerebrospinal fluid leaks and cephaloceles. *Laryngoscope.* 1990;100:857–862.

65. Ng M, Maceri DR, Levy MM, Crockett DM. Extracranial repair of pediatric traumatic cerebrospinal fluid rhinorrhea. *Arch Otolaryngol Head Neck Surg.* 1998;124:1125–1130.

66. Papay FA, Maggiano H, Dominquez S, et al. Rigid endoscopic repair of paranasal sinus cerebrospinal fluid fistulas. *Laryngoscope.* 1989;99:1195–1201.

67. Park J-I, Strelzow VV, Firedman WH. Current management of cerebrospinal fluid rhinorrhea. *Laryngoscope.* 1983;93:1294–1300.

68. Schoentgen C. Management of post-traumatic cerebrospinal fluid (CSF) leak of anterior skull base: 10 years experience. *Acta Otolaryngol.* 2013;133(9):944–950.

69. Wetmore RF, Duhaime AC, Klausner RD. Endoscopic repair of traumatic CSF rhinorrhea in a pediatric patient. *Int J Pediatr Otorhinolaryngol.* 1996;36:109–115.

70. Yoon JH, Lee JG, Kim SH, Park IY. Microscopical surgical management of cerebrospinal fluid rhinorrhea with free grafts. *Rhinology.* 1995;33:208–211.

71. Dunn CJ, Goa KL. Fibrin sealant; a review of its use in surgery and endoscopy. *Drugs.* 1999;58:863–886.

72. Gnjidic Z, Tomac D, Negovetic L, et al. Fibrin sealants in the management of cerebrospinal fistulae. *Biomed Prog.* 1994;7:39–42.

73. Friedman JA, Ebersold MJ, Quast LM. Post-traumatic cerebrospinal fluid leakage. *World J Surg.* 2001;25(8):1062–1066.

Frontal Bone and Frontal Sinus Injuries

David A. Shaye, E. Bradley Strong

BACKGROUND

The frontal sinus is protected by thick cortical bone. High-velocity impacts can result in frontal sinus fracture and brain injury. These complex injuries pose many surgical challenges and can be associated with long-term sequelae such as mucocele and meningitis. Optimal management strategies remain controversial. Treatment goals should include protection of the intracranial contents, avoidance of short- and long-term complications, restoration of an aesthetic frontal contour, and maintenance of sinus function when possible. A treatment algorithm is presented based on injury to three anatomic regions: the anterior table, the frontal recess, and the posterior table/dura.

ANATOMY

Although not present at birth, the frontal sinus aerates by extension of the ethmoid air cells into the frontal bone. This process usually begins at 2 years of age and the sinus is completely developed by about the age of 15 (Fig. 1.7.1). The degree of frontal sinus development is variable, with up to 11% of people having only a unilateral frontal sinus and 4% of people having no frontal sinuses at all. The anterior table bone averages 4 mm in thickness; while the posterior table is thinner, providing less protection to the anterior cranial fossa (Fig. 1.7.2). The intersinus septum often divides the frontal sinus into two sides, each of which drains into their respective frontal sinus outflow tract. The frontal sinus drainage pathway has an hourglass shape (Fig. 1.7.3), with the infundibulum above, true ostia in the middle (1–3 mm), and frontal recess below.[1]

ETIOLOGY AND INCIDENCE

Frontal sinus fractures comprise approximately 5%–15% of maxillofacial injuries.[1,2] The force required to fracture the frontal bone is greater than for any other facial bone.[1] Improvements in vehicle safety, such as seatbelts and airbags, have significantly decreased the incidence of frontal sinus fractures.[1,3] The majority of patients are young males (average 30 years) who sustain high-velocity injuries such as: motor vehicle collisions (52%), interpersonal violence (26%), and recreation or industrial accidents (14%).[1,4,5] One-third of these injuries are isolated anterior table fractures; two-thirds involve some combination of the anterior and posterior tables as well as the nasofrontal recess; while isolated posterior table fractures remain quite rare (<2%).[1,5,6] The majority of patients (75%) who sustain frontal sinus injuries will have associated craniofacial fractures.[1,7]

HISTORY AND PHYSICAL EXAMINATION

Due to the high velocity nature of these injuries, the initial evaluation should focus on airway control and hemodynamic stability. A complete head and neck examination should rule out injury to the brain, spine, orbits, and facial skeleton; including the frontal sinus. Patients with frontal sinus fractures often complain of forehead pain and swelling. Physical findings may include paresthesias, epistaxis, diplopia, forehead abrasions, lacerations, and hematoma.

Fractures of the posterior table place patients at increased risk of dural tear, cerebrospinal fluid (CSF) rhinorrhea, and meningitis.[8] The most common clinical presentation of CSF rhinorrhea is intermittent bloodstained, or clear watery anterior nasal discharge, salty postnasal drainage, and headache. If rhinorrhea is present, it can be evaluated with a "halo test," whereby the fluid is allowed to drop onto filter paper. If CSF is present, it will diffuse faster than blood and result in a clear halo around the blood. A more definitive diagnosis can be made using a beta-2 transferrin assay. With its high sensitivity (99%) and specificity (97%), this biochemical assay is viewed as the gold standard for diagnosis of CSF rhinorrhea.[9] Disadvantages of the test include: expense, labor-intensive fluid collection, and waiting period for results (approximately 3–5 days).[10]

RADIOGRAPHY

The gold standard radiographic examination for traumatic injuries of the facial skeleton is a thin cut (≤1 mm) computed tomography (CT) scan. To help improve diagnostic accuracy, these images should be reformatted into coronal, sagittal, and 3-dimensional reconstructions. The axial images are preferred for evaluation of the anterior and posterior table (Fig. 1.7.4); sagittal images for the frontal sinus outflow tract and skull base (Fig. 1.7.5); and the coronal images for the orbital roof/sinus floor (Fig. 1.7.6). Three-dimensional reconstructions (Fig. 1.7.7) offer a comprehensive view of the injury. They are helpful to assist in surgical planning, facilitate patient education, and delineate the size/location of bone fragments, which can reduce the need for soft tissue dissection.

SURGICAL APPROACHES

The major surgical approaches to the frontal sinus include: laceration, trephination, percutaneous, endoscopic brow, direct forehead/suprabrow, upper blepharoplasty, endonasal sinusotomy, and coronal.

Lacerations

When lacerations are present, they should be used to assist with fracture visualization/reduction as well as hardware placement. While lacerations can be extended for greater access, caution should be used. This may result in more pronounced facial scaring and paresthesias. Small fractures can be treated through lacerations alone. But the actual exposure requirements necessary to complete the repair can only be assessed intraoperatively. Therefore, consent for other surgical approaches should always be obtained.

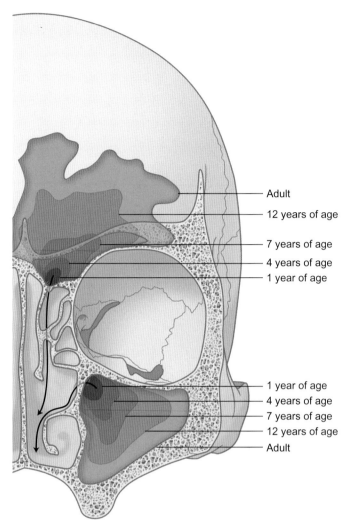

Fig. 1.7.1 Frontal sinus development.

Adult
12 years of age
7 years of age
4 years of age
1 year of age

1 year of age
4 years of age
7 years of age
12 years of age
Adult

Trephination

Frontal sinus trephination is a technique that offers added visualization and access to the frontal sinus. A 1.0–1.5 cm curved skin incision midway between the medial canthus and glabella is made just inferior to the brow (Fig. 1.7.8). Incisions within the brow itself are not recommended due to the risk of alopecia and injury to the supratrochlear/supraorbital neurovascular bundles. To reduce the risk of visible scar formation or webbing, a "V" can be inserted to break up the incision line. Careful dissection down to the frontal bone is performed with a guarded needle tip electrocautery. The frontal sinus location is confirmed with a CT scan or the use of intraoperative navigation. A small cutting bur is used to create a 4–5 mm frontal sinusotomy (Fig. 1.7.9), the mucosa is opened, and a 30 degree endoscope is used to visualize the sinus. A Valsalva maneuver can be performed to better localize a CSF leak. If more lateral visualization is required, a flexible pediatric bronchoscope can be used.

Percutaneous

Several authors have described case reports or small case series of percutaneous fracture reduction for primary repair.[11–13] This involves stab incisions to visualize the bone segments, and percutaneous screws for fracture reduction.

Endoscopic Brow

Endoscopic brow approaches, while developed for brow-lifting procedures,[14,15] have been adapted for primary and secondary repair of anterior table frontal bone fractures.[16–18] Using brow-lift instrumentation, a 3–5-cm parasagittal "working" incision (Fig. 1.7.10) is placed 3 cm posterior to the hairline directly above the fracture. Limited use of electrocautery will reduce the risk of alopecia. The incision is taken down to bone and a brow-lift elevator is used for subperiosteal dissection to the level of the fracture. Through a second 1–2-cm "endoscope" incision (placed approximately 6 cm medial to the working incision), a 4 mm 30 degree endoscope within a rigid endosheath is introduced for visualization. A large guard on the endosheath will help with tissue elevation and maintenance of the optical cavity. Careful subperiosteal dissection (Fig. 1.7.11) is performed over the fracture deformity under endoscopic visualization, with care to identify and preserve the supraorbital and supratrochlear neurovascular bundles.

Direct Forehead/Suprabrow

Large lacerations can provide adequate access for open reduction and internal fixation of some fractures. Significant extension of such lacerations should be avoided for aesthetic reasons. However, a direct approach, whereby an incision is placed within a horizontal rhytid over the fracture, is effective in patients with deep rhytids. Direct transcutaneous supra- and infrabrow incisions have also been described.[19] Paresthesias related to these approaches resolve in most patients,[20] however the authors believe that incisions placed directly above the brow have a higher risk of long-term paresthesias and visible scarring.

Upper Blepharoplasty

An upper blepharoplasty incision will allow access to fractures of the superior orbital rim and inferior frontal bone. This approach has been cited more commonly for sinus surgery,[21] CSF leak repair,[22] skull base surgery,[23–25] and orbital roof fractures.[26] An incision is placed in the supratarsal crease at least 10–12 mm above the eyelid margin. It can be extended from the supraorbital notch to just outside the lateral canthus as necessary for access. The incision is initially carried through the skin and orbicularis oculi muscle, allowing identification of the orbital septum. The orbital septum should not be violated, as this will expose orbital fat and the levator palpebrae superioris. At this point, upward traction can be applied to the brow, transposing the incision over the bony orbital rim. An electrocautery with a microtip needle (on a low setting) is then used to dissect directly onto the frontal bone. Once the rim is palpated, the electrocautery can be used to incise the periosteum and expose the frontal bone in a subperiosteal plane.

Endonasal Sinusotomy

A transnasal endoscopic frontal sinusotomy (or Draf III procedure) is commonly used for management of chronic frontal sinusitis, mucoceles, frontal sinus trauma, and frontal sinus tumors.[27] It provides access to the frontal recess as well as the anterior and posterior table of the frontal sinus. The procedure begins with an endoscopic ethmoidectomy and identification of the ethmoid skull base and lamina papyracea (Fig. 1.7.12A). Utilizing angled endoscopes (30, 45, or 70 degree depending on surgeon preference) and through cutting instrumentation, the floor, posterior wall, and roof of the agger nasi cell are removed. The frontal recess has now been dissected and an endoscopic view of the frontal sinus is achieved. The same procedure is then performed on the contralateral side until the bilateral frontal sinus ostia are visible. A 2 × 2 cm superior septectomy is then performed to gain bilateral access to the floor of the frontal sinus (Fig. 1.7.12B). The posterior limit of

Text continued on p. 95

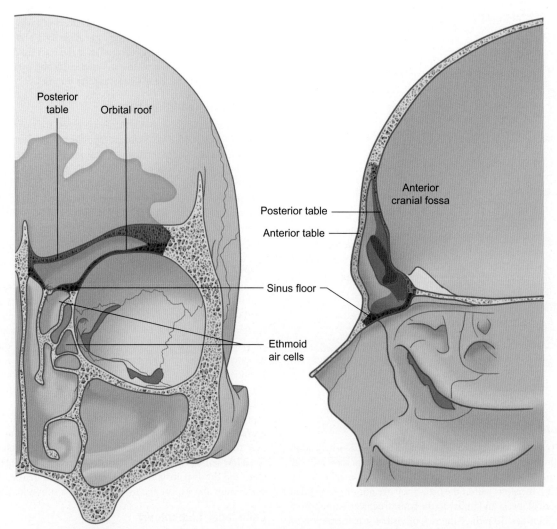

Fig. 1.7.2 Anterior and lateral views of the frontal sinus demonstrating a thick anterior table and relatively thin posterior table. The floor of the sinus forms the medial portion of the orbital roof. The posterior table forms a portion of the anterior cranial fossa. The anterior table forms part of the forehead, brow, and glabella.

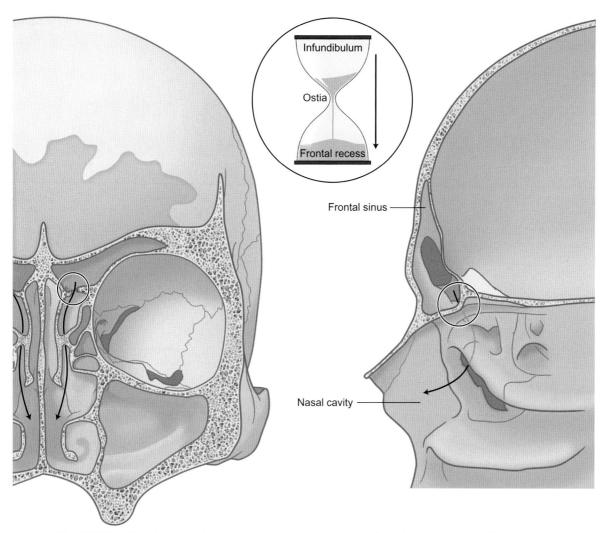

Fig. 1.7.3 The frontal sinus drainage pathway has an hourglass configuration with the infundibulum above and the frontal recess below.

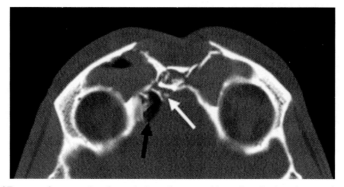

Fig. 1.7.4 Axial CT scan of a complex frontal sinus fracture. Note the displaced posterior table bone fragments (*white arrow*) and pneumocephalus (*black arrow*).

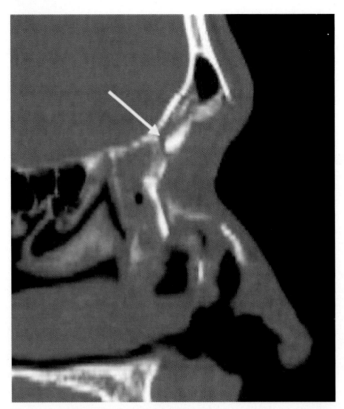

Fig. 1.7.5 Sagittal CT scan of a complex frontal sinus fracture. Note the involvement of the frontal sinus outflow tract.

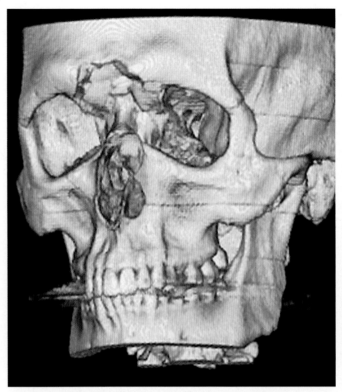

Fig. 1.7.7 Three-dimensional reconstruction of a complex frontal sinus fracture. The 3-dimensional representation gives the surgeon a better understanding of the size and location of the bone fragments. This can reduce the need for soft tissue dissection during surgery.

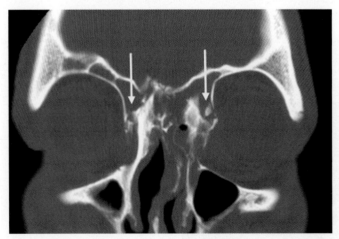

Fig. 1.7.6 Coronal CT scan of a complex frontal sinus fracture. Note the involvement of the medial orbital wall and the frontal sinus outflow tract (*white arrows*).

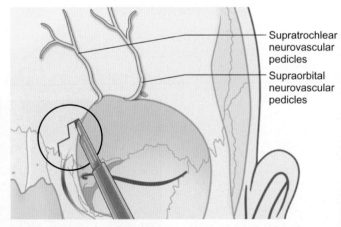

Supratrochlear neurovascular pedicles

Supraorbital neurovascular pedicles

Fig. 1.7.8 Incision for a frontal sinus trephination, placed midway between the medial canthus and the glabella, and approximately 1 cm inferior to the brow. The incision is best hidden when placed inferior to the forehead curvature.

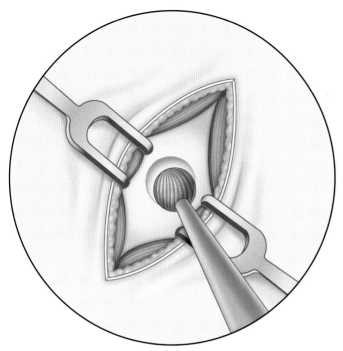

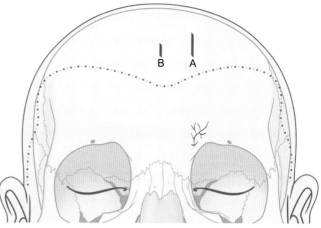

Fig. 1.7.10 Illustration of the "working" incision (A) and the "endoscope" incision (B) used for endoscopic repair of anterior table frontal sinus fractures.

Fig. 1.7.9 Illustration of a cutting bur being used to trephinate the frontal sinus. Care should be used to avoid posterior table injury.

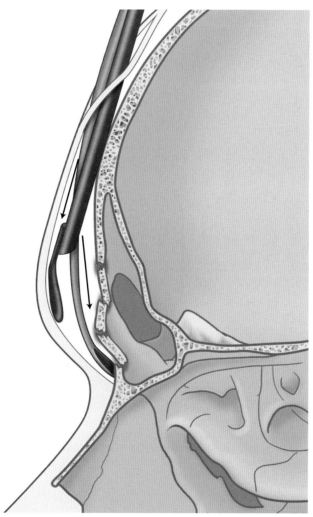

Fig. 1.7.11 Endoscopic subperiosteal dissection to expose the anterior table frontal sinus fracture.

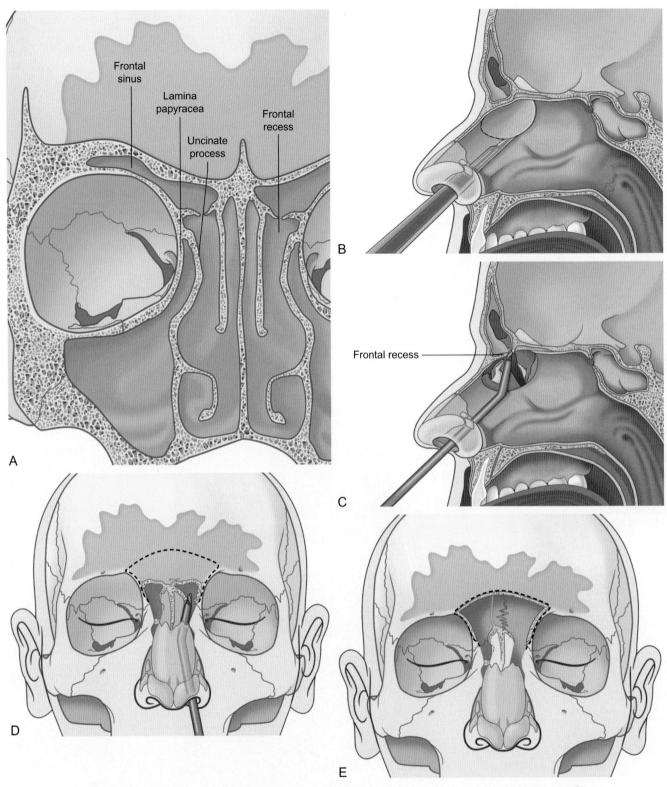

Fig. 1.7.12 (A) Coronal illustration of the anterior ethmoid sinuses, frontal sinus, and anterior skull base. (B) Illustration of an anterior septectomy used to visualize the anterior skull base bilaterally. (C) Illustration of a high-speed diamond bur being used to remove the floor of the frontal sinus. (D) Illustration of a high-speed diamond bur being used to remove the frontal process of the maxilla, identifying the periosteum of the overlying skin. (E) Illustration of completed frontal sinusotomy with the entire frontal sinus floor removed, forming a single common drainage pathway into the nose.

this window should align with the anterior aspect of the middle turbinate. The septal window is lowered until the opposite frontal recess and upper half of the opposing middle turbinate is visible. The septal mucosa is harvested and preserved as it may later be used for mucosal grafting of the exposed bone of the frontal beak.[28] Utilizing a high-speed, angled 4 mm diamond bur, the bone of the septum is removed to identify the floor of the frontal sinus (Fig. 1.7.12C). The posterior limit of this dissection is the first olfactory neuron. The axilla of the middle turbinate (i.e., frontal process of the maxilla) is demucosalized and drilling proceeds from lateral to medial, removing the bone of the axilla and identifying the periosteum of the underlying skin (Fig. 1.7.12D). This marks the lateral limit of the dissection. The floor of the frontal sinus is then removed to create a large horseshoe-shaped neostium. The nasofrontal beak is thinned utilizing a 70 degree bur and 30 degree endoscope. The frontal intersinus septum is partially removed to create a median drainage pathway for the frontal sinus (Fig. 1.7.12E). The exposed bone of the frontal beak may be left bare, dressed with Silastic sheeting, or grafted with septal mucosa harvested from the creation of the septal window.

Coronal Incision

The coronal incision is still considered the "gold standard" for management of significant frontal sinus injuries. However, as less invasive approaches are adopted, it is less commonly used. The approach provides uncompromised access to the anterior table, frontal recess, posterior table, and anterior cranial fossa. The coronal approach can be used for primary fracture repair, as well as treatment of secondary deformities. Unfortunately, it carries a significant risk of iatrogenic sequelae such as alopecia, paresthesias, facial nerve injury, and visible scarring. Therefore this approach is usually reserved for complex injuries requiring open manipulation and hardware application.

The coronal incision is marked out at least 4–6 cm behind the hairline. The hair can be banded and need not be shaved. The incision may be a peaked line (Fig. 1.7.13) or "zig-zag" (Fig. 1.7.14). The zig-zag incision assists with scar camouflage; taking advantage of the hair's inferior alignment which covers the transverse arms of the scar. The scalp is opened in thirds to minimize blood loss. Hemostasis during the initial scalp incision is addressed with limited use of bipolar cautery (minimizing damage to hair follicles), local sutures, or hemostatic clips according to surgeon preference.

An intimate knowledge of the temporal anatomy is required to preserve the temporal branch of the facial nerve, minimize alopecia, and reduce the risk of temporal hollowing (Fig. 1.7.15). If use of the pericranial flap is not required, the pericranium can be incised and elevated along with the scalp in a subperiosteal plane. If a pericranial flap is needed for dural repair or frontal sinus obliteration, the scalp is elevated first; leaving the pericranium on the bone. The pericranium is then elevated as a separate vascularized flap (Fig. 1.7.16). Inferior dissection should identify and preserve the supraorbital and supratrochlear neurovascular pedicles (Fig. 1.7.17). These pedicles may exit from a notch in two-thirds of cases or a foramen in one-third of cases. True foramina can be outfractured with a 2 mm osteotome to free the contents of the foramen and gain access to the orbital roof and medial wall (Fig. 1.7.18).

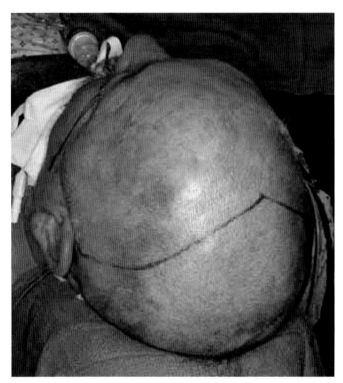

Fig. 1.7.13 Traditional peaked line coronal incision.

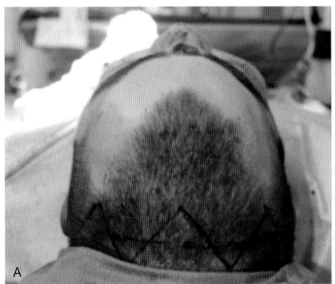

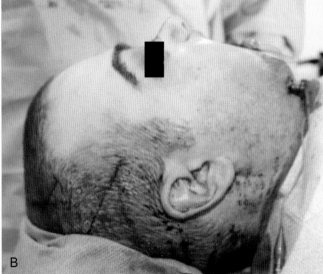

Fig. 1.7.14 "Zig-zag" coronal incision, which hides the horizontal limbs of the scar within hair.

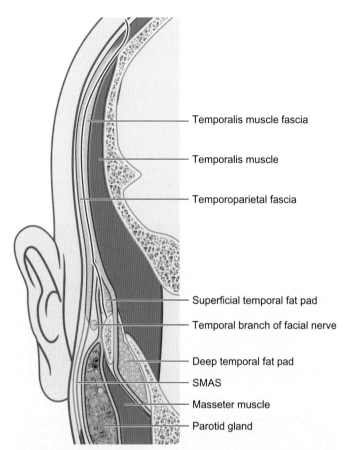

Fig. 1.7.15 Anatomy of the temporal scalp region. The incision plane is shown in red.

- Temporalis muscle fascia
- Temporalis muscle
- Temporoparietal fascia
- Superficial temporal fat pad
- Temporal branch of facial nerve
- Deep temporal fat pad
- SMAS
- Masseter muscle
- Parotid gland

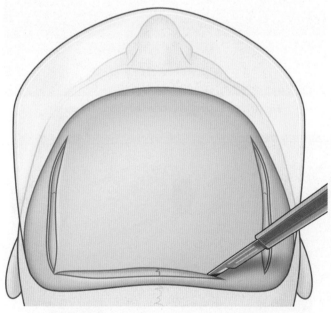

Fig. 1.7.16 Incision to elevate a pericranial flap.

Laterally, the dissection continues below the temporal line, leaving the temporalis muscle fascia (deep temporal fascia) intact. The temporoparietal fascia is carefully elevated to preserve the temporal branch of the facial nerve (Fig. 1.7.15). If the zygomatic arch requires exposure, the superficial layer of the temporalis muscle fascia is incised approximately 2 cm above the arch and the dissection continues between the fascia and the superficial temporal fat pad. This is a dense dissection

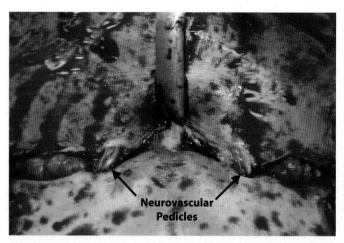

Fig. 1.7.17 Supraorbital rim and neurovascular bundles, after turn-down of coronal flap.

Neurovascular Pedicles

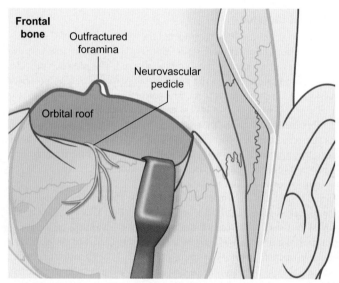

Frontal bone

Outfractured foramina

Neurovascular pedicle

Orbital roof

Fig. 1.7.18 Release of the supratrochelar neurovascular pedicle using an osteotome.

plane that does not elevate easily. Once the zygomatic arch is exposed, the periosteum is incised on the upper border (to protect the temporal branch of the facial nerve) and a periosteal elevator is used to expose the bony arch.

After fracture repair, the closure is performed in layers, suturing and re-suspending the temporal soft tissue layers to prevent postoperative ptosis. The galea aponeurosis is realigned with absorbable suture and the skin is carefully closed with atraumatic technique to prevent alopecia. Drains and a pressure dressing can be used according to surgeon preference.

TREATMENT STRATEGIES

Commonly accepted treatment strategies include: primary repair, secondary camouflage, frontal sinus salvage, obliteration, cranialization, and ablation (Reidel procedure).

Primary Repair
Coronal Incision

While less invasive approaches are preferred when possible, the coronal incision gives unparalleled access for more severe frontal sinus, brain,

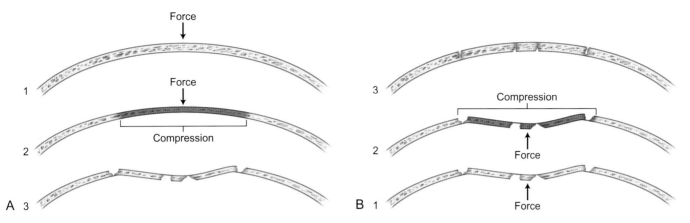

Fig. 1.7.19 (A) Force applied to the convex surface of the frontal bone results in compression of the bone, followed by release and fracture into a concave shape. (B) Reduction of a frontal bone fracture can require significant force to pull the bone segment back through the compression phase and into a convex shape.

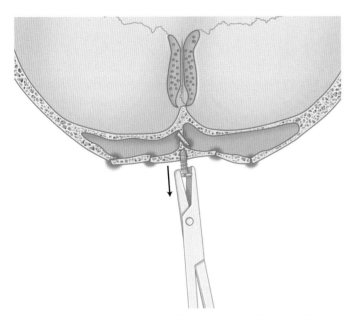

Fig. 1.7.20 A bone screw can be placed to assist with application of a perpendicular force and reduction of the anterior table bone fragments.

and skull base injuries. Even with a coronal incision, fracture reduction can be challenging. When the convex surface of the frontal bone fractures, it goes through a compression phase, before becoming concave (Fig. 1.7.19). Fracture reduction requires enough force to pull the bone fragments back through the compression phase. It may be necessary to remove a bone fragment to release the tension and reduce the fracture. If comminution exists or bone segments overlap, a small bone hook may be insinuated between the fragments to assist with elevation. Another technique is to place a 1.5 mm screw in a depressed segment, grasp the screw with a heavy hemostat, and pull upward (with controlled force) to reduce the bone fragments (Fig. 1.7.20). The majority of bone fragments should be kept in place, allowing for a more accurate repair. If the sinus is opened, a 30 degree endoscope can be placed through a bone defect to inspect the sinus outflow tract. Once the anterior table bone fragments are reduced, 1.0–1.3 mm microplates are used to stabilize the fracture segments. Micromesh can be used to cover any small gaps and reduce the risk of postoperative embossment, which may be visible through the skin.

Direct Percutaneous

Direct percutaneous approaches to the anterior table have been described.[29–31] However, they are technically challenging and hardware application is not possible. This approach has significant risk of failure (≥20%) due to fracture comminution or inability to mobilize the fractured bone.[32,33]

Endoscopic Brow

While open reduction and internal fixation of anterior table fractures via an endoscopic brow approach has been described,[34–36] it is technically challenging. Although hardware can be passed through the working incision, and percutaneous stab incisions can be used for fracture reduction/fixation; the authors feel this approach is most applicable for secondary camouflage techniques that require no fracture manipulation (see "Secondary Camouflage" below).

Direct Forehead/Suprabrow

Direct forehead and suprabrow incisions/lacerations provide less access than a coronal incision; however, they can be adequate for repair of limited appropriately selected anterior alone table fractures. Fracture reduction and hardware application can generally be achieved solely through the incision or laceration.

Upper Blepharoplasty

The upper blepharoplasty incision is extremely well hidden and offers visualization of the inferior frontal bone. Superior and medial visualization is often limited by the skin envelope and supraorbital neurovascular bundle. An endoscope can be helpful to visualize the distal extent of the fracture. Hardware can be inserted through the eyelid incision. Screws can be applied through the eyelid incision or through a percutaneous "stab" incision. The addition of a frontal sinus trephination can provide greater access to both anterior and posterior table fractures. Limited injuries may be amenable to open reduction without fixation.

Endonasal Sinusotomy

Transnasal endoscopic fracture management continues to be studied and is gaining acceptance.[37] Grayson et al.[38] published a series of 46 frontal sinus fractures successfully repaired via an endonasal approach. A Draf IIb approach was used in 80% of patients, with only one patient requiring a revision procedure for stenosis and outflow obstruction. Forty (87%) of these patients had isolated posterior table injuries. However, 5 patients had anterior table fractures and one had a combined anterior and posterior table injury. All anterior table fracture patients had acceptable aesthetic outcomes.

While surgical techniques continue to improve, acute repair of frontal sinus fractures is technically challenging and should be reserved for surgeons with significant endoscopic sinus surgery experience. However, complex fractures of the frontal sinus and sinus outflow tract can be managed effectively with an endoscopic Draf III approach (Fig. 1.7.12).[39,40] The principle advantages of this approach is avoidance of an external incision and the ability to maintain a patent frontal sinus outflow tract that can be followed endoscopically in the clinic.

Transnasal endoscopic treatment of patients with *isolated anterior table* injuries should be carefully considered. The risk of frontal bone contour deformity must be weighed against potential for iatrogenic injury. If observed, many of these patients will require no surgical intervention.[41,42] If there is a deformity after all swelling has resolved, secondary camouflage is a viable option (see below). Primary repair can also be achieved through an upper blepharoplasty or direct approach without the risks of iatrogenic injury to the skull base or postoperative sinusitis secondary to scarring and outflow obstruction.

The use of balloon dilation for treatment of anterior table fractures has also been described.[43,44] While such case reports have been successful, the technique has not gained popularity. The authors feel that the iatrogenic risks associated with this technique (particularly applying pressure to the thin posterior table) far outweigh the potential benefits.

Secondary Camouflage

Secondary camouflage of frontal sinus deformities can be performed using titanium mesh, porous polyethylene sheeting, or a patient-specific implant for camouflage onlay.[45–47] These materials can be placed using a variety of approaches including coronal, direct forehead/suprabrow, upper blepharoplasty, and endoscopic brow depending on the fracture location and surgeon preference. If an endoscopic brow approach is used, the implant of choice is inserted through the working incision, and positioned over the defect (Fig. 1.7.21). A 25-gauge needle can be used to locate the optimal position for a 2 mm, transcutaneous stab incision. This is used to apply a 4–7 mm positioning screw stabilizing the implant (Fig. 1.7.22). If additional stabilization is required, a second screw is applied.

Frontal Sinus Salvage

Injury to the sinus floor, anterior ethmoid region, or sinus ostia may result in scarring and obstruction of the sinus outflow tract.[48–50] Unfortunately, outflow tract obstruction cannot be accurately evaluated in the acute setting. For patients felt to be at lower risk of frontal recess stenosis and obstruction, observation and frontal sinus salvage is an option. The frontal sinus salvage procedure (i.e., endonasal sinusotomy) is performed only in the minority of patients who are found to have stenosis and outflow tract obstruction after healing. The procedure is used to recanalize the frontal recess and aerate the sinus. The rationale for this more conservative approach include: significant improvements in CT imaging over the last 10 years,[51,52] major advances in sinus surgery that allow surgeons to reliably treat the frontal sinus via an endonasal approach, and limiting any surgical intervention to only those patients who have shown they will require it.[53–56]

While there are no prospective studies that evaluate the degree of frontal recess disruption with the risk of long term stenosis, several authors have looked at the overall rate of stenosis after frontal recess injury. In 2002 Smith et al.[57] published the first prospective study evaluating conservative management of frontal recess injuries. They treated 7 patients with anterior table and frontal recess fractures; performing open repair of the anterior table fracture and observing the frontal recess injury. Five patients ultimately had well-aerated sinuses (mean

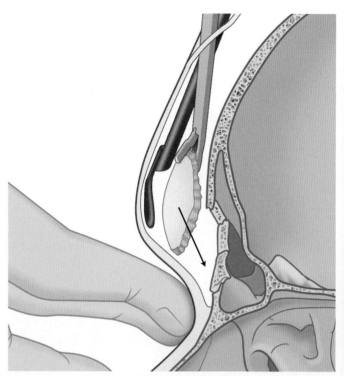

Fig. 1.7.21 Porous polyethylene implant is inserted and placed over the fracture.

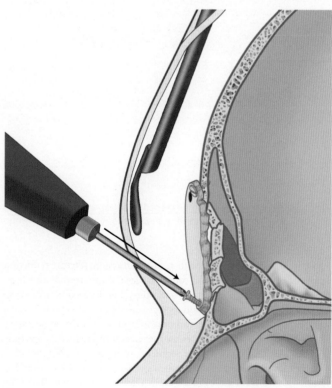

Fig. 1.7.22 A screw is placed through a stab incision and used to stabilize the implant.

follow-up 17 months), while 2 developed frontal sinusitis. After attempts at medical management, both sinusitis patients required an endonasal sinusotomy. The sinusotomies remained aerated at 21 and 25 months, respectively. Emara et al.[54] published a similar study in 2014 evaluating 17 patients with frontal recess injuries. They found 13 patients had well-aerated sinuses and 4 had mild mucosal thickening (mean follow-up 20 months). No opacification was found and no further surgical management was required. Jafari et al.[58] evaluated 8 similar patients and found that 7 of 8 (88%) were aerated at 6 weeks.

It should be emphasized that this "observational" approach to frontal recess injuries is a relatively new paradigm and should be adopted by surgeons who have significant experience in both open and endoscopic frontal sinus surgery. Patients should also be reliable and able to provide long-term follow-up. Irrespective of the course of treatment, patients should be educated about the signs and symptoms of chronic frontal sinusitis and mucocele formation as this can occur many years after treatment.

Frontal Sinus Obliteration

Historically, frontal sinus obliteration has been a mainstay of treatment when the frontal recess is severely disrupted. The endoscopic Draf III, used for both acute repair and secondary salvage, has significantly reduced (and may someday eliminate) the need for obliteration. Sinus obliteration is generally performed through a coronal incision. It requires meticulous removal of all sinus mucosa, obstruction of the outflow tract, and obliteration of the sinus cavity with autologous material (i.e., fat, muscle, fascia, bone, etc.). However, because complete removal of *all* sinus mucosa is extremely challenging, there is a long-term risk of mucocele formation. Patients must therefore be educated about the signs and symptoms of a mucocele formation and have long-term follow-up.

A coronal flap is elevated, the pericranial flap is preserved, and the frontal sinus fracture is identified. Anterior table bone fragments should be carefully removed and kept moist on gauze on a side table. It is helpful to maintain the orientation of the fragments with a drawing (Fig. 1.7.23). The remainder of the anterior table must be removed to visualize the entire sinus cavity. This can be accomplished using several techniques. Historically a "6-foot penny Caldwell" X-ray was obtained and placed directly onto the patient's frontal bone to outline the sinus. Current techniques include: (1) intraoperative navigation, which requires a thin cut CT and intraoperative registration; (2) transillumination (Fig. 1.7.24); and (3) mechanical palpation (Fig. 1.7.25) – in which one tine of a bipolar cautery is placed through the anterior table defect and "walked" around the internal periphery of the sinus. The outer tine is then visualized externally and used to mark the outline of the sinus on the frontal bone. Regardless of the method, the outline of the anterior table is then pre-plated with 2–3 microplates (1.0–1.3 mm) that span the planned osteotomy cuts (Fig. 1.7.26). All but one screw is removed from each plate. They are left in the surgical field, but rotated superiorly away from the osteotomy line (Fig. 1.7.27). The frontal sinus osteotomy is then performed using a side cutting bur (Midas Rex B-1, Medtronic Inc., Minneapolis MI) to "postage stamp" small holes at the periphery of the sinus (Fig. 1.7.28), angling the drill internally to avoid intracranial violation (Fig. 1.7.29). A protective footplate is then applied, and the side cutting bur is used to join the perforations and complete the osteotomy (Fig. 1.7.30). The orbital rims and glabellar regions are osteotomized approximately 5 mm superior to the junction of the nasal bones. Finally, the intersinus septum is osteotomized and the remaining anterior table bone is removed.

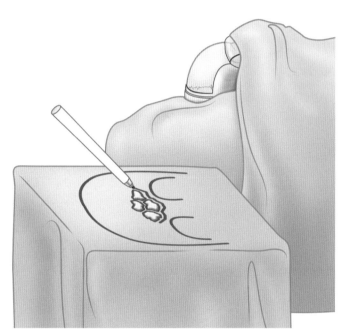

Fig. 1.7.23 An illustration can be used to orient bone fragments that are removed from the fractures site, thus assuring an accurate placement at the end of the procedure.

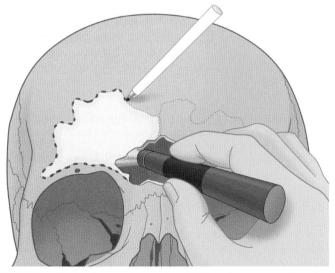

Fig. 1.7.24 Transillumination can be used to highlight the margin of the sinus.

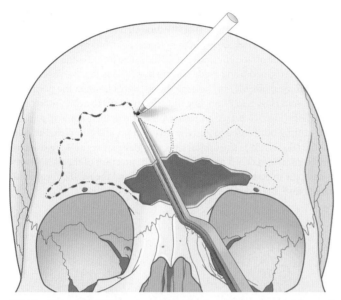

Fig. 1.7.25 A bipolar cautery can be used to outline the periphery of the sinus. One tine is placed on each side of the anterior table and the outer tine is used to mark the distal aspect of the sinus.

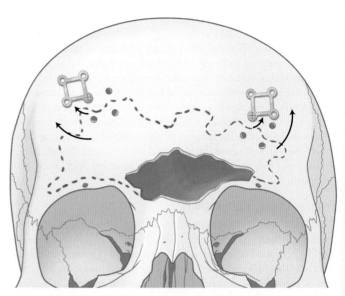

Fig. 1.7.27 Microplates need not be removed to perform the frontal sinusotomy, but can be rotated superiorly and left in place until the bone flap is replaced.

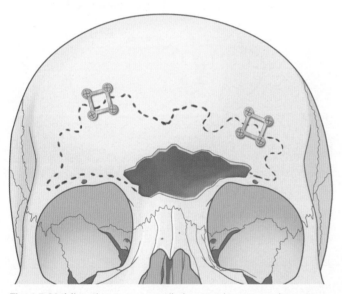

Fig. 1.7.26 Microplates are preapplied across the proposed osteotomy site, thus maintaining the precise location of the bone flap once the procedure is complete.

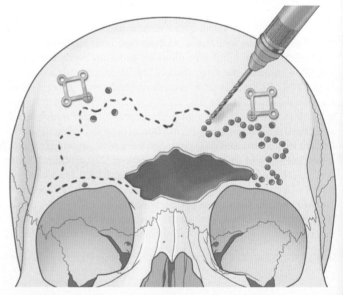

Fig. 1.7.28 A drill can be used to place perforations along the osteotomy line. This allows the surgeon to "feel" the drill pass through the out-table bone, assuring that the osteotomy line is accurate.

Once the entire sinus is exposed, all sinus mucosa is meticulously removed using a 1–6 mm diamond bur with irrigation. Particular attention is paid to the supraorbital and lateral sinus recesses, as well as the posterior surface of the anterior table. The frontal recess mucosa is elevated and inverted into the ostia, thereby occluding the frontal recess. Temporalis muscle fascia can be placed in the infundibulum, followed by placement of an outer table bone graft to hold it in place. The bone graft can be rigidly fixated if necessary. The remainder of the frontal sinus is filled with autologous material according to surgeon preference (fat, cancellous bone, muscle, pericranium, or spontaneous osteoneogenesis with auto-obliteration).[7,59] If abdominal fat is used the graft is harvested as a single piece with minimal electrocautery. Finally, the anterior table fragments are meticulously replaced to reconstruct the premorbid frontal contour.

Frontal Sinus Cranialization

Cranialization of the frontal sinus is performed when the posterior table bone is severely disrupted or needs to be removed for control of CSF leak. A formal craniotomy is not necessary as the procedure can be performed through the sinus cavity. However, neurosurgical assistance is strongly recommended. After elevation of the coronal flap the frontal sinus is completely exposed by removing all free bone fragments from the anterior and posterior tables. The sinus fragments are drilled free of mucosa, and oriented on a side table using an illustration (Fig. 1.7.23).

It is important to maintain the integrity of the pericranial flap. It can be used for dural repair and control of CSF leak. Posterior table fragments that are adherent to the dura are freed with a Penfield elevator. The dura is inspected for tears and then elevated behind stable bone at the periphery of the sinus. Malleable retractors are used to protect the brain and Kerrison rongeurs or a drill can be used to make the sinus cavity flush with the anterior cranial fossa (Fig. 1.7.31).

Lacerations of the dura can be repaired with interrupted 5-0 nylon sutures in combination with the neurosurgical team. Dural graft material is sometimes necessary. Each frontal sinus infundibulum is occluded as described under "sinus obliteration" and the pericranial flap can then be used to cover the frontal recess, fill dead space, and/or repair dural tears (Fig. 1.7.32). Anterior table bone fragments are then used to reconstruct the anterior table using microplates. If a pericranial flap remains pedicled, a small bony defect or kerf must be fashioned in the anterior table to allow passage of the pericranial flap without cutting off its blood supply (Fig. 1.7.32 inset). Micromesh can be helpful to smooth any bony irregularities or defects. The use of antibiotics after dural

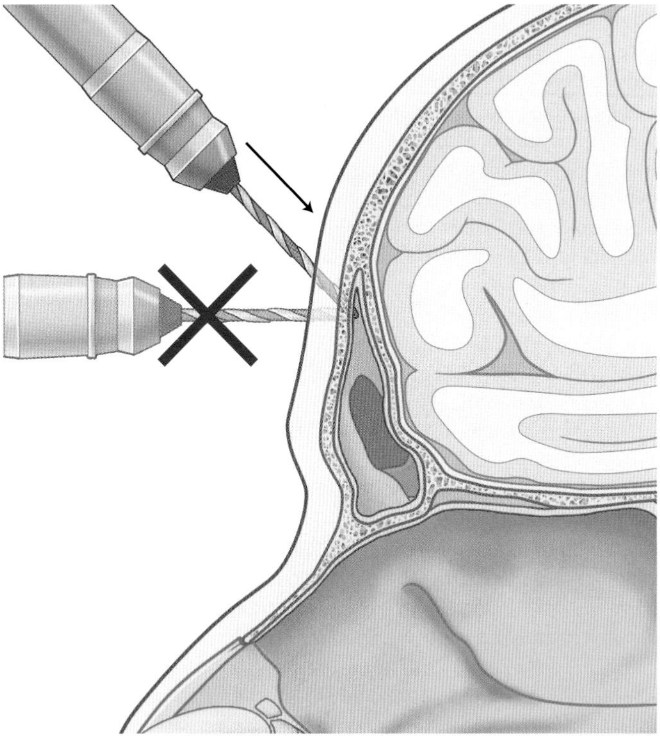

Fig. 1.7.29 The drill should be angled toward the sinus cavity to avoid intracranial penetration.

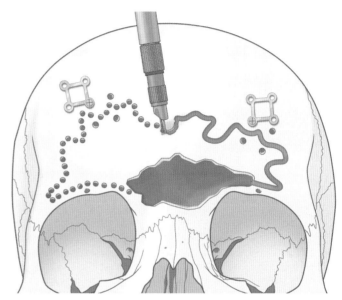

Fig. 1.7.30 A side cutting drill can then be used to join the perforations and complete the osteotomy.

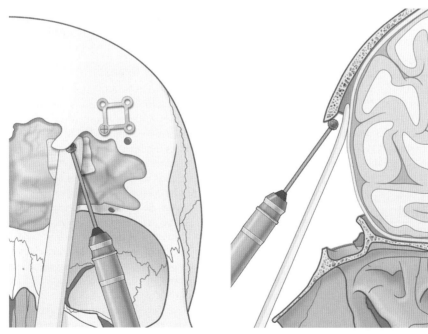

Fig. 1.7.31 A brain retractor can be used to protect the dura while the posterior table bone is drilled flush with the sinus walls, floor, and anterior cranial fossa.

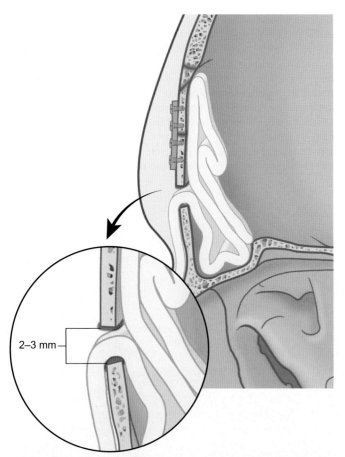

Fig. 1.7.32 The pericranial flap can be used for dural repair and coverage of the frontal recess. When inserting the pericranial flap, a small defect should be fashioned in the anterior table bone to allow passage of the pericranial flap intracranially without cutting off the blood supply.

disruption remains controversial and they are used according to surgeon preference; however, there is no conclusive evidence that antibiotics decrease the risk of meningitis in the setting of traumatic CSF leaks.[60]

Ablation

Frontal sinus ablation (i.e., "Reidel procedure) is used for management of severe frontal bone osteomyelitis.[61] The anterior table and a portion of the orbital rims are removed through a coronal incision, eliminating the infected bone and the potential space.[62,63] This results in a significant cosmetic deformity that is repaired in a second stage 6–12 months later. Patient-specific implants are often used for reconstruction. These can be fabricated from porous polyethylene, Polyetheretherketone, or other biocompatible alloplasts. Free tissue transfer may be required in more extreme settings.[64]

TREATMENT ALGORITHM

Selecting an appropriate treatment strategy involves intimate knowledge of the patient, the deformity, and the risk/benefit of the various surgical approaches. While maintaining a functional frontal sinus is optimal, it may not always be possible. However, it is imperative to create a "safe" sinus. This will reduce the risk of long-term sequelae. Optimal treatment strategy can be determined by evaluating the structural integrity of three anatomical parameters: (1) anterior table, (2) frontal recess, and (3) posterior table/dura. These findings can then be applied to the treatment algorithm presented in Fig. 1.7.33).

Anterior Table Fractures

While anterior table fractures can result in aesthetic deformities, most surgeons believe there is little risk of mucocele formation.[41,65,66] Anterior table fractures are categorized into three groups: *mild*, *moderate*, and *severe*.

Mild (≤4 mm displacement): Following an anterior table frontal bone fracture, facial swelling usually obscures the deformity. Patients cannot make an informed decision about the risk–benefit of surgery until after the edema has resolved. Fortunately, mild fractures can be observed with little risk of aesthetic deformity. Della Torre et al.[42] reported that only 4 of 96 patients treated conservatively for frontal sinus fractures had long-term external deformities, none of which opted for secondary surgical treatment. Kim et al.[67] evaluated a series of anterior table fractures treated nonoperatively and assessed the frequency of external deformity. Patients with computed tomography "step offs" that were less than 4 mm had no incidence of long-term external deformity. If the patient is seen acutely and a delayed repair is planned, the rationale and indications for such an approach must be discussed (i.e., risk of iatrogenic injury may be greater than the traumatic deformity itself). The patient must also understand that the fracture cannot be reduced once it has healed; a camouflage technique would be required (see "Secondary Camouflage" above).

Moderate (4–6 mm displacement and moderate fracture area with mild comminution): Moderate fractures present little risk of mucocele formation; however, the risk of an aesthetic deformity increases with the degree of fracture displacement. These fractures encompass a disparate group of injuries with many different treatment options, and little evidence to indicate the optimal approach. *Primary repair* should be considered for injuries with: (1) large lacerations which provide direct access, (2) inferior fractures that are accessible via an upper blepharoplasty approach, (3) patients with deep rhytids for whom a direct brow incision is appropriate, and (4) patients who may have limited follow-up. *Secondary camouflage* should be considered for moderate fractures where the sequelae of surgical access may outweigh the benefit of primary repair. This allows the swelling to resolve and the patient can make an informed decision about the risks and benefits of surgery.

Severe (>6 mm displacement, large fracture area with severe comminution): Severe fractures present a higher risk of external deformity. These injuries are generally managed acutely with primary repair.[6,41,58]

Nasofrontal Recess

Bony displacement and comminution of the nasofrontal recess can result in outflow obstruction and mucocele formation. The authors group these injuries into two major categories: (1) *mild to moderate* displacement/comminution – which ranges from nondisplaced fractures to injuries resulting in narrowing of the frontal recess without obstructing the lumen and (2) *severe* displacement/comminution – which include injuries that result in complete collapse of the frontal recess.

Mild to moderate: Patients with mild to moderate nasofrontal recess injuries can be observed and treated with medical management (nasal steroid and irrigations). A CT scan is repeated at approximately 6 weeks and 12 months. If the sinus remains aerated, continued observation is appropriate. If the patient has minimal symptoms and mild mucosal thickening, medical management should be continued. Progression of symptoms or sinus opacification is an indication for endonasal sinusotomy.

Severe: Severe nasofrontal recess injuries are a poor prognostic sign for long-term aeration of the sinus. While there are no prospective studies assessing long-term patency after such injuries, it is assumed that the vast majority of these patients will scar and occlude without

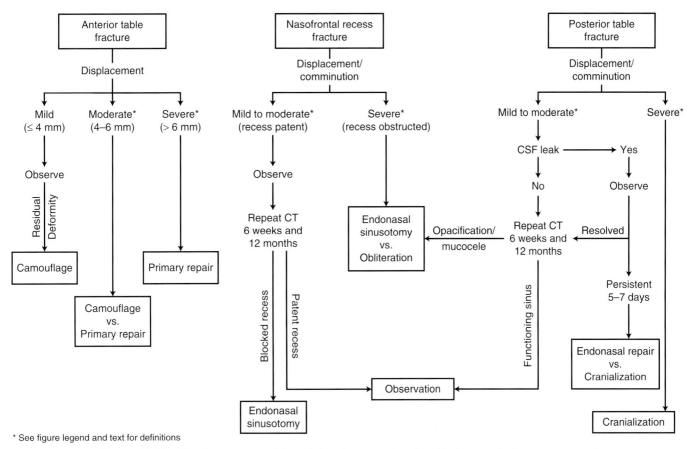

* See figure legend and text for definitions

Fig. 1.7.33 Algorithm for treatment of frontal sinus fractures. Anterior table fracture displacement grouped as (1) mild (<4 mm), (2) moderate (4–6 mm), (3) severe (>6 mm). Nasofrontal recess injuries grouped as (1) mild/moderate (injuries resulting in narrowing of the frontal recess without obstructing the lumen) and (2) severe (injuries that result in collapse of the frontal recess). Posterior table fractures are grouped as (1) mild/moderate (includes fractures with up to 4 mm of displcement, small amounts of intracranial air, and mild to moderate communution) and (2) severe (includes fractures with > 4 mm of displacement, involvment of large areas of the posterior table, significant pneumocephalus, as well as dural disruption and CSF rhinorrhea).

surgical intervention. To avoid the long-term risk of mucocele formation, an endonasal sinusotomy and maintenance of the sinus cavity is the preferred treatment. However, if this is not technically feasible for the surgeon, a sinus obliteration would be required.

Posterior Table Fractures

Posterior table injury is poorly defined in the literature. Previous authors have attempted to describe the degree of posterior table displacement as an indication of the severity of injury; assuming that greater displacement would correlate with increased risk of postoperative complications. "Significant disruption" has been defined as "greater than 2 mm"[6] or "greater than one table width."[4] The lack of prospective data analyzing these injuries offers little direction, however any surgical intervention must be weighed against the risk of long-term complications such as CSF leak, meningitis, and mucocele formation.[7,55,56]

As with frontal recess fractures, many surgeons are now taking a more conservative approach to management of these injuries. The authors group these injuries into two major categories: (1) *mild to moderate* displacement/comminution – ranges from nondisplaced fractures to injuries with displacement up to 3–4 mm, small amounts of intracranial air, and mild to moderate posterior table comminution, and (2) *severe* displacement/comminution – includes injuries with >4 mm of displacement involving large areas of the posterior table, severe pneumocephalus,

and clear dural disruption with CSF rhinorrhea. These severe posterior table fractures break down the barrier between the sinus and anterior cranial fossa resulting in a higher risk of meningitis and long-term morbidity.[7]

Mild to moderate: If there is no CSF leak and there are no other injuries that would require surgical intervention (i.e., intracranial bleeding, severe frontal recess involvement, etc.), patients can be observed and treated with medical management. A CT scan is repeated at 6 weeks and 12 months. If the sinus remains aerated, continued observation is appropriate. If the patient has minimal symptoms and mild mucosal thickening, medical management should be continued. Progression of symptoms, sinus opacification, or mucocele formation are indications for surgical management. Maintaining the sinus cavity with an endonasal sinusotomy is the preferred treatment. If this is not technically feasible for the surgeon, an obliteration would be required.

Patients noted to have a CSF leak should be observed for approximately 5–7 days, as the majority of leaks will resolve spontaneously.[8] If the leak does not resolve, surgical treatment is indicated. This can be accomplished via an endonasal sinusotomy and repair or sinus cranialization depending on surgeon preference. If an endonasal approach is selected, careful preoperative assessment of the frontal sinus anatomy is performed. Midline injuries are most accessible, while far lateral injuries may require the addition of an upper blepharoplasty incision and lateral sinusotomy for adequate instrumentation.[21]

Severe: Severe posterior table fractures may not be amenable to endoscopic or other minimally invasive treatment. In these cases, definitive treatment of the sinus is via a coronal incision and cranialization.

COMPLICATIONS AND LONG-TERM FOLLOW UP

Short-term complications may include wound infection, facial nerve injury, supraorbital/supratrochlear nerve injury, and contour irregularities. First-generation cephalosporins are used in the perioperative setting. Prophylactic postoperative antibiotics (even in the presence of dural injury) are controversial. Postoperative wound infections are managed with culture-directed antibiotics and local wound care. Facial nerve paresis or paralysis should be documented and monitored. If the paresis appears permanent, contralateral chemodenervation can be performed to improve symmetry. Sensory deficits related to the supraorbital and supratrochlear nerves should be observed, as the majority will resolve over time. Contour irregularities related to hardware or bone defects should be observed for a matter of months to allow delineation of the full deformity. While larger incisions can be used for revision, minimally invasive or endoscopic approaches are often adequate for hardware removal or contour camouflage.

Long-term complications may include sinusitis, mucocele, and mucopyocele. These can occur months to years after treatment. It is imperative that patients are educated about signs/symptoms of these complications including mucopurulent nasal drainage, nasal obstruction, headache, and progressive orbitofacial deformity. Common symptoms of meningitis should also be discussed (i.e., fever, chills, sweats, stiff neck, photophobia, etc.). Follow-up CT scans in the acute setting are indicated as discussed above while long-term CT follow-up is generally reserved for symptomatic patients.

EXPERT COMMENTARY

Frontal sinus fracture management is controversial. There is always the question of how much to do and how to do it. Consulting large series in the literature documenting traditional approaches is extremely helpful [1–3]. The more recently described endoscopic approaches have the potential to reduce morbidity and maintain sinus function.

It is useful to divide fractures into those that involve the anterior table, posterior table, or both; as well as the amount of displacement involving each [4]. Evaluation of the nasofrontal duct is also critical. A higher-risk group of patients are those with posterior table disruption, cerebrospinal fluid (CSF) leak, and severe frontal recess injury. They have a higher incidence of infection due to their transgression of the sinuses and penetration of the CSF and brain. More aggressive management is indicated in this patient population. Finally, Rodriguez et al. [1] have defined a single step "salvage operation" to treat severely infected frontal sinuses using free tissue transfer.

References
1. Rodriguez ED, Stanwix MG, Nam AJ, et al. Twenty-six-year experience treating frontal sinus fractures: a novel algorithm based on anatomical fracture pattern and failure of conventional techniques. *Plast Reconstr Surg.* 2008;122(6):1850–1866.
2. Manson PN, Stanwix M, Yaremchuk M, et al. Frontobasilar fractures: anatomy, classification and clinical significance. *Plast Reconstr Surg.* 2009;124:2096–2106.
3. Rodriguez ED, Stanwix MG, Nam AJ, et al. Definitive treatment of persistent frontal sinus infections: elimination of dead space and sinonasal communication. *Plast Reconstr Surg.* 2009;123(3):957–967.
4. Stanwix MG, Nam AJ, Manson PN, et al. Computed tomographic diagnostic criteria for frontal sinus fractures. *J Oral Maxillofac Surg.* 2010;68(11):2714–2722.

REFERENCES

1. Nahum AM. The biomechanics of maxillofacial trauma. *Clin Plast Surg.* 1975;2(1):59–64.
2. Strong EB, Pahlavan N, Saito D. Frontal sinus fractures: a 28-year retrospective review. *Otolaryngol Head Neck Surg.* 2006;135(5):774–779.
3. Rontal ML. State of the art in craniomaxillofacial trauma: frontal sinus. *Curr Opin Otolaryngol Head Neck Surg.* 2008;16(4):381–386.
4. McGraw-Wall B. Frontal sinus fractures. *Facial Plast Surg.* 1998;14(1):59–66.
5. Rohrich RJ, Hollier LH. Management of frontal sinus fractures: changing concepts. *Clin Plast Surg.* 1992;19(1):219–232.
6. Papel ID. *Facial plastic and reconstructive surgery.* 3rd ed. New York: Thieme; 2009.
7. Wallis A, Donald PJ. Frontal sinus fractures: a review of 72 cases. *Laryngoscope.* 1988;98(6 Pt 1):593–598.
8. Phang SY, Whitehouse K, Lee L, et al. Management of CSF leak in base of skull fractures in adults. *B J Neurosurg.* 2016;1–9.
9. Warnecke A, Averbeck T, Wurster U, et al. Diagnostic relevance of beta2-transferrin for the detection of cerebrospinal fluid fistulas. *Arch Otolaryngol Head Neck Surg.* 2004;130:1178–1184.
10. Meco C, Oberascher G, Arrer E, et al. Beta-trace protein test: new guidelines for the reliable diagnosis of cerebrospinal fluid fistula. *Otolaryngol Head Neck Surg.* 2003;129:508–517.
11. Kim KS, Kim ES, Hwang JH, Lee SY. Transcutaneous transfrontal approach through a small peri-eyebrow incision for the reduction of closed anterior table frontal sinus fractures. *J Plast Reconstr Aesthetic Surg.* 2010;63:763–768.
12. Yoo A, Eun SC, Baek RM. Transcutaneous reduction of frontal sinus fracture using bony tapper device. *J Craniofac Surg.* 2012;23:1835–1837.
13. Kim NH, Kang SJ. A simple aesthetic approach for correction of frontal sinus fracture. *J Craniofac Surg.* 2014;25:544–546.
14. Perenack JD. The endoscopic brow lift. *Atlas Oral Maxillofac Surg Clin North Am.* 2016;24:165–173.
15. Drolet BC, Phillips BZ, Hoy EA, et al. Finesse in forehead and brow rejuvenation: modern concepts, including endoscopic methods. *Plast Reconstr Surg.* 2014;134:1141–1150.
16. Graham HD III, Spring P. Endoscopic repair of frontal sinus fracture: case report. *J Craniomaxillofac Trauma.* 1996;2(4):52–55.
17. Strong EB, Kellman RM. Endoscopic repair of anterior table–frontal sinus fractures. *Facial Plast Surg Clin North Am.* 2006;14(1):25–29.
18. Lappert PW, Lee JW. Treatment of an isolated outer table frontal sinus fracture using endoscopic reduction and fixation. *Plast Reconstr Surg.* 1998;102(5):1642–1645.
19. Lee Y, Choi HG, Shin DH, et al. Subbrow approach as a minimally invasive reduction technique in the management of frontal sinus fractures. *Arch Plast Surg.* 2014;41:679–685.
20. Noury M, Dunn RM, Lalikos JF, et al. Frontal sinus repair through a frontalis rhytid approach. *Ann Plast Surg.* 2011;66:457–459.
21. Knipe TA, Gandhi PD, Fleming JC, Chandra RK. Transblepharoplasty approach to sequestered disease of the lateral frontal sinus with ophthalmologic manifestations. *Am J Rhinol.* 2007;21:100–104.
22. Chu EA, Quinones-Hinojosa A, Boahene KD. Trans-blepharoplasty orbitofrontal craniotomy for repair of lateral and posterior frontal sinus cerebrospinal fluid leak. *Otolaryngol Head Neck Surg.* 2010;142:906–908.
23. Bly RA, Morton RP, Kim LJ, Moe KS. Tension pneumocephalus after endoscopic sinus surgery: a technical report of multiportal endoscopic skull base repair. *Otolaryngol Head Neck Surg.* 2014;151:1081–1083.
24. Ramakrishna R, Kim LJ, Bly RA, et al. Transorbital neuroendoscopic surgery for the treatment of skull base lesions. *J Clin Neurosci.* 2016;24:99–104.
25. Moe KS, Kim LJ, Bergeron CM. Transorbital endoscopic repair of cerebrospinal fluid leaks. *Laryngoscope.* 2011;121:13–30.
26. Matsuzaki K, Enomoto S, Aoki T. Treatment of orbital roof blow-up fracture using a superior blepharoplasty incision. *Orbit.* 2015;34:166–171.
27. Weber R, Draf W, Kratzsch B, et al. Modern concepts of frontal sinus surgery. *Laryngoscope.* 2001;111:137–146.

28. Illing EA, Woodworth BA. Management of frontal sinus cerebrospinal fluid leaks and encephaloceles. *Otolaryngol Clin North Am.* 2016;49:1035–1050.

29. Kim KS, Kim ES, Hwang JH, Lee SY. Transcutaneous transfrontal approach through a small peri-eyebrow incision for the reduction of closed anterior table frontal sinus fractures. *J Plast Reconstr Aesthetic Surg.* 2010;63:763–768.

30. Yoo A, Eun SC, Baek RM. Transcutaneous reduction of frontal sinus fracture using bony tapper device. *J Craniofac Surg.* 2012;23:1835–1837.

31. Kim NH, Kang SJ. A simple aesthetic approach for correction of frontal sinus fracture. *J Craniofac Surg.* 2014;25:544–546.

32. Spinelli G, Lazzeri D, Arcuri F, Agostini T. Closed reduction of the isolated anterior frontal sinus fracture via percutaneous screw placement. *Int J Oral Maxillofac Surg.* 2015;44:79–82.

33. Strong EB, Buchalter GM, Moulthrop TH. Endoscopic repair of isolated anterior table frontal sinus fractures. *Arch Facial Plast Surg.* 2003;5:514–521.

34. Egemen O, Ozkaya O, Aksan T, et al. Endoscopic repair of isolated anterior table frontal sinus fractures without fixation. *J Craniofac Surg.* 2013;24:1357–1360.

35. Graham HD 3rd, Spring P. Endoscopic repair of frontal sinus fracture: case report. *J Craniomaxillofac Trauma.* 1996;2:52–55.

36. Mensink G, Zweers A, van Merkesteyn JP. Endoscopically assisted reduction of anterior table frontal sinus fractures. *J Craniomaxillofac Surg.* 2009;37:225–228.

37. Steiger JD, Chiu AG, Francis DO, Palmer JN. Endoscopic-assisted reduction of anterior table frontal sinus fractures. *Laryngoscope.* 2006;116:1978–1981.

38. Grayson JS, Jeyarajan H, Illing EA, et al. Changing the surgical dogma in frontal sinus trauma: transnasal endoscopic repair. *Int Forum Allergy Rhinol.* 2017;109.

39. Gross CW, Harrison SE. The modified Lothrop procedure: indications, results, and complications. *Otolaryngol Clin North Am.* 2001;34:133–137.

40. Hajbeygi M, Nadjafi A, Amali A, Saedi B. Sadrehosseini SM. Frontal sinus patency after extended frontal sinusotomy Type III. *Iran J Otorhinolaryngol.* 2016;28:337–343.

41. Kim DW, Yoon ES, Lee BI, et al. Fracture depth and delayed contour deformity in frontal sinus anterior wall fracture. *J Craniofac Surg.* 2012;23:991–994.

42. Della Torre D, Burtscher D, Kloss-Brandstatter A, et al. Management of frontal sinus fractures – treatment decision based on metric dislocation extent. *J Craniomaxillofac Surg.* 2014;42:1515–1519.

43. Yoo MH, Kim JS, Song HM, et al. Endoscopic transnasal reduction of an anterior table frontal sinus fracture: technical note. *Int J Oral Maxillofac Surg.* 2008;37:573–575.

44. Hueman K, Eller R. Reduction of anterior frontal sinus fracture involving the frontal outflow tract using balloon sinuplasty. *Otolaryngol Head Neck Surg.* 2008;139:170–171.

45. Kim KK, Mueller R, Huang F, Strong EB. Endoscopic repair of anterior table: frontal sinus fractures with a Medpor implant. *Otolaryngol Head Neck Surg.* 2007;136:568–572.

46. Strong EB, Kellman RM. Endoscopic repair of anterior table–frontal sinus fractures. *Facial Plast Surg Clin North Am.* 2006;14:25–29.

47. Arcuri F, Baragiotta N, Poglio G, Benech A. Post-traumatic deformity of the anterior frontal table managed by the placement of a titanium mesh via an endoscopic approach. *Br J Oral Maxillofac Surg.* 2012;50:e53–e54.

48. Harris L, Marano GD, McCorkle D. Nasofrontal duct: CT in frontal sinus trauma. *Radiology.* 1987;165:195–198.

49. Heller EM, Jacobs JB, Holliday RA. Evaluation of the frontonasal duct in frontal sinus fractures. *Head Neck.* 1989;11:46–50.

50. Landsberg R, Friedman M. A computer-assisted anatomical study of the nasofrontal region. *Laryngoscope.* 2001;111:2125–2130.

51. Landsberg R, Friedman M. A computer-assisted anatomical study of the nasofrontal region. *Laryngoscope.* 2001;111:2125–2130.

52. Mahmutoglu AS, Celebi I. Akdana Bet al. Computed tomographic analysis of frontal sinus drainage pathway variations and frontal rhinosinusitis. *J Craniofac Surg.* 2015;26:87–90.

53. Illing EA, Woodworth BA. Management of frontal sinus cerebrospinal fluid leaks and encephaloceles. *Otolaryngol Clin North Am.* 2016;49:1035–1050.

54. Conger BT Jr, Illing E, Bush B, Woodworth BA. Management of lateral frontal sinus pathology in the endoscopic era. *Otolaryngol Head Neck Surg.* 2014;151:159–163.

55. Emara TA, Elnashar IS, Omara TA, et al. Frontal sinus fractures with suspected outflow tract obstruction: a new approach for sinus preservation. *J Craniomaxillofac Surg.* 2015;43:1–6.

56. Freeman JL, Winston KR. Breach of posterior wall of frontal sinus: management with preservation of the sinus. *World Neurosurg.* 2015;83:1080–1089.

57. Smith TL, Han JK, Loehrl TA, Rhee JS. Endoscopic management of the frontal recess in frontal sinus fractures: a shift in the paradigm? *Laryngoscope.* 2002;112:784–790.

58. Jafari A, Nuyen BA, Salinas CR, et al. Spontaneous ventilation of the frontal sinus after fractures involving the frontal recess. *Am J Otolaryngol.* 2015;36:837–842.

59. Rodriguez ED, Stanwix MG, Nam AJ, et al. Twenty-six-year experience treating frontal sinus fractures: a novel algorithm based on anatomical fracture pattern and failure of conventional techniques. *Plast Reconstr Surg.* 2008;122(6):1850–1866.

60. Ratilal BO, Costa J, Pappamikail L, Sampaio C. Antibiotic prophylaxis for preventing meningitis in patients with basilar skull fractures. *Cochrane Database Syst Rev.* 2015;(4):CD004884.

61. Raghavan U, Jones NS. The place of Riedel's procedure in contemporary sinus surgery. *J Laryngol Otol.* 2004;118:700–705.

62. Mohr RM, Nelson LR. Frontal sinus ablation for frontal osteomyelitis. *Laryngoscope.* 1982;92:1006–1015.

63. Olson NR. Frontal sinus ablation. *Arch Otolaryngol Chicago, Ill.: 1960).* 1982;108:749.

64. Rodriguez ED, Stanwix MG, Nam AJ, et al. Definitive treatment of persistent frontal sinus infections: elimination of dead space and sinonasal communication. *Plast Reconstr Surg.* 2009;123(3):957–967.

65. Delaney SW. Treatment strategies for frontal sinus anterior table fractures and contour deformities. *J Plast Reconstr Aesthetic Surg.* 2016;69:1037–1045.

66. Egemen O, Ozkaya O, Aksan T, et al. Endoscopic repair of isolated anterior table frontal sinus fractures without fixation. *J Craniofac Surg.* 2013;24:1357–1360.

67. Kim DW, Yoon ES, Lee BI, et al. Fracture depth and delayed contour deformity in frontal sinus anterior wall fracture. *J Craniofac Surg.* 2012;23:991–994.

Endoscopic Approaches to Frontal and Maxillary Sinus Fractures

Christopher R. Roxbury, Kofi D.O. Boahene, Bradford A. Woodworth, Douglas D. Reh

BACKGROUND

The paranasal sinuses are aerated spaces in the middle and upper third of the face that develop during the first and second decades of life in the frontal, ethmoid, maxillary, and sphenoid bones. The theoretical role of these structures in facial trauma is to provide shock absorption and dispersal of forces in order to prevent more severe injuries to critical anatomical structures such as the brain and eyes.[1,2]

The frontal sinuses, located in the frontal bone, are paired cavities that are present at birth in only 12% of neonates.[3] These sinuses typically form their adult shape by age 12, and continue to fully aerate into early adulthood.[4] Due to protection from thick cortical bone anteriorly, the frontal sinus is least likely to sustain a fracture, accounting for 5%–15% of all maxillofacial injuries.[1,5] As a result, frontal sinus fractures typically result from high-impact mechanisms, such as motor vehicle collisions and assault.[6] These fractures are typically classified by their location, and may involve the anterior table or outer wall of the frontal sinus, the posterior table or inner wall of the frontal sinus, or both. Disruption of the inferior portion of the frontal sinus may compromise the frontal sinus outflow tract or frontal recess. As a result, long-term sequelae of these fractures may include chronic frontal sinusitis, mucocele, mucopyocele, and intracranial complications.

The maxillary sinuses are paired cavities in the maxilla that are located inferior to the orbits bilaterally. They are the largest sinuses present at birth, and aerate in an inferolateral direction to extend laterally to the zygomatic recess and inferiorly to the level of the nasal floor by age 12.[3] While the majority of maxillary sinus fractures are inconsequential and do not require surgical repair, the maxillary sinus roof is the orbital floor, and fractures in this region may result in orbital injury.

Traditional open surgical approaches to the mid- and upper face have been extensively described in the literature and provide good access to fractures in this region. Traditional approaches to the frontal sinus included osteoplastic flaps or sinus obliteration via a bicoronal incision[5–9] as well as cranialization.[6,10–12] Open approaches to the orbital floor included transconjunctival and transcaruncular approaches.[13–18]

With advances in nasal endoscopy and endoscopic instrumentation, less invasive approaches to these fractures are now feasible. While these approaches may offer a less invasive means to manage frontal and orbital floor fractures, evidence to date is limited to case reports and case series. Moreover, long-term outcomes in these patients have yet to be established. Regardless, a growing body of evidence suggests that endoscopic approaches have acceptable safety and efficacy, and represent a promising means to manage these injuries with decreased morbidity and better cosmesis than traditional approaches.[19–24] These endoscopic approaches will be discussed further in this chapter.

SURGICAL ANATOMY

The frontal sinuses are paired sinuses present in the frontal bone separated by a variable intersinus septum. The anterior table of the frontal sinus is the bone just deep to the skin and subcutaneous tissue of the brow. The posterior table of the frontal sinus is the bone just anterior to the dura mater of the frontal lobe. The anterior table (4–12 mm) is significantly thicker than the posterior table (0.1–4.8 mm).[1] The anatomy of the frontal sinus and frontal recess, which is shaped like an inverted funnel, is highly variable.[25–28] The anteroposterior (A-P) distance of the frontal recess is perhaps the most important anatomical consideration, with a distance of at least 5 mm required in order to adequately instrument the area endoscopically.[29] When considering endoscopic approaches it is important to understand that the frontal recess is bordered laterally by the lamina papyracea of the orbit, medially by the vertical lamella of the middle turbinate, and lateral lamella of the cribriform plate, anteriorly by the frontal beak, and posteriorly by the posterior table and anterior skull base. The configuration of the frontal recess is highly variable, and may be restricted by ethmoid pneumatization. Pneumatization anteriorly is typically by agger nasi or supra-agger nasi cells, which may extend into the frontal sinus itself. Pneumatization posteriorly is typically by air cells superior to the bulla ethmoidalis, or suprabullar cells. These suprabullar cells may also extend superiorly into the frontal sinus and laterally above the orbit. Finally, frontal septal cells are anterior ethmoid cells that pneumatize medially and may be contiguous with the frontal sinus septum, pushing the frontal drainage pathway laterally.[30] These cells may also be described as types 1–4 frontal cells.[25–28] A computed tomography (CT) of the sinuses showing frontal recess anatomy is provided (Fig. 1.8.1).

The maxillary sinus is located just lateral to the nasal cavity and, most importantly relative to facial trauma, shares its superior border with the orbital floor. Endoscopically, the maxillary sinus is approached via the osteomeatal complex, which is generally well visualized by gentle medialization of the middle turbinate endonasally. The key anatomical structures when approaching the maxillary sinus include the maxillary line, which is the junction of the hard maxillary bone and the lacrimal bone, and the uncinate process. The uncinate process is a thin, sickle-shaped bone that is typically removed at the beginning of any approach to the maxillary sinus in order to visualize the natural ostium of the sinus. This ostium must be identified and widened in continuity with the maxillary antrostomy in order to prevent mucociliary recirculation, which may lead to chronic maxillary sinusitis.[31]

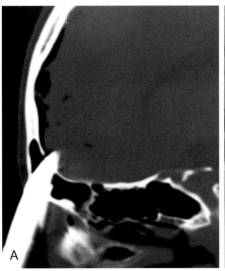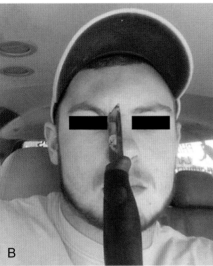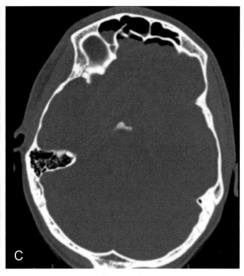

Fig. 1.8.1 Sagittal CT scan (A), A-P view (B) of penetrating knife injury through the anterior and posterior tables of the frontal sinus. Axial CT scan reveals fractures once the knife is removed. (Copyright Bradford A. Woodworth, MD.)

CLINICAL PRESENTATION

In a large retrospective cohort study, frontal sinus fractures most commonly occurred in males, with an average age of 30 years. Fractures most commonly involved both the anterior and posterior tables, followed by the anterior table alone. Only 3% were isolated posterior table fractures, and only 2% involved the frontal recess alone.[7] As frontal fractures are associated with high-impact mechanisms of injury, clinical evaluation must consider other associated fractures, injuries to the skull base, and intracranial injuries. Physical examination should begin with a primary trauma survey. In patients with frontal sinus fractures, focused physical examination should include any contour deformity of the glabella and brow, and a cranial nerve examination. Forehead paresthesias may be present if fractures involve the supraorbital and/or supratrochlear nerves. Any lacerations should be noted, and may be considered as potential ports for direct surgical approaches.[32] Anterior rhinoscopy should be performed as an overview assessment for any nasal septal deviation, injury, or hematoma. A more comprehensive nasal endoscopic examination should be offered to assess for cerebrospinal fluid (CSF) leak, particularly in patients with known posterior table injury. In these cases, it is important to obtain consultation with a neurosurgeon for operative planning.

Orbital floor fractures are typically due to trauma to the globe and periorbita, with common mechanisms of injury being motor vehicle accidents and personal assaults. Assessment of patients with orbital floor fractures after primary trauma survey should include a thorough evaluation of the eye and orbit. Physical examination should include gross visual fields and assessment of extraocular motion. Malar paresthesias are common in these patients. They result from injury to the infraorbital nerve as it travels through the infraorbital groove and foramen, which is a weak spot in the orbital floor and a common area for fractures to occur. The patient should also be assessed for enophthalmos, although this typically develops in a delayed fashion. Cosmetic deficits such as contour deformity of the midface or midface instability, as well as the possibility of dental involvement, should also be considered. An ophthalmology consultation should be considered where available in all patients suffering an orbital fracture.

RADIOLOGICAL EVALUATION

The maxillofacial CT scan is the gold standard for the radiological assessment of any maxillofacial fracture. This scan should be performed with thin slices, no greater than 1 mm spacing, to achieve the appropriate resolution for assessment of paranasal sinus fractures. Bone windows are important to determine the location and extent of fractures, and soft tissue windows should also be examined to assess for injury to the surrounding soft tissue structures.

Similar to all fractures, frontal sinus fractures should be examined in the axial, coronal, and sagittal planes. Of these planes, the axial and sagittal provide the most important information. These planes allow the examiner to determine the location of the fracture with respect to the anterior and posterior tables as well as any potential for the fracture to occlude the frontal recess. Displacement and comminution of the frontal bones may also be assessed in these planes and have a significant impact on management. For instance, nondisplaced, noncomminuted fractures may be managed expectantly, particularly when isolated to the anterior table. Conversely, more displaced, comminuted fractures and those that involve the posterior table are typically managed surgically.

Maxillary sinus fractures are also assessed using a maxillofacial CT scan. These fractures must be visualized in all three planes and location of the fractures with respect to the orbit is of the utmost importance. As with frontal sinus fractures, the degree of displacement and comminution also play a role in management. Orbital floor fractures are typically repaired either urgently in cases of orbital entrapment, or electively in larger fractures that may result in enophthalmos.

SURGICAL INDICATIONS

Absolute indications for repair of frontal sinus fractures include overt evidence of CSF leak or involvement of the frontal recess with concern for future frontal sinus outflow obstruction that could lead to chronic frontal sinusitis and/or mucocele formation. Whereas fractures in patients presenting with CSF leak should be repaired within 48 hours to reduce the risk of complications such as pneumocephalus and meningitis,[33] fractures involving the frontal recess without evidence of intracranial involvement may be repaired on an elective basis. A relative indication for repair of frontal sinus fractures is contour deformity of the glabella and the resultant cosmetic defect. These repairs are typically performed once acute edema has resolved to obtain an appropriate cosmetic result.

Indications for repair of maxillary sinus fractures include orbital floor fractures with evidence of entrapment and/or those involving greater than 50% of the orbital floor. Such fractures have the potential to cause long-term sequelae such as ophthalmoplegia, diplopia, and visual deficits. Cosmetic deformity, such as enophthalmos, is also a concern in these cases. While surgical repair of these fractures is indicated, the timing of repair remains controversial and ranges from emergent repair to outpatient repair on an elective basis.[34]

TRANSNASAL ENDOSCOPIC APPROACH TO FRONTAL SINUS FRACTURES

While endoscopic-assisted approaches to both the anterior and posterior tables have been described in the literature,[22,35–38] the transnasal endoscopic approach will be described here (Figs. 1.8.2 and 1.8.3). Endoscopic reduction of anterior table fractures should be performed within 10 days before significant healing to avoid difficulty in closed reduction

of the segments.[24] Operative intervention for posterior table injuries depends on the extent of the fractures and presence of CSF leak. Significant injuries should be addressed in a timely fashion (also usually within 10 days) when the patient's condition is stable for anesthesia. While small linear fractures with CSF leak could be managed conservatively, it should be noted CSF leaks can present years after conservative management or previous open procedures.

A Draf 2b frontal sinusotomy is typically performed for transnasal reduction of anterior and posterior table fractures, but a Draf 3 procedure may be required to create a common frontal sinus cavity with wide exposure for bilateral or significantly comminuted fractures.[22] A 70-degree scope should be used for visualization and dissection of the frontal sinus as fractures usually extend laterally.[39] An isolated, displaced segment of the posterior table can be manually reduced with curved suction or frontal curettes after removing the surrounding mucosa. If there is significant comminution, fragments should be meticulously removed from adhered dura using bipolar cauterization. No manipulation is necessary for linear cracks where mucosa can just be removed from the surrounding area and repair initiated without reduction. Anterior table fracture segments can be manually reduced with curved suction or frontal curettes. Skull base repair for posterior table defects can be performed using a variety of grafts and flaps. Overlay grafts or

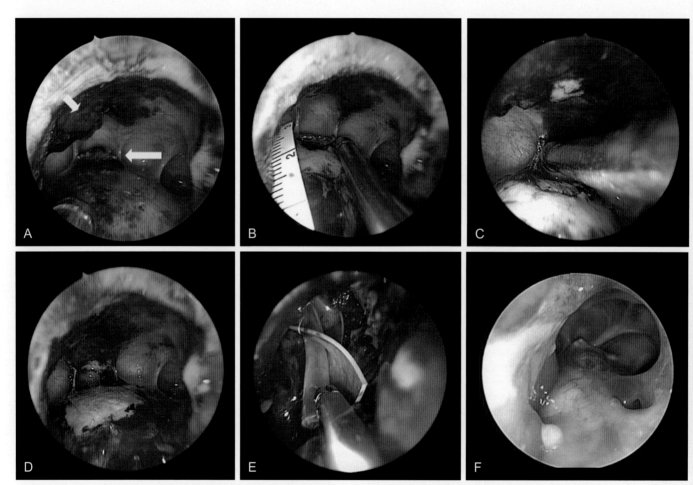

Fig. 1.8.2 Transnasal 70-degree endoscopic views of the endoscopic surgical repair. The anterior (*short arrow*) and posterior (*long arrow*) table fractures are visualized (A). Mucosa is removed around the defect and the length up the posterior table and diameter of the defect are measured (B). The anteriorly displaced segment of posterior table bone is placed back into position (C). A porcine small intestine submucosal graft (Biodesign ®, Cook Medical, Bloomington, IN) is placed in overlay fashion (D). Gelfoam packing and Silastic stent are inserted to support the repair (E). The healed patent frontal sinus is shown at 3 months (F). (Copyright Bradford A. Woodworth, MD.)

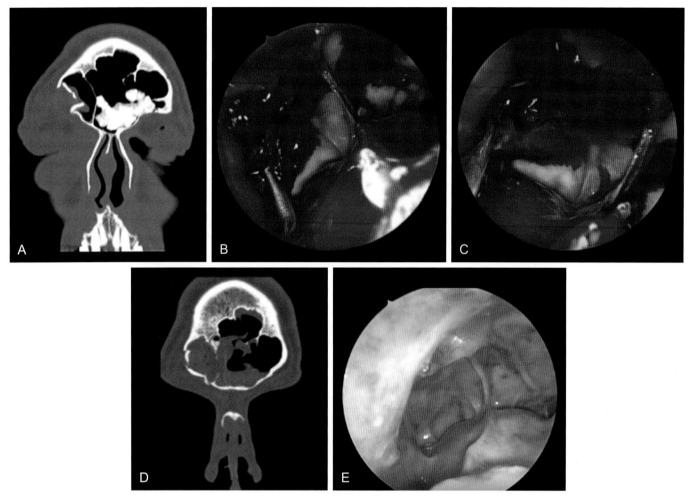

Fig. 1.8.3 Coronal CT scan of a patient with projectile injury resulting in displaced anterior table fracture who also had a contralateral frontal sinus osteoma. While a Draf 2b would have been sufficient to reduce the fracture, a Draf 3 was performed to remove the osteoma as well. Transnasal 70-degree endoscopic view after the Draf 3 was performed and osteoma removed (B). The frontal curette is used to reduce the fracture segments (C) with excellent reduction on postoperative CT scan (D). Endoscopic view of the Draf 3 at 3 months reveals a well-healed cavity (E). (Copyright Bradford A. Woodworth, MD.)

nasoseptal flaps (NSF) can be used when segments are reduced or simple cracks are present.[40] However, when fragments are removed and there is a significant defect, underlay epidural repair should be inserted first. Nasoseptal flaps can be harvested as previously described and can cover up to 3 cm of ipsilateral posterior table defects.[41] Supportive packing should be inserted, such as gel foam and rolled Silastic stents carved to fit in the frontal sinus. If a Draf 3 is performed, mucosal grafts covering the anterior aspect can reduce long-term risk of stenosis.[20,42] A Merocel sponge inside a sterile non-latex glove finger positioned within the middle meatus also provides support to the gelfoam placed in the frontal sinus. Spacers and frontal sinus stents are removed approximately 2 weeks postoperatively.

Indications and Contraindications to Endoscopic Repair of Frontal Sinus Fractures

An algorithm for endoscopic management of frontal sinus fractures has recently been developed by Grayson et al.[24] and is shown in Figs. 1.8.4 and 1.8.5.[24] It is important to note that because this technique is fairly new, there are no large outcomes studies available yet to ascertain long-term results. However, the authors feel that recent studies on this technique have shown that it is a safe, minimally invasive and effective procedure that can be used for repair of frontal sinus fractures.[24] The only absolute contraindication to endoscopic repair of frontal sinus fractures is the need to perform a craniotomy due to other injuries. Relative contraindications include the presence of lacerations that would provide easy portals of access to open repair of the fracture or lack of ability to endoscopically visualize the fracture (either due to bleeding or herniation of orbital tissues obstructing endoscopic visualization). Of course, as with any approach lack of surgeon experience is a relative contraindication. Fractures involving the posterior table in patients requiring a craniotomy may be better candidates for cranialization rather than an endoscopic repair, and cranialization may be performed if primary repair fails. The authors do not advocate the use of obliteration techniques as a patent frontal sinus outflow tract can typically be created through the techniques described above.

ENDOSCOPIC APPROACHES TO REPAIR OF ORBITAL FLOOR FRACTURES

Endoscopic exposure to the orbital floor typically requires an expanded maxillary antrostomy. A traditional maxillary antrostomy in which the uncinate is removed and the natural ostium of the maxillary sinus is

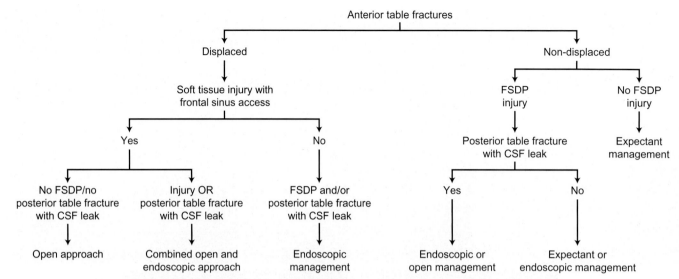

Fig. 1.8.4 Anterior table fracture repair algorithms. CSF = cerebrospinal fluid leak; FSDP = frontal sinus drainage pathway.

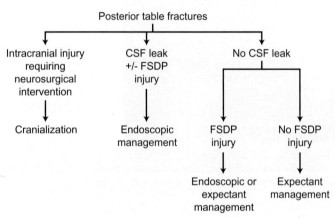

Fig. 1.8.5 Posterior table fracture repair algorithm. CSF = cerebrospinal fluid leak; FSDP = frontal sinus drainage pathway.

widened does not provide adequate access to the fracture. Rather, a mega-antrostomy or endoscopic medial maxillectomy should be performed depending on the location and extent of fractures. Medial fractures or those that require less manipulation may be accessed via a mega-antrostomy, whereas larger, comminuted, and more lateral fractures require the access of a medial maxillectomy or a sublabial Caldwell-Luc approach.[43]

Using an angled endoscope and curved dissectors, the mucosa of the maxillary roof is removed to expose the fracture. Once the fracture is exposed, the bone causing entrapment is removed using forceps. If instruments are unable to reach bone fragments via the maxillary antrostomy, a sublabial approach with osteotomy of the anterior maxillary sinus may be added for improved lateral exposure. A forced duction test is performed to assess the adequacy of bone removal. Orbital contents may then gently be replaced back into the orbit using gentle pressure from a balloon.[44,45] The orbital floor may then be reconstructed. A wide variety of reconstructive materials have been described, including MedPore, polydioxanone and titanium. Specific materials are discussed elsewhere in this book.

POSTOPERATIVE COURSE

The postoperative course after endoscopic management of frontal and orbital floor fractures depends on the extent and severity of the injury itself as well as the presence of other comorbid injuries. In general, patients should be treated with perioperative antibiotics consisting of a single dose prior to surgery.[46] Patients with frontal sinus fractures and concomitant CSF leak may be treated with longer courses of antibiotics to prevent meningitis, although this remains controversial.[47] Patients undergoing orbital floor fracture repair must have close follow-up to ensure that entrapment has resolved and that there is no postoperative hematoma leading to visual deficits.

In all patients undergoing endoscopic transnasal approaches, postoperative debridement is crucial to maintain nasal hygiene and prevent stenosis, particularly in the case of frontal recess manipulation. In cases of frontal sinus surgery in which stents are placed, these are typically left in place for 1–3 weeks, with removal based on extent of postoperative scarring and crusting. All patients are encouraged to perform nasal irrigations daily to help loosen crusts and assist with in-office debridement.

COMPLICATIONS

Complications of frontal sinus fractures can be classified as early or delayed. Early complications can occur in the perioperative period, whereas delayed complications may occur years or decades after the injury. The most feared early complications are intracranial infectious complications such as meningitis, encephalitis, subdural empyema, and brain abscess. These are typically prevented by early repair of frontal sinus fractures, particularly complex fractures involving the posterior table with associated CSF leak.[33] Delayed complications consist of cosmetic concerns and frontal recess obstruction. Cosmetic concerns include frontal contour deformity, which is notable after the edema associated with the initial injury resolves. Frontal recess obstruction may lead to chronic frontal sinusitis, or in cases of total obstruction, mucocele formation. Over time, mucoceles may expand and cause problems via mass effect on the eye or brain, or may become infected mucopyoceles that could serve as a nidus for intraorbital or intracranial infections. The major advantage of the endoscopic approach is clearance of the frontal sinus drainage pathway which obviates the need for long-term radiological follow-up and risk of long-term mucocele formation. Importantly, current Draf 2B and 3 techniques have high rates of success so that the likelihood of frontal sinus closure long-term is much lower than the risk of mucocele formation with open procedures.[20,42]

Complications of orbital floor fractures may also be classified as early or delayed. Early complications may include entrapment of the extraocular musculature, diplopia, and/or decreased visual acuity. Intra-orbital bleeding from either an arterial or venous source can lead to retrobulbar hematoma, which could create increased intraocular pressure, ischemic optic neuropathy and subsequent blindness. The most common delayed complication of orbital floor fractures is enophthalmos. In patients undergoing external approaches to reconstruction, ectropion and scar are common,[48] whereas patients undergoing an endoscopic approach are at risk for chronic maxillary sinusitis due to mucociliary recirculation if the operative approach does not fully incorporate the natural os of the maxillary sinus.

CONCLUSION

Midface trauma commonly occurs because of high-speed motor vehicle collisions and assault. The paranasal sinuses provide a means by which to dissipate forces and decrease the risk of injury to vital structures such as the eye and brain. However, fractures of the paranasal sinuses can present both cosmetic and functional consequences. While open approaches to repair of frontal and maxillary sinus fractures have traditionally been utilized to prevent these consequences with great success, the advent of endoscopic transnasal approaches to these injuries may provide a means by which to achieve similar results with less morbidity.

EXPERT COMMENTARY

Modern diagnosis and treatment of facial injuries and their complications must involve consideration for nasal and sinus endoscopy in appropriate circumstances; this may either be provided by the surgeons themselves or by consultation with an expert.

Today, many of our problems in facial injury repair are being solved more simply in terms of the operative approaches, but with sophisticated equipment for more minimally invasive surgery. Indeed orbital floor fractures, medial wall orbital fractures, and frontal sinuses and their complications may be able to be managed with endoscopic procedures. The repair of cerebrospinal (CSF) leaks, for instance, by endoscopic surgery is considerably less morbid and frequently equally effective with endoscopic procedures. Therefore, endoscopic diagnosis and treatment must be offered to the appropriate patients, and it may be provided by the suitably trained primary surgeon, or by consultation with experts skilled in these disciplines. Here the basic principles and results are discussed, so that we may benefit from these new opportunities for solutions.

REFERENCES

1. Nahum AM. The biomechanics of maxillofacial trauma. *Clin Plast Surg.* 1975;2:59–64.
2. Kellman RM, Schmidt C. The paranasal sinuses as a protective crumple zone for the orbit. *Laryngoscope.* 2009;119:1682–1690.
3. Shah RK, Dhingra JK, Carter BL, et al. Paranasal sinus development: a radiographic study. *Laryngoscope.* 2003;113:205–209.
4. Wolf G, Anderhuber W, Kuhn F. Development of the paranasal sinuses in children: implications for paranasal sinus surgery. *Ann Otol Rhinol Laryngol.* 1993;102:705–711.
5. Strong EB, Sykes JM. Frontal sinus and naso-orbital-ethmoid complex fractures. In: Papel ID, ed. *Facial Plastic and Reconstructive Surgery.* 2nd ed. New York: Thieme Medical Publishers, Inc; 2002:754–758.
6. Wallis A, Donald PJ. Frontal sinus fractures: a review of 72 cases. *Laryngoscope.* 1988;98:593–598.
7. Strong EB, Pahlavan N, Saito D. Frontal sinus fractures: a 28-year retrospective review. *Otolaryngol Head Neck Surg.* 2006;135:774–779.
8. McGraw-Wall B. Frontal sinus fractures. *Facial Plast Surg.* 1998;14:59–66.
9. Rohrich RJ, Hollier LH. Management of frontal sinus fractures: changing concepts. *Clin Plast Surg.* 1992;19:219–232.
10. Donald PJ. Frontal sinus ablation by cranialization: report of 21 cases. *Arch Otolaryngol.* 1982;108:142–146.
11. Luce EA. Frontal sinus fractures: guidelines to management. *Plast Reconstr Surg.* 1987;80:500–510.
12. Rodriguez ED, Stanwix MG, Nam AJ, et al. Twenty-six year experience treating frontal sinus fractures: a novel algorithm based on anatomical fracture pattern and failure of conventional techniques. *Plast Reconstr Surg.* 2008;122:1850–1866.
13. Goldberg RA, Lessner AM, Schorr N, et al. The transconjunctival approach to the orbital floor and orbital fat. A prospective study. *Ophthal Plast Reconstr Surg.* 1990;6:241–246.
14. Garcia GH, Goldberg RA, Shorr N. The transcaruncular approach in repair of orbital fractures: a retrospective study. *J Craniomaxillofac Trauma.* 1998;4:7–12.
15. Goldberg RA, Mancini R, Demer JL. The transcaruncular approach: surgical anatomy and technique. *Arch Facial Plast Surg.* 2007;9:443–447.
16. Lane KA, Bilyk JR, Taub D, et al. "Sutureless" repair of orbital floor and rim fractures. *Ophthalmology.* 2009;116:135–138.
17. Novelli G, Ferrari L, Sozzi D, et al. Transconjunctival approach in orbital traumatology: a review of 58 cases. *J Craniomaxillofac Surg.* 2011;39:266–270.
18. Nguyen DC, Shahzad F, Snyder-Warwick A, et al. Transcaruncular approach for treatment of medial wall and large orbital blowout fractures. *Craniomaxillofac Trauma Reconstr.* 2016;9:46–54.
19. Woodworth BA, Schlosser RJ, Palmer JN. Endoscopic repair of frontal sinus cerebrospinal fluid leaks. *J Laryngol Otol.* 2005;119:709–713.
20. Conger BT Jr, Riley K, Woodworth BA. The Draf III mucosal grafting technique: a prospective study. *Otolaryngol Head Neck Surg.* 2012;146:664–668.
21. Jones V, Virgin F, Riley K, et al. Changing paradigms in frontal sinus cerebrospinal fluid leak repair. *Int Forum Allergy Rhinol.* 2012;2:227–232.
22. Chaaban MR, Conger B, Riley KO, et al. Transnasal endoscopic repair of posterior table fractures. *Otolaryngol Head Neck Surg.* 2012;147:1142–1147.
23. Illing EA, Woodworth BA. Management of frontal sinus cerebrospinal fluid leaks and encephaloceles. *Otolaryngol Clin North Am.* 2016;49:1035–1050.
24. Grayson JW, Jeyarajan H, Illing EA, et al. Changing the surgical dogma in frontal sinus trauma. *Int Forum Allergy Rhinol.* 2017;7:441–449.
25. Bent JP, Cuilty-Siler C, Kuhn FA. The frontal cell as a cause of frontal sinus obstruction. *Am J Rhinol.* 1994;8:185–191.
26. Kuhn FA, Javer AR. Primary endoscopic management of the frontal sinus. *Otolaryngol Clin North Am.* 2001;34:59–75.
27. Wormald PJ. The agger nasi cell: the key to understanding the anatomy of the frontal recess. *Otolaryngol Head Neck Surg.* 2003;129:497–507.
28. Lund VJ, Stammberger H, Fokkens WJ, et al. European position paper on the anatomical terminology of the internal nose and paranasal sinuses. *Rhinol Suppl.* 2014;24:1–34.
29. Chiu AG, Schipor I, Cohen NA, et al. Surgical decisions in the management of frontal sinus osteomas. *Am J Rhinol.* 2005;19:191–197.
30. Wormald PJ, Hoseman W, Callejas C, et al. The international frontal sinus anatomy classification (IFAC) and classification of the extent of endoscopic frontal sinus surgery (EFSS). *Int Forum Allergy Rhinol.* 2016;6:677–696.
31. Messerklinger W. *Endoscopy of the Nose.* Baltimore, MD: Urban Schwartzenberg: 1978:123.
32. Matras H, Kuderna H. Management of upper midfacial injuries. *J Oral Surg.* 1977;35:809–817.

33. Bellamy JL, Molendik J, Reddy SK, et al. Severe infectious complications following frontal sinus fracture: the impact of operative delay and perioperative antibiotic use. *Plast Reconstr Surg.* 2013;132:154–162.

34. Nguyen A, Ho T, Czerwinski M. Safety of outpatient isolated orbital floor fracture repair. *J Craniofac Surg.* 2016;27:1686–1688.

35. Lappert PW, Lee JW. Treatment of an isolated outer table frontal sinus fracture using endoscopic reduction and fixation. *Plast Reconstr Surg.* 1998;102:1642–1645.

36. Chen DJ, Chen CT, Chen YR, et al. Endoscopically assisted repair of frontal sinus fracture. *J Trauma.* 2003;55:378–382.

37. Steiger JD, Chiu AG, Francis DO, et al. Endoscopic-assisted reduction of anterior table frontal sinus fractures. *Laryngoscope.* 2006;116:1978–1981.

38. Strong EB. Endoscopic repair of anterior table frontal sinus fractures. *Facial Plast Surg.* 2009;25:43–48.

39. Conger BT Jr, Illing E, Bush B, et al. Management of lateral frontal sinus pathology in the endoscopic era. *Otolaryngol Head Neck Surg.* 2014;151:159–163.

40. Hadad G, Bassagasteguy L, Carrau RL, et al. A novel reconstructive technique after endoscopic expanded endonasal approaches: vascular pedicle nasoseptal flap. *Laryngoscope.* 2006;116:1882–1886.

41. Virgin F, Baranano CF, Riley K, et al. Frontal sinus skull base defect repair using the pedicled nasoseptal flap. *Otolaryngol Head Neck Surg.* 2011;145:338–340.

42. Illing EA, Cho do Y, Riley KO, et al. Draf III mucosal graft technique: long-term results. *Int Forum Allergy Rhinol.* 2016;6:514–517.

43. Otori N, Haruna S, Moriyama H. Endoscopic endonasal or transmaxillary repair of orbital floor fracture: a study of 88 patients treated in our department. *Acta Otolaryngol.* 2003;123:718–723.

44. Yamaguchi N, Arai S, Mitani H. Endoscopic endonasal technique of the blowout fracture of the medial orbital wall. *Oper Tech Otolaryngol Head Neck Surg.* 1992;2:269–274.

45. Jin HR, Shin SO, Choo MJ, et al. Endonasal endoscopic reduction of blowout fracture of the medial orbital wall. *J Oral Maxillofac Surg.* 2000;58:847–851.

46. Mundinger GS, Borsuk DE, Okhah Z, et al. Antibiotics and facial fractures: evidence-based recommendations compared with experience-based practice. *Craniomaxillofac Trauma Reconstr.* 2015;8:64–78.

47. Friedman JA, Ebersold MJ, Quast LM, et al. Persistent posttraumatic cerebrospinal fluid leakage. *Neurosurg Focus.* 2000;9:e1.

48. Cheung K, Voineskos SH, Avram R, et al. A systematic review of the endoscopic management of orbital floor fractures. *JAMA Facial Plast Surg.* 2013;15:126–130.

Orbital Fractures

Bartlomiej Kachniarz, Michael Grant, Amir H. Dorafshar

BACKGROUND

Orbital fractures are among the most common facial fractures, and their associated cost to the healthcare system has been on the rise. Surgical repair of orbital fractures has been shown to add a day of hospitalization and an average of $22,000 in hospital charges for the average trauma patient.[1] Treatment of orbital trauma at high-volume specialized eye centers has been shown to reduce cost compared to management at other hospitals.[2] The incidence and etiology of orbital fractures vary greatly with geography, demographics, and socioeconomic factors, such as rates of violence and access to automobile safety technology.[3,4] Among the civilian population within the United States, 38% of orbital fractures result from motor vehicle collisions, followed closely by 34% from assault; falls and sport injuries account for another 15% and 7%, respectively. Sixty-eight percent of orbital fracture patients are male and over half are aged between 18 and 44. Approximately 1 in 4 orbital fractures in the United States are managed surgically.[1]

SURGICAL ANATOMY

A thorough understanding of orbital anatomy is key to achieving optimal clinical outcomes and minimizing postoperative complications. The bony orbit is approximately 30 mL in volume and 35–40 mm in length. The orbital floor is composed of the maxillary, zygomatic, and palatine bones. The thin medial wall includes the orbital plate of the ethmoid bone, lacrimal bone, frontal process of the maxillary bone, and the lesser wing of the sphenoid (Fig. 1.9.1). The posterior maxillary wall is frequently used as a bony landmark for the orbital apex, beyond which dissection should be avoided to minimize the risk of injury to the optic nerve.

The orbit includes six muscles responsible for extraocular movements. The four rectus muscles originate at the posterior orbit at a fibrous ring called the annulus of Zinn. The inferior rectus runs along the orbital floor and attaches approximately 6.5 mm inferior to the limbus. It must be evaluated for entrapment or rounding on computed tomography (CT) following orbital trauma. The inferior oblique muscle has its origin at the maxillary bone, just lateral to the opening of the nasolacrimal duct, and inserts on the lateral aspect of the globe. Its origin may come in the way of surgical access, particularly during combined floor and medial wall fracture repair. The anterior and posterior ethmoidal arteries run along the frontoethmoidal suture line at the superior border of the medial orbital wall, and must likewise be protected during dissection. The anterior ethmoidal artery lies approximately 24 mm from the lacrimal crest; the posterior ethmoidal artery may be found 36 mm from the lacrimal crest and approximately 6 mm from the orbital apex.

CLINICAL PRESENTATION

As with any injury, a detailed patient history should be taken upon presentation following orbital trauma. Evidence of head or neck injury, loss of consciousness, nausea, and vomiting are all particularly relevant in facial trauma patients. Muscle entrapment or increased orbital pressure may trigger the oculocardiac reflex, leading to syncope, nausea, vomiting, or even life-threatening arrhythmias.[5] The clinical history should include perception of a clear understanding of the mechanism of injury; a direct blow to the orbit or high-energy trauma should raise the suspicion for globe injury or other associated injuries. In fact, the mechanism of injury has been found to be a better predictor of visual prognosis than the specific pattern of facial fractures.[6] The age, baseline vision acuity and occupational history will likewise factor into the surgical management of an orbital fracture. Although focus is generally placed on preserving primary and downward gaze, patients should be asked about any activities that require prolonged upward gaze or extensive extraocular movement. A young heavy machinery operator, baseball outfielder, or pilot may warrant more aggressive surgical intervention to minimize the risk of posttraumatic diplopia.

The initial physical examination of any trauma patient should focus on ensuring adequate ventilation, hemodynamic stability, and prompt assessment of any life-threatening injuries. Once stable, every patient should undergo at least a basic eye exam, pending more thorough ophthalmologic evaluation. An initial eye exam in the emergency room should at the least include visual acuity testing, extraocular movements, pupillary exam, and an external exam. Evidence of diminished visual acuity, proptosis, or afferent pupillary defect all raise the suspicion for orbital compartment syndrome, which should prompt an emergent cantholysis to decompress the orbit. Bradycardia and defects in extraocular motility should raise concern for muscle entrapment. True muscle entrapment is rare in the adult population owing to diminished orbital wall bone elasticity, and significant periorbital edema may sometimes limit extraocular movements. Forced duction testing may be performed at the bedside to rule out entrapment. The external exam should assess any point tenderness, bony step-offs, crepitus, and sensory deficits; trauma to the infraorbital nerve may frequently lead to dysesthesia. Globe position should be assessed for inferior displacement, enophthalmos, or exophthalmos. A flat anterior chamber, misshapen pupil, or circumferential subconjunctival hemorrhage should raise the suspicion for globe injury.[7] Lateral or medial canthal deformity may indicate either zygomatic involvement or a naso-orbital ethmoid fracture, respectively.

Full ophthalmological evaluation and clearance is critical for all orbital fracture patients prior to surgical repair. In addition to the aforementioned basic eye exam, ophthalmological evaluation should include

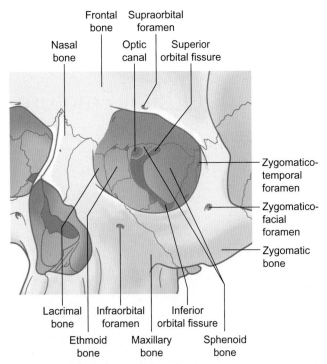

Nasal bone · Frontal bone · Supraorbital foramen · Optic canal · Superior orbital fissure · Zygomatico-temporal foramen · Zygomatico-facial foramen · Zygomatic bone · Lacrimal bone · Infraorbital foramen · Inferior orbital fissure · Ethmoid bone · Maxillary bone · Sphenoid bone

Fig. 1.9.1 Orbital bone anatomy. (Reproduced from Love LP, Farrior EH. Periocular anatomy and aging. Facial Plast Surg Clin North Am 2010;18(3):411–417.)

a more thorough assessment of visual acuity, globe pressure, visual fields, a slit lamp ocular exam, and a retinal exam. Approximately 22%–29% of orbital fracture patients will present with concomitant ocular injuries.[8,9] In one series, 79% of open globe injuries resulted in blindness.[6] Several studies have demonstrated higher incidence of globe injuries associated with blow-out fractures compared to fractures with rim involvement.[8,10]

Any evidence of muscle entrapment on exam should warrant early surgical intervention within 24–48 hours. Several studies have demonstrated increased risk of late diplopia with delayed repair in the setting of muscle entrapment. It has been postulated that true muscle incarceration leads to occlusion of the artery running in the central portion of the inferior rectus muscle, resulting in scarring and fibrosis within the muscle.[11–13] Persistent bradycardia and hemodynamic instability secondary to the oculocardiac reflex are additional indications for immediate surgical repair. Additionally, many authors advocate immediate repair of large wall defects that result in early enophthalmos on presentation.[11]

The timing of surgical repair of orbital fractures in the setting of concomitant globe injury remains controversial. On one hand, early intervention risks further trauma to a ruptured globe, compromising long-term vision outcomes. On the other hand, delaying repair of facial fractures may be detrimental to long-term cosmetic outcomes. Within the reconstructive surgery literature, many authors support careful early repair of orbital fractures with associated globe injury, particularly in the setting of high-energy penetrating trauma, where return of visual acuity is unlikely.[6,14]

In the absence of globe injury or indications for immediate repair, many authors advocate repair of orbital fractures within a 2-week window.[15–17] The degree of scarring and adhesions tend to increase after 2 weeks, complicating and decreasing the effectiveness of surgical repair because of fixed scar tissue. Conversely, waiting several days following

initial injury may help with resolution of periorbital edema, which might otherwise complicate access during repair. Some feel that the immediate post-injury period is more vulnerable to spasm in the circulation to the optic nerve.

RADIOLOGICAL EVALUATION

Thin-cut non-contrast CT of the orbits and face are the gold standard imaging modality for detecting orbital fractures. Cuts of 1–2 mm are generally recommended for adequate visualization, and the entire face should be imaged to assess for other associated facial injuries. Three-dimensional reconstructions may be helpful in assessing craniofacial fracture patterns following trauma. The orbital floor is best visualized on coronal and sagittal views, while the medial orbital wall is best seen on axial and coronal cuts. The sagittal view is particularly useful for assessment of the posterior ledge for orbital floor implant support. The coronal view provides good visualization of the orbital soft tissues and may be used to assess fat herniation or muscle entrapment. Rounding of the inferior rectus muscle has been associated with late enophthalmos if left untreated.[18]

CLASSIFICATION

Orbital wall fractures are generally categorized based on involvement of the orbital floor, roof, or medial wall. Considering the specific fracture pattern is critical in selecting the appropriate surgical approach and implant. Isolated orbital floor fractures are most frequently repaired with an onlay implant with or without an orbital rim component. In isolated medial orbital wall fractures, the inferonasal bone strut is frequently preserved, serving as support for implant reconstruction. Traditional onlay reconstruction is an option if surrounding bone is strong enough to support an implant. In cases of poor exposure or lack of sturdy support surrounding the fracture segments, an inlay technique may be used.[19] Porous polyethylene may be inserted into the ethmoid sinuses after reduction of orbital contents. Lastly, in the setting of an intact medial orbital wall fracture fragment, the defect may be repaired via endoscopic repositioning.[20] The orbital contents are reduced, and the wall reconstructed by rotating the fracture fragment into stable position.

Combined medial wall and orbital floor fractures present a unique set of challenges. They are frequently associated with loss of the inferonasal bony strut support (a shallow bulge), hindering secure implant placement and increasing the risk of enophthalmos and diplopia.[21] Further, dissection adequately exposing both the orbital floor and medial wall is frequently complicated by the origin of the inferior oblique muscle near the lacrimal fossa. Several implant choices exist for combined orbital floor and medial wall fractures. Some authors support the use of a rim-fixed orbital floor implant with a medial wing; single wraparound sheets are also available to cover both defects with one implant.[22] Alternatively, each defect may be reconstructed separately, with two individual floor and medial wall implants.[23]

Orbital fractures may additionally be categorized as either pure blow-out fractures or those involving the orbital rim. Two primary mechanisms have been described to explain isolated orbital wall fractures without associated rim involvement.[24,25] The hydraulic theory holds that a blow to the orbital contents transiently increases the intraorbital pressure, leading to outfracture of the orbital wall. According to the buckling theory, a high-energy impact to the orbital rim is directly transmitted to the more fragile orbital wall, leading to the fracture. Many authors contend that both theories are likely at play in most orbital floor fractures. Given the anatomy of the medial orbit and neighboring ethmoid air cells, the hydraulic theory is likely most pertinent in medial orbital wall fractures.[26] A third possibility is that the globe itself is driven posteriorly, fracturing the orbital walls when the globe diameter exceeds the diameter of the orbit.

SURGICAL INDICATIONS

Indications for surgical repair remain controversial and are largely based on predicting long-term cosmetic and visual sequalae of orbital trauma. The aforementioned cases of persistent bradycardia, optic nerve compression, periorbital muscle entrapment, and enophthalmos greater than 2 mm on initial presentation warrant early surgical repair within 24–48 hours. In the absence of indications for acute intervention, patients may be reevaluated and scheduled for surgery within 1–2 weeks. Evidence of extraocular movement restriction or diplopia, particularly in primary and downward gaze, are indications for repair when limitation of muscle movement can be proven. Certain patient populations dependent on intact extraocular motility, such as athletes, pilots, or heavy machinery users, may warrant more aggressive intervention. Significant globe malposition or orbital rim involvement leading to bony step-offs and disfigurement should likewise be reduced to prevent long-term cosmetic sequelae.

Predicting which injury patterns will lead to long-term enophthalmos and visual restrictions remains challenging. Fractures involving 50% of the orbital floor area are frequently used as a cut-off for non-surgical management. Fractures up to 3 cm^2 have been managed conservatively with optimal outcomes.[27] The medial wall appears to be less forgiving, warranting repair for defects over 2 cm.[2,28] Other imaging findings predictive of long-term globe malposition include rounding of the inferior rectus muscle on CT imaging.[18]

SURGICAL TECHNIQUES

Repair of orbital wall fractures is performed under general anesthesia after infiltration of the surgical site with a local analgesic. Several commonly used surgical approaches exist to expose the orbital floor and medial wall (Fig. 1.9.2). The subtarsal approach involves a cutaneous incision just below the tarsal plate, along a natural crease line. The orbicularis oculi muscle is dissected, and the orbital rim approached in the preseptal plane. The closely related infraorbital rim incision involves a cutaneous incision directly overlying the orbital rim. The latter approach has come out of favor due to less favorable scar placement. Some of the benefits of the subtarsal approach include lower risk of lower lid malposition and ectropion, as well as easier exposure without the need for a lateral canthotomy.[29,30]

The subciliary approach includes an incision several millimeters below the lash line. Dissection is then either continued directly through the orbicularis oculi muscle, or carried in a step fashion in the subcutaneous plane for a few millimeters before muscle division just below the tarsal plate. The rim is then exposed in a preseptal plane. A major disadvantage of the subciliary approach is the high risk of scar contracture leading to ectropion. Extensive subcutaneous dissection may even lead to skin necrosis.[31,32]

The transconjunctival approach involves a mucosal incision through the conjunctiva below the level of the tarsus[33,34] (Fig. 1.9.3). The rim is then exposed via either a preseptal or retroseptal dissection plane (Video 1.9.1). The transconjunctival approach has gained popularity in recent years due to its lower risk of ectropion and lack of cutaneous scar. Some authors have even noted favorable results without the use of suture.[35] One downside is its limited exposure, frequently requiring the use of lateral canthotomy for larger fractures.[36,37]

A related approach frequently used for exposure of the medial orbital wall is the transcaruncular approach[38] (Fig. 1.9.4). It involves an

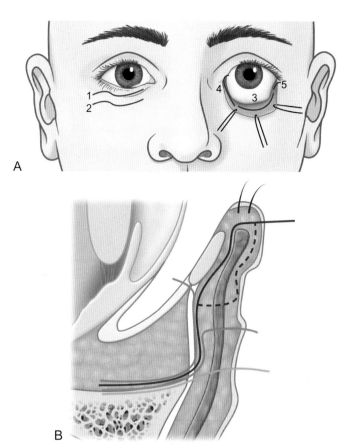

Fig. 1.9.2 Common surgical approaches used for exposure of the orbit. (A) 1, Subtarsal; 2, infraorbital; 3, transconjunctival; 4, transcaruncular; 5, transconjunctival with lateral skin incision. (B) Sagittal view of orbital anatomy. *Solid red,* subciliary nonstepped; *dotted red,* subciliary stepped; *blue,* transconjunctival; *dark green,* subtarsal; *light green,* infraorbital. (Reproduced from Kothari NA, Avashia YJ, Lemelman BT, et al. Incisions for orbital floor exploration. J Craniofac Surg 2012;23(7 Suppl 1):1985–1989.)

approximately 12 mm vertical incision through the caruncle along the medial conjunctiva. Some authors advocate placing the incision more laterally between the caruncle and plica semilunaris, in a retrocaruncular fashion.[39] This technique preserves the Horner muscle, as well as the inferior oblique muscle in 89% of cases. Blunt dissection is performed onto the bone posterior to the lacrimal crest, and continued in the subperiosteal plane. The initial incision may be extended superiorly toward the superior tarsal plate for increased exposure. It may likewise be extended inferiorly and combined with the transconjunctival approach for access to large combined orbital floor and medial wall fractures.[40]

Finally, some surgeons have adopted endoscopic techniques to repair orbital floor and medial wall fractures.[41,42] The fracture site and implant placement may arguably be better assessed under direct visualization with an endoscope. For some medial wall fractures, the fracture fragment may even be repositioned after orbital content reduction, obviating the need for implant placement.[20] The lack of periorbital incisions minimizes the risk of ectropion or unfavorable scarring. An obvious downside of endoscopic repair is that it requires access to, and experience with, endoscopic sinus surgery instrumentation.

Prior to implant placement, all bone fragments and blood are removed from the maxillary sinus, and irrigation of the sinus should demonstrate free passage of fluid into the nose. Numerous implant materials have been used in recent years for orbital wall reconstruction. They have largely supplanted autografting owing to their lack of donor site

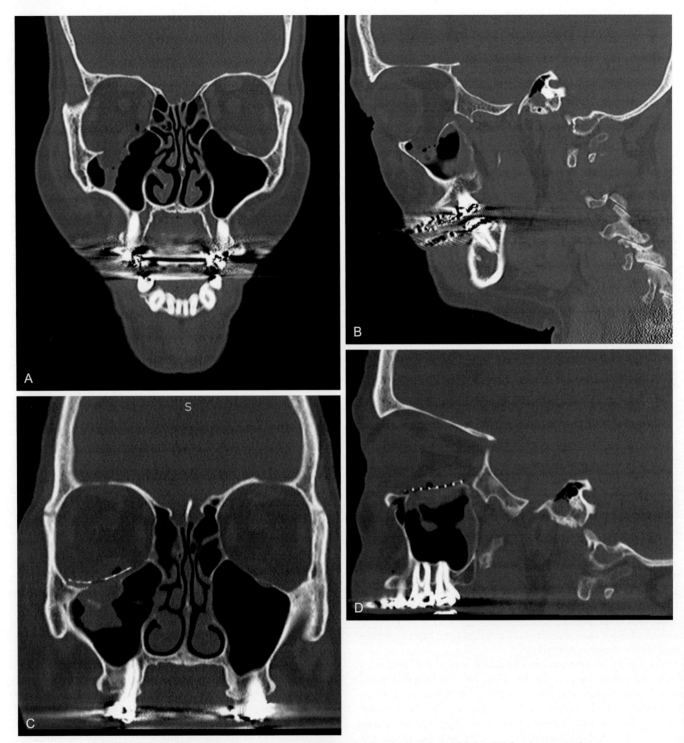

Fig. 1.9.3 Repair of orbital floor fracture with Medpor titanium implant (see Video 1.9.1 for demonstration of operative procedure). (A–B) Preoperative coronal and sagittal views on CT scanning. (C–D) Postoperative coronal and sagittal CT view demonstrating adequate reduction and implant resting on posterior ledge. (Courtesy Dr. Amir H. Dorafshar.)

morbidity and more accurate anatomic reconstruction.[43] Several common biocompatible materials are presently in use and may be broadly categorized based on their elasticity and porosity. Nylon, for example, has been used in the form of a nonporous flexible sheet.[22,44] A titanium metal mesh provides greater rigidity and shape retention, while more porous materials like polyethylene may offer improved tissue ingrowth

and integration.[45,46] Combination products of the two providing a firm porous scaffold are also available.

Selection of the appropriate implant may be aided by preoperative virtual fitting software.[47] The software utilizes axial orbital CT scan data to mirror the unfractured orbital template onto the fractured side. Digital models of various commercially available preformed anatomic

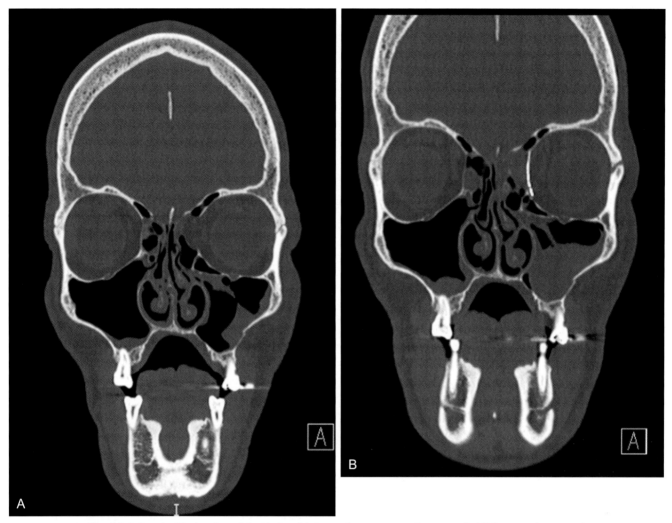

Fig. 1.9.4 Repair of isolated medial orbital wall fracture via transcaruncular approach. (A) Preoperative coronal CT. (B) Postoperative coronal CT demonstrating reduction of fracture. (Courtesy Dr. Amir H. Dorafshar.)

implants are then loaded and used to find the best match for the mirrored orbital wall. Superimposing the defect shape is then used to plan cuts along the implant and placement of fixation screws. The software may even be used in cases of bilateral orbital fractures; standardized models may be used in place of mirroring, with custom adjustments to ensure anatomic reduction and symmetry.

In addition to off-the-shelf anatomic designs (Fig. 1.9.5), new strategies are emerging to design custom implants preoperatively; both polyethylene and titanium have been used for fabrication of patient-specific implants.[48,49] The implant shape is extrapolated by mirroring intact bony structures on the contralateral uninjured side. This is most feasible in cases of delayed orbital reconstruction within 1–2 weeks, although the speed of custom implant fabrication in the United States continues to improve rapidly. Although the technology carries a higher cost, it offers the advantage of more accurate reproduction of the complex three-dimensional shape of the orbital walls. Further, it in many cases reduces operative times by obviating the need for intraoperative implant shaping. Finally, the software used for implant design may be used for operative planning, including optimizing exposure and deciding on strategies to best secure the implant. Some surgeons have even used the CT data for intraoperative navigation.

POSTOPERATIVE COURSE

Postoperatively, all patients should undergo forced duction testing prior to leaving the operating room to rule out extraocular muscle impingement. Forced duction testing is performed by gently grasping the limbus with a pair of forceps and assessing globe passive range of motion in all directions. Likewise, many surgeons advocate postoperative CT imaging to assess implant placement and reduction of orbital contents. Repeat imaging is particularly helpful if intraoperative imaging navigation was not used, or if diplopia is present which was not present preoperatively. Light perception should be checked immediately after recovery from anesthesia; many surgeons admit patients overnight for close light perception checks and monitoring for development of retrobulbar hematoma. Corneal exposure is another concern in the postoperative period, as periorbital edema may lead to temporary lagophthalmos. Temporary stitch tarsorrhaphy may prevent exposure keratitis in the immediate postoperative period and may be easily removed at bedside prior to discharge. Lubricating ophthalmic drops are frequently prescribed for outpatient therapy. Swelling may be reduced with head-of-bed elevation and ice application. Patients should avoid any nose blowing and heavy lifting for at least 2 weeks postoperatively.[7] The use of prolonged

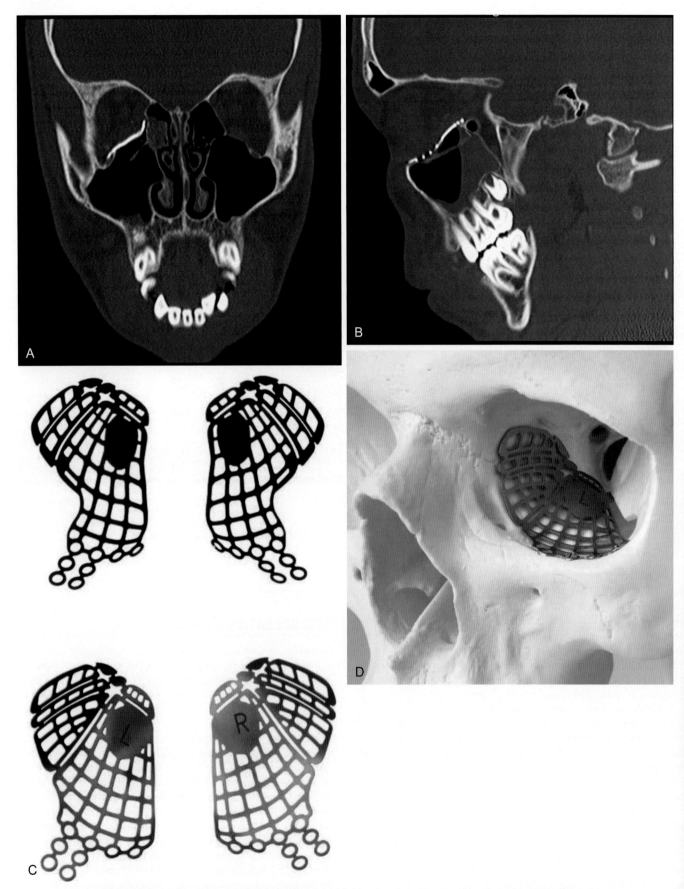

Fig. 1.9.5 Use of preformed anatomically shaped orbital implant for reconstruction of combined medial wall and floor fracture. (A) Postoperative coronal view demonstrating preformed implant. (B) Postoperative sagittal CT view demonstrating implant resting on posterior ledge. (C–D) Examples of Synthes preformed orbital implants. (Panels C–D courtesy Synthes MatrixORBITAL™. MatrixMIDFACE Preformed Orbital Plates Booklet.)

postoperative antibiotics has been explored by several authors and has not been shown to impact rates of surgical site infection.[50] Antibiotics beyond a perioperative regimen are generally not recommended, although the practice remains controversial.

ACUTE COMPLICATIONS

Risks of common complications following reconstruction should be discussed with patients preoperatively. Dysesthesia in the infraorbital nerve distribution, for instance, is reported in approximately 55% of patients. The incidence of persistent diplopia following repair varies widely in the literature, ranging from 8% to 52%.[7,51] The variable results may at least partially be explained by differences in definition of clinically significant symptoms. Double vision following surgical reduction may be caused by muscle ischemia, scarring, or persistent entrapment by the implant or fracture fragments. CT imaging may be helpful in evaluating physical muscle impingement. Extraocular muscle paresis may also be neurogenic in nature, which frequently resolves spontaneously over time. In some cases, diplopia may develop after weeks or even months following surgery secondary to development of adhesions between the orbital implant and extraocular muscles.

Among the most serious complications following orbital trauma, vision loss has been reported in approximately 7.1%–7.9% of patients presenting with orbital fractures. Acute vision loss following surgery is much less common, occurring in less than 0.4% of patients. The most common mechanism is retrobulbar hemorrhage leading to orbital compartment syndrome and compression of the optic nerve. Most surgeons monitor postoperative patients overnight for any symptoms of orbital compression, such as sudden pain, swelling, loss of light perception, or proptosis. Clinical concern for retrobulbar hematoma should prompt an emergent bedside canthotomy. The lateral canthal tendon may be accessed via a transverse cutaneous incision; when performing the canthotomy, care should be taken to release both the superior and inferior limbs of the tendon. Postoperative blindness may also be caused by direct nerve injury or from retinal arteriolar occlusion from excessive dissection over the posterior ethmoid foramen. Ophthalmic arterial spasm may likewise lead to vision loss.

Correlating a constellation of postoperative complaints with orbital anatomy can be essential to early diagnosis and intervention. Implant or fracture fragment impingement on the superior orbital fissure may lead to superior orbital fissure syndrome. This condition is characterized by involvement of cranial nerve passing through the superior orbital fissure; these include superior and inferior divisions of the oculomotor nerve, the trochlear nerve, branches of the ophthalmic nerve, as well as the abducens nerve. Injury to the extraocular motor nerves leads to ophthalmoplegia, ptosis, and pupil dilation. Compression of ophthalmic branches of the trigeminal nerve leads to impaired lacrimal gland function and numbness along the eyelid and forehead or nose, cheek, and upper lip. Orbital apex syndrome is characterized by involvement of the optic nerve and vision loss, in addition to the cranial nerve dysfunction seen in superior orbital fissure syndrome. Surgical intervention is generally warranted in cases of anatomic compression secondary to either hemorrhage or impingement. In the absence of a surgical indication, medical management includes high-dose intravenous steroids followed by an oral taper regimen.

LONG-TERM COMPLICATIONS

Long term complications following orbital trauma include persistent enophthalmos and diplopia, which occur in 27% and 8%–52% of patients, respectively. Diplopia may present late as adhesions between the healing fracture site, implant, and extraocular muscles develop. As the surgical access incision heals, contracture may lead to lower eyelid malposition. Ectropion has been reported in 12.9% of patient who underwent orbital repair via subciliary incisions. The rates are lower for subtarsal and rim incisions. Placing transconjunctival incisions too close to the eyelid margin similarly may lead to entropion. Careful incision placement may reduce the risk of lower lid malposition secondary to contracture.

Evidence-based medicine (EBM) content available in Appendix 1 (online only)

Continued

EXPERT COMMENTARY—cont'd

events also contribute to the deformity: the supratarsal sulcus deformity, for instance, is caused by prolapse of extraconal fat away from the upper lid orbital septum. Fat prominence here against the upper lid is restored by pushing up on the intraconal compartment from the floor just behind the globe, forcing the soft tissue upward, which pushes the extraconal upper lid orbital fat against the orbital septum causing a pleasing fullness to occur as in prior to injury. Fat atrophy is generally *not* a significant component of the standard (90%) unoperated orbital fracture, so the issue is then restoring the soft tissue to its proper position, moving the soft tissue volume into its normal position. (Fat atrophy occurs in about 10% of unoperated orbital fractures, but may be more frequent in the multiply operated patient – this has *not* been studied.)

As correction techniques advanced, surgeons began using not only bone grafts but artificial materials such as polyethylene and titanium to stabilize soft tissue/orbital wall replacement, as subsequent resorption was minimized.

Allen Putterman, MD gave us the idea that you should "separate the analysis of the muscle injury from the volume change." The musculofibrous ligament system (MFL), identified by Leo Koorneef, MD, unifies the concept of how the interconnected soft tissue results in the various clinical symptoms by extending throughout the soft tissue of the orbit, running through the fat and connecting all the extraocular muscles with the walls of the orbit and the globe. In blow-out fractures, an extraocular muscle can be incarcerated by trapping the MFL system alone, or the fat; generally this is the occurrence rather than trapping the extraocular muscle itself, and this process may be correctly identified in good CT scans.

The theory of an orbital muscle compartment syndrome was raised, however it was eventually concluded that, unlike lower extremities, extraocular muscle has no dense fascia surrounding it, and therefore it is unlikely to create an isolated true compartment syndrome, but there is often a generalized rise in intraorbital pressure within the whole orbit, so physicians must be aware of and manage this phenomenon.

The mechanisms of diplopia which are surgically correctable are: change in origin or path of the extraocular muscle because of its adherence; entrapment or sagging of this muscle; true MFL incarceration; and, more rarely, incarceration of the muscle itself.

Several studies have explored the correlation of enophthalmos and diplopia with rounding of extraocular muscles in CT scans, theorizing that it must be related to disruption of the ligaments that keep that muscle in an elliptical shape.

It has subsequently proven that the original concept of Converse was true, that a "sagging" muscle, one with an abnormal or misaligned path, could itself cause double vision.

Orbital shape is a crucial concept in reconstructive surgery: the shape of the orbital soft tissue is dictated by the absolute volume of the orbit and by its shape – the subtle curves of the walls which are generated by the precise reconstruction of the orbital buttress system. The curves (shape) of the orbital walls have to be reproduced to get the best result in terms of appearance.

The positioning of the orbital walls follows the positioning of the orbital rim correctly, and allows one to reconstruct the missing orbital wall as accurately as possible with the curves necessary to reproduce the normal shape of the respective wall. Finding the posterior "ledge," the intact bone of the wall in the posterior portion of the orbit, allows one to angle and position the respective wall correctly between the orbital rim and the posterior "ledge."

If possible, one should avoid orbital incisions in the "critical area" of the lower lid: the subciliary junction of the anterior lamella, tarsal plate, and posterior lamella. If you keep your incision outside of that area you avoid damaging or denervating the pretarsal orbicularis, weakening facial nerve innervation and creating fibrosis, both of which normally constitute the mechanisms of reduced vertical (upward) support of the lid allowing inferior lower lid positioning, scleral show or ectropion.

Finally, realigning and reattaching the periorbital soft facial tissue on the bone as it was preinjury will prevent an unwelcome change in appearance; the facial soft tissue will "sag" if not properly reattached to the facial skeleton, producing soft tissue ptosis and a poor appearance.

3D modeling and CT segmental analysis can decrease frustration in achieving orbital fracture alignment. Many patients are relatively similar in orbital shape and volume across races in the key parts of the orbit that fracture. Orbital fracture defects can therefore be organized into several common patterns and treated with some commonly designed plates, or better by intraoperative CT analysis, or a patient-specific computer-designed preoperatively molded plate. Significant improvements in plate design and application have occurred as new generations of surgeons have completed training and built on the work of earlier colleagues.

This knowledge and these techniques improve results of orbital fracture treatment, and make the attainment of preinjury function and appearance a possibility following orbital injury.

REFERENCES

1. Ko MJ, Morris CK, Kim JW, et al. Orbital fractures: national inpatient trends and complications. *Ophthal Plast Reconstr Surg.* 2013;29(4):298–303.
2. Koo JJ, Wang J, Thompson CB, et al. Impact of hospital volume and specialization on the cost of orbital trauma care. *Ophthalmology.* 2013;120(12):2741–2746.
3. Hwang K, You SH, Sohn IA. Analysis of orbital bone fractures: a 12-year study of 391 patients. *J Craniofac Surg.* 2009;20(4):1218–1223.
4. Duma SM, Jernigan MV. The effects of airbags on orbital fracture patterns in frontal automobile crashes. *Ophthal Plast Reconstr Surg.* 2003;19(2):107–111.
5. Kim BB, Qaqish C, Frangos J, Caccamese JF. Oculocardiac reflex induced by an orbital floor fracture: report of a case and review of the literature. *J Oral Maxillofac Surg.* 2012;70(11):2614–2619.
6. Vaca EE, Mundinger GS, Kelamis JA, et al. Facial fractures with concomitant open globe injury: mechanisms and fracture patterns associated with blindness. *Plast Reconstr Surg.* 2013;131(6):1317–1328.
7. Boyette JR, Pemberton JD, Bonilla-Velez J. Management of orbital fractures: challenges and solutions. *Clin Ophthalmol.* 2015;9:2127–2137.
8. He D, Blomquist PH, Ellis E. Association between ocular injuries and internal orbital fractures. *J Oral Maxillofac Surg.* 2007;65(4):713–720.
9. Kreidl KO, Kim DY, Mansour SE. Prevalence of significant intraocular sequelae in blunt orbital trauma. *Am J Emerg Med.* 2003;21(7): 525–528.
10. Brown MS, Ky W, Lisman RD. Concomitant ocular injuries with orbital fractures. *J Craniomaxillofac Trauma.* 1999;5(3):48.
11. Burnstine MA. Clinical recommendations for repair of isolated orbital floor fractures: an evidence-based analysis. *Ophthalmology.* 2002;109(7):1213.
12. Liao JC, Elmalem VI, Wells TS, Harris GJ. Surgical timing and postoperative ocular motility in type B orbital blowout fractures. *Ophthal Plast Reconstr Surg.* 2015;31(1):29–33.
13. Iliff N, Manson PN, Katz J, et al. Mechanisms of extraocular muscle injury in orbital fractures. *Plast Reconstr Surg.* 1999;103(3):787–799.
14. Li KK, Teknos TN, Lauretano A, Joseph MP. Traumatic optic neuropathy complicating facial fracture repair. *J Craniofac Surg.* 1997;8(5):359.
15. Hawes MJ, Dortzbach RK. Surgery on orbital floor fractures: influence of time of repair and fracture size. *Ophthalmology.* 1983;90(9):1066–1070.
16. Dubois L, Steenen SA, Gooris PJJ, et al. Controversies in orbital reconstruction – II. Timing of post-traumatic orbital reconstruction: a systematic review. *Int J Oral Maxillofac Surg.* 2015;44(4):433–440.
17. Damgaard OE, Larsen CG, Felding UA, et al. Surgical timing of the orbital "blowout" fracture: a systematic review and meta-analysis. *Otolaryngol Head Neck Surg.* 2016;155(3):387–390.

18. Matic DB, Tse R, Banerjee A, Moore CC. Rounding of the inferior rectus muscle as a predictor of enophthalmos in orbital floor fractures. *J Craniofac Surg.* 2007;18(1):127–132.

19. Kim Y, Kim TG, Lee JH, et al. Inlay implanting technique for the correction of medial orbital wall fracture. *Plast Reconstr Surg.* 2011;127(1):321–326.

20. Lee T, Lee HM, Lee JM, Nam JG. Endoscopic reduction of orbital medial wall fracture using rotational repositioning of the fractured: lamina papyracea fragment. *J Craniofac Surg.* 2014;25(2):460–462.

21. Biesman BS, Hornblass A, Lisman R, Kazlas M. Diplopia after surgical repair of orbital floor fractures. *Ophthal Plast Reconstr Surg.* 1996;12(1):16. discussion 17.

22. Nunery WR, Tao JP, Johl S. Nylon foil "wraparound" repair of combined orbital floor and medial wall fractures. *Ophthal Plast Reconstr Surg.* 2008;24(4):271–275.

23. Su GW, Harris GJ. Combined inferior and medial surgical approaches and overlapping thin implants for orbital floor and medial wall fractures. *Ophthal Plast Reconstr Surg.* 2006;22(6):420–423.

24. Raflo GT. Blow-in and blow-out fractures of the orbit: clinical correlations and proposed mechanisms. *Ophthalmic Surg.* 1984;15(2):114–119.

25. Ahmad F, Kirkpatrick NA, Lyne J, et al. Buckling and hydraulic mechanisms in orbital blowout fractures: fact or fiction? *J Craniofac Surg.* 2006;17(3):438–441.

26. Rhee JS, Kilde J, Yoganadan N, Pintar F. Orbital blowout fractures: experimental evidence for the pure hydraulic theory. *Arch Facial Plast Surg.* 2002;4(2):98–101.

27. Kunz C, Sigron GR, Jaquiéry C. Functional outcome after non-surgical management of orbital fractures – the bias of decision-making according to size of defect: critical review of 48 patients. *Br J Oral Maxillofac Surg.* 2013;51(6):486–492.

28. Sung YS, Chung CM, Hong IP. The correlation between the degree of enophthalmos and the extent of fracture in medial orbital wall fracture left untreated for over six months: a retrospective analysis of 81 cases at a single institution. *Arch Plast Surg.* 2013;40(4):335–340.

29. Holtmann B, Wray RC, Little AG. A randomized comparison of four incisions for orbital fractures. *Plast Reconstr Surg.* 1981;67(6):731–737.

30. Ridgway EB, Chen C, Colakoglu S, et al. The incidence of lower eyelid malposition after facial fracture repair: a retrospective study and meta-analysis comparing subtarsal, subciliary, and transconjunctival incisions. *Plast Reconstr Surg.* 2009;124(5):1578–1586.

31. Appling WD, Patrinely JR, Salzer TA. Transconjunctival approach vs subciliary skin-muscle flap approach for orbital fracture repair. *Arch Otolaryngol Head Neck Surg.* 1993;119(9):1000–1007.

32. Kothari NA, Avashia YJ, Lemelman BT, et al. Incisions for orbital floor exploration. *J Craniofac Surg.* 2012;23(7 suppl 1):1985–1989.

33. Tenzel RR, Miller GR. Orbital blow-out fracture repair, conjunctival approach. *Am J Ophthalmol.* 1971;71(5):1141–1142.

34. Tessier P. The conjunctival approach to the orbital floor and maxilla in congenital malformation and trauma. *J Maxillofac Surg.* 1973;1(1):3–8.

35. Ho VH, Rowland JP, Linder JS, Fleming JC. Sutureless transconjunctival repair of orbital blowout fractures. *Ophthal Plast Reconstr Surg.* 2004;20(6):458–460.

36. Kushner GM. Surgical approaches to the infraorbital rim and orbital floor: the case for the transconjunctival approach. *J Oral Maxillofac Surg.* 2006;64(1):108–110.

37. Goldberg RA, Lessner AM, Shorr N, Baylis HI. The transconjunctival approach to the orbital floor and orbital fat: a prospective study. *Ophthal Plast Reconstr Surg.* 1990;6(4):241–246.

38. Choi M, Flores RL. Medial orbital wall fractures and the transcaruncular approach. *J Craniofac Surg.* 2012;23(3):696–701.

39. Shen Y, Paskowitz D, Merbs SL, Grant MP. Retrocaruncular approach for the repair of medial orbital wall fractures: an anatomical and clinical study. *Craniomaxillofac Trauma Reconstr.* 2015;8(2):100–104.

40. Lee CS, Yoon JS, Lee SY. Combined transconjunctival and transcaruncular approach for repair of large medial orbital wall fractures. *Arch Ophthalmol.* 2009;127(3):291–296.

41. Cheong E, Chen C, Chen Y. Endoscopic management of orbital floor fractures. *Facial Plast Surg.* 2009;25(1):8–16.

42. Strong EB, Kim KK, Diaz RC. Endoscopic approach to orbital blowout fracture repair. *Otolaryngol Head Neck Surg.* 2004;131(5):683–695.

43. Ellis E, Tan Y. Assessment of internal orbital reconstructions for pure blowout fractures: cranial bone grafts versus titanium mesh. *J Oral Maxillofac Surg.* 2003;61(4):442–453.

44. Park DJJ, Garibaldi DC, Iliff NT, et al. Smooth nylon foil (SupraFOIL) orbital implants in orbital fractures: a case series of 181 patients. *Ophthal Plast Reconstr Surg.* 2008;24(4):266–270.

45. Browning CW, Walker RV. Polyethylene in posttraumatic orbital floor reconstruction. *Am J Ophthalmol.* 1961;52:672–677.

46. Choi TJ, Burm JS, Yang WY, Kang SY. A wrapping method for inserting titanium micro-mesh implants in the reconstruction of blowout fractures. *Arch Plast Surg.* 2016;43(1):84–87.

47. Mahoney NR, Peng MY, Merbs SL, Grant MP. Virtual fitting, selection, and cutting of preformed anatomic orbital implants. *Ophthal Plast Reconstr Surg.* 2017;33(3):196–201.

48. Kozakiewicz M. Computer-aided orbital wall defects treatment by individual design ultrahigh molecular weight polyethylene implants. *J Craniomaxillofac Surg.* 2014;42(4):283–289.

49. Scolozzi P, Momjian A, Heuberger J, et al. Accuracy and predictability in use of AO three-dimensionally preformed titanium mesh plates for posttraumatic orbital reconstruction: a pilot study. *J Craniofac Surg.* 2009;20(4):1108–1113.

50. Wladis EJ. Are post-operative oral antibiotics required after orbital floor fracture repair? *Orbit.* 2013;32(1):30–32.

51. Gart Michael S., Gosain Arun K. Evidence-based medicine: orbital floor fractures. *Plast Reconstr Surg.* 2014;134(6):1345–1355.

Nasal Fractures

Leslie Kim, Matthew G. Huddle, Ryan M. Smith, Patrick Byrne

BACKGROUND

Nasal bone fractures are the most common type of facial bone fracture, accounting for at least half of all adult facial fractures.[1] The annual incidence of nasal bone fracture ranges from 0.053% to 0.37%, with peak incidence in adolescence or early adulthood.[2] Most nasal fractures are due to accidents (41%), with assault (31%) and sports (29%) also prominent etiologies.[2] Nasal bone fractures are frequently associated with cartilaginous and soft tissue injuries. Fractures of nearby facial bones may also occur, with orbital blowout and zygomaticomaxillary complex (ZMC) fractures being most common.[3]

SURGICAL ANATOMY

The nasal bones are paired, and attach to the nasal process of the frontal bone superiorly, frontal process of the maxilla laterally, upper lateral cartilages inferiorly, contralateral nasal bone medially, and septum internally. The septum is made up of the quadrangular cartilage anteriorly, perpendicular plate of the ethmoid superiorly, the vomer posteroinferiorly, and the crest of the maxillary and palatine bones inferiorly.

The blood supply of the external nose is robust and receives contributions from the internal carotid artery via the dorsal nasal branch of the ophthalmic artery and the external carotid artery via the lateral nasal and septal branches of the facial artery.

Sensation of the nasal dorsum is derived from the ophthalmic branch of the trigeminal nerve, while the nasal sidewalls are innervated by the maxillary branch of the trigeminal nerve.

CLINICAL PRESENTATION

History

Upon encountering a patient with nasal trauma, it is important to first establish the timing and mechanism of injury. The history is likely to provide clues to the pattern and severity of the fractures. A lateral blow to the nose, such as from an assault or being elbowed during a sports game, tends to result in lateral displacement of the nasal pyramid. On the other hand, a frontal blow, such as from a fall or from steering wheel impact in a motor vehicle crash, is more likely to result in frontal depression of the nasal bones with potential impaction of the nasal bones and nasal septum.

It is important to inquire about associated symptoms such as nasal airway obstruction, change in external appearance of nose, and epistaxis. Trauma resulting from a high force of impact or the presence of unusual symptoms including clear rhinorrhea, vision changes, diplopia, facial numbness, trismus, and/or change in occlusion should prompt investigation for other concomitant fractures. It is also important to establish any prior history of nasal trauma or nasal surgery as these patients are more likely to require secondary reconstruction after initial management of their fracture.

Physical Examination

The goal of the physical examination is to determine the extent and severity of the injury in order to counsel the patient appropriately regarding optimal management and outcome expectations. Examination should begin with a visual inspection for nasal deformity or deviation and noting any soft tissue injuries. Photo documentation of the external appearance of the nose is important for preoperative and postoperative counseling of the patient (Fig. 1.10.1). It is often helpful to compare the external appearance to a photograph from prior to the injury.[4]

Gentle palpation of the nasal dorsum should be performed in order to evaluate for the extent of displacement, depression, or lateralization of the nasal bones. The keystone region, the junction between the nasal bones and upper lateral cartilages, should also be palpated as trauma may result in disruption of this critical support region, leading to middle vault collapse. The nasal tip should be palpated to assess for potential loss of septal support.

An internal nasal examination with anterior rhinoscopy and nasal endoscopy should be performed to evaluate for septal fracture, septal hematoma, epistaxis, and clear rhinorrhea. A septal hematoma, if identified, must be drained as quickly as possible to avoid septal cartilage loss. Severe epistaxis may require additional management such as nasal packing. The presence of clear rhinorrhea necessitates further evaluation for a cerebrospinal fluid leak, such as with a beta-2 transferrin assay and high-resolution facial computed tomography (CT) scan to assess for a skull base fracture.

A complete physical examination must include investigation for physical signs of other facial bone fractures. A thorough examination of the head and neck should include palpation of the entire facial skeleton, assessment of extraocular motility, visual acuity, facial movements and sensation, and thorough evaluation for dental injury or pain, trismus, and malocclusion. The presence of any of these associated injuries should prompt further investigation with imaging.

RADIOLOGICAL EVALUATION

Isolated nasal fractures are primarily diagnosed through history and physical examination; therefore, the role of radiology in the diagnosis and management of nasal bone fractures is controversial. Plain radiographs are not helpful in the management of routine nasal bone fractures and should not be ordered.[5] Plain films are unable to distinguish between acute and old fractures and there is often poor correlation between the radiological findings and the presence of external deformity.[6]

Facial CT has been shown to demonstrate superior diagnostic accuracy when compared to conventional radiography in the detection of

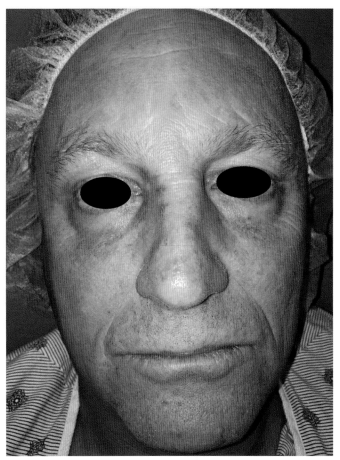

Fig. 1.10.1 Preoperative photograph demonstrating bilateral nasal bone fractures with deviation of the nasal dorsum.

nasal bone fractures.[7,8] In a review of 503 cases, only 82% of nasal bone fractures were correctly identified by plain films taken in both lateral and Waters views versus 100% by facial CT.[8] Despite the high positive predictive value of CT in detecting nasal bone fractures, the presence of a nasal bone fracture on CT scan has not been shown to reliably predict the need for surgical management.[9] The use of a CT, however, does document the direction and degree of bone and septal displacement.

Although CT is described as the gold standard modality of imaging for nasal bone fractures, some studies have suggested that high-resolution ultrasonography is as sensitive and specific, and may be particularly beneficial in pregnant women and children due to its absence of ionizing radiation.[10,11] However, the main disadvantage of ultrasonography is that it is operator-dependent.

Imaging, in general, may be beneficial in cases with equivocal physical exam findings or suspected associated injuries such as naso-orbito-ethmoid (NOE), orbital, and/or zygomaticomaxillary complex (ZMC) fractures. However, experienced clinical assessment remains the gold standard in determining the need for surgery.

CLASSIFICATION

Most clinical classification schemes are based on the degree and direction of force suspected to result in nasal injuries. Nasal fractures can be broadly divided into two types: those that result from a lateral blow and those that result from frontal impact.[12] Lateral impact injuries are more common than frontal injuries, as greater force is typically required to cause the latter.[13]

The lateral force fracture may range from a slight depression of a unilateral nasal bone to full lateral deviation of the nasal bridge due to bilateral nasal bone fractures (medial displacement of the ipsilateral nasal bone and lateral displacement of the contralateral nasal bone) with or without accompanying septal fracture. Disruption of the keystone region is less common. Treatment tends to be relatively simple, requiring centralization of the deviated nasal bones and septum.

According to Stranc and Robertson,[12] frontal impact injuries can be divided into three categories depending on the depth of the injury in the coronal plane. *Plane 1* injuries do not extend a line joining the lower end of the nasal bones to the anterior nasal spine. The force is predominantly transmitted to the cartilaginous framework and the inferior tip of the nasal bones, leading to deviations in the nasal septum and injury to the upper lateral cartilages while the nasal bones remain largely central. *Plane 2* injuries are more extensive but still limited to the nose. Flattening or splaying apart of the nasal bones as well as mucoperichondrial tears, more extensive overriding fractures of the septum, and loss of central support can be seen. *Plane 3* injuries are essentially NOE fractures; increased comminution of the nasal bones with fracture extension into adjacent bony structures is seen. Injuries to the nasal septum are often severe, with associated telescoping of septal fragments and structural collapse.

Murray et al.[13] describe an alternate classification scheme based on seven pathological types of fractures that resulted when various weights were dropped on cadavers' noses. Their study demonstrates that nasal fracture patterns are not consistently predicted by the amount and vector of the applied force. This system emphasizes that if the nose is deviated more than one-half its width from the midline, then the bony septum is involved; therefore, mere manipulation of the nasal bones alone will likely lead to recurrent deformation and need for secondary reconstruction.

Many other clinical classification schemes have since been proposed, most of which attempt to categorize trauma based on the extent of injury to the nasal bones and septum: simple vs. comminuted, unilateral vs. bilateral, degree of deviation, and degree of septal injury.[14,15] Most emphasize the importance of adequate septal repair in optimizing nasal fracture management and in minimizing the need for secondary surgery.

SURGICAL INDICATIONS

Surgical intervention following nasal trauma is warranted only if there is a change to the appearance and/or function of the nose after injury. Nasal fracture repair is typically elective, and may be deferred based on patient preference or condition.

Pediatric nasal trauma warrants special consideration. The pediatric nasal skeleton is more cartilaginous and flexible, and less prone to bony comminution.[16] However, the pediatric nasal septum – which plays a crucial role as a growth center for nose and midface – is more vulnerable to injury. In general, conservative treatment of nasal fractures in the pediatric population is recommended, with close observation and closed treatment of fractures as the mainstay. Although many surgeons favor delaying septoplasty and open reduction methods until after the adolescent growth spurt, early intervention may be indicated if there is severe nasal airway obstruction or external deformity that may result in adverse facial growth and/or problems with sleep disturbance and quality of life.[17]

SURGICAL TECHNIQUES

Timing of Repair

The timing of nasal fracture repair is dependent on the degree of injury and the amount of associated soft tissue edema. In the uncommon circumstance that a patient presents with an acute fracture within hours of injury with minimal associated edema, immediate fracture reduction might be performed. More typically, patients present with significant edema that obscures underlying nasal landmarks. In these instances, patients should be reassessed 3–5 days later after severe swelling subsides to determine need for reduction.[14]

Fracture reduction is ideally performed 1–2 weeks following the injury, in order to obtain maximal accuracy and stability.[4,18] Pediatric patients should be managed within 7–10 days given their tendency to heal more rapidly. After about 2–3 weeks it becomes more difficult to manipulate the healing nasal bones, although some report successful outcomes with manipulation up to 5 weeks following injury, particularly in patients with thinner bones or more comminuted fractures.[2]

Considerations for Anesthesia

The use of local versus general anesthesia for acute nasal bone fracture reduction is somewhat controversial. Benefits of local anesthesia include avoidance of the risks of general anesthesia and decreased associated costs and resources. General anesthesia is particularly advantageous in children and less cooperative or anxious adults, and for fractures that may require more extensive or open manipulation. However, the timing of treatment is often dependent on operating room and personnel availability.

A number of studies have compared the outcomes of local versus general anesthesia for the closed treatment of nasal fractures.[19–23] Current literature suggests that 79–90% of patients are satisfied after closed manipulation overall.[19] Several studies demonstrate equivalent functional and cosmetic results from both patient and surgeon perspectives as well as equivalent reoperation rates after closed reduction.[19–21] However, at least one study demonstrates higher rates of reoperation with septoplasty, septorhinoplasty, or rhinoplasty in patients treated under local anesthesia (17%) versus general anesthesia (3%).[22] A recent systematic review with meta-analysis of the limited literature suggests that although there is a trend towards better outcomes with general anesthesia, there are no significant differences between anesthesia modalities for nasal airway outcome, anesthetic experience, or number of revision procedures.[23]

The literature is relatively inconclusive and considerations for anesthesia are ultimately dependent on surgeon and patient preferences. It is the authors' preference to perform surgical intervention in an ambulatory surgical center under brief general anesthesia as it optimizes airway control and allows for unhindered nasal examination and more accurate and complete manipulation.

Local anesthesia, in either setting, may be provided by both topical and infiltrative agents. A 1:1 mixture of 4% topical lidocaine and oxymetazoline can be applied intranasally via pledgets for mucosal decongestion, vasoconstriction, and topical anesthesia. Infiltrative anesthesia with 1% lidocaine with 1:100,000 epinephrine can be administered both externally and internally. Infiltrative blocks can also be applied to the infraorbital and dorsal nasal nerves although generalized infiltration of the external dorsum has been found to be significantly less painful for patients.[24]

The operative set-up is shown in Fig. 1.10.2.

Closed Reduction (Figs. 1.10.3–1.10.7)

After anesthesia is achieved, a typical closed reduction begins with assessment of the bony nasal pyramid. A force opposite to the vector of trauma must be applied to achieve fracture reduction. The Boies elevator is commonly used intranasally to elevate depressed nasal bones while using a bimanual technique to palpate externally and assess for osseous movement. The Walsham or Asch forceps may be helpful in

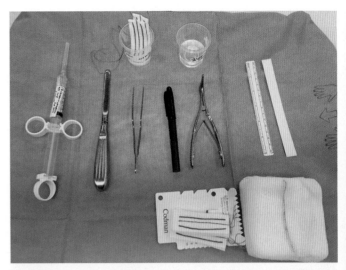

Fig. 1.10.2 Operative set-up for closed reduction of nasal bone fracture, including cotton pledgets, topical decongestant, local anesthetic in control syringe, Boise elevator, bayonet forceps, marking pen, nasal speculum, ruler, and sterile gauze.

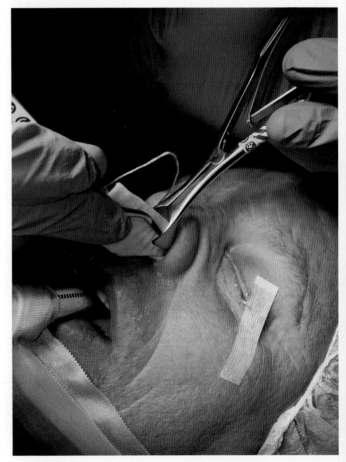

Fig. 1.10.3 Topical decongestant-soaked cotton pledgets are placed in the nasal passages using a bayonet forceps and nasal speculum.

the reduction of impacted and depressed nasal bones. Frequently, an audible and palpable "pop" will be observed as the bony fractures are reduced.

Attention to the nasal septum is critical, as nasal bone deformities will likely recur if a septal injury is not adequately addressed. Reduction

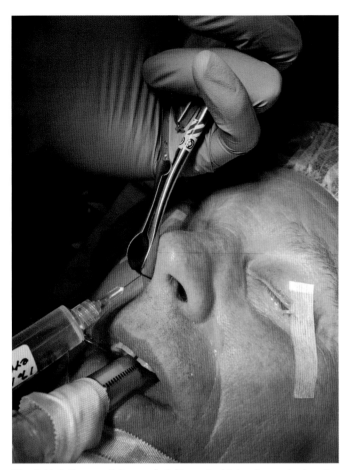

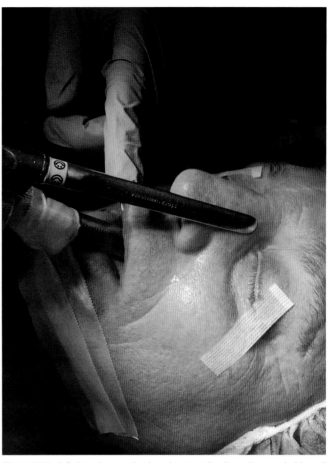

Fig. 1.10.4 The nasal dorsum is infiltrated with local anesthetic using a nasal speculum and control syringe.

Fig. 1.10.5 A Boies elevator is placed externally along the nasal sidewall to measure the length required to reduce the fracture.

of the fractured nasal septum is achieved by relocating the displaced septum back towards the midline and into the vomerine groove.[14] This can be accomplished with the Boies elevator or the Asch forceps by applying blunt pressure opposite to the direction of deviation with concurrent elevation of the nasal pyramid. The nose is then reexamined for correction of deviation and deformity, with further manipulation performed until adequate reduction is achieved.

Stabilization

All reduced fractures benefit from postoperative stabilization with external and/or internal splinting (Fig. 1.10.8). External splinting provides support to reduced nasal bones and cartilage and may aid in postoperative swelling and skin adherence to the underlying framework, particularly after an open procedure.[25] Extranasal splinting is most commonly performed with Steri-Strip™ adhesives (3M, Maplewood, MN) and application of an aluminum or thermoplastic Denver Splint® (Summit Medical, St. Paul, MN).

The internal nose can be stabilized with septal splints and/or intranasal packing. Doyle™ nasal splints (Boston Medical Products, Inc., Shrewsbury, MA) help provide septal stabilization after reduction and may help prevent synechiae after substantial manipulation, particularly if intranasal lacerations are present. Focused intranasal packing may be helpful when placed directly underlying severely comminuted or depressed nasal bones to prevent collapse after reduction. Both absorbable and non-absorbable packing may be used. Absorbable options include NasoPore® (Polyganic, Groningen, The Netherlands) and layered Gelfoam®

(Pfizer Inc., New York, NY) and non-absorbable options include Merocel® (Medtronic, Inc., Minneapolis, MN) and rolled Telfa™ (Medtronic, Inc., Minneapolis, MN). Recent studies suggest that NasoPore® may be superior to Merocel® as a nasal packing material with regards to pain, bleeding, as well as nasal obstruction.[26,27]

Open Reduction

Recognition and management of nasal septal fractures is critical to the successful management of nasal fractures. Therefore, the extent of septal injury typically determines the proper approach to correction. Open reduction is indicated in extensive fractures in which the nasal pyramid deviation exceeds one-half the width of the nasal bridge[13] (suggests involvement of the bony septum), fracture dislocations of the caudal septum, severe or complex septal injuries that extend posteriorly across the perpendicular plate of the ethmoid, and fractures that are irreducible with closed techniques.[14,18,28]

Open reduction techniques include septoplasty, osteotomies, and full septorhinoplasty.[15,18] The septum is most typically approached through a hemitransfixion or Killian incision on the side of the dislocation. Limited inferior and posterior septal resection and reconstruction may be performed in order to realign the septum. Caudal septal dislocations may be addressed in a closed fashion using full transfixion incisions with suture fixation to the midline nasal spine using figure-of-eight sutures. More severe caudal septal fracture-dislocations may require a limited open septorhinoplasty with structural cartilage grafting. Radical elevation and resection of cartilage or bone is avoided where

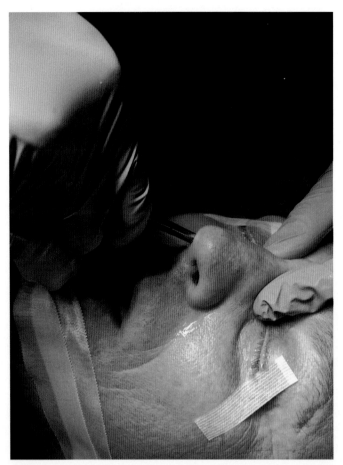
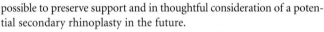

Fig. 1.10.6 The Boies elevator is placed inside the nasal passage and beneath the nasal bone while manual palpation is maintained with the opposite hand. Firm traction is applied to reduce the fracture.

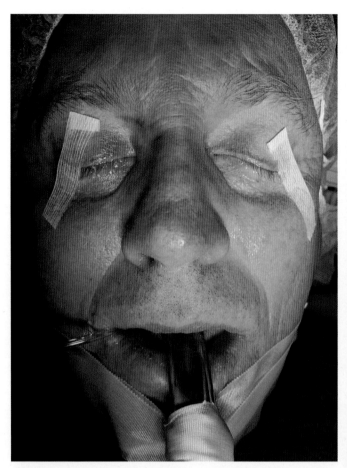

Fig. 1.10.7 Closed reduction of bilateral nasal bone fractures shows an improvement in dorsal symmetry and correction of the nasal deviation.

possible to preserve support and in thoughtful consideration of a potential secondary rhinoplasty in the future.

Limited completion osteotomies may be useful to mobilize the nasal bones, particularly in patients who have greenstick or impacted fractures.[15] If the dorsum remains deviated, release of the upper lateral cartilages from the septum may assist in unbuckling and realigning the middle vault.[18] As some degree of external and internal stabilization is provided by the skin–soft tissue envelope and periosteal and mucosal attachments of the nasal skeleton, excessive undermining is generally avoided to limit further destabilization. In most instances, a full formal septorhinoplasty is also typically delayed for at least a few months given the potential for unpredictable healing in the acute setting.

POSTOPERATIVE COURSE

External and intranasal splints are typically removed 5–7 days after surgery. Most surgeons traditionally prescribe antibiotics with coverage for *Staphylococcus* for patients – particularly those with nasal packing – for prophylaxis against Toxic Shock Syndrome (TSS). However, the evidence for this practice is poor, with incidence of TSS in patients with intranasal packing estimated to be quite rare (less than 20 per 100,000), and antibiotics have not been shown to have a significant protective effect.[29,30]

At the first follow-up, around 1 week after surgery, the patient should be evaluated for residual nasal obstruction and/or deformity. If these issues are evident early after initial closed reduction, consideration might be made for immediate open repair. Otherwise, follow-up should extend for at least 3 months following surgery to allow for resolution of edema. Definitive secondary septorhinoplasty, if needed, is usually delayed 3–6 months to allow time for healing and bony stabilization.

COMPLICATIONS

Medical complications following nasal trauma and nasal fracture repair include epistaxis, septal hematoma, septal perforation, intranasal synechiae, and cerebrospinal fluid leak. The most common complication, however, is poor reduction with persistent deformity and/or nasal obstruction. The incidence of post-reduction nasal deformity requiring subsequent rhinoplasty or septorhinoplasty is estimated to be between 14% and 50%.[14] Appropriate and thoughtful selection of reduction techniques, particularly with regards to the nasal septum, can minimize the need for reoperation. Despite this, patient satisfaction rates following nasal fracture repair remain relatively high, ranging between 68% and 87% for nasal cosmesis and 64% and 86% for nasal breathing.[2]

EXPERT COMMENTARY

Nasal fractures, which are the most common fracture, often go untreated or undertreated, or are managed in emergency rooms with no or poor imaging, and closed or *no* procedures, leading to underappreciation of the diagnosis and deformity, and to inadequate management. Often, the philosophy is advanced

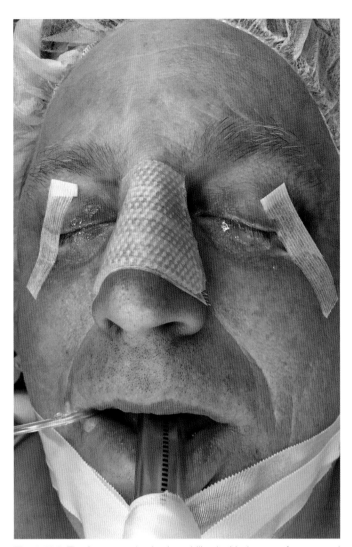

Fig. 1.10.8 The fracture reduction is stabilized with the use of an external nasal cast.

EXPERT COMMENTARY—cont'd

that a single late secondary procedure can achieve restoration of the preinjury architecture and structure, which may or may not be achievable because of the absence of "setting the stage" with a proper initial reduction.

While most significant fractures of the face are treated open, nasal fractures are still (for the majority) treated closed, limiting the alignment achieved and especially its confirmation through open reduction.

So what can be done to improve the results with this most under-imaged and undertreated fracture?

First a good physical examination and a good quality CT scan provide all the information necessary to make a diagnosis and a treatment plan. The extent of the fracture and the direction and the degree of displacement in two directions *must* be quantified for each (or both) of the common displacements observed: (1) lateral and (2) posterior displacement alone or in combination. In lateral displacements the nose is pushed to one side, and in posterior displacements the nose is pushed posteriorly. Both types of displacements are frequently observed simultaneously, in varying proportions. Then, injury to the septum must be assessed and quantified. Commonly, a laterally displaced nasal fracture has a "reverse C-shaped" dislocation of the septum. With posterior nasal displacements, the septal injury becomes more complicated, with multiple overlapping segments, foreshortening, and up-tilting of the nose. The skin contracts to fit the reduced skeletal volume, fixing the skin volume and thus the deformity.

Currently, the standard of care is an initial closed reduction, followed by late secondary surgery for residual deformity and aesthetics. Appropriate existing lacerations can occasionally be used to achieve a partial or complete open reduction, improving the accuracy of the reduction by visualizing the displaced bones and the cartilages (the latter do not show in CT scans.). When open reduction is not possible, the exact knowledge of the patterns of the fragments gained by physical examination and CT guide the closed maneuvers necessary to achieve the maximal alignment of cartilage and bone structures.

And don't wait too long, or the fracture healing will obstruct the reduction. I do closed nasal reductions under general anesthesia, because I found that I was seldom able to achieve sufficient local anesthesia or patient cooperation in the face of apprehension. Less commonly, my attempt at closed reduction under local was accompanied by an unanticipated profuse nasal hemorrhage precipitated by the manipulation of the reduction maneuvers. This event can make aspiration and airway issues a possibility, especially in a sedated patient, and so I do these with the patient intubated, nasally vasoconstricted, and it takes me 5 minutes or less, but I do a good job. I can complete the fractures thoroughly, which is often *not* able to be done under local anesthesia, which otherwise yields recurrent or persistent deformity. Whatever is incomplete after the initial closed reduction may be managed open by late secondary rhinoseptoplasty.

For laterally displaced nasal fractures, I complete the fracture on each side, and if the unilateral nasal bone is unfractured or greensticked, I make sure to complete the fracture by a reduction maneuver or an osteotome (2 mm percutaneously as in a rhinoplasty). When the lateral fractures are replaced in the midline (and stay where placed – an indication that the fractures have been properly completed), I reduce the septum with an Asch forcep completing the fractures. I reduce the higher septum and the lower septum with separate reduction maneuvers, and I am certain before this to determine the position of the cribiform plate by palpation with a cotton applicator. Two reduction maneuvers replace the septum in the midline, completing the fractures. Doyle splints hold the septum in position, and are anchored anteriorly with a 2/0 nylon through the hole and NOT through the splint, which tears the silicone.

For posteriorly impacted fractures, I elevate the depressed fracture, and stabilize it with one of several maneuvers: (1) internal Mirocel® packs to support the depressed nasal bone segments under the nasal bones; (2) less commonly, percutaneous nasal compression bolsters placed as used for molding NOE fractures will control the width of the nose and add some lost nasal height by narrowing the base width of the nose; (3) rarely I perform cartilage or bone grafting of the dorsum and columella.

Finally, realize that some "bad nasal fractures" are occasionally Type I NOE fractures in their early stages, and the unilateral depressed pyriform rim is actually *not* a nasal fracture even though it masquerades as a unilateral laterally dislocated nasal fracture. A good result can *only* be achieved by an open reduction intraorally of the medial buttress of the maxilla which is greensticked and incompletely fractured. This fracture is corrected through a gingival buccal sulcus incision, reducing the pyriform rim with a small right-angle clamp placed medial and posterior to the displaced pyriform aperture. Elevate this with the clamp, and the fracture rises into position.

REFERENCES

1. Renner GJ. Management of nasal fractures. *Otolaryngol Clin North Am.* 1991;24(1):195–213.
2. Basheeth N, Donnelly M, David S, et al. Acute nasal fracture management: a prospective study and literature review. *Laryngoscope.* 2015;125(12):2677–2684.

3. Hwang K, You SH, Lee HS. Outcome analysis of sports-related multiple facial fractures. *J Craniofac Surg*. 2009;20(3):825–829.

4. Fomon S, Schattner A, Bell JW, et al. Management of recent nasal fractures. *AMA Arch Otolaryngol*. 1952;55(3):321–342.

5. Clayton MI, Lesser TH. The role of radiography in the management of nasal fractures. *J Laryngol Otol*. 1986;100(7):797–801.

6. Nigam A, Goni A, Benjamin A, et al. The value of radiographs in the management of the fractured nose. *Arch Emerg Med*. 1993;10(4):293–297.

7. Baek HJ, Kim DW, Ryu JH, et al. Identification of nasal bone fractures on conventional radiography and facial CT: comparison of the diagnostic accuracy in different imaging modalities and analysis of interobserver reliability. *Iran J Radiol*. 2013;10(3):140–147.

8. Hwang K, You SH, Kim SG, et al. Analysis of nasal bone fractures; a six-year study of 503 patients. *J Craniofac Surg*. 2006;17(2):261–264.

9. Peterson B, Doerr T. Utility of computed tomography scans in predicting need for surgery in nasal injuries. *Craniomaxillofac Trauma Reconstr*. 2013;6(4):221–224.

10. Mohammadi A, Ghasemi-Rad M. Nasal bone fracture – ultrasonography or computed tomography? *Med Ultrason*. 2011;13(4):292–295.

11. Javadrashid R, Khatoonabad MJ, Shams N, et al. Comparison of ultrasonography with computed tomography in the diagnosis of nasal bone fractures. *Dentomaxillofac Radiol*. 2011;40(8):486–491.

12. Stranc MF, Robertson GA. A classification of injuries of the nasal skeleton. *Ann Plast Surg*. 1979;2(6):468–474.

13. Murray JAM, Maran AGD. A pathologic classification of nasal fractures. *Injury*. 1986;17:338–344.

14. Rohrich RJ, Adams WP Jr. Nasal fracture management: minimizing secondary nasal deformities. *Plast Reconstr Surg*. 2000;106(2):266–273.

15. Ondik MP, Lipinski L, Dezfoli S, Fedok FG. The treatment of nasal fractures: a changing paradigm. *Arch Facial Plast Surg*. 2009;11(5):296–302.

16. Verwoerd CDA, Verwoerd-Verhoef HL. Rhinosurgery in children: basic concepts. *Facial Plast Surg*. 2007;23:219–230.

17. Wright RJ, Murakami CS, Ambro BT. Pediatric nasal injuries and management. *Facial Plast Surg*. 2011;27:483–490.

18. Staffel JG. Optimizing treatment of nasal fractures. *Laryngoscope*. 2002;112(10):1709–1719.

19. Rajapakse Y, Courtney M, Bialostocki A, et al. Nasal fractures: a study comparing local and general anesthesia techniques. *ANZ J Surg*. 2003;73:396–399.

20. Waldron J, Mitchell DB, Ford G. Reduction of fractured nasal bones; local versus general anaesthesia. *Clin Otolaryngol Allied Sci*. 1989;14(4):357–359.

21. Khwaja S, Pahade AV, Luff D, et al. Nasal fracture reduction: local versus general anaesthesia. *Rhinology*. 2007;45(1):83–88.

22. Courtney MJ, Rajapakse Y, Duncan G, et al. Nasal fracture manipulation: a comparative study of general and local anaesthesia techniques. *Clin Otolaryngol Allied Sci*. 2003;28(5):472–475.

23. Al-Moraissi EA, Ellis E. Local versus general anesthesia for the management of nasal bone fractures: a systematic review and meta-analysis. *J Oral Maxillofac Surg*. 2015;73(4):606–615.

24. Cook JA, Murrant NJ, Evans K, et al. Manipulation of the fractured nose under local anesthesia. *Clin Otolaryngol Allied Sci*. 1992;17(4):337–340.

25. Ozucer B, Yildirim YS, Veyseller B, et al. Effect of postrhinoplasty taping on postoperative edema and nasal draping: a randomized clinical trial. *JAMA Facial Plast Surg*. 2016;18(3):157–163.

26. Yi CR, Kim YJ, Kim H, et al. Comparison study of the use of absorbable and nonabsorbable materials as internal splints after closed reduction for nasal bone fracture. *Arch Plast Surg*. 2014;41(4):350–354.

27. Wang J, Cai C, Wang S. Merocel versus nasopore for nasal packing: a meta-analysis of randomized control trials. *PLoS ONE*. 2014;9(4):e93959.

28. Mondin V, Rinaldo A, Ferlito A. Management of nasal bone fractures. *Am J Otolaryngol*. 2005;26(3):181–185.

29. Gioacchini FM, Alicandri-Ciufelli M, Kaleci S, et al. The role of antibiotic therapy and nasal packing in septoplasty. *Eur Arch Otorhinolaryngol*. 2014;271(5):879–886.

30. Jacobson JA, Kasworm EM. Toxic shock syndrome after nasal surgery. Case reports and analysis of risk factors. *Arch Otolaryngol Head Neck Surg*. 1986;112(3):329–332.

Naso-orbito-ethmoid (NOE) Fractures

Craig Birgfeld

BACKGROUND

The naso-orbito-ethmoid (NOE) region of the central face is defined by the orbits laterally, the glabella superiorly and the nose inferiorly. It is a particularly challenging region of the face to reconstruct due to its aesthetic prominence, its 3-dimensional contour and the delicate associated structures involved in the region. NOE fractures occur from direct blunt force trauma to the central face, such as striking the dashboard in a motor vehicle collision (MVC). While isolated NOE fractures accounted for only (5.8%)[1] of all facial fractures at a busy trauma center, they are a frequent component of associated midface fractures[2] and must be accurately diagnosed and treated to attain anatomic fracture reduction.

SURGICAL ANATOMY

The NOE complex is comprised of the frontal process of the maxilla, internal angular process of the frontal bone, the ethmoid sinuses, and the lacrimal bone (Fig. 1.11.1). As such, it contributes to the shape and volume of the medial orbits, the contour of the inferior orbital rim, the patency of the pyriform aperture, and the support of the nasal dorsum. Additionally, it serves as the drainage of the frontal sinus and the attachment of the medial canthal tendon and the trochlea, and the location of the nasolacrimal apparatus are associated structures (Fig. 1.11.2).

CLINICAL PRESENTATION

Patients present after blunt force trauma to the central face. They will often complain of diplopia, nasal airway obstruction, and alteration of physical appearance. They may report numbness of the central face and forehead, epiphora,[3] and CSF rhinorrhea.[4]

After a complete ATLS evaluation with particular attention paid to the C-spine,[5] a focused craniofacial examination is performed. Begin with inspection of the eyes, noting telecanthus, rounding of the palpebral fissure, and lid malposition. If avulsion of the medial canthal tendon is suspected, the examiner can use forceps to pull on the tendon, noting presence or absence of a firm stop (Video 1.11.1). Assess visual acuity and test extraocular muscle integrity looking for entrapment. Measure globe position noting enophthalmos or exophthalmos. The presence of an orbital fracture merits an ophthalmological consultation to rule out injury to the eye, visual system, and retina.[6]

The examiner should note asymmetry of the nose and presence of a saddle nose deformity (Fig. 1.11.3). Sequentially, assess nasal airway patency and perform a speculum exam noting integrity of the septum, nasal perforation, and presence of a septal hematoma, which requires prompt drainage.[7] The presence of a collapsed/telescoped septal fracture

may require dorsal or caudal nasal cantilever bone grafting to maintain nasal support. Proceed next with gentle palpation of the craniofacial skeleton noting point tenderness, crepitus, and bony step-offs.

RADIOLOGICAL EVALUATION

If, after physical exam, an NOE fracture is suspected, one should obtain a fine cut (0.5 mm) maxillofacial computed tomography (CT) scan extending from vertex through menton. Plain films are of no utility.[8] Axial and coronal views are both required and additional sagittal and 3D views may be helpful if orbital involvement is extensive and/or the fractures are complicated. The skull should be included to assess for viable split calvarial bone graft harvest sites for possible nasal and orbital reconstruction.

CLASSIFICATION

The severity of NOE fractures is determined by CT scan evaluation based on either the Manson or Gruss classification system. In the Gruss classification, severity is graded into five types based on the presence of increasingly difficult surrounding midface fractures (Table 1.11.1).[9] As severity increases, additional surgical maneuvers such as orbital repositioning or bone grafting may be required. In the Manson classification system, focus is placed on the medial canthal tendon. Severity is graded into three types based on the degree of comminution of the NOE segment and the integrity of the medial canthal attachment (Fig. 1.11.4).[10] Similarly, with increasing severity, the Manson classification system predicts additional surgical maneuvers such as open reduction internal fixation, transnasal wires, and medial canthoplasty.

SURGICAL INDICATIONS

Once an NOE fracture is diagnosed, the surgeon must decide whether an operative intervention is warranted. Generally, this decision is based on amount of displacement and degree of comminution. A nondisplaced, nonmobile NOE fracture can be treated nonoperatively. A minimally impacted, large segment NOE fracture may be treated with closed reduction and splint stabilization[11] (Fig. 1.11.5), whereas a displaced, comminuted NOE fracture may require operative fixation via one or multiple surgical approaches (Fig. 1.11.6).

In addition to displacement and comminution, the effects of the NOE fracture on various facial features are taken into consideration when deciding operative management. With regards to the orbit, NOE fractures affect orbital volume, medial canthal position, and inferior rim support. As the ethmoid bulge is diminished, orbital volume increases which can lead to enophthalmos and such fractures should be treated with bone graft or alloplastic implant to the medial orbital wall.

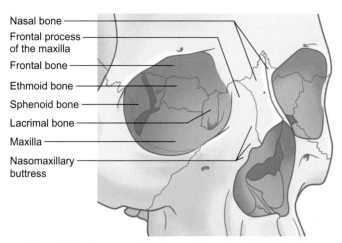

Nasal bone
Frontal process of the maxilla
Frontal bone
Ethmoid bone
Sphenoid bone
Lacrimal bone
Maxilla
Nasomaxillary buttress

Fig. 1.11.1 Anatomy of the naso-orbito-ethmoid (NOE) region.

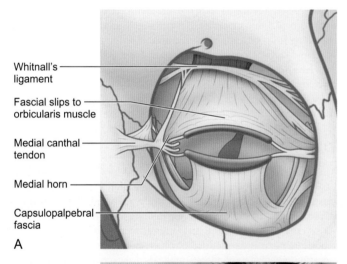

Whitnall's ligament
Fascial slips to orbicularis muscle
Medial canthal tendon
Medial horn
Capsulopalpebral fascia

A

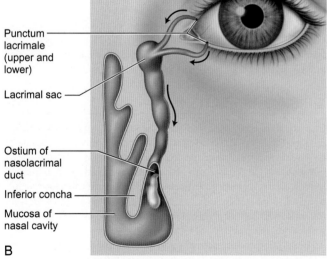

Punctum lacrimale (upper and lower)
Lacrimal sac
Ostium of nasolacrimal duct
Inferior concha
Mucosa of nasal cavity

B

Fig. 1.11.2 Attachment of the medial canthal tendon to the NOE segment and passage of the nasolacrimal apparatus through the NOE segment.

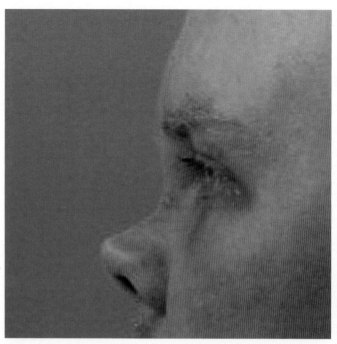

Fig. 1.11.3 Saddle nose deformity with loss of dorsal nasal support.

TABLE 1.11.1	**Gruss Classification of NOE Injuries**
Type 1:	Isolated bony NOE injury
Type 2:	Bony NOE injury and central maxilla
2a:	Central maxilla only
2b:	Central maxilla and one lateral maxilla
2c:	Central and bilateral lateral maxillae
Type 3:	Extended NOE injury
3a:	With craniofacial injuries
3b:	With LeFort II and III fractures
Type 4:	NOE injury with orbital displacement
4a:	With oculo-orbital displacement
4b:	With orbital dystopia
Type 5:	NOE injury with bone loss

NOE, naso-orbito-ethmoid. Note Gruss in his original publication refers to "naso-ethmoid-orbital injury."
Source: From Gruss JS. Naso-ethmoid-orbital fractures: classification and role of primary bone grafting. Plast Reconstr Surg 1985;75:303–317.

Rotation of the NOE segment can change the 3-dimensional ogee of the naso-orbital region and create a bony step-off at the inferior rim. This rotation can also lead to telecanthus as can comminution or detachment of the medial canthal tendon, all of which require surgical intervention to reestablish normal intercanthal distance (35–40 mm in adults).[12]

With regards to the nose, NOE fractures can affect the patency of the airway and the stability of the nasal tip and dorsum. Fracture segments that impact into the pyriform can narrow the airway. If obstruction is noted on exam, then the segment must be reduced and fixated to reestablish the normal lateral pyriform contour. With severe comminution and concomitant septal fracture, loss of dorsal support can

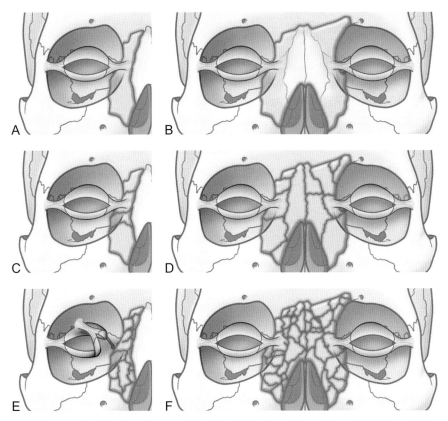

Fig. 1.11.4 Manson classification of naso-orbito-ethmoid fractures. Type I injury (A–B): large single segment with medial canthal tendon attached. Type II (C–D): comminuted NOE segment but medial canthal tendon retains attachment to a bony segment which can be treated with ORIF. Type III injury (E–F): avulsion of the medial canthal tendon which requires canthoplasty with transnasal wire to repair. (Reproduced from Markowitz BL, Manson PN, Sargent L, et al. Management of the medial canthal tendon in nasoethmoid orbital fractures: the importance of the central fragment in classification and treatment. Plast Reconstr Surg 1991;87:843–53.)

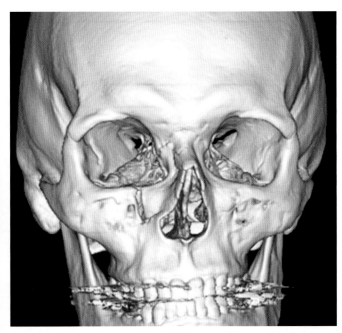

Fig. 1.11.5 Large fragment right NOE fracture (Manson I) amenable to closed reduction.

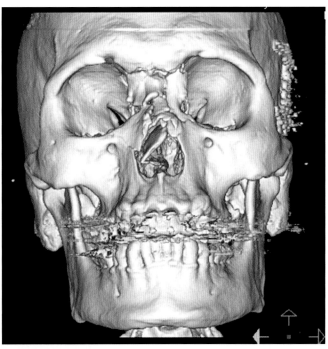

Fig. 1.11.6 Comminuted NOE (Manson II) requiring multiple surgical approaches for repair.

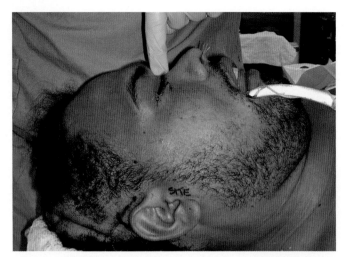

Fig. 1.11.7 Loss of dorsal nasal support due to comminuted NOE fracture (CT in Fig. 1.11.6) and concomitant septal fracture (Gruss 2).

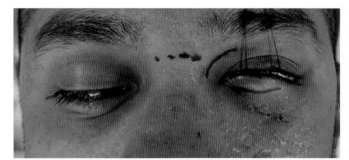

Fig. 1.11.8 Example of Lynch incision for access to nasofrontal junction in combination with a lower lid incision for access to the orbital rim.

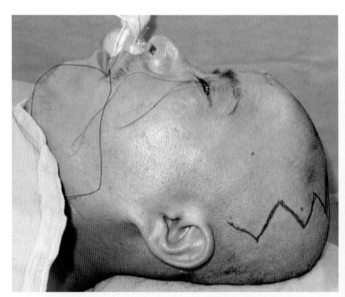

Fig. 1.11.9 Example of coronal incision. Begin at least 1 cm above temporal hairline and use zig-zag incision to optimize camouflage within the hair.

lead to a saddle nose deformity (Fig. 1.11.7), which is difficult, if not impossible, to correct secondarily once the soft tissue envelope contracts and must therefore be treated acutely.[13]

NOE fractures are commonly associated with other facial fractures such as midface fractures, ZMC fractures, and especially frontal sinus fractures. It is paramount to identify and treat the NOE component of these multilevel fractures in order to attain an anatomic reduction.[2] While most isolated NOE fractures do not cause compromise of frontal sinus drainage by blocking the nasofrontal outflow, obstruction of the nasofrontal outflow tracts by comminuted NOE fractures may increase the risk of mucocele formation with associated frontal sinus fractures. One must first disimpact and fixate the NOE component before obliterating or cranializing the frontal sinus to avoid mucocele formation.

SURGICAL TECHNIQUES

Surgical treatment of NOE fractures focuses on restoration of normal anatomy with minimal incisions and soft tissue stripping. However, attaining a perfect anatomic reduction must not be compromised in an effort to reduce exposure. A gingivobuccal sulcus incision alone may be adequate to treat a large segment NOE impacted at the pyriform. Addition of a lower eyelid incision can help attain reduction along the inferior orbital rim. A short vertical linear incision at the radix or the horizontal alone portion of the Converse "open sky" incision (Fig. 1.11.8) may suffice for a minimally displaced, large segment NOE fragment at the nasofrontal junction. However, often a coronal incision (Fig. 1.11.9) is needed to establish anatomical reduction in severely impacted and comminuted fractures. This also allows access to the medial orbital wall and the frontal sinus if involved. Additionally, access for calvarial bone graft harvest is afforded if dorsal nasal reconstruction is warranted.

Begin with the lower eyelid incisions, dissecting the delicate tissue carefully before edema sets in. Then turn the coronal flap in the subgaleal plane, leaving the temporalis muscles in place. Expose the fracture at the nasofrontal (NF) junction, then make the gingivobuccal sulcus incision to expose the medial maxillary buttress. Disimpact the fracture with Asch forceps placed in the nose. Place cephalad traction on a plate at the NF junction (Fig. 1.11.10) or an orbital spanning plate (Video 1.11.2) to establish vertical position. Rotate the segment using a clamp on the pyriform until the orbital rim is reduced, then fixate the rim and medial buttress. If comminution exists (Manson type II), make sure the canthal bearing fracture fragment is included in the fixation

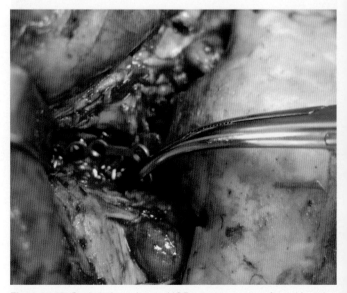

Fig. 1.11.10 Cephalad traction on NOE segment at nasofrontal junction to obtain vertical reduction at nasion.

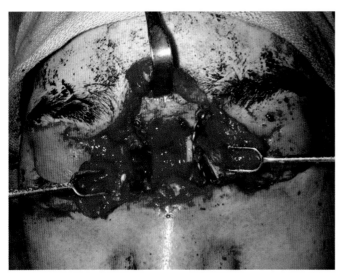

Fig. 1.11.11 Comminuted NOE fragment on left (Manson type II) is captured within the plate to reposition medial canthal tendon medially.

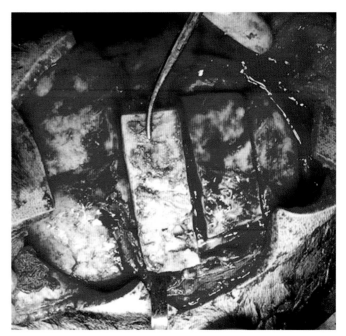

Fig. 1.11.12 Harvest of split calvarial bone graft.

(Fig. 1.11.11). If the tendon is avulsed (Manson type III), perform a medial canthoplasty with transnasal wires or a canthal barb. One way to perform a transnasal wire entails using a wire-passing drill bit to create two parallel tunnels from the contralateral orbit, across the ethmoid sinus to the intended location of the affected medial canthal tendon. A wire is then passed cephalad and caudal to the avulsed medial canthal tendon. The two ends of the wire are then passed through the drill holes and are twisted down in the unaffected orbit until the avulsed canthus is elevated and medialized to its proper position (overcorrected slightly). With comminuted fractures, the surgeon may need to twist the wire down to a titanium plate in the unaffected orbit to stabilize its position. To use the canthal barb, drill a single hole from the unaffected orbit to the intended medial canthal position. Then pass the Keith needle through the avulsed canthal tendon until the barb catches the canthus. Pass the wire through the hole and loop it around a screw placed in the superomedial aspect of the unaffected orbit, providing tension until the avulsed canthus is in a slightly overcorrected position. Then tighten the screw to maintain the wire's position. Again, placement of a titanium plate into the contralateral orbit may be necessary in comminuted fractures.

If there is loss of nasal support (Gruss type II), then a split calvarial bone graft is harvested (Fig. 1.11.12), shaped, and secured to the nasal frontal junction *below* the frontal prominence. Placement of this graft too high upon the frontal bone will efface the radix and give an unnatural appearance to the nasal profile (Fig. 1.11.13). An external rhinoplasty approach may be used to ensure the alar cartilages are centralized above the tip of the cantilevered bone graft.[14]

POSTOPERATIVE COURSE

Postoperative care depends on the operative intervention performed. A single dose of intravenous antibiotics with sinus flora coverage followed by an additional 24 hour course is indicated,[15] but prolonged therapy has no proven benefit.[16–19] If a coronal incision is used, a JP drain is placed for 48 hours. If orbital grafts or implants are placed, Frost sutures are utilized for 48 hours to reduce scleral edema. The nose is packed for 24 hours and if a septal fracture is treated, Doyle splints are placed for 3–4 weeks. External nasal splints are used to redrape the soft tissue around the medial canthi (Fig. 1.11.14). Begin

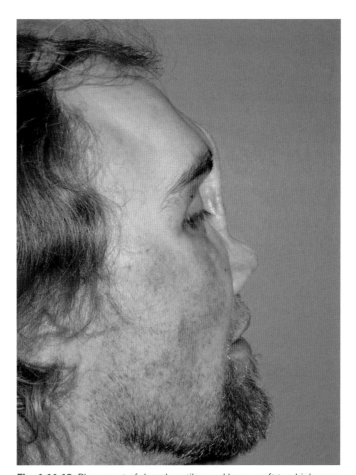

Fig. 1.11.13 Placement of dorsal cantilevered bone graft too high upon the frontal bone does not correct the saddle nose deformity nor restore proper nasal aesthetics.

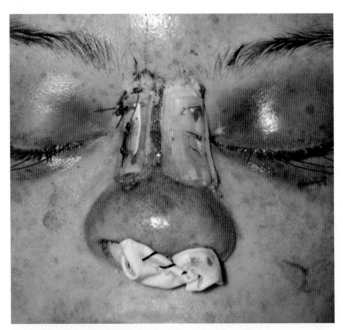

Fig. 1.11.14 Nasal packing and external nasal splints allows redraping of soft tissue around the medial canthal tendons.

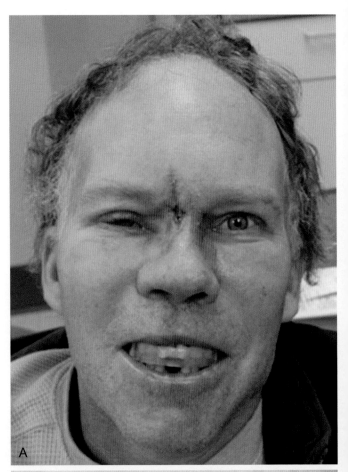

A

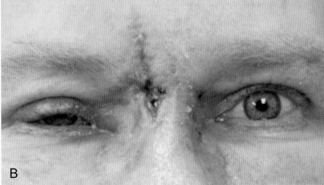

B

Fig. 1.11.15 Pressure necrosis from external nasal splints and exposure of underlying hardware at site of glabella laceration.

by placing xeroform gauze on the skin along the nasal sidewalls down to the medial canthal attachment. Then, trim Doyle nasal splints to the size and shape of the patient's nasal sidewalls. Place the Doyle splints over the xeroform gauze and secure them with a silk suture passed through the splint, across the nasal base (through the fractures), then through the contralateral splint. Typically two horizontal mattress sutures are required. If this is not performed, then the patient will appear to have persistent telecanthus even if the canthi are adequately reduced and fixated with the operative canthoplasties.

ACUTE COMPLICATIONS

Acute complications from NOE repair center around vision, hemorrhage, and soft tissue-related issues. If the orbit is manipulated, and especially if an implant is placed along the floor or medial wall, then injury to the globe and/or optic nerve is possible. An intraoperative or immediate postoperative CT scan can confirm anatomic placement of an orbital implant and frequent postoperative vision checks are mandatory to detect alterations in vision due to injury or impingement. While transient diplopia is common for a week or two after surgery, persistent, non-improving diplopia merits investigation to rule out entrapment of orbital contents under or around the implant.

Epiphora is common after NOE fracture due to swelling and possibly injury to the nasolacrimal apparatus. While routine probing and stenting during acute fracture care is not recommended,[20] dacrocysto-rhinostomy (DCR) may be needed later.[3] Epistaxis is also common, and typically controlled with Afrin and nasal packing. But, persistent or uncontrollable epistaxis warrants consideration of injury to the anterior ethmoid arteries. Lastly, careful repair of soft tissue incisions and lacerations ensure optimal aesthetic results. Care must be taken to limit pressure of nasal packing and splints to avoid soft tissue necrosis (Fig. 1.11.15), especially on and around the nose.

LONG-TERM COMPLICATIONS

Long-term complications of NOE fractures such as persistent telecanthus, enophthalmos, saddle nose deformity, and airway obstruction occur due to failure to recognize fracture patterns, failure to anatomically reduce fracture segments, and undercorrection (Fig. 1.11.16). Common mistakes and their sequelae are listed in Table 1.11.2. These can be difficult if not impossible to correct secondarily and therefore anatomic reduction at the first operation should be the goal.[21,22] Remember, the pyriform aperture cannot be too patent, the NOE segments cannot be too anterior, and the canthi cannot be too medially corrected.

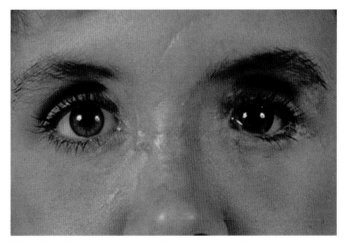

Fig. 1.11.16 Persistent telecanthus, rounded palpebral fissures and epiphora due to malreduction of bilateral NOE fractures.

TABLE 1.11.2 Common Mistakes and Their Sequelae

Mistake	Sequelae
Lack of anterior reduction of NOE segment	Saddle nose deformity
Lack of lateral reduction of NOE segment	Airway obstruction
Lack of medial reduction of NOE segment at canthus	Telecanthus, rounded palpebral fissure, epiphora
	Saddle nose deformity
Imprecise placement of medial canthal wire	Blocked nasolacrimal duct, requiring DCR
Lack of fixation of medial canthal wire in contralateral orbit	Persistent telecanthus
Failure to redrape medial canthal soft tissue with external nasal splints	Appearance of telecanthus despite normal intercanthal distance

DCR, dacrocystorhinostomy.

EXPERT COMMENTARY

Four large trauma systems have defined the classification and treatment of naso-orbital-ethmoid fractures: Manson, Markowitz and Sargent, Shock Trauma, Baltimore (and later Sargent, Chattanooga [1–4]); Gruss, Sunnybrook, Toronto, and later Harborview, Seattle. From these experiences patterns of injury have been defined leading to patterns of treatment. Fractures are either partial or complete, large piece or comminuted, unilateral or bilateral and isolated to the nasoethmoid area or extended to other areas such as the orbit, maxilla or frontal bone.

Classification of the fractures helps organize the most expeditious treatment necessary, and limits incisions to the fewest necessary [1–3]. Isolated NOE fractures rarely cause nasofrontal outflow tract obstruction, and rarely should anything be done primarily to the frontal sinus or the lacrimal system, such as prophylactic intubation or stenting [2]. The frontal sinus seldom needs treatment or stenting in the absence of direct frontal sinus involvement [2].

NOE fractures are diagnosed by their appearance, and by physical examination, particularly a bimanual examination [4]. An inferiorly alone displaced Type 1 NOE [2] fracture (greensticked at the nasofrontal junction) is actually usually misdiagnosed as a nasal fracture, since it displaces the pyriform rim posteriorly. Treating it therefore as a nasal fracture is ineffective, and treatment must be accomplished intraorally, raising the supporting buttress of the nose, the pyriform rim. The best incisions for local exposure of the NOE complex are the short vertical incision over the radix and, better, the horizontal limb alone of the Converse "open sky" approach (do *not* use the extensions, as they cause scar hypertrophy and deformity). Complete dislocations of Type I single segment fractures may frequently be managed with gingival buccal sulcus and lower eyelid incisions alone, especially if the nasofrontal attachment fracture is greensticked (incomplete and not dislocated), or fractured but undisplaced.

The bimanual examination is the best physical sign for confirming the diagnosis of complete nasoethmoid fractures (4) as the "eyelid traction test" is of little clinical value and will miss all but the most complete fractures.

When the comminution extends under the canthal insertion, the tendon must be stripped to do the bone reduction, and it must then be secondarily re-attached. We use a separate set of wires for each canthus, passed through the nose and medial canthal bone attachments and tied over a screw in the frontal bone [1,2]. The nasal bones should be reassembled with wires, and then junctional rigid fixation around the periphery of this wired complex is used to stabilize the entire reassembled NOE complex as excessive plate use adds to the thickness of the nose and detracts from the appearance. Dorsal nasal bone grafts smooth the appearance and add nasal height correction, and caudal (columellar) bone grafts correct the nasal length and base dimensions. Caudal bone grafts help lengthen the nose, and are necessary in the event of the collapsed, foreshortened nose with the telescoped septum.

Much attention should be directed toward reattaching the soft tissue when it has been removed in primary repairs. We use compression bolsters to mold the soft tissue to the bone, controlling edema and scar tissue thickening. The tissue in what Converse called the "naso-orbital valley" must be reapplied to the sidewall of the nose creating a right-angle between the medial maxilla and the nasal sidewall, otherwise the space fills with blood and remodels with scar tissue creating the appearance of an unrepaired nasoethmoid fracture despite what may be a good bone repair. Sargent [5] actually currently uses sutures from the dermis to the nasal sidewall to reattach the soft tissue to the nasal skeleton.

Nasoethmoid repair is a combination of bone and soft tissue reduction and stabilization, and specific maneuvers need to be directed toward each tissue component to achieve good results.

References

1. Manson P, Markowitz B, Mirvis S, et al. Toward CT-based facial fracture treatment. *Plast Reconstr Surg.* 1990;85:202–212.
2. Markowitz B, Manson P, Sargent L, et al. Management of the medial canthal tendon in nasoethmoid orbital fractures: the importance of the central fragment in treatment and classification. *Plast Reconstr Surg.* 1991;87:843–853.
3. Manson PN. Dimensional analysis of the facial skeleton. In: *Problems in Plastic Surgery.* Philadelphia: J.B. Lippincott Co.; 1991.
4. Paskert J, Manson PN. The bimanual examination for assessing instability in nasoethmoid orbital fractures. *Plast Reconstr Surg.* 1989;83:165.
5. Sargent LA. Hypertelorism repair. In: Prein J, Ehrenfeld M, Manson P, Futran N, eds. *Rigid Fixation of the Craniofacial Skeleton.* Vol. 2. Stuttgart: Thieme; 2019 (in press).

REFERENCES

1. Birgfeld CB, Hopper RA, Gruss JS. Facial fractures from Harborview Medical Center Trauma Registry (Harborview Medical Center, Seattle WA, unpublished data, 2004–2009).

2. Buchanan EP, Hopper RA, Suver DW, et al. Zygomaticomaxillary complex fractures and their association with naso-orbito-ethmoid fractures: a 5-year review. *Plast Reconstr Surg.* 2012;130:1296–1304.

3. Ali MJ, Gupta H, Honavar SG, Naik MN. Acquired nasolacrimal duct obstructions secondary to naso-orbito-ethmoidal fractures: patterns and outcomes. *Ophthal Plast Reconstr Surg.* 2012;28:242–245.

4. Maxwell JA, Goldware SI. Use of tissue adhesive in the surgical treatment of cerebrospinal fluid leaks. Experience with isobutyl 2-cyanoacrylate in 12 cases. *J Neurosurg.* 1973;39:332–336.

5. Mulligan RP, Mahabir RC. The prevalence of cervical spine injury, head injury, or both with isolated and multiple craniomaxillofacial fractures. *Plast Reconstr Surg.* 2010;126:1647–1651.

6. Holt GR, Holt JE. Incidence of eye injuries in facial fractures: an analysis of 727 cases. *Otolaryngol Head Neck Surg.* 1983;91:276–279.

7. Sayin I, Yazici ZM, Bozkurt E, Kayhan FT. Nasal septal hematoma and abscess in children. *J Craniofac Surg.* 2011;22:e17–e19.

8. Johnson DH Jr, Colman M, Larsson S, et al. Computed tomography in medial maxilla-orbital fractures. *J Comput Assist Tomogr.* 1984;8:416–419.

9. Gruss JS. Naso-ethmoid-orbital fractures: classification and role of primary bone grafting. *Plast Reconstr Surg.* 1985;75:303–317.

10. Markowitz BL, Manson PN, Sargent L, et al. Management of the medial canthal tendon in nasoethmoid orbital fractures: the importance of the central fragment in classification and treatment. *Plast Reconstr Surg.* 1991;87:843–853.

11. Evans GR, Clark N, Manson PN. Identification and management of minimally displaced nasoethmoidal orbital fractures. *Ann Plast Surg.* 1995;35:469–473.

12. Freihofer HP. Inner intercanthal and interorbital distances. *J Maxillofac Surg.* 1980;8:324–326.

13. Sargent LA. Nasoethmoid orbital fractures: diagnosis and treatment. *Plast Reconstr Surg.* 2007;120:16S–31S.

14. Potter JK, Muzaffar AR, Ellis E, et al. Aesthetic management of the nasal component of naso-orbital ethmoid fractures. *Plast Reconstr Surg.* 2006;117:10e–18e.

15. Bratzler DW, Houck PM, Surgical Infection Prevention Guideline Writers. Antimicrobial prophylaxis for surgery: an advisory statement from the National Surgical Infection Prevention Project. *Am J Surg.* 2005;189:395–404.

16. Andreasen JO, Jensen SS, Schwartz O, Hillerup Y. A systematic review of prophylactic antibiotics in the surgical treatment of maxillofacial fractures. *J Oral Maxillofac Surg.* 2006;64:1664–1668.

17. Chole RA, Yee J. Antibiotic prophylaxis for facial fractures: a prospective, randomized clinical trial. *Arch Otolaryngol Head Neck Surg.* 1987;113:1055–1057.

18. Soong PL, Schaller B, Zix J, et al. The role of postoperative prophylactic antibiotics in the treatment of facial fractures: a randomised, double-blind, placebo-controlled pilot clinical study. Part 3: Le Fort and zygomatic fractures in 94 patients. *Br J Oral Maxillofac Surg.* 2014;52:329–333.

19. Mottini M, Wolf R, Soong PL, et al. The role of postoperative antibiotics in facial fractures: comparing the efficacy of a 1-day versus a prolonged regimen. *J Trauma Acute Care Surg.* 2014;76:720–724.

20. Gruss JS, Hurwitz JJ, Nik NA, Kassel EE. The pattern and incidence of nasolacrimal injury in naso-orbital-ethmoid fractures: the role of delayed assessment and dacryocystorhinostomy. *Br J Plast Surg.* 1985;38:116–121.

21. Herford AS, Ying T, Brown B. Outcomes of severely comminuted (type III) nasoorbitoethmoid fractures. *J Oral Maxillofac Surg.* 2005;63:1266–1277.

22. Merkx MA, Freihofer HP, Borstlap WA, van 't Hoff MA. Effectiveness of primary correction of traumatic telecanthus. *Int J Oral Maxillofac Surg.* 1995;24:344–347.

Orbitozygomaticomaxillary Complex Fractures

Alan S. Herford, Meagan Miller, Daniel Cantu

BACKGROUND

Because of its prominent position, the zygoma is one of the more frequently injured facial bones. The zygomatic bone is an essential structure of the midface and serves as a foundation, contributing greatly to both form and function. Fractures of the zygoma occur independently and in association with fractures to adjacent bones, such as Le Fort fractures. Since the zygoma constitutes most of the lateral orbital wall and part of the orbital floor, these fractures are sometimes referred to as orbital (orbito-) zygomaticomaxillary complex fractures (OZMC fractures).[1]

INCIDENCE AND ETIOLOGY

In a study of 362 patients, the age group presenting with zygomatic fractures most heavily represented was between 20 and 29 years of age, at 41% of the patient population, followed by the group between 30 and 39 years of age, at 18% of the patient population.[2] In a separate study conducted by Ozyazgan et al., 689 patients with midface fractures were evaluated.[3] Males constituted 81% and females 19% of these patients.[3] Throughout the majority of the literature most of the patients presented between 20 and 40 years old. The most common causes leading to OZMC fractures are motor vehicle collisions, assaults, falls and sporting injuries.[4] Some variations in incidence and pattern occur with age and geographic location.

SURGICAL ANATOMY

The zygoma or cheek bone is an important foundation structure of the craniofacial skeleton; it is the most anterolateral projection of the midface. This lateral structural pillar helps dissipate forces along the cranial base. In doing so, it provides significant strength and stability to the midface. The zygoma presents as a thick quadrangular bone and constitutes most of the lateral and inferior orbital walls.[1] Its strength comes from its five projections. These projections articulate with the frontal, sphenoid, temporal, maxillary bones, and inferior orbital rim (Fig. 1.12.1) forming the zygomaticofrontal, zygomaticosphenoid, zygomaticotemporal, and zygomaticomaxillary sutures, and inferior orbital rim respectively. Fractures usually occur at or near these five articulations. The articulation at the frontal bone is strongest, often fracturing incompletely, or greensticking. The frontal process of the zygoma may also be displaced behind the zygomatic process of the frontal bone, and thus, impacted.[5]

A comprehensive knowledge and understanding of the surgical anatomy of the orbit is necessary when treating OZMC fractures, as the orbit is frequently involved (Figs. 1.12.2–1.12.4). The lateral orbital wall is formed by both the orbital process of the zygoma and the greater wing of the sphenoid bone. The zygomaticosphenoid suture, the greater wing of the sphenoid, and the zygomatic arch serve as key anatomical landmarks to ensure proper reduction and are especially helpful in treating comminuted fractures.

Another key anatomical landmark is the zygomaticofrontal suture – the site where the frontal bone and the lateral orbital wall meet. This area is usually at least 4 mm thick. The zygomatic arch, which lies lateral to the zygoma, includes the temporal process of the zygoma and the zygomatic process of the temporal bone. In the area where it inserts to the body of the zygoma it is commonly 4 mm or more in thickness. The area of the zygoma that extends medially towards the infraorbital foramen can be as thin as 2 mm. These thicknesses are pertinent as thinner areas correlate with a higher likelihood of fracture and comminution.

The second division of the trigeminal nerve also branches to the zygomatic-facial and temporal branches that exit the foramina in the body and frontal process of the zygoma, and provide sensory innervation in the area adjacent to the zygoma, including a segment of the lateral cheek and anterior temporal region, respectively. Another branch of the maxillary nerve, the infraorbital nerve, exits via the infraorbital foramen after coursing the orbital floor. This nerve provides sensation to the anterior cheek, bilateral nose, upper lip, and through a separate branch in the bone, the anterior maxillary teeth.

Pertinent facial and mimetic muscles in this area include the temporalis, zygomaticus major and minor, the levator labii superioris, and the masseter. The zygomaticus major, minor, and labii superioris are all innervated by cranial nerve VII and are all muscles of facial expression. The temporalis muscle attaches to the zygomatic arch and posterior portion of the body of the zygoma. These muscles and fascia are displaced inferiorly with fractured fragments due to their attachments. The masseter attaches along the inferior zygomatic arch around the temporal surface of the zygoma and plays a role in the inferior displacement of the zygoma following fracture.

Other anatomic landmarks of relevance include Lockwood's suspensory ligament, Whitnall's tubercle, and the lateral canthal tendon. The vertical position of the globe is largely determined by the attachment of Lockwood's suspensory ligament and the lateral canthal tendon to the lateral orbital wall. The lateral canthal tendon is attached to Whitnall's tubercle, which is located below the zygomaticofrontal articulation and is positioned on the inner medial portion of the frontal process of the zygoma. Inferiorly displaced fractures of the OZMC may result in inferior displacement of the lateral canthus.

CLINICAL PRESENTATION

OZMC fractures are most commonly attributed to motor vehicle collisions, assaults, falls, and sports injuries. Patients presenting from such trauma should be first evaluated for life-threatening injuries and stabilized. Careful evaluation must be taken of both bony and soft tissue components of the injury. It is critical to evaluate the status of cranial

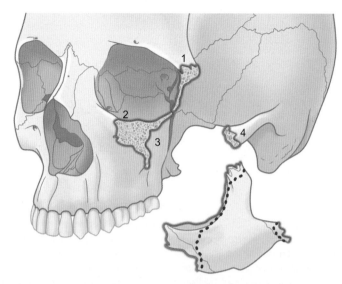

Fig. 1.12.1 Disarticulated zygoma showing attachment sites with the frontal, maxillary, and temporal bones.

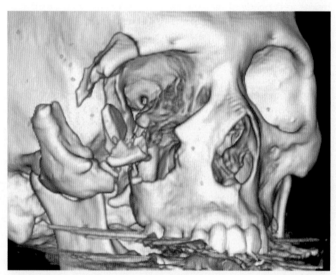

Fig. 1.12.2 Three-dimensional reconstruction showing fracture with comminution of the zygoma and orbit.

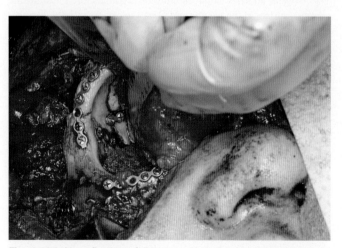

Fig. 1.12.3 Note fixation of the zygoma to the nondisplaced greater wing of the sphenoid bone. The orbital floor has been reconstructed with titanium mesh.

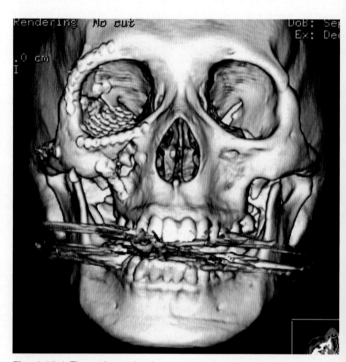

Fig. 1.12.4 Three-dimensional reconstruction showing postoperative results following open reduction and internal fixation.

nerves II to VI, eyelids, lacrimal apparatus, canthal tendons, globe, visual function and acuity, diplopia, and retina. An ophthalmology consultation should be considered whenever injury to any part of the ophthalmic apparatus is present. It is also important to record the history: the nature, force, and direction of the causative trauma. The direction of trauma is important as differing directions of impacts create different presentations. Assault usually results in direct lateral blows that typically present with inferomedial fracture and posterior displacement. A direct blow to the side of the head may result in an isolated zygomatic arch fracture. Trauma from a frontal direction often leads to a fracture with posterior and inferior displacement. More severe impact forces cause disruption of muscle attachments and ligaments, creating lateral displacement and more comminution. Displaced fractures may lead to facial flattening on the affected site which is often best appreciated from a superior "bird's eye" view. This is due to a depression of both the malar eminence and infraorbital rim. Enophthalmos may also be evident especially from an inferior or "worm's eye" view with the globe positioned inferiorly, posteriorly, and medially. The palpebral fissure may be altered due to the inferior position of the zygoma with its attachment of the lateral canthus. In higher energy fractures, the displacement of the zygomatic body is lateral, and the midface is widened on that side.

Patients with OZMC fractures often present with pain, epistaxis, diplopia, subconjunctival hemorrhage, and periorbital edema and ecchymosis.[6] OZMC fractures typically involve the orbital floor and normally travel through the infraorbital foramen and groove of the infraorbital nerve. Because of this, many patients present with decreased or absent sensation in the areas of distribution of both the zygomaticotemporal and infraorbital nerve. These areas include the cheek, lateral nose, maxillary anterior teeth, and ipsilateral upper lips. Trismus may be present whenever medial displacement causes impingement of the body on the coronoid process of the mandible or may be due to contusion of the masseter muscle. This manifests as limited opening and range of motion of the mandible. Downward displacement of the zygoma of that side can present with an antimongoloid slant of the palpebral fissure because of displacement of the lateral canthus, enophthalmos because of orbital enlargement, and a more pronounced supratarsal fold of the upper eyelid.[6] On clinical examination, physical palpation should be completed and must include the orbital rim, zygomaticofrontal suture, zygoma, zygomaticomaxillary interface, and zygomatic arch. These areas should be assessed for any bone separation, step-offs or tenderness, as these would suggest further radiographical evaluation and indicate the presence of a fracture.

Patients with isolated arch fractures usually have trismus and limited mouth opening. These patients normally present with pain and decreased mandibular motion, but no orbital signs. A depression is often observed over the fracture; however, this may be masked if there is significant edema in the area.

Patients should have a thorough orbital examination, including evaluation of extraocular muscle movements noting incomplete excursion as possible entrapment of the globe. An ophthalmology examination prior to surgery may be necessary based on initial examination and suspected visual loss or globe injury.[7] A study by Barry et al. found 23 patients out of 138 to have ocular injuries.[8] The most common include diplopia, enophthalmos, retina and pupil injuries (traumatic mydriasis). Jamal et al. evaluated 98 patients and found that 66.6% sustained minor ocular injuries. Studies have shown major ocular injuries such as ruptured globe, retinal hemorrhage or detachment and hyphema occur in approximately 10% of these patients, whereas the incidence of traumatic optic neuropathy is approximately 6%.[7]

RADIOLOGICAL EVALUATION

Computed tomography (CT) is the gold standard in the identification and imaging of OZMC fractures. Fracture patterns, as well as displacement and comminution, are readily appreciated on CT. CT also allows for the visualization of soft tissue damage that is sometimes not clinically evident. Often three views – the axial, coronal, and sagittal – and a 3-dimensional reformatted CT scan provide the best imaging for evaluating OZMC fractures. The axial and the 3D views aid in determining the anterior/posterior position of the zygoma and the degree of displacement and rotation. For evaluation of the orbit, the coronal and sagittal views provide the most useful information regarding the internal orbital bony and soft tissue anatomy, especially when determining whether an orbital floor repair will be required and the extent of

such repair. Attention should be given to the orbital volume as well as any herniation of orbital contents. Soft tissue windows are useful to evaluate extraocular muscles and to evaluate for herniation of soft tissues into the maxillary sinus. Computed tomography is not only important in identifying the fracture patterns; it is also an important tool in treatment planning, resulting in more adequate treatment and consequently better prognosis. Finally, intraoperative and postoperative CT scans can evaluate the effectiveness of the reduction.

For more complex injuries, including those that present with severe comminution, intraoperative CT may be useful to evaluate the reduction of the repositioned zygoma. The status of the orbital floor can be evaluated following reduction of the zygoma to determine whether the orbital floor should be accessed to avoid postoperative enophthalmos.

CLASSIFICATION

Classification of OZMC fractures is of utmost importance as it sets the foundation for proper treatment planning and in so doing achieves the best possible prognosis. Classification systems have been described in order to predict which fractures would remain stable after certain points of open reduction. These systems of classification have evolved to provide uniformity in diagnosis and treatment. Previous classification systems depended on the direction of displacement seen in a Waters view radiograph. As imaging and techniques improved, so did the classification of these fractures. Manson et al. proposed classifying fractures based on segmentation and displacement patterns. They described low-energy, middle-energy, and high-energy injuries. Low-energy injuries are those with minimal to no displacement. Medium-energy injuries compromise the majority of injuries and present with fracture of all articulations along with moderate displacement. High-energy injuries presented with involvement of the lateral orbit, lateral displacement, and segmentation of the zygomatic arch. Gruss et al. proposed a classification system that expanded the existing system and stressed the importance of recognizing and treating fractures of the zygomatic arch in association with those of the zygomatic body.[9] They also stressed the importance of identifying and treating segmentation, comminution, and lateral bowing of the zygomatic arch. Zingg et al. reviewed 1025 fractures and classified zygomatic injuries into three types – Types A, B, and C.[10] Type A fractures were low-energy incomplete fractures involving only one articulation, either the zygomatic arch, infraorbital rim, or lateral orbital wall. Type B fractures, or monofragment fractures, were complete, nonsegmented fractures with displacement along all four articulations; and Type C included comminuted multifragment fractures, including fragmentation of the zygomatic body.

Classification techniques are helpful to standardize terminology and to aid in developing a surgical plan and in selecting approaches. Common among these classification systems is that as the amount of displacement and comminution increases, the role of open reduction and fixation increases.

SURGICAL INDICATIONS

Treatment of each OZMC fracture should be individualized.[11] Management of these fractures depends on the degree of displacement at each articulation and its predicted aesthetic and functional deficits. Treatment may range from observation of or barely displaced fractures to extensive reconstruction of the zygoma, orbit, and zygomatic arch in severe fractures with lateral displacement at each buttress.[1,5] The selection of incisions and fixation areas for OZMC fractures ultimately depend on the degree of comminution and stability of the zygoma and its associated structures. Some zygoma fractures are amenable to less invasive treatment with minimal reduction and limited surgical approaches.

The availability of intraoperative CT has the potential to limit the need for additional incisions once the reduction has been confirmed. Each incision considered for access of the fractured zygoma carries with it inherent risks and complications. Incisions providing exposure with less risk should be utilized first. For example, a transoral surgical approach offers good visibility with minimal surgical risk. The upper lid, lower lid, and coronal approaches each carry increasing risk for more visible scarring.

Disruption and displacement of the orbital floor with no or poor reconstruction may result in postoperative enophthalmos. If the orbital floor component does not require repair, a lower eyelid incision may not be required. Over half of zygoma fractures can be treated without internal orbital reconstruction and therefore lend themselves to a less invasive surgical approach.[12] A study by Ellis and Reddy found that in patients with minimal or no soft tissue herniation and minimal disruption of the internal orbit, reduction of the points of the rim of the zygoma alone was adequate.[13] Shumrick and colleagues found that by utilizing preoperative CT they could avoid orbital exploration in 70% of their patients with OZMC fractures.[12] Their criteria for internal orbital reconstruction were cases where greater than 50% of the orbital floor was comminuted and where associated soft tissue prolapse into the sinus was present.

In order to restore proper facial width, height, and projection, especially in patients sustaining multiple/comminuted facial fractures, it can be desirable to expose and plate the zygomatic arch. This important horizontal buttress is better approached through a coronal approach, which also aids in the visualization and reduction of the superior articulations of the zygoma and lateral internal orbit (Fig. 1.12.5).

SURGICAL TECHNIQUES

A surgical plan should be based on both clinical examination and preoperative CT (Fig. 1.12.6). An initial determination should be made as to whether the internal orbit requires reconstruction as part of the treatment.[13] CT should be evaluated for the presence of herniation of periorbital soft tissues. The degree of fracture displacement and comminution are crucial in the determination of both the approach to be taken and the number of points used for fixation. Whenever displacement exceeds 5 mm, multiple approaches for confirmation of alignment and fixation are mandatory. In these cases, the infraorbital rim and zygomaticofrontal suture approaches are indicated in addition to the zygomaticomaxillary buttress approach.[14]

Proper reduction is the most important principle when dealing with fractures; stabilization is inadequate in the absence of adequate reduction. Different approaches have been taken. Some authors advocate techniques emphasizing 3-point visualization and liberal fixation.[15,16] Ellis and Kittidumkerng presented an algorithm that includes a sequential surgical approach beginning with the zygomaticomaxillary buttress, lateral orbit, and infraorbital rim[17] (Fig. 1.12.7).

The intraoral zygomaticomaxillary buttress approach is usually considered first as it helps to minimize scarring and provides excellent access to both the zygomaticomaxillary buttress and visualization of the inferior orbital rim[14] (Fig. 1.12.8). The orbital rim and lateral orbit are palpated for any step-offs that may remain. If existing lacerations are present, these can always be incorporated or substitute for the approaches for reduction. If there are no useful lacerations, the zygomaticofrontal and zygomaticosphenoid sutures are exposed via the lateral 2 cm of an upper blepharoplasty incision in the supratarsal fold and subperiosteal dissection is performed at the lateral orbital rim. The area is exposed and an elevator or sound is placed opposite the lateral malar eminence on the posterior portion of the inside of the maxillary sinus applying pressure to complete the fractures and achieve the

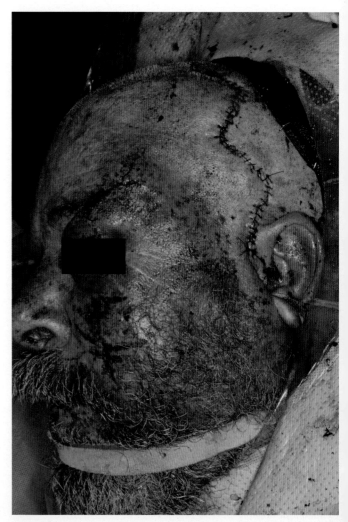

Fig. 1.12.5 Postoperative results following wound closure after coronal approach.

reduction (Video 1.12.1). A Caroll–Girard screw can be placed into the malar eminence to facilitate reduction either transcutaneously or through the intraoral incision, providing a "handle" to rotate and reduce the zygoma. This technique is especially helpful for severely displaced fractures and fractures that are difficult to mobilize. Once the fracture has been reduced, rigid internal fixation is accomplished using miniplates as they provide stability of reduction and have low complication rates. These are easily adaptable and prevent tension and flexion movements.[17,18] These plates have replaced wire fixation in all but the Z–F suture, where they are palpable and visible. Wire fixation was previously used but unsatisfactory results were common as they permitted displacement and small fragments could not always be fixated.[19,20] Biodegradable materials have gained some acceptance in the intraoral approach, as this area is a low load-bearing area.[21]

Once reduction and fixation are completed the patient is examined for symmetry of the malar prominence and vertical height of the inferior orbital rim to that of the opposing uninjured side. Symmetry is usually obtained when the reduction of the zygoma, orbital floor, and zygomatic arch are completed.[5] For comminuted fractures and those with missing bone it is helpful to evaluate the reduction at the zygomaticosphenoid area in the orbit. The anterior lip of the greater wing of the sphenoid is less commonly fractured and provides a valuable aid in assessing the adequacy of the reduction with the orbital process of the zygoma.

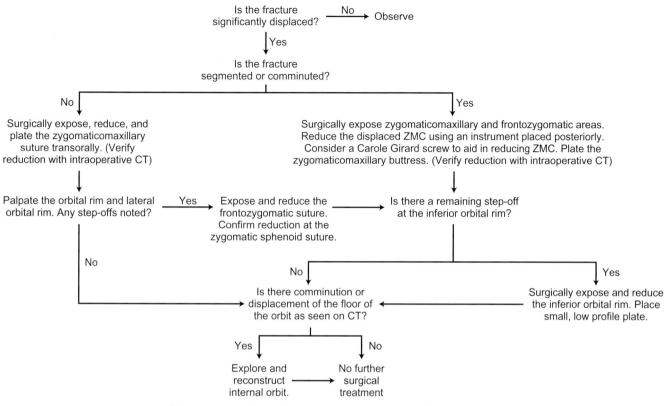

Is the fracture significantly displaced? — No → Observe

↓ Yes

Is the fracture segmented or comminuted?

No ↓

Surgically expose, reduce, and plate the zygomaticomaxillary suture transorally. (Verify reduction with intraoperative CT)

↓

Palpate the orbital rim and lateral orbital rim. Any step-offs noted? — Yes → Expose and reduce the frontozygomatic suture. Confirm reduction at the zygomatic sphenoid suture.

No

Yes ↓

Surgically expose zygomaticomaxillary and frontozygomatic areas. Reduce the displaced ZMC using an instrument placed posteriorly. Consider a Carole Girard screw to aid in reducing ZMC. Plate the zygomaticomaxillary buttress. (Verify reduction with intraoperative CT)

↓

Is there a remaining step-off at the inferior orbital rim?

No

Yes →

Surgically expose and reduce the inferior orbital rim. Place small, low profile plate.

Is there comminution or displacement of the floor of the orbit as seen on CT?

Yes ↓   No ↓

Explore and reconstruct internal orbit. → No further surgical treatment

Fig. 1.12.6 Algorithm of treatment considerations for OZMC fractures.

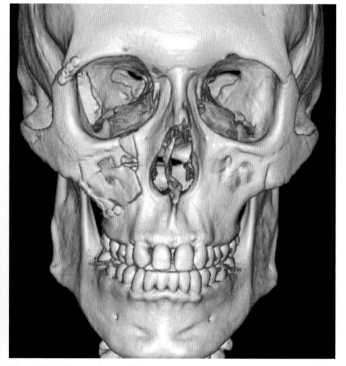

Fig. 1.12.7 Two-point stabilization to restore and maintain the position of the zygoma. The zygomaticomaxillary buttress was fixated first and was followed by plating of the zygomaticofrontal buttress second.

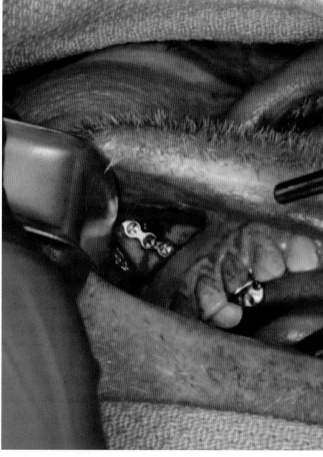

Fig. 1.12.8 One-point fixation of the zygomaticomaxillary buttress via an intraoral vestibular approach.

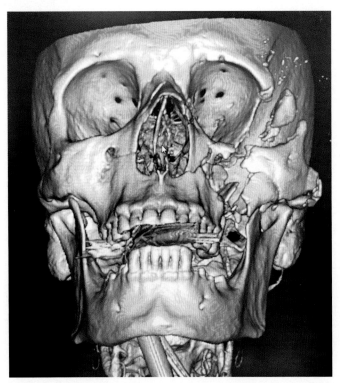

Fig. 1.12.9 Severely comminuted and displaced OZMC fracture resulting from a high-energy injury.

For OZMC fractures that require orbital reconstruction and those that require alignment of the inferior orbital rim, a lower eyelid incision is performed to gain access to those areas of the fracture. Commonly used incisions include subciliary, midtarsal, and transconjunctival incisions. The benefit of the transconjunctival incision is the absence of a cutaneous scar, and there is a lower risk of ectropion and scleral show postoperatively. It can be extended via a transcaruncular or lateral canthotomy to provide additional access medially or laterally, respectively, when needed. A small bone plate is placed along the inferior orbital rim. Using CT preoperatively one can often determine if the internal orbit should be addressed (Fig. 1.12.9), and if so, it would be reconstructed after the orbital rim fractures of the zygoma had been reduced and stabilized (Figs. 1.12.10–1.12.12).

It is important to consider forces on the OZMC complex when assessing the stability of the reduction and the need for fixation. These forces include those created by the masseter and temporalis muscles, which cause rotational displacement. In cases where plating is indicated, this fixation should provide the necessary strength to overcome these forces. The location of fixation and the number of sites that are stabilized depend on the fracture pattern, location, vector displacement, and degree of instability.[22,23] For comminuted, high-energy fractures, a fourth point of fixation may be required in order to restore proper facial width, projection, and stability.

After the zygoma has been repositioned, the reduction of the fracture should be confirmed. This may be performed with intraoperative CT or manual palpation of the zygoma or visualization of each of the points of alignment of the zygoma with adjacent bones. Additionally, it is important to assess the stability of the zygoma by placing firm pressure to detect any instability.

Zygoma reductions may benefit from the resuspension of the lateral canthus (Fig. 1.12.13). Resuspension of the soft tissues of the malar eminence is recommended in order to minimize traction on the infraorbital tissue and subsequent ectropion or increased scleral

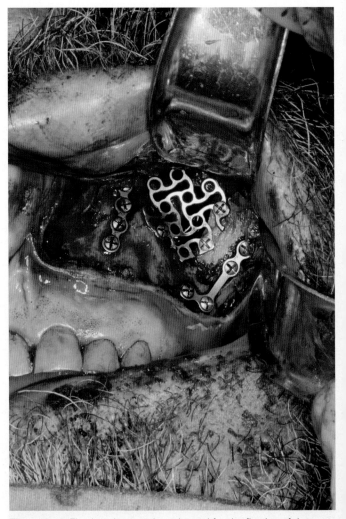

Fig. 1.12.10 Fixation plates and mesh used for the fixation of the zygomaticomaxillary buttress area.

show.[24,25] Resuspension of the suborbicularis oculi fat pad (SOOF) to the inferior orbital rim is also helpful to avoid a tear trough deformity postoperatively.[26]

For isolated zygomatic arch fractures that require treatment, access can be either transoral, as in the Keene or Lothrop approaches, or through a temporal incision known as a Gillies approach (Fig. 1.12.14). For comminuted arch fractures and those that are associated with multiple facial fractures, a coronal incision is used to visualize and reconstruct the arch (Fig. 1.12.15). The arch can be an important landmark to ensure projection of the midface.[9] It is important to remember that the arch is more straight than arched and when the arch is properly reduced, the alignment in the internal orbit of the greater wing of the sphenoid with the orbital process of the zygoma is achieved. If the anterior lip of the greater wing of the sphenoid is fractured, then the intact posterior portion of the greater wing of the sphenoid is the point that needs to be the point of alignment for the rest of the fragments of the sphenoid and orbital process of the zygoma and lateral orbital rim.

POSTOPERATIVE COURSE

Proper follow-up and postoperative care are essential for a favorable long-term prognosis. Fractures of the zygomatic complex often result in disruption of the maxillary sinus and bone fragments in the sinus.

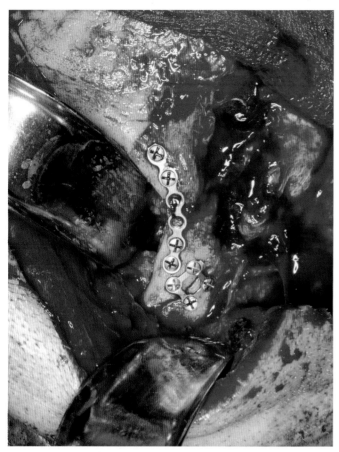

Fig. 1.12.11 Properly reduced and fixated OZMC fracture.

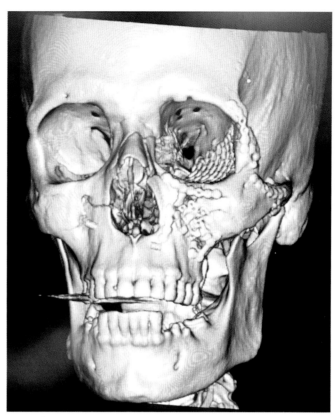

Fig. 1.12.12 Postoperative results of reduction and fixation of facial fracture. This required three-point fixation and orbital floor reconstruction.

Loose bone fragments should be removed at the time of fracture reduction and the patency of the maxillary sinus into the nose can be confirmed with irrigation. Fractures of the sinus may benefit from antibiotics and decongestants can be provided to minimize potential complications and infection. Although there is currently no definitive scientific evidence favoring a certain antibiotic regime, traditional antibiotics used include ampicillin, amoxicillin, cephalosporins, or clindamycin. Nasal spray decongestants and over-the-counter decongestants, such as pseudo-ephedrine, can also be recommended.[6]

Recommended postoperative care includes careful observation, follow-up, and cleaning of wounds and incisions. Intraoral hygiene includes brushing the teeth. Proper monitoring of these incisions for signs of infection and prompt treatment if infection does arise is of paramount importance. Ocular and orbital examinations are also crucial to ensure the absence of visual complications. Visual acuity must be assessed and complications such as corneal abrasion must be excluded. Double vision and its occurrence and cause must be determined.

Finally, postoperative imaging should be considered to document that proper reduction was obtained. This allows for additional surgical treatment and discussion if warranted. For patients that undergo closed reduction of an isolated arch fracture an external splint (guard) may be used to protect the temporal region and maintain the position of the repositioned arch and prevent displacement.

ACUTE COMPLICATIONS

Although complications are uncommon, when they do occur they may either present early postoperatively or may be visible in the later stages of the healing process. The treating surgeon must be well versed in the recognition of the signs and symptoms to be able to adequately identify and manage complications in a timely manner. The most common complications include common surgery sequelae – pain, numbness, dehiscence of incisions, unsuccessful loosening or disruption of fixation, infection, and hematoma. More site-specific complications include trismus, ectropion, eyelid ptosis, infraorbital nerve paresthesia, enophthalmos, diplopia, epiphora, hyphema, optic neuropathy, superior orbital fissure syndrome, and retrobulbar hemorrhage.[6,14] Because the maxillary sinus is always involved, acute sinusitis and obstruction have the potential to infect the hardware and create abscess and sepsis.[6]

Trismus is a potential complication. It can present both preoperatively and postoperatively. When it does present postoperatively, it is usually transient and resolves over time after proper reduction. In these cases, patients may benefit from jaw physiotherapy to regain their preinjury maximal mouth opening. Preoperative trismus can also persist postoperatively, and when it does it is due either to the zygomatic body impinging on the coronoid process of the mandible or because of fibrous or bony ankylosis of the coronoid to the zygomatic arch. Coronoidectomy may be indicated when this occurs in the absence of improvement with physiotherapy.

Another potential early complication is infraorbital paresthesia. The probability that this occurs is largely dependent on the patient's presentation. Nondisplaced fractures present with a lower incidence of paresthesia and have a more favorable prognosis and faster healing time. Medial displacement of the zygoma can "pinch" the nerve between fracture fragments, and the nerve impingement must be freed specifically by clearing the nerve foramen by zygoma reduction.

Enophthalmos and diplopia are two frequently seen orbital complications related to changes in orbital volume. Enophthalmos is mainly

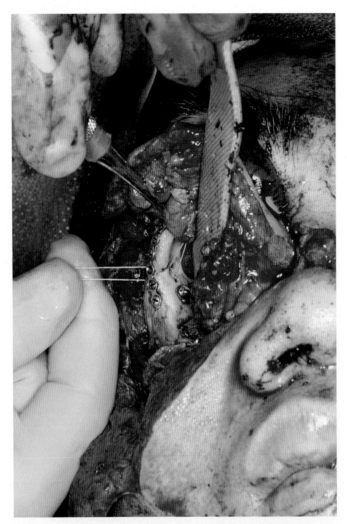

Fig. 1.12.13 Resuspension of the avulsed lateral canthus.

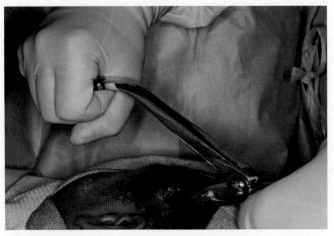

Fig. 1.12.14 Gentle reduction of the zygomatic arch fracture through a Gillies approach.

attributed to an increase in orbital volume and less frequently occurs from orbital fat atrophy. It is vital that proper replication of the original anatomy is obtained as minor changes in zygoma position can result in significant changes in orbital volume. The incidence and severity of diplopia is directly related to the patient's initial muscle presentation.

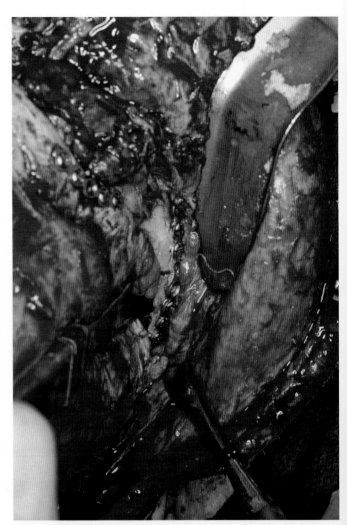

Fig. 1.12.15 Reduction and fixation of the zygomatic arch to restore adequate facial projection. Note the arch is not bowed, but rather straight.

Patients who require orbital floor repair will frequently have postoperative diplopia that spontaneously resolves with the dissipation of edema or hematoma. Whenever diplopia is caused by the entrapment or damage due to anatomical structures such as extraocular muscles, repeat surgery and muscle exploration or release may be indicated. It is extremely important to verify proper orbital floor plate placement by performing a forced-duction test intraoperatively to ensure good mobility of the eye and to verify that no entrapment is present. Free full globe movement and excursion should be noted before exploration, after reduction of soft tissue and replacement into the orbit, and after the placement of orbital floor or wall reconstruction materials. When performing OZMC repairs through a periorbital approach, gentle retraction of the orbital contents allows for good visualization and accurate fixation and helps to minimize the resulting soft tissue trauma. This reduces the likelihood of postoperative diplopia and periorbital muscle injury. Persistent postoperative restricted gaze that remains unresolved may require ophthalmological intervention and eye muscle surgery.

OZMC fractures may present with trauma to the eye. This trauma may result in hyphema – bleeding that extends into the anterior chamber (Fig. 1.12.16). When this is encountered, stabilization and maintenance of ocular tension is necessary. Depending on the case, one can treat this pharmacologically through the use of corticosteroids, beta-blockers, cycloplegics, carbonic anhydrase inhibitors, osmotic agents, and/or

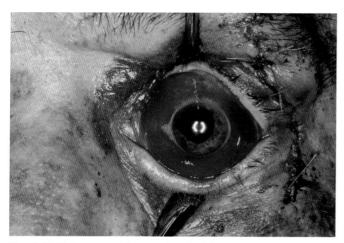

Fig. 1.12.16 Presence of subconjunctival hemorrhage and hyphema associated with multiple facial fractures.

systemic antifibrinolytics. Some cases require surgical intervention. Another potential complication is optic neuropathy. Optic neuropathy may range from a mild visual deficit to complete vision loss. Any level of visual loss or optic neuropathy warrants immediate ophthalmologic consultation and imaging of the optic nerve. Whenever there is preoperative presentation of either hyphema or optic neuropathy, it is crucial to address and treat these issues completely prior to fracture repair.

Superior orbital fissure syndrome or Rochon–Duvigneaud syndrome can present as another complication whenever a fracture involves the superior orbital fissure. The complete syndrome includes diplopia, paralysis of extraocular muscles, ptosis, ophthalmoplegia, a fixed dilated pupil, forehead anesthesia, and proptosis, but partial presentations are frequent. Whenever loss of vision or blindness is encountered in conjunction with these symptoms this is known as orbital apex syndrome or Jacod syndrome.

LONG-TERM COMPLICATIONS

Long-term complications can result from any of the previously mentioned acute complications that persist and do not resolve. Whenever access to a fracture is obtained through or below the lower eyelid, ectropion, entropion, scleral show, and sagging of the lateral canthus or the lateral lid margin are possible complications. The incidence of such deformities varies but in one study was found to be 20% at 6 weeks after surgery.[17] For fractures that require wide subperiosteal exposure the facial soft tissue may descend inferiorly resulting in loss of anterior malar projection, accentuation of the nasolabial fold, increased scleral show, and ectropion.

Functional consequences of zygoma fractures include diplopia, impaired range of ocular motility, hypesthesia of the infraorbital nerve, and mandibular hypomobility.[27] Cosmetic consequences of zygoma fractures include loss of malar projection, enophthalmos, and hypophthalmos.

There is also the possibility of malposition creating a facial asymmetry state following malunion. This asymmetry can be due to inadequate intraoperative reduction or failed or insufficient stabilization. Persistent inferior and posterior rotation of the zygoma will result in a clinically evident malar insufficiency. Treatment of high-energy injuries may result in malunion with decreased zygomatic projection and increased facial width. Proper intraoperative and postoperative imaging allows early recognition and corrective intervention with ultimately improved results and prognosis. Secondary reconstruction of the OZMC will be discussed later in this book.

CONCLUSION

OZMC fractures are challenging fractures to treat. They are a heterogenous group of fractures with potentially devastating changes in appearance, visual function and sensation, and require varying degrees of surgical exposure and fixation. Development of a treatment plan that incorporates CT scan findings allows for a thoughtful, stepwise approach to treat these complex fractures.

EXPERT COMMENTARY

Zygomatic fractures are one of the most common injuries and come in a variety of types, both isolated and occurring with other fractures. Many are simple; in fact, about 25% of zygoma fractures are so minimally displaced that they do not need to be operated on.

And of course, there are the isolated arch fractures, which come in two types. (1) A "W"-shaped deformity, depressed inward and compressing the coronoid process of the mandible, which needs to be reduced slowly, forcefully and precisely by placing an elevator underneath the point of maximal depression, and hearing it slowly and gently click into reduction – overdoing it or moving the arch back and forth with multiple reduction maneuvers will destroy the solidity of the reduction and precipitate the need for an open reduction. (2) The arch has a single fracture inwardly depressed just anterior to the glenoid fossa – just put an elevator underneath the point of maximal depression, and repeat the gentle but forceful maneuver listening for it to click into place.

Some 35% of zygoma fractures are "greensticked" or incomplete at the zygomaticofrontal suture. Therefore, they do not need to have the incomplete suture opened unless its solidity opposes the reduction. The zygoma is depressed medially and posteriorly. Simply opening this fracture intraorally, putting an elevator in the maxillary sinus and pressing beneath the body of the zygoma laterally (not up into the orbit) will again slowly and precisely lever it into position. The alignment may be confirmed intraorally by viewing the inferior orbital rim above the infraorbital nerve, and by examining the zygomaticomaxillary buttress which should come into perfect alignment. One may view the orbital floor through the maxillary sinus to confirm that it is in alignment, and again, it may (confirmed by the study of Ellis [1]) not benefit from an open reduction of the floor.

Another 35% of zygoma fractures are complete, inwardly and posteriorly displaced with the frontal process dislocated and either free or partially incomplete; the latter come in two varieties: one which is angulated and nearly complete but not freely movable, and one which is locked and pinned behind the zygomatic process of the frontal bone. In either case, dealing with this articulation first simplifies the reduction process – otherwise much time and frustration is spent trying to reduce the zygoma unsuccessfully from other vantage points. If the frontal process of the zygoma is anterior, go through the lateral limb alone of an upper blepharoplasty incision (1 cm, moving the exposure around to view various areas) and drive an osteotome through the zygomaticofrontal (ZF) suture aiming into the temporal fossa, making sure that that partially complete fracture is complete. The osteotome may be levered up and down to ensure completion of the fracture. Then, proceed within the maxillary sinus, with the Kelly clamp under the body pushing the zygoma into position, watching the articulations of the zygomaticomaxillary (ZM) buttress and the inferior orbital rim. Place an elevator under the arch through a closed approach and proceed to reduce the arch with the same technique used for the isolated arch fracture. At this point, go back to the ZF suture, place a wire through drill holes, which then prevents most displacement, but the other articulations can be adjusted into position and do the ZM buttress first or the inferior orbital rim, then address the other intraoral buttress. It is not necessary

Continued

EXPERT COMMENTARY—cont'd

to plate the ZF suture, as plates are both visible and palpable and often deserve removal. Finally, the internal orbit needs to be done, and do not be surprised if a very medially impacted zygoma with slight prominence of the globe before reduction has a giant floor defect and needs a challenging internal orbital reconstruction. Find the intact "ledges" within the orbit, and bend a plate to approximate them, not overlap them, and do not forget to make the "inferomedial bulge" with a subtle extra curvature constriction.

Five percent of isolated zygoma fractures (and many Le Fort fractures [2]) are high-energy zygoma fractures, where the arch is laterally displaced, with complete fractures at all of the buttresses. It is not possible to closed-reduce this arch, but it must be opened through a coronal incision with a direct reduction. After putting a wire in the ZF suture and provisionally making sure the fractures at the other zygomatic articulations are complete and freely movable, bring the components of the arch into the right medial to lateral position, which moves the body of the zygoma anteriorly correcting the retrusion. As the arch comes into the proper medial position (the central part of the arch should be flat, remember) the orbital process of the zygoma will come into alignment with the undisplaced greater wing of the sphenoid (beware the fractured laterally displaced anterior lip of the greater wing of the sphenoid, which, if used as the point of alignment, causes lateral malposition of the arch). The other buttresses may then be addressed. One may wish to temporarily provisionally align fractures with wires, which are flexible enough to permit fine adjustments in position, and then to later convert the wire fixation to plates and screws where desired.

Finally, incisions for exposure need to be closed in the same layers encountered in their creation: the temporal aponeurosis in the open arch approach, the incision through the periosteum over the ZF suture, the inferior orbital rim incision in the periosteum (which is easier if one marks this with a short silk suture on each side at the time of incising it) and the buccinator muscle incision intraorally. And do not forget to resuspend the superior origin of the zygomaticus major and minor muscles by grasping their periosteal insertions and suturing them to the infraorbital rim fixation plate.

References

1. Ellis E III, Reddy L. Status of the internal orbit after reduction of zygomaticomaxillary complex fractures. *J Oral Maxillofac Surg.* 2004;62:275–283.
2. Manson P, Clark N, Robertson B, et al. Subunit principles in midface fractures: the importance of sagittal buttresses, soft tissue reductions and sequencing treatment of segmental fractures. *Plast Reconstr Surg.* 1999;103:1287–1306.

 Evidence-based medicine (EBM) content available in Appendix 1 (online only)

REFERENCES

1. Wang S, Xiao J, Liu L, et al. Orbital floor reconstruction: a retrospective study of 21 cases. *Oral Surg Oral Med Oral Pathol Oral Radiol Endod.* 2008;106:324–330.
2. Perrot DH, Kaban LB. Acute management of orbitozygomatic fractures. *Oral Maxillofac Surg Clin North Am.* 1993;51(3):275–279.
3. Ozyazgan I, Gunay GK, Eskitascioglu T, et al. A new proposal of classification of zygomatic arch fractures. *J Oral Maxillofac Surg.* 2007;65:462–469.
4. Matsuniga RS, Simpson W, Toffal PH. Simplified protocol for treatment of malar fractures: based on 1220 case eight-year experience. *Arch Otolarygol.* 1977;103:535.

5. He D, Blomquist PH, Ellis E 3rd. Association between ocular injuries and internal orbital fractures. *J Oral Maxillofac Surg.* 2007;65:713–720.
6. Miloro M, Ghali GE, Larsen P, Waite P. *Peterson's Principles of Oral and Maxillofacial Surgery.* 3rd ed. 2012:2054–2136 [Chapter 21].
7. Jamal BT, Pfahler SM, Lane KA, et al. Ophthalmic injuries in patients with zygomaticomaxillary complex fractures requiring surgical repair. *J Oral Maxillofac Surg.* 2009;67(5):986–989.
8. Barry C, Coyle M, Hickey Dwyer M, et al. Ocular findings in patients with orbitozygomatic complex fractures: a retrospective study. *J Oral Maxillofac Surg.* 2008;66:888–892.
9. Gruss JS, Van Wyck L, Phillips JH, Antonyshyn O. The importance of the zygomatic arch in complex midfacial fracture repair and correction of posttraumatic orbitozygomatic deformities. *Plast Reconstr Surg.* 1990;85:878.
10. Zingg M, Laedrach K, Chen J, et al. Classification and treatment of zygomatic fractures: a review of 1,025 cases. *J Oral Maxillofac Surg.* 1992;50:778.
11. Ellis E. Zygomatic fracture. In: Laskin DM, Abubaker AO, eds. *Decision making in Oral and Maxllofacial Surgery.* Chicago, IL: Quintessence Publishing; 2007:63–65.
12. Shumrick KA, Kersten RC, Kulwin DR, Smith CP. Criteria for selective management of the orbital rim and floor in zygomatic complex and midface fractures. *Arch Otolaryngol Head Neck Surg.* 1997;123:378–384.
13. Ellis E III, Reddy L. Status of the internal orbit after reduction of zygomaticomaxillary complex fractures. *J Oral Maxillofac Surg.* 2004;62:275–283.
14. Olate S, Monteiro Lima S Jr, Sawazaki R, et al. Surgical approaches and fixation patterns in zygomatic complex fractures. *J Craniofac Surg.* 2010;21:4.
15. Makowski G, Van Sickels J. Evaluation of results with three-point visualization of zygomaticomaxillary complex fractures. *Oral Surg Oral Med Oral Pathol Oral Radiol Endod.* 1995;80:624–628.
16. Karlan MS, Cassisi NJ. Fracture of zygoma. *Arch Otolaryngol.* 1979;105:320–327.
17. Ellis E 3rd, Kittidumkerng W. Analysis of treatment for isolated zygomaticomaxillary complex fractures. *J Oral Maxillofac Surg.* 1996;54:386–400.
18. Beccelli R, Carboni A, Cerulli G, et al. Delayed and inadequately treated malar fractures: evolution in the treatment, presentation of 77 cases, and review of the literature. *Aesthetic Plast Surg.* 2002;26:134–138.
19. Lund K. Fractures of the zygoma: a follow-up study on 62 patients. *J Oral Surg.* 1971;29:557–560.
20. Pozatek ZW, Kaban LB, Guralnick WC. Fractures of the zygomatic complex: an evaluation of surgical management with special emphasis on the eyebrow approach. *J Oral Surg.* 1973;31:141–148.
21. Enislidis G, Pichomer S, Kainberger F, et al. Lactosorb panel and screw for repair of large orbital floor defects. *J Craniomaxillofac Surg.* 1997;25:316–321.
22. Hollier LH, Thornton J, Pazmino P, Stal S. The management of orbitozygomatic fractures. *Plast Reconstr Surg.* 2003;111:2386.
23. Schilli W. Treatment of zygoma fractures. *Oral Maxillofac Surg Clin North Am.* 1990;2(1):155–169.
24. Manson PN, Grivas A, Rosenbaum A, et al. Studies on enophthalmos II. The measurement of orbital injuries and their treatment by quantitative computed tomography. *Plast Reconstr Surg.* 1986;77:203–214.
25. Phillips JH, Gruss JS, Wells MD, Chollett A. Periosteal suspension of the lower eyelid and cheek following subciliary exposure of facial fractures. *Plast Reconstr Surg.* 1991;88:145.
26. Freeman MS. Transconjunctival sub-orbicularis oculi fat (SOOF) pad lift blepharoplasty: a new technique for the effacement of nasojugal deformity. *Arch Facial Plast Surg.* 2000;2:16–21.
27. Ellis E. Discussion: the concept and method of closed reduction and internal fixation: a new approach for the treatment of simple zygoma fractures. *Plast Reconstr Surg.* 2013;132(5):1241–1242.

Le Fort Fractures

Colin M. Brady, Lauren T. Odono, Mark Urata

BACKGROUND

Injury to the midface can have significant aesthetic and functional sequelae. The bony skeleton serves as a framework that aids in respiratory, ocular, vocal, olfactory, and digestive functions. Normal anatomy and symmetry of the midface is integral to social recognition and perception.

Injury to the midface can involve a complex constellation of the skeletal anatomy: the maxillary and zygomatic processes of the frontal bone, nasal bones, bones of the orbit, zygomas, ethmoids, vomer, pterygoid plates, maxilla, and palate. Both conceptually and practically, a fundamental understanding of the horizontal and vertical structural pillars of the midface skeleton is critical to understanding the diagnosis and management of these injuries. Failure to restore the structural pillars after injury can lead to inadequate projection, height, and width, resulting in a short, retruded, and widened face. The anatomical patterns if these structural pillars are compromised following the application of frontal or lateral injury forces at varied levels within the midface have been shown to be predictable, and are termed Le Fort fractures.

INCIDENCE

Young men are the most commonly affected population with an age range of 16–40, with the highest incidence between the ages of 21 and 25. Males are more commonly affected, with a 4:1 male to female ratio.[1,2]

ETIOLOGY

Maxillary fractures are most commonly associated with motor vehicle and motorcycle collisions, followed by assault. They often occur in conjunction with facial lacerations, other facial fractures, spinal and neurological injuries, and polysystem trauma.[3,4]

Specifically, Le Fort I fracture type patterns occur secondary to a force vector directed at or below the infraorbital foramen and above include the maxillary arch, resulting in a floating palatal and maxillary segment containing the alveolus and teeth. Le Fort II type fractures occur in the setting of a force directed at the level of the nasal bones. The fracture leads to mobility of the central midface through the orbits in a pyramidal pattern. Concomitant brain injuries are more commonly observed than in laterally directed forces. Finally, the Le Fort III type fractures result from a force vector delivered at the orbital level frequently laterally, resulting in craniofacial dysjunction from the skull base.[5] Le Fort III type injuries are frequently more extensive and complete on one side.

Who Was René Le Fort?

In 1901, René Le Fort published his landmark work in a three-part experiment using 32 cadavers. The cadaver heads were subjected to various traumatic force vectors, the soft tissue envelope removed and fracture patterns observed within the craniofacial skeleton. First, Le Fort observed that the skull was rarely fractured if the face was fractured. Secondly, he observed that facial fracture patterns were reproducible, and occurred across three weak levels, or "linea minoris resistentiae" of the midface skeleton when the injury force was directed in an anterior to posterior vector. The most common patterns were termed Le Fort I, II, and III fractures, occurring in "weak areas" of the midface, defining the original Le Fort classification system.[6] The classification scheme established a simple and efficient vocabulary promoting improved dialogue amongst practitioners. Though the frequency of multivector high-energy injuries has increased, resulting in midface fractures of less predictability which are more comminuted and frequently vary from side to side, these classically described major fracture patterns of injury are still applicable today.

Difference Between Surgical Le Fort Osteotomies and "Impure" Le Fort Type Injuries

Pure Le Fort fractures (single fragment and bilaterally symmetrical) are rare in the present day due to the increase in frequency of multivector high-energy mechanisms of injury. Presently, these classically described bilateral symmetric patterns form a loose classification system, and were not even purely observed in Le Fort's experiments, and are almost relegated to surgically planned exacting osteotomies performed for correction of midface craniofacial dyscrasias.[5–7] In contrast, in the traumatic setting, Le Fort fractures are often asymmetric and associated with other midface fractures. They may even occur unilaterally. Single fragment (greensticked and incomplete) Le Fort III fractures are occasionally observed, and display minimal displacement and malocclusion. Though René Le Fort did not describe a "hemi-Le Fort" injury pattern in his original classification scheme, the nomenclature serves to provide expedient and comprehensible discourse between radiologists and surgeons alike.

Midfacial Buttresses and Their Role in Craniofacial Reconstruction

The midface "buttress" system transmits and absorbs the kinetic energy of injury forces when applied to the facial skeleton. The midface serves an important role functionally and cosmetically. The vertical pillars, which are comprised of the pterygomaxillary, nasofrontal, and zygomaticomaxillary buttresses, primarily provide protection from vertically directed force or stress vectors (Figs. 1.13.1 and 1.13.2). Masticatory forces are transmitted through the skull base, mainly through the vertical buttresses. The horizontal pillars, which are comprised of the supraorbital bar, infraorbital rims, and zygomatic arches, support the transverse facial dimension and contribute supplemental orthogonal support to the buttress vertical pillars (Fig. 1.13.3). These major buttresses are further supported by the thin lateral nasal walls, nasal septum, and the maxillary walls, and although weak, they serve to resist frontal and

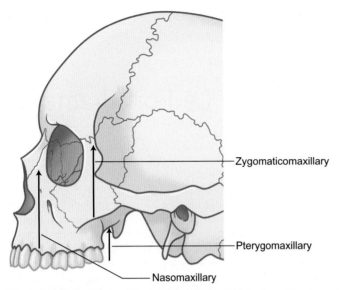

Fig. 1.13.1 Sagittal view of the vertical buttresses of the face. (Courtesy Lauren Odono, DDS.)

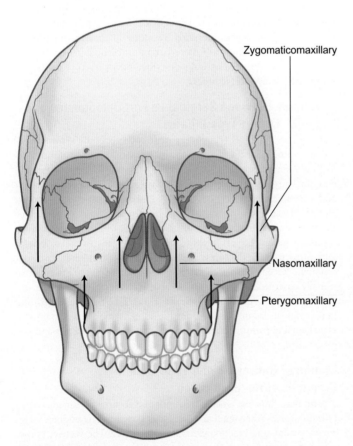

Fig. 1.13.2 Anterior view of the vertical buttresses of the face. (Courtesy Lauren Odono, DDS.)

laterally directed forces. The buttress system resists external forces and prevents disruption of the facial skeleton until a critical force level is reached, resulting in fracture. Posterior to the buttress system are the skull base superiorly and the medial and lateral pterygoids inferiorly, completing a craniofacial framework with minimal sites of anatomic weakness and therefore predictable resistance to fracture patterns.[5–8]

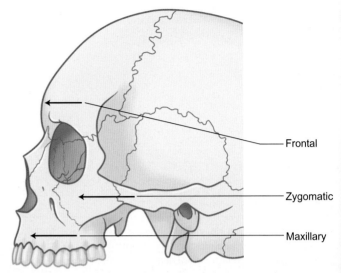

Fig. 1.13.3 Horizontal buttresses of the face. (Courtesy Lauren Odono, DDS.)

An in-depth understanding of the concepts of the buttress support system will aid in the: (1) diagnosis and treatment planning of complex facial fractures; (2) simplification of the complex interrelationship of the facial bones; and (3) placement of screws and plates in regions of adequately dense bone, allowing for the restoration of facial dimensions and profile, width and height and projection, establishing support for the nose, teeth, and globes.

SURGICAL ANATOMY

The skeletal anatomy of the cranial and midface skeleton is depicted in Figs. 1.13.4–1.13.6.

CLINICAL PRESENTATION

History

The diagnostic evaluation and work-up for the midface starts with a thorough history. Special attention to past medical history may reveal previous trauma, bone disease, osteoporosis, neoplasms both primary and metastatic, preexisting dental pathologies and interventions, nutritional and metabolic disorders, endocrinopathies, and psychiatric conditions which might influence both the etiology, timing of surgery, and choice of treatment stratagem for the relevant fracture types.

Ascertaining the etiology of the injury, specifically its force and velocity, can help the practitioner confirm the ultimate midface fracture pattern. Similarly, the vector of injury forces often serves as a predictive indicator of the ultimate fracture profile. For example, traumatic forces directed anteriorly may result in the classically described bilateral, symmetric midface Le Fort II fractures, whereas multidirectional or laterally oriented injury forces may lead to a nonclassic, asymmetric fracture pattern.[4]

Often overlooked and frequently underappreciated is the impact of the patient's premorbid dental history and occlusion on surgical decision-making and outcomes. Old photographs of the patient's facial profiles, contours, lip–tooth relations and prominence of the eyes are essential. The surgeon should be aware of any history of dental interventions, extractions, cosmetic and reconstructive dental rehabilitation, use of orthodontic appliances, significant carious and/or periodontal disease. Perturbations of the premorbid occlusion should be initially screened by asking if the patient feels that their bite is abnormal. If available,

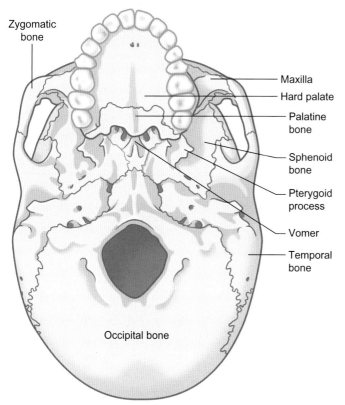

Fig. 1.13.4 Inferior view of the skull – skeletal anatomy. (Courtesy Lauren Odono, DDS.)

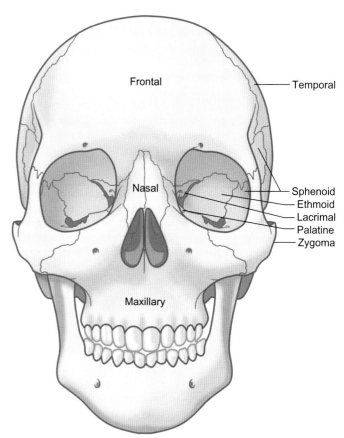

Fig. 1.13.6 Anterior view of the skull – skeletal anatomy. (Courtesy Lauren Odono, DDS.)

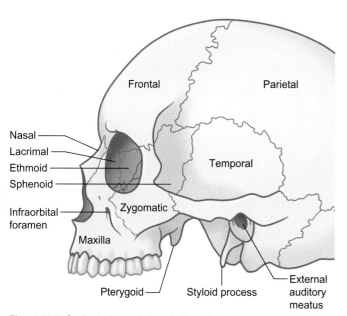

Fig. 1.13.5 Sagittal view of the skull – skeletal anatomy. (Courtesy Lauren Odono, DDS.)

premorbid photographs can be reviewed to better elucidate the patient's baseline bite. In the patient who is completely or partially edentulous, the status of their dentures should be ascertained. For the patient engaged in phased orthodontic care, a preoperative discussion with the orthodontist may help guide treatment modalities.

Physical

Given the force that is often required to create significant midface fracture patterns and the potential for airway compromise and associated polysystem trauma, the assessment begins always with the ABCs of trauma care and Advanced Trauma Life Support protocols. Once the patient is stabilized, facial symmetry should be evaluated to distinguish the obvious deformities of the skull, soft tissue injuries, and lacerations. Presence of rhinorrhea or otorrhea should be assumed to be cerebrospinal fluid (CSF) until proven otherwise. If a patient is able to answer questions, any metallic or salty-tasting discharge can be indicative of CSF drainage.[9]

Bimanual palpation of the entire craniofacial skeleton should be performed to identify any step-offs or bony irregularities. Signs of orbital trauma such as periorbital ecchymosis subconjunctival hematoma and edema are suggestive of orbital fracture and should be appreciated. "Raccoon eyes" or a "Battle" sign may be present and are indicative of anterior, middle or posterior cranial base fractures. Visual acuity, extraocular muscle function, the presence and extent of subconjunctival hemorrhage, diplopia, strabismus, pupil size, shape, and reaction to light should all be evaluated. In a study by Al-Qurainy et al. it was shown that 90% of patients with midface fractures presented with some degree of ocular injury, 15% had decrease in vision, 12% had severe injuries, and 16% had moderate injuries. Thus, facial fractures involving the bony orbit should have an ophthalmological evaluation.[1,10–12]

The integrity and stability of medial canthal ligament should be evaluated by palpation. Physical findings of medial canthal disruption include epiphora, increased intercanthal distance, and rounding of the eyelid commissure and lacrimal lake. If detachment is suspected, a bow-string test can initially be performed by placing one finger on the medial canthal tendon followed by pulling the eyelid laterally with the clinician's other hand. Lack of resistance or movement of the underlying bony platform upon lateral stress is indicative of a fracture of the area and loss of medial canthal integrity. Paskert and Manson advocated an alternate version of the bimanual exam characterized by placement of a Kelly clamp intranasally while assessing the stability of the central fragment by a finger placed externally in the region of the medial canthal attachment.[13] The provider should also consider that soft tissue avulsion/laceration in region of the medial lid and canthus may portend an underlying injury to the lacrimal apparatus that will need to be formally evaluated.

Maximum incisal opening should be assessed to determine the extent of zygoma involvement. Decreased incisal opening can be a result of trismus, however it can also be caused by impingement on the coronoid process by a zygoma fracture. Intraoral examination should include assessment of soft tissue integrity, status of dentition and periodontium with evaluation of the teeth for subluxation, malposition dental fracture, and most importantly, occlusion. Gingival lacerations predict tooth, alveolar, and palate fractures, and contribute to malocclusion. A number of malocclusive bite patterns can be seen, the nature of which is largely dependent on the pattern of and laterality of presenting midface fracture.[5]

Le Fort I

Malocclusion and segmental mobility are the most obvious indicators of an isolated Le Fort I level or palatal or alveolar fracture. Fractures of the maxilla are typically displaced posteriorly, resulting in premature contact of posterior teeth and an anterior open-bite (Fig. 1.13.7). The

maxilla should be assessed by placing an index finger and thumb as posteriorly as possible on the maxilla, ideally posterior to the maxillary tuberosities, followed by attempting to displace the maxilla in all three dimensions (Fig. 1.13.8B). Mobility of the maxilla in the superior and inferior direction can also be assessed by firmly grasping the premaxilla,

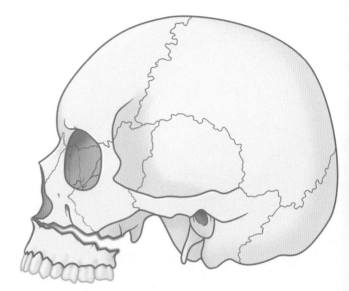

Fig. 1.13.7 Le Fort I fracture resulting in an anterior open-bite. (Courtesy Lauren Odono, DDS.)

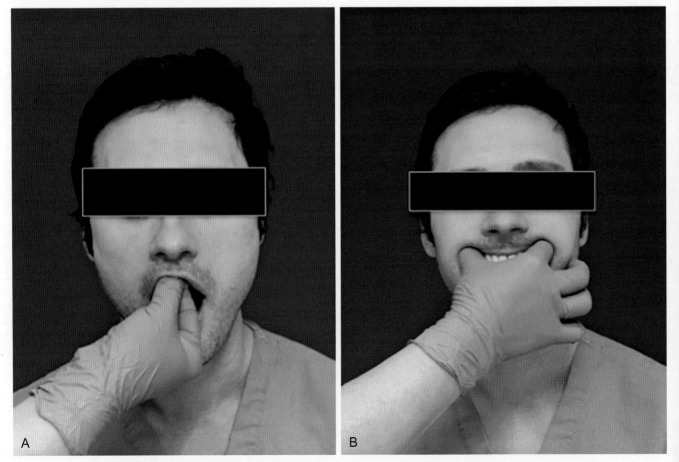

Fig. 1.13.8 Assessing Le Fort I level maxillary instability: (A) anterior–posterior maxillary instability; (B) transverse maxillary instability. (Courtesy Mark Urata, MD DDS.)

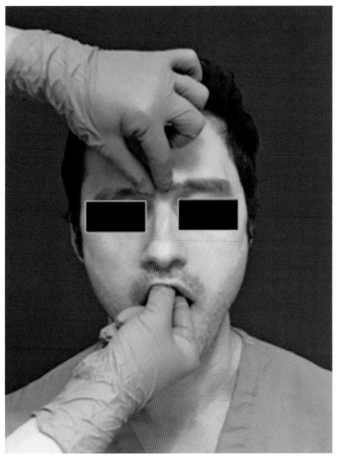

Fig. 1.13.9 Assessing Le Fort II level instability. (Courtesy Mark Urata, MD DDS.)

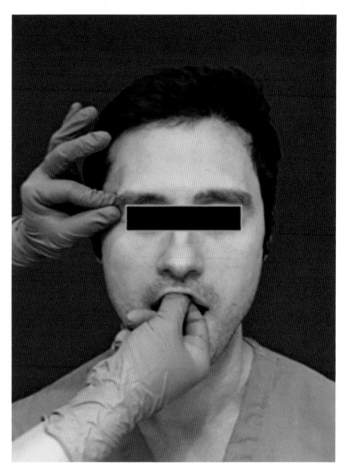

Fig. 1.13.10 Assessing Le Fort III level instability. (Courtesy Mark Urata, MD DDS.)

holding and supporting the skull to prevent excessive movement (Fig. 1.13.8A). Transverse discrepancies in the arch should also be evaluated by attempting to expand and compress the maxillary arch and comparing these dimensions to the mandibular arch width. Palatal ecchymosis is a common finding in maxillary fractures. Pharyngeal lacerations should be assessed for retropharyngeal bleeding and are common in palatal fractures.[14]

Le Fort II

The Le Fort II fracture pattern is typically more grossly clinically apparent. Significant periorbital, perinasal, malar, maxillary, and upper lip swelling may be present. Fractures at the nasofrontal region may present with CSF rhinorrhea or epistaxis. Involvement of the orbital floor and rim may result in significant soft tissue ecchymosis, dystopia, entrapment, and conjunctival or globe injury. Extension through the maxillary wall may result in infraorbital nerve paresthesia. Gingivobuccal vestibular soft tissue swelling and ecchymosis is common. The injury complex can be evaluated by mobilizing the maxilla with thumb and forefinger as previously discussed for Le Fort I level injury, while concomitantly palpating the nasofrontal junction and orbital rims (Fig. 1.13.9). Le Fort II fracture patterns are either high through the nasofrontal junction centrally, or low through the mid/lower nose.

Le Fort III

Le Fort III level injuries can result in complete craniofacial dysjunction and be associated with raccoon eyes on exam. A strong clinical suspicion for concomitant skull base injury should be maintained. CSF rhinorrhea

or otorrhea may be present and should be evaluated with beta-2 transferrin as the most specific diagnostic modality.[15] A Le Fort III fracture can be assessed with mobilization of the maxilla as previously described while simultaneously palpating the nasofrontal and zygomaticofrontal sutures for instability (Fig. 1.13.10).

RADIOLOGICAL EVALUATION

There is limited applicability for plain film radiography in the evaluation of midface Le Fort level fractures. If utilized for craniofacial skeletal evaluation outside of the midface, nonspecific radiographic opacifications of the maxillary sinuses on Waters and Caldwell views may be seen.

The gold standard for radiographic evaluation is thin-slice helical computed tomography (CT). Midface fractures are confirmed by axial, coronal, and sagittal views. The degree of comminution, bone loss, and detailed images of the fracture patterns can be assessed and juxtaposed to surrounding soft tissue structures. 3D reconstruction, when utilized, can aid in visualizing the complex 3D anatomical orientation of fracture fragments that occur in Le Fort injuries and facilitate reconstructive planning.[16–20]

CLASSIFICATION

Le Fort I pattern fractures are characterized by a transverse fracture extending from the pyriform aperture, propagating laterally across the maxillary wall involving medial, anterior, and lateral components, and ending posteriorly at, or through, the level of the pterygoid plates (Figs. 1.13.11–1.13.13). This results in mobilization of the lower third of the midface, whilst the upper two-thirds remains intact. The force is typically delivered above the maxillary teeth, causing a palatal/alveolar separation from the upper maxilla.[1,8,21]

Le Fort II fractures are pyramidal in shape, involving the central portion of the midface while the lateral orbits and zygoma remain intact. The line of fracture extends bilaterally through the nasofrontal junction, medial orbital wall, inferior orbital rim, along the maxilla, through the dental alveolus anteriorly and posteriorly at the level of the maxillary tuberosity into the pterygoid plates (Figs. 1.13.14 and 1.13.15). Only Le Fort II fractures violate the inferior orbital rim, causing the highest incidence of infraorbital nerve hypesthesia due to the

proximity to the infraorbital foramen. Bones of the maxilla below the Le Fort II line of fracture can be intact, however they are often comminuted with other fracture patterns occurring in the Le Fort II segment. The force is typically delivered centrally at the level of the nasal bones, resulting in the separation of the central maxilla from the surrounding facial skeleton.[8] Brain injuries are more frequent in central Le Fort II injury patterns.

Le Fort III fractures generally consist of a combination of fractures that involve the palatine bones, the maxilla, the pterygoid plates, the nasal bones, lacrimal bone, and zygomas; they essentially separate the face along the base of the skull. The fracture pattern extends through the nasofrontal suture along the medial wall of the orbit, through the inferior orbital fissure and the lateral orbital wall to the

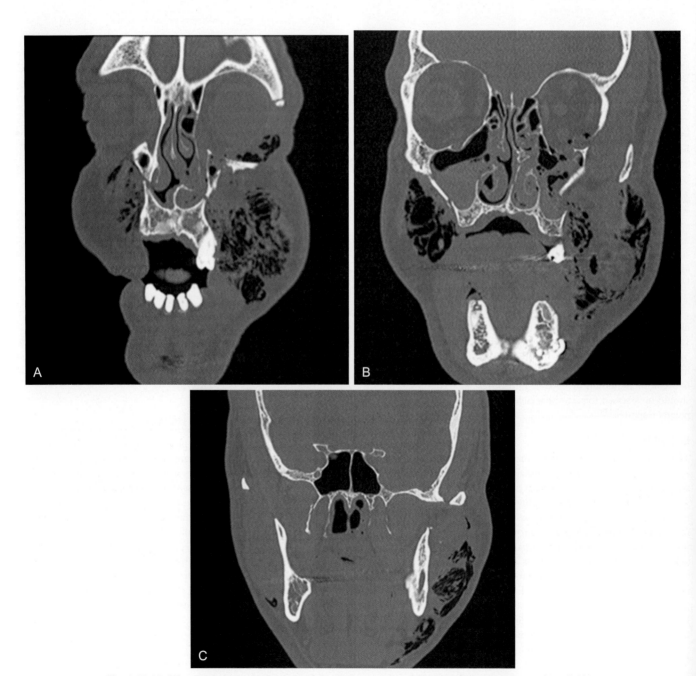

Fig. 1.13.11 CT coronal view – Le Fort I fracture: (A) fracture through the pyriform aperture and medial buttress bilaterally; (B) progressing through the lateral buttress bilaterally; and (C) ending posteriorly in the pterygoid plates. (Courtesy Mark Urata, MD DDS.)

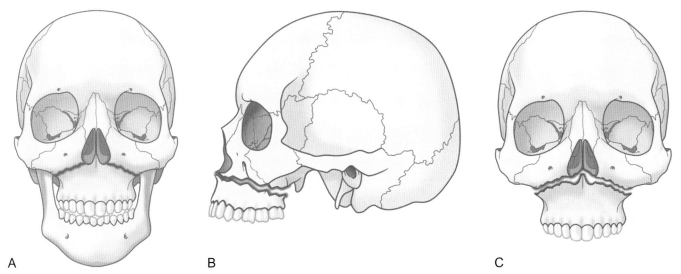

Fig. 1.13.12 Le Fort I fracture pattern: (A) coronal view, nondisplaced; (B) sagittal view illustrating propagation posteriorly through pterygoids; (3) coronal view with maxillary dysjunction. (Courtesy Lauren Odono, DDS.)

zygomaticofrontal suture. In addition, the zygomaticotemporal suture is separated. The fracture extends across the sphenoid bone resulting in dysjunction at the pterygoid plates (Figs. 1.13.16 and 1.13.17). The septum is separated from the cribriform plate of the ethmoid. Pure Le Fort III fractures are rare, and in actuality, most are ZMC fractures in conjunction with Le Fort I and II fractures lending the appearance of a comminuted "Le Fort III." The force is delivered from the orbital level, resulting in craniofacial dysjunction. The fracture is generally more comminuted and more extensive on the side of force application.[1,8,21]

Although Le Fort described the patterns of these fractures as pure, bilateral, and symmetric, they are rarely found in isolation in their classic forms. Le Fort fractures are often caused by oblique, high-energy force vectors, lending to asymmetric involvement of each hemifacial unit. When two patterns or different categories of Le Fort fractures are involved in a single patient, the higher Le Fort classification is often applied when naming the fracture (Fig. 1.13.18).

SURGICAL INDICATIONS

In patients presenting with complex midface fracture patterns, the patient should first be stabilized with special attention to establishing a stable patent airway and treating other associated and perhaps life-threatening injuries. Significant hemorrhage, often nasal in origin, should be initially managed by nasal packing or balloon tamponade with anterior–posterior nasal packing in moderate to severe cases. If ineffective, vascular embolization in the interventional radiology suite may rarely be required. In the setting of significant central midface retrusion with airway compromise, manual midface mobilization and placement in maxillomandibular fixation (MMF) can assist in stabilizing a patent airway.[22–24]

All complex midface fractures are essentially unstable. Only in the rare setting of a patient with a Le Fort type fracture pattern without malocclusion or displacement or too ill to undergo elective general anesthetic should no intervention be entertained. In these patients a soft diet only or nasogastric tube feeding can be recommended with the potential for suboptimal long-term function and aesthetics. Even in the aforementioned population, closed reduction and application of MMF is usually feasible to employ.[8,9,25,26]

For those patients with evident malocclusion and displacement of fracture fragments, an open approach is advocated if feasible given the patient's overall injury complex and candidacy for elective general anesthesia. The surgical techniques are outlined in later sections.

SURGICAL GOALS/TECHNIQUES

Le Fort I

The treatment goals for Le Fort I fractures are to restore the relationship of the fractured dental segments to their correct anatomical position and relationship to the cranial base, midface structures and the dentition of the mandible. Successful reconstruction should involve preservation of bone, restoration of facial contour, recovery of continuity of the alveolar height, and reconstitution of the width, projection, and dental arch of the maxilla.

The standard approach to reduction and fixation of Le Fort I fractures is via an upper transoral vestibular incision, 1 cm above the attached gingiva. In rare instances of high or irregular fracture patterns, a coronal facial degloving in isolation or in combination with the vestibular approach may be helpful, but is generally not required. The incision is made in the mobile mucosa 5–10 mm above the attached gingiva from first molar to first molar. In patients who do not have a significantly impacted maxillary segment, midline frenulum and sulcal tissues may remain intact while the vestibular buccal incision is opened on either side for exposure. Local anesthesia with epinephrine is infiltrated prior to incision. A subperiosteal dissection is then performed to expose the four anterior vertical buttresses of the maxilla and fracture lines bilaterally. The infraorbital nerve should be identified and protected.[6,7,21,27,28]

The pull of the medial and lateral pterygoid muscles contribute to the displacement of fractures in an inferior and posterior direction, resulting in a classic anterior open-bite deformity, shortening and retrusion of the Le Fort I segment. Le Fort I fractures can also present as immovable, free-floating, or impacted maxillary segments. Necessary reduction must be performed prior to fixation and can be achieved through numerous modalities such as maxillomandibular fixation, Rowe disimpaction forceps, or by drilling a small hole through the thick bone of the anterior nasal spine and threading a wire loop providing traction

Text continued on p. 159

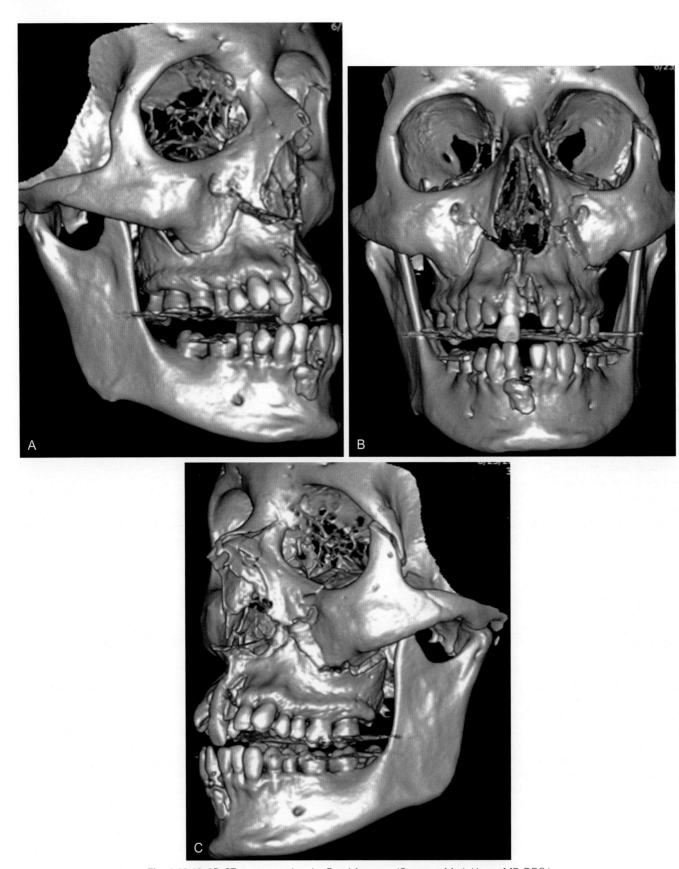

Fig. 1.13.13 3D CT reconstruction: Le Fort I fracture. (Courtesy Mark Urata, MD DDS.)

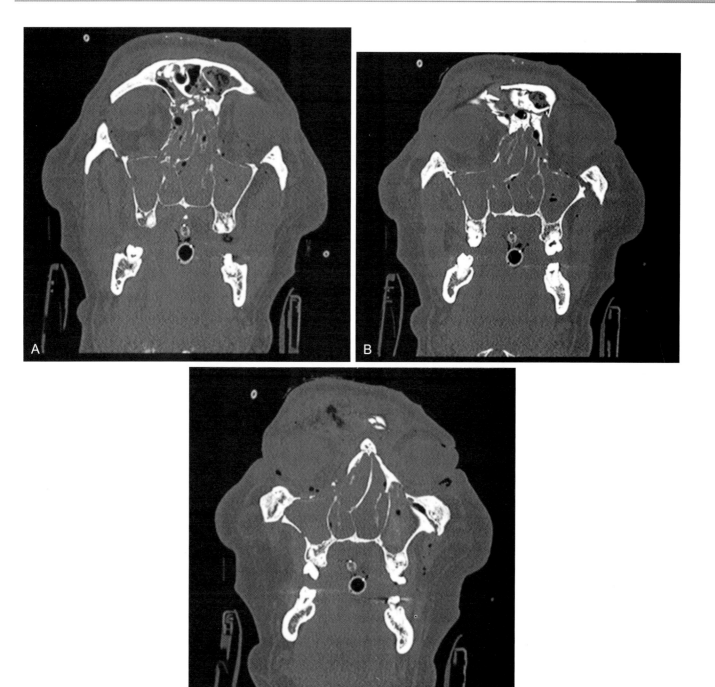

Fig. 1.13.14 CT coronal view – Le Fort II fracture: (A–C) progression of the pyramidal fracture pattern extending through the nasofrontal suture, infraorbital rim, maxilla, and ending posteriorly at the pterygoid plates. (Courtesy Mark Urata, MD DDS.)

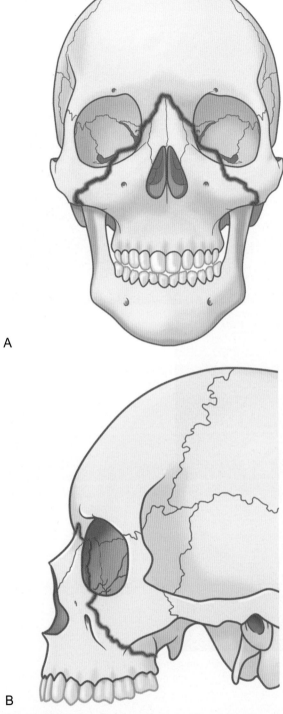

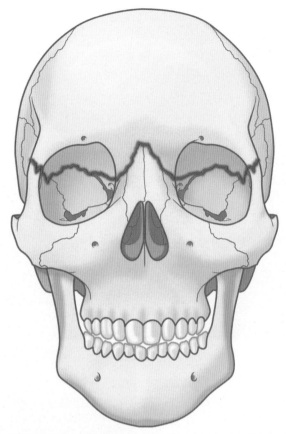

Fig. 1.13.16 Le Fort III fracture pattern. (Courtesy Lauren Odono, DDS.)

Fig. 1.13.15 Le Fort II fracture pattern: (A) coronal; (B) sagittal views. (Courtesy of Lauren Odono, DDS.)

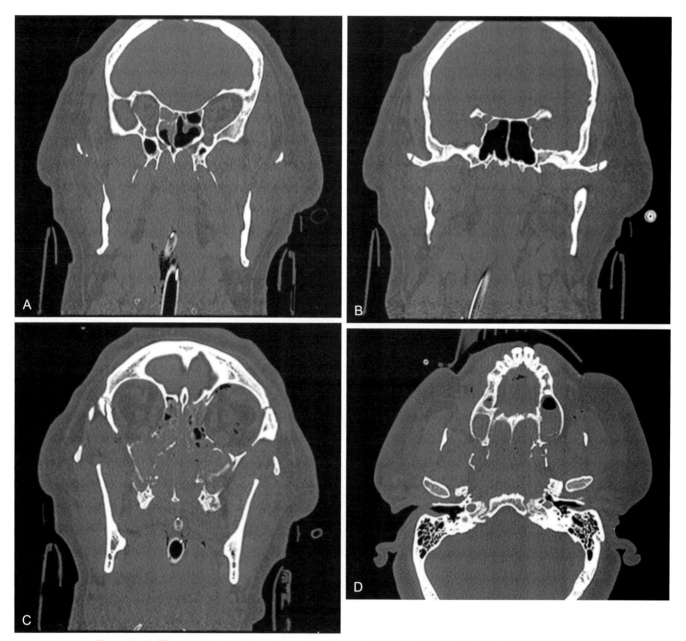

Fig. 1.13.17 CT cross-sections Le Fort III fracture: (A–C) coronal images illustrating fracture through the zygomaticofrontal suture; (D–F) transverse cross-sections through the pterygoid plates;

Continued

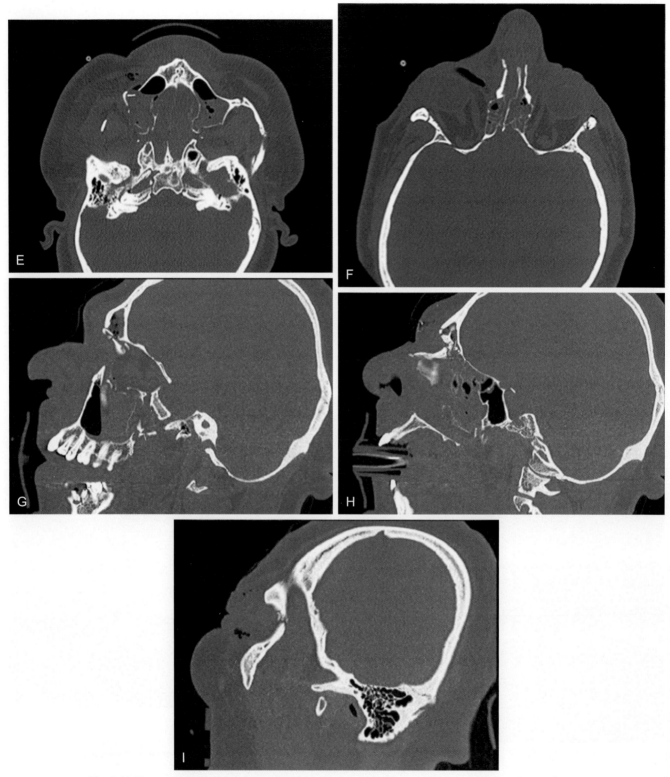

Fig. 1.13.17, cont'd (G–I) sagittal images detailing fracture of the nasofrontal suture. (Courtesy Lauren Odono, DDS.)

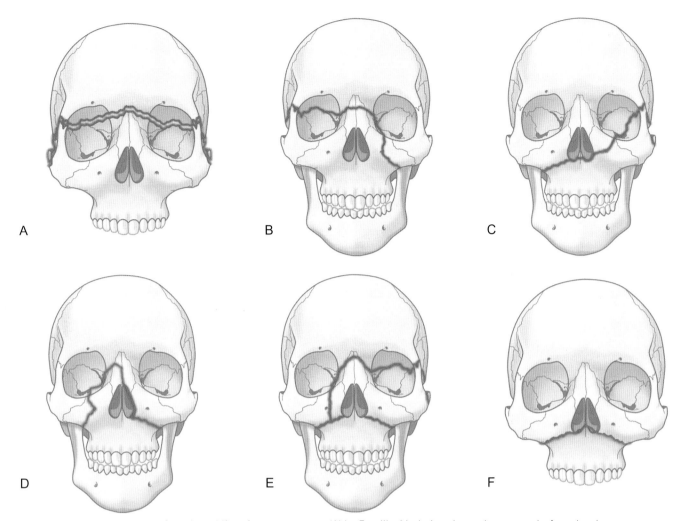

Fig. 1.13.18 Complex midface fracture patterns: (A) Le Fort III with dysjunction at the zygomaticofrontal and zygomaticotemporal sutures; (B) combined Le Fort III/II; (C) combined Le Fort III/I; (D) Le Fort II/I; (E) Le Fort III, II, and I; (F) Le Fort I with impaction. (Courtesy Lauren Odono, DDS.)

to reduce the fractured segments. If treatment has been delayed, or in partially complete or "greensticked" incomplete fractures, osteotomies are sometimes necessary to complete fractures to mobilize the Le Fort I segment. Following reduction the patient's maxilla is placed in MMF with the mandible to stabilize the reduced segments during osteosynthesis fixation.

Osteosynthesis utilizing plates and screws at the four anterior vertical maxillary buttresses allows for fixation and stabilization in three dimensions, which in turn will allow for increased survival of bone and bone grafts. Internal fixation is commonly achieved using 1.5–2.0 mm profile miniplates. L- or Y-shaped plates are placed along the medial and lateral buttresses, which have the highest bone stock and density, providing stable areas for screw anchorage. Proper stabilization and adaptation of plates prevents midface collapse, excess mechanical stress, and microfractures of the bone (Fig. 1.13.19).[6–8,21,29] Additionally, adequate internal fixation usually eliminates the need for postoperative MMF, in turn facilitating soft diet, exercise, range of motion and hygiene, decreasing costs of care and the convalescent interval.

Comminuted fractures of the maxilla should be addressed with longer and higher profile plates to bridge the fragments. Bone fragments should be retained and repositioned if possible. Loose, unstable bony fragments stripped of their periosteal sleeve even if essentially "floating," should be first repositioned and rarely removed as they may supplement

contour. When comminution results in large defects across the Le Fort buttress areas exceeding several millimeters, bone grafting should be implemented in conjunction with internal fixation to prevent possible plate fatigue, rupture or displacement of plates due to significant masticatory forces.[30,31]

When an alveolar component is involved in the maxillary fracture, care should be taken to maintain blood supply to the alveolar segments.

Upon closing the incision, if the midline has been opened, an "alar-cinch" suture should be placed to avoid widening of the alar bases. If the midline maxillary frenulum has been left intact, an alar repositioning suture is not required. The vestibular incision is general closed with resorbable vicryl or chromic sutures, suturing the muscular and mucosal layers.

Le Fort II and III

Wide surgical exposure is often necessary when approaching Le Fort II and III fractures to ensure proper reduction and stabilization. Transcutaneous and/or coronal incisions can be used to approach the craniofacial junction and upper midface fractures.

Deciding between approaches is determined by surgeon's preference, pattern and constellation of fractures present, and the amount of associated displacement.

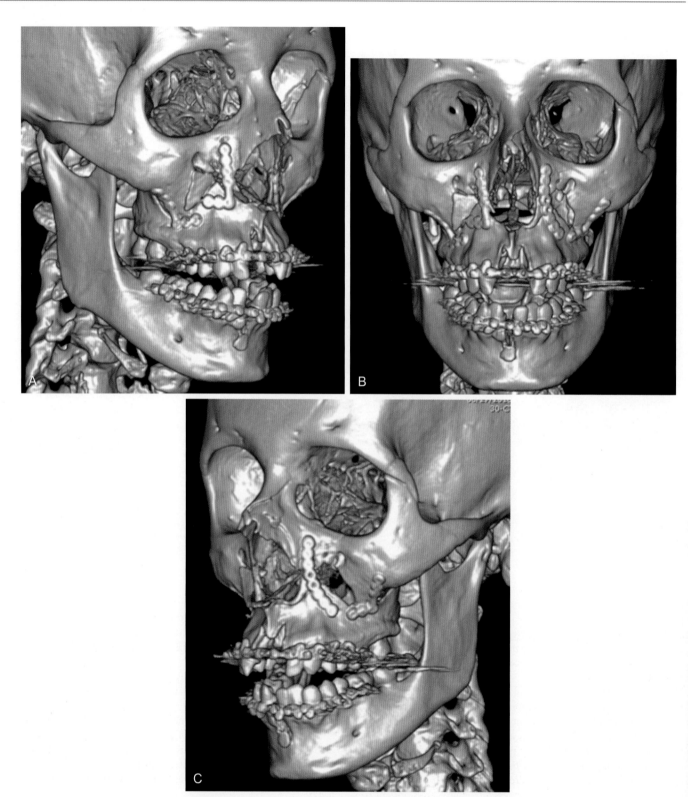

Fig. 1.13.19 3D CT reconstruction: open reduction internal fixation (ORIF) of a Le Fort I fracture. (Courtesy Lauren Odono, DDS.)

The coronal incision allows for wide exposure in the subperiosteal plane of the supraorbital rims, frontal process of the zygoma, glabella, zygomatic arches, and the superior, medial, and lateral orbital walls. The cutaneous incision is made from posterior or anterior to the helix root to the vertex of the skull and down to the contralateral helical root usually in a sinusoidal or zig-zag pattern through the hair. Special consideration should be taken in men with male-patterned baldness, with the incision extending further posteriorly over the vertex, allowing for preservation of hair vitality, facilitating skin closure, and improving esthetics.

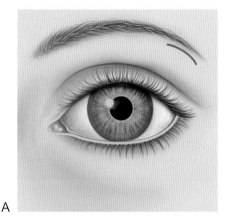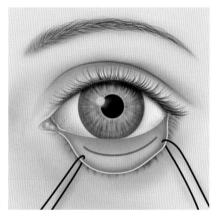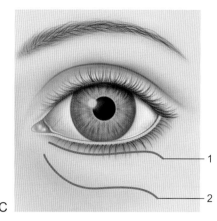

Fig. 1.13.20 Approaches to orbital alignment/reconstruction following midface trauma: (A) lateral brow incision to access the zygomaticofrontal suture; (B) transconjunctival incision to approach the orbital rim and floor; (C) subciliary (1) and infraorbital (2) approaches. (Courtesy Lauren Odono, DDS.)

When utilizing the coronal approach, it is essential to preserve the temporal branch of the facial nerve by completing the dissection to the arch by incising through the anterior layer of the deep temporal fascia at two finger-breaths superior to the zygomatic arch remaining in the deep temporal fat pad with the nerve reflected anteriorly. Release of the supraorbital nerve may be required to complete the exposure of the medial and lateral orbital walls along with the orbital roof.[7,8,28,32,33]

An upper blepharoplasty or lateral brow incision can sometimes be used to expose the zygomaticofrontal suture, thus avoiding a coronal incision. Obtaining symmetrical control in the reduction of bilateral fractures, specifically in the zygomatic arches, is near impossible via this technique and as such is not generally advocated (Fig. 1.13.20A).

Access to the orbital floor can be obtained via transconjunctival, subciliary/midtarsal, and less desirably, infraorbital approaches. Lid anatomy, presence of lacerations, patient age, and orbicular muscle tone are all factors to take into account when choosing which approach to utilize (Figs. 1.13.20B–C).

The transconjunctival approach was made popular by Tessier in 1973. The incision is made pre-septal or post-septal through the conjunctiva, paralleling the gray line. A lateral canthotomy and inferior cantholysis can be utilized to gain further lateral exposure. Both ectropion and entropion are possible complications from the transconjunctival approach.

The subciliary or lower blepharoplasty incision is made 2–3 mm inferior to the gray line of the lower eyelid, parallel to and along the length of the lower eyelid margin. This approach is contraindicated in older patients with great lid and orbicular laxity to prevent significant risk of ectropion.

The infraorbital incision, which was first described by Converse et al. in 1944, consists of a transcutaneous incision 4.5 mm below the gray line in eyelid skin, over the infraorbital rim. The approach also allows for excellent access to the surrounding areas and the orbital floor, however the complications include more visible scarring, development of lymphedema, poor healing, and possible distortion of the lower eyelid making this approach of limited utility except where there is a pre-existing laceration in the same location.[1,11,27,34–39]

In Le Fort II or III fractures combined with a Le Fort I component, the transoral vestibular incision is added for exposure and fixation at the Le Fort I level.

Adequate reduction following exposure is the key to restoration of midface width, height, and projection. This can be performed with gentle manipulation with reduction clamps, disimpaction forceps or in cases of delayed management, with osteotomies. Greenstick or incomplete fractures may also require a completion osteotomy if proper reduction is unattainable.

It should be noted that although establishment of premorbid occlusion with intermaxillary fixation (IMF)/MMF or wire ligature is important prior to fracture stabilization with plates and screws, it cannot be relied upon to necessarily reduce and restore central midface alignment and projection on its own without formal internal osteosynthesis fixation. Instead, restoration of occlusion should be considered a preparatory adjunct to achieving ultimate adequate internal fixation with plates and screws.[26]

The surgeon must carefully consider plate thickness at each required location for fixation accounting for the thickness of the soft tissue envelope in order to prevent palpability and/or visibility. Sequencing of fixation in Le Fort II and III fractures is largely dependent on the injury profile, degree of displacement and comminution.

In isolated central midface Le Fort II injuries, the frontonasal junction is fixated bilaterally with 1.3–1.5 mm profile plates, followed by the infraorbital rims with similar low profile osteosynthesis. Stronger 1.5–2.0 miniplates are utilized to fixate medial and lateral maxillary buttresses inferiorly at the Le Fort I level.

In Le Fort III, craniofacial dysjunction, the approach outlined by Gruss et al. is often utilized to restore the outer framework and facial width prior to central glabellar fixation. In this approach, the root of the zygomatic arch, and the zygomaticofrontal sutures are stabilized first acting as a foundation for the craniofacial construct, and utilizing the zygomaticosphenoidal suture alignment to control the width and lateral position of the zygoma.[8,32,33]

Palatal Fractures

Palatal, gingival or lip lacerations, displacement of alveolar segments, palatal ecchymosis or changes in occlusion on clinical examination can indicate a possible palatal fracture and must be investigated. Palatal fractures are often seen in conjunction with Le Fort fractures with a rate of 8–13% and are rarely present as isolated fractures. To confirm the diagnosis of a palatal fracture, the best images to view are coronal cuts from a CT scan.[40–43]

The classification of palatal fractures is based on the anatomic location of the palatal fracture. The Hendrickson classification system is outlined below[43]:

Type I: alveolar fracture

Type Ia: anterior alveolus; containing only incisor teeth and associated alveolus

Type Ib: posterolateral; contains premolars, molars and associated alveolus

Type II: sagittal fracture, a split of the palatal midline; typically occurs in second or third decade because of lack of ossification of the midline palatal suture

Type III: parasagittal fracture; most common fracture pattern in adults (63%) because of thin bone parasagittally; fracture pattern differs from Type I fracture by inclusion of maxillary canine

Type IV: para-alveolar fracture; occurs palatal to the maxillary alveolus and incisors

Type V: complex comminuted fracture; multiple fractured segments

Type VI: transverse fracture, rare; involves a division in the coronal plane

Treatment of palatal fractures is dependent on the presence or absence of dentition, associated facial fractures and type of palatal fracture. Treatment can include utilization of acrylic splints, rigid internal fixation and application of arch bars. Rigid internal fixation is rarely indicated for palatal fractures. The major disadvantage of rigid internal fixation is the lack of occlusal control at the time of fixation, secondary to the inability to place patients in MMF in advance. The latter may risk inadequate reduction of the maxillary height and transverse width. When utilized, internal rigid fixation proceeds via transoral technique with an incision on the palate to access the fracture, elevation of greater palatine flaps, reduction of palatal fracture fragments, followed by the placement of fixating plates and screws. It should be remembered that vascularization of the maxilla is achieved via the ascending pharyngeal and palatal mucosal blood supply, and must be taken into consideration to ensure that the entire maxillary blood supply is not compromised when placing access incisions on the palate. Maxillomandibular fixation should be utilized in dentate patients. The utilization of occlusal splints can add additional stabilization in severely comminuted palatal fractures. In edentulous patients, existing dentures can be used to place the patient in maxillomandibular fixation. If dentures are not readily accessible, a Gunning splint can be fabricated. If either of the options previously mentioned is unattainable, internal rigid fixations for sagittally oriented palatal fractures should be utilized. Necrosis of fracture segments due to compromised vascularity and development of palatal fistulas are all possible complications of palatal fractures.[41–45]

POSTOPERATIVE COURSE

In the infrequent incidence of closed treatment only, the length of MMF is not well studied and largely up to surgeon preference determined by the comminution of the fracture. Anecdotally, 4–6 weeks of traditional MMF followed by 2 weeks in guiding elastics is a reasonable approach.[26]

As noted, complex pattern midface fixation is ideally achieved via open osteosynthesis with plate/screw fixation. Patients with stable occlusion following internal stabilization do not need to remain in MMF postoperatively. By avoiding extended postoperative MMF, a patient is better able to maintain proper oral hygiene and nutrition. Four weeks of soft diet is recommended. In the setting of palatal, panfacial, or comminuted fractures, MMF may be utilized for up to 3 weeks postoperatively, followed by 2 or more weeks of guiding elastics.

Antibiotics

Practice patterns for prophylactic antibiosis amongst surgeons who treat midface pathology are markedly variable and poorly documented in the surgical literature. With a paucity of high-level evidence-based medicine and expert consensus, the management of antibiotics in the setting of fractures of the craniofacial skeleton remains an area of significant controversy.

In one of the larger reviews of the literature to date, Mundinger et al. sought to compare evidence-based recommendations regarding antibiotic prophylaxis in facial fracture management with expert-based practice. A systematic review of 44 relevant studies in the literature was performed and studies were divided by facial thirds. Overall, studies were found to be of poor quality, and thus precluded formal statistical analysis. The percentages of prescribers administering pre-, peri-, and postoperative antibiotics in fractures of the midface were 47.1%, 100%, and 70.6%, respectively. Despite the significant proportion of practitioners still prescribing pre- and postoperative antibiotics, no evidence to support the validity of such practices exists in the scientific literature. Though conclusions were limited, there seemed to be a consensus that perioperative antibiotic use alone is recommended for midface fracture management. Based on the study quality of the series in the literature, higher-level studies are warranted to better guide practice patterns in the administration of antibiotics for fractures of the craniofacial skeleton and the midface.[46]

ACUTE COMPLICATIONS

Loss of Airway

Midface trauma may result in the displacement of cartilaginous or bony structures, hematoma formation or edema, which in turn can cause nasopharyngeal obstruction and make nasal intubation difficult. Displaced hard palatal fractures and an edematous velum and uvula may lead to oropharyngeal obstruction. Nevertheless, the airway can often be controlled in the emergency department by airway adjuncts.[9,47–49]

If preoperative intubation is required, involvement of the cranial base should be assessed when feasible. When involvement is observed, orotracheal intubation is the preferred method. Orotracheal intubation is performed in 75% of patients who sustain severe facial trauma requiring airway management, with less than 12% of patients requiring surgical tracheotomy.[9,47–49]

When surgical intervention is required, the clinician must carefully consider the method of airway management. Orotracheal intubation can interfere with obtaining MMF, which is often utilized intraoperatively to reproduce premorbid occlusion. As a result, nasotracheal intubation is generally advocated during operative intervention. If the cranial base is involved, a fiberoptic endoscope can be used to safely pass a nasotracheal tube. If an orotracheal tube must be used, it should be passed around the last tooth or through an edentulous area to permit MMF.[9,47,48]

An alternative form of airway management that can facilitate intraoperative MMF and fracture exposure is submental intubation. Described by Hernandez Altemir in 1986, the technique involves passing the orotracheal tube through the submental area, medial to the mandible, anterior to the lingual nerve and facial artery.[50] Advantages to submental intubation include excellent access to the nasal and oral cavities during surgery with few complications.

Bleeding

Blood supply to the maxilla is via the internal maxillary arteries, along with the superior and posterior alveolar arteries, supplying the hard and soft palates. The nasopalatine artery traverses through the incisive foramen, supplying the mucoperiosteum of the anterior palate. The greater palatine and internal maxillary arteries along with the retromaxillary venous plexus can lead to life-threatening bleeding in midface fractures.

If bleeding emanates from the septal wall, the anterior and posterior ethmoidal arteries that supply the anterior aspect of the septum are often the source vessels. Posteriorly, nasopalatine branches of the sphenopalatine artery are implicated.

Though uncommon, significant hemorrhage, generally manifested as epistaxis, should be initially managed by nasal packing. In moderate to severe cases, balloon tamponade may be utilized with Fogarty or Foley catheters. If ineffective, vascular embolization of select branches of the internal maxillary artery in the interventional radiology suite may be required. IMF with fracture reduction is frequently effective and can be combined with ligation of the facial and superficial temporal arteries unilaterally or bilaterally for emergency treatment.[9,22–24]

Infection

Bony instability is most commonly seen with loosening of screws, plates or unstable bone grafts, or poor application of IMF, and is most often implicated in postoperative infection. If the fracture is not healed, treatment consists of exchanging hardware or bone graft with drainage and debridement. Infections can also be the result of contaminated foreign materials, soft tissue lacerations, odontogenic infection or hematomas.

CSF Rhinorrhea

Midface trauma is associated with the highest rate of CSF leaks in injuries of the craniofacial skeleton. CSF may emanate from a dural tear, manifesting as CSF rhinorrhea or otorrhea, and is secondary to bony disruption at the cribriform plate, sphenoidal, ethmoidal and frontal sinuses, or temporal bone/mastoid region. A leak is most commonly noted acutely but may be recognized in a delayed fashion days to weeks after the inciting trauma. On clinical examination, CSF presents as straw-colored or clear drainage. Several diagnostic procedures can be used if a CSF leak is suspected: (1) the "halo" test; (2) fluid characterization with minimal sediment and glucose level around 45 mg/dL; and (3) a more specific send-out analysis detecting CSF beta-2 transferrin (Box 1.13.1). Following recognition, CSF precautions are recommended and include avoidance of straining, sneezing, and nose blowing.

CSF leak in midface trauma can predispose the patient to meningitis. The use of prophylactic antibiosis remains controversial, though there is some low level evidence suggesting a decreased incidence of meningitis when prophylaxis is used once a leak is recognized. If utilized, the antibiotic chosen varies from between institutions and is based on present antibiograms.[15,51–53]

Visual Disturbances

Visual disturbances are one of the most significant complications of significant midface trauma. Traumatic diplopia, enophthalmos, and blindness can all occur.

Diplopia

The incidence of diplopia following midface trauma is variable, reported between 3.4% and 20%, and the pathology is secondary to interference of action of the extraocular muscles. Interference can be secondary to significant periorbital edema, hemorrhage, displacement of the globe, or muscle entrapment. Extraocular motility should be examined carefully

---

> ## BOX 1.13.1 Diagnostic Procedures to Evaluate for Posttraumatic CSF Leak
>
> - Beta-2-transferrin laboratory analysis
> - CT scan with 0.5 mm coronal cuts of the cribiform plate
> - Tilt test with positive halo sign
> - Application of fluorescent dyes and direct visualization of leakage via trans-nasal endoscopy
> - Concentration of glucose between drainage compared with patient's serum
>
> Courtesy Mark Urata, MD DDS

---

by both the initial evaluating team and an ophthalmologist. If there is concern for restriction of directional gaze, a forced duction test should be performed by placing local anesthetic in the cul-de-sac of the lower lid, and using a toothed forceps to mobilize the globe in all cardinal directions. If resistance is present, a high index of suspicion for entrapment should be maintained and exploration considered. Forced duction testing should also be performed following orbital reconstruction/fixation to ensure that iatrogenic muscular entrapment has not been introduced by reduction or materials.

The timing of treatment for diplopia remains controversial and largely dependent on the presumed causality. Acute traumatic entrapment or enophthalmos requires expedient intervention, whilst diplopia presumed secondary to edema and/or hemorrhage can be monitored closely for resolution in the first 7 days with or without the administration of steroids.[11,12,20,27,37,38,54,55]

Enophthalmos

Posttraumatic enophthalmos is generally attributed to: (1) attenuation, contraction, or disruption of periorbital tissues and ligaments; or (2) enlargement of the bony orbit. The most common cause of enophthalmos is the lateral and inferior displacement of the body of the zygoma, resulting in increased orbital volume. The reconstruction of the zygoma must be realized in three dimensions to restore orbital volume, guided by realignment of the zygomaticosphenoidal sutures and infraorbital rims. Dulley et al. stress the importance of prevention with regard to the management of enophthalmos, noting a 72% incidence when treatment is delayed longer than 6 months compared to 20% when repair is performed within 2 weeks of injury.[56] The importance of early intervention is further supported by the finding that 40% of patients undergoing delayed management required multiple surgical interventions.

If the recognition is acute, management occurs by reduction and fixation of fracture fragments restoring the normal orbital volume. If delayed, correction proceeds by periorbital release of cicatricial tissue, osteotomies and repositioning of nonanatomic bony segments. Rigid fixation and bone grafts may be utilized to resituate a laterally and inferiorly displaced zygomatic segment and cranial bone grafting or synthetic constructs may be utilized to reconstruct the orbital floor or wall support and elevate the globe. Delayed reconstruction is difficult and slight overcorrection of anterior globe prominence (but not vertical overcorrection of the globe) is generally recommended to account for inevitable relapse. Multiple procedures may be required to achieve an optimal result.[37,38,54–61]

Blindness

With an incidence of 0.3%–3%, blindness is the most devastating ophthalmic complication of midface trauma. Thin-sliced helical CT may show edema of the optic nerve or fracture of the optic canal.

The most common etiology of posttraumatic blindness is retrobulbar hemorrhage (RBH) occurring in less than 1% of all midface trauma. RBH typically occurs acutely with the first few hours after trauma or postoperatively, however, it may present hours to days after the inciting event. An increase in retrobulbar pressure causes occlusion of the ciliary arteries, which are responsible for the blood supply to the optic nerve head and retina, resulting in ischemia, causing optic neuropathy. Decreased visual acuity, proptosis, and pain are signs and symptoms associated with retrobulbar hematoma (Box 1.13.2). Additionally, papilledema, ophthalmoplegia, and increased ocular pressures may be seen.

Conservative management can be initiated to dilate intraocular vessels, decrease intraocular pressures, limit inflammation and edema via administration of supplemental oxygen, mannitol, acetazolamide

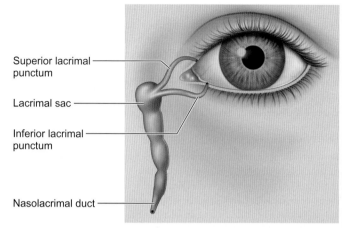

Fig. 1.13.21 Anatomy of the lacrimal system. (Courtesy Lauren Odono, DDS.)

Superior lacrimal punctum

Lacrimal sac

Inferior lacrimal punctum

Nasolacrimal duct

sodium, or methylprednisolone sodium succinate. Symptoms should improve within 30–45 minutes, or surgical intervention should be initiated. The sooner a retrobulbar hematoma is decompressed, the better the prognosis. Surgical treatment via lateral canthotomy allows rapid access to eliminate the elevated pressure and evacuate the developing hematoma. After local anesthetic is injected to the area, the blade of a tissue scissors is placed on the lateral orbital rim, cutting at a 45-degree angle posteroinferiorly. An alternative to lateral canthotomy is a lateral brow incision followed by subperiosteal dissection.[62–68]

If blindness occurs at the time of trauma, it is unlikely that it will return. Penetrating trauma with subsequent loss of vision has a poorer prognosis than loss of vision secondary to blunt trauma.

Superior orbital fissure syndrome was first described by Hirschfeld in 1858. Contents of the superior orbital fissure include the inferior division of cranial nerve III, cranial nerves IV and VI, lacrimal nerve, frontal nerve (V_1), ophthalmic vein, and the superior ophthalmic vein. Symptoms are secondary to depletion of the fissure's contents. Depending on the degree of involvement, symptoms may include: (1) loss of corneal reflex; (2) decreased sensation over the forehead; (3) a fixed and dilated pupil; (4) alteration of pupillary reflex and accommodation to direct light; and less commonly, (5) proptosis as a direct result of pressure, hemorrhage or decreased muscle tone (Box 1.13.3). Clinical symptoms guide treatment, and decompression is warranted if and when orbital compartment syndrome is suspected.

Orbital apex syndrome includes all symptoms of superior orbital fissure syndrome with the addition of injury to the optic nerve, often resulting from a fracture propagating through the optic canal.[69–73]

LONG-TERM COMPLICATIONS

Malunion

Malunion following midface trauma is often the result of improper reduction and fixation, treatment delay or significant comminution, which in turn can lead to facial asymmetry, malocclusion, ocular dystopia, enophthalmos, obstruction of the nasolacrimal ducts, and/or impingement of the infraorbital nerves. As revisional surgery to correct malunion can prove difficult to execute, the clinician's evaluation should determine whether the sequelae are primarily functional or aesthetic in nature.

If the resulting defect is functionally limiting, revisional osteotomies, leveling and symmetrizing bone grafts should be utilized. If aesthetic

in nature, one might consider less complicated overlay autologous, alloplastic, or synthetic grafting to restore facial symmetry.[3,27,35,62,74–76]

Malocclusion

As previously discussed, an anterior open-bite is the most common form of malocclusion encountered in patients with Le Fort fractures, resulting from the posterior and inferior pull of the pterygoid muscles on the maxilla lending to premature posterior occlusal contact during bite (see Fig. 1.13.7).

Postoperatively, chronic malocclusion can occur following inadequate reduction and anatomic fixation resulting in malunion or nonunion, or from delayed treatment. When recognized in follow-up, preexisting hardware removal, revisional osteotomies, and bone grafting with rigid fixation may be required to correct the occlusal deformity.[76]

Nonunion

Nonunion, though rare in the midface, can occur as a result of compromised blood supply, movement of segments, nutritional deficiencies, inaccurate positioning or infection. When it occurs, it is approached in the manner previously discussed for malunion with revisional osteotomies and bone grafting.[25,35,62,74,76,77]

Nasolacrimal Injury

The lacrimal system may be disrupted during midface trauma, most commonly when there is a naso-orbito-ethmoidal (NOE) component to the fracture pattern. Disruption anywhere from the puncta to the egress of the nasolacrimal duct beneath the inferior turbinate can lead to epiphora, with 80% of the lacrimal secretions associated with the inferior canaliculus (Fig. 1.13.21). Gruss et al. noted that disruption of the nasolacrimal system is not the sole cause of posttraumatic or postoperative epiphora, but is instead largely due to lid malposition or obstruction in the bony lacrimal canal.

Evaluation should proceed initially with close visual inspection evaluating the puncta for discharge and the lacrimal sac for engorgement. Where there is a high index of suspicion for injury, Jones I and II tests are used to evaluate the patency of the lacrimal system. The Jones I test proceeds via injection of 2% fluorescein dye into the conjunctival sac, observing if there is dye present in the nose after 5 minutes. Five percent cocaine is placed on a cotton-tipped applicator and onto the inferior turbinate to observe dye. If no dye is present, the Jones II test should then be initiated. The Jones II test aids in determining the location of the obstruction. A microcannula is inserted into the inferior canaliculus allowing for the injection of saline to flush the fluorescein dye from the lacrimal sac. If dye containing saline is observed in the nose, then a partial blockage was relieved by the injection. If there is reflux fluid present from the opposite punctum, it is indicative of an obstruction existing at or below the level of the nasolacrimal sac. In the presence of an obstruction distal to the lacrimal sac a dacryocystorhinostomy (DCR) should be performed. The DCR can be safely performed 3–4 months after initial reconstruction if a nasolacrimal blockage was not recognized at the time of initial trauma.[27,76,78–80]

EXPERT COMMENTARY

The hallmarks of diagnosis of Le Fort maxillary fractures are maxillary mobility and malocclusion. There are three types of Le Fort fractures without maxillary mobility, two common and one uncommon. The most common is the greensticked but incompletely fractured Le Fort fracture, and it can occur at any Le Fort level, I, II or III, with the symptoms varying with the level of occurrence. To understand Le Fort fractures, one must read the original translation by Paul Tessier of Le Fort's original experiments [1] to realize the myriad patterns and variations, as painstakingly described by René Le Fort, a French orthopedic surgeon. At his retirement ceremony this work was not mentioned, yet today it is the only thing for which he is remembered [1].

Incomplete Le Fort I fractures present with malocclusion, which may be subtle with no maxillary mobility. Or Le Fort fractures may be impacted, the second most common presentation resulting in their immobility. Le Fort II fractures present with again malocclusion and perhaps a unilateral zygoma, and again the malocclusion may be subtle. Le Fort III single segment incomplete fractures are the least common type of immobile Le Fort fracture, and present with a very subtle malocclusion, half to one cusp. I became acquainted with these thanks to Norman Rowe in his writings and in his book [2], and I am sure I missed the first ones of these I saw (as he did) by not being careful to check the occlusion accurately with the condyle seated in the fossa. Subtle malocclusion may sometimes be corrected with arch bars and elastic traction alone, as in the barely displaced single fragment Le Fort III fracture, but may come to osteotomy, preferably at the Le Fort I level despite the level of the fracture, as I dislike "rocking" fractures loose with "Rowe disimpaction forceps" for Le Fort level II and III fractures, as fractures may be produced that travel though the orbit to unfavorable locations, like the optic foramen, creating blindness. An incomplete fracture that is subtly displaced, is not loose, and not mobilized will easily tract the mandible condyles out of the fossa when placed in IMF, and when the IMF is released the patient is healed but in malocclusion and the condyles reseat themselves in the fossa (the patient drops into an open-bite with malocclusion).

Split palate, and alveolar fractures of the maxilla and mandible may also confuse the occlusion pattern, but these are usually easily recognized by gingival lacerations, and a deviation in the arch form [3–5].

Given that the usual description of Le Fort fractures has been oversimplified into Le Fort I, II, and III, what should the system be that is used to characterize the exact pattern of fragments, so one can organize the treatment to be prescribed?

Years ago, I designed a description [6] that accurately tells me the superior level of the fracture on each side, the pattern of the segment bearing the maxillary dentition, and the presence of alveolar or palatal fractures. Add to this the presence or absence of the NOE using the Markowitz classification [7], a description of the mandible fractures, the frontal bone/frontal sinus fractures, and a comprehensive description of the individual fragments is then given, which may be plugged into any one of several patterns of treatment organization, and an order of treatment developed [3,8–10].

My favorite order of treatment is to divide the face into functional units of the orbit, the occlusion, the frontal bone, and the mandible and to deal with each unit as described, proceeding from intact landmarks to the anterior facial skeleton, assembling the units in sequence as described. Finally the units are linked together, and we have maxillary and perhaps panfacial fracture treatment [3].

References

1. LeFort René. Experimental study of fractures of the upper and lower jaw, Parts I and II. In: McDowell F, ed. *Source Book of Plastic Surgery*. Baltimore, MD: Williams & Wilkins; 1977:360–377.
2. Rowe NL, Killley HC. *Fractures of the Facial Skeleton*. 2nd ed. London: E&S Livingston, Inc; 1968.
3. Manson P, Clark N, Robertson B, et al. Subunit principles in midface fractures: the importance of sagittal buttresses, soft tissue reductions and sequencing treatment of segmental fractures. *Plast Reconstr Surg*. 1999;103:1287–1306.
4. Hendrickson M, Clark N, Manson PN, et al. Palatal fractures: classification, patterns, and treatment with rigid internal fixation. *Plast Reconstr Surg*. 1998;101(2):319–332.
5. Manson PN, Clark N, Robertson B, et al. Comparative management of panfacial fractures. In: Hultman C Scott, ed. *50 Studies Every Plastic Surgeon Should Know*. Boca Raton, FL: CRC Press; 2015:123–132.
6. Kelly KJ, Manson PN, Vander Kolk CA, et al. Sequencing LeFort fracture treatment (Organization of treatment for a panfacial fracture). *J Craniofac Surg*. 1990;1(4):168–178.
7. Markowitz BL, Manson PN, Sargent L, et al. Management of the medial canthal tendon in nasoethmoid orbital fractures: the importance of the central fragment in classification and treatment. *Plast Reconstr Surg*. 1991;87(5):843–853.
8. Manson P, Markowitz B, Mirvis S, et al. Toward CT-based facial fracture treatment. *Plast Reconstr Surg*. 1990;85:202–212.
9. Manson P, Glassman D, Vander Kolk C, et al. Rigid stabilization of sagittal fractures of the maxilla and palate. *Plast Reconstr Surg*. 1990;85:711–717.
10. Manson PN. Dimensional analysis of the facial skeleton. *Prob Plast Reconstr Surg Surg*. 1991;1(2):213–238.

REFERENCES

1. al-Qurainy IA, Stassen LF, Dutton GN, et al. The characteristics of midfacial fractures and the association with ocular injury: a prospective study. *Br J Oral Maxillofac Surg*. 1991;29(5):291–301.
2. Davidoff G, Jakubowski M, Thomas D, Alpert M. The spectrum of closed-head injuries in facial trauma victims: incidence and impact. *Ann Emerg Med*. 1988;17(1):6–9.
3. Cook HE, Rowe M. A retrospective study of 356 midfacial fractures occurring in 225 patients. *J Oral Maxillofac Surg*. 1990;48(6):574–578.
4. Shere JL, Boole JR, Holtel MR, Amoroso PJ. An analysis of 3599 midfacial and 1141 orbital blowout fractures among 4426 United States Army Soldiers, 1980–2000. *Otolaryngol Head Neck Surg*. 2004;130(2):164–170.
5. Manson PN, Hoopes JE, Su CT. Structural pillars of the facial skeleton: an approach to the management of Le Fort fractures. *Plast Reconstr Surg*. 1980;66(1):54–62.
6. Manson PN, Clark N, Robertson B, et al. Subunit principles in midface fractures: the importance of sagittal buttresses, soft-tissue reductions, and sequencing treatment of segmental fractures. *Plast Reconstr Surg*. 1999;103(4):1287–1306, quiz 307.
7. Kelly KJ, Manson PN, Vander Kolk CA, et al. Sequencing LeFort fracture treatment (Organization of treatment for a panfacial fracture). *J Craniofac Surg*. 1990;1(4):168–178.
8. Manson PN. Some thoughts on the classification and treatment of Le Fort fractures. *Ann Plast Surg*. 1986;17(5):356–363.
9. Harris T, Rice S, Watts B, Davies G. The emergency control of traumatic maxillofacial haemorrhage. *Eur J Emerg Med*. 2010;17(4):230–233.
10. al-Qurainy IA, Dutton GN, Ilankovan V, et al. Midfacial fractures and the eye: the development of a system for detecting patients at risk of eye injury – a prospective evaluation. *Br J Oral Maxillofac Surg*. 1991;29(6):368–369.

11. al-Qurainy IA, Stassen LF, Dutton GN, et al. Diplopia following midfacial fractures. *Br J Oral Maxillofac Surg.* 1991;29(5):302–307.

12. Dutton GN, al-Qurainy I, Stassen LF, et al. Ophthalmic consequences of mid-facial trauma. *Eye (Lond).* 1992;6(Pt 1):86–89.

13. Paskert JP, Manson PN. The bimanual examination for assessing instability in naso-orbitoethmoidal injuries. *Plast Reconstr Surg.* 1989;83(1):165–167.

14. Mosby EL, Markle TL, Zulian MA, Hiatt WR. Technique for rigid fixation of Le Fort and palatal fractures. *J Oral Maxillofac Surg.* 1986;44(11):921–922.

15. Gorogh T, Rudolph P, Meyer JE, et al. Separation of beta2-transferrin by denaturing gel electrophoresis to detect cerebrospinal fluid in ear and nasal fluids. *Clin Chem.* 2005;51(9):1704–1710.

16. Alder ME, Deahl ST, Matteson SR. Clinical usefulness of two-dimensional reformatted and three-dimensionally rendered computerized tomographic images: literature review and a survey of surgeons' opinions. *J Oral Maxillofac Surg.* 1995;53(4):375–386.

17. Gillespie JE, Isherwood I, Barker GR, Quayle AA. Three-dimensional reformations of computed tomography in the assessment of facial trauma. *Clin Radiol.* 1987;38(5):523–526.

18. Gillespie JE, Quayle AA, Barker G, Isherwood I. Three-dimensional CT reformations in the assessment of congenital and traumatic cranio-facial deformities. *Br J Oral Maxillofac Surg.* 1987;25(2):171–177.

19. Manson PN, Markowitz B, Mirvis S, et al. Toward CT-based facial fracture treatment. *Plast Reconstr Surg.* 1990;85(2):202–212, discussion 213–214.

20. Hopper RA, Salemy S, Sze RW. Diagnosis of midface fractures with CT: what the surgeon needs to know. *Radiographics.* 2006;26(3):783–793.

21. McRae M, Frodel J. Midface fractures. *Facial Plast Surg.* 2000;16(2):107–113.

22. Buchanan RT, Holtmann B. Severe epistaxis in facial fractures. *Plast Reconstr Surg.* 1983;71(6):768–771.

23. Hassard AD, Kirkpatrick DA, Wong FS. Ligation of the external carotid and anterior ethmoidal arteries for severe or unusual epistaxis resulting from facial fractures. *Can J Surg.* 1986;29(6):447–449.

24. Lanigan DT, Hey JH, West RA. Major vascular complications of orthognathic surgery: hemorrhage associated with Le Fort I osteotomies. *J Oral Maxillofac Surg.* 1990;48(6):561–573.

25. Poncet JL, Conessa C, Brinquin L. [Evaluation of the severity and early complications of cranio-facial trauma]. *Rev Prat.* 2003;53(9):1033–1040.

26. Haug RH, Prather J, Bradrick JP, Indresano AT. The morbidity associated with fifty maxillary fractures treated by closed reduction. *Oral Surg Oral Med Oral Pathol.* 1992;73(6):659–663.

27. al-Qurainy IA. Convergence insufficiency and failure of accommodation following midfacial trauma. *Br J Oral Maxillofac Surg.* 1995;33(2):71–75.

28. Gruss JS, Bubak PJ, Egbert MA. Craniofacial fractures. An algorithm to optimize results. *Clin Plast Surg.* 1992;19(1):195–206.

29. Fan X, Li J, Zhu J, et al. Computer-assisted orbital volume measurement in the surgical correction of late enophthalmos caused by blowout fractures. *Ophthal Plast Reconstr Surg.* 2003;19(3):207–211.

30. Bloomquist DS, Feldman GR. The posterior ilium as a donor site for maxillo-facial bone grafting. *J Maxillofac Surg.* 1980;8(1):60–64.

31. Tessier P, Kawamoto H, Matthews D, et al. Taking bone grafts from the anterior and posterior ilium–tools and techniques: II. A 6800-case experience in maxillofacial and craniofacial surgery. *Plast Reconstr Surg.* 2005;116(5 suppl):25S–37S, discussion 92S–94S.

32. Gruss JS. Complex nasoethmoid-orbital and midfacial fractures: role of craniofacial surgical techniques and immediate bone grafting. *Ann Plast Surg.* 1986;17(5):377–390.

33. Gruss JS, Van Wyck L, Phillips JH, Antonyshyn O. The importance of the zygomatic arch in complex midfacial fracture repair and correction of posttraumatic orbitozygomatic deformities. *Plast Reconstr Surg.* 1990;85(6):878–890.

34. Erling BF, Iliff N, Robertson B, Manson PN. Footprints of the globe: a practical look at the mechanism of orbital blowout fractures, with a revisit to the work of Raymond Pfeiffer. *Plast Reconstr Surg.* 1999;103(4):1313–1316, discussion 7–9.

35. Browning CW. Alloplast materials in orbital repair. *Am J Ophthalmol.* 1967;63(5):955–962.

36. Converse JM, Firmin F, Wood-Smith D, Friedland JA. The conjunctival approach in orbital fractures. *Plast Reconstr Surg.* 1973;52(6):656–657.

37. Converse JM, Smith B. Enophthalmos and diplopia in fractures of the orbital floor. *Br J Plast Surg.* 1957;9(4):265–274.

38. Curi L, Marinelli LF. [Surgical treatment of fractures of the floor and rim of the orbit with enophthalmos and diplopia]. *Valsalva.* 1963;39:376–384.

39. Freihofer HP. [Secondary post-traumatic periorbital reconstructions]. *Fortschr Kiefer Gesichtschir.* 1994;39:58–61.

40. Chen CH, Wang TY, Tsay PK, et al. A 162-case review of palatal fracture: management strategy from a 10-year experience. *Plast Reconstr Surg.* 2008;121(6):2065–2073.

41. Denny AD, Celik N. A management strategy for palatal fractures: a 12-year review. *J Craniofac Surg.* 1999;10(1):49–57.

42. Goldberg MH. Palatal fractures. *Plast Reconstr Surg.* 1998;102(3):920.

43. Hendrickson M, Clark N, Manson PN, et al. Palatal fractures: classification, patterns, and treatment with rigid internal fixation. *Plast Reconstr Surg.* 1998;101(2):319–332.

44. Hoppe IC, Halsey JN, Ciminello FS, et al. A single-center review of palatal fractures: etiology, patterns, concomitant injuries, and management. *Eplasty.* 2017;17:e20.

45. Kumaravelu C, Thirukonda GJ, Kannabiran P. A novel adjuvant to treat palatal fractures. *J Oral Maxillofac Surg.* 2011;69(6):e152–e154.

46. Mundinger GS, Borsuk DE, Okhah Z, et al. Antibiotics and facial fractures: evidence-based recommendations compared with experience-based practice. *Craniomaxillofac Trauma Reconstr.* 2015;8(1):64–78.

47. Crosby E. Airway management after upper cervical spine injury: What have we learned? *Can J Anaesth.* 2002;49(7):733–744.

48. Manninen PH, Jose GB, Lukitto K, et al. Management of the airway in patients undergoing cervical spine surgery. *J Neurosurg Anesthesiol.* 2007;19(3):190–194.

49. Nandyala SV, Marquez-Lara A, Park DK, et al. Incidence, risk factors, and outcomes of postoperative airway management after cervical spine surgery. *Spine.* 2014;39(9):E557–E563.

50. Hernandez Altemir F. The submental route for endotracheal intubation. A new technique. *J Maxillofac Surg.* 1986;14(1):64–65.

51. Crawford C, Kennedy N, Weir WR. Cerebrospinal fluid rhinorrhoea and Haemophilus influenzae meningitis 37 years after a head injury. *J Infect.* 1994;28(1):93–97.

52. Loew F, Pertuiset B, Chaumier EE, Jaksche H. Traumatic, spontaneous and postoperative CSF rhinorrhea. *Adv Tech Stand Neurosurg.* 1984;11:169–207.

53. Poletti-Muringaseril SC, Rufibach K, Ruef C, et al. Low meningitis-incidence in primary spontaneous compared to secondary cerebrospinal fluid rhinorrhoea. *Rhinology.* 2012;50(1):73–79.

54. Hartmann N, Haase W. [Diplopia, enophthalmos and motility disorders in isolated orbital floor fractures]. *Klin Monbl Augenheilkd.* 1987;191(2):116–119.

55. Hwang K, Huan F, Hwang PJ. Diplopia and enophthalmos in blowout fractures. *J Craniofac Surg.* 2012;23(4):1077–1082.

56. Dulley B, Fells P. Long-term follow-up of orbital blow-out fractures with and without surgery. *Mod Probl Ophthalmol.* 1975;14:467–470.

57. Balaji SM. Surgical correction of severe enophthalmos caused by bullet injury. *Indian J Dent Res.* 2016;27(4):445–449.

58. Crumley RL, Leibsohn J. Enophthalmos and diplopia in orbital floor fractures. *Trans Pac Coast Otoophthalmol Soc Annu Meet.* 1976;57:105–109.

59. Konrade KA, Clode AB, Michau TM, et al. Surgical correction of severe strabismus and enophthalmos secondary to zygomatic arch fracture in a dog. *Vet Ophthalmol.* 2009;12(2):119–124.

60. Manson PN, Clifford CM, Su CT, et al. Mechanisms of global support and posttraumatic enophthalmos: I. The anatomy of the ligament sling and its relation to intramuscular cone orbital fat. *Plast Reconstr Surg.* 1986;77(2):193–202.

61. Mathog RH, Hillstrom RP, Nesi FA. Surgical correction of enophthalmos and diplopia. A report of 38 cases. *Arch Otolaryngol Head Neck Surg.* 1989;115(2):169–178.

62. Dimov Z, Abramov G, Dimov K, et al. [Complications in Le Fort facial fractures combined with craniocerebral trauma]. *Khirurgiia (Sofiia).* 1999;55(5):35–37.

63. Hislop WS, Dutton GN. Retrobulbar haemorrhage: Can blindness be prevented? *Injury.* 1994;25(10):663–665.

64. Kallela I, Hyrkas T, Paukku P, et al. Blindness after maxillofacial blunt trauma. Evaluation of candidates for optic nerve decompression surgery. *J Craniomaxillofac Surg.* 1994;22(4):220–225.

65. Manfredi SJ, Raji MR, Sprinkle PM, et al. Computerized tomographic scan findings in facial fractures associated with blindness. *Plast Reconstr Surg.* 1981;68(4):479–490.

66. Ord RA. Post-operative retrobulbar haemorrhage and blindness complicating trauma surgery. *Br J Oral Surg.* 1981;19(3):202–207.

67. Rosdeutscher JD, Stadelmann WK. Diagnosis and treatment of retrobulbar hematoma resulting from blunt periorbital trauma. *Ann Plast Surg.* 1998;41(6):618–622.

68. Wu N, Yin ZQ, Wang Y. Traumatic optic neuropathy therapy: an update of clinical and experimental studies. *J Int Med Res.* 2008;36(5):883–889.

69. Gasco J, Hooten K, Ridley RW, et al. Neuronavigation-guided endoscopic decompression of superior orbital fissure fracture: case report and literature review. *Skull Base.* 2009;19(3):241–246.

70. Murakami I. Decompression of the superior orbital fissure. *Am J Ophthalmol.* 1965;59:803–808.

71. Niho S, Murakami K, Kimura S. [Transethmoidal route to the optic foramen. Decompression of the superior orbital fissure]. *Ganka.* 1967;9(4):256–267.

72. Niho S, Niho M, Niho K. Decompression of the optic canal by the transethmoidal route and decompression of the superior orbital fissure. *Can J Ophthalmol.* 1970;5(1):22–40.

73. Wang X, Li YM, Huang CG, et al. Endoscopic transmaxillary transMuller's muscle approach for decompression of superior orbital fissure: a cadaveric study with illustrative case. *J Craniomaxillofac Surg.* 2014;42(2):132–140.

74. Jackson IT, Adham M, Bite U, Marx R. Update on cranial bone grafts in craniofacial surgery. *Ann Plast Surg.* 1987;18(1):37–40.

75. Marx RE. Bone harvest from the posterior ilium. *Atlas Oral Maxillofac Surg Clin North Am.* 2005;13(2):109–118.

76. Morris LM, Kellman RM. Complications in facial trauma. *Facial Plast Surg Clin North Am.* 2013;21(4):605–617.

77. Tessier P. Complications of facial trauma: principles of late reconstruction. *Ann Plast Surg.* 1986;17(5):411–420.

78. Gentry LR, Manor WF, Turski PA, Strother CM. High-resolution CT analysis of facial struts in trauma: 2. Osseous and soft-tissue complications. *AJR Am J Roentgenol.* 1983;140(3):533–541.

79. Gruss JS, Hurwitz JJ, Nik NA, Kassel EE. The pattern and incidence of nasolacrimal injury in naso-orbital-ethmoid fractures: the role of delayed assessment and dacryocystorhinostomy. *Br J Plast Surg.* 1985;38(1):116–121.

80. Harris GJ, Fuerste FH. Lacrimal intubation in the primary repair of midfacial fractures. *Ophthalmology.* 1987;94(3):242–247.

1.14

Mandible Fractures

Lauren T. Odono, Colin M. Brady, Mark Urata

BACKGROUND

The earliest descriptions referencing the management of mandible fractures date back to Ancient Egypt (1650 BC) in which the pathology was described as incurable, inevitably resulting in infectious complications, and leading ultimately to demise. Hippocrates would revolutionize the management with his introduction of the concepts of reduction and stabilization with circumdental wiring and external bandages for stabilization, similar to the technique of "bridle wiring" still used today.[1,2]

Through the centuries, a number of techniques to achieve closed reduction and stabilization of the various fracture patterns were introduced. In early times, external bandaging came into popularity with the introduction of the Barton Bandage. This would quickly fall out of favor, however, due to resulting "bird face" deformities and malunion in the setting posterior deformational forces.[3] Subsequently, a number of extra- and intraoral appliances would be introduced. Early designs were primitive, vice-like, and only moderately effective in gaining proper occlusion and adequate immobilization to promote union.[4,5] It would be Gunning who would first utilize a customized intraoral splint for immobilization in combination with a head-piece that allowed for relative intermaxillary fixation (IMF).[6–8] A modified version of Gunning's approach to achieve IMF is still applicable today in the management of mandible fractures in edentulous individuals.

In patients with intact dentition, the mid- to late 19th century would bring the rise of advances in monomaxillary wiring, arches and custom-designed metal splint techniques; but without additional fixation, these methods were found to provide inadequate immobilization to promote bony union.[5,9]

There are conflicting reports as to whether it was Gilmer or Guglielmo Salicetti who was the first to utilize the modern concept of IMF in the reduction and stabilization of the traumatic mandible. Each supported the use of individual transdental wires on mandibular and maxillary dentition, which were subsequently ligated in an opposing fashion to provide stability and restore occlusion.[10] Gilmer would eventually expound upon this concept, introducing the modern day concept of IMF by fixation of full arch bars to the maxilla and mandible that could subsequently be stabilized with opposing ligatures.[11]

As evidenced by the aforementioned management strategies, early management of the mandibular trauma was approached with closed reduction and immobilization with varied success. It was not until the late 19th century that the first reports of open reduction, internal fixation techniques were published. In 1869, the Thomas principle introduced an intraoral approach to mandibular open reduction followed by transosseous wire osteosynthesis using coil-like silver wire, which could be tightened periodically to achieve bony union.[12] Modifications of transosseous wiring techniques would be frequently utilized in the primary management of mandibular trauma until the 1960s

despite criticism that these methods lacked rigid stability across the fracture site.

The incidence of suboptimal unions and complications with wire/rod/splint technologies spurred early efforts to devise plate and screw fixation systems. In 1888, Schede would report the first usage of formal plate fixation across the fracture site, in the form of a steel plate stabilized by four screws. In the early part of the 20th century, Mahe, Ivy and Cole experimented with a combination of plates made of either steel or silver, combined with screw and/or wire fixation to stabilize the fractures. These early plate designs were ultimately abandoned due to a significant incidence of infection and surrounding tissue corrosion.[12]

Despite early setbacks, recognition of the merits of rigid fixation in the promotion of primary bone healing furthered ingenuity in the engineering, materials, and fabrication of these systems. An understanding that plate fixation in the dynamic craniofacial skeleton is a different entity to that of the extra-axial skeleton eventually made way for the development of a number of fixation technologies: rigid versus semi-rigid fixation, locking versus nonlocking plates, threaded versus tapered plates, and bicortical versus monocortical fixation. An in-depth familiarity with this diverse armamentarium is critical to the successful management of the spectrum of mandibular trauma. In the sections that follow we will discuss the anatomy, classification, diagnosis, work-up, and management of fractures of the mandibular angle, ramus, body, and symphysis, highlighting best practice recommendations.

EPIDEMIOLOGY

The causes of mandible fractures are diverse and include: motor vehicle collisions (MVCs), assaults, falls, sports- and industrial-related injuries, ballistic injuries, and pathologic fractures. Taking all-comers, approximately 75% of mandible fractures are caused by MVC and assault, 7% are due to falls, 7% and 4% are due to industrial- and sports-related injuries, respectively, and the remainder are due to pathological, ballistic, and other miscellaneous causes (Fig. 1.14.1).[13,14] The most common etiology is variable depending on the socioeconomic status of the patient and the population being examined. For example, in rural or developing countries, MVC remains the most common cause of mandibular trauma; whereas in certain urban settings of developed nations, assault and interpersonal violence can account for much of the mandibular trauma presenting to trauma centers.[15]

An increasingly frequent and previously underrecognized cause of mandible fracture is pathological fracture associated with dental implantation. As indications for and access to restorative dentistry are ever-increasing, a wider range of patients are now the recipients of implant technologies and by extension at risk for unfavorable fractures. Greenstein et al. noted the following predisposing factors to implant-associated fractures: (1) poor bony stock (osteoporosis); (2) stress/strain at site of implant placement; and (3) trauma.[16] An understanding of these

Causes of mandible fractures

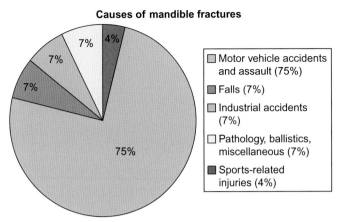

- Motor vehicle accidents and assault (75%)
- Falls (7%)
- Industrial accidents (7%)
- Pathology, ballistics, miscellaneous (7%)
- Sports-related injuries (4%)

Fig. 1.14.1 Causes of mandible fractures by percentage.[13,14]

Location of mandible fractures

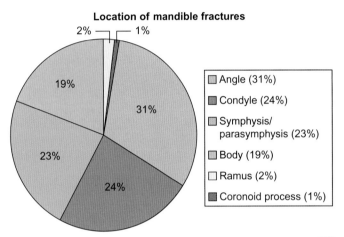

- Angle (31%)
- Condyle (24%)
- Symphysis/parasymphysis (23%)
- Body (19%)
- Ramus (2%)
- Coronoid process (1%)

Fig. 1.14.2 Anatomic location of mandible fractures by percentage.[14,15]

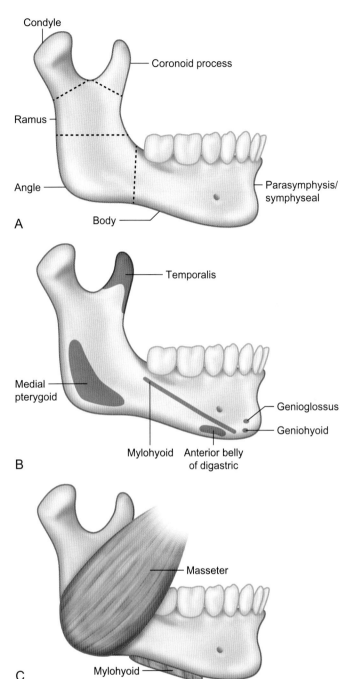

Fig. 1.14.3 (A) Classification of mandible fractures by anatomical boundaries; (B) lingual aspect of the mandible with muscle attachments; (C) buccal aspect of the mandible with muscle attachments.

risks and considerations for the management thereof are important for both the oral surgeon placing implants and the trauma surgeon who manages traumatic fractures in an increasing population of patients who may also have had dental rehabilitation.

The incidence of mandible fractures by anatomical location is as follows: angle (31%), condyle (24%), symphysis and parasymphysis (23%), body (19%), ramus (2%), and coronoid process (1%) (Fig. 1.14.2).[14,15] In addition, a number of studies have looked at the association between causality and fracture location. In fractures secondary to MVC, the body is the most common site of injury. In those associated with assault the angle and body are most commonly involved. Boole et al. found that fractures after motorbike accidents most commonly involved the condyle or ramus.[17]

When considering the incidence of concomitant facial fractures, 15% of individuals were found to have another facial fracture in addition to the mandible fracture. The number of fractures per mandible has also been analyzed retrospectively with a reported mean of 1.65. Several authors have extrapolated that between 40% and 50% of patients presenting with mandibular trauma have more than one fracture.[17,18]

The surgeon managing complex mandibular trauma should also be versed in the risk of nonmaxillofacial trauma that can be associated with the mandibular fractures. The incidence of non-bony facial injuries has been reported to range from 15% to 34% in a review of UK and North American Trauma Databases, respectively.[17,19] As expected, the mechanism of injury is an important predictor of the presence or absence of other injuries. Mandible fractures secondary to assault were most commonly isolated. In contrast, mandible fractures secondary to an MVC were associated with nonmaxillofacial injuries in 46% of patients reviewed.[20] The risk of concomitant cervical spine injury has been reported to range from 2.6% to 6.5%.[17] An understanding and appreciation for the mechanism of injury and the possibility of associated polysystem trauma is an important preoperative consideration for the trauma surgeon with respect to clearance and timing of fracture repair.

SURGICAL ANATOMY

See Fig. 1.14.3.

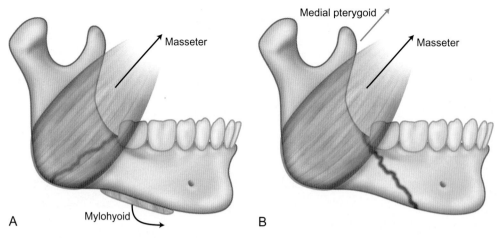

Fig. 1.14.4 (A) Horizontally unfavorable fracture; (B) horizontally favorable fracture.

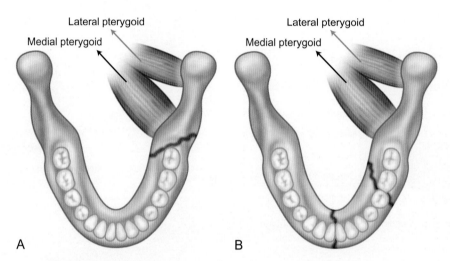

Fig. 1.14.5 (A) Vertically unfavorable fracture; (B) vertically favorable fracture.

CLASSIFICATION

Though a myriad of classification schemes have been presented in the maxillofacial trauma literature, there is no single system globally accepted by practitioners by which to standardize communication. The most commonly referenced scheme is classification by anatomic region: symphysis, body, angle, ramus, condyle, coronoid, and alveolus.[21] These anatomic units are often further subclassified into favorable and unfavorable patterns. Favorableness is determined by the direction of a fracture line when viewed on radiographs in the horizontal or vertical plane. The displacing forces of the muscles of mastication influence the favorableness of mandible fractures (Fig. 1.14.4). Horizontally favorable fracture lines resist upward displacing forces. A vertically favorable fracture line resists the medial pull of the medial pterygoid on the proximal fragment when viewed in the vertical plane (Fig. 1.14.5). The following defines each subunit by its anatomy and elucidates relevant favorable and unfavorable fracture patterns.

Symphysis

The symphyseal region of the mandible is defined as the region between the roots of the central incisors, running from the alveolar process through the inferior border of the mandible in a vertical orientation (Fig. 1.14.6).

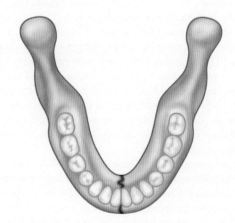

Fig. 1.14.6 Symphysis of the mandible fracture.

Parasymphysis

The parasymphysis region of the mandible is defined as the area between the lateral roots of the canines and the distal aspect of the lateral incisors, extending from the alveolar process to the inferior border of the mandible (Fig. 1.14.7). Linear and oblique fracture orientations are characteristic in this region. The combined action of the digastric and suprahyoid muscles on a bilateral fracture can pull on the distal fragment inferiorly in an unfavorable fracture, placing the patient at risk of acute upper airway obstruction.

Body

The body region of the mandible is defined as the line coincident with the anterior border of the masseter muscle to the canine. The buccal and lingual cortices of this area are well-defined. Fractures typically follow a linear pattern, however, in the incidence of high-energy trauma, comminution can be seen (Fig. 1.14.8). Fractures of the body of the mandible are usually seen in combination with fractures on the contralateral side of the mandible or with ipsilateral fractures of the condyle or ramus.

Angle

The angle region of the mandible is defined as a triangular area bounded by the anterior border of the masseter muscle to the posterosuperior attachment of the masseter muscle, usually distal to the third molar area. The angle of the mandible is thinner than the body of the mandible. Most fractures of the angle occur in the location of the third molar and extend to the antegonial notch anterior to the true angle. The masseter, temporalis, and medial pterygoid muscle attachments to the ramus cause displacement of the proximal segment of the angle of the mandible in a superior and medial direction when the fracture is horizontally and vertically unfavorable, respectively (Fig. 1.14.9). Alternately, these muscles can serve to secondarily stabilize the proximal and distal bony segments in fracture patterns that are vertically and horizontally favorable. The more anterior a fracture occurs along the angle/body, the more the superior displacement of the fracture is counteracted by the pull of the mylohyoid muscle downward.

Combining the input and focus of a number of other classification schemes, Kruger presents a comprehensive four-category system (Table 1.14.1).[22]

CLINICAL PRESENTATION

The diagnostic work-up of mandible trauma starts with a thorough history. Special attention to past medical history may reveal previous trauma, bone disease, osteoporosis, neoplasms both primary and

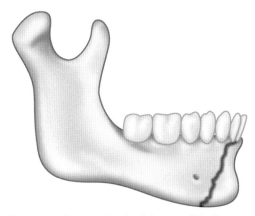

Fig. 1.14.7 Parasymphysis of the mandible fracture.

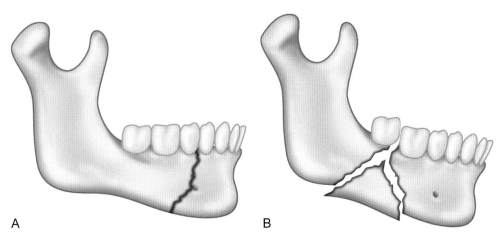

A   B

Fig. 1.14.8 (A) Body of the mandible fracture; (B) comminuted body of the mandible fracture.

TABLE 1.14.1	**Kruger and Schilli Classification of Mandible Fractures**		
Relation to External Environment	**Types of Fractures**	**Dentition of the Jaw With Reference to the Use of Splints**	**Localization**
• Simple or Closed • Compound or Open	• Incomplete • Complete • Green stick • Comminuted	• Sufficiently dentulous jaw • Edentulous or insufficiently dentulous jaw • Primary and mixed dentition	• Fractures of the symphysis region between the canines • Fractures of the canine region • Fractures of the body of the mandible between the canine and angle of the mandible • Fractures of the angle of the mandible in the third molar region • Fractures of the mandible ramus between the angle of the mandible and the sigmoid notch • Fractures of the coronoid process • Fractures of the condylar process

Source: Kruger E. *Oral and maxillofacial traumatology*. Chicago. IL: Quintessence; 1982.

metastatic, pre-existing dental pathologies and interventions, nutritional and metabolic disorders, endocrinopathies, and psychiatric conditions that might influence both the etiology, timing of surgery, and choice of treatment stratagem for the relevant fracture. Preoperative temporomandibular joint (TMJ) dysfunction should be elucidated in the history and clearly documented in the preoperative evaluation if present, as it can have a profound impact on setting accurate patient expectations for postsurgical outcomes.

Ascertaining the velocity of the injury can help understand and predict the fracture patterns, as high- and low-speed impacts each manifest differently. As noted previously, assaults (low-velocity injuries) tend to cause isolated fractures, often nondisplaced, whereas high-speed MVCs are often associated with multiple fractures that are more likely to be displaced and comminuted.

The type of object also plays a role in the presenting fracture pattern. Blunt objects tend to cause multiple fractures due to the propagation and dispersion of forces throughout the jaw. Sharp or more well-defined objects isolate the injury forces to a single location within the jaw resulting in a localized comminuted fracture.

Similarly, the vector of injury forces often serves as a predictive indicator of the ultimate fracture profile. For example, traumatic forces directed anteriorly at the symphysis may result in associated bilateral condylar fractures and an anterior open-bite (Fig. 1.14.10).[23] Coup–contracoup patterns are often seen in high-velocity injuries when a force fracturing the parasymphysis may cause a concomitant contralateral angle fracture, and so forth (Fig. 1.14.11).

Often overlooked and frequently underappreciated is the impact on surgical decision-making and outcomes of the patient's premorbid dental history and occlusion. The surgeon should be aware of any history of dental interventions, extractions (especially third molars), cosmetic and reconstructive dental rehabilitation, use of orthodontic appliances, significant carious and/or periodontal disease. Perturbations of the premorbid occlusion should be initially screened by asking if the patient feels that their bite is abnormal. If available, premorbid photographs can be reviewed to better elucidate the patient's baseline bite. In the patient who is completely or partially edentulous, the status of their dentures should be ascertained. For the patient engaged in phased orthodontic care, a preoperative discussion with the orthodontist may help guide treatment modalities.

PHYSICAL EXAMINATION

The physical examination should consist of palpation and inspection. The four classic signs of inflammation, pain, swelling, redness and localized heat, are highly indicative signs of a mandible fracture. Fractured dentition, gingival bruising, lacerations, mobility of teeth, decreased incisal opening and malocclusion are common intraoral findings associated with mandible fractures. Alteration of sensation to the lower lip and chin is pathognomonic of a fracture of the mandible posterior to the mental foramen. However, nondisplaced fractures of the parasymphysis, body or angle rarely give rise to numbness in the distribution of the inferior alveolar nerve. Gingival tissue should be inspected for

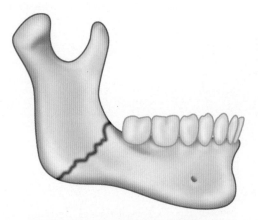

Fig. 1.14.9 Angle of the mandible fracture.

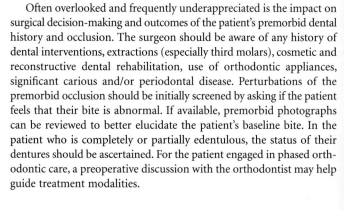

Fig. 1.14.10 Symphyseal fracture with bilateral subcondylar fractures.

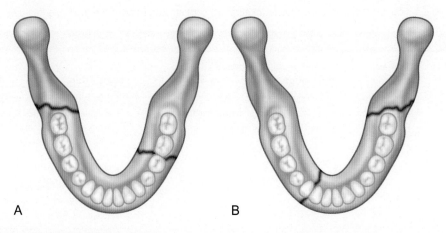

Fig. 1.14.11 (A) Right angle and left body of the mandible fractures; (B) right parasymphysis and left angle of the mandible factures.

bruising or lacerations. Trauma causing bleeding, a hematoma, and discontinuity of skin or mucosa may indicate an injury to the underlying mandible. Sublingual ecchymosis is the most common pathognomonic sign of a fracture of the mandible, especially of the symphyseal, parasymphyseal or body regions. Depending on the direction and degree of displacement of a mandible fracture, the fractured segments can be visualized directly through the laceration. Forces that are strong enough to fracture or even loosen teeth have the ability to fracture the mandible. Fractured teeth should be evaluated along with any steps or irregularities within the dental arch. Missing teeth or fragments of teeth that have not been accounted for should be considered as swallowed, displaced into localized soft tissue, or aspirated. Abrasions, contusions, and lacerations of the gingiva and adjacent soft tissues should be examined for damage to vital structures. Mobility of fractured teeth should be assessed to determine risk of aspiration. Though alteration of occlusion can indicate displacement of teeth and fracture of dentoalveolar structures, it is highly suggestive of a mandible fracture. Changes in occlusion can be a result of fractures of the alveolar process, fractured teeth, mandible fracture, trauma to the muscles of mastication, temporomandibular joint effusion or dislocation. A posterior crossbite can be due to fractures of the parasymphysis region and condyle, causing bilateral splaying of the posterior mandible. An anterior open-bite with a posterior pre-mature contact can be indicative of an angle fracture, a condylar fracture or fracture of the maxilla. A posterior open-bite can indicate a fracture of the symphysis, parasymphysis, or alveolar process. Skin on the face of the affected area should be inspected for lacerations, hematoma and swelling, for example, a wound under the chin is a common site of laceration typically indicating symphyseal, parasymphysis, and/or subcondylar fractures. Asymmetries of a patient's face are indications of the possibility of a mandible fracture and abnormal facial contours of the mandible should be assessed. Bilateral parasymphysis fractures can cause a retruded chin. Bilateral body and subcondylar fractures can cause the downward displacement of the anterior mandible, leading to an elongated face. A fracture along the body or ramus of the mandible can lead to a flattened appearance on the lateral face.

RADIOLOGICAL EXAMINATION

Box 1.14.1 outlines the most common radiographic studies utilized in the diagnosis of mandible fractures. The panoramic radiograph (panorex) can be extremely useful in the initial evaluation of the patient with mandibular trauma. It is advantageous in that it allows a survey of all relevant anatomic subunits of the mandible in a single study, is comparatively cost-effective, and generally provides acceptable detail if taken by a skilled technician.[24] There are several drawbacks, however, to this diagnostic approach: (1) panoramic radiography requires the patient to be upright or prone making this an unfeasible approach for most trauma patients; (2) medial condylar and buccal-lingual bony displacement is difficult to characterize; (3) resolution is poor when evaluating the

symphysis, dentoalveolar arches, and the TMJ; and (4) though accessible in all dental, oral surgery, and orthodontic offices, the equipment is often not available in hospital-based radiology departments.[25]

Though panoramic radiography may not be readily available, most of the information on the location and vector of displacement can ultimately be garnered by a plain film mandible series inclusive of the following views: (1) Caldwell posteroanterior (PA) radiograph; (2) lateral oblique radiograph; (3) mandibular occlusal view; (4) periapical view; (5) reverse Towne's view. The advantage of the Caldwell PA is the clear demonstration of symphyseal fractures and the ability to discern medial or lateral displacement of fractures of the ramus, angle, body, and symphysis. The disadvantage of the PA view is that the condylar region is not well visualized. The lateral oblique view is easy to obtain and may be helpful in the diagnosis of angle, ramus, and posterior body fractures. The condylar, symphyseal, and premolar regions are often obscured. The occlusal view is helpful in determining the extent of medial and lateral displacement of body fractures. The reverse or modified Towne's view is helpful in elucidating the degree of medial displacement of the condyle. Anterior condylar displacement can be evaluated with transcranial TMJ views, although these are less often utilized by clinicians.[24]

With the advent of helical computerized tomography (CT) offering better resolution, more expedient scan intervals, and decreased radiation exposure, trauma practice patterns have shifted to the more liberal utility of CT scanning in the evaluation of the polytrauma patient. Similarly, these practice patterns have been extended to include the evaluation of trauma within the craniomaxillofacial skeleton, and as such, helical CT with the addition of 3D reformatting has largely supplanted plain-film radiography as the diagnostic gold standard in the acute setting. CT of the craniofacial skeleton provides detailed resolution, and the ability to rapidly and accurately assess the fracture location, vector, and degree of displacement.[25,26]

SURGICAL INDICATIONS

The indications dictating the chosen management strategy are best subdivided into nonoperative versus closed versus open reduction techniques (Table 1.14.2).

Indications for Soft Diet Only

Nonoperative treatment of a mandible fracture with observation only and mechanical soft diet modification is considered in greenstick

---

BOX 1.14.1 Common Radiographic Studies

- Panoramic radiograph
- Caldwell posteroanterior
- Lateral oblique
- Mandibular occlusal view
- Periapical view
- Reverse Towne's view
- Computerized tomography

TABLE 1.14.2 Indications for Surgical Management of Mandible Fractures

Closed Reduction	Open Reduction
• Nondisplaced favorable fractures	• Displaced unfavorable fractures of the angle/body/parasymphysis
• Grossly comminuted fractures	• Concomitant fractures of the craniofacial skeleton
• Fractures with extensive soft tissue injury	• Malunion
• Edentulous mandible fractures	• Nonunion
• Pediatric mandible fractures	• Contraindications to maxillomandibular fixation
• Condylar fractures	• Displaced bilateral condylar fracture with midface fractures
	• Edentulous maxilla opposite a mandibular fracture

fractures or incomplete fractures without pain, functional disruption, malocclusion or pathology.

Indications for Closed Reduction

Closed reduction may be utilized for nondisplaced, favorable fractures, grossly comminuted fractures, and fractures exposed by significant loss of overlying soft tissue. In the nondisplaced, favorable fracture, destabilizing, asymmetric muscle pull on either side of the fracture is not a concern and as such rigid fixation is not required to prevent significant motion of the reduced segments during bone healing and consolidation. In grossly comminuted fractures, the bony fragments are too small to individually fixate, and attempting to do so would disrupt often-intact periosteal blood supply. Surgeons often treat these fracture patterns as a "bag of bones" and utilize closed techniques with establishment of premorbid occlusion to prevent the loss of periosteal integrity that would be associated with an open approach. In patients with poor overlying soft tissue coverage, whether due to associated soft tissue trauma or adjunctive treatment modalities (e.g. radiotherapy) often utilized in patients with pathologic fractures in the setting of cancer, closed techniques should be considered to prevent the increased risk of hardware exposure associated with open fixation. Closed reduction techniques may also be utilized in the intraoperative setting for establishment of the premorbid occlusion prior to rigid fixation, used as a tension band, and for stabilization of dentoalveolar fractures (Box 1.14.2). Utility in the setting of the edentulous mandible, pediatric fractures, and coronoid and condylar process fractures is beyond the scope of this chapter.

Indications for Open Reduction

Control over the proximal segment is the overriding factor in selecting an open reduction for a surgical option. Displaced unfavorable angle fractures where the proximal segment is displaced superiorly or medially and reduction is unattainable with simple manipulation, require open reduction internal fixation (Fig. 1.14.12). Displaced unfavorable fractures of the body or parasymphysis region of the mandible due to asymmetric muscle pull of the geniohyoid, digastric, genioglossus, and mylohyoid on the fracture fragments also favor an open approach (Fig. 1.14.13). Delayed treatment or soft tissue interposition preventing proper reduction warrants open technique.

The advantages of open reduction are the ability of the patient to return to function expediently, and a more exacting reduction and approximation of bony segments. In 1978, Champy defined regions of the mandible with smaller degrees of force that would require only a miniplate with monocortical screws for stable fixation across the angle, parasymphysis, and symphyseal of the mandible.[27] These Champy lines coincide with the tension bands of the mandible. Tension bands across a mandible fracture are of utmost importance. Due to muscle actions and the differential forces being distributed across the mandible, stabilizing the areas of tension will allow the forces to be distributed equally over the fracture surface and alleviate asymmetric displacement. The disadvantages of open reduction are potentially damage to adjacent teeth and nerves, rejection of hardware, prolonged anesthesia, increased risk of infection, increased in-hospital time and cost as well as intraoral and extraoral scarring. The surgical approaches to mandible fractures are discussed further in the following section.

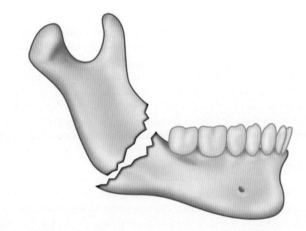

Fig. 1.14.12 Superior displacement of the proximal segment of an angle of the mandible fracture.

> **BOX 1.14.2   Indication for Intraoperative Maxillomandibular Fixation**
>
> - Intraoperative fixation
> - Temporary fragment stabilization in emergency case prior to definitive treatment
> - Fixation of avulsed and alveolar crest fragments
> - Use as a tension band

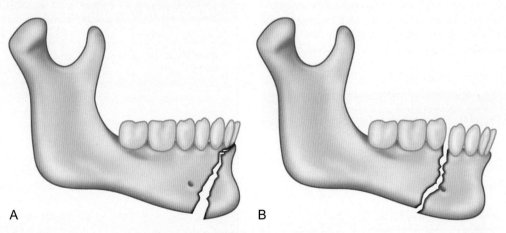

A   **B**

Fig. 1.14.13 (A) Displaced parasymphyseal mandible fracture; (B) displaced body of the mandible fracture.

SURGICAL APPROACHES/TECHNIQUES

Maxillomandibular Fixation Techniques

Reestablishing proper occlusion, stability and immobilization of fracture segments are all principles of maxillomandibular fixation (MMF).

Arch bars are typically placed two teeth proximal to the fracture, typically from first molar to first molar. 24-gauge wire is recommended for circumdental components, while 24- or 26-gauge wires are typically used for intermaxillary fixation. Adapting the arch bar to the dentition allows for the maximal arch bar to tooth contact and decreases the sag in the arch bar. One significant disadvantage of placing arch bars and circumdental wires is the increased risk of accidental skin puncture to the practitioner, increasing the chance of transmission of viral hepatitis and HIV.[28]

IMF screws can typically be applied with local anesthesia. IMF screws are self-tapping, measuring 8–12 mm in length and inserted into bone in a transmucosal fashion. A scalpel can also be used to incise gingiva prior to placement of the IMF screw. In addition, pilot holes can be drilled to facilitate placement of IMF screws. Root apices and the mental foramen should be closely observed to avoid placement of IMF screws in these locations resulting in iatrogenic injury. IMF is then achieved using 24-gauge wire. Advantages of IMF screws is the ease of their application, decreased risk of transmission of viral hepatitis or HIV, avoidance of damage to the attached gingiva and decreased surgical time, which leads to an overall decrease in cost. Screws can be retrieved under local anesthesia, however, mucosa will usually grow over the screws requiring an incision and minimal dissection to locate the screws. The absence of a tension band effect, which can be obtained with arch bars, is one of the disadvantages of IMF screws. Another disadvantage of IMF screws is the possibility of interference with the placement of plates during open reduction internal fixation.[29]

Similar to traditional arch bars, hybrid systems are measured and cut to the length of the patient's jaws. Hybrid system screws should be observed to avoid iatrogenic encroachment on the periodontal ligament, tooth fracture or pulpal injury. The hybrid system is typically fixated using 6 mm screws in attempts to decrease iatrogenic injury to the dentition. An advantage of the hybrid system would be in patients with severe periodontal disease where placement of traditional arch bars is not possible. Time efficiency compared to the applications of traditional arch bars is a significant advantage of the hybrid system. Mucosal overgrowth along with the potential for the loosening of fixation screws are drawbacks of the hybrid system.[30]

Symphysis and Parasymphysis

Approach

In most cases, fractures of the anterior mandible are easily accessible via intraoral incisions. A local anesthetic with vasoconstrictors is used to infiltrate the mucosa in the area of the mandibular pathology. A curvilinear incision is made with the lip retracted, perpendicular to mucosa. Approximately 1 cm of attached mucosa should be left to decrease the risk of recession across the anterior teeth. The mentalis muscle is incised perpendicular to bone, ensuring that a flap of muscle is attached for closure. A subperiosteal dissection is carried posteriorly to the mental neurovascular bundle, which is usually identified below the second premolar between the inferior border of the mandible and the alveolar ridge. Once the fracture is identified and reduced, the remaining pedicle of the mentalis muscle is reapproximated, followed by mucosal closure. A supportive adhesive bandage may then be applied to the skin to decrease the risk of a chin droop or "witch's chin" deformity than can occur with mentalis laxity.

Technique

Symphyseal and parasymphysis fractures can be managed in three ways. For simple nondisplaced fractures, closed reduction with arch bars with maxillomandibular fixation alone can be utilized to reestablish and maintain premorbid occlusion (Fig. 1.14.14). Fractures can be opened, reduced, and fixated with one of two techniques: (1) plate and screw fixation (Fig. 1.14.15) or (2) lag screws (Fig. 1.14.16). Two miniplates can be used across the Champy lines of tension or a single bone plate at the inferior border of the mandible with an arch bar serving as the tension band (Fig. 1.14.17). Reduction forceps at the superior or inferior border can be used to aid in the reduction of difficult fractures prior to plating (Fig. 1.14.18).

Body and Angle

Approach

Angle and body fractures may be managed via an intraoral approach or with a transbuccal trochar system. Local anesthetics with vasoconstrictors are administered to the areas followed by a perpendicular incision through mucosa. Once through mucosa the remaining soft tissue is incised perpendicular to bone. Similar to the approach to the anterior mandible, approximately 5–10 mm of mucosa away from the mucogingival junction should remain to aid in closure. The most proximal portion of the incision should not extend past the occlusal plane, avoiding violation of the buccal fat pad. Visualization and angling of instrumentation can be difficult when attempting to access fractures via an intraoral approach, resulting in inadequate visualization of complete fracture anatomy and subsequent inappropriate fixation. In these situations, a percutaneous transbuccal trochar affords a conduit by which to allow the perpendicular introduction of drills and screws during surgical fixation.[31]

When the intraoral and transbuccal approaches do not allow for sufficient visualization and reduction of fractures of the angle and body, the Risdon approach can be utilized. Risdon first described the submandibular approach in 1934, with a skin incision 2 cm below the angle of the mandible, 4–5 cm in length. The skin incision should be made in a skin crease to hide the scar. Following incision through the dermis, subcutaneous fat and superficial fascia are dissected to reach the platysma muscle, which is sharply dissected to reach the superficial layer of the deep cervical fascia. Care must be taken to avoid injury to the marginal mandibular nerve.[31,32] Dingman and Grabb discussed the course of the marginal mandibular branch of the facial nerve finding that the nerve passed above the inferior border of the mandible proximal to the antegonial notch 81% of the time. The nerve took a downward course in 19% of the patients, with the lowest being 1 cm below the inferior border.[33] Dissection is carried through the deep cervical fascia to bone, using a nerve stimulator to determine the location of the marginal mandibular branch. Once down to the inferior border of the mandible, the submandibular gland and capsule is often encountered with the possibility of observing the lower pole of the parotid gland. Once the masseter is seen and the pterygomasseteric sling is located, it is sharply divided at the inferior border to expose the mandible, all the while carefully retracting the nerve fibers superiorly. Periosteum, nerve and muscle are retracted superiorly aiding in the visualization of the fracture site. The facial vessels may need to be ligated if the vessels are not easily mobilized out of the surgical field. Dissecting the stylomandibular ligament and medial pterygoid from the inferior and posterior borders of the mandible may aid in the closure and increase the visibility of the fracture and surgical field.

Technique

Body and angle fractures of the mandible are often difficult to manage due to adjacent structures. For open treatment, both rigid and nonrigid

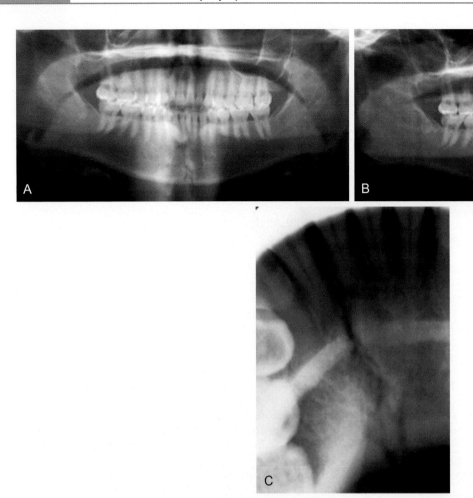

Fig. 1.14.14 Case 1: Symphyseal fracture. 32 y.o. male s/p MVC. (A) Initial panorex illustrating nondisplaced symphyseal fracture. (B) Management via closed reduction and IMF via arch bars with transition to heavy elastics after 2 weeks. (C) Occlusal view following closed reduction and IMF.

fixation stratagems are utilized. If rigid fixation is chosen, plate and screw fixation with a 2-plate technique is most commonly employed (Figs. 1.14.19 and 1.14.20). One miniplate with monocortical screws at the superior border and one miniplate with bicortical screws at the inferior border of the mandible are placed (Figs. 1.14.21 and 1.14.22). Additionally, a rigid plate can be placed at the inferior border with circumdental wires serving as a tension band (Fig. 1.14.23). Great care must be taken to avoid the inferior alveolar, mental nerve, and tooth roots.[34–39]

Nonrigid fixation via Champy technique is most commonly employed in fractures of the angle. This approach allows for micromotion between segments and promotes secondary bone healing through an intermediate phase of callous formation prior to ossification. Due to the conservative dissection with less tissue stretching and periosteal stripping, the use of Champy plates has shown a decrease in operative time and less postoperative discomfort while resulting in equivalent rates of bony union. Miniplate osteosynthesis of Champy technique can be performed intraorally with a single plate to the lateral body of the angle of the mandible. An incision is made through mucosa down to bone to access the fracture. The miniplate is typically placed on the oblique ridge with the application of monocortical screws. With the placement of monocortical fixation, the roots of the teeth are avoided.[34,35,40,41]

Evidence-Based Medicine: Is One Technique Superior to the Other for Angles?

Ellis compared the two techniques and emphasized the superiority of a Champy plate in the treatment of angle fractures, while utilizing a 2-plate technique increased the rate of infection. Mehra and Haitham showed that using fewer plates resulted in less periosteal stripping, causing less disruption to the blood supply. In a study by Boulox, Chen, and Threadgill, it was found that the use of a small 2.0 mm titanium plate with monocortical screws for nonrigid fixation was as effective as the use of a large 2.3–2.7 mm plate with bicortical screws. Ellis and Walker advocate the use of a single noncompression Champy miniplate as a consistently reliable technique for the treatment of an angle fracture. Eighty-one patients were treated, no patients were placed into MMF postoperatively, and all were allowed to return to function immediately.[34,40–43]

Although multiple studies have advocated for the use of the Champy plate technique, it is important that the clinician adequately consider their patient population. Factors such as smoking, substance abuse, and metabolic comorbidities may all affect the postoperative course and as such the choice of fixation technique. Ultimately, the surgical approach and plating technique is at the discretion of the operating clinician.

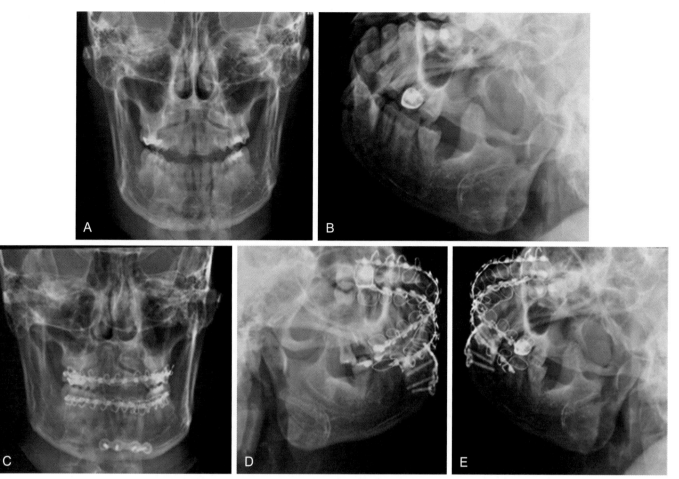

Fig. 1.14.15 Case 2: Parasymphyseal fracture. 45 y.o. male s/p assault. (A–B) Initial AP and lateral oblique plain films illustrating left parasymphyseal fracture. (C–E) Management via ORIF with inferior border plate/ screw fixation and arch bars as a tension band.

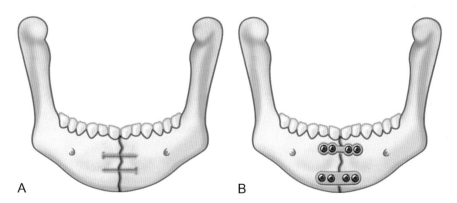

Fig. 1.14.16 (A) Lag screws to the symphysis of the mandible. (B) Two plates to the symphysis of the mandible.

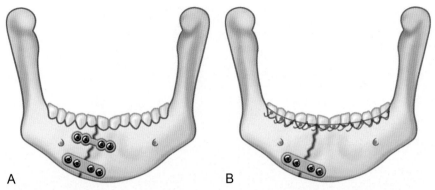

Fig. 1.14.17 (A) Internal fixation with two plates to the parasymphysis of the mandible. (B) Internal fixation with one bone plate to the inferior border with arch bar as tension band to the parasymphysis of the mandible.

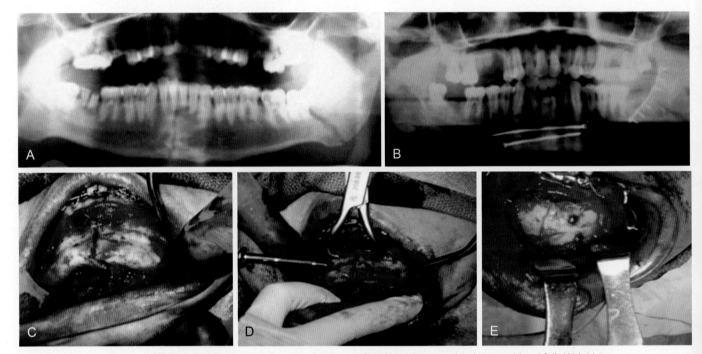

Fig. 1.14.18 Case 3: Symphyseal fracture: lag screw fixation. 55 y.o. male s/p ground level fall. (A) Initial panorex illustrating nondisplaced symphyseal fracture. (B) Management via lag screw fixation. (C) Gingivobuccal surgical exposure of symphyseal fracture. (D) Open reduction of fracture fragments. (E) Following lag screw fixation.

Evidence-Based Medicine: Extraction or Retention of the Tooth in the Line of Fracture?

In a study by Ellis, studying 402 patients with fractures in the angle of the mandible, teeth in the line of fracture were removed in 75% of cases. Postoperative complications occurred in 19.5% when the tooth was retained and 19% when the tooth was removed. Additionally, postoperative infection occurred in 19.1% with retained teeth in the line of fracture and 15.8% when teeth in the line of fracture were extracted. Ellis showed no statistically significant difference in complications, whether teeth in the line of fracture were extracted or retained. This is in accord with the findings of other smaller case series to answer the same question.[44]

There are many other factors (such as patient cooperation and oral hygiene) to consider in the decision to remove teeth in the line of fracture. The location of fracture is important in determining the decision to remove teeth (Box 1.14.3). Fractures of the angle of the mandible

> **BOX 1.14.3   Indications for Removal of Teeth in the Line of Fracture**
>
> - Gross mobility
> - Periapical pathology
> - Significant periodontal disease
> - Fractured roots
> - Partially erupted 3rd molars with pericoronitis or associated cyst

are more prone to infection than any other mandible fracture. On occasion a tooth in the line of fracture can make reduction easier or more difficult if the tooth is displaced. If the tooth needs to be removed, removal may often be delayed until internal fixation has been achieved, however, care should be taken when removing the tooth at this point as the fracture can become displaced upon attempted removal. The

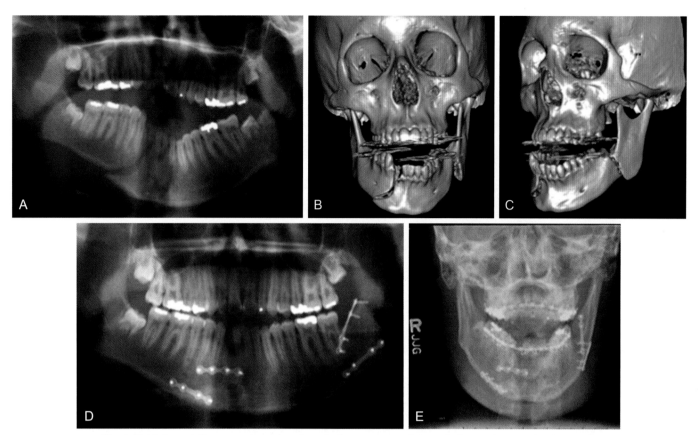

Fig. 1.14.19 Case 4: Parasymphyseal and angle fracture: two plate technique. 18 y.o. male s/p assault. (A) Initial panorex illustrating displaced right parasymphyseal and left angle fracture. (B–C) 3D reformatted CT showing the injury complex. (D) Panorex following ORIF with two plate/screw fixation at both the parasymphysis and angle. (E) PA mandible film following ORIF.

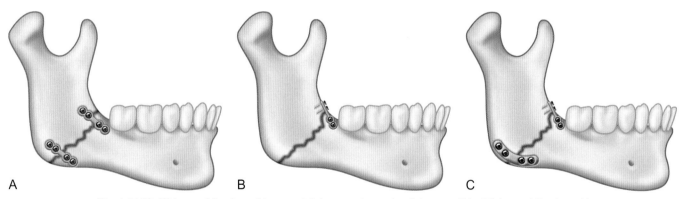

Fig. 1.14.20 (A) Internal fixation with two miniplates to the angle of the mandible. (B) Internal fixation with Champy plate to the angle of the mandible. (C) Internal fixation with one miniplate and one bone plate to the angle of the mandible.

condition of teeth left in the line of fracture should be monitored postoperatively. Kahnberg and Ridell studied 185 teeth left in the line of fractures. Using clinical and radiographic findings, 59% of patients recovered without complications.[45,46]

Comminuted Fractures

Comminuted fractures of the mandible have been treated with numerous methods, including closed reduction and MMF, external pin fixation and open reduction and internal fixation. The treatment of these fractures remains controversial due to the theory that the blood supply to these segments is periosteal and risks circulatory compromise with excessive soft tissue stripping or manipulation resulting in sequestration and infection. Due to the complexity of comminuted fractures, with telescoped segments in three dimensions, causing widening in the mediolateral direction along with collapse of the anteroposterior dimensions, open reduction with internal fixation is often utilized. With a large displacement of segments, resulting in facial distortion, comminuted mandible fractures should be reconstructed to restore pretraumatic dimensions and orientation of the facial skeleton along with proper facial symmetry and proportion. Restoration of these facial proportions is often difficult to achieve with closed reduction alone. Although proper occlusion may be obtained via MMF, rotation of mandibular fragments often occurs and these bony segments are rarely reduced in to proper anatomical reduction, with the risk of causing facial widening. In these cases, reconstruction plates are used to span the area of comminution and restore the facial form and continuity of the mandible during the phases of scarring and healing (Fig. 1.14.24). Plate application can prevent facial collapse and retains the projection of the mandible if

secondary bone grafting is needed. Segments of comminution can be treated as free bone grafts and fixated to the reconstruction plate with locking screws, or stabilized with wires or miniplates.[47,48]

Comminuted mandible fractures may be associated with soft tissue defects both intra- and extraorally. In these cases MMF or an external fixator device are often utilized as the index method of fracture fixation. For moderate intraoral soft tissue defects, complex closure with buccal myomucosal flaps may allow for tenable coverage following debridement of macerated or nonviable mucosa. The larger the defect to be spanned via this method, the shallower the resulting buccal vestibule, which can create difficulties for long-term dental restoration. For large intraoral defects, free tissue transfer with one of a myriad of fasciocutaneous flap options may be required. For moderate extraoral soft tissue deficiencies, local tissue rearrangement with rotational or advancement flaps may similarly be necessary. For those patients with large extraoral soft tissue defects, free tissue transfer to provide tension-free viable coverage should be considered.

POSTOPERATIVE COURSE

For long-term success of any treatment of a mandible fracture, the postoperative management is imperative. Follow-up appointments are extremely important to reinforce proper diet, and progression of function. All methods of internal fixation should have a goal of early restoration of full function, including diet, speech and airway.

Soft Diet

Placing patients on a soft diet serves to reduce fracture motion and reduce the bite force. A soft diet is recommended for approximately 4 weeks postoperatively. It is important to avoid full masticatory function throughout this time. Supplemental liquid nutrition is of importance in patients who will be placed in MMF for an extended period of time.

Postoperative IMF: Wire vs. Elastics

MMF serves to restore premorbid occlusion, provides stability and aids in reduction. There is much debate in the literature as to the benefit of continued MMF following internal fixation. Many clinicians believe that postoperative MMF can be beneficial, especially in cases with multiple fractures. Advantages of postoperative MMF include decreased mobility during callous formation, promotion of oral mucosal epithelial seal, and occlusal stability, especially in the setting of nonrigid fixation. In addition, continuing MMF for a short interval postoperatively, 1–2 weeks, serves as a reinforced tension band. Once released from MMF, patients can be transitioned to guiding elastics. Guiding elastics can be

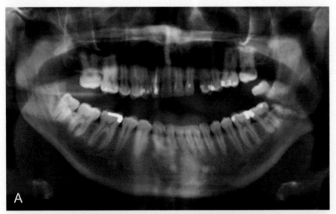

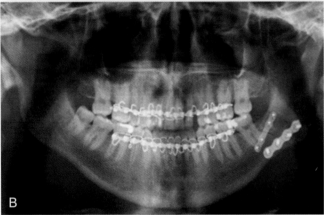

Fig. 1.14.21 Case 5: Angle fracture: two plate technique. 24 y.o. M s/p assault. (A) Initial panorex illustrating displaced left angle fracture through mesial root of left third molar. (B) Management via extraction of left third molar in the line of fracture, followed by two plate fixation (1.5 mm profile inferior border, 1.0 mm profile superior-oblique tension band).

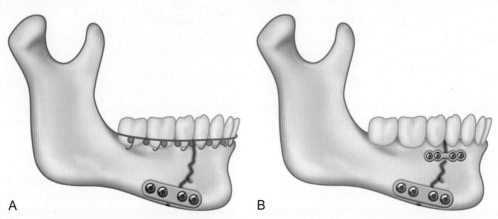

Fig. 1.14.22 (A) Internal fixation with one bone plate to the inferior border with arch bar as tension band to the body of the mandible. (B) Internal fixation with two plates to the body of the mandible.

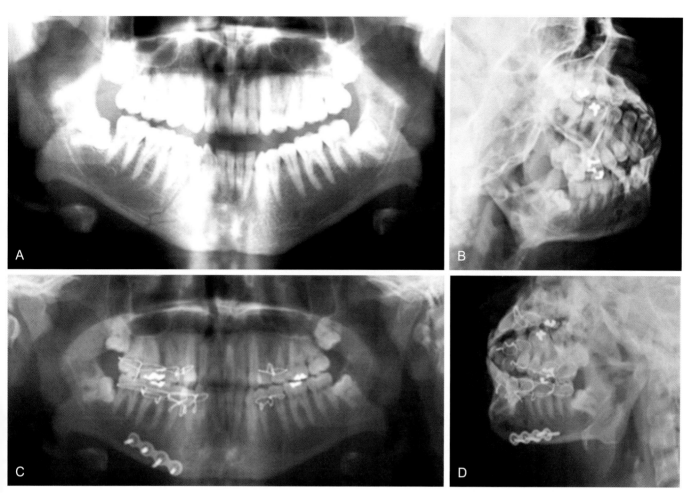

Fig. 1.14.23 Case 6: Body fracture. 45 y.o. male s/p assault. (A–B) Initial panorex and lateral oblique plain film illustrating right oblique body fracture. (C–D) Management via ORIF with inferior border plate/screw fixation and circumdental wires as a tension band.

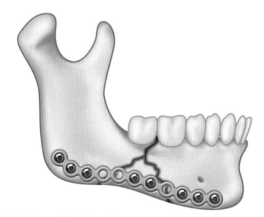

Fig. 1.14.24 Internal fixation with reconstruction plate to the comminuted body of the mandible.

utilized if there is a discrepancy in occlusion and serve to functionally train a patient into the proper occlusion. With comminuted fractures, MMF will aid in the reestablishment of the occlusion and ensure that occlusal forces do not disturb the open repair and reconstruction of the mandible. Retained MMF can also prove beneficial in the presence of concomitant alveolar fractures, aiding in stability and undisturbed bony healing. Increased gingival trauma, inadequate oral hygiene and

delay in the mobility of the temporomandibular joint are disadvantages of continued MMF. The duration and utilization of postoperative MMF is at the discretion of the clinician. If employed postoperatively, the current trend amongst surgeons has been to limit the amount of time in MMF compared to traditional mantra, with most using wire MMF for no longer than 2 weeks with a rapid transition to elastics or free swing. Despite these trends, there is no high-level evidence supporting the utilization of MMF postoperatively in patients who have undergone rigid or nonrigid internal fixation.[49,50]

Antibiotics

There are no current standards for the prescription and administration of antibiotics in the pre-, peri-, and postoperative settings regarding the management of mandible fractures. Furthermore practice patterns amongst surgeons who treat mandibular pathology are vastly variable and largely undocumented in the surgical literature. With a paucity of high-level evidence-based medicine and expert consensus, the management of antibiotics in the setting of fractures of the craniofacial skeleton, and more specifically the mandible, remains an area of significant controversy.

Despite this, it has become clear that the overall trend in the administration of antibiotics across pre-, peri-, and postoperative intervals is one of "less is more." In a prospective, randomized, double-blind trial of 30 patients, Abubaker and Rollert concluded that the use of postoperative oral antibiotics in uncomplicated fractures of the mandible had no benefit in reducing the incidence of infections.[28]

In one of the larger reviews of the literature to date, Mundinger et al. sought to compare evidence-based recommendations regarding antibiotic prophylaxis in facial fracture management with expert-based practice. A systematic review of 44 relevant studies in the literature was performed and studies were divided by facial thirds. As previously referenced, overall, studies were found to be of poor quality thus precluding formal statistical analysis. The percentages of prescribers administering pre-, peri-, and postoperative antibiotics in fractures of the mandible were 68.8%, 94.1%, and 64.7%, respectively. Despite the significant proportion of practitioners still prescribing postoperative antibiotics, no evidence to support the validity of such practices exists in the scientific literature. Though conclusions were limited, there seemed to be a consensus that pre- and peri- but not postoperative antibiotic use is recommended for comminuted mandible fractures, specifically.[51]

The utility of prophylactic antibiosis in the pre- and perioperative settings for noncomminuted fractures of the mandible based on anatomic subunit remains controversial and inadequately studied.[52,53] What is clear, however, is that higher-level studies are required to better guide practice patterns in the administration of antibiotics for fractures of the craniofacial skeleton and of the mandible.

COMPLICATIONS

Complications following treatment of mandibular fractures are not common. There are numerous factors affecting the rate of complications in the management of mandible fractures: teeth in the line of fracture, socioeconomic status, compromised metabolism, substance abuse, and the level of patient compliance. With the mandible being the only mobile bone in the facial region, with less support and blood supply than the maxilla, there is an increase in unstable fractures, and therefore an increase in complications. Studies have found a relationship between the severity of the mandibular fracture and the rate of associated complications.[32,54]

Acute Complications
Infection

The presence of oral flora is a unique risk factor for complications in the management of mandible fractures. Direct wound contamination can occur from any surgical intervention. An acute infection typically requires incision and drainage, in addition to immobilization of the fractures with MMF and extraction of any involved teeth. Fracture segments should be debrided of sequestrum, reapproximated, and rigid fixation placed. Depending on the extent of the infection a simple passive rubber drain can be left postoperatively. The most common organisms found in mandible fractures are *Staphylococcus*, *Streptococcus*, *Klebsiella*, and *Actinomyces*. Infections occurring within the first 2 weeks (early infections) are typically due to soft tissue problems and as long as the hardware is stable can be treated by drainage. If loose hardware is present, it should be replaced. Infections occurring after 2 weeks are more likely associated with dental pathology or inadequate fixation, requiring replacement of hardware with a larger plate for fixation. Empiric antibiosis in conjunction with surgical management should cover commensurate oral and skin flora. All wounds should be cultured, and choice of antibiotic tailored to subsequent sensitivities.[55,56]

Plate Exposure

Hardware exposure following internal fixation can be indicative of ischemia, infection, excess tension in the closure of the overlying soft tissues, or infection of the hardware itself. In the author's experience, this may particularly be the case in tobacco abusers, and the patient should be counseled to quit smoking preoperatively whenever feasible. An acute exposure is most commonly due to the soft tissue factors outlined above. In this setting, management may include prompt washout, inspection of hardware, debridement of any nonviable tissue, and reapproximation. Hardware salvage of this type is only indicated in a compliant patient population, when plates and screws are not loose, when the plate exposure interval has been minimal and there is no evidence of gross infection. When one of more of the latter is present, removal of the exposed hardware is necessary. If the bony segments are stable following hardware removal, additional intervention may not be necessary, and the soft tissues are managed as discussed. If removal is required during the bone healing/consolidation phase, then washout followed by placement of a new reconstruction plate or application of an external fixator may be required. If overlying soft tissues cannot be adequately debrided and closed in a tension-free manner, local flap/tissue transfer may be required to attain durable soft tissue coverage.

Long-Term Complications
Malunion

Although bony union is present in a malunion, it is in an abnormal orientation with unsatisfactory reduction. A finding of malunion may be secondary to improper MMF prior to final rigid fixation, or fractures with delayed presentation and no treatment. Treatment malunion requires an opening osteotomy at the previous fracture site, repositioning and reestablishing of proper premorbid occlusion followed by rigid fixation.

Nonunion

A nonunion occurs when there is a lack of osseous union between two or more fractured segments following the usual healing and consolidation interval. The incidence of nonunion following treatment of a mandible fracture is dependent upon the type of fixation utilized: 0.1%–2.4% following closed reduction and MMF, 0.7%–4.5% following interosseous wiring, and 0.9%–3.9% following rigid plate fixation. Although infection is the most common cause of a nonunion, there are many other factors that may contribute, including decreased mobility, patient noncompliance, inadequate reduction, alcoholism, nutritional deficiency, lack of stability, severity of the injury, as well as metabolic deficiencies. The management of clinical nonunion requires open technique, removal of interpositional sequestrum if present, anatomic reduction of fracture fragments, and application of a reconstruction bar to achieve rigid fixation with or without immediate or delayed bone grafting (Fig. 1.14.25).[57,58]

Osteomyelitis

Osteomyelitis can be defined as an inflammation of the bone marrow with a tendency to progress, often involving periosteal tissues and adjacent cortical plates. Patients often present with pain, fever, malaise, trismus, swelling and erythema of overlying tissues, fistulas, paresthesia of the inferior alveolar nerve, and adenopathy. The incidence of osteomyelitis in the mandible tends to be higher due to the poorly vascularized, dense cortical plate of the mandible and the primary source of blood supply arising from the inferior alveolar neurovascular bundle. Infections are often of mixed species with the primary pathogens being streptococci, *Bacteroides* and peptostreptococci. Although a definitive antimicrobial therapy should be decided after final culture and sensitivities are known, treatment of osteomyelitis usually consists of dual-drug therapy of penicillin and metronidazole or single-drug therapy with clindamycin. Antibiotic therapy alone is rarely curative, therefore surgical intervention and sequestrectomy is utilized. Necrotic bone or poorly vascularized bony sequestra should be debrided to promote blood flow. Clinical judgment is paramount when determining the

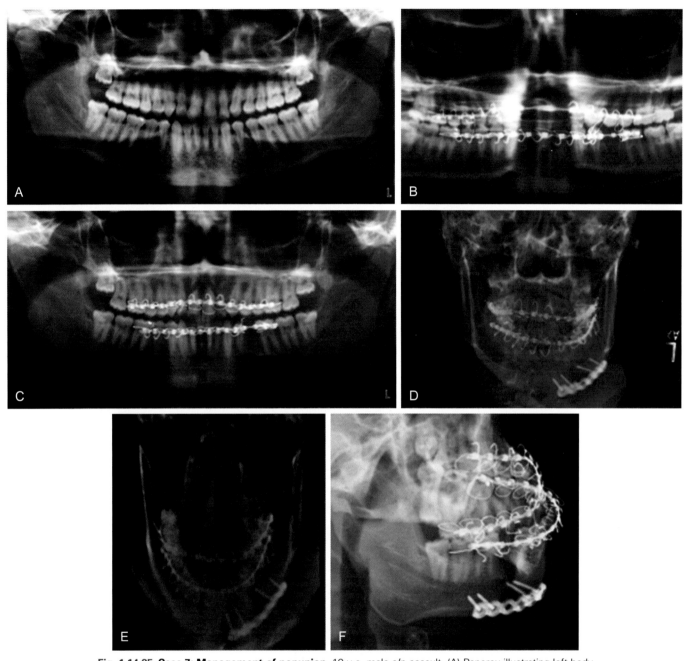

Fig. 1.14.25 **Case 7: Management of nonunion**. 19 y.o. male s/p assault. (A) Panorex illustrating left body fracture (B) treated with closed reduction, initial arch bar fixation, and plan for ORIF. Patient was noncompliant and lost to follow-up. (C) Panorex showing symptomatic nonunion of left body. (D–F) Postoperative films following management with application of a reconstruction plate and maintenance of arch bars as a tension band.

extent of bone that should be removed, which is usually determined once well-vascularized bone is encountered. Patients will commonly need to be placed in MMF in addition to the placement and/or exchange of rigid fixation. Osteomyelitis requires 6 weeks of systemic antibiotics with a peripherally inserted central catheter.[59–61]

Increased Facial Width

Facial widening can occur if the rigid fixation in a mandible is incorrectly placed. The fracture pattern of a concomitant symphysis and condylar fracture is most commonly associated with facial widening. Muscle pull from the suprahyoid and tongue in a symphysis fracture may result in the lingual tipping of the buccal segments and lateral flaring of the gonial angles (Fig. 1.14.26). Although the buccal cortex of a symphysis fracture may remain intact, the lingual cortex is separated. Overtightening of the maxillomandibular fixation wires and bilateral subcondylar fractures may also result in flaring. Some authors have suggested that symmetric medialized pressure to the gonial angles during reduction and fixation can decrease the chance of facial widening.[43,62]

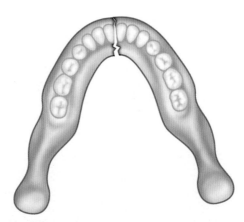

Fig. 1.14.26 Symphyseal fracture with flaring at the gonial angles causing facial widening.

EXPERT COMMENTARY

This detailed and thorough chapter by authors with ideal multiple specialty training combines dental/oral surgical expertise with plastic surgery approaches to produce a comprehensive multispecialty approach to injuries of one of the most challenging facial bones. My own knowledge and skill in mandible fracture treatment was improved by CT evaluation of each fracture in multiple planes, so that I knew the precise path and fragments involved in the injury. Painfully, I studied occlusion, dental anatomy, and made models of each patient, learning from each patient about the varied patterns of the ways the teeth fit together. These models helped me determine a plan and to evaluate results in each case, and served as a record of the injury, which more than occasionally were facts to convince patients of what findings were present after the injury and not the result of treatment. Learning to apply Erich arch bars skillfully and rapidly, tight enough to stabilize the fracture, but not overtight so as to adversely rotate the fracture segments lingually or palatally requires skill and experience, and can be mastered only with frequent episodes of learning. I prefer joining the little pieces of the fracture to the big pieces, using small fixation devices, then adjusting the big pieces, trying to align both the external and internal cortices of the mandible to guard against rotation, splaying or opening of the lingual aspect of the fracture. Remember the advice of Edward Ellis with symphysis/parasymphysis fractures to watch for the gap in the anterior cortex as the posterior (lingual) cortex is approximated as a sign of proper reduction, and remember that more complicated and multiple fractures may require larger and longer plates to guarantee the proper shape of the mandible in reconstruction. Widening and rotation for mandibular fragments may not be prevented by small plates which have no ability to shape the dimensions of the mandibular arch. Beware extension of floor of mouth lacerations accompanying anterior mandibular fractures toward the pharynx,

which communicate with the deep spaces of the neck and can easily lead to severe deep neck infections. These should be cleansed, closed, and the deep spaces drained. Replacement of comminuted devitalized bone fragments, while often successful, has a high (40%) rate of infection, and early debridement/removal should be pursued when infection occurs. The aggressive advice of Brian Alpert to further stabilize the infected mandible fracture with larger more stable plates and considering immediate bone grafting in the face of infection seems initially not to be logical, but has been successful if stabilization, washout, antibiotics, and large plate stabilization are pursued, and should at least be considered. Finally, take the patient out of occlusion and look at the angulation of the teeth and the shape and dimensions of the dental arch after achieving the first screw of the open reduction. Adjustments are easily and predictably made at this time.

Hygiene is important, and I do not hesitate to take the patient with complicated fractures back to the operating room or to the dental clinic for hygiene maneuvers for a "wash out" to clean the teeth, irrigate the oral and nasal mucous membranes and brush the teeth, removing the IMF wires, ranging the mandible, checking the occlusion and making certain that wires are tight, arch bars stable, replacing loose or broken wires, achieving hygiene and confirming that laceration repair and incision closure are optimal, and that incisions remain water tight and that plates are not exposed. Postoperative films can confirm mandibular reduction. Finally, begin function of the patient with arch bars in place, so that they can be used to subtly adjust position of the teeth and guide initial motion with light training elastics. Check the patient frequently once/twice a week, upon discharge, so that hygiene is confirmed, and problems can be detected and managed while they are reversible.

 Evidence-based medicine (EBM) content available in Appendix 1 (online only)

REFERENCES

1. Hippocrates. *Oeuvres Completes (English Translation by Withnington).* Cambridge: Cambridge University Press; 1928.
2. Gahhos F, Ariyan S. Facial fractures: Hippocratic management. *Head Neck Surg.* 1984;6(6):1007–1013.
3. Barton JR. A systematic bandage for fractures of the lower jaw. *Am Med Recorder Phila.* 1819;2:153.
4. Parkhill C. A new apparatus for the treatment of fractures o the inferior maxilla. *JAMA.* 1894;23:467.
5. Covey EM. The interdental splint. *Richmond Med J.* 1866;1:81.
6. Fraser-Moodie W. Gunning and his splint. *Br J Oral Surg.* 1869;7:112.
7. Gunning TB. Treatment of fractures of the lower jaw by interdental splints. *Br J Dent Sci.* 1866;9:481.
8. Romm S. Thomas Brian Gunning and his splint. *Plast Reconstr Surg.* 1986;78(2):252–258.
9. Moon H. Mechanical appliances for treatment of fracture of the jaws. *Br J Dent Sci.* 1874;17:303.
10. Salicetti G. Cirurgia. 1275.
11. Gilmer TL. Fractures of the inferior maxilla. 1881-1882;2:14,57,112.
12. Dorrance GM. The history of treatment of fractured jaws; 1941. Washington, DC.
13. Adi M, Ogden GR, Chisholm DM. An analysis of mandibular fractures in Dundee, Scotland (1977 to 1985). *Br J Oral Maxillofac Surg.* 1990;28(3):194–199.
14. Telfer MR, Jones GM, Shepherd JP. Trends in the aetiology of maxillofacial fractures in the United Kingdom (1977–1987). *Br J Oral Maxillofac Surg.* 1991;29(4):250–255.

15. Chrcanovic BR, Abreu MH, Freire-Maia B, Souza LN. 1,454 mandibular fractures: a 3-year study in a hospital in Belo Horizonte, Brazil. *J Craniomaxillofac Surg.* 2012;40(2):116–123.

16. Greenstein G, Cavallaro J, Romanos G, Tarnow D. Clinical recommendations for avoiding and managing surgical complications associated with implant dentistry: a review. *J Periodontol.* 2008;79(8): 1317–1329.

17. Boole JR, Holtel M, Amoroso P, Yore M. 5196 mandible fractures among 4381 active duty army soldiers, 1980 to 1998. *Laryngoscope.* 2001;111(10): 1691–1696.

18. Kapoor AK, Srivastava AB. Maxillofacial fracture: an analysis of 320 cases. In: Jacobs JR, ed. *Maxillofacial Trauma: an International Perspective.* New York: Praeger; 1983.

19. Lee KH. Interpersonal violence and facial fractures. *J Oral Maxillofac Surg.* 2009;67(9):1878–1883.

20. James RB, Fredrickson C, Kent JN. Prospective study of mandibular fractures. *J Oral Surg.* 1981;39(4):275–281.

21. Salem JE, Lilly GE, Cutcher JL, Steiner M. Analysis of 523 mandibular fractures. *Oral Surg Oral Med Oral Pathol.* 1968;26(3):390–395.

22. Sastry SM, Sastry CM, Paul BK, et al. Leading causes of facial trauma in the major trauma outcome study. *Plast Reconstr Surg.* 1995;95(1): 196–197.

23. Kruger GO. *Textbook of Oral Surgery.* 4th ed. St. Louis: Mosby; 1974.

24. Kruger E. *Oral and Maxillofacial Traumatology.* Chicago. IL: Quintessence; 1982.

25. Roth FS, Kokoska MS, Awwad EE. The identification of mandibular fractures by helical computed tomography and panorex tomography. *J Craniofac Surg.* 2005;16:394.

26. Johnson DH Jr. CT of maxillofacial trauma. *Radiol Clin North Am.* 1984;22(1):131–144.

27. Champy M, Lodde JP, Schmitt R, et al. Mandibular osteosynthesis by miniature screwed plates via a buccal approach. *J Maxillofac Surg.* 1978;6(1):14–21.

28. Abubaker AO, Rollert MK. Postoperative antibiotic prophylaxis in mandibular fractures: a preliminary randomized, double-blind, and placebo-controlled clinical study. *J Oral Maxillofac Surg.* 2001;59(12):1415–1419.

29. West GH, Griggs JA, Chandran R, et al. Treatment outcomes with the use of maxillomandibular fixation screws in the management of mandible fractures. *J Oral Maxillofac Surg.* 2014;72(1):112–120.

30. Park KN, Oh SM, Lee CY, et al. Design and application of hybrid maxillomandibular fixation for facial bone fractures. *J Craniofac Surg.* 2013;24(5):1801–1805.

31. Kale TP, Baliga SD, Ahuja N, Kotrashetti SM. A comparative study between transbuccal and extra-oral approaches in treatment of mandibular fractures. *J Maxillofac Oral Surg.* 2010;9(1):9–12.

32. Furr AM, Schweinfurth JM, May WL. Factors associated with long-term complications after repair of mandibular fractures. *Laryngoscope.* 2006;116(3):427–430.

33. Dingman RO, Grabb WC. Surgical anatomy of the mandibular ramus of the facial nerve based on the dissection of 100 facial halves. *Plast Reconstr Surg Transplant Bull.* 1962;29:266–272.

34. Ellis E 3rd. A prospective study of 3 treatment methods for isolated fractures of the mandibular angle. *J Oral Maxillofac Surg.* 2010;68(11):2743–2754.

35. Ellis E 3rd. Treatment methods for fractures of the mandibular angle. *Int J Oral Maxillofac Surg.* 1999;28(4):243–252.

36. Ellis E 3rd. Treatment of mandibular angle fractures using the AO reconstruction plate. *J Oral Maxillofac Surg.* 1993;51(3):250–254, discussion 5.

37. Ellis E 3rd, Graham J. Use of a 2.0-mm locking plate/screw system for mandibular fracture surgery. *J Oral Maxillofac Surg.* 2002;60(6):642–645, discussion 5–6.

38. Ellis E 3rd, Karas N. Treatment of mandibular angle fractures using two mini dynamic compression plates. *J Oral Maxillofac Surg.* 1992;50(9): 958–963.

39. Ellis E 3rd, Walker L. Treatment of mandibular angle fractures using two noncompression miniplates. *J Oral Maxillofac Surg.* 1994;52(10): 1032–1036, discussion 6–7.

40. Ellis E 3rd, Walker LR. Treatment of mandibular angle fractures using one noncompression miniplate. *J Oral Maxillofac Surg.* 1996;54(7):864–871, discussion 71–72.

41. Potter J, Ellis E 3rd. Treatment of mandibular angle fractures with a malleable noncompression miniplate. *J Oral Maxillofac Surg.* 1999;57(3):288–292, discussion 92–93.

42. Bouloux GF, Chen S, Threadgill JM. Small and large titanium plates are equally effective for treating mandible fractures. *J Oral Maxillofac Surg.* 2012;70(7):1613–1621.

43. Mehra P, Murad H. Internal fixation of mandibular angle fractures: a comparison of 2 techniques. *J Oral Maxillofac Surg.* 2008;66(11):2254–2260.

44. Ellis E 3rd. Outcomes of patients with teeth in the line of mandibular angle fractures treated with stable internal fixation. *J Oral Maxillofac Surg.* 2002;60(8):863–865, discussion 6.

45. Kahnberg KE. Surgical extrusion of root-fractured teeth – a follow-up study of two surgical methods. *Endod Dent Traumatol.* 1988;4(2): 85–89.

46. Kahnberg KE, Ridell A. Prognosis of teeth involved in the line of mandibular fractures. *Int J Oral Surg.* 1979;8(3):163–172.

47. Smith BR, Teenier TJ. Treatment of comminuted mandibular fractures by open reduction and rigid internal fixation. *J Oral Maxillofac Surg.* 1996;54(3):328–331.

48. Dai J, Shen G, Yuan H, et al. Titanium mesh shaping and fixation for the treatment of comminuted mandibular fractures. *J Oral Maxillofac Surg.* 2016;74(2):337.e1–337.e11.

49. Pattar P, Shetty S, Degala S. A prospective study on management of mandibular angle fracture. *J Maxillofac Oral Surg.* 2014;13(4):592–598.

50. Gaspar G, Brakus I, Kovacic I. Conservative orthodontic treatment of mandibular bilateral condyle fracture. *J Craniofac Surg.* 2014;25(5):e488–e490.

51. Mundinger GS, Borsuk DE, Okhah Z, et al. Antibiotics and facial fractures: evidence-based recommendations compared with experience-based practice. *Craniomaxillofac Trauma Reconstr.* 2015;8(1):64–78.

52. Lovato C, Wagner JD. Infection rates following perioperative prophylactic antibiotics versus postoperative extended regimen prophylactic antibiotics in surgical management of mandibular fractures. *J Oral Maxillofac Surg.* 2009;67(4):827–832.

53. Strong EB, Buchalter GM, Moulthrop TH. Endoscopic repair of isolated anterior table frontal sinus fractures. *Arch Facial Plast Surg.* 2003;5(6):514–521.

54. Senel FC, Jessen GS, Melo MD, Obeid G. Infection following treatment of mandible fractures: the role of immunosuppression and polysubstance abuse. *Oral Surg Oral Med Oral Pathol Oral Radiol Endod.* 2007;103(1):38–42.

55. Brasileiro BF, Passeri LA. Epidemiological analysis of maxillofacial fractures in Brazil: a 5-year prospective study. *Oral Surg Oral Med Oral Pathol Oral Radiol Endod.* 2006;102(1):28–34.

56. Schon R, Gutwald R, Schramm A, et al. Endoscopy-assisted open treatment of condylar fractures of the mandible: extraoral vs intraoral approach. *Int J Oral Maxillofac Surg.* 2002;31(3):237–243.

57. Bochlogyros PN. Non-union of fractures of the mandible. *J Maxillofac Surg.* 1985;13(4):189–193.

58. Melmed EP, Koonin AJ. Fractures of the mandible. A review of 909 cases. *Plast Reconstr Surg.* 1975;56(3):323–327.

59. Ogasawara T, Sano K, Hatsusegawa C, et al. Pathological fracture of the mandible resulting from osteomyelitis successfully treated with only intermaxillary elastic guiding. *Int J Oral Maxillofac Surg.* 2008;37(6):581–583.

60. Quadu G, Miotti A, Rubini L. [Chronic osteomyelitis of the mandible with pathologic fracture. Case report]. *G Stomatol Ortognatodonzia.* 1983;2(3):99–100.

61. Jauhar P, Handley T, Hammersley N. A pathological fracture of the mandible due to osteomyelitis following a full dental clearance. *Dent Update.* 2016;43(2):168–170, 73, 75.

62. Wagner WF, Neal DC, Alpert B. Morbidity associated with extraoral open reduction of mandibular fractures. *J Oral Surg.* 1979;37(2):97–100.

Fractures of the Condylar Process of the Mandible

Edward Ellis III, Daniel Perez

BACKGROUND

Approximately 11%–50% of all facial fractures and 30%–40%% of all mandibular fractures (MFs) are fractures of the mandibular condyle.[1,2] Most are not caused by direct trauma, but follow indirect forces transmitted to the condyle from a blow elsewhere, usually in the body or symphysis region. They are often the result of rapid deceleration injuries such as when the chin of an unrestrained passenger in a car strikes the dashboard, the bicycle rider who lands on their chin, or a patient who falls on their face.

SURGICAL ANATOMY AND CLINICAL PRESENTATION

The four main components of the temporomandibular joint that are important when considering condylar process fractures are the condylar process itself, the glenoid fossa of the temporal bone, including the articular eminence, the intraarticular disk, and the lateral pterygoid muscle. For purposes of this chapter, it will be assumed that the glenoid fossa and temporal articulations are uninjured.

Because the lateral pterygoid muscle inserts mostly onto the pterygoid fovea of the condyle, when a fracture occurs below this level, contraction of the muscle causes the condylar fragment to be displaced anteromedially. For the same reason, condylar fractures are associated with impaired translational movement of the condyle along the articular eminence because the lateral pterygoid muscle is no longer connected to the distal portion of the mandible (Fig. 1.15.1). Although rotation can occur, lack of translation produces a characteristic deviation of the chin on opening toward the side of a unilateral condylar fracture (Fig. 1.15.2). Displacement of the condylar process produces a loss in the anatomic height of the ramus, which allows premature contact of the ipsilateral most distal tooth (Fig. 1.15.3). The point of contact acts as a fulcrum and produces a characteristic open-bite on the side opposite of a unilateral fracture (Fig. 1.15.3). Bilaterally displaced fractures of the condylar processes produce a symmetric anterior open-bite (Fig. 1.15.4).[3,4]

Some patients who sustain mandibular injury may present with pain in the joint and a malocclusion where the mandible comes forward on the side of the injury or they may not be able to bring the teeth together on that side and yet a fracture of the condylar process cannot be identified on imaging. In such instances, one should suspect a contusion/hematoma within the affected joint.

RADIOLOGICAL EVALUATION

The vast majority of condylar process fractures in adults can be identified using plain radiographs. It is important to get at least two radiographs 90° to the other. For instance, the combination of panoramic and Towne's projections offer most of what might be needed to prescribe treatment in the vast majority of patients (Fig. 1.15.5). Plain films are not as useful for pediatric condylar process fractures because the bone is less dense, the condylar neck is much shorter, and often the fractures are through the condylar head, which are not revealed well with plain films. On the other hand, if the surgeon routinely treats condylar process fractures in children closed, the need for more detailed imaging (CT) may not be warranted given the need for more radiation to do so.

The main limitation of plain radiographs is that they do not give three-dimensional details of the fracture. Computed tomography (CT) is almost universally available today and most patients will already have a scan performed by the emergency department before a surgical consultation is made. CT gives extremely good detail of the position of the fracture(s) and the displacement of the segments. It is especially good for intraarticular fractures (Fig. 1.15.6). CT scans cannot show the position of the intraarticular disk but the need to have that information available for treatment planning purposes is a hotly debated topic (discussed later). Should one desire more information on the position of the disk, a magnetic resonance imaging (MRI) scan would be needed as this is the imaging modality that provides the best view of the disk and other soft tissues within the joint.

TERMINOLOGY

Controversy exists with respect to terminology and classification of condylar process fractures. Practitioners in Europe and North America may refer to the same entity with different words. For the purpose of this chapter and to clarify the vocabulary, it is important to make a distinction between the following terms:

Displacement. Displacement refers to the relationship of the fractured ends of the bones to one another. Often arbitrarily broken down into mild, moderate and severe displacement, it can be used for fractures throughout the skeleton whereas "dislocation" and "luxation" (see below) can be used only for fractures that involve a joint. The amount of displacement and its direction can be quantified by measuring the angle the condylar process makes with the ramus of the mandible in both the sagittal and coronal planes (Fig. 1.15.5). A fracture that is displaced 90 degrees medially is one that is also dislocated because the articular surfaces will no longer have much contact. The relationship of the fractured ends can be further classified as those with medial and those with lateral override (displacement) of the segments (Fig. 1.15.7).

Dislocation (aka Luxation). Dislocation refers to the lack of relationship of the articular surfaces to one another. It usually indicates that the articulating surface of the mandibular condyle is mostly not contacting the articulating surface of the glenoid fossa (Fig. 1.15.8). To be dislocated, the fracture would have to be severely displaced (see above).

Subluxation. Sometimes the term subluxation is used to describe a partial separation of the articular surfaces but the condyle is not completely dislodged outside of the glenoid fossa. The difference between subluxation and dislocation (and luxation) is a matter of degree in that the articulating surfaces are not contacting.

Diacapitular (fractures). This is another European term that is used when the fracture line starts at the articular surface, goes through the head of the condyle and may extend outside the capsule. So it extends from within the capsule to outside the capsule (Fig. 1.15.9). These types of fractures are also known as *intracapsular fractures*, especially in North America. However, it has been shown that in a large number of "intracapsular" fractures, the fracture extends inferior to the capsule on the medial aspect. The name "intracapsular" therefore may be anatomically incorrect in such cases.[5]

CLASSIFICATION OF CONDYLAR PROCESS FRACTURES

There are many classification systems in the literature.[6–10] Classification systems are used for two main purposes. One is to categorize injuries so their treatment may be studied. For this purpose, the classification system must be very complete (Table 1.15.1). Unfortunately, most classification systems used to adequately classify condylar process fractures for purposes of research are complex, cumbersome, and have very little clinical usefulness. The other purpose of a classification system is to help decide between the possibilities for treatment. Such systems do not have to be as complex and the ones that are used the most today by clinicians to classify condylar process fractures are based on the level or anatomic position of the fracture(s) (i.e., head, neck, subcondylar) (Fig. 1.15.10) and the magnitude and direction of displacement of the fragments (Fig. 1.15.5).

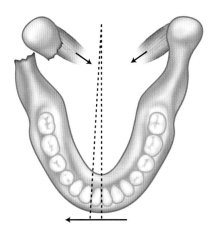

Fig. 1.15.1 Illustration showing fractured mandibular condyle on the right side. Note how the contraction of the lateral pterygoid muscle, which is attached at the pterygoid fovea of the condyle, displaces the condylar head anteromedially. This illustration also shows why the mandible deviates toward the side of a unilateral condylar fracture when a patient opens their mouth. Contraction of the lateral pterygoid muscle on the nonfractured side moves the condyle anteriorly. Because the lateral pterygoid muscle on the fractured side is no longer connected to the distal portion of the mandible, the fractured side mandible cannot move anteriorly, so the unbalanced asymmetric action of the lateral pterygoid muscle on the nonfractured side causes the mandible to deviate toward the fractured side.

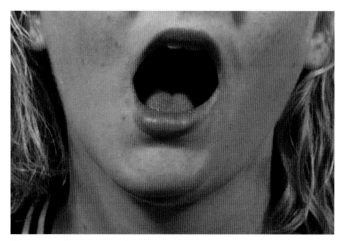

Fig. 1.15.2 Photograph of a patient with deviation to the right side when opening their mouth. This patient was treated for a right mandibular condylar process fracture and has a good occlusion but persistent deviation on opening toward the side of the fracture.

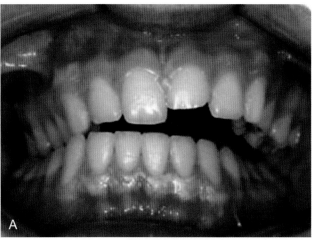

Premature contact on fractured side

Deviation of mandible toward fractured side (rt)

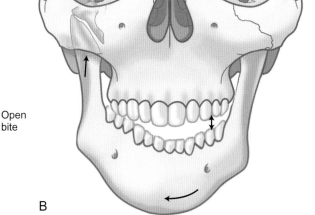

Open bite

Fig. 1.15.3 (A) Occlusion of a patient with a fresh condylar process fracture on the right. Note the premature occlusion on the right side, deviation of the mandible to the right, and a left open-bite. (B) Illustration showing how a right condylar process fracture allows the right ramus to move upward causing the premature contact of teeth on that side, deviation of the mandible to that side, and the contralateral open-bite.

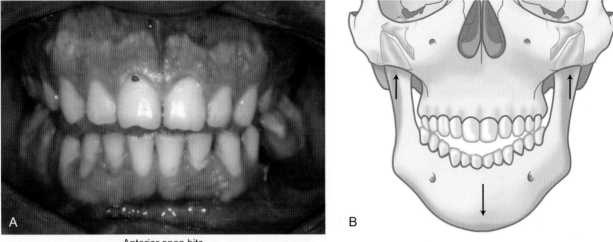

Anterior open bite

Fig. 1.15.4 (A) Occlusion of a patient with fresh bilateral condylar process fractures. Note the premature occlusion on the terminal molars and the anterior open-bite. (B) Illustration showing how bilateral condylar process fractures allow the mandibular rami to move upward, causing premature occlusion on the posterior teeth and an anterior open-bite.

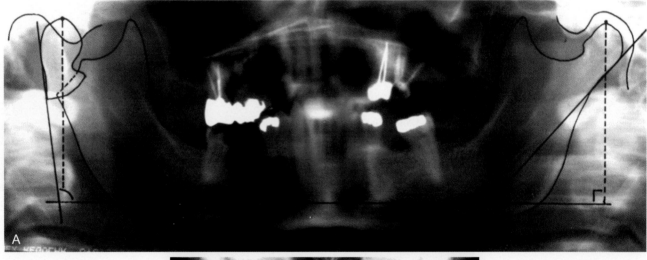

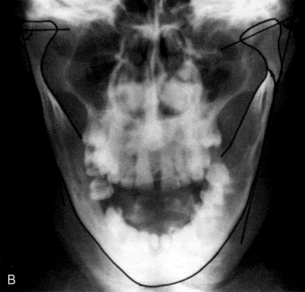

Fig. 1.15.5 Panoramic and Towne's radiographs of condylar process fractures. Note that the angle between the ramus and the condylar process can be quantified in both views.

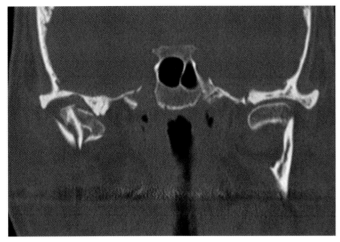

Fig. 1.15.6 CT scan of a patient with bilateral condylar process fractures. The condyle on the right is comminuted whereas the condyle on the left is luxated 90 degrees medially. Plain radiographs would not show this degree of detail.

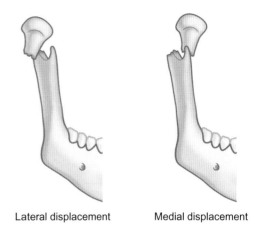

Lateral displacement   Medial displacement

Fig. 1.15.7 Illustration showing lateral and medial displacement (override) of the fractured ends of a condylar process fracture.

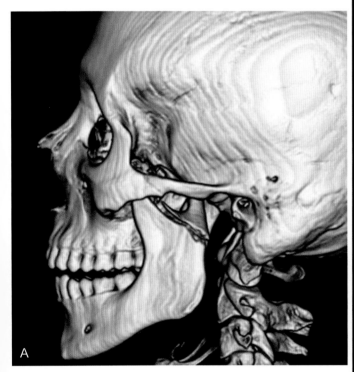

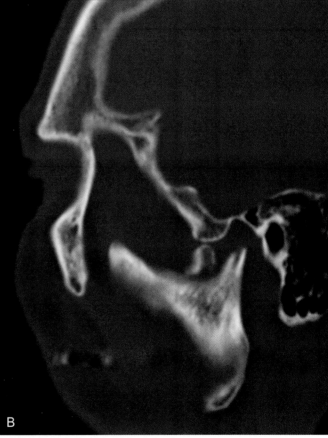

Fig. 1.15.8 CT scans of two completely dislocated condylar process fractures. Note that the articulating surface of the condyle is not in contact with the articulating surface of the glenoid fossa.

Level of the Fracture

The "level" or anatomical position of the fracture is a method of broadly classifying fractures. Although a debated issue is the exact anatomic position of the divisions, a simple method is to divide condylar process fracture into three types: condylar head, condylar neck, and subcondylar region (Fig. 1.15.10). A condylar head fracture is one at the level of the joint capsule, so the fracture is essentially intracapsular or possibly diacapitular. The neck of the condylar process is from the joint capsule above to the level of the sigmoid notch below. Anything lower than that is considered a subcondylar fracture. The main usefulness of such a classification is that it directly correlates with the possibility of placing

TABLE 1.15.1   The AO/ASIF Classification

SPECIFIC LEVEL 3 CONDYLAR PROCESS SYSTEM		SUBREGIONS			
Parameters	Code and Description	Process	Head	Neck	Base
Location	M ¼ Medial to the pole zone/P ¼ within or lateral to the pole zone		x		
Fragmentation	0 ¼ None/1 ¼ fragmented minor/2 ¼ fragmented major		x	x	x
Vertical apposition	0 ¼ Complete/1 ¼ partial/2 ¼ lost		x		
Sideward displacement	0 ¼ None/1 ¼ partial/2 ¼ full			x	x
	Direction a ¼ anterior/p ¼ posterior and m ¼ medial/l ¼ lateral			x	x
Angulation	0 ¼ None (up to 5 degrees)/1 ¼ > 5–45 degrees/2 ¼ > 45 degrees			x	x
	Direction a ¼ anterior/p ¼ posterior and m ¼ medial/l ¼ lateral			x	x
Displacement head fragment/fossa	0 ¼ No displacement/1 ¼ displacement/2 ¼ dislocation	x			
	Direction a ¼ anterior/p ¼ posterior and m ¼ medial/l¼ lateral	x			
Displacement caudal fragment/fossa	0 ¼ No displacement/1 ¼ displacement	x[a]			
	Direction a ¼ anterior/p ¼ posterior and l ¼ lateral	x[a]			
Distortion of condylar head	0 ¼ orthotopic/1 ¼ dystopic	x			
Overall loss of ramus height	0 ¼ No change of height/1 ¼ loss of height/2 ¼ increase of height	x			

[a]Only in case of neck or base fracture.
From Neff A, Cornelius CP, Rasse M, et al. The comprehensive AOCMF classification system: condylar process fractures – level 3 tutorial. Craniomaxillofac Trauma Reconstr 2014;7(Suppl 1):S44–S58.

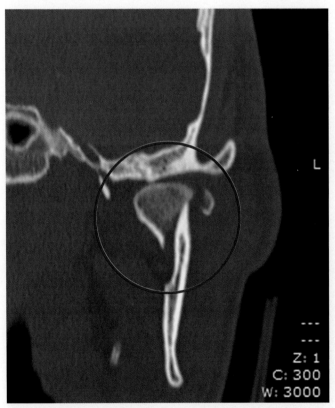

Fig. 1.15.9 CT of a diacapitular fracture. Note that the fracture line begins on the articular surface, goes through the head of the condyle and may extend outside the joint capsule on the medial side.

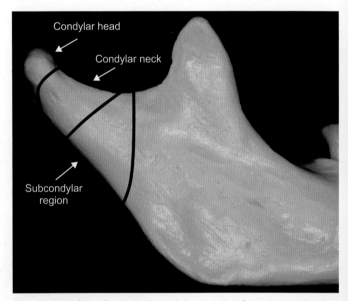

Fig. 1.15.10 Classification of condylar process fractures by location (head, neck, subcondylar).

stable bone plate osteosynthesis across the fracture. For example, most condylar neck and all subcondylar fractures are amenable to stabilization with standard 2.0 mm bone plate osteosynthesis whereas intracapsular fractures through the condylar head are often not treated open by most surgeons except those skilled in temporomandibular joint surgery.

TREATMENT OF CONDYLAR PROCESS FRACTURES

Most condylar process fractures require treatment. There are some cases, however, where observation may be indicated, for instance, a patient with a condylar process fracture that is nondisplaced or minimally displaced, but who can bring their teeth into a normal occlusion. Such patients can be placed on a soft diet and monitored. When treatment is deemed necessary, there are options that have to be considered. The main decision is whether to treat the fracture open or closed.

Deciding on Open or Closed Treatment

The age-old question is whether or not condylar fractures should be treated open or closed. This question will never be answered because it is the wrong question. What we should instead be asking is whether there are some condylar fractures that would obtain predictably better outcomes when treated open. And if that is the case, how do we identify them?

In selecting open or closed treatment, one must first understand the goals of treatment. The outcomes that are sought when treating patients with condylar fractures are the following[11]:
1. Maintenance of pretrauma occlusion
2. Pain-free function
3. Normal range of mandibular motion (interincisal opening > 40 mm, 9–12 mm lateral and protrusive excursions)
4. Maintenance of facial symmetry

If the clinician feels that closed treatment can achieve the above outcomes, it would make no sense to perform open surgery because all surgical procedures have known risks (i.e., bleeding, infection, nerve damage, facial scars, etc.). On the other hand, if the clinician feels that they can better achieve the above outcomes with open treatment than with closed treatment, then they should consider open treatment. However, they have to weigh the risks of open treatment against the potential benefits of that treatment. This is often an experiential question because some surgeons are very facile in safely performing open treatment whereas others may do so very infrequently and are not as sure of their abilities to safely do so.

The literature is not very useful in helping an individual surgeon decide about what treatment to provide an individual patient. A fair synthesis of the entire world literature on the topic of condylar fracture treatment would be: While *objective* measures of outcomes vary with the level of the fracture (head, neck, subcondylar), the amount of displacement and/or dislocation, the presence of bilateral vs. unilateral condylar fractures, and whether or not they were treated open or closed, most patients with condylar fractures have few *subjective* complaints after treatment, irrespective of the above factors. One must keep this in mind when making treatment decisions for patients who present with condylar fractures. But knowing this may not be useful in making individual treatment decisions because each fracture, patient, and surgeon is different.

There are prerequisites to *closed* treatment that are important to understand.[12]
1. The patient must have a good complement of teeth, especially posterior teeth on the side(s) of the fracture(s). Without them, there will be a significant loss of posterior vertical dimension and an increase in the mandibular plane angle. The loss of posterior vertical dimension can also make future prosthetic reconstruction difficult because there will be no room between the retromolar pad and the maxillary tuberosity to accommodate the thickness of a denture base. Open treatment in patients without good posterior teeth will be better able to maintain the posterior vertical dimension and interarch space.
2. The patient must be cooperative. They must wear their elastics, frequently verify their occlusion, do their functional exercises, and return often for follow-up. If one does not feel that a patient will be cooperative, then closed treatment may fail to achieve the above outcomes; open treatment might be more favored.
3. The surgeon must be willing to see the patient often to assess treatment and alter functional therapy as necessary. There is no question that patients treated closed require more visits to assure the occlusion is being maintained and the physiotherapy is being performed adequately. If the surgeon is unwilling to see the patient more often, open treatment might be a more favorable option.

There are also pre-requisites to *open* treatment that are important to understand.
1. The surgeon must be capable of *safely* performing open reduction and internal fixation (ORIF) of a condylar process fracture.

2. Stable internal fixation must be applied to the fragments to assure no loss of stability during the postoperative healing period. If the fixation fails, loose hardware in this area will likely cause inflammation/infection for which more surgery will be needed. Therefore, one should only perform open surgery when the fragments are large enough to adequately stabilize with internal fixation devices and when the quality of the bone is adequate to maintain a stable screw–bone interface. The very young and the osteoporotic elderly female may have bone that is not capable of maintaining screw–bone interface stability.

Considerations for Open Reduction and Internal Fixation

Most condylar process fractures can be treated closed with satisfactory outcomes. This is especially true of unilateral condylar fractures that satisfy the prerequisites for closed treatment listed above. This is also true of severely displaced unilateral fractures, high or low. However, there are some conditions where open treatment facilitates the overall care of the patient. These conditions include the following:
1. *Bilateral condylar process fractures.* When a patient has both condylar processes fractured, especially when they are displaced, it will be difficult to *predictably* achieve the above desirable outcomes using closed techniques. The reason for this is that the biomechanics become unfavorable.[13] If one considers that under the power stroke of mastication the mandible functions as a Class III lever system (Fig. 1.15.11A), when the fulcrum (condyle) is removed (by displacing the condyles), contraction of the elevator muscles causes premature contact of the terminal molars, resulting in an anterior open-bite (Fig. 1.15.11B). While closed treatment can often achieve the pretrauma occlusion and does so in the majority of patients, it is not predictable. Some patients obtain good outcomes, some do not. It is not possible to determine which patients will have a good outcome with closed treatment of bilateral condylar fractures and which will not. Therefore, ORIF of at least one of the condylar fractures will greatly increase the predictability of a favorable outcome.
2. *Associated maxillary fracture(s).* When a patient has condylar fracture(s) associated with a free-floating maxilla from fractures superior to the maxillary dentition, especially when there is comminution of the articulations of the maxilla with the zygomas along the Le Fort I level, ORIF of the condyle(s) will facilitate repositioning the maxilla. By performing open treatment of the condylar fractures, as well as any other mandibular fracture(s), the case becomes an isolated midface fracture. The treatment then is simplified by simply mobilizing the maxilla, placing it into maxillomandibular fixation (MMF) with the mandible, and rotating the maxillomandibular complex until first bone contact, followed by passive fixation across the Le Fort I level. When both condyles are fractured, both must be treated open or there might be deviation of the entire maxillomandibular complex (maxilla and mandible) to the side of the nontreated condyle fracture.
3. *Edentulous condylar fractures.* Edentulous patients who do not wear a prosthesis (dentures) and are unconcerned that their chin has shifted to one side of the face do not require any treatment at all. But for those who do wear a dental prosthesis, treatment will be needed for most condylar fractures, especially those with displacement. If not treated, the mandibular retromolar area will collapse vertically against the maxillary tuberosity, eliminating any reconstructive space for a dental prosthesis. As noted above, one of the prerequisites for a good outcome with closed treatment is posterior teeth to maintain the vertical dimension of the ramus. With patients who have no teeth, maintaining the position of the mandible is difficult when there is/are condylar fracture(s). Using the patient's

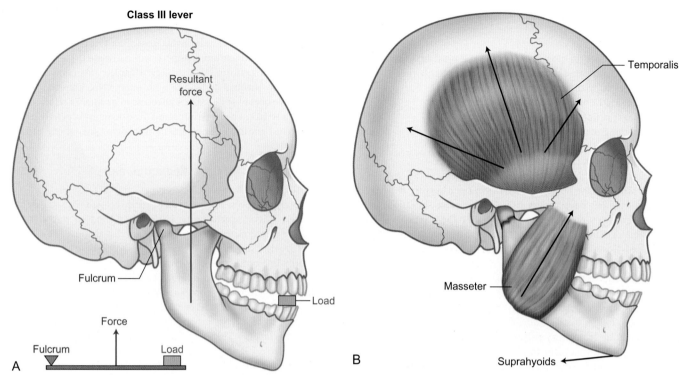

Fig. 1.15.11 Illustration of the biomechanics involved with bilateral condylar process fractures. (A) A Class III lever system where the resultant muscle force from the elevator muscles is between the fulcrum (TMJ) and the load (teeth). (B) A fractured mandibular condyle removes the fulcrum (TMJ), allowing the elevator muscles to move the ramus upward, causing premature contact on the terminal molars and a resultant anterior open-bite.

dental prosthesis may help but the jaws must be wired into MMF with the prostheses in place because functional therapy is not possible without a "handle" on the jaws that teeth usually provide. It has never been demonstrated whether closed treatment using removable dental prostheses can truly maintain the posterior vertical dimension. Open reduction and internal fixation of condylar fractures in the edentulous patient immediately reconstructs the vertical dimension of the ramus and maintains it.

Method of Closed Treatment

The literature is full of closed techniques that can be used to treat condylar fractures. They include periods of MMF, functional therapy, or most frequently a combination of both. For those advocating a period of MMF, the duration ranges from a day or two all the way to 6 weeks. A method that has worked well for us over the years is the following[14]:

1. *Application of arch bars.* It is much more predictable in achieving a successful occlusal outcome when arch bars are used instead of bone fixation appliances. The reason for this is that orthodontic adaptations such as extrusion of some teeth and intrusion of others are often required to maintain the pretrauma occlusion while the skeletal adaptations, like forming a new articulation, are progressing.[15] Using elastics with appliances attached directly to the teeth facilitates the needed orthodontic adaptations.

2. *Open reduction and internal fixation of all other noncondylar fractures.* It is important that any noncondylar fracture(s) be treated with *rigid* internal fixation so that no motion across them will occur during the functional therapy of the condylar process fracture.

3. *Removal of MMF and examining the occlusion.* Typically, the mandible will deviate toward the side of the condylar fracture (Fig. 1.15.12A).

This is of no consequence and occlusal guidance commences the following day.

4. *Placement of elastics p.r.n.* The next day, assessment of the occlusion is performed. Most commonly, there will be a premature contact posteriorly on the side of the condylar process fracture with deviation to that side and possibly a contralateral open-bite (Fig. 1.15.3). If there is a malocclusion, elastics are applied to assist the neuromusculature in obtaining the proper occlusion. For unilateral fractures, this is typically one elastic on the side of the condylar fracture applied in a Class II manner, to help draw the mandible anteriorly when the patient closes the mouth. Occasionally, a second one is necessary (Fig. 1.15.12B). One should apply as much elastic guidance as is necessary to allow the patient to obtain their normal occlusal relationship when they occlude. The goal, however, is to use as little as necessary to facilitate active use of the mandible. For bilateral fractures, elastics are usually required bilaterally in a Class II vector, and often supplementation with vertical elastics in the anterior. While the patient sleeps, they should apply sufficient elastics to maintain MMF throughout the night.

5. *Postsurgical physiotherapy.* Patients are encouraged to use their jaws as much as possible beginning on the first postoperative day. They are instructed in physiotherapeutic exercises to increase range of mandibular motion, which they should employ at least four times a day. Exercises consist of maximum opening of the mouth, attempting to do so without deviation toward the side of fracture. The patient should also be shown how to use lateral excursive exercises to both the right and left sides. Finally, protrusive excursions should be practiced, again attempting to do so without deviation of the mandible to one side or the other. During the exercises, eating, and oral hygiene procedures, the patient can remove the elastics. The

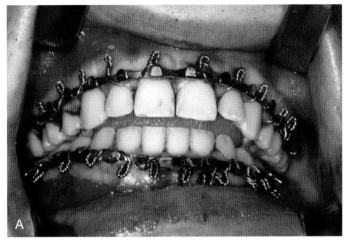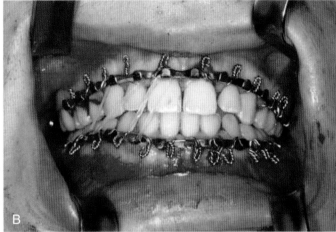

Fig. 1.15.12 Intraoperative photographs of a patient who is being treated for a right unilateral condylar process fracture. Note the premature occlusion on the right, the deviation of the mandible to the right, and the left anterior open-bite. This patient required two Class II elastics to bring the mandible into the proper occlusion.

elastics are then reapplied, and the patient is shown how to determine they are biting in the proper occlusal relationship in a mirror, using as few elastics as possible. Patients with unilateral fractures may always have some degree of deviation toward the side of fracture on wide opening or protrusion (Fig. 1.15.2). Typically, patients will be able to obtain the above treatment goals in 4–5 weeks.

6. *Weaning the patient from the elastics.* After 2 or 3 weeks of this treatment, the patient should be able to obtain their pretraumatic occlusion without the constant use of elastics. The elastics are withdrawn more and more over the next 2–3 weeks so that they are used only while sleeping for another 2–3 weeks. Once the use of elastics is no longer necessary for the patient to obtain their pretraumatic occlusion, they can be discontinued (Fig. 1.15.13). The arch bars should be left in place, however, for a few weeks beyond that time so that if the patient has some difficulty with occlusion later, elastics can be easily reapplied.

7. *Removal of arch bars.* Most commonly, arch bars are left in place for 6–8 weeks for unilateral and 3–4 months for bilateral condylar process fractures. Once the patient can consistently assume their normal occlusion without the use of elastics, the arch bars can be removed.

Method for Open Treatment

When the decision is made to treat the patient's condylar process fracture with ORIF, the following steps are followed[14]:

1. Application of arch bars.
2. Open reduction and internal fixation of all other non-condylar fractures.
3. Removal of MMF and examining the occlusion. Typically, the mandible will deviate toward the side of the condylar fracture.
4. Placement of interarch elastics. If using a transfacial approach to the condylar fracture, elastics are placed between the upper and lower arch bars to provide the proper occlusal relationship. Elastics are used instead of wires during open treatment of the condylar process fractures because the mandibular ramus must frequently be distracted inferiorly to retrieve a medially displaced condylar process. When using a transoral approach to the condylar fracture, elastics are unnecessary because one will have direct visualization of the occlusion.
5. Open reduction and stable internal fixation of condylar process fracture. The surgeon should use whichever surgical approach they prefer (see below). The condylar process should be properly reduced

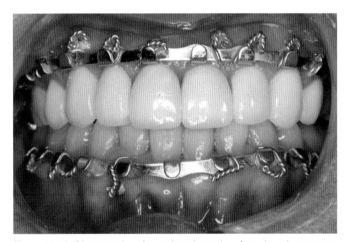

Fig. 1.15.13 Photographs of a patient 6 weeks after closed treatment of a right condylar process fracture using one Class II elastic on the right side. She has been able to obtain a normal occlusion without elastics for 2 weeks so the arch bars are no longer required.

and stabilized. The use of either a single strong bone plate employing 2.0 mm self-threading screws or two standard miniplates that employ 2.0 mm screws is adequate fixation (Fig. 1.15.14).

6. Occlusal verification. The occlusion is checked to assure the mandible rotates properly into occlusion with the maxilla.
7. Closure. If a transfacial approach has been used, the incision is closed in layers, taking care to hermetically close the parotid capsule if the surgical approach violates the gland.
8. Occlusal guidance. The next day, assessment of the occlusion is performed. Most commonly there will be a slight posterior open-bite on the side of the condylar process fracture secondary to edema in the TMJ. This will resolve within a week. If the posterior open-bite is still present at the end of one week, light vertical elastics are applied to close the bite. Elastics should be placed only if there is a malocclusion, and as few as necessary are employed. The goal is to use as few as required to facilitate active use of the mandible.
9. Postsurgical physiotherapy. Same as described above for closed treatment.
10. Removal of arch bars. Once the patient can consistently assume their normal occlusion without the use of elastics, the arch bars

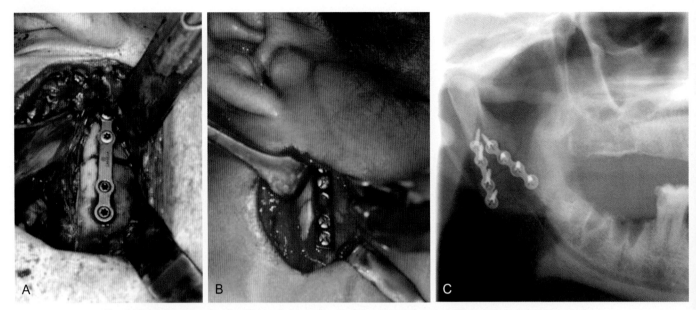

Fig. 1.15.14 Photographs of sufficient fixation of a condylar process fracture. (A) A single 4-hole plate employing 2.0 mm screws. Note that the plate is wider than a standard miniplate. (B) A small mandibular compression plate using 2.0 mm screws. (C) Two standard miniplates using 2.0 mm screws.

can be removed. Most commonly, arch bars are left in place for 4–6 weeks for condylar process fractures treated open.

Surgical Approaches for ORIF of Condylar Process Fractures

Like most fractures, there are different surgical approaches that can be used. The choice depends as much on experience of the surgeon or other factors but the position of the fracture and the choice of fixation scheme may also help direct the surgical approach.

Retromandibular Approach

The retromandibular technique has the advantage that it is a direct dissection to the condylar neck region. This facilitates the reduction of condylar neck and subcondylar fractures and the application of bone plate fixation to them. The disadvantages are that the dissection is thought to be difficult because it is a dissection through the parotid gland with the branching VII nerve. Once mastered, it is a safe and relatively fast surgical approach.

The incision for the retromandibular approach begins 0.5 cm below the lobe of the ear and continues inferiorly 2.5–3 cm (Fig. 1.15.15A). Another incision is then made through the scant platysma muscle found in this location and the parotid capsule (Fig. 1.15.15B). At this point, blunt dissection begins in an anteromedial direction towards the posterior border of the mandible (Fig. 1.15.15C). The marginal mandibular and cervical branches of the facial nerve will frequently be encountered during this dissection. When the buccal and/or marginal mandibular branches are located, they should be dissected free. Once the nerves are retracted, one can readily expose the pterygomasseteric sling at the posterior border of the mandible. The periosteum along the posterior border of the mandible and partially around the mandibular angle is incised from as far superiorly as is reachable to as far inferiorly around the gonial angle as is possible (Fig. 1.15.15D). The masseter muscle is then stripped from the ramus. The fractured condylar fragment is then identified (Fig. 1.15.15E), reduced and stabilized. The wound is closed in layers.

Submandibular Approach

The submandibular approach to the condylar process has the advantage that most surgeons are familiar with the approach because it is used for many other problems besides condylar fractures. The disadvantage, when treating condylar process fractures, is that one is distant from the area of injury. This makes it difficult to reduce condylar fractures, especially those that are medially displaced. Plating them requires a transcutaneous trocar for instrumentation.

The incision is 1.5–2 cm inferior to the mandibular border. The initial incision is carried through skin and subcutaneous tissues to the level of the platysma muscle. Retraction of the skin edges reveals the underlying platysma muscle. Division of the fibers (Fig. 1.15.16A) is performed and reveals the white superficial layer of deep cervical fascia. The submandibular salivary gland can also be visualized through the fascia, which helps form its capsule. Dissection through the superficial layer of deep cervical fascia is the step that requires the most care because the facial vein and artery are usually encountered when approaching the area of the premasseteric notch of the mandible, as may the marginal mandibular branch of the facial nerve (Fig. 1.15.16B). If the facial vessels are in the way, they can be isolated, clamped, divided, and ligated. Dissection continues until the only tissue remaining on the inferior border of the mandible is the pterygomasseteric sling. The pterygomasseteric sling is sharply incised with a scalpel along the inferior border (Fig. 1.15.16C) and the lateral surface of the mandibular ramus is stripped of the masseter muscle in a subperiosteal plane. Further dissection superiorly should reveal the fractured condylar process (Fig. 1.15.16D). After ORIF of the condylar fracture, a layered closure is performed.

Preauricular Approach

The preauricular approach to the temporomandibular joint (TMJ) is relatively easy to expose surgically, although the amount of exposure obtained is not great. The structure that limits the amount of exposure is the branching facial nerve. The advantage of the preauricular approach is that most surgeons who do TMJ surgery are familiar with it. The

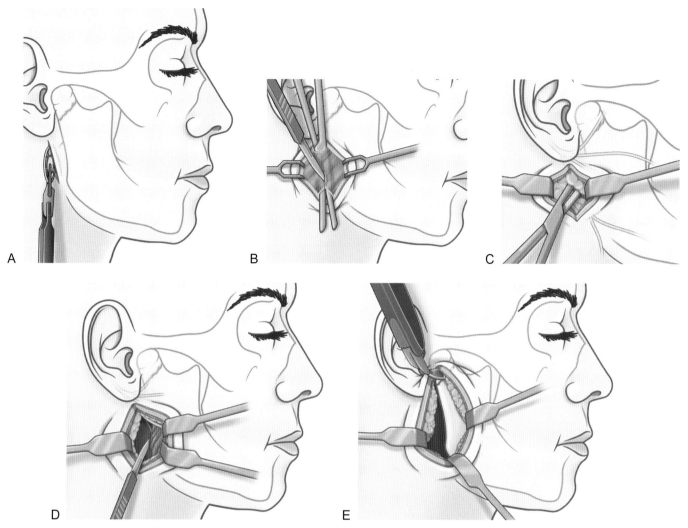

Fig. 1.15.15 The retromandibular approach to the condylar process. (A) Incision through skin and subcutaneous tissues. (B) Incision through SMAS and parotid capsule. (C) Blunt dissection through the parotid gland. (D) Incision through the pterygomasseteric sling along the posterior border. (E) Exposure of the fracture. (Adapted from Ellis E, Zide MF. Surgical approaches to the facial skeleton. 2nd ed. Philadelphia: Lippincott Williams & Wilkins; 2006.)

disadvantage is that it only provides good access to intracapsular and condylar neck fractures. Fractures below the neck of the condyle are difficult to stabilize because exposure of the subcondylar region is poor with this approach.

The incision is made through skin and subcutaneous connective tissues (including temporoparietal fascia) to the depth of the temporalis fascia (superficial layer) (Fig. 1.15.17A). Dissection with sharp scissors commences along the cartilaginous auditory canal below the zygomatic arch and to the glistening outer layer of temporalis fascia above the zygomatic arch (Fig. 1.15.17B). The tissue is dissected and retracted anteriorly at the depth of the superficial (outer) layer of temporalis fascia. The superficial temporal vessels and auriculotemporal nerve are retracted anteriorly in the flap. The entire flap is retracted anteriorly, and blunt dissection at this depth (just superficial to the capsule of the TMJ) proceeds anteriorly until the articular eminence is exposed. The entire TMJ capsule should then be revealed. The temporal branches of the facial nerve are located within the substance of the retracted flap (Fig. 1.15.17C). If a condylar neck fracture is being treated, dissection proceeds inferiorly until just below the capsule (Fig. 1.15.17C) at which point an incision is made through the periosteum and dissection of

the condyle neck proceeds (Fig. 1.15.17D). The distal fragment is then identified and a subperiosteal dissection of the masseter muscle inferiorly exposes the posterior border and lateral surface of the ramus. If an intraarticular fracture is being treated, the capsule is opened and entrance into the lower joint space is performed. The condylar head is identified and the fragment stripped of as much capsule as needed to perform the reduction and fixation. One should take care to maintain the attachment of the lateral pterygoid muscle as it may be the only blood supply remaining on the condylar fragment. The fracture is then reduced and stabilized. A layered closure is then performed.

Intraoral Approach

The intraoral approach is the easiest approach to perform because there are no tissue layers to dissect in approaching the bone. There is only the fusion of the oral mucosa, buccinator muscle, and the periosteum through which one incises. The scar will remain hidden within the oral cavity, which is very important for many patients. The other advantage is that there are no major anatomic structures that have to be negotiated. The main disadvantage is the limited amount of visibility provided and the technical difficulties of reducing and stabilizing the condylar

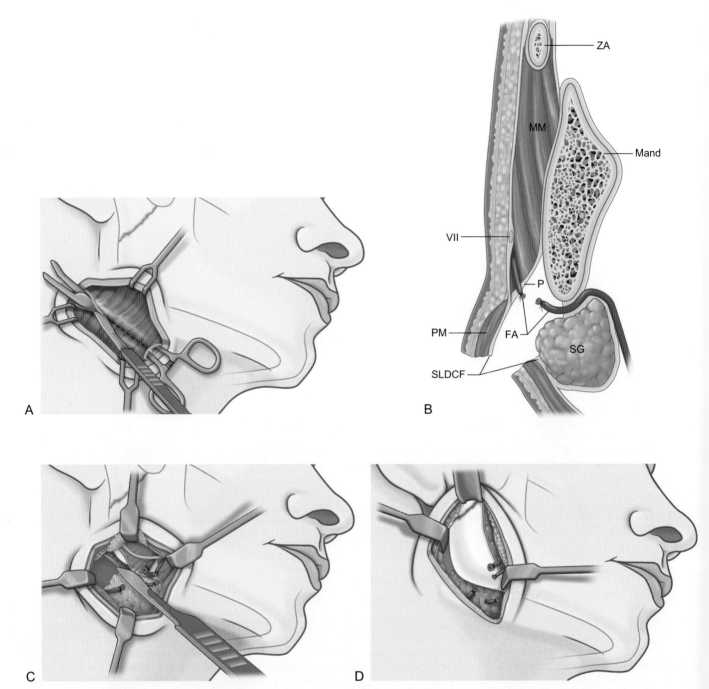

Fig. 1.15.16 The submandibular approach to the condylar process. (A) Incision through platysma. (B) Cross-sectional anatomy in the area. (C) Incision through pterygomasseteric sling. (D) Exposure of the fracture. (Adapted from Ellis E, Zide MF. Surgical approaches to the facial skeleton. 2nd ed. Philadelphia: Lippincott Williams & Wilkins; 2006.)

process. The use of an endoscope can greatly facilitate visibility and instruments designed for this approach facilitate reduction and fixation. A right-angle drill and screwdriver make the application of fixation devices easier than using a transbuccal trocar.

After instillation of local anesthetic with a vasoconstrictor along the incision line as well as between the masseter muscle and the ramus, an incision is made through mucosa, buccinator muscle, and periosteum from the depth of the coronoid notch along the external oblique ridge to the second molar. Subperiosteal dissection exposes the entire lateral surface of the ramus (Fig. 1.15.18A). The condylar process is located

and the soft tissues inferior to the joint capsule are dissected off the fragment to facilitate reduction. If the fragment is displaced medially, downward traction on the posterior mandible can help pull the fragment into a more vertical position. Once the fragment is clearly visible and dissected, it is reduced into position and held there by using an instrument. If using an endoscope for assistance, it can be placed through the same intraoral incision (Fig. 1.15.18B) or alternately through a small incision in the submandibular region (Fig. 1.15.18C). Once the fracture is plated, a single-layered closure of the oral mucosa is then performed.

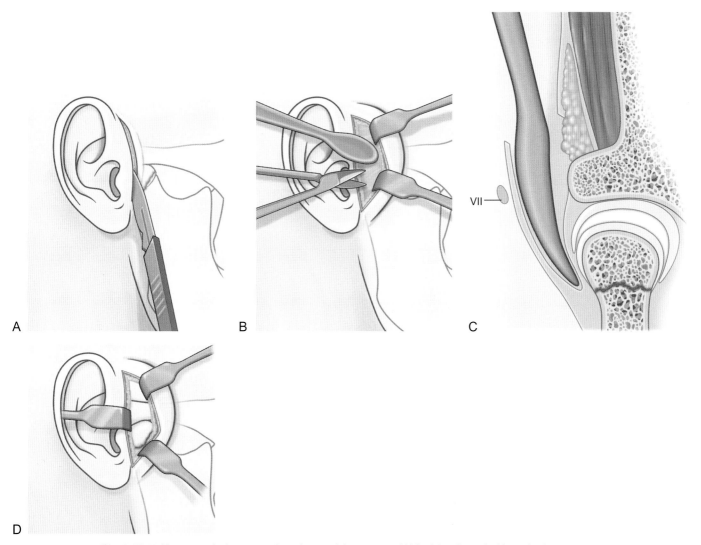

Fig. 1.15.17 The preauricular approach to the condylar process. (A) Incision through skin and subcutaneous tissues. (B) Dissection along the superficial layer of the temporalis fascia. (C) Cross-sectional anatomy in the area. Note that branches of the facial nerve should be lateral to the path of dissection. (D) Exposure of the fracture. (Adapted from Ellis E, Zide MF. Surgical approaches to the facial skeleton. 2nd ed. Philadelphia: Lippincott Williams & Wilkins; 2006.)

What About the Articular Disk?

The articular disk is an important component of normal TMJ anatomy. Several questions might be asked about the relationship between a condylar fracture and the articular disk. The answers to these questions are important because they may provide some information about what treatment should be provided to patients with condylar fractures and/or intraarticular injuries.

The first question that should be asked is whether or not the articular disk or its attachments are injured when a patient sustains a condylar process fracture. Studies using MRI and TMJ arthroscopy have shown that injuries to the intraarticular structures can occur not just in patients who sustain condylar process fractures but also to those who have sustained noncondylar mandibular fractures.[16–26] These studies have shown effusions, hemarthroses, perforations of the disc, displacement of the disc, and tears to the capsular attachments of the disc in some patients with condylar fractures – especially those with gross displacement/dislocation and those with intracapsular fractures. When the condylar process is fractured and grossly displaced and/or dislocated, the articular disc tends to become displaced in the same direction with the condylar head.[21–23,26]

The second question that should be asked is, given that intra-articular injuries can occur with condylar process fractures, should our treatment address the intra-articular injuries? For instance, should the articular disc be repositioned when performing open treatment of the condylar process fracture? There are advocates of such treatment,[22,26,27] especially for displaced intracapsular fractures. However, most surgeons do not surgically address the intraarticular injuries and instead confine their treatment to closed treatment or open treatment of the condylar process without entering the joint capsule. Open reduction and internal fixation has been shown to bring the articular disk into a more normal position in most cases.[22,23,26]

Treating the intraarticular injuries with benign neglect has been done for centuries and overall most patients recover quite well. There are good reasons to *not* address the intraarticular injuries. First, identification of such injuries requires MRI scans, which are not routinely obtained with the treatment of condylar process fractures. Second, if

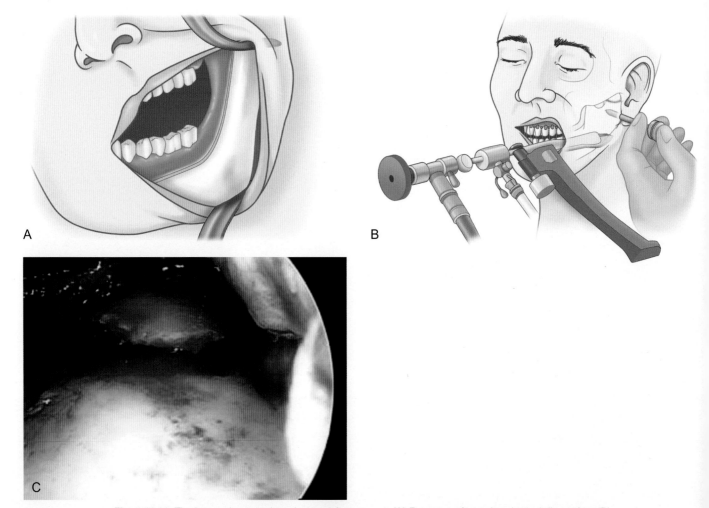

A

B

C

Fig. 1.15.18 The intraoral approach to the condylar process. (A) Exposure after subperiosteal dissection. (B) Use of an endoscope inserted through the transoral incision and insertion of a transbuccal trochar. (C) Exposure of a condylar process fracture as viewed through an endoscope. (Panels A and C adapted from Ellis E, Zide MF. Surgical approaches to the facial skeleton. 2nd ed. Philadelphia: Lippincott Williams & Wilkins; 2006.)

MRIs showed displacement of the disc, it is not always possible to know if this was a consequence of the injury or a preexisting problem. Studies have shown a high incidence of displaced TMJ discs in the general population (approximately one-third).[28–30] Third, performing disc repositioning surgery requires an intraarticular operation which can disrupt the remaining blood supply to the head of the condyle which after fracture only comes from the TMJ capsule and the lateral pterygoid muscle.[15] Last, repositioning the disc assumes that patients will do better than those who do not have disc repositioning. There is not much evidence to support this assumption. For the average surgeon, especially those who do not routinely perform TMJ surgery, addressing any intraarticular injuries will likely not occur with any frequency when treating condylar process fractures.

TRAUMA-DERIVED TEMPOROMANDIBULAR DISORDERS

Temporomandibular disorders (TMD) are very common in developed countries and are multifactorial in cause.[31,32] Stress, anxiety, malocclusion, internal derangements, muscle spasms, eating and functional habits among others have been identified as important factors in TMD. Such

factors can be considered as causing microtrauma to the joint. Condylar or noncondylar mandibular fractures would be considered forms of macrotrauma to the TMJ and have been implicated as an important factor with intraarticular TMDs.[33,34]

Animal studies have shown condylar trauma results in biochemical changes within the TMJ, cartilage degeneration and intraarticular adhesions.[35,36] The long-term effect of such TMJ changes on jaw function is not clear and although most clinicians are aware of the association between mandibular trauma and the later development of TMD there have been few systematic studies. When one considers how common TMDs are in the general population and how relatively rare macrotrauma to the TMJ is, it is hard to implicate trauma as a major cause of TMDs.[32]

The majority of patients respond well to TMJ trauma and adapt with very few complaints long term. However, it is important to realize that trauma may play an important role in the onset of acute TMDs or may exacerbate an already preexistent and perhaps dormant TMD.

TMJ trauma has been implicated as an important etiological factor in TMJ ankylosis, especially in untreated or poorly treated patient populations.[37–40] While the most common cause of TMJ ankylosis is condylar fracture, the incidence of TMJ ankylosis from condylar fracture is very low (<.05%).[41,42]

EXPERT COMMENTARY

This chapter, whose senior author is the master of principlization and problem solving in the mandible as well as other facial injuries, is my favorite literature on the subject. Clearly, briefly written and well organized, the chapter distills an overwhelming volume of literature into a minimal number of well-defined principles. What one learns quickly is that picking the treatment is as much about picking the complications as the results. The condyle also is a more brittle piece of bone, has more consistent microfractures than the literature would indicate, making it a poor candidate for stability after open reduction, and is prone therefore to screw loosening and repeat displacement following open reduction, especially in non-cooperative patients. These problems are far more frequent than in other mandibular locations treated with internal fixation. Resorption is also frequent, especially if the head is stripped to accomplish the reduction, and I have several patients in whom the head has entirely resorbed over 1 year, leaving the plate sticking up by itself. Personally, I went to immediate replacement with a costochrondral bone graft [1–3] in situations of high comminution like gunshot wounds, or when the head was replaced as a free graft, as it is better bone, and more likely to survive.

I have not seen closed treatment maintain the vertical height of the ramus as well as open techniques, and occlusal adjustments are frequently necessary but well tolerated. Whether they are better than occlusal adjustments is a subject for discussion. The idea of treating one condyle alone in bilateral fractures with fractures of the horizontal mandible has never made much sense to me.

In patients who require anterior elastics, some support for the arch bar to bone with skeletal wires prevents/minimizes extrusion of anterior teeth, which without them is inevitable.

There ought to be patient instructions available on diet, exercise of the mandible, occlusion and elastics and the goals and self-monitoring of the occlusion. At Shock Trauma, we had a book for patients which covered: "Let's Face this Together" by P. Azman and P. Manson.

Note Ellis's advice on the superiority of arch bars, and how they do orthodontics to help restore occlusion, and especially how long the bars must stay on after the initial perception of stability. Personally, I have had far more problems with malocclusion from early discontinuance of IMF with loss of control of the occlusion, than I have had stiffness, and I firmly believe in a period of rest for both the bone and the soft tissue immediately after treatment in IMF. Poor application of arch bars or poorly setting up the occlusion are some of the most frequent causes of problems I have seen, especially in those who infrequently treat fractures of the mandible. I use a Penrose drain in areas where I have transected the parotid, and in the retromandibular incision I do not go through the parotid but mobilize it anteriorly and superiorly.

One of the best mandible surgeons I know is Anthony Tufaro, who trained in three specialties and who does condylar open reductions like a head and neck surgeon, with two approaches – a simultaneous preauricular and a retromandibular exposure with visualization and protection of the facial nerve – allowing him to generate the inferior distraction which facilitates the reduction, and which gives him precise control of all of the variables that haunt the more limited approaches to the condyle [4].

Finally, precise application and management of Erich arch bars, the addition of skeletal wires where necessary especially anteriorly, occlusal monitoring weekly, patient education, and rigid supervision of the patient will improve the results dramatically, as will obtaining dental records and old models in challenging cases. At the end of the case, and often after placing one screw on each side of the plate, I will frequently take the patient out of occlusion and, with the condyles clearly and solidly seated into its proper position in the fossa, check the occlusion and thus the accuracy of the temporary reduction. The sound of the "click" as all of the teeth come together precisely at once cannot be mimicked by any other sound.

References

1. Serletti J, Crawley W, Manson PN. Autogenous reconstruction of the temporomandibular joint. *J Craniofac Surg.* 1993;4:28–34.
2. Evans G, Clark N, Manson P. Technique of costochondral graft placement. *J Craniofac Surg.* 1994;5:340–343.
3. Azman P, Manson P. *Let's Face It Together.* Miemss Publication for Patient Education and Distribution; 1986.
4. Tufaro AP. Open reduction of condylar fractures. J Craniofac Trauma Reconstr. in press.

* Evidence-based medicine (EBM) content available in Appendix 1 (online only)

REFERENCES

1. Chrcanovic BR. Surgical versus non-surgical treatment of mandibular condylar fractures: a metaanalysis. *Int J Oral Maxillofac Surg.* 2015;44:158–179.
2. Zachariades N, Mezitis M, Mourouzis C, et al. Fractures of the mandibular condyle: a review of 466 cases. Literature review, reflections on treatment and proposals. *J Craniomaxillofac Surg.* 2006;34:421–432.
3. Walker RV. Traumatic mandibular condyle fracture dislocations. *Am J Surg.* 1960;100:850–863.
4. Rudderman RH, Mullen RL. Biomechanics of the facial skeleton. *Clin Plast Surg.* 1992;19:11–21.
5. Loukota RA, Eckelt U, DeBond L, Rasse M. Subclassification of fractures of the condylar process of the mandible. *Br J Oral Maxillofac Surg.* 2005;43:72–73.
6. Lindahl L. Condylar fractures of the mandible: I. Classification and relation to age, occlusion, and concomitant injuries of teeth and teeth-supporting structures, and fractures of the mandibular body. *Int J Oral Surg.* 1977;6:12–21.
7. Spiessl B, Schroll K. Gelenkfortsatz und gelenkkopfchenfracturen [Fractures of the condylar neck and head]. In: Higst H, ed. *Spezielle Frakture und Luxationslehre [Textbook of Specialized Fractures and Dislocations].* BD. I/I. Stuttgart: Thieme; 1972:36–42.
8. Cornelius CP, Audigé L, Kunz C, et al. The comprehensive AOCMF classification system: mandible fractures – level 2 tutorial. *Craniomaxillofac Trauma Reconstr.* 2014;7(suppl 1):S15–S30.
9. Cornelius C-P, Audigé L, Kunz C, et al. The comprehensive AOCMF classification system: mandible fractures – level 3 tutorial. *Craniomaxillofac Trauma Reconstr.* 2014;7(suppl 1):S31–S43.
10. Neff A, Cornelius CP, Rasse M, et al. The comprehensive AOCMF classification system: condylar process fractures – level 3 tutorial. *Craniomaxillofac Trauma Reconstr.* 2014;7(suppl 1):S44–S58.
11. Walker RV. Discussion: Open reduction of condylar fractures of the mandible in conjunction with repair of discal injury: a preliminary report. *J Oral Maxillofac Surg.* 1988;46:262.
12. Ellis E, Kellman RM, Vural E. Subcondylar fractures. *Facial Plast Surg Clin North Am.* 2012;20:365–382.
13. Talwar RW, Ellis E, Throckmorton GS. Adaptations of the masticatory system after bilateral fractures of the mandibular condylar process. *J Oral Maxillofac Surg.* 1998;56:430–439.
14. Ellis E. Condylar process fractures of the mandible. *Facial Plast Surg.* 2000;16:193–205.
15. Ellis E, Throckmorton GS. Treatment of mandibular condylar process fractures: biological considerations. *J Oral Maxillofac Surg.* 2005;63:115–134.
16. Goss AN, Bosanquet AG. The arthroscopic appearance of acute temporomandibular joint trauma. *J Oral Maxillofac Surg.* 1990;48:780–783, discussion 784.
17. Jones JK, Van Sickels JE. A preliminary report of arthroscopic findings following acute condylar trauma. *J Oral Maxillofac Surg.* 1991;49:55–60.

18. Ozmen Y, Rischbach R, Lenzen J. MRI assessment of disc position following surgical and nonsurgical treatment of condylar fractures. *Dtsch Z Mund Kiefer Gesichts Chir.* 1995;19:277–280.

19. Ozmen Y, Mischkowski RA, Lenzen J, Fischbach R. MRI examination of the TMJ and functional results after conservative and surgical treatment of mandibular condyle fractures. *Int J Oral Maxillofac Surg.* 1998;27:33–37.

20. Sullivan SM, Banghart PR, Anderson Q. Magnetic resonance imaging assessment of acute soft tissue injuries to the temporomandibular joint. *J Oral Maxillofac Surg.* 1995;53:763.

21. Choi B-H. Magnetic resonance imaging of the temporomandibular joint after functional treatment of bilateral condylar fractures in adults. *Int J Oral Maxillofac Surg.* 1997;26:344–347.

22. Choi B-H, Yi J-H. MRI examination of the TMJ after surgical treatment of condylar fractures. *Int J Oral Maxillofac Surg.* 2001;30:296–299.

23. Schneider A, Zahnert D, Klengel S, et al. A comparison of MRI, radiographic and clinical findings of the position of the TMJ articualr disc following open treatment of condylar neck fractures. *Br J Oral Maxillofac Surg.* 2007;45:534–537.

24. Tripathi R, Sharma N, Dwivedi AN, Kumar S. Severity of soft tissue injury within the temporomandibular joint following condylar fracture as seen on magnetic resonance imaging and its impact on outcome of functional management. *J Oral Maxillofac Surg.* 2015;73:2379.e1–2379.e7.

25. Yang X, Yao Z, He D, et al. Does Soft tissue injury affect intracapsular condylar fracture healing? *J Oral Maxillofac Surg.* 2015;73(11):2169–2180.

26. Zheng J, Zhang S, Yang C, et al. Assessment of magnetic resonance images of displacement of the disc of the temporomandibular joint in different types of condylar fracture. *Br J Oral Maxillofac Surg.* 2016;54:74–79.

27. Chuong R, Piper MA. Open reduction of condylar fractions of the mandible in conjunction with repair of discal injury: a preliminary report. *J Oral Maxillofac Surg.* 1988;46:257–263.

28. Katzberg RW, Westesson PL, Tallents RH, Drake CM. Anatomic disorders of the temporomandibular joint disc in asymptomatic subjects. *J Oral Maxillofac Surg.* 1996;54:147–153.

29. Tasaki MM, Westesson PL, Isberg AM, et al. Classification and prevalence of temporomandibular joint disk displacement in patients and symptom-free volunteers. *Am J Orthod Dentofacial Orthop.* 1996;109:249–262.

30. Larheim TA, Westesson P-L, Sano T. Temporomandibular joint disk displacement: Comparison in asymptomatic volunteers and patients. *Radiology.* 2001;218:428–432.

31. Greene CS. Etiology of temporomandibular disorders. *Semin Orthod.* 1995;1:222–228.

32. Al-Hashmi A, Al-Azri A, Al-Ismaily M, Goss AN. Temporomandibular disorders in patients with mandibular fractures: a preliminary comparative case-control study between South Australia and Oman. *Int J Oral Maxillofac Surg.* 2011;40:1369–1372.

33. Luz JG, Jaeger RG, de Araujo VC, de Rezende JR. The effect of indirect trauma on the rat temporomandibular joint. *Int J Oral Maxillofac Surg.* 1991;20:48–52.

34. Pullinger AG, Seligman DA. Trauma history in diagnostic groups of temporomandibular disorders. *Oral Surg Oral Med Oral Pathol.* 1991;71:529–534.

35. Li L, Wang L, Sun Y, et al. Establishment and histological evaluation of a goat traumatic temporomandibular joint model. *J Oral Maxillofac Surg.* 2015;73:943–950.

36. Li Z, Li ZB. Mandibular condylar growth in growing rats after experimentally displaced condylar fracture with associated attachment damage and disc displacement: an observation by polychrome sequential labeling. *J Oral Maxillofac Surg.* 2012;70:896–901.

37. El-Sheikh MM. Temporomandibular joint ankylosis: the Egyptian experience. *Ann R Coll Surg Engl.* 1999;81:12–18.

38. Guven OA. Clinical study on TMJ ankylosis. *Auris Nasus Larynx.* 2000;27:27–33.

39. He D, Ellis E, Zhang Y. Etiology of temporomandibular joint ankylosis secondary to condylar fractures: The role of concomitant mandibular fractures. *J Oral Maxillofac Surg.* 2007;66:77–84.

40. He D, Cai Y, Yang C. Analysis of temporomandibular joint ankyloses caused by condylar fracture in adults. *J Oral Maxillofac Surg.* 2014;72:763.e1–763.e9.

41. Gupta VK, Mehrotra D, Malhotra S, et al. An epidemiologic study of temporomandibular ankyloses. *Natl J Maxillofac Surg.* 2012;3:25–30.

42. Anyanechi CE. Temporomandibular joint ankylosis caused by condylar fractures: a retrospective analysis of cases at an urban teaching hospital in Nigeria. *Int J Oral Maxillofac Surg.* 2015;44:1027–1033.

Complications of Mandibular Fractures

Brian Alpert, Lewis C. Jones

THE PROBLEM

The mandible is a complex structure involved in many functions. It is a hoop-like bone which gives form to the lower face. It supports the lower teeth, tongue, lips, and some of the muscles of facial expression. Through it runs the sensory innervation of the chin and lower lip. It is suspended in space by paired muscles of mastication which functionally move the jaw through mastication, expression, and speech. It articulates with the skull base through paired diarthrodial joints with interposed menisci. It is involved with facial form and appearance, mastication and movement, speech, sensation, and expression. As such, it is one of the most unforgiving structures, certainly bones, in the body as any alteration of one or more of these functions is not likely to be ignored.

NATURE OF COMPLICATIONS

There are complications of injury: traumatic loss of a tooth, severance of an inferior alveolar nerve. There are complications that occur with proper treatment: approach scars, paresis, infection. There are complications of inadequate or inappropriate treatment: infection, delayed, nonunion or malunion from inadequate reduction and/or fixation. There are surgical misadventures: pithing the nerve with a screw during the process of applying fixation. There are complications of no treatment: malunion, nonunion, infection. Treatment is designed to minimize or overcome the potential complications of injury, not introduce additional ones.

EVOLUTION OF COMPLICATIONS

In the 19th and early 20th century, the measure of success for mandibular fractures was functional union. One accepted infection, loss of teeth, sequestration of bone, paresthesia, etc. as the complications of injury. Suppuration of open fractures, exfoliation of teeth, bone fragments, were all considered part of the process. One only has to read the accounts of treatment and outcomes during the 19th century to see how far we have come.[1,2]

The great advance to avoid and/or treat infection was immobilization of the jaws. Gunning and Bean utilized gutta percha splints.[3] Lewis Gilmer introduced maxillomandibular fixation (MMF).[4] These closed techniques of immobilization – later with the addition of skeletal pins[5] – formed the basis of mandibular fracture treatment prior to antibiotics. Indeed, the great giants of maxillofacial trauma care were masters of the closed reduction. They knew how to reduce and immobilize the mandible without resorting to open reduction and internal fixation (ORIF). The first edition of the Kazanjian and Converse classic text *The Surgical Treatment of Facial Injuries* is replete with descriptions of the closed techniques for the management of mandibular fractures.[6]

The Antibiotic Era

With the advent of antibiotics, ORIF of open fractures in the tooth-bearing region emerged as a supplement to MMF. Stainless steel wire was used to maintain alignment, particularly for proximal control. By this time, the main complication in a properly managed mandibular fracture (MMF alone or MMF+ORIF or skeletal pin fixation) was "infection," usually related to a tooth or dead bone. Nonunion, delayed and malunion often resulted. It was not uncommon to have prolonged periods of treatment, often lasting a year or more. Initial management – MMF+ORIF or X-fix – followed by "infection" with drainage, followed by debridement of nonvital teeth and/or bone, waiting 3–6 months after the cessation of drainage before bone grafting amounted to a year off one's life.

Additionally, complications of condylar fractures in the form of ankylosis, malocclusion, and acquired retrognathia occurred. All required surgical correction.

As can be seen, complications of this era were primarily complications of injury or of "proper" treatment. Unless one failed to use adequate MMF with a "wire" ORIF or performed ORIF on a comminuted fracture (contraindicated prior to rigid fixation), operator error was most unusual.

The different areas of the mandible were not equal with respect to the incidence of complications. Angle fractures with teeth in the line of fracture were most prone to complication, with almost one-third having them.[7] This occurred irrespective of whether they were done open or closed or whether the teeth involved were removed or retained. It remains true today.[8]

It should be noted that treatment times, even for successful outcomes, often extended to 2 or 3 months as fractures were often not firm at 6 or 8 weeks. Following MMF, it was necessary to "rehabilitate" the jaw opening, a process often taking several more weeks.

Rigid Fixation

Rigid fixation (RIF) was introduced in Europe in the mid 1970s and North America in the mid 1980s. There were three distinct lineages: the AO, with reduction and rigid immobilization with stainless steel plates and screws – usually applied transfacial;[9] the Luhr Vitalium system, also rigid immobilization but primarily transoral; and the transoral miniplate system of semirigid fixation popularized by Champy.[10,11]

All of these systems allowed for convalescent function – life without MMF. RIF had the potential of dramatically shortening the course of treatment. However, its use was highly technique-sensitive with a steep learning curve. Thus, the incidence of complications increased dramatically due to operator error. Complications related to inadequate reduction – "the OIF" (open internal fixation … *without* the reduction) (Figs. 1.16.1–1.16.3), inadequate fixation (Figs. 1.16.4–1.16.7) and surgical misadventure (Fig. 1.16.8) began to appear. Indeed, by the early 1990s

Text continued on p. 210

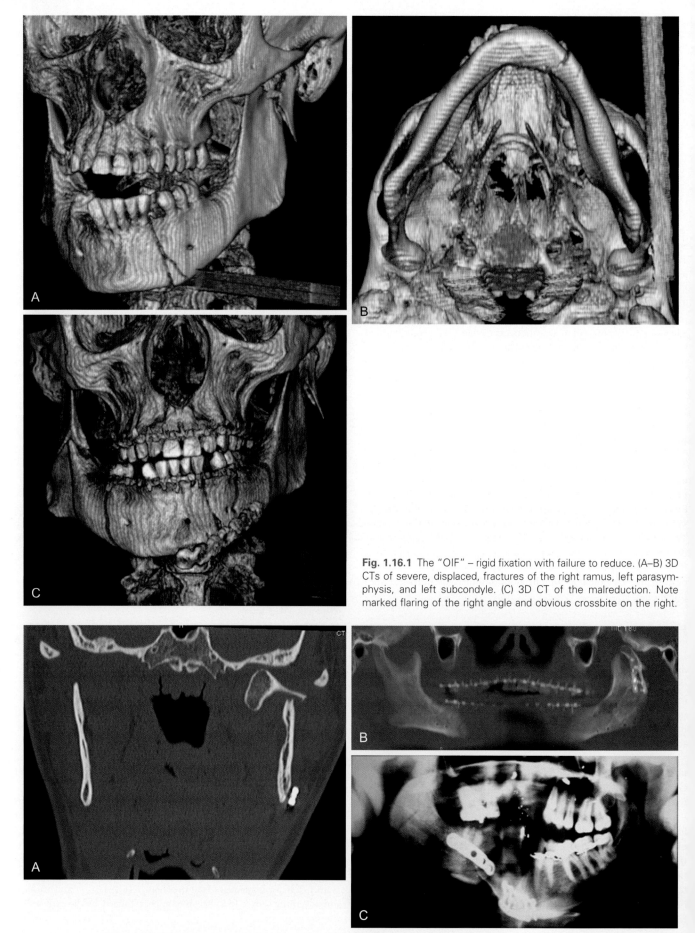

Fig. 1.16.1 The "OIF" – rigid fixation with failure to reduce. (A–B) 3D CTs of severe, displaced, fractures of the right ramus, left parasymphysis, and left subcondyle. (C) 3D CT of the malreduction. Note marked flaring of the right angle and obvious crossbite on the right.

Fig. 1.16.2 Malreduction of a displaced condylar fracture. (A) CT of displaced condylar fracture. (B) CT and panoramic view demonstrating malreduction. (C) Panoramic X-ray of OIF.

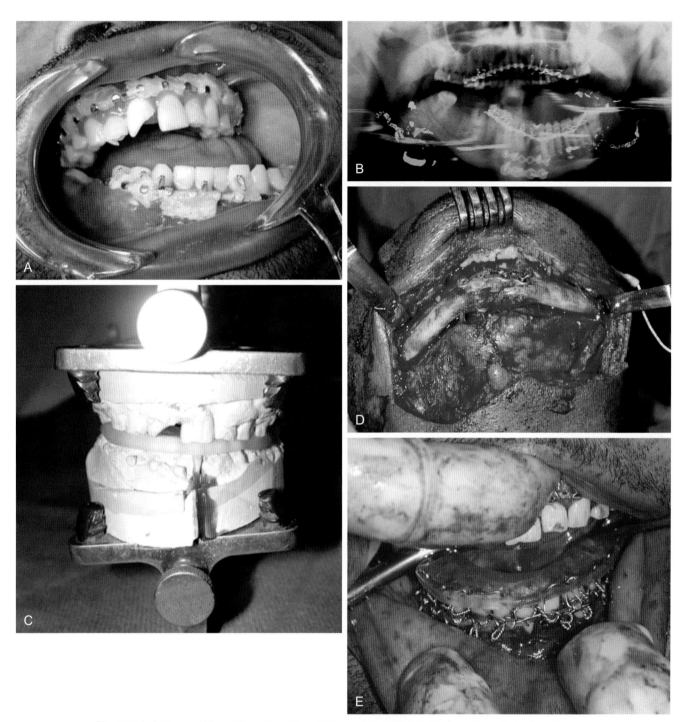

Fig. 1.16.3 A 31-year-old man 3 weeks status post gunshot wound to the face. He had significant hemorrhage and required embolization of his lingual arteries. Arch bars were applied following OIF of his symphysis, planning to reduce the bilateral angle fractures closed. It was not possible to bring his teeth into occlusion with elastics so he was referred for definitive treatment. (A) X-ray demonstrating presenting occlusion. (B) Panoramic X-ray. Note coils from embolization. Molds of his teeth were made, sectioned, and reassembled into correct occlusion. A splint was fabricated. (C) Mounted, sectioned models with splint. (D) Fractures exposed through neck. Note OIF of symphysis fracture. The left angle was draining pus. (E) Acrylic splint fixed to mandibular teeth confirming correct alignment.   *Continued*

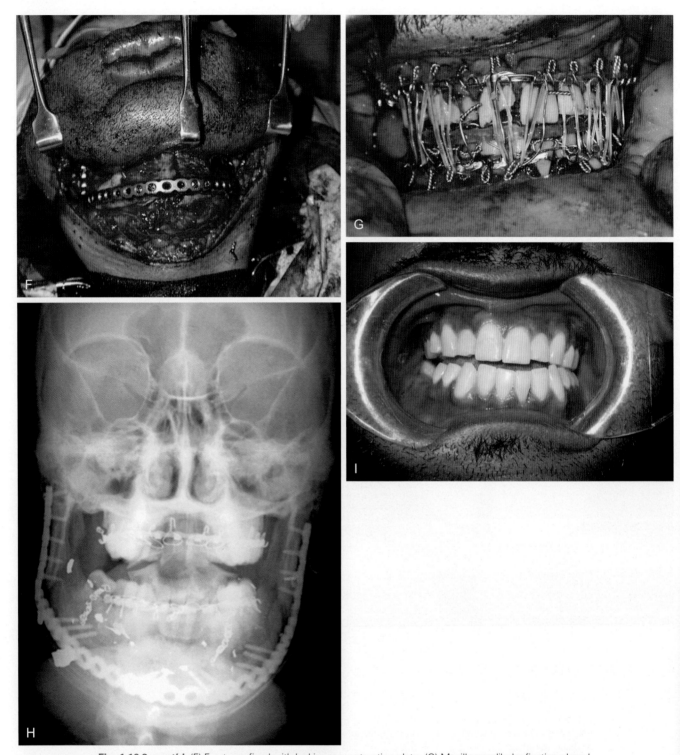

Fig. 1.16.3, cont'd (F) Fractures fixed with locking reconstruction plate. (G) Maxillomandibular fixation placed. (H) Postoperative X-ray. (I) Postoperative occlusion. Note slight anterior open-bite later corrected with a Le Fort I osteotomy.

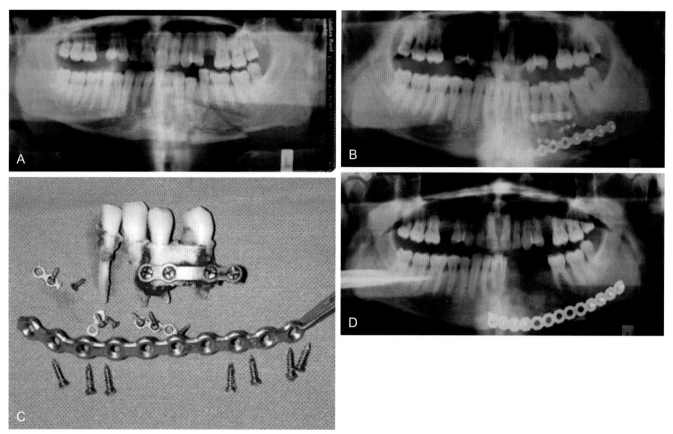

Fig. 1.16.4 Comminuted parasymphysis fracture inadequately managed with a combination of miniplates and a 2.0 locking plate. (A) Preoperative panoramic X-ray. (B) Post reduction panoramic X-ray. (C) Debrided failed fixation, bone, and teeth. (D) Postoperative panoramic X-ray. (Courtesy Dr. Mark Engelstad.)

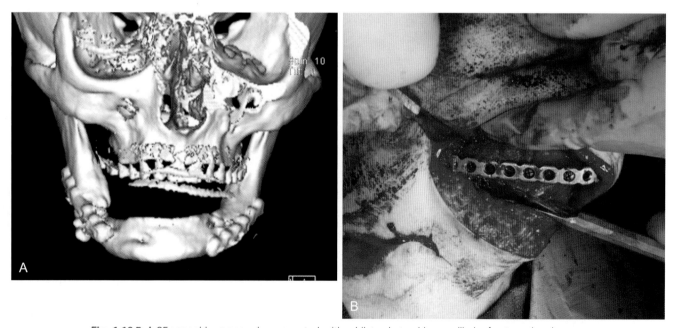

Fig. 1.16.5 A 35-year-old woman who presented with a bilateral atrophic mandibular fracture already operated twice. It was first fixed with miniplates, later with two plates on each fracture. Both fractures were mobile. (A) CT of failed fixation. (B–C) Fracture sites grafted.   *Continued*

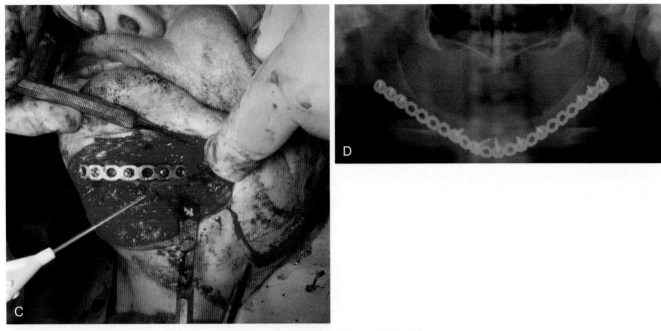

Fig. 1.16.5, cont'd (D) Postoperative X-ray.

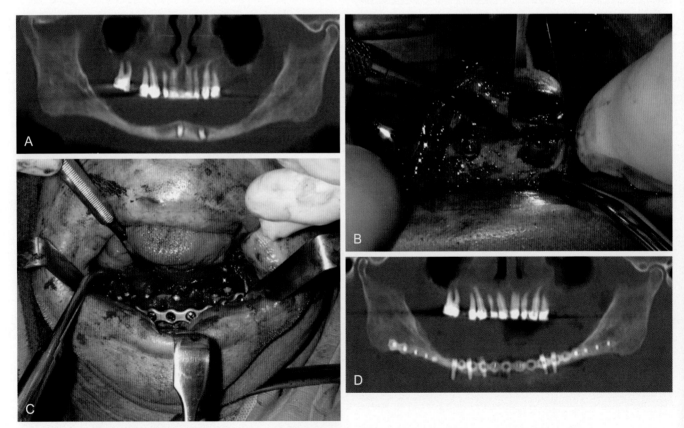

Fig. 1.16.6 A 71-year-old man with pathological fracture of his atrophic mandible secondary to failing dental implants. The treatment plan called for removal of the implants, RIF of the mandible with a 2.0 locking plate, bone graft, and new implants through a transoral approach. (A) Atrophic mandible. (B) Exposure of failing implants. (C) Application of 2.0 plate, implants, and particulate bone graft. (D) Panoramic radiograph.

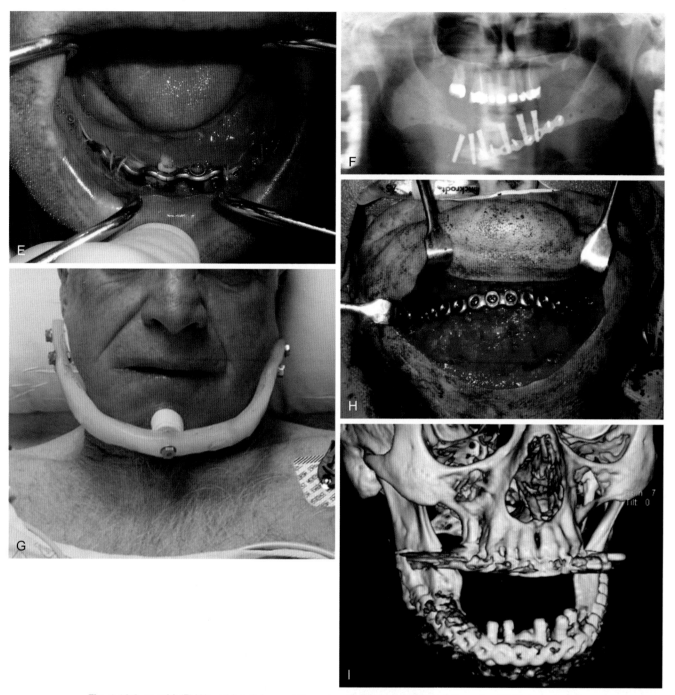

Fig. 1.16.6, cont'd (E) Wound breakdown at 2 weeks. (F) Fracture of plate at 6 weeks. (G) Plate removed, external fixator applied. (H) Following healing of oral wound, external fixator removed and larger locking reconstruction plate applied through neck with additional bone graft. (I) 3D CT. Note dental implants still in place and functional.

Continued

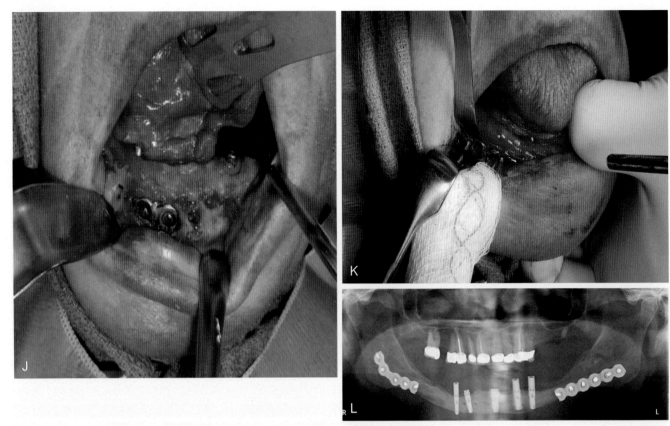

Fig. 1.16.6, cont'd (J) Four years later, patient returns with exposed plate intraorally. (K) Plate further exposed surgically, sectioned on either side, and removed. (L) Post-removal X-ray.

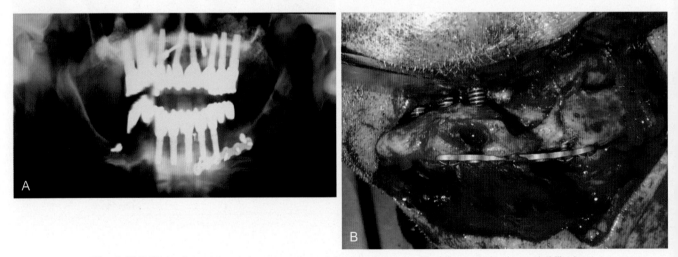

Fig. 1.16.7 Bilateral condylar and parasymphyseal fracture in man with full-mouth implant rehabilitation managed with MMF screws and locking miniplate for parasymphyseal fracture. Parasymphysis plate failed with loss of the dental implant. (A) Image of failing construct. (B) Simplification with inferior border miniplate.

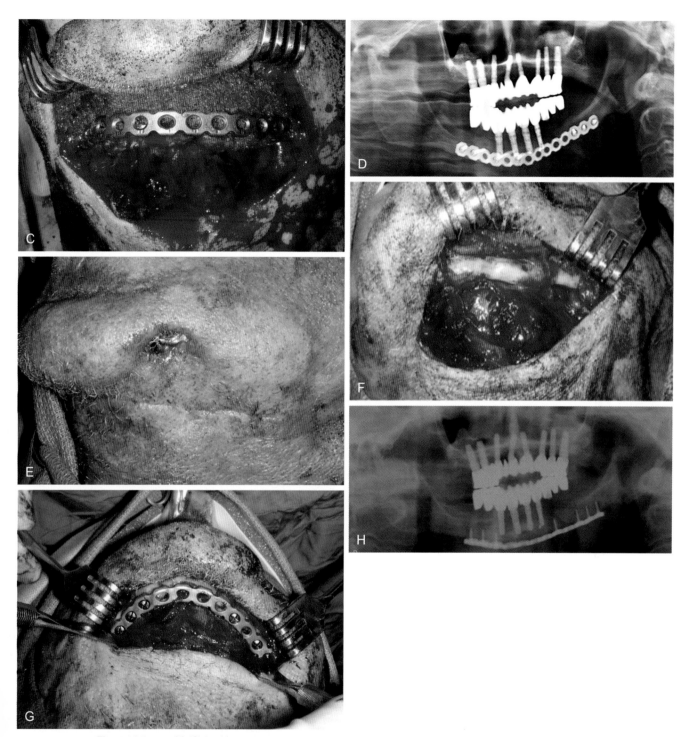

Fig. 1.16.7, cont'd (C) Locking reconstruction plate and tibial bone graft. (D) Image of construct. (E) Patient returns 4 years later with exposed hardware. (F) Plate removed, nonunion discovered. (G) Locking reconstruction plate placed over inferior border to allow closure. (H) Image of construct.

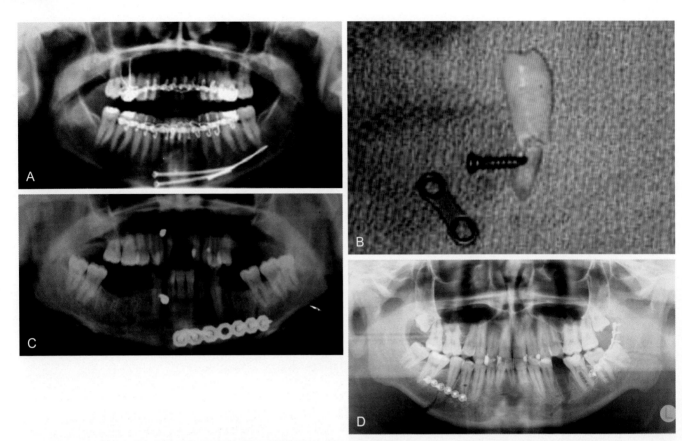

Fig. 1.16.8 Surgical misadventures. (A) Broken drill in mandibular medullary spaces lost during attempted lag screw placement. (B) Tooth root pithed and fractured during attempted screw placement. (C) MMF screws placed into tooth roots. (D) Root pithed from MMF screw.

operator error was the number one cause of mandibular fracture complications. Quite obviously, RIF is very unforgiving. When done poorly, one has a rigidly fixed mistake. The latest series of misadventures are related to the use of IMF screws. Bone-anchored arch bars will most likely be next. Not all believe that RIF and convalescent function is cost-effective with respect to the increased cost, potential for complications, and patient acceptance.[12]

INCIDENCE OF COMPLICATIONS

As has been noted, this largely depends on what one considers a complication. Some feel that minor complications – loss of teeth, exposure of hardware, exfoliation of bone and modest delay to union – do not count, so long as union and some semblance of functional occlusion is achieved. Others consider complications to include anything that delays union or results in a suboptimal result. For example, transoral miniplate fixation of angle fractures has a 22% *minor* complication rate – exposure of hardware, loose screws, wound dehiscence – which can be simply managed in an office setting and do not affect the final outcome. The same treatment has a low (2%) *major* complication rate requiring return to the OR and major surgery in the form of application of additional RIF and/or bone graft.[13]

Quite obviously, complications can depend on the one evaluating them. If that individual only considers union as an outcome, other complications will not be recognized.

It should be noted that studies involving complications of mandibular fractures are difficult to compare since some areas of the mandible are more prone to complications than others. Open fractures of the angle involving a tooth are most prone whereas closed fractures outside

the tooth-bearing area are least prone. Other areas fall in between. In large series, all areas are included so the incidence may vary dramatically. Indeed, infection rates for ORIF of mandibular fractures have been reported to range from 3% to 30%.[7,13–25] The most meaningful studies of the incidence of complications for varying treatments of mandibular fractures have been the angle fracture studies done by Ellis and coworkers.[13,15–18,22,25] They compared different specific treatments of these fractures with comparable patient populations and similar surgical teams. As such, they compared "apples to apples vs. apples to oranges vs. considering all to be fruit." These studies have clearly defined the incidence of complications of mandibular angle fractures with varying treatments.

ETIOLOGIC FACTORS IN MANDIBULAR FRACTURE COMPLICATIONS

Multiple authors note an increased incidence of complications in the immunocompromised, i.e., diabetics, patients with AIDS, etc.[26–29] substance abusers,[28,30–36] and smokers.[31,37,38] This has certainly been our almost-50-year experience. Delay in treatment has been studied extensively and not found to be a factor in the development of complications.[31,36–42] One condition that seems to overshadow all of these other factors is the severity of the fracture(s). *The more complex the injury, the more likely there will be complications.*[26,27,31,38,43–45]

Role of Antibiotics in Preventing Infective Complications

Antibiotic coverage during convalescence has not made any difference in the emergence of infections.[30,31,37,46] Mandibular fractures in the tooth-bearing area, which are open by definition, are covered with antibiotics from the time they are seen and evaluated. This coverage along with intraoperative intravenous antibiotics seems to be the general standard today. Many surgeons have substituted chlorhexidine rinses for oral antibiotics in the postoperative period.

INFECTION, DELAYED, NON- AND MALUNION, HARDWARE EXPOSURE, HARDWARE FAILURE

Infection

Osteomyelitis is properly defined as an inflammation of bone and marrow with a tendency to progression. In the mandible it would be characterized by chills, fever, leukocytosis, adenopathy, paresthesia, malaise, and a moth-eaten appearance on X-ray. Infected fractures are not osteomyelitis in the true sense. There are no chills, fever or leukocytosis. Dead bone, sequestration, and drainage does not make an osteomyelitis. In Europe, they use the term "osteitis."

Infected fractures result from inadequate fixation of an already contaminated open fracture. (Closed fractures, even those managed with ORIF, rarely become infected.) Historically, infected fractures were managed by removing associated teeth (which helped), placing the patient on antibiotics (which did nothing) and waiting for radiographic evidence of sequestrum formation (generally following 3 or 4 weeks of drainage). At that time, the fracture site was debrided of dead bone – and hardware or wire if present. MMF was continued. One waited for 2 or 3 months following the cessation of drainage before grafting the area – obviously a long course of treatment. Over the years we learned that antibiotics did nothing. Only removal of the etiology – dead bone, dead tooth, loose hardware – and rigid splinting would end the drainage (Fig. 1.16.9).

This protocol involved removal of involved teeth, if any, replacing inadequate (failed) fixation with new fixation in the form a larger, longer plate with better anchorage (three screws on either side of the defect) or stable skeletal pin fixation. Thus, infected fractures, treated or untreated, are managed by removal of involved teeth, debridement of nonviable bone, removal of loose hardware, if present, and application of more adequate fixation.[9,47–52] Today this would likely be a locking reconstruction plate (LRP), an "internal fixator," well anchored with at least three screws on either side of the fracture (Figs. 1.16.4, 1.16.10, 1.16.11).

When debridement results in a defect between the bone ends, a bone graft is necessary, as with rigid fixation there is no micromovement to stimulate bone formation. There is no need to delay bone grafting. *Bone grafting can be done even with fractures draining purulence.* The modern protocol of removal of failed fixation, debridement, and application of an internal fixator (reconstruction plate) plus bone graft works,[53] irrespective of the approach – intraoral (Fig. 1.16.11) or extraoral (Figs. 1.16.3 and 1.16.10) – and the patient is functional during the entire period of convalescence. The graft of choice is particulate marrow from the tibia or hip. If a portion becomes exposed through wound breakdown, a few flakes may be lost. With a block, which becomes exposed, one may lose the entire graft. This has been one of the most significant advances in infected fracture care and has stood the test of time.

Delayed union and nonunion are managed similarly: debridement if necessary and a definitive internal fixator, with bone graft if there is no contact between the ends (Fig. 1.16.12).

Teeth in the Line of Fracture

As previously noted, teeth involved in infected fractures are removed. Indeed, this is the first thing one should consider with an infected mandibular fracture. If the tooth is loose, has associated drainage, or if roots are surrounded by radiolucency on X-ray, it is removed.

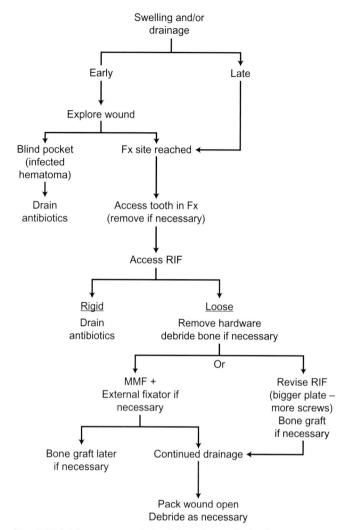

Fig. 1.16.9 Management of the infected mandibular fracture treated with RIF.

The question still arises regarding the advisability of removing all teeth in the line of fractures prophylactically. Numerous studies over the past 50 years have demonstrated that one *does not* decrease morbidity by removing a sound tooth in the line of fracture.[41,54] One removes teeth that interfere with reduction or, by virtue of existing disease (periodontal, periapical, etc.), would be removed anyway. Sound teeth generally assist in the reduction and serve to minimize the defect at the fracture site.

Malunion

Malunion is one of the more common complications of mandibular fractures today. The etiology is usually operator error or inability to achieve proper reduction (Figs. 1.16.1–1.16.3, 1.16.13), although it sometimes occurs in properly managed fractures (Fig. 1.16.12). This commonly results in an acquired malocclusion – the patient's teeth do not come together as before – and/or loss of facial form. Midline deviation, prominence or loss of mandibular angle definition, tilted occlusal plane, etc. may also be manifestations of malunion. *The treatment is not necessarily based on the site(s) of deformity but where best corrected.* The patient should be approached and worked up as for any dentofacial deformity (DFD), with correction done with standard approaches.

Text continued on p. 216

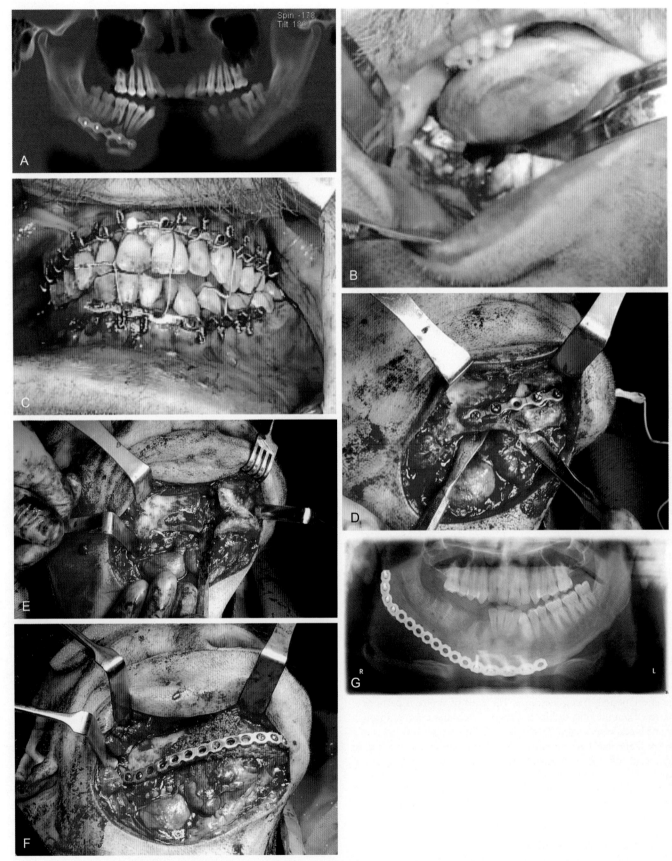

Fig. 1.16.10 A 29-year-old man with bilateral mandibular fracture managed elsewhere one year ago. He has been draining through the neck wound for 2 months, his teeth are loose, and the jaw is mobile. He was managed with debridement of the failed fixation and dead bone, application of a heavy locking reconstruction plate (LRP), and tibial bone graft. He healed uneventfully. (A) Image of failed fixation. (B) Involved teeth removed, oral mucosa closed. (C) MMF placed. (D) Failed fixation. (E) Defect following debridement. (F) LRP plus tibial bone graft. (G) Image of healed reconstruction.

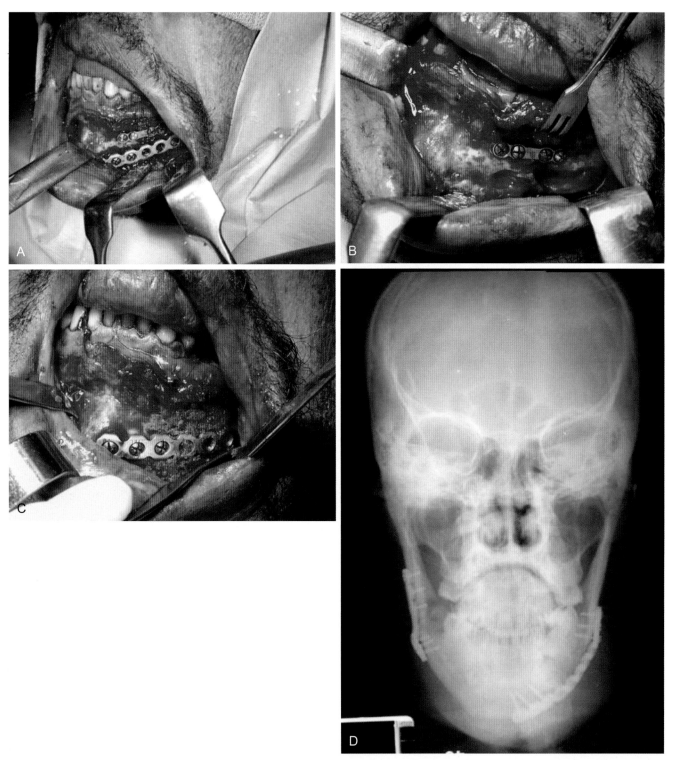

Fig. 1.16.11 Infected parasymphyseal fracture 7 weeks post ORIF with reconstruction plate and 2.0 tension band. The wound was draining intraorally and both plates were floating in granulation tissue. (A) Loose plates. (B) Reconstruction plate lifted off. Note defect. (C) Larger LRP applied and defect grafted with tibial bone graft. (D) PA radiograph of reconstruction.

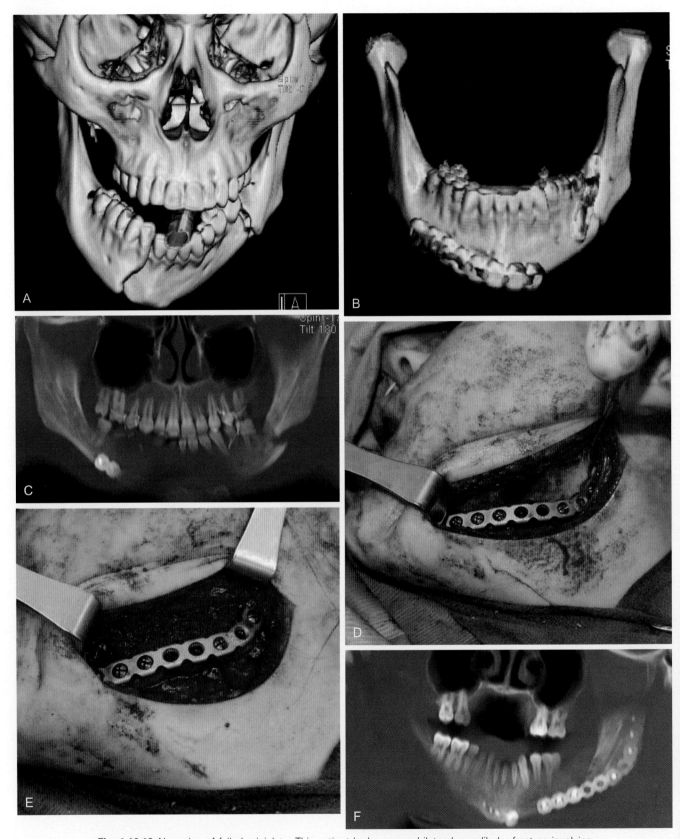

Fig. 1.16.12 Nonunion of failed miniplate. This patient had a severe bilateral mandibular fracture involving the right parasymphysis and left angle. Both were managed intraorally with a locking reconstruction plate on the parasymphysis and a "Champy style" miniplate on the angle. (A) Preoperative 3D CT. (B) Postoperative 3D CT. The patient returned 10 weeks later with swelling and intraoral drainage over the left angle. The miniplate, which had fractured, was removed. MMF was applied with IV loops. She returned 2 weeks later demanding the MMF be released. (C) CT-generated panoramic view demonstrating displacement of left angle. (D) Application of LRP. (E) Defect grafted. (F) CT of reconstruction.

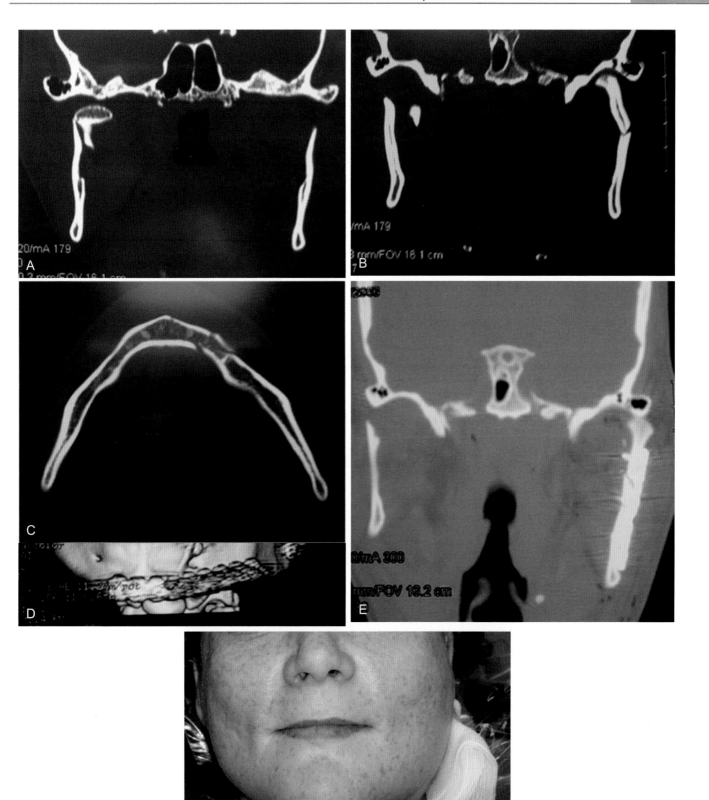

Fig. 1.16.13 Facial widening secondary to malreduction of a bilateral condylar and parasymphyseal fracture. (A–C) CTs demonstrating bilateral condyles and parasymphysis fracture. (D–E) Postoperative images. Note condyle laterally displaced. (F) Note prominent left angle in clinical photo.

There are some specific fracture patterns that are prone to malunion, with malocclusion and loss of facial form. These are bilateral condylar fractures (acquired retrognathia and/or open-bite) and bilateral condylar fractures with a symphyseal fracture, commonly known as the "guardsman fracture" (facial widening).

Hardware Exposure

Hardware exposure can be a simple or difficult problem depending on location and, most importantly, what is the condition of the bone

(fracture) underneath. As previously noted, with transorally placed miniplates used in the management of angle fractures, exposure and screw loosening is quite common yet the fracture is generally healed underneath, even after 2 or 3 weeks. Plate exposure in the symphyseal region following transoral approach will often granulate over with irrigations and proper hygiene. If it does not, it must be removed to allow healing (Fig. 1.16.6). If the fracture is unstable, alternative fixation – MMF, placing alternative internal fixation, skeletal pins, K-wire, etc. – is required (Figs. 1.16.6, 1.16.7, 1.16.14). Advancing flaps to cover

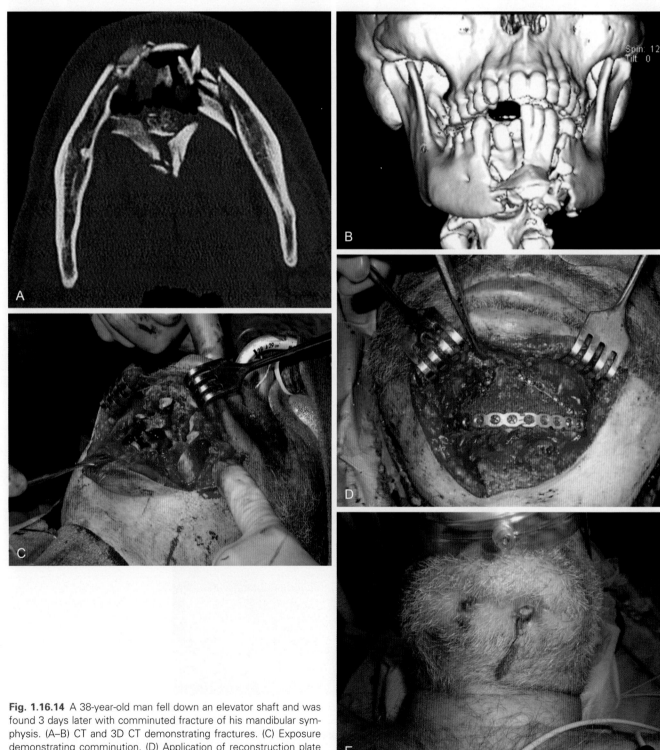

Fig. 1.16.14 A 38-year-old man fell down an elevator shaft and was found 3 days later with comminuted fracture of his mandibular symphysis. (A–B) CT and 3D CT demonstrating fractures. (C) Exposure demonstrating comminution. (D) Application of reconstruction plate and primary bone graft. (E) Wound breakdown at 7 weeks.

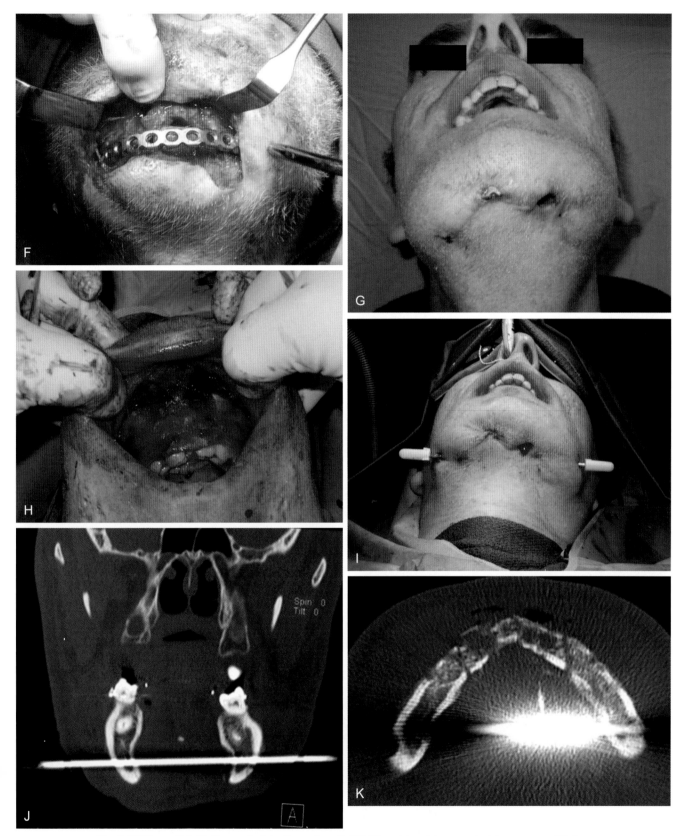

Fig. 1.16.14, cont'd (F) Removal of teeth, and graft. (G) Wound breakdown and plate exposure 16 days later. (H) Removal of LRP. (I) Application of heavy "K-wire" across mandibular bodies. (J–K) CTs of construct.

a plate exposed in the mouth is an exercise in futility. If it does not granulate over spontaneously it must be removed. External exposure is another story. Again, if the bone is healed underneath, simply remove the hardware, freshen the wound edges adjacent to the exposure and close it. If the plate is still needed, the conservative approach would be to place the patient in MMF and apply an external fixator if necessary. Following soft tissue healing, the plate and screws could be reapplied if necessary – generally longer, heavier, and with more screws for anchorage.

We have had limited success with opening the area widely, removing the plate and screws, scrubbing and resterilizing them and placing them back on the mandible if the construct was stable and no screws were loose. An appropriate local flap would be advanced to close the wound and cover the hardware (Fig. 1.16.15). We have also had success with replacing the plate with one of a different configuration and advancing a local flap to cover it (Fig. 1.16.7).

Hardware Failure

When first introduced to the theory and practice of rigid internal fixation it was stressed that there was a race between hardware failure – loosening of the screws and/or fracture of the plate – and the achievement

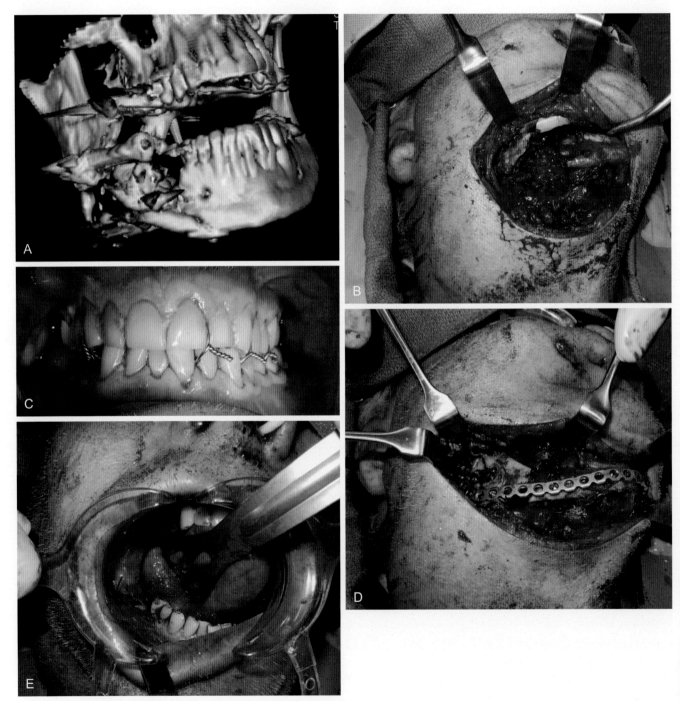

Fig. 1.16.15 A 63-year-old man sustained a gunshot wound to the face resulting in a comminuted fracture of the mandible. (A) 3D CT demonstrating comminuted fracture. (B) Fracture exposed. (C) MMF with embrasure wires. (D) ORIF with locking reconstruction plate.

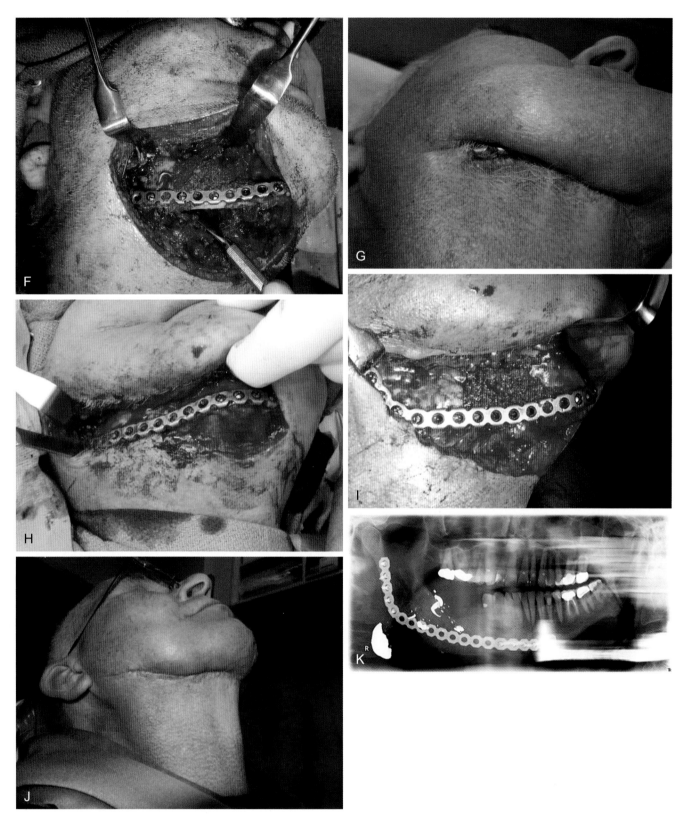

Fig. 1.16.15, cont'd (E) Intraoral closure. (F) Bone graft to defect. (G) Plate dehiscence at 8 weeks. (H) Wound reopened, defect noted. (I) Plate reapplied, defect regrafted. (J) Healed neck wound. (K) Postoperative panoramic X-ray.

of union. If the construct was properly selected and applied, union would win the race. This concept is still valid and must be considered when an internal fixation scheme fails. Was the plate of adequate size for the task? Was the screw anchorage appropriate? Was it properly applied? Obviously, not all hardware failure is iatrogenic. Properly executed RIF occasionally fails (Figs. 1.16.11 and 1.16.12).

Hardware failure is managed by treating the result of the hardware failure – infection, delayed or non-union – by removing the failed fixation and applying a larger, stronger, better anchored internal fixation device, debriding the area and doing a primary reconstruction by grafting if necessary[9,47–53] (Figs. 1.16.5, 1.16.7, 1.16.10–1.16.12). Alternatively, MMF and/or an external fixator can be applied and the area allowed to "dry up" with reconstruction later (Figs. 1.16.6, 1.16.14).

PARESTHESIA/PARESIS

Paresthesia in the mental nerve distribution commonly occurs with fractures of the angle and body region when the inferior alveolar canal is disrupted. Sensation generally returns but not always. In rare cases, painful dysesthesia remains.[55] Further, when fractures of the symphysis and parasymphysis are exposed through the transoral approach, there will often be temporary paresthesia – days, weeks, even months (from stretching of the neurovascular bundle). It is important to document any paresthesias or paresis preoperatively so the surgeon is not blamed. Temporary or permanent paresis of the marginal mandibular nerve is a complication of submandibular and retromandibular surgical approaches for ORIF.

COMPLICATIONS OF CONDYLAR FRACTURES

Malocclusion is perhaps the most common long-term complication of condylar fractures. Closed treatment (brief periods of MMF followed by physiotherapy and training elastics) generally avoids the problem. When it has occurred, DFD work-up and correction is indicated. Trismus (inadequate opening) is a sequela particularly following treatment with MMF. If mouth stretching with opening appliances (Therabite) is unsuccessful, forced opening under anesthesia, often supplemented with bilateral transoral coronoidectomy, gains the necessary opening, which can be maintained with exercise. The procedure essentially lengthens the temporalis muscle attachment allowing full opening.

Ankylosis of the temporomandibular joint following condylar fractures is a rare complication in the developed world. It generally happens when there has been splaying of the mandible at a symphysis or parasymphysis fracture allowing contact of the distal edge of an intracapsular condylar fracture with the articular surface of the arch. It may also be seen following prolonged periods of maxillomandibular fixation with intracapsular fractures (Fig. 1.16.16). Avoidance of these is related to both proper reduction of associated fractures and early and vigorous function.

The management of ankylosis of the temporomandibular joint is beyond the scope of this chapter, however custom total joint prostheses fabricated on stereolithic models are currently in vogue and appear to give more predictable results than traditional gap or intrapositional arthroplasty or costochondral grafting.

PATIENT NONCOMPLIANCE

Noncompliance has been a historic excuse for treatment failure and complications. In the days prior to RIF, when MMF was an integral part of mandibular fracture care, cutting oneself out of MMF would occasionally lead to complications. Today, failure to follow soft diet instructions with miniplate, semi-rigid fixation of a mandibular fracture

would be an obvious cause of hardware failure. Failure in this case was caused by inadequate fixation for that particular patient. One has to select an appropriate technique for that patient. Obviously, there is a difference between the middle class woman with a minimally displaced angle fracture and the "warrior" who sustains a similar injury in a fight. One has to consider "screwing in the compliance" with fixation which will be adequate for that particular individual.[34] Failure from too much fixation is a rare occurrence indeed. Failure from not enough fixation is common.

Noncompliance can be most significant with condylar fractures – those injuries and their treatment producing trismus. If the patient does not exercise and stretch their opening muscles of mastication, they tend to experience limited opening which is a significant problem. RIF with convalescent function as opposed to prolonged periods of MMF has done much to limit this restricted opening, and noncompliance in doing jaw opening exercises is a significant problem.

There are devices to assist rehabilitation of opening, such as the Therabite, tongue blades, Molt mouth props, etc., but the patient has to be diligent and work hard. Close supervision is mandatory with announced weekly goals for interincisal opening. Examination under anesthesia and forced opening is sometimes necessary to at least see what can be achieved with exercise and effort. Occasionally, bilateral coronoidectomies will release the restriction. This maneuver seems to lengthen the temporalis muscle attachments, allowing further opening and a "fresh start" and goal for opening exercises.

CONCLUSION

RIF has revolutionized craniomaxillofacial surgery by both fixing skeletal structures in their proper positions (not possible with non-rigid techniques) and allowing for convalescent function. It has allowed the surgeon to achieve more optimal results when managing complex mandibular fractures that were not possible before RIF. With the management of these complex injuries come complications that are inherent to the complex injury as well as the treatment. Management of these complications should likewise be facilitated by RIF. There is much truth in the statement that the treatment of failed RIF is a bigger plate and more screws.

EXPERT COMMENTARY

This chapter is one of the finest of its type, providing seasoned, relevant information based on a half-century of consistent experience. The most common mistakes by non-oral surgeons are poor, unstable application of arch bars, and faulty application of IMF devices, leading to instability and failure to establish the preinjury occlusion. In difficult cases, dental models are helpful. Next, not realizing the complex 3-dimensional anatomy of the fracture/not appreciating areas of comminution, which lead to instability, as fixation must be several good screws in both directions beyond the fractured area. In complex, multiple fractures, fixation should be strong enough to hold the mandible in the specific shape of its normal architecture, not just hold the ends of the bone in approximation. Finally, secure suturing techniques such as layers of non-absorbable sutures (interrupted + running lock) to prevent dehiscence in intraoral incisions/lacerations minimizes wound separation. Be aware of the "promise" of soft tissue integrity from absorbable sutures, especially chromic, and do not hesitate to use non-absorbable sutures. Don Tilghman taught me to use interrupted permanent and running permanent locked sutures together when I was really concerned about a wound or incision staying together intraorally. I would take them out after mandibular and soft tissue healing. My strong recommendation is that rest initially is always more important than too early mobilization.

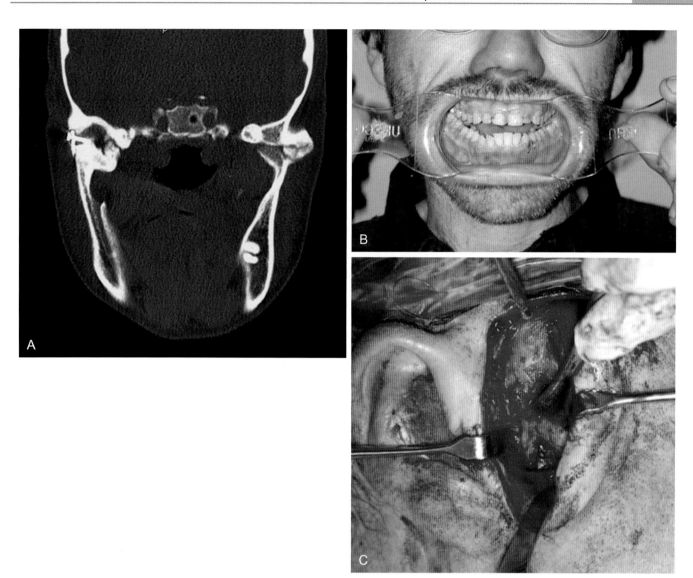

Fig. 1.16.16 TMJ ankylosis secondary to inadequate ORIF of condylar fracture followed by 9 weeks of MMF. (A) CTs of bilateral TMJ ankylosis. Note screw in right joint. (B) Maximal opening. (C) Note screw in joint.

REFERENCES

1. Gunning T. Treatment of fracture of the lower jaw by interdental splints: I–III. *Am J Dent Sci.* 1868;2:214–220.
2. Lattimer JK, Bartlett CE, Humphrey WM. An historic case of jaw fracture. *J Am Dent Assoc.* 1968;76(1):102–106.
3. Pollock RA. Management of jaw injuries in the American Civil War: the diuturnity of Bean in the South, Gunning in the North. *Craniomaxillofac Trauma Reconstr.* 2011;4(2):85–90.
4. Gilmer T. A case of fracture of the lower jaw with remarks on treatment. *Arch Dent.* 1887;4:388–390.
5. Converse JM, Waknitz FW. External skeletal fixation in fractures of the mandibular angle. *J Bone Joint Surg.* 1942;24(1):154–160.
6. Kazanjian V, Converse JM. Fractures of the mandible. In: *The Surgical Treatment of Facial Injuries*. London: Bailliere, Tindall and Cox; 1949:85–145.
7. Wagner WF, Neal DC, Alpert B. Morbidity associated with extraoral open reduction of mandibular fractures. *J Oral Surg (Am Dent Assoc 1965).* 1979;37(2):97–100.
8. Seemann R, Perisanidis C, Schicho K, et al. Complication rates of operatively treated mandibular fractures – the mandibular neck. *Oral Surg Oral Med Oral Pathol Oral Radiol Endod.* 2010;109(6):815–819.
9. Spiessl B. *Internal Fixation of the Mandible. Adherence of AO/ASIF Principles*. Berlin: Springer; 1989.
10. Luhr H. *Compression Plate Osteosynthesis Through the Luhr System. Oral Maxillofac Traumatol*. Chicago, IL: Quintessence; 1982:319–347.
11. Champy M, Pape HD, Gerlach KL, Lodde JP. The Strasbourg miniplate osteosynthesis. In: Kruger E, Schilli W, eds. *Oral and maxillofacial traumatology*. Vol. 2. Chicago, IL: Quintessence; 1986:19–43.
12. Shetty V, Atchison K, Leathers R, et al. Do the benefits of rigid internal fixation of mandible fractures justify the added costs? Results from a randomized controlled trial. *J Oral Maxillofac Surg.* 2008;66(11):2203–2212.
13. Ellis E 3rd, Walker LR. Treatment of mandibular angle fractures using one noncompression miniplate. *J Oral Maxillofac Surg.* 1996;54(7):864–871, discussion 871–872.
14. Anderson T, Alpert B. Experience with rigid fixation of mandibular fractures and immediate function. *J Oral Maxillofac Surg.* 1992;50(6):555–560, discussion 560–561.
15. Ellis E 3rd. Treatment of mandibular angle fractures using the AO reconstruction plate. *J Oral Maxillofac Surg.* 1993;51(3):250–254, discussion 255.
16. Ellis E 3rd, Ghali GE. Lag screw fixation of mandibular angle fractures. *J Oral Maxillofac Surg.* 1991;49(3):234–243.

17. Ellis E 3rd, Karas N. Treatment of mandibular angle fractures using two mini dynamic compression plates. *J Oral Maxillofac Surg.* 1992;50(9):958–963.

18. Ellis E 3rd, Sinn DP. Treatment of mandibular angle fractures using two 2.4-mm dynamic compression plates. *J Oral Maxillofac Surg.* 1993;51(9):969–973.

19. Iizuka T, Lindqvist C, Hallikainen D, Paukku P. Infection after rigid internal fixation of mandibular fractures: a clinical and radiologic study. *J Oral Maxillofac Surg.* 1991;49(6):585–593.

20. Kearns GJ, Perrott DH, Kaban LB. Rigid fixation of mandibular fractures: does operator experience reduce complications? *J Oral Maxillofac Surg.* 1994;52(3):226–231, discussion 231–232.

21. Lazow SK. A mandible fracture protocol. *J Oral Maxillofac Surg.* 2002;60(1):133–134.

22. Passeri LA, Ellis E 3rd, Sinn DP. Complications of nonrigid fixation of mandibular angle fractures. *J Oral Maxillofac Surg.* 1993;51(4):382–384.

23. Reinhart E, Reuther J, Michel C, et al. [Treatment outcome and complications of surgical and conservative management of mandibular fractures]. *Fortschr Kiefer Gesichtschir.* 1996;41:64–67.

24. Tu HK, Tenhulzen D. Compression osteosynthesis of mandibular fractures: a retrospective study. *J Oral Maxillofac Surg.* 1985;43(8):585–589.

25. Ellis E 3rd, Walker L. Treatment of mandibular angle fractures using two noncompression miniplates. *J Oral Maxillofac Surg.* 1994;52(10):1032–1036, discussion 1036–1037.

26. Gordon PE, Lawler ME, Kaban LB, Dodson TB. Mandibular fracture severity and patient health status are associated with postoperative inflammatory complications. *J Oral Maxillofac Surg.* 2011;69(8):2191–2197.

27. Malanchuk VO, Kopchak AV. Risk factors for development of infection in patients with mandibular fractures located in the tooth-bearing area. *J Craniomaxillofac Surg.* 2007;35(1):57–62.

28. Senel FC, Jessen GS, Melo MD, Obeid G. Infection following treatment of mandible fractures: the role of immunosuppression and polysubstance abuse. *Oral Surg Oral Med Oral Pathol Oral Radiol Endod.* 2007;103(1):38–42.

29. Ward NH 3rd, Wainwright DJ. Outcomes research: mandibular fractures in the diabetic population. *J Craniomaxillofac Surg.* 2016;44(7):763–769.

30. Domingo F, Dale E, Gao C, et al. A single-center retrospective review of post-operative infectious complications in the surgical management of mandibular fractures: post-operative antibiotics add no benefit. *J Trauma Acute Care Surg.* 2016;81(6):1109–1114.

31. Furr AM, Schweinfurth JM, May WL. Factors associated with long-term complications after repair of mandibular fractures. *Laryngoscope.* 2006;116(3):427–430.

32. Lamphier J, Ziccardi V, Ruvo A, Janel M. Complications of mandibular fractures in an urban teaching center. *J Oral Maxillofac Surg.* 2003;61(7):745–749, discussion 749–750.

33. Passeri LA, Ellis E 3rd, Sinn DP. Relationship of substance abuse to complications with mandibular fractures. *J Oral Maxillofac Surg.* 1993;51(1):22–25.

34. Schiel H, Hammer B, Ehrenfeld M, Prein J. [Therapy of infected mandibular fractures]. *Fortschr Kiefer Gesichts Chirurg.* 1996;41:170–173.

35. Serena-Gomez E, Passeri LA. Complications of mandible fractures related to substance abuse. *J Oral Maxillofac Surg.* 2008;66(10):2028–2034.

36. Webb LS, Makhijani S, Khanna M, et al. A comparison of outcomes between immediate and delayed repair of mandibular fractures. *Canad J Plast Surg.* 2009;17(4):124–126.

37. Gutta R, Tracy K, Johnson C, et al. Outcomes of mandible fracture treatment at an academic tertiary hospital: a 5-year analysis. *J Oral Maxillofac Surg.* 2014;72(3):550–558.

38. Odom EB, Snyder-Warwick AK. Mandible fracture complications and infection: the influence of demographics and modifiable factors. *Plast Reconstr Surg.* 2016;138(2):282e–289e.

39. Biller JA, Pletcher SD, Goldberg AN, Murr AH. Complications and the time to repair of mandible fractures. *Laryngoscope.* 2005;115(5):769–772.

40. Czerwinski M, Parker WL, Correa JA, Williams HB. Effect of treatment delay on mandibular fracture infection rate. *Plast Reconstr Surg.* 2008;122(3):881–885.

41. Ellis E 3rd. Outcomes of patients with teeth in the line of mandibular angle fractures treated with stable internal fixation. *J Oral Maxillofac Surg.* 2002;60(8):863–865, discussion 866.

42. Lee UK, Rojhani A, Herford AS, Thakker JS. Immediate versus delayed treatment of mandibular fractures: a stratified analysis of complications. *J Oral Maxillofac Surg.* 2016;74(6):1186–1196.

43. Mathog RH, Toma V, Clayman L, Wolf S. Nonunion of the mandible: an analysis of contributing factors. *J Oral Maxillofac Surg.* 2000;58(7):746–752, discussion 752–753.

44. Moreno JC, Fernandez A, Ortiz JA, Montalvo JJ. Complication rates associated with different treatments for mandibular fractures. *J Oral Maxillofac Surg.* 2000;58(3):273–280, discussion 280–281.

45. Munante-Cardenas JL, Facchina Nunes PH, Passeri LA. Etiology, treatment, and complications of mandibular fractures. *J Craniofac Surg.* 2015;26(3):611–615.

46. Schaller B, Soong PL, Zix J, et al. The role of postoperative prophylactic antibiotics in the treatment of facial fractures: a randomized, double-blind, placebo-controlled pilot clinical study. Part 2: Mandibular fractures in 59 patients. *Br J Oral Maxillofac Surg.* 2013;51(8):803–807.

47. Alpert B. Complications in mandibular fracture treatment. In: Manson P, ed. *Cranio-Maxillofacial Trauma: Problems in Plastic and Reconstructive Surgery.* Vol. 1. Philadelphia: Lippincott; 1991:253–289.

48. Alpert B. Management of complications of mandibular fracture treatment. In: Manson P, ed. *Operative Techniques in Plastic and Reconstructive Surgery.* Vol. 4. Philadelphia: Saunders; 1998:325–333.

49. Alpert B. Complications in the treatment of facial trauma. *Oral Maxillofac Clin North Am.* 1999;11(2):255–272.

50. Alpert B, Kushner GM, Tiwana PS. Contemporary management of infected mandibular fractures. *Craniomaxillofac Trauma Reconstr.* 2008;1(1):25–29.

51. Beyer M, Prein J. Management of infection and non-union in mandibular fractures. *Oral Maxillofacial Clin North Am.* 1990;2:187–194.

52. Prein J. *Manual of Internal Fixation in the Cranio-facial Skeleton.* Berlin: Springer-Verlag; 1998.

53. Benson PD, Marshall MK, Engelstad ME, et al. The use of immediate bone grafting in reconstruction of clinically infected mandibular fractures: bone grafts in the presence of pus. *J Oral Maxillofac Surg.* 2006;64(1):122–126.

54. Neal DC, Wagner WF, Alpert B. Morbidity associated with teeth in the line of mandibular fractures. *J Oral Surg (Am Dent Assoc 1965).* 1978;36(11):859–862.

55. Marchena JM, Padwa BL, Kaban LB. Sensory abnormalities associated with mandibular fractures: incidence and natural history. *J Oral Maxillofac Surg.* 1998;56(7):822–825, discussion 825–826.

Temporal Bone Fractures

Heather M. Weinreich, Andrew Lee, John P. Carey

The force required to fracture the temporal bone is substantial and can lead to vascular injury, hearing loss, vertigo or imbalance, facial nerve injury, and cerebral spinal fluid (CSF) leaks. This chapter will discuss the epidemiology of temporal bone trauma, the pathophysiology as well as complications, and current recommendations for management.

BACKGROUND

Incidence

Temporal bone fractures occur in 1%–9% of all head injuries, in 5% of all skull fractures, but in 36% of skull base fractures.[1–3] Fractures are more common in males[4–6] with an average age of 32–41 years in adults[5–7] and 4–7 years in children.[7,8]

ETIOLOGY

Motor vehicle collisions (MVCs) are the primary mechanism of injury, followed by assaults, falls, and gunshot wounds (GSWs).[5,9,10] Falls and violence are making up an increasing proportion of injuries. A recent series found that falls accounted for the majority of injuries,[1] while in another series, violence was estimated to be as high as 70%.[11] Among children, mechanisms include falls, crush or blunt injuries, MVCs, and GSWs.[8]

Approximately 1875 lb of force is required to fracture the temporal bone.[12] Transverse fractures caused by frontal or occipital forces require more energy than longitudinal fractures that occur with lateral force.[13] Fractures associated with GSWs occur at far lower energies (0.3 kJ) than with falls (5 kJ).[13] Damage from a GSW is dependent on the projectile's kinetic energy, the weapon's caliber, and the plasticity of the bullet. Low-velocity projectiles deflect off of bone, leading to non-linear and unpredictable paths, while high-velocity projectiles penetrate bone, leading to crush injuries and cavity formation.

TEMPORAL BONE ANATOMY

The temporal bone consists of the squamous, petrous, tympanic and mastoid portions (Fig. 1.17.1). The squamous portion articulates with the frontal, parietal, and occipital bones to form the lateral skull. The petrous bone is wedge-shaped, extending anteromedially, and contains the otic capsule (OC), carotid canal, and facial nerve. The tympanic ring abuts the petrous portion and is posterior to the mandibular condyle. The mastoid portion contains the vertical facial nerve.

CLINICAL PRESENTATION

History and Physical Examination

A complete head and neck exam is performed to confirm airway stability, neurological status, soft tissue injury, craniofacial fractures, and cranial nerve status. Life-threatening injuries are addressed first. Mortality in these individuals is 10%.[11,14] Almost half report loss of consciousness (LOC)[15] and in children, LOC, altered mental status (AMS), headache, and nausea/vomiting are common findings.[16] Intracranial injuries are seen in up to 79% of temporal bone fractures.[1,2,4,5,17] Common injuries include subdural hematoma[4] and subarachnoid hemorrhage,[1] with 17%–30% of patients requiring surgical neurological intervention.[6,15]

Hemotympanum, hearing loss, vertigo, and nystagmus are strong predictors of temporal bone fractures.[15] Other suggestive findings include external auditory canal (EAC) lacerations, otorrhagia, and tympanic membrane (TM) perforation.[5] Classically, the examiner may appreciate ecchymosis over the mastoid tip ("Battle's sign"), hemotympanum or periorbital ecchymosis ("raccoon eyes").

Otorrhagia is common, and the presence of a "halo sign" (clear fluid ring external to internal blood ring when ear fluid drains onto filter paper) can signal a leak of cerebrospinal fluid (CSF). Significant bleeding can indicate a carotid injury. Prompt packing, imaging, and consultation with vascular surgery, interventional neuroradiology, or neurosurgery are necessary.

Presence of nystagmus can suggest OC trauma. The direction of the nystagmus can provide a clue as to which labyrinth may be affected with nystagmus beating towards the intact ear. Once the patient's C-spine is cleared, head impulse testing to assess semicircular canal function and Dix–Hallpike testing for benign paroxysmal positioning vertigo (BPPV) are performed. Presence of direction changing, pendular, or vertical nystagmus that does not suppress with visual input may suggest central findings and should be further investigated.

As soon as the patient is cooperative, a facial nerve exam should be consistently documented. It is critical that each of the five branches of the facial nerve is examined. Temporal bone fractures generally affect all five branches of the facial nerve, and examination should note the degree of brow elevation, eye closure (minimal and maximal effort), nasal ala flaring/nasolabial fold symmetry, and oral commissure symmetry with efforts at smiling, lip pursing, and frowning.

Hearing Test

Hearing loss is the most common complaint, with up to 80% of patients experiencing it.[14,18,19] A 512 Hz tuning fork exam can distinguish a conductive hearing loss (CHL) from a sensorineural hearing loss (SNHL). An audiogram should be obtained 4–6 weeks following injury.

Radiological Evaluation

Computed tomography (CT) is the best modality for assessing temporal bone fractures (Fig. 1.17.2). Opacification of air cells and pneumocephalus can suggest a fracture. Pneumolabyrinth suggests OC involvement and is found in up to 8% of fractures.[4,5,20] A head, maxillofacial, or cervical CT can detect a fracture without the need for a dedicated

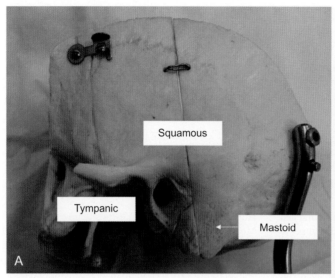
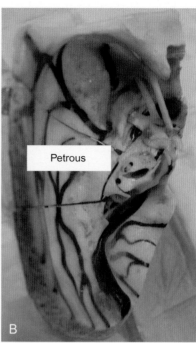

Fig. 1.17.1 Temporal bone. (A) Lateral view. (B) Skull base, superior view.

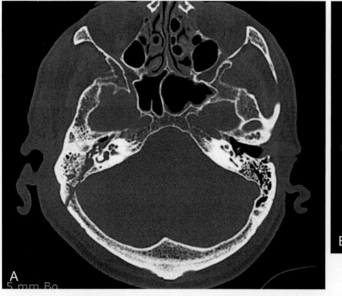
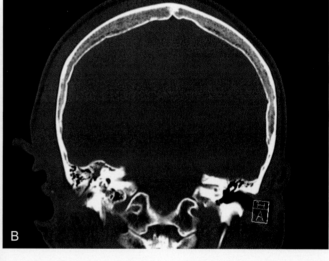

Fig. 1.17.2 (A) Axial CT image of the temporal bone showing right-sided longitudinal fracture through the mastoid resulting in ossicular chain disruptions and opacification within middle ear and mastoid air cells. (B) Coronal CT image of right-sided temporal bone fracture extending through tegmen lateral to the otic capsule.

temporal bone scan. The sensitivity and specificity of a maxillofacial CT scan in cases of blunt head trauma and associated vascular injury are greater than 90% and imply a negative predictive value of >95%.[21] A separate HRCT can add cost, radiation exposure, and time to a work-up without significantly changing management. However, if standard imaging does not show a fracture but physical exam suggests its presence, or if management dictates the superior anatomical information offered by HRCT, then a dedicated temporal bone CT should be obtained. In cases where surgical management is considered or an unreliable clinical exam is present, a HRCT scan provides adjuvant information that changes treatment.

HRCT should include proper filters for bone edge detection and reconstructions from small fields of view with minimal slice thickness (e.g. 0.5 mm) and spacing (ideally 0 mm). Scans obtained with spiral technique or from multidetector scanners using 0.5 mm³ or smaller voxels allow for reconstructions in any plane without loss of resolution. For pediatric patients, low-dose radiation protocols may be used; however, evaluation of small structures may be difficult.[22] The evolution of flat panel CT is a promising development that may offer even higher resolution of bony anatomic detail with lower total radiation dose.[23] No matter the technique used for HRCT, the clinician should review the images and correlate physical findings with imaging (Box 1.17.1).

BOX 1.17.1 Items to Assess on Temporal Bone Imaging

- Location and direction of temporal bone fracture
- Violation of otic capsule: cochlea, vestibule, semicircular canals, vestibular aqueduct
- Ossicular integrity: malleus, incus, stapes
- Facial nerve canal: internal auditory canal, fallopian canal, geniculate fossa, tympanic, mastoid
- Tegmen: tympani, mastoideum
- Vascular: carotid canal (petrous, cavernous), venous sinus (transverse, sigmoid, jugular bulb)

Fractures involving vascular structures should be examined with CT angiography as the stroke rate for carotid artery injury is 31%–33% in this population.[24] Findings include vessel wall irregularity, changes in vessel caliber, abnormal outpouching, and occlusion of a vessel or a contrast blush indicating extravasation of blood. The gold standard is catheter angiography. In a retrospective review, 38% of patients with temporal bone fractures who underwent angiography had abnormal findings, including pseudoaneurysm, carotid dissection, and vasospasm.[9]

CLASSIFICATION OF TEMPORAL BONE FRACTURES

Temporal bone fractures have traditionally been described as transverse, longitudinal, or mixed with respect to the petrous apex. Conceptually, transverse temporal bone fractures have fracture lines that run perpendicular to the long axis of the petrous bone, ending in the foramen magnum. Longitudinal fractures extend anteromedially to end generally in the foramen ovale or foramen lacerum. Roughly 80% of fractures are classified as longitudinal while 20% are transverse.[5,18,20] CHL is more likely in longitudinal fractures while SNHL and facial nerve injuries are more likely in transverse fractures.[18]

With the advent of HRCT, many fractures do not fit precisely into this classical pattern. Two alternative classifications have been proposed – OC sparing (OCS) versus OC violating (OCV)[25] and petrous versus nonpetrous fractures.[26]

OCV fractures involve the labyrinth and can present with SNHL, CSF otorrhea, and facial nerve paralysis. OCV fractures are 7–25 times more likely to develop SNHL, 4–8 times more likely to have a CSF leak, and 2–5 times more likely to develop facial paralysis.[19,27]

Petrous fractures include OC as well facial nerve and carotid injuries. Nonpetrous fractures include injury to the mastoid (bone) and/or tympanic ring with potential damage to the ossicular chain and facial nerve.

MANAGEMENT, SURGICAL INDICATIONS, AND TECHNIQUES

Temporal bone fractures rarely require surgical intervention. Exceptions exist for persistent CHL, facial nerve injury, CSF leaks with or without encephaloceles, and control of hemorrhage. In the acute period, otic drops help clear debris from the EAC. In a systematic review, Villalobos et al. found prophylactic antibiotics did *not* reduce the rate of meningitis in patients with skull base fractures.[28]

Conductive Hearing Loss

CHL can occur in up to 58% of fractures,[14,29] with an estimated 27% in the pediatric population.[16] The most frequent cause of a CHL is hemotympanum. Treatment is observation, with the majority of patients improving to normal or near normal hearing levels.[14,29,30] About 25% of CHL may persist beyond 6 weeks.[18] The majority of traumatic TM

perforations will heal within 3–5 months.[30] In cases of persistent CHL without TM perforation or hearing loss greater than 30 dB, ossicular chain disruption should be considered. Ossicular abnormalities are found in 43% of patient with CHL,[10] and the majority of ossicular pathology is related to the incus.[30]

Hollinger et al.[13] speculate that ossicular disruption is due to a transient deformation of tegmen tympani, pushing the incus inferiorly and tilting the stapes towards the promontory. Disarticulation of the incudostapedial joint and complete dislocation of the incus occurs. In cases of penetrating trauma, Hollinger et al.[13] speculate the pressure wave created by a projectile causes a high frequency vibration within the chain leading to ossicular damage.

Ossicular fracture is more unusual. Tailored multiplanar reconstructions (MPRs) coupled with even higher-resolution techniques like flat-panel CT allow the neuroradiologist and otolaryngologist to visualize the entire ossicular chain to localize damage[31] (Fig. 1.17.3).

Middle ear exploration can be offered in cases of persistent CHL and if hearing is not severely impaired in the contralateral ear. The ideal time to explore is unknown. Early intervention may be premature; however, the longer one waits, the greater likelihood of ossicular chain fixation. Outcomes for surgical repair are good, with most patients improving by 20 dB to near or normal hearing levels.[32]

Cranial Nerve Injury and Facial Nerve Paralysis

Cranial nerves VI, VII, VIII, and the lower cranial nerves including XII, can be injured in temporal bone trauma.[17,33] Cranial nerve injuries can be difficult to assess due to life-threatening injuries and/or AMS. Almost 60% of deficits are documented greater than seven days after injury, with 15% identified more than a month later.[34]

The facial nerve is the most commonly injured nerve, with a reported prevalence of 5%–54%.[10,14,18,35] About 4% are bilateral injuries as a result of bilateral temporal bone fractures.[36]

Contusion, edema, and hematoma of the nerve sheath are found in 86% of fractures with facial paralysis, while frank nerve section is rare.[37] The ganglion and perigeniculate region is the most commonly injured site, followed by the vertical segment.[10,29,30,37]

In GSWs, facial nerve injury rates have been reported to be between 15% up to 75%.[17,33] Mechanical trauma and thermal injury can cause destruction to the nerve.[17] The vertical segment and its exit at the stylomastoid foramen are common sites of injury[17,33] (Fig. 1.17.4).

Timing and Prognosis

About 30% of patients experience immediate paralysis,[5] which may suggest transection or direct injury to the nerve. A delayed onset has a better prognosis, with injury likely from edema or compression.[38] Electrophysiology and imaging have surpassed topographic testing for assessing the nerve and location of injury. Electroneuronography (ENOG) can be performed 72 hours post injury to allow for Wallerian degeneration and can quantify the percentage of functional axons present. If degeneration of >90% of functional axons is seen in the first 2 weeks after injury, surgical decompression may be warranted. Darrouzet et al. stress that usage of electromyography (EMG) has a greater value in traumatic paralysis.[37] ENOG obtained 3 weeks post injury may not show activity; however, activity may be present on the EMG, indicating reinnervation, whereas fibrillation potentials suggest denervation injury.

Treatment

Management of facial paralysis includes observation, steroid treatment, and surgical decompression. Delayed paralysis should be observed, and observation should be strongly considered even in immediate paralysis. Over 90% with delayed paralysis and 75% with immediate paralysis will gain near or complete recovery.[14] In cases of neurapraxia, total

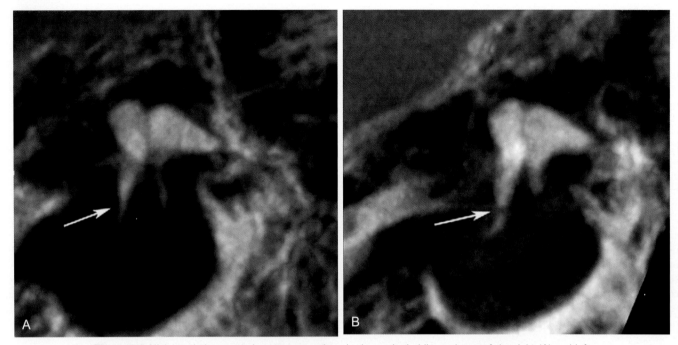

Fig. 1.17.3 High-resolution secondary reconstructions in the sagittal oblique planes of the right (A) and left (B) malleus demonstrate an intact manubrium (*white arrow*) on the right and a fracture of the manubrium (*white arrow*) on the left. (From Tan M, Ullman N, Pearl MS, et al. Fracture of the manubrium of the malleus. Otol Neurotol 2016;37(8):e254–255.)

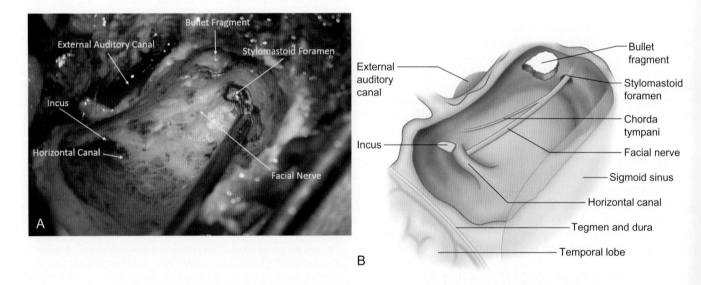

Fig. 1.17.4 Patient with GSW to right temporal bone with resulting facial nerve paralysis. (A) Intraoperative view of bullet fragment involving external auditory canal. Second bullet fragment (not shown) was located at stylomastoid foramen with resulting damage to facial nerve. (B) Illustration of intraoperative view.

recovery should be expected within 5–6 weeks.[37] The indication for steroids is not clear. If risks are low, a trial is reasonable.

Decompression

Frank nerve injury, as with a clear-cut fracture of the fallopian canal having bony fragments impinging on the nerve, may warrant surgical decompression. Most literature supports decompression within 2 weeks of injury,[35] with a few case series reporting good outcomes when performed 3 months out from injury.[39] CT imaging, clinical examination, and electrophysiology are the best tools to determine if surgery is

advisable. MRI can detect ischemia, edema, and presence of an intraneural hematoma.

Approaches to the nerve depend on location of injury and hearing status. The surgeon should be prepared to explore the entire length of the nerve. The middle fossa approach allows for access to the internal auditory canal, labyrinthine segment, and geniculate ganglion, while the transmastoid approach allows access to tympanic and mastoid segments. In cases of complete hearing loss, a translabyrinthine approach may be considered. Removal of all bone with or without opening of the facial nerve sheath with removal of fibrous tissue, bone spicules or hematoma can be performed. The tightest bony constriction around the facial nerve is at the labyrinthine segment, so the middle fossa approach is often needed for effective decompression.

Repair techniques and mechanisms for facial reanimation are beyond the scope of this chapter. If there is doubt about a transection, only a decompression should be performed, given that the results of an anastomosis will be at best scored House–Brackmann grade III/VI.[35] If less than 1 cm of nerve is missing, an attempt can be made to perform an end-to-end repair. If primary repair is not possible, a jump or interposition graft can be considered. A House–Brackmann III–IV is a realistic outcome.[10,37]

A recent systematic review performed by Nash et al.[38] examined facial nerve outcomes as related to treatment. In the analysis, 66% of patients, regardless of initial facial nerve exam (e.g. complete, delayed) achieved full return of function with observation alone. Similarly, 67% of patients treated with steroids alone achieved full function. Only 23% of surgical patients returned to a HB I with the majority being intermediate (HB II–V). Immediate paralysis was a poor indicator overall. With partial paralysis, the likelihood of patients returning to full function was good for all modes of therapy but greater for observation and steroids.

CSF Leak and Meningitis

Rates of CSF leak with temporal bone fractures range from 12% to 45%.[2,5,18,19] The majority of CSF leaks occur within 2 days of injury but can occur years later. The majority of cases resolve spontaneously and can be managed conservatively with bed rest, stool softeners, and medications (e.g. acetazolamide). With a robust leak, a lumbar drain may divert CSF allowing fracture sites to heal, but there is a risk of increasing pneumocephalus if CSF pressure is lowered in the face of fractures admitting intracranial air, and this could further promote meningitis.

The rate of meningitis among patients with a fracture and CSF leak is about 7% as compared to those with a fracture and no leak (1%).[14] In the presence of a concurrent ear infection and persistent leak beyond 7 days, the risk increases by 23%.[14] Common pathogenic organisms include *Streptococcus pneumoniae*, *Serratia marcescens*, and *Staphylococcus aureus*.[17] Conflicting literature exists regarding usage of prophylactic antibiotics. In a large series, Brodie et al.[14] concluded that in the context of CSF leak and temporal bone fracture, data do support usage of antibiotics. Some advocate that the risk of meningitis extends far beyond the acute period even after a leak has stopped. The otic capsule heals not with a callus but with a fibrous layer,[40] which provides a potential avenue for infection.

A persistent leak can be from significant loss of bone and dura, increased intracranial pressure, or incomplete healing of the labyrinthine bone. Surgical approach is dependent upon location of the leak, size of the defect, and status of hearing. Before performing surgery, an audiogram should be obtained and hearing loss discussed with the patient. Transmastoid and middle fossa approaches have been discussed extensively in the literature. If the temporal bone is extensively damaged, the only solution may be to close off the ear canal.

Tympanic Ring Fractures

Tympanic ring fractures are seen in 40%–59% of temporal bone trauma and are associated with force pushing the mandibular condyle posteriorly.[20,41] The fracture can be seen in Pöschl, axial, or coronal views.[42] Ear canal stenosis (Fig. 1.17.5), temporal-mandibular joint dysfunction, and prolapse of the mandibular condyle into the EAC are complications.

Treatment can be challenging, and early identification is critical. The EAC should be examined for edema, lacerations or anterior bulging.[41] Packing the EAC is beneficial as it provides hemostasis and can be used as a stent. Merocels™ or other expandable wicks are atraumatic in their insertion and allow for instillation of topical antibiotic drops. Treatment includes canalplasty ± soft tissue excision with and without skin grafting.

LONG-TERM COMPLICATIONS

Overall quality of life is affected by temporal bone trauma. A majority of patients find that their social lives, relationships, and work are affected

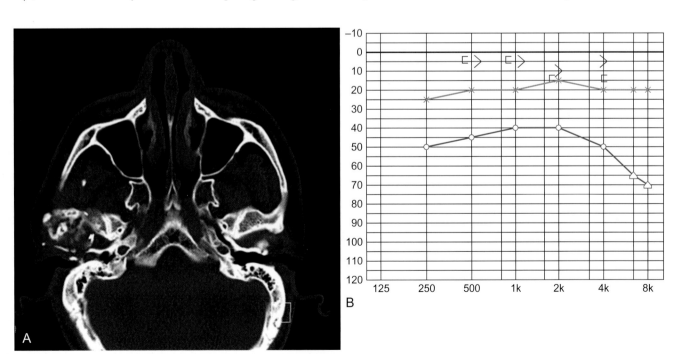

Fig. 1.17.5 (A) Axial CT scan of patient with history of right-sided mandibular and tympanic ring fracture with resulting ear canal stenosis. (B) Audiogram of same patient showing conductive hearing loss from ear canal stenosis.

by the fracture more than one year from their trauma.[5] Over half of patients have issues with tinnitus and hearing loss, and 44% continued to have balance problems. Over 75% of patients described their hearing and balance issues as disabling.

Sensorineural Hearing Loss

SNHL ranges from 31%–57% in temporal bone fractures[10,14] but is lower in children.[16] Fracture, hemorrhage into the cochlea,[43] or direct trauma to the ossicular chain can damage the organ of Corti.[44] Cochlear concussion can cause progressive bilateral SNHL.[29] A perilymphatic fistula (PLF), degenerative changes to the cochlea, and autoimmune reactions secondary to trauma can also cause SNHL.[44] Tinnitus can develop from direct damage to the auditory pathway or from abnormal somatosensory input from the neck or trigeminal system.

Cochlear hemorrhage will appear bright on pre-gadolinium T1-weighted MRI imaging. Fast imaging employing steady-state acquisition sequence (FIESTA) can detect nerve compression, transection, or injury. Pneumolabyrinth can cause hearing loss, tinnitus, ear fullness, and dizziness.[4]

With OCV fractures, hearing loss is likely permanent, and the rate of future hearing loss, especially among older patients, may be more rapid.[44] A conventional, contralateral routing of signal (CROS), Bi-CROS hearing aid or osseointegrated implant can be offered.

In cases of severe to profound bilateral SNHL, cochlear implantation should be considered if imaging demonstrates a patent cochlea and presence of a cochlear nerve. In cases of bilateral fractures involving the internal auditory canal, an auditory brainstem implant can be considered. However, published reports show poor results.[45]

Vertigo

Vertigo is a common complication with temporal bone fractures. Direct trauma to the labyrinth, vestibular aqueduct, vestibular nerves, perilymphatic fistula, superior semicircular canal dehiscence, and BPPV can be causes. The most common type of vertigo, BPPV, is characterized by sudden onset of vertigo, triggered by movement and thought to be due to free-floating otoliths within the endolymphatic space of the semicircular canals. Labyrinthine concussion can produce a temporary dysfunction with a short recovery period. Fistualization of the bony labyrinth, direct injury to the membranous labyrinth or endolymphatic duct can lead to disturbances in fluid balance.[46] Symptoms of aural fullness, tinnitus, fluctuating hearing loss and episodic vertigo as well as evaluation with electrocochleography may suggest the diagnosis.

In the acute phase, vestibular suppressants should be initiated. Usage of these medications for extended periods limit central compensation. Benzodiazepines should be avoided due to their addictive potential. Vestibular rehabilitation should be the mainstay of treatment. BPPV can be treated with repositioning maneuvers.

About 10%–30% of patients without complicated temporal bone fractures may continue to be vertiginous due to poor central compensation.[47] Evaluation for traumatic brain injury, migraine or persistent postural-perceptual dizziness should be considered before subjecting patients to use of long-term vestibular suppressants.

Encephaloceles

Encephaloceles can form decades after the trauma. Surgical management depends on the size and location of the encephalocele. Repair should be considered with cases of chronic otitis media, CSF leaks or increased risk of meningitis. A middle fossa approach provides exposure to anterior encephaloceles that involve tegmen tympani, the ossicular chain or for large dehiscences of the middle fossa floor. A transmastoid approach is good for small defects especially those involving the posterior fossa.

Cholesteatoma

Trauma either by direct fracture or by foreign body (e.g. GSW) can implant squamous material, leading to cholesteatoma development. Entrapment of epithelium before callus formation, widening or diastasis of suture lines, and TM perforation allow for cholesteatoma development[48] (Fig. 1.17.6). Development of cholesteatoma can occur over a time range from 6 months to 10 years.[49]

CONCLUSION

Prevalence of temporal bone fractures has decreased over the past 50 years. Various classification schemes have been proposed, with those identifying critical structures being more useful. CT remains the imaging modality of choice. Hearing loss remains the most common complication, with CHL being most common and resolving spontaneously. Facial nerve paralysis continues to be one of the most dreaded consequences; however, a recent review of the literature supports favorable outcomes with observation in the majority of cases.

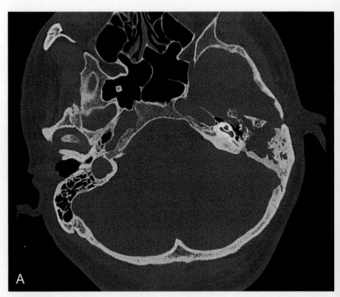

Fig. 1.17.6 (A) Axial CT of temporal bone in patient with history of a left temporal bone fracture showing erosive soft tissue density in left temporal bone consistent with cholesteatoma.

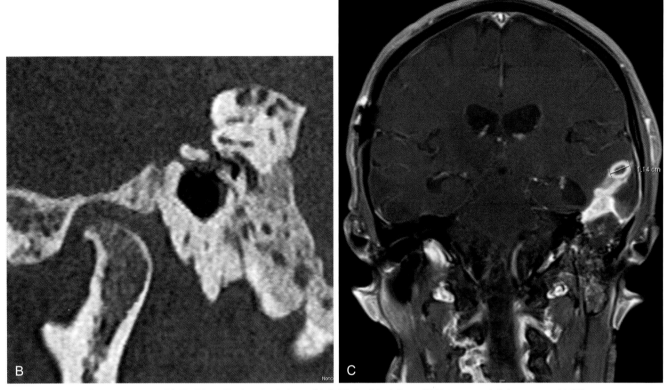

Fig. 1.17.6, cont'd (B) Magnified sagittal view of left EAC with defect. (C) T-1 postgadolinium coronal MRI showing soft tissue within mastoid with enhancement extending into left temporal lobe consistent with cholesteatoma and intracranial abscess.

EXPERT COMMENTARY

Fractures of the temporal bone have patterns, with the mechanism, symptoms, and prognosis proportional to the patterns. While the detailed management of these injuries in terms of their interpretation, management, and outcomes prediction is a matter for a specialist, each practitioner managing facial injuries will see these occasionally, and the recognition, consultation, and patient management must be included with the patient's other injuries.

Here specialist authors have written a clear and concise chapter describing the identification, findings, therapeutics, and prognosis so that the details of the management may easily be included with the treatment of the rest of the patient's facial injuries.

These important cranial base fractures of the middle cranial fossa have patterns and symptoms clearly defining them from other facial injuries, such as condyle fractures with laceration and bleeding into the ear canal. It is easy to memorize the patterns and prognosis that will repay the facial injuries surgeon with grateful patients for guidance in consultation and overall management.

Temporal bone fractures represent one pattern of skull base fracture, described in a reference on how the skull breaks and responds to blunt injury [1].

Reference

1. Manson PN, Stanwix M, Yaremchuk M, et al. Frontobasilar fractures: anatomy, classification and clinical significance. *Plast Reconstr Surg.* 2009;124:2096–2116.

REFERENCES

1. Schubl SD, Klein TR, Robitsek RJ, et al. Temporal bone fracture: Evaluation in the era of modern computed tomography. *Injury.* 2016;47(9):1893–1897.
2. Rafferty MA, McConn Walsh R, Walsh MA. A comparison of temporal bone fracture classification systems. *Clin Otolaryngol.* 2006;31(4):287–291.
3. Nicol JW, Johnstone AJ. Temporal bone fractures in children: A review of 34 cases. *J Accid Emerg Med.* 1994;11(4):218–222.
4. Choi HG, Lee HJ, Lee JS, et al. The rates and clinical characteristics of pneumolabyrinth in temporal bone fracture. *Otol Neurotol.* 2015;36(6):1048–1053.
5. Montava M, Mancini J, Masson C, et al. Temporal bone fractures: Sequelae and their impact on quality of life. *Am J Otolaryngol.* 2015;36(3):364–370.
6. Asha'ari ZA, Ahmad R, Rahman J, et al. Patterns of intracranial hemorrhage in petrous temporal bone fracture. *Auris Nasus Larynx.* 2012;39(2):151–155.
7. Chan J, Putnam MA, Feustel PJ, et al. The age dependent relationship between facial fractures and skull fractures. *Int J Pediatr Otorhinolaryngol.* 2004;68(7):877–881.
8. Frisenda JL, Schroeder JW Jr, Ryan ME, et al. Cost effective use of audiograms after pediatric temporal bone fractures. *Int J Pediatr Otorhinolaryngol.* 2015;79(11):1926–1931.
9. Ahmed KA, Alison D, Whatley WS, et al. The role of angiography in managing patients with temporal bone fractures: A retrospective study of 64 cases. *Ear Nose Throat J.* 2009;88(5):922–925.
10. Yetiser S, Hidir Y, Gonul E. Facial nerve problems and hearing loss in patients with temporal bone fractures: Demographic data. *J Trauma.* 2008;65(6):1314–1320.
11. Alvi A, Bereliani A. Acute intracranial complications of temporal bone trauma. *Otolaryngol Head Neck Surg.* 1998;119(6):609–613.
12. Travis LW, Stalnaker RL, Melvin JW. Impact trauma of the human temporal bone. *J Trauma.* 1977;17(10):761–766.
13. Hollinger A, Christe A, Thali MJ, et al. Incidence of auditory ossicle luxation and petrous bone fractures detected in post-mortem multislice computed tomography (MSCT). *Forensic Sci Int.* 2009;183(1–3):60–66.
14. Brodie HA, Thompson TC. Management of complications from 820 temporal bone fractures. *Am J Otol.* 1997;18(2):188–197.
15. Kahn JB, Stewart MG, Diaz-Marchan PJ. Acute temporal bone trauma: Utility of high-resolution computed tomography. *Am J Otol.* 2000;21(5):743–752.
16. Waissbluth S, Ywakim R, Al Qassabi B, et al. Pediatric temporal bone fractures: A case series. *Int J Pediatr Otorhinolaryngol.* 2016;84:106–109.
17. Shindo ML, Fetterman BL, Shih L, et al. Gunshot wounds of the temporal bone: A rational approach to evaluation and management. *Otolaryngol Head Neck Surg.* 1995;112(4):533–539.
18. Nosan DK, Benecke JE Jr, Murr AH. Current perspective on temporal bone trauma. *Otolaryngol Head Neck Surg.* 1997;117(1):67–71.
19. Dahiya R, Keller JD, Litofsky NS, et al. Temporal bone fractures: Otic capsule sparing versus otic capsule violating clinical and radiographic considerations. *J Trauma.* 1999;47(6):1079–1083.
20. Wood CP, Hunt CH, Bergen DC, et al. Tympanic plate fractures in temporal bone trauma: Prevalence and associated injuries. *AJNR Am J Neuroradiol.* 2014;35(1):186–190.
21. Dempewolf R, Gubbels S, Hansen MR. Acute radiographic workup of blunt temporal bone trauma: Maxillofacial versus temporal bone CT. *Laryngoscope.* 2009;119(3):442–448.
22. Nauer CB, Rieke A, Zubler C, et al. Low-dose temporal bone CT in infants and young children: Effective dose and image quality. *AJNR Am J Neuroradiol.* 2011;32(8):1375–1380.
23. Majdani O, Thews K, Bartling S, et al. Temporal bone imaging: Comparison of flat panel volume CT and multisection CT. *AJNR Am J Neuroradiol.* 2009;30(7):1419–1424.
24. Miller PR, Fabian TC, Croce MA, et al. Prospective screening for blunt cerebrovascular injuries: Analysis of diagnostic modalities and outcomes. *Ann Surg.* 2002;236(3):386–393, discussion 393–395.
25. Kelly KE, Tami TA. Temporal bone and skull trauma. In: Jackler RK, Brackmann D, eds. *Neurotology.* St. Louis, MO: Mosby; 1994:340.
26. Ishman SL, Friedland DR. Temporal bone fractures: Traditional classification and clinical relevance. *Laryngoscope.* 2004;114(10):1734–1741.
27. Little SC, Kesser BW. Radiographic classification of temporal bone fractures: Clinical predictability using a new system. *Arch Otolaryngol Head Neck Surg.* 2006;132(12):1300–1304.
28. Villalobos T, Arango C, Kubilis P, et al. Antibiotic prophylaxis after basilar skull fractures: A meta-analysis. *Clin Infect Dis.* 1998;27(2):364–369.
29. Lambert PR, Brackmann DE. Facial paralysis in longitudinal temporal bone fractures: A review of 26 cases. *Laryngoscope.* 1984;94(8):1022–1026.
30. Grant JR, Arganbright J, Friedland DR. Outcomes for conservative management of traumatic conductive hearing loss. *Otol Neurotol.* 2008;29(3):344–349.
31. Tan M, Ullman N, Pearl MS, et al. Fracture of the manubrium of the malleus. *Otol Neurotol.* 2016;37(8):e254–e255.
32. Conoyer JM, Kaylie DM, Jackson CG. Otologic surgery following ear trauma. *Otolaryngol Head Neck Surg.* 2007;137(5):757–761.
33. Haberkamp TJ, McFadden E, Khafagy Y, et al. Gunshot injuries of the temporal bone. *Laryngoscope.* 1995;105(10):1053–1057.
34. Kampshoff JL, Cogbill TH, Mathiason MA, et al. Cranial nerve injuries are associated with specific craniofacial fractures after blunt trauma. *Am Surg.* 2010;76(11):1223–1227.
35. Chang CY, Cass SP. Management of facial nerve injury due to temporal bone trauma. *Am J Otol.* 1999;20(1):96–114.
36. Elicora SS, Dinc AE, Biskin S, et al. Bilateral facial paralysis caused by bilateral temporal bone fracture: A case report and a literature review. *Case Rep Otolaryngol.* 2015;2015:306950.
37. Darrouzet V, Duclos JY, Liguoro D, et al. Management of facial paralysis resulting from temporal bone fractures: Our experience in 115 cases. *Otolaryngol Head Neck Surg.* 2001;125(1):77–84.
38. Nash JJ, Friedland DR, Boorsma KJ, et al. Management and outcomes of facial paralysis from intratemporal blunt trauma: A systematic review. *Laryngoscope.* 2010;120(7):1397–1404.
39. Quaranta A, Campobasso G, Piazza F, et al. Facial nerve paralysis in temporal bone fractures: Outcomes after late decompression surgery. *Acta Otolaryngol.* 2001;121(5):652–655.
40. Zehnder A, Merchant SN. Transverse fracture of the temporal bone. *Otol Neurotol.* 2004;25(5):852–853.
41. Burchhardt DM, David J, Eckert R, et al. Trauma patterns, symptoms, and complications associated with external auditory canal fractures. *Laryngoscope.* 2015;125(7):1579–1582.
42. Zayas JO, Feliciano YZ, Hadley CR, et al. Temporal bone trauma and the role of multidetector CT in the emergency department. *Radiographics.* 2011;31(6):1741–1755.
43. Schuknecht HF. Mechanism of inner ear injury from blows to the head. *Ann Otol Rhinol Laryngol.* 1969;78(2):253–262.
44. Bergemalm PO. Progressive hearing loss after closed head injury: A predictable outcome? *Acta Otolaryngol.* 2003;123(7):836–845.
45. Medina M, Di Lella F, Di Trapani G, et al. Cochlear implantation versus auditory brainstem implantation in bilateral total deafness after head trauma: Personal experience and review of the literature. *Otol Neurotol.* 2014;35(2):260–270.
46. Shea JJ Jr, Ge X, Orchik DJ. Traumatic endolymphatic hydrops. *Am J Otol.* 1995;16(2):235–240.
47. Friedman JM. Post-traumatic vertigo. *Med Health R I.* 2004;87(10):296–300.
48. Freeman J. Temporal bone fractures and cholesteatoma. *Ann Otol Rhinol Laryngol.* 1983;92(6 Pt 1):558–560.
49. Brookes GB, Graham MD. Post-traumatic cholesteatoma of the external auditory canal. *Laryngoscope.* 1984;94(5 Pt 1):667–670.

Dentoalveolar Trauma

Matthew E. Lawler, Corbett A. Haas, Zachary S. Peacock

BACKGROUND

Dentoalveolar trauma represents a significant proportion of facial injuries. Treatment of dentoalveolar trauma has been documented as early as the era of Hippocrates, who described the use of dental splinting with bridal wires.[1,2] Although many advances have occurred, the basic principles of fixation of loose teeth or bony segments to allow for hard and soft tissue healing are still paramount.

The incidence and prevalence of injuries to the dentoalveolar complex are difficult to determine. Dentoalveolar injuries are often treated in an office setting and largely underreported.[3] Across the globe, dental injury affects nearly one-third of preschool children in the primary dentition. Trauma to the teeth due to a fall is the most common facial injury in this age group.[4] Subsequently, 25% of children in the mixed dentition sustain dental trauma most commonly due to sports injuries. Lastly, 25% of adults sustain a traumatic injury to permanent teeth.[5] There is a large variance in the incidence of injuries depending on race, socioeconomic status, age, sex, geographic location, anatomic factors (e.g. class II dental relationship) and medical conditions (seizures, gait or balance disturbances). These injuries can occur in isolation or in association with craniofacial fractures and/or orthopedic injuries.[6] Fortunately, the overall incidence of craniofacial injuries is decreasing in developed regions due to advances in motor vehicle safety, traffic laws, reduction in intoxicated driving, and improved safety equipment for athletes (e.g. mouth guards and face masks).[3,7] Injuries as a result of interpersonal violence, falls during daily life activities, and sports-related injuries have become more common than those from motor vehicle collisions.[7–9]

The mechanism of dentoalveolar injury is either direct trauma to the teeth or secondary to a blow to the chin resulting in the mandibular dentition being forced into the maxillary dentition. Direct injury most commonly affects the maxillary central incisors, which protrude beyond the other teeth.[3] Predisposing conditions include class II malocclusion (overjet >4 mm), labially inclined central incisors, and lip incompetence.[10] Children are more likely to sustain damage to the underlying periodontal structures (i.e., luxation or avulsion of teeth) than adults, who are more likely to sustain tooth or alveolar bone fractures.[3] The presence of the developing secondary dentition, smaller less pneumatized maxillary sinuses, and less dense bone make the pediatric alveolar bone more pliable and resistant to fracture.[9,11]

SURGICAL ANATOMY

When considering the anatomy of dentoalveolar injuries, distinction must be made between primary and adult dentition as well as between teeth and the periodontium. A complete deciduous dentition includes two primary molars, a canine, and lateral and central incisors in each quadrant for a total of 20 teeth. The adult dentition includes three molars, two premolars, a canine and lateral and central incisors in each quadrant for a total of 32 teeth. At age 6, the adult first molars erupt posterior to the primary second molars, starting the 'mixed dentition' phase. A well-defined pattern of primary tooth exfoliation and adult tooth eruption ensues leaving one with mixed dentition until the last primary tooth exfoliates around 12 years of age (Fig. 1.18.1).[12]

All teeth are composed of enamel, dentin, dental pulp, and cementum (Fig. 1.18.2). The periodontium is the structures that support the teeth, including the periodontal ligament, alveolar bone, and the overlying gingiva. As the name suggests, dentoalveolar injuries involve either or both dental structures along with alveolar bone. The term is oversimplified as injuries can include fractures through enamel, dentin, and exposure of the pulpal tissues and typically involve disruption of the periodontal ligament and lacerations of the overlying gingival mucosa.

Dental Anatomy

Enamel, *dentin*, and *cementum* are the calcified structures of the dentition made up of 96%, 70%, and 50% inorganic mineral components, respectively.[13–15] Enamel, the hardest substance in the human body, is the outer surface of the crown of a tooth, with high compressive strength and brittle nature. It is acellular and lacks reparative capacity. Cementum is the outer layer of the root, extending from the cementoenamel junction (CEJ) to the root apex. Cementoblasts remain on the surface and are entrapped as new matrix is formed. The cells, deriving nutrition from the adjacent vascularized periodontal ligament, provide ability for some self-repair after injury. Beneath enamel and cementum lies dentin, with a low compressive but high tensile strength due to greater organic content, providing support for the overlying crown. The internal wall of dentin is lined with odontoblasts with cytoplasmic extensions spanning the length of the dentinal layer through dentinal tubules that can respond to external insults with additional dentin formation over time. Dental fractures extending to this layer tend to be associated with hypersensitivity, likely due to hydrodynamic forces through the dentinal tubules.

Pulpal tissue is the neurovascular bundle of the tooth contained within the pulp chamber and root canals. It comprises the central portion of the tooth and is easily visible on dental films. In primary and new permanent teeth there are extensions of the pulp towards the occlusal surface called pulp horns increasing the likelihood of pulp exposure in pediatric dental fractures.

Periodontal Anatomy

The periodontal ligament (PDL, Fig. 1.18.3) is a set of connective tissue fibers that secure the tooth to the adjacent alveolar bone. It provides for physiologic mobility and helps support the tooth against compressive forces through its insertion into cementum (via Sharpey's fibers). It is seen on dental radiographs and orthopantomograms as the radiolucent line between the tooth and the cortical margin of the adjacent

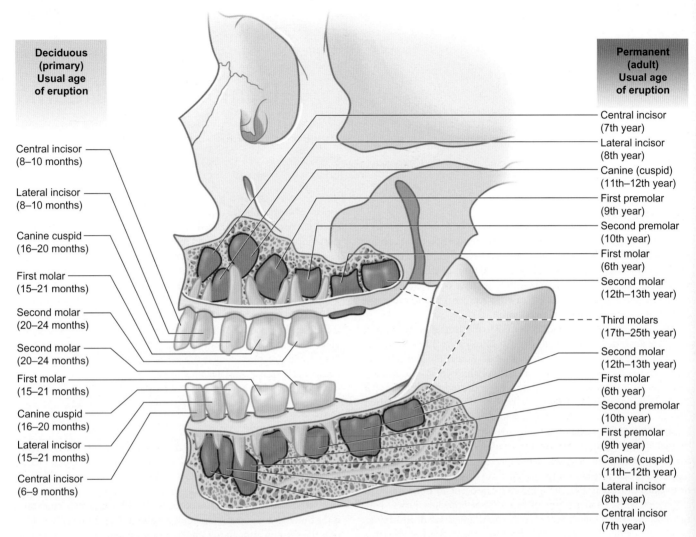

Deciduous (primary) Usual age of eruption

Central incisor (8–10 months)

Lateral incisor (8–10 months)

Canine cuspid (16–20 months)

First molar (15–21 months)

Second molar (20–24 months)

Second molar (20–24 months)

First molar (15–21 months)

Canine cuspid (16–20 months)

Lateral incisor (15–21 months)

Central incisor (6–9 months)

Permanent (adult) Usual age of eruption

Central incisor (7th year)

Lateral incisor (8th year)

Canine (cuspid) (11th–12th year)

First premolar (9th year)

Second premolar (10th year)

First molar (6th year)

Second molar (12th–13th year)

Third molars (17th–25th year)

Second molar (12th–13th year)

First molar (6th year)

Second premolar (10th year)

First premolar (9th year)

Canine (cuspid) (11th–12th year)

Lateral incisor (8th year)

Central incisor (7th year)

Fig. 1.18.1 Erupted deciduous teeth with developing succedaneous tooth buds and associated age of eruption. (From Norton NS. Oral cavity. In: Norton NS, editor. Netter's head and neck anatomy for dentistry. Philadelphia, PA: Saunders; 2007. p.360.)

alveolar bone known as the lamina dura (see Fig. 1.18.8). The PDL is highly vascular, providing blood supply to the adjacent cementum. Osteoblasts and cementoblasts are within the PDL, allowing for reparation of alveolar bone and cementum. The viability of the PDL and associated cells after trauma is important in the prognosis of the injured tooth. Loss of the PDL leads to ankylosis of the tooth to the bone or external resorption of the tooth.[16]

Alveolar bone supports teeth in the maxilla and mandible. It consists of buccal/facial and lingual/palatal cortices that surrounding trabecular bone along with a cortical alveolar lining (lamina dura) comprising the tooth socket. The cortical plates are supported by Haversian systems and are thinnest in the maxillary teeth and thickest over the posterior mandibular teeth. The status of the less-supported buccal/facial plate following injury or extraction of a tooth can determine the need for bone grafting prior to dental implant placement to replace the tooth. All measures should be taken to preserve as much alveolar bone as possible after dentoalveolar trauma.

Gingiva is the soft tissue lining that overlies the alveolar bone and surrounds the dentition (Fig. 1.18.3). It is made of epithelial and deeper connective tissue components. The reduced enamel epithelium surrounds an erupting tooth and forms a complex attachment at the cementoenamel junction of the tooth thereby sealing the deeper periodontal structures from the oral environment.[15] In a healthy state there exists 1–3 mm of a gingival sulcus between the attachment of the gingiva to tooth structure and the visible portion of the tooth (free gingival margin). This mucosa immediately adjacent to the teeth is highly keratinized and tightly bound to the underlying alveolar bone. Unlike the buccal mucosa or that of the floor of the mouth it is immobile and provides protection during masticatory function. On the facial aspect of the maxilla and the facial and lingual aspects of the mandible the attached gingiva extends several millimeters and forms a junction with the unattached mucosa (mucogingival junction, Fig. 1.18.4). On the palatal aspect of the maxilla the mucosa remains keratinized and tightly bound to the hard palate. It is important to maintain and properly position the keratinized gingiva after dentoalveolar trauma.

CLINICAL PRESENTATION

Examination of the injured face can be daunting. One should avoid focusing on the obvious injuries and perform a detailed history and systematic physical exam in a focused and efficient manner.

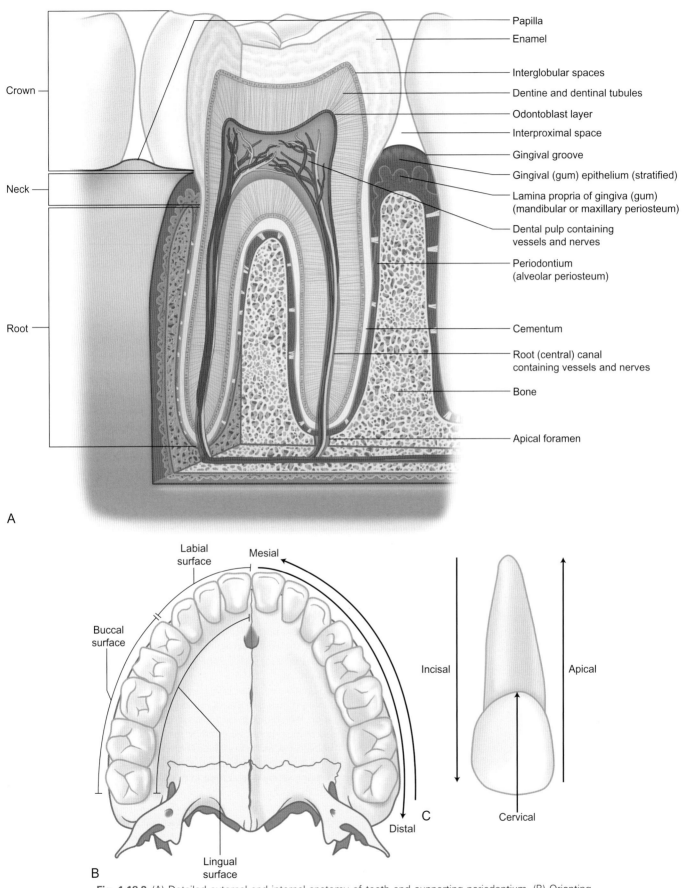

Fig. 1.18.2 (A) Detailed external and internal anatomy of tooth and supporting periodontium. (B) Orienting terminology describing surfaces of teeth. (C) Terminology describing position within a tooth. Posterior teeth do not have incisal edges but rather occlusal surfaces. (From Norton NS. Oral cavity. In: Norton NS, editor. Netter's head and neck anatomy for dentistry. Philadelphia, PA: Saunders; 2007. (A) p.361, (B) p.360, (C) Adapted from p.363.)

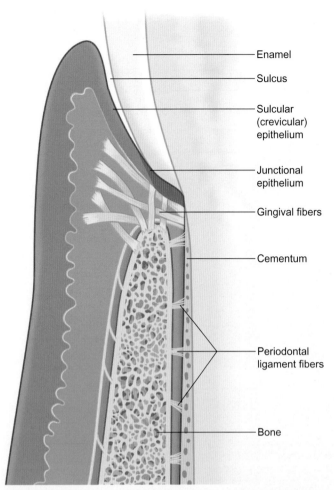

— Enamel

— Sulcus

— Sulcular (crevicular) epithelium

— Junctional epithelium

— Gingival fibers

— Cementum

— Periodontal ligament fibers

— Bone

Fig. 1.18.3 Anatomy of supporting periodontal structures highlighting the extensive connective tissue network of gingival fibers and periodontal ligament fibers. (Modified from Rose LF, Minsk L. Dental implants in the periodontally compromised dentition. In: Rose LF, Mealy BL, editors. Periodontics: medicine, surgery and implants. St. Louis, MO: Mosby; 2004. Fig. 1.18.26-1.)

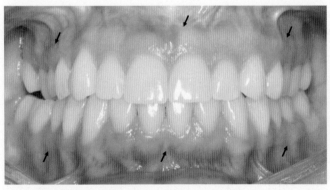

Fig. 1.18.4 Healthy dentition and gingiva with border of mucogingival junction (*arrows*) between keratinized (attached) tissue closest to teeth and loose alveolar mucosa extending into the vestibule.

Injuries to the teeth and supporting structures should be evaluated urgently as many injuries require diagnosis and treatment in a limited timeframe.

A complete history surrounding the injury must be obtained, including the mechanism, onset, duration, and associated symp-toms. It is imperative to consider that patients with dentoalveo-lar trauma may have concomitant head, cervical spine or airway injury and patients should be evaluated appropriately (see Chapter 1.1, Assessment of the patient with traumatic facial injury, for details).[17–20]

A detailed dental history including previous treatments (prosthetics, gingival surgery, orthodontia) and the patient's perception of their premorbid occlusion should be obtained. In cases of tooth avulsion, the clinician must determine how long the tooth has been avulsed, what type of medium the tooth has been stored in, and if it is a primary or permanent tooth. It is recommended to request preinjury facial photographs to determine the patient's native occlusion, facial symmetry, and contours. If the patient has undergone orthodontic treatment, photographs and dental models should be sought to help establish the native occlusion.

A comprehensive and methodical physical exam should be performed on every patient with dentoalveolar trauma. Once appropriate interventions are performed to stabilize the patient with life-threatening injuries as part of the primary survey, the clinician performs a detailed maxillofacial examination as part of the secondary survey. In patients with bilateral mandibular fractures and tooth avulsions/fractures a detailed airway and pulmonary evaluation are also important as mandibular fractures can compromise the airway due to loss of soft tissue support and risk of aspiration of avulsed teeth or tooth fragments.

An accurate maxillofacial examination is only possible following adequate exposure, which includes cleaning the patient's face and wound. Given the vascularity of the maxillofacial region, blood and debris from even minor soft tissue lacerations can misrepresent the severity of injury. Proper cleaning and examination of wounds may require sedation or general anesthesia to ensure patient comfort. A standard set of photographs should be obtained of patients sustaining facial trauma (Fig. 1.18.5), including anterior, lateral, submental, intraoral, and wound photographs. These photos provide a baseline examination for medicolegal purposes, allow for a visual tool to describe treatment to the patient, and aid the clinician in forming the definitive treatment plan. This chapter will focus on the examination of the oral cavity and mandibular function.

Extraoral exam: Initial evaluation of the dentition should start with asking the patient to open and close their jaw. Deviation of the mandible with opening, premature occlusion (i.e., teeth hitting early preventing the remaining teeth from coming together) with shifting of the mandible, limitation in mouth opening, and pain when biting should be recognized. Next, measurements of the maximal incisal opening (MIO) and lateral excursive movements should be performed.

Intraoral soft tissue exam: A detailed and systematic soft tissue examination is then performed, starting with inspection for abrasion, ulceration, lacerations, hematoma, swelling, and pre-existing pathology. All lacerations should be carefully inspected for the presence of foreign body (e.g. dental restorations, tooth fragments, bone, or debris).[21] Gingival lacerations should raise suspicion for dentoalveolar fractures or dental luxations. Laceration in the floor mouth should raise suspicion of salivary duct injury. The submandibular gland should be massaged to confirm expression of clear saliva from the opening of Wharton's duct to help rule out salivary duct injury (Fig. 1.18.6). Hematoma within the floor of mouth is often associated with dentoalveolar or mandibular fractures. The tonsillar pillars and uvula should also be examined for symmetry as any deviation could indicate airway compromise.

Intraoral hard tissue exam (bone): The hard tissue exam includes evaluation of the maxillary, mandibular, alveolar, and palatal bone.

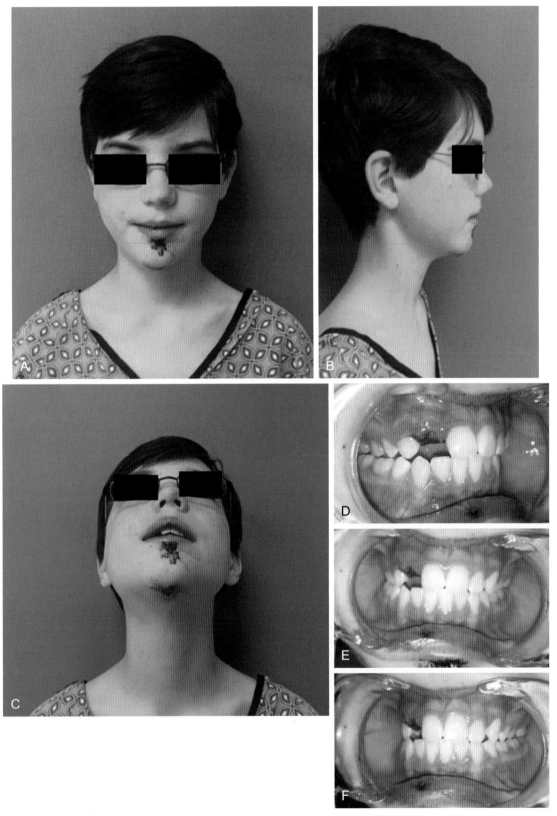

Fig. 1.18.5 Clinical photography. Standard frontal (A), lateral (B), submental (C), and intraoral (D – right lateral, E – frontal, F – left lateral) photographs are obtained for every patient with maxillofacial trauma. These photographs serve to aid in treatment planning, and documentation for medicolegal purposes as well as for patient education. We suggest using a standardized background (blue), and taking intraoral photographs in the patient's maximal intercuspation position (MIP) if possible. These photos demonstrate a full-thickness lip laceration as well as an intrusion injury of the permanent maxillary left lateral incisor.

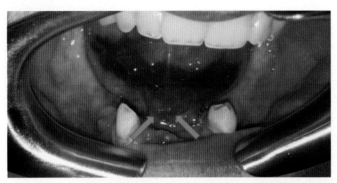

Fig. 1.18.6 A 66-year-old patient 5 days following a traumatic mandibular symphyseal fracture with resulting large floor of mouth hematoma and edema. Also visible are the bilateral submandibular (Wharton's) ducts (*arrows*).

as well as the dentition. Fractures of the mandible or dentoalveolar segment often result in interdental step-offs, increased dental spacing, mobility of dentoalveolar segments (two or more teeth moving as a unit). More subtle findings may include crepitus, bleeding from the gingival sulcus, gingival lacerations or floor of mouth ecchymoses.[3]

Intraoral hard tissue exam (dentition): The surgeon must first account for all preexisting teeth, teeth fragments or restorations. If there is avulsion or loss of a sizeable portion of a tooth, the fragment should be assumed to be in the oral cavity, airway, or GI tract until proven otherwise. Radiographs of the head, neck, chest, and abdomen (KUB) should be obtained to locate displaced teeth unable to be located to rule out aspiration. An understanding of the types of restorations (e.g. fixed/removable prostheses, implants, crowns, fillings, and orthodontic appliances) is useful in determining the extent of the injury and account for displacement. Be aware of indirect dental injury with forced occlusion of teeth from a superiorly directed force on the chin resulting in crown and/or root fractures of the posterior dentition.

Next, each remaining tooth and restoration should be evaluated systematically (see Classification section). Transillumination of visible light along the long axis of the tooth can identify subtle dental injuries to enamel. Each tooth should be evaluated for mobility, both individually or along with its adjacent teeth (indicating a dentoalveolar fracture). Mobility of an individual tooth can indicate luxation of the entire tooth or a root fracture that can require dental radiographs to diagnose. The clinician should then evaluate the alignment of the dental arches. Teeth are most commonly displaced in a buccolingual direction due to the vector of trauma perpendicular to the tooth's long axis.[3] A tilting of the occlusal plane can indicate luxation or intrusion injuries, but may indicate maxillary or mandibular fracture. Each tooth should be tested for mobility in all dimensions with care not to avulse loose teeth or dentoalveolar segments. A commonly used mobility index is the Miller classification, in which tooth mobility is evaluated using two hard objects (e.g. two tongue depressors). If a tooth is nondisplaced but mobile, this may indicate either preexisting periodontal disease or a crown/root fracture. Dental fractures more coronally positioned generally have more mobility.

Intraoral occlusal exam: The patient is instructed to carefully bring their teeth into occlusion with the clinician evaluating the movement. Premature occlusal contacts could indicate fracture or luxation injuries. The patient is then guided into their premorbid occlusion if tolerated. This allows the clinician to determine the complexity of restoring the patient's dentition. Interferences of the palatal cusps of the molars with

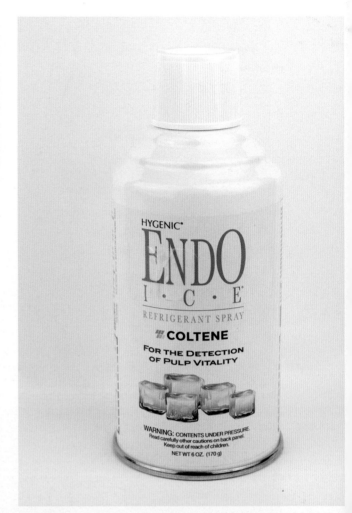

Fig. 1.18.7 Cold testing of dental pulp vitality is performed by applying Hygenic® Endo-Ice® Pulp Vitality Refrigerant Spray – 6 oz Spray Can – Coltene/Whaledent (Alstatten, Switzerland) to a cotton tipped applicator and placing it on a tooth to assess for pain response (mild pain for 1–2 seconds that stops with removal of cold stimulus).

a seemingly intact mandible could indicate a palatal fracture with change in the transverse width of the maxilla.

Tooth percussion and vitality testing: An injury to a tooth and periodontal ligament without displacement is referred to as a subluxation. Subluxated teeth have increased mobility or pain to percussion relative to adjacent teeth. Percussion is performed by applying a vertical or horizontal force using a blunt object (e.g. the back end of a dental mirror or tongue blade) and can determine damage to the PDL. A subluxated tooth will also have a change in the quality of sound produced by percussion from the normal sharp metallic sound to a dull resonance.[22] Dental injuries can disrupt the neurovascular bundle at the apex of teeth. Tooth vitality testing measures the ability of the nerve fibers of the tooth to relay information to the trigeminal system. This is performed routinely by dentists and endodontists using different methods with varying sensitivity, including thermal (hot or cold), electric, pulse oximetry, and laser Doppler flowmetry (Fig. 1.18.7).[3,23–25] Within the first several weeks after dental trauma vitality testing is not reliable and is typically done after several weeks to months to determine the need for endodontic treatment for non-vital teeth.

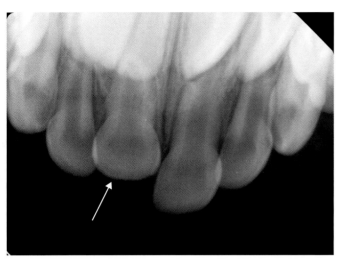

Fig. 1.18.8 Maxillary occlusal film of a 3-year-old patient who sustained a mechanical fall and intrusion of his maxillary right central incisor (*arrow*) into the permanent tooth bud.

RADIOLOGICAL EVALUATION

The last two decades have seen a dramatic advance in head and neck imaging. The advent of digital radiographs and cone beam computed tomography (CBCT) has revolutionized the way many hospital and community-based clinicians utilize imaging. The goal of imaging is to evaluate the tooth roots, pulp canals, and periodontium for preexisting disease and traumatic injury. In children, radiographs also serve to evaluate the development of the tooth roots and location of the succedaneous tooth buds relative to injuries. Imaging can also be used post treatment to confirm tooth or bone reduction and position of hardware. This section will serve as a guide for use of different types of imaging available. The availability of imaging modalities varies widely in the emergency room setting, but most centers have facial films and computed tomography (CT).

Intraoral radiographs: Intraoral radiographs are high-resolution two-dimensional radiographs that include bitewings, periapical, and occlusal film used by dentists and dental specialists. Bitewings evaluate tooth crowns and alveolar bone to detect caries and periodontal disease. They have little utility in the setting of trauma. Periapical radiographs (PA) show the crowns and roots of 1–4 teeth. They show the periodontal ligament, and alveolar bone around the tooth. Multiple angles may be needed to detect a root fracture. PA films can be used to confirm reduction following splinting of avulsed and luxated teeth by comparing the position of the tooth root to the surrounding cortical margin of the socket (lamina dura). Occlusal films are taken perpendicular to the occlusal plane of the maxilla and mandible and are larger than PAs (Fig. 1.18.8). They are easier to obtain than periapical radiographs in the trauma setting as they do not require that the film or sensor be placed into the lingual or palatal tissue. They can be used to identify crown/root fractures, luxation injuries, and are useful in detection of radiopaque foreign bodies or tooth fragments in the surrounding soft tissue (e.g. floor of mouth, lips, vestibule).

Orthopantomogram (OPG) and computed tomography (CT): The orthopantomogram (panoramic radiograph or panorex) is a useful tool to evaluate for mandibular fractures associated with dentoalveolar fractures, especially if the clinician suspects a condylar, ramus, or angle fracture (Fig. 1.18.9). Although OPGs can detect dentoalveolar trauma, they do not provide the diagnostic accuracy and resolution of periapical or occlusal radiographs. In addition, panoramic radiographs are better

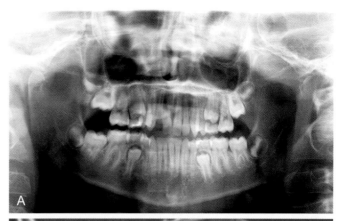

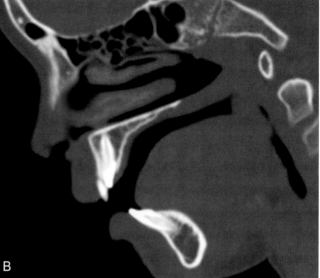

Fig. 1.18.9 Panoramic imaging of a child in the mixed dentition with an intruded maxillary left lateral incisor (A) with bilateral mandibular condylar fractures. The tooth intrusion is better appreciated on the sagittal CT cut showing intrusion of the tooth with the apex near the nasal floor (B).

tolerated by the trauma patient, however severe distortion or ghost images result from improper positioning, particularly in the anterior maxillary and mandibular arches.

Conventional and CBCT scans are now considered the gold standard for diagnosis of facial fractures. However, with dentoalveolar trauma these scans often show distorted anatomy due to patient movement, foreign bodies, or dental restorations. Because they are more available in the emergency room setting and easily tolerated, CT scans are often obtained to evaluate dentoalveolar trauma. CBCT provides high-resolution images of the dentoalveolar structures with less radiation and are now commonly found in the outpatient setting.

CLASSIFICATION

Multiple classification systems have been used to describe dentoalveolar trauma to facilitate diagnosis, communication, and treatment. A systematic review of the literature in 2006 identified 54 distinct classification systems based on the mechanism, location, severity, and therapeutic options.[26] Many of these classification systems are variations of one another, resulting in confusion within the literature and difficulty with epidemiological studies.

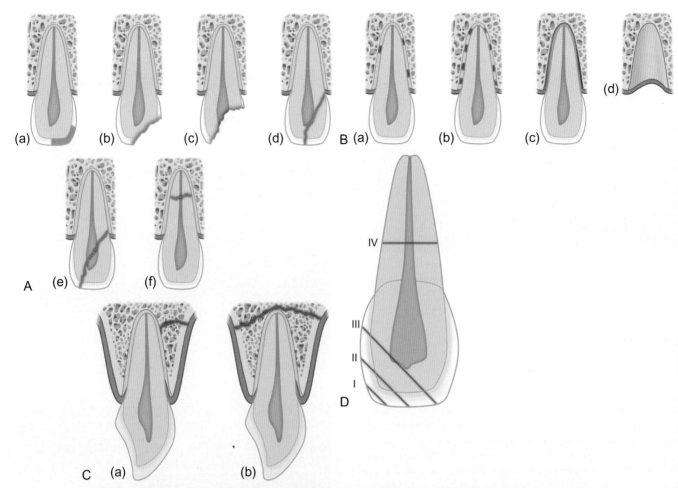

Fig. 1.18.10 A pictorial representation of the Andreasen classification system. (A) Tooth injuries including (a) enamel infraction, (b) uncomplicated crown fracture, and (c) complicated crown fracture involving the dental pulp. Uncomplicated crown-root fractures (d) do not include the dental pulp, and complicated crown-root fractures (e) include the dental pulp. Isolated horizontal root fractures (f) do not include the coronal tissue. (B) Periodontal injuries include (a) concussion, (b) subluxation, (c) luxation, and (d) avulsion. (C) Alveolar process injuries include (a) a single wall fracture (buccal or lingual plate, or (b) the entire alveolar process. (D) Diagram of Ellis classification system: enamel (I), enamel and dentin (II), enamel/dentin into the pulpal tissue (III), and root structures (IV). (From Leathers RD, Gowans RE. Management of alveolar and dental fractures. In: Miloro M, editor. Peterson's principles of oral and maxillofacial surgery. 2nd ed. Hamilton: BC Decker; 2004. (A) p.388; (B) p.389; (C) p.390; (D) p.387.)

The two most widely used classifications are those of Andreasen (32%) and Ellis (14%).[26–29] The Andreasen classification includes a broad spectrum of injuries and was the first system adopted by the World Health Organization (WHO). Injuries are classified based on anatomic location (tooth/pulp, periodontium, alveolar bone, and gingiva/mucosa) and severity of the injury (Fig. 1.18.10).

The Ellis classification, described in 1962, is a numeric system initially used exclusively in the anterior dentition but is now applied to the entire dentition.[28] It describes the severity of tooth fractures: Class I fractures are through enamel only; Class II fractures transverse enamel and dentin; Class III propagate through the pulp; and Class IV indicates fractures through the tooth root. Root fractures can further be subdivided into mesioangular (II), horizontal (III), and vertical (IV) fractures (Fig. 1.18.10D).

MANAGEMENT

Treatment of dentoalveolar injuries is tailored to the structures involved as well as the severity of injury. Most injuries need operative intervention to correct the deformity or restore the tooth typically from multiple specialties (e.g. surgeon, endodontist, general dentist). The authors follow the treatment guidelines proposed by the International Association of Dental Traumatology (IADT), which have been adapted to an interactive public access website.[30] This website provides evidence-based treatment algorithms based on the Andreasen classification of dentoalveolar injuries.

The goal of treatment of a dentoalveolar injury is to restore the premorbid masticatory function and esthetics. The majority of these injuries are best managed in a well-equipped ambulatory dental clinic. Despite the time-sensitive nature of many dentoalveolar images, more severe injuries are managed first per Advanced Trauma Life Support (ATLS) protocols. All attempts are made to preserve native teeth and supporting bone, however hopeless teeth should be identified and either removed in the emergency setting or deferred to preserve space and alveolar bone. The extraction can be carried out by a clinician capable of preservation of alveolar bone or optimizing the ridge for dental implants. Minimal to no alveolar bone should be removed in the acute setting, as the intraoral structures are well vascularized and even a small amount of overlying gingiva can allow the clinician to preserve a fractured dentoalveolar segment.

Injuries to the Dentition

Injuries isolated to the crown of a tooth (Ellis Class I and II fractures) are treated with composite (resin) restorations and can be deferred to a general dentist (Fig. 1.18.11). The clinician must ensure that there is no mobility of the tooth or associated percussion tenderness that would indicate a displacement injury and damage to the PDL. If large pieces of enamel or dentin are retrieved they can often be replaced via dental bonding. These fragments should be stored in an isotonic solution and given to the patient if bonding is not possible at that time.

Dental injuries with exposure of the pulp (Ellis Class III fractures) require timely treatment. Dental fractures in children more likely lead to pulp exposure due to the closer proximity of the pulp to the tooth surface. Treatment of the pulp involves "pulp capping" (i.e., placement of a medicament in the coronal aspect of the pulp) and coverage with a composite resin restoration to preserve the vitality of the teeth. This is especially important in younger patients with incompletely developed tooth roots (open apices) requiring further development. Calcium hydroxide and mineral trioxide aggregate (MTA) are two common agents used for this purpose. If the tooth has a closed apex (beyond 8 or 9 years of age for incisors), endodontic (root canal) treatment is typically required.

Dental fractures can also involve the root (Ellis Class IV fractures), either extending from the crown or isolated within the root. There may or may not be associated pulp exposure. These injuries can have varied prognoses and the definitive treatment can be complex and beyond the

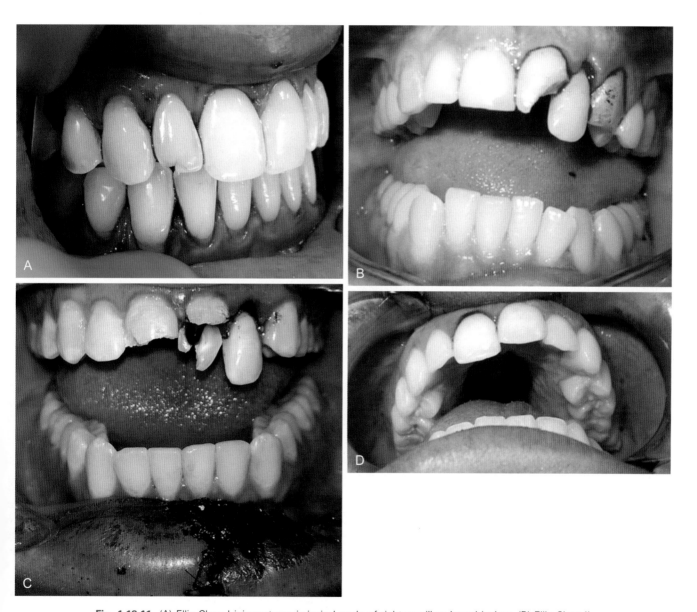

Fig. 1.18.11. (A) Ellis Class I injury at mesio-incisal angle of right maxillary lateral incisor. (B) Ellis Class II injury of left maxillary central incisor and left maxillary canine with associated extrusion injury of left lateral incisor. Characteristic bleeding in the gingival sulcus denotes injury to the periodontal ligament fibers. (C) Ellis Class II fracture involving right maxillary central incisor. Ellis Class III fracture with loose fragment of the left maxillary central incisor. Left maxillary lateral incisor with extrusion injury. (D) Luxation injury involving right maxillary central incisor. *Continued*

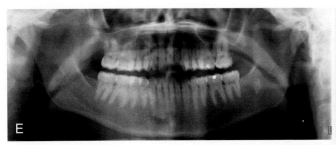

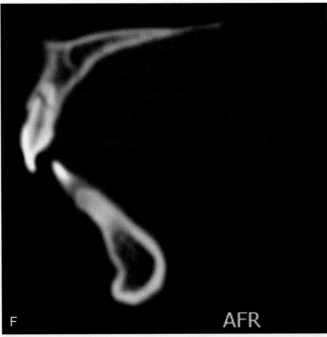

Fig. 1.18.11, cont'd A root fracture in this tooth is difficult to appreciate on orthopantomogram, (E) but is easily identified on the sagittal view of a maxillofacial CT scan (F), taken to identify other facial injuries.

scope of emergency care. In general, root fractures that are closer to the crown of the tooth have a worse prognosis. Fractures of the apical third of the root can be splinted as if it was a displaced tooth and the coronal root and crown may stabilize and/or remain vital in some cases. Loose fragments should be stabilized or removed (and given to the patient in an isotonic solution) and definitive treatment deferred to the general dentist. This may involve a combination of root canal therapy, crown lengthening, root repositioning, orthodontic extrusion and final restorative therapy. In the interim the patient should be placed on a soft diet and prescribed chlorhexidine (0.12%) oral rinse. Root fractures with pulp exposure typically require at least endodontic therapy if the tooth can be salvaged.

Displaced Dentition

Managing displaced teeth represents a major component of dentoalveolar injuries, particularly in children. Displacement can range from mild tooth mobility to complete avulsion. Blunt injury to a tooth that results in tenderness to percussion, but no mobility or displacement, is known as a concussion injury (compression of the PDL). The neurovascular supply typically remains intact. No intervention is needed, but the patient should be limited to a soft diet for 7–10 days. Subluxation refers to a blunt injury resulting in tooth mobility without displacement. Treatment is tailored to patient comfort and can be performed as an outpatient by a general dentist. If the patient is occluding prematurely on the tooth (due to edema within the PDL), relief can be provided by selective removal of enamel. If a permanent tooth is subluxed, a flexible acid-etched resin secured splint (braided 26-gauge wire secured to the teeth with dental composite resin) may also be placed for comfort but is not necessary. Any splint placed should maintain physiological tooth mobility. The vitality of the dental pulp should be assessed over 1–3 months by a dentist, with endodontic treatment if necrosis ensues. No treatment is needed for subluxed primary teeth.

Luxation is displacement of a tooth beyond its alveolar socket. Forces applied in a direction in line with the long axis of the tooth can result in either an extrusion or intrusion injury (Figs. 1.18.12A–B). Extrusion results in displacement of the tooth in an occlusal direction, often with exposure of root structure and resulting in occlusal prematurity. After adequate local anesthesia, the tooth and socket should be cleaned with saline and the tooth repositioned into its socket with digital pressure. The tooth should then be secured using a flexible, acid-etched resin bonded splint (Fig. 1.18.12C). Prior to splint placement the patient can often assist with identifying the appropriate position of the tooth. The patient should be asked to bring their teeth together to determine if the prematurity has been relieved and it aligns with adjacent teeth. Post-reduction radiographs should also be obtained to ensure accurate repositioning. The splint should allow for physiological mobility and remain in place for 2 weeks. The patient should remain on a soft diet while the splint is in place and should be followed by a general dentist or endodontist for monitoring of the pulpal vitality over 1–3 months (Figs. 1.18.12D–E). Endodontic treatment is typically required; 64% and 96% extrusion and intrusion injuries result in pulpal necrosis, respectively.[31] Primary teeth with minimal displacement (<3 mm) can be left alone if spontaneous realignment will occur, otherwise the tooth should be extracted, as needed for displacement >3 mm.

Intrusion represents displacement of the tooth in an apical direction into the alveolar bone leaving the crown shortened and immobile (see Figs. 1.18.5 and 1.18.16). There is always an associated alveolar bone fracture as a wider portion of the tooth is driven into a narrower part of the socket. In some cases there is complete intrusion with the crown buried in the gingiva. Adjunct imaging should be performed to ensure there has not been displacement into the nasal cavity or maxillary sinus. Management is dependent on the degree of displacement and the root development. Mature teeth with closed apices with greater than 3 mm displacement should be repositioned and splinted with a flexible acid-etched resin bonded splint for 2 weeks (up to 4 weeks if the displacement is significant and significant mobility is present after repositioning). With less than 3 mm of intrusion, the tooth can be allowed to spontaneously re-erupt over 2–3 weeks. If no movement occurs the tooth should be repositioned and splinted to prevent ankyloses (direct connection of the tooth to the alveolar bone). In immature teeth with

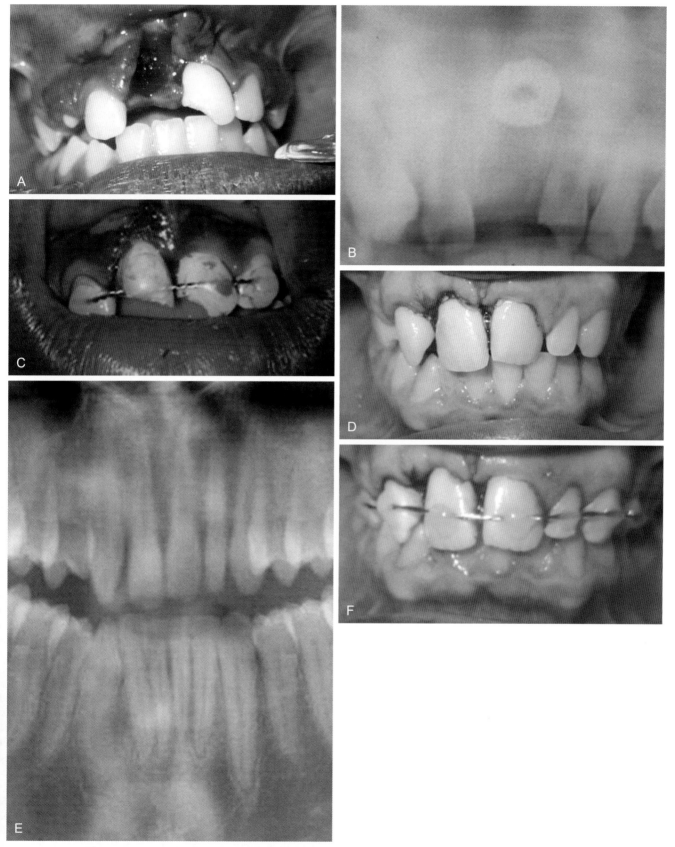

Fig. 1.18.12 Intrusion and extrusion injuries. (A) Right maxillary central incisor intrusion injury with crown completely buried in gingiva. There is an associated Ellis Class II injury of the left maxillary central incisor. (B) Orthopantomogram demonstrates superior displacement of tooth. (C) The intruded tooth was mobilized with a dental elevator and forceps, repositioned and splinted into place. It was found to have associated Ellis Class II fracture. (D) Extrusion injury involving right maxillary central incisor. (E) Orthopantomogram shows inferior displacement of the tooth. (F) Following repositioning with digital pressure a flexible, an acid-etched resin splint was placed.

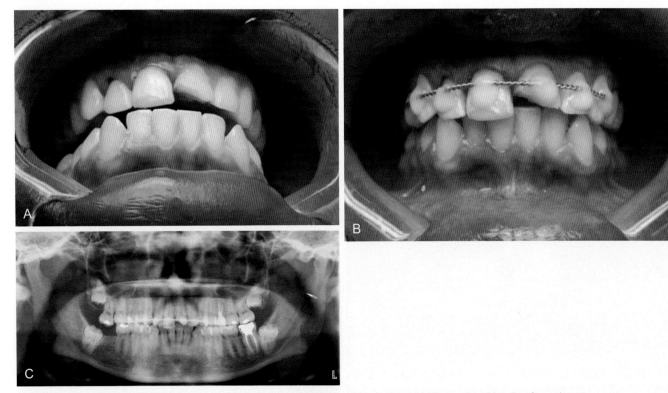

Fig. 1.18.13 Luxation injury. (A) Palatal and incisal luxation of a lateral incisor, minor bleeding from the surrounding gingival sulcus, and Ellis Class II fracture of the maxillary right central incisor. (B) The tooth was reduced manually and splinted with a braided 26-gauge wire (see also Video 1.18.1) and secured with acid-etched resin bonding. (C) Post-reduction radiograph showing adequate reduction within the socket with reestablished overbite and overjet relationship.

incomplete root development (open root apex), spontaneous re-eruption can be allowed with up to 7 mm of intrusion with orthodontic repositioning performed if no movement within 3 weeks. Intrusive displacement of primary teeth can result in damage to the developing permanent tooth bud. If impingement on a permanent tooth is found radiographically, the displaced tooth should be extracted. Otherwise the primary tooth can be left to spontaneously re-erupt.

Displacement in any direction other than axial is referred to as lateral luxation (Fig. 1.18.13). Most commonly, lateral luxation occurs with a blow to the facial surface of the incisors displacing them to the palatal/lingual and is associated with an alveolar bone fracture on the side of displacement. Adequate local anesthesia must be provided and the affected area cleaned with saline. The tooth should be repositioned with digital pressure, although dental forceps may be required to disengage the tooth from the fractured bony element to allow for proper positioning. A flexible acid-etched resin bonded splint should be placed for 1–2 weeks and the patient should see a general dentist to monitor pulpal vitality. Lateral luxation of primary teeth can be left alone for spontaneous realignment if not interfering with occlusion. Severely displaced primary teeth should be extracted.

Avulsion refers to complete displacement of the tooth out of the socket (Fig. 1.18.14). Timely treatment is paramount to improving the prognosis of the tooth. The goal is to preserve the vitality of the cells of the PDL. In the rare case in which prehospital treatment can be performed or when a patient has called prior to arrival, instruction should be given to reinsert the tooth as soon as possible. The root of the tooth should not be handled and should be gently rinsed with cold saline or water prior to insertion. If reinsertion is not tolerated, the tooth should be stored in an isotonic solution during transport.

Commercially available storage media include Hank's Balanced Salt Solution (Fig. 1.18.14E). Alternatively, the tooth can be held between the buccal mucosa and molars or stored in cow's milk. Water should never be used as it will lead to hydrolysis of the cells of the PDL. If the patient presents having already reinserted the tooth, appropriate imaging should be performed to ensure complete seating and a flexible bonded splint placed for 1–2 weeks. Immature teeth (incomplete root development) replaced immediately may revascularize and endodontic therapy may be avoided. Mature teeth will need endodontic treatment 7–10 days after injury. Avulsed primary teeth should never be replaced given the risk for ankylosis and disturbance of the eruption of the permanent teeth.

Injured patients often present with the avulsed tooth in a container. In this case, treatment depends on the maturity of the tooth and the duration of the extraoral dry time. When a mature tooth with a closed apex has been stored in an appropriate medium for less than 60 minutes the tooth should be handled only by the crown and the root surface gently cleansed with saline. After adequate local anesthesia, the socket should be irrigated thoroughly and examined to rule out alveolar bone fracture. Any fracture present should be reduced. The tooth should then be replanted with digital pressure and secured with a flexible acid-etched, resin bonded splint for 1–2 weeks. Tooth position should be confirmed with a dental radiograph. Endodontic therapy should be performed 7–10 days from the injury and prior to splint removal. If the tooth is immature with an open apex it should be soaked in a minocycline or doxycycline solution for 5 minutes prior to reinsertion. Occasionally, endodontic therapy may be avoided given the potential for revascularization, but pulp vitality should be monitored for 1– months.

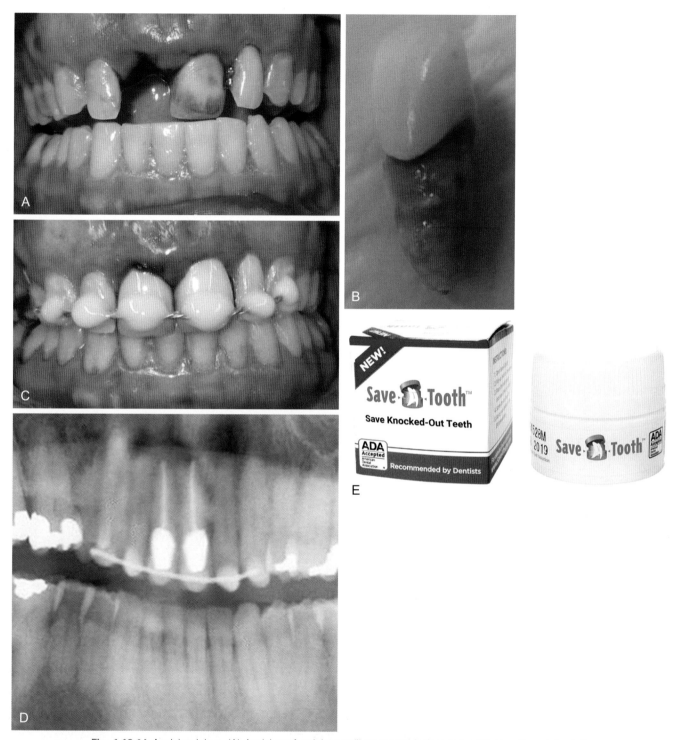

Fig. 1.18.14 Avulsion injury. (A) Avulsion of a right maxillary central incisor and palatal luxation of the left central incisor. (B) Tooth recovered from napkin brought in by patient within 60 minutes of injury. (C) Teeth were replanted and repositioned and secured with a flexible splint. (D) Postoperative orthopantomogram confirms positioning of teeth (endodontic treatment existed pre-injury). (E) Save-a-Tooth solution™ (Phoenix-Lazarus Inc.) containing a balanced salt solution medium optimal for tooth preservation.

Teeth (mature and immature) with more than 60 minutes of extraoral dry time have a poor prognosis due to necrosis of the PDL. Ankylosis followed by resorption is expected and the goal of therapy is temporary restoration of dentition and maintenance of alveolar bone for secondary reconstruction. Necrotic tissue should be removed from the root surface and the tooth soaked in a 2% fluoride solution for 20 minutes. After adequate anesthesia the socket should be cleaned and examined with any fractures reduced and the tooth replanted and secured with a flexible bonded splint for 1–2 weeks. Postop imaging should be obtained to confirm ideal positioning. Ideally endodontic therapy should be performed while the tooth is out of the mouth but this is not typically practical in an emergency department. Root canal therapy should be performed 7–10 days following the injury and prior to splint removal.

Following reinsertion of any avulsed tooth, tetanus immunization should be assured. Also, appropriate antibiotic coverage should be provided. Doxycycline is considered the preferred agent, but should be avoided in children less than 12 years of age due to staining of the developing dentition. Amoxicillin is the next alternative.[32]

Alveolar Injuries

Fractures through the alveolar bone only are known as alveolar segment or dentoalveolar fractures (Fig. 1.18.15). These may extend through the sockets of the associated teeth and can be associated with a concomitant dental injury within the fractured segment. Most commonly, the segment contains multiple teeth and although the alveolar segment

is mobile, the teeth within are firmly seated in bone and move as a unit. These injuries should be considered a maxillofacial fracture rather than a dental fracture and the same principles of reduction and fixation should be applied. After adequate local anesthesia, the fractured segment should be irrigated, manually repositioned and secured using a rigid splint. The most common fixation method is with Erich arch bars. After the segment has been repositioned the arch bar should be adapted to the affected arch extending at least two teeth adjacent to the fractured segment. Apply circumdental wires (26-gauge) to the adjacent teeth first and then secure the fractured segment to the arch bar using the full complement of dentition within the fractured segment for increased stability (Fig. 1.18.16). Post-reduction imaging should confirm appropriate position and the segment should remain in fixation for 4 weeks. Concomitant dental injuries should be treated independently, such as applying an acid-etched resin bonded splint for luxated teeth within a

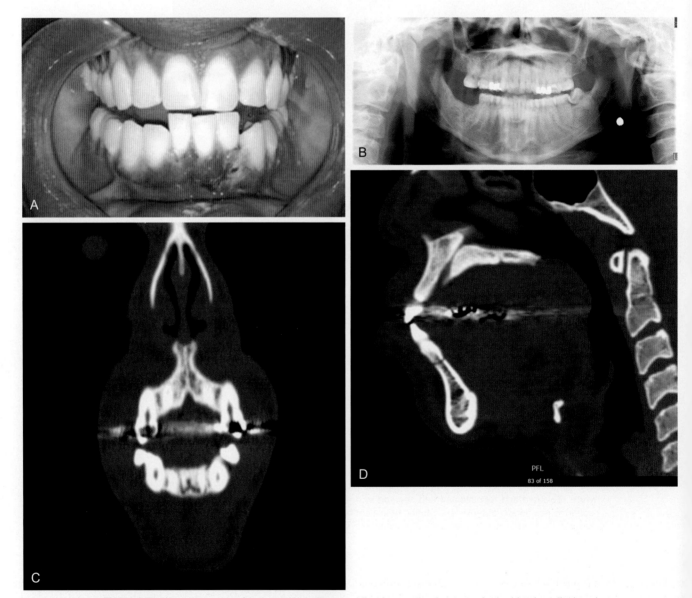

Fig. 1.18.15 Alveolar process fractures. (A) A 30-year-old male sustained an assault resulting in a displaced fracture segment containing the right mandibular central, left mandibular central, and lateral incisors. (B) An orthopantogram showed displacement of the segment superiorly, but fracture the tooth roots. (C–D) CT images show the fractured alveolar segment in the coronal (C) and sagittal planes (D).

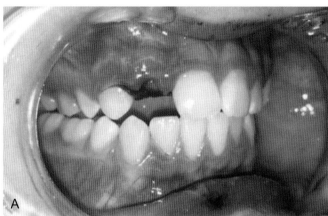
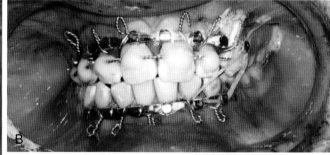
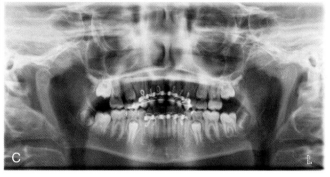

Fig. 1.18.16 Combined mandibular fracture and dental injury. A 13-year-old boy who sustained a bicycle accident with subsequent complete intrusion of his maxillary right lateral incisor and bilateral subcondylar fractures (clinical photos are shown in Fig. 1.18.5). (A) Preoperative malocclusion with dental interferences posteriorly preventing full dental intercuspation (due to the condylar fractures). The lateral incisor was intruded below the gingiva. (B) Post-reduction view of the lateral incisor splinted with braided 26-gauge wire secured with acid-etched resin. An anterior arch bar was placed for guiding elastics for management of the condylar fractures. (C) Post-reduction radiograph showing adequate reduction of the right lateral incisor.

fractured dentoalveolar segment. Gingival lacerations are often associated with the injuries and should be sutured with an absorbable material. The goal is to maintain keratinized tissue around teeth typically avoiding advancement flaps that bring non-keratinized, mobile alveolar mucosa adjacent to teeth.

SURGICAL TECHNIQUES

Splinting of Teeth

Armamentarium: local anesthetic, cheek retractors, dental etch (30%–40% phosphoric acid), dental prime and bonding agents, curing light, 26-gauge wire.

See Video 1.18.1.

Reduction and Fixation of Dentoalveolar Fractures

Armamentarium: local anesthetic, cheek retractors, Erich arch bars, 26-gauge wires.

See Video 1.18.2.

ACUTE COMPLICATIONS

Because the majority of dentoalveolar fractures are treated in an outpatient and community setting, there are few data on the incidence of complications associated with treatment. Several complications can arise in the first 1–2 weeks of management, including malocclusion from inadequate reduction of teeth or alveolar segments, hardware failure, local site infection, and soft tissue necrosis. With close follow-up (2–3 days after treatment) the majority of acute complications can be mitigated or eliminated. During this follow-up, the integrity of the dental

splint or arch bar should be evaluated, as well as mobility of the teeth within the hardware. Any premature occlusal contact or malocclusion should raise suspicion for inadequate reduction or improper positioning and be corrected as soon as possible as increased occlusal force can lead to malunion, nonunion, or tooth loss.

The patient should also be encouraged to follow up with an appropriate dental specialist for endodontic or restorative treatment in the acute setting and treatment planning for replacement of teeth as necessary. Any evidence of infection during follow-up should be treated with incision, drainage and antibiotics. Gingival inflammation or compromise should be treated with chlorhexidine (0.12%) mouth rinse twice a day until inflammation subsides or areas of bony exposure granulate.

LONG-TERM COMPLICATIONS

Long-term complications from dentoalveolar trauma arise from improper positioning of the fractured segments, or complications associated with hard and soft tissue healing. The fate of the pulpal and periodontal tissues varies according to type and severity of injury and time until reduction (especially in the case of dental avulsion). In luxation, intrusion, and avulsion injuries the most common complication is necrosis of the dental pulp. This will usually present as a delayed discoloration of a tooth, and lack of response to stimulus on vitality testing. Patients with pulp necrosis require root canal treatment to prevent infection and esthetic complications.

As the pulp and periodontium respond to an insult there are several reactions that can occur. Hyperemia of the pulp chamber that occurs in response to trauma can be reversible and the vitality restored or irreversible leading to pulpal necrosis. Pulpal hemorrhage can occur, resulting in discoloration of the tooth due to the presence of hemosiderin within the dentinal tubules. Discoloration can occur in the presence or absence of pulp necrosis. Other reactions of the pulpal tissue include calcific metamorphosis and internal resorption months to years after injury. Calcific metamorphosis results in a narrowing or obliteration of the pulp chamber with additional dentin formation leading the tooth to appear opaque and/or yellow in color. Internal resorption can occur in a slow or rapid fashion resulting in destruction of the tooth structure initiating from the pulpal tissue. This process can be seen by a pink hue of the tooth or with increased size or abnormal shape of the pulp chamber on a radiograph. Internal resorption can be arrested with an endodontic treatment if detected early

Another common complication after damage to the PDL is secondary external resorption. Avulsed and intruded teeth are most commonly associated with both pulpal necrosis and resorption. External root resorption results from irreversible damage to the PDL.[30] If external resorption is suspected, a prompt referral to an endodontist is indicated, but the most common result is eventual need for extraction of the tooth.

Displacement of primary teeth can lead to damage to developing tooth buds. This can manifest as discoloration, malformation, or failure of eruption of the permanent tooth.[33,34] Treatment of these complications may require multiple dental specialists.

Posttreatment malocclusion can result due to a variety of factors. Depending on the severity of the malocclusion, treatment could include occlusal adjustment (i.e., selective tooth reduction), orthodontics, prosthodontics, extractions with dental implant placement, or surgical correction with osteotomies. These complex cases require multispecialty (prosthetic, orthodontic, and surgical) collaboration.

Loss of alveolar bone following trauma or dental extractions creates functional and prosthetic challenges. While the details of rehabilitation techniques are not within the scope of this chapter, clinicians who treat dentoalveolar trauma should understand the basic concepts of functional and prosthetic rehabilitation. Deficits in alveolar bone height and width commonly occur following tooth loss or traumatic avulsion. These deficits should be recognized at the time of the injury and the patient can be informed of the need for secondary bone grafting to allow dental implant placement and/or prosthetic rehabilitation. Advances in endosteal dental implants have led to a trend toward less bone grafting and innovative ways of overcoming a deficit in alveolar bone such as short implants and guided bone regeneration. These advances minimize treatment time, donor site morbidity, and recent studies have shown comparable outcomes to traditional approaches.[35-37]

EXPERT COMMENTARY

Most books on dental injury, alveolar fractures, and occlusion are long, detailed, and difficult for non-dental trained clinicians to understand. Yet, the principles of treatment are often simpler than anticipated, and may (and should be) pursued at the time of primary treatment. The principles described in this well-written and accurate chapter should be employed by all clinicians managing facial fractures, and improved care will result [1,2].

References

1. Manson P, Clark N, Robertson B, et al. Subunit principles in midface fractures: the importance of sagittal buttresses, soft tissue reductions and sequencing treatment of segmental fractures. *Plast Reconstr Surg*. 1999;103:1287–1306.
2. Hendrickson M, Clark N, Manson P. Sagittal fractures of the maxilla: classification and treatment. *Plast Reconstr Surg*. 1998;101:319–332.

REFERENCES

1. Leathers RD, Gowans RE. Management of alveolar and dental fractures. In: Miloro M, Ghali GE, Larsen P, Waite P, eds. *Peterson's Principles of Oral and Maxillofacial Surgery*. 3rd ed. Shelton, CT: PMHP-USA; 2012.
2. Shayne's Dental Site. History of dentistry, Greco-Roman dentistry (AD 350–750). Available at: http://www.dental-site.itgo.com/grecoroman.htm. Accessed August 12, 2016.
3. Abubaker AO, Papadopoulos H, Giglio JA. Diagnosis and management of dentoalveolar injuries. In: Fonseca R, Marciani RD, Turvey T, eds. *Oral and Maxillofacial Surgery*. 2nd ed. St. Louis: Saunders; 2000.
4. Lida S, Matsuya T. Pediatric maxillofacial injuries: their aetiological characters and fracture patterns. *J Craniomaxillofac Surg*. 2002;30:237–241.
5. Zaleckiene V, Peciuliene V, Brukiene V, Drukteinis S. Traumatic dental injuries: etiology, prevalence and possible outcomes. *Stomatologija*. 2014;16:7–14.
6. Kraft A, Abermann E, Stigler R, et al. Craniomaxillofacial trauma: synopsis of 14,654 cases with 35,129 injuries in 15 years. *Craniomaxillofac Trauma Reconstr*. 2012;5:41–50.
7. Mock C, Quansah R, Krishnan R, et al. Strengthening the prevention and care of injuries worldwide. *Lancet*. 2004;363:2172–2179.
8. Telfer MR, Jones GM, Shepherd JP. Trends in the aetiology of maxillofacial fractures in the United Kingdom (1977–1987). *Br J Oral Maxillofac Surg*. 1991;29:250–255.
9. Imahara SD, Hopper RA, Wang J, et al. Patterns and outcomes of pediatric facial fractures in the United States: a survey of the National Trauma Data Bank. *J Am Coll Surg*. 2008;207:710–716.
10. Andreasen JO. Classification, etiology and epidemiology. In: *Traumatic Injuries of the Teeth*. 2nd ed. Copenhagen: Munksgaard; 1981.
11. Baumann A, Troulis MJ, Kaban LB. Facial Trauma II: dentoalveolar injuries and mandibular fractures. In: Kaban LB, Troulis MJ, eds. *Pediatric Oral and Maxillofacial Surgery*. Amsterdam: Elsevier; 2004.
12. Norton NS. Oral cavity. In: Norton NS, ed. *Netter's Head and Neck Anatomy for Dentistry*. 2nd ed. Philadelphia, PA: Saunders; 2012.
13. Gwinnett AJ. Structure and composition of enamel. *Oper Dent*. 1992;5(s):10–17.
14. Goldberg M, Kulkarni AB, Young M, Boskey A. Dentin: structure, composition and mineralization: the role of dentin ECM in dentin formation and mineralization. *Front Biosci (Elite Ed)*. 2011;3: 711–735.
15. Nanci A, Bosshardt DD. Structure of periodontal tissues in health and disease. *Periodontol 2000*. 2006;40(1):11–28.
16. Trope M. Root resorption of dental and traumatic origin: classification based on etiology. *Pract Periodontics Aesthet Dent*. 1998;10:515–522.
17. Sobin L, Kopp R, Walsh R, et al. Incidence of concussion in patients with isolated mandible fractures. *JAMA Facial Plast Surg*. 2016;18(1):15–18. doi:10.1001/jamafacial.2015.1339. Published online October 8, 2015.
18. Afrooz PN, Grunwaldt LJ, Zanoun RR, et al. Pediatric facial fractures: occurrence of concussion and relation to fracture patterns. *J Craniofac Surg*. 2012;23(5):1270–1273.
19. Elahi MM, Brar MS, Ahmed N, et al. Cervical spine injury in association with cranial maxillofacial fractures. *Plast Reconstr Surg*. 2008;121:201–208.
20. Jamal BT, Diecidue R, Qutob A, Cohen M. The pattern of combined maxillofacial and cervical spine fractures. *J Oral Maxillofac Surg*. 2009;67(3):559–562.
21. Andreasen JO. Classification, etiology and epidemiology. In: Andreasen JO, ed. *Traumatic Injuries of the Teeth*. 2nd ed. Copenhagen: Munksgaard; 1981.
22. Rowe NL, Killey HC. The clinical examination of fractures of the middle third of the facial skeleton involving the dentoalveolar component. In: Rowe NL, Killey HC, eds. *Fractures of the Facial Skeleton*. 2nd ed. Baltimore: Williams & Wilkins; 1970:345.
23. Evans D, Reid J, Strang R, Stirrups D. A comparison of laser Doppler flowmetry with other methods of assessing the vitality of traumatized anterior teeth. *Endod Dent Traumatol*. 1990;15(6):284–290.

24. Munshi A, Hegde A, Radhakrishnan S. Pulse oximetry: a diagnostic instrument in pulpal vitality testing. *J Clin Pediatr Dent.* 2003;26(2):141–145.
25. Alghaithy RA, Qualtrough AJ. Pulp sensibility and vitality tests for diagnosing pulpal health in permanent teeth: a critical review. *Int Endod J.* 2016;doi:10.1111/iej.12611.
26. Feliciano KMPC, De Franca Caldas A Jr. A systematic review of the diagnostic classifications of traumatic dental injuries. *Dent Traumatol.* 2006;22:71–76.
27. Andreasen JO. Etiology and pathogenesis of traumatic dental injuries: a clinical study of 1298 cases. *Scand J Dent Res.* 1970;78:329–342.
28. Ellis RG. *The Classification and Treatment of Injuries to the Teeth of Children.* Chicago: Year Book Publishers; 1945.
29. Garcia-Godoy F. A classification for traumatic injuries to primary and permanent teeth. *J Pedod.* 1981;5:295–297.
30. Andreasen JO. Dental trauma guide. Resource Centre for Rare Oral Diseases and Department of Oral and Maxillo-Facial Surgery at the University Hospital of Copenhagen. Edited July 1, 2014. http://www.dentaltraumaguide.org/Default.aspx. Accessed October 31, 2016.
31. Leathers RD, Gowans RE. Office-based management of dental alveolar trauma. *Atlas Oral Maxillofac Surg Clin North Am.* 2013;21:185–197.
32. Hinckfuss SE, Messer LB. An evidenced-based assessment of the clinical guidelines for replanted avulsed teeth. Part II: prescription of systemic antibiotics. *Dent Traumatol.* 2009;25(2):158–164.
33. Andreasen JO, Sundstrom B, Ravn JJ. The effect of traumatic injuries to primary teeth on their permanent successors. I. A clinical and histologic study of 117 injured permanent teeth. *Scand J Dent Res.* 1971;79:219.
34. Andreasen JO, Ravn JJ. The effect of traumatic injuries to primary teeth on their permanent successors. II. A clinical and radiographic follow-up study of 213 injured teeth. *Scand J Dent Res.* 1971;79:284.
35. Alani A, Austin R, Djemal S. Contemporary management of tooth replacement in the traumatized dentition. *Dent Traumatol.* 2012;28(3):183–192.
36. Vega LG, Gielincki W, Fernandes RP. Zygoma implant reconstruction of acquired maxillary bony defects. *Oral Maxillofac Surg Clin North Am.* 2013;25:223–239.
37. Thoma DS, Zeltner M, Husler J, et al. EAO Supplement Working Group 4 – EAO CC 2015 Short implants versus sinus lifting with longer implants to restore the posterior maxilla: a systematic review. *Clin Oral Implants Res.* 2015;26(suppl 11):154–169.

Management of Panfacial Fractures

Gerhard S. Mundinger, Joseph S. Gruss, Richard A. Hopper

BACKGROUND

A panfacial craniofacial injury refers to fractures present simultaneously in the cranio-orbital (upper third), orbitozygomaticomaxillary (middle third), as well as the mandibular (lower third) portions of the craniofacial skeleton (Fig. 1.19.1). This requirement of panfacial injuries to have fractures present in all three levels of the face is not consistently used among trauma studies, with some authors including patients with severe injury in only two levels.[1] The incidence of panfacial injury ranges from 0.8% to 3% in large craniofacial fracture series, and can occur from a number of mechanisms, including blunt, penetrating, and avulsive mechanisms in all age groups.[2] These injuries present challenges in surgical management to avoid long-term sequelae of inadequate correction, including increased facial width, enophthalmos, facial retrusion, and malocclusion (Figs. 1.19.2 and 1.19.3).[3] The purpose of this chapter is to provide an algorithm for management of these panfacial injuries in order to optimize outcomes.

SURGICAL ANATOMY

Due to the multiple components and steps in acute surgical correction of panfacial fractures, it is imperative always to remember the overall goals of increasing facial projection, decreasing facial width, restoring functional and symmetric globe position, and restoring optimal occlusion. These goals can be lost during the focus on individual fractures during a prolonged surgery, after which each individual fracture may appear well reduced, but the overall esthetic result is suboptimal. Understanding, identifying, and restoring reliable transverse and vertical facial buttresses rather than reducing single fracture lines is paramount to achieving a favorable three-dimensional outcome (Fig. 1.19.4).[4–6]

CLINICAL PRESENTATION

Patients with panfacial injuries have sustained a degree of trauma that results in multiple potential associated injuries. All patients must undergo full multidisciplinary ACLS staged assessment to rule out other associated life-threatening conditions before focusing on the specific facial injuries.[7–9] Intracranial, cervical spine, thoracic, abdominal, and severe extremity injuries must be ruled out or treated before the patient will be stable enough for craniofacial reconstruction.[10,11] Although many facial injuries can be surgically treated acutely at the time of presentation before swelling occurs, panfacial injuries typically require days, and in rare cases weeks, before stabilization allows clearance for the craniofacial team to treat the facial injuries. Life-threatening acute facial bleeding will require a staged escalating algorithm for treatment in these patients along a spectrum from compressing and packing to interventional radiology embolization.[12]

RADIOLOGICAL EVALUATION

Due to the high incidence of internal carotid injuries in high sub-cranial fractures, it is our protocol to perform CT angiography on all panfacial injuries.[12,13] High-definition, thin-slice CT scans with three dimensional reconstructions are invaluable in evaluation, surgical planning, and subsequent long-term management of panfacial fractures. Additionally, intraoperative CT scanning, when available, can be useful for assuring accurate placement of orbital implants at the time of surgery (Fig. 1.19.5).[14] Although stereotactic navigation and computer generated models are useful in secondary corrections of complex cases, they are not usually readily available for acute treatment.

PRESURGICAL PREPARATION

Prior to commencing surgical treatment of a panfacial injury, preoperative considerations include perioperative airway management, cervical spine precautions, anesthetic/transfusion plans, surgical team composition, as well as preparation for anticipated adjunctive techniques, such as pericranial flaps, bone graft donor sites, and need for free-tissue reconstruction. A number of options for airway management are available and should be considered, including oral, nasal, submental, and tracheal airways. The entire team should identify the key milestones of treatment at the beginning of surgery, as well as a plan to cycle team members to prevent fatigue and optimize efficiency.

SURGICAL TECHNIQUES

When considering the sequence for fracture reduction and fixation, it is important follow a vertical and horizontal system of reconstruction as guided by the vertical and horizontal facial buttresses. A number of systems (top-down vs. bottom-up; outside to inside vs. inside to outside, etc.) have been proposed.[4,15–17] Each approach has merits, and most experienced trauma teams will be comfortable with more than one sequence of treatment which they will interchange depending on the specific pattern and differential degrees of injury in the regions of the face. For this chapter, we will describe the 11 steps of a top-down, outside-to-inside approach that is the most commonly used at our institutions (Table 1.19.1). It is important to emphasize that most panfacial injuries will require autologous bone grafts and/or vascularized pericranial flaps at some step of the surgery, therefore care must be taken to ensure that these resources are available during prepping and draping of the patient and during the initial dissection.

Step 1: Expose All Treatable Fractures

The cranium, nasofrontal, zygomatic arch, lateral orbital rims, and medial orbital wall regions can be best exposed with a coronal incision. Lower

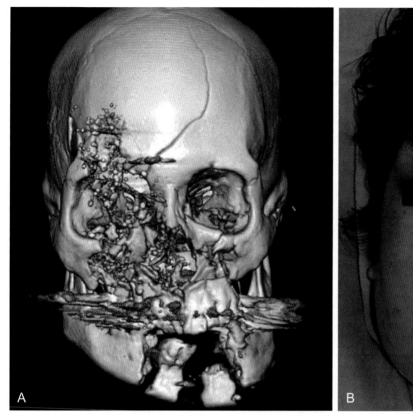 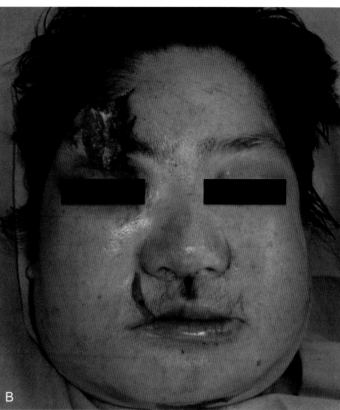

Fig. 1.19.1 True panfacial injury, involving all three of the facial thirds, resulting from a gunshot. Note the increased facial width and height.

TABLE 1.19.1 An 11-Step, Top-Down, Inside-Out Algorithm for Treatment of Panfacial Injuries

Step	Action
1	Expose all treatable fractures
2	Establish skullbase and fronto-orbital bandeau references
3	Position the zygomas
4	Isolate and reconstruct the orbits
5	Address the nasomaxillary region
6	Set the vertical facial height
7	Set the first arch width
8	Establish and maintain centric occlusion
9	Estimate centric relation
10	Step back and reconsider the big picture
11	Move closer and consider the details

eyelid incisions facilitate orbital floor exposure as well as visualization of the upper transverse and vertical facial buttresses. Upper and lower gingivobuccal sulcus incisions will allow access to the transverse buttresses of the maxilla and anterior mandible. Posterior mandible skin incisions such as the Risdon approach or retromandibular approach may be required for complex angle or condylar fractures in order to achieve reliable reconstruction of the posterior vertical buttress of the mandible ramus (Fig. 1.19.6). Parasagittal palate incisions may be required to reestablish the posterior maxillary width if a reliable mandible arch is not available as a reference. Incisions should be tailored to individual

patient patterns of hair loss and preexisting lacerations, which can provide excellent access and should always be considered in surgical planning.

Step 2: Establish Skullbase and Fronto-Orbital Bandeau References

The anterior skullbase and fronto-orbital region serves as a reliable reference in all but the most severe panfacial fractures. Fractures in this region should be plated and the supraorbital bar reduced and fixated to serve as the foundation for reconstruction of subcranial skeleton. If this reconstruction is done inaccurately, it will create a domino effect of a series of malreduced subcranial fractures. The goals of skullbase and frontal treatment include sealing the sinuses from the cranium,[18] prevention of pulsatile enophthalmos by rigid correction of the superior orbit, and preservation/correction of orbital volume. It is paramount to ensure that bone grafts to the superior orbit are not positioned too low, and are rigidly fixated (Fig. 1.19.7). Sphenoid fractures are an indication of high velocity injury, and require reduction to decompress the orbital apex as well as create a reliable reference for reduction of the zygomas.[19] Rigid fixation of anterior cranial base or orbital roof grafts is required to prevent inferior migration from pulsation of the brain postoperation, as well as to allow salvage of the grafts in case of intracranial infection and the need for a surgical washout. Cranial bone segments should maximize bone-to-bone contact at as much of the perimeter of the fracture segments as possible. This may necessitate leaving bony gaps at other portions of the fracture in order to optimize contact elsewhere. This is preferable to positioning calvarial bone at the center of the skull defect with equal circumferential spacing, which is essentially creating a sequestra and will lead to nonunion, resorption, and/or infection. A small intentional bony gap is left, however, between the superior orbital rim and the frontal craniotomy bone in the cases

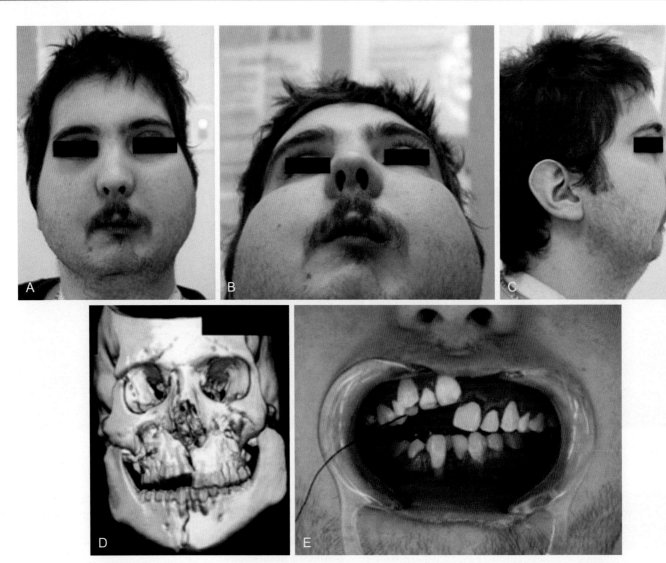

Fig. 1.19.2 Sequelae of untreated panfacial fractures one year after injury due to comorbidities preventing surgical treatment. Untreated panfacial injuries result in increased facial width at the zygomatic and mandible levels, enophthalmos, chin point retrusion, and severe malocclusion.

where a pericranial flap is placed through the gap to provide soft tissue seal of the anterior cranial fossa.

Step 3: Position the Zygomas

Once the skullbase and frontal bone is reconstructed, accurate positioning of the zygomas is crucial to restoring midfacial width and projection, but is challenging given the tendency of the zygoma to pivot around all of its four articulations (Fig. 1.19.8).[20] It is important to be cognizant of temporal bone fractures extending onto the zygomatic arch, and sphenoid impaction, both of which can result in inaccurate zygoma positioning. The zygomatic arch is a hyperbola, rather than a true arch or straight line, and therefore should project linearly in a sagittal plane from the temporal bone before curving sharply at the zygomatic body (Fig. 1.19.9).[21] In complex cases, plating of the arch at the junction of the temporal skullbase or sphenoid reduction is required for accurate zygoma positioning.

Step 4: Isolate and Reconstruct the Orbits

Following restoration of midfacial width and projection by positioning the zygomas, the orbits are explored and a plan for reconstruction made. Restoring orbital floor and medial wall position with grafts or

implants at this point in the reconstruction sequence affords excellent exposure, and may be the best chance for access to this region before plating other segments that can subsequently limit access when facial width is decreased to the normal anatomic position. Orbital graft or implant position and freedom from implying soft tissue contents, however, must always be rechecked at the end of the case with direct visualization (often challenging due to the swelling), forced duction test, and/or intraoperative CT scan.

Step 5: Address the Nasomaxillary Region

Fractures in the nasomaxillary region typically have a superior component close to the nasofrontal junction, and an inferior component closer to the inferior orbital rim. In severely comminuted or displaced cases, spanning plates are necessary. The twisted, curvilinear shape in this region is created in the spanning plate, which is then pulled subperiosteally, anterior to the medial canthus, from the coronal incision to the lower lid incision. It is important to first correct the sagittal rotation of the zygomas and naso-orbital ethmoid (NOE) segments before compressing the facial width. The increased facial width will not be corrected without addressing the rotation deformity first, regardless of the degree of compression. Our usual sequence in this complex

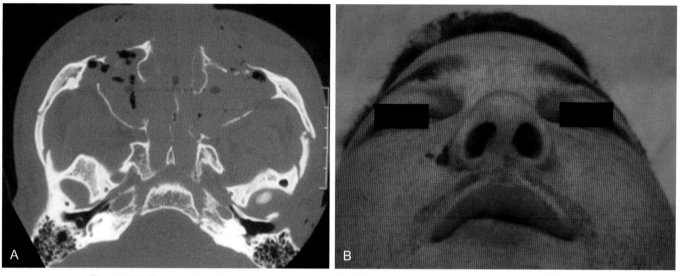

Fig. 1.19.3 The broad goals of treatment of panfacial injuries are to restore increased facial width and decreased facial projection. Facial impaction and widening is evident on CT imaging (A) and is clinically most appreciated in the submental view (B).

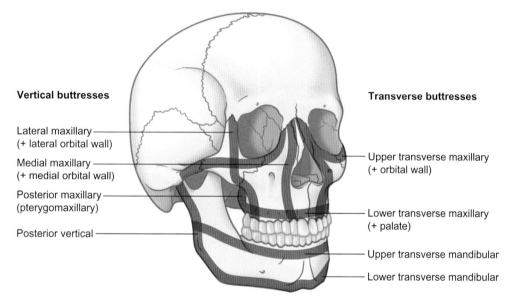

Vertical buttresses

Lateral maxillary
(+ lateral orbital wall)

Medial maxillary
(+ medial orbital wall)

Posterior maxillary
(pterygomaxillary)

Posterior vertical

Transverse buttresses

Upper transverse maxillary
(+ orbital wall)

Lower transverse maxillary
(+ palate)

Upper transverse mandibular

Lower transverse mandibular

Fig. 1.19.4 The transverse and vertical buttresses of the face guide fracture reduction and are sites of strong bone suitable for placement of fixation hardware. (Reproduced with permission from Hopper RA, Salemy S, Sze RW. Diagnosis of midface fractures with CT: What the surgeon needs to know. RadioGraphics 2006;26:783–793.)

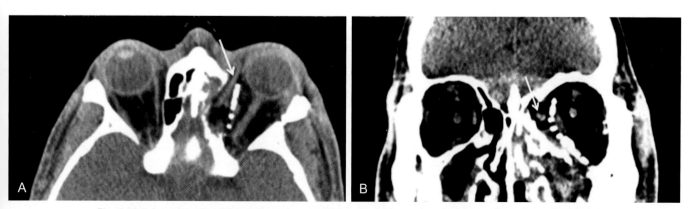

Fig. 1.19.5 Intraoperative CT imaging, when available, can aid in precise placement of reconstructive hardware. This is particularly useful for orbital implants to mitigate improper placement, as illustrated here in a patient where the orbital implant was between the medial rectus muscle (*arrow*) and globe, which would lead to severe postoperative diplopia.

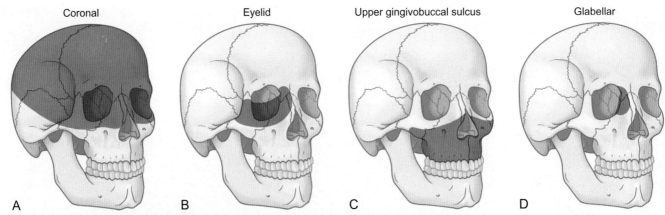

| Coronal | Eyelid | Upper gingivobuccal sulcus | Glabellar |

A   B   C   D

Fig. 1.19.6 Common upperface and midface craniofacial incisions and regions that can be accessed through them. Coronal (A), eyelid (B), upper gingivobuccal sulcus (C), glabellar (D). (Modified with permission from Hopper RA, Salemy S, Sze RW. Diagnosis of midface fractures with CT: What the surgeon needs to know. RadioGraphics 2006;26:783–793.)

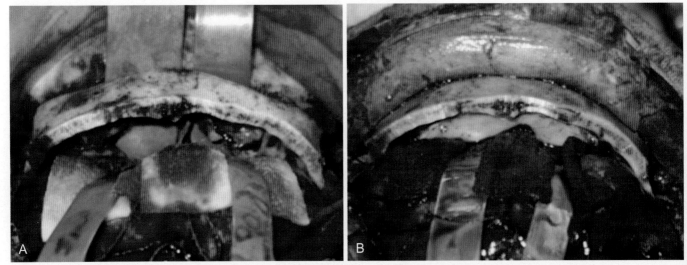

A   B

Fig. 1.19.7 In cases of severe comminution or bony loss, reconstruction of the orbital roofs back to the middle cranial fossa can be achieved with titanium implants but the pulsations of the brain can lead to inferior displacement. Split calvarial bone grafts that are rigidly fixated and placed higher than anatomical position not only prevent pressure on the globe, but also provide a rigid separation of the intracranial cavity and subcranial sinuses that can better withstand irrigation and salvage in the case of postoperative infection and reoperation.

region is to fixate the premolded spanning plate to the zygoma, use elevators through the mouth incisions to derotate the segments, then compress the facial width, and fixate the spanning plate to the frontal bone. Percutaneous digital compression of the plate in the region anterior to the medial canthus just prior to frontal bone fixation will give the optimum anterior control of the NOE segment (Fig. 1.19.10). It is critical to recognize that NOE fractures in combination with zygomaxillary complex fractures (Gruss type 4 NOE)[22] are extremely disruptive to the upper transverse facial curve, leading to appreciable facial flattening and lengthening if unrecognized or inadequately corrected. It is paramount not to miss medial canthal disruption, or to avulse partially injured medial canthal structures.[23] Transnasal compression wires and barb suture repositioning of the canthus superiorly and posteriorly are useful for correcting posterior rotation of nasoethmoid fracture segments/

medial canthal avulsions, which can also be molded to the bone by the application of a well-padded transnasal skin bolster at the conclusion of the case.[24]

Step 6: Set the Vertical Facial Height

Reduction and plating of fractures in the preceding steps establishes restoration of the upper facial horizontal buttresses, thereby setting the facial width at the level of the orbits. Fixation of the first vertical buttress of the face below the orbits will restore the facial height, and is required to establish centric relation of the occlusion. The most reliable vertical buttress (given the fracture pattern and areas of bone loss) should be identified, reduced, and plated. The main choices for vertical fixation include the posterior vertical mandibular (ramus and condyle), medial maxillary (nasomaxillary), and lateral maxillary (zygomaticomaxillary)

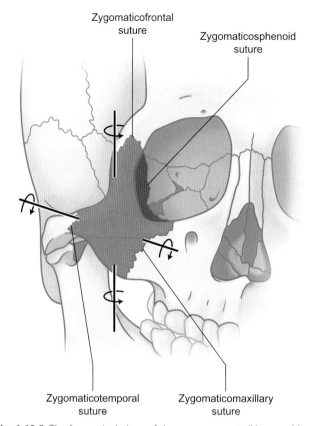

Fig. 1.19.8 The four articulations of the zygoma must all be considered for accurate reduction. (Reproduced with permission from Hopper RA, Salemy S, Sze RW. Diagnosis of midface fractures with CT: What the surgeon needs to know. RadioGraphics 2006;26:783–793.)

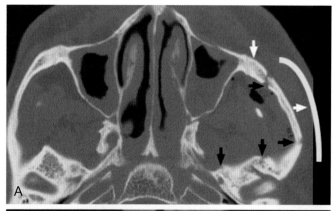

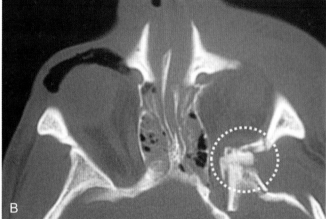

Fig. 1.19.9 (A) The zygomatic arch is a hyperbola (*yellow line*, mirrored from the contralateral unfractured side), not a straight line, and should be reconstructed to restore this shape (*black arrows*: sites of fracture; *white arrows*: direction of fracture displacement). (B) Sphenoid fractures (*dotted circle*) can greatly influence zygoma positioning, and need to be telescoped out to achieve appropriate zygoma position and arch form.

buttresses. In many panfacial cases, the midface is so comminuted that open treatment of a condylar fracture is required to establish vertical facial height.

Step 7: Set the First Arch Width

In many panfacial fractures there is lack of continuity of both the maxillary and mandibular arches . In order to eventually set centric occlusion, the most reliable arch form to reconstruct must be reduced and fixation completed. In cases of severe maxillary segmentation, treatment of multiple mandible fractures reestablishing bigonial width may be the most reliable first arch. In other cases, mandible damage may require maxillary palatal reduction and fixation in order to determine premorbid arch width. For the maxilla, plates can be placed at the anterior piriform aperture and roof of the hard palate, and for the mandible, standard plate positioning can be utilized to stabilize tooth-bearing segments. It is important to recognize that mandibular width can be increased by bigonial splaying, leading to a wide and lingually splayed arch form (Fig. 1.19.11). Mandible splaying can be corrected with bigonial angle pressure to correct arch width during fixation. Preoperative model surgery to fashion a splint in cases of severe comminution and alveolar bone disruption can greatly aid in establishing arch width, and should be considered when feasible.

Step 8: Establish and Maintain Centric Occlusion

Establishment of centric occlusion gives the best functional maxilla–mandibular occlusal relationship given multiple fractured segments.

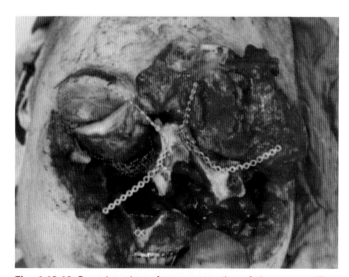

Fig. 1.19.10 Spanning plates for reconstruction of the nasomaxillary region.

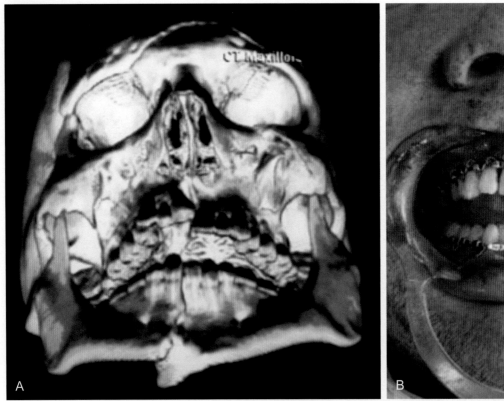
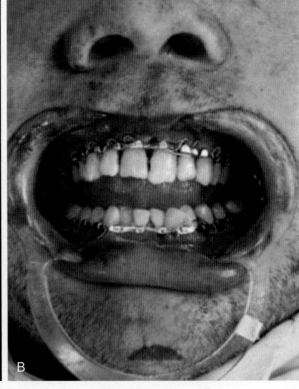

Fig. 1.19.11 (A) A patient with a palatal split and symphyseal mandible fracture resulting in increased maxillary and mandible arch width. (B) The maxilla has been corrected through anterior alveolar and posterior palatal platings, but the mandible fixation has been inadequate in restoring mandible arch width, resulting in posterior crossbites. The mandible was subsequently reduced with bigonial pressure and refixation to restore a functional occlusion.

Intermaxillary fixation sets the arch width of the most severely damaged arch to the reconstructed arch. All arch segments are held in position with standard plate fixation. At the end of this step, the maxilla and mandible are in optimal intercuspation occlusion (centric occlusion) but are not connected in 3-dimensional space relative to the skullbase (not in centric relation).

Step 9: Estimate Centric Relation

Precisely identifying centric relation can be challenging in panfacial injury, given fracture displacement of the condylar process and glenoid fossa. Centric relation should be estimated using the most reliable reconstructed vertical buttress as a guide (Step 7), while maintaining the patient in established occlusion (Step 8). The maxillary–mandibular occlusal unit established in Step 8 is repositioned and fixated to the most reliable buttress that establishes the best centric relation with the skull base. In some cases this is by reconstructing the relationship of the posterior mandible vertical buttress of the condyle to the temporal bone, and in other cases it is the relationship of the medial or lateral maxillary buttresses to the anterior cranial base. Once the most reliable vertical buttress has been identified, the patient's centric occlusal unit is rotated into centric relation until there is optimal bone contact along the buttress. Once the reference buttress is plated, remaining fractures can then be plated sequentially from this buttress. Autologous bone grafts can be used to fill in existing fracture gaps to maintain estimated centric relation, or gaps can be spanned with plates if soft tissue coverage is inadequate or there is gross contamination. Gaps and bony step-offs more remote from the functional occlusal segments are expected in most cases, and attempts at perfect reduction of nonfunctional segments can result in less functional outcomes and paradoxically more

distorted anatomy. By altering sides of plating away from occlusal segments, shifting of centric relation can be minimized. This is analogous to changing a flat tire on a car, where wheel bolts should be replaced by alternatively tightening opposite, rather than adjacent, bolts to avoid an unbalanced wheel.

Step 10: Step Back and Reconsider the Big Picture

The art of panfacial treatment lies in consideration of the larger functional and final esthetic outcome after initial treatment. Long-term problems and revisional surgeries may often be avoided by stepping back and reconsidering the larger goals of treatment, and by thoughtful reflection on the goals of management. Does the fixation make sense? Is the facial width compressed at all levels? Is the vertical height appropriate? Has facial projection been restored? Is the face compartmentalized into upper, middle, and lower units with restored barriers between the frontal sinus and brain, and midface sinuses and oral cavity? Has occlusal function been maximized to the greatest extent possible given the injuries?

Step 11: Move Closer and Consider the Details

Accurate reduction and fixation sets the foundation for reconstruction of panfacial injuries. Additional work beyond bone reconstruction of the craniofacial skeleton is important to avoid common and noticeable sequelae. Panfacial injuries and surgical approaches to the midface result in increased laxity of the midfacial soft tissues because of necessary dissection of the suspensory ligaments. The periosteal envelope of the face must be resuspended to holes in the inferior and lateral orbital rim with large resorbable sutures to avoid cheek ptosis, and an overly long and aged-appearing face with time (Fig. 1.19.12).[25] Similarly, lateral canthoplasties can aid in accurate positioning of the lateral canthus to the lateral orbit if they have been released during the dissection. The temporalis muscle and deep temporal fascia should also be resuspended to avoid temporal hollowing. Nasal profile and projection should be critically evaluated, especially in nasoethmoid fractures, and corrected with cantilever bone grafts and soft tissue splints to improve nasal definition if there is lack of support with manual pressure (Fig. 1.19.13). The outer parietal cortex can be harvested for this purpose with good results.

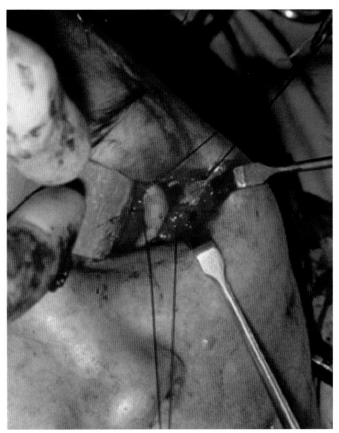

Fig. 1.19.12 Resuspension of the cheek periosteum to the inferior and lateral orbital rim to avoid cheek ptosis following extensive facial dissection.

POSTOPERATIVE COURSE

Multidisciplinary team care following panfacial fracture treatment can minimize the risks of ophthalmological, airway, or infectious complications. Due to the increased risk of deep space infections following a prolonged surgery, repeat washouts of contaminated and devitalized soft tissues are frequently necessary to avoid delayed wound healing and facial scarring in cases with extensive soft tissue injuries. In the absence of confirmed infections, perioperative antibiotics should be discontinued within 48 hours of surgery, as no benefit has been associated with prolonged prophylactic antibiotic treatment. Some studies of upper face fractures have demonstrated an increased rate of antibiotic-resistant infections with prolonged prophylactic antibiotic treatment.[26] In cases with severe soft-tissue loss such as gunshot wounds, early free flap reconstruction should be considered during the same hospitalization after initial reduction and fixation of fracture segments as described above.

ACUTE COMPLICATIONS

Acute complications following panfacial fracture treatment include surgical site infection, abscess formation, cerebrospinal fluid (CSF) leaks, malunion, and nonunion of fracture segments. CSF leaks stem from dural tears, which may be unmasked by reduction of fracture segments. These may be directly visualized and repaired intraoperatively at the time of fracture fixation, or may develop postoperatively. Most can be managed conservatively and will resolve within the immediate postoperative period, but large or persistent leaks may need further neurosurgical intervention (i.e., shunting or reexploration) to achieve resolution.

LONG-TERM COMPLICATIONS

Long-term complications of panfacial fractures include plate exposure and extrusion, temporal hollowing, malocclusion, orbital dystopia, frontal sinus mucocoeles, and discrepancies in facial width, projection, and length with malunions or nonunions. In contrast to acute complications, these long-term complications can be minimized by accurate reduction and fixation of fracture segments with adequate soft tissue plate coverage at the time of the initial repair. Malunions are treated with either refracture and repositioning or with onlay camouflage implants if they are functionally or esthetically significant. Nonunion treatment depends on the location. In the zygomatic arch, for example,

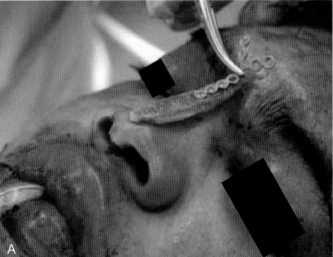
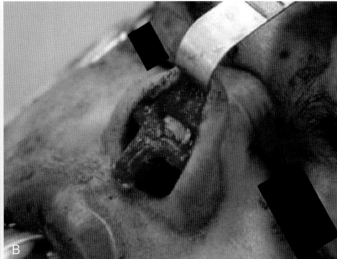

Fig. 1.19.13 Restoration of dorsal nasal support using a cantilever split calvarial bone graft with an open tip rhinoplasty approach to place the lower lateral cartilages over the tip of the bone graft.

nonunions can be mildly symptomatic and left untreated, whereas mandible nonunions usually lead to functional occlusion problems, infections, and pain. Plate exposures can be managed with plate removal once fractures have healed at approximately 6 weeks post repair. This is most common in the palate and in the upper ginigivobuccal sulcus in edentulous patients with dentures. Occasionally, patients may develop pain localized to a particular plate, in which case selective plate removal may achieve resolution. Temporal hollowing may be corrected with serial micro-fat grafting, dermal-fat grafts or alloplast implants beneath the temporalis. Persistent malocclusion may require single or double jaw surgery to maximize occlusal contact and mouth opening, and severe residual deformities may benefit from microsurgical reconstruction.[27] Discussion of these treatments is beyond the scope of this chapter, but the treating surgeon should be aware of options for treatment of long-term complications and be able to discuss these treatment options for patients suffering panfacial fractures.

CASE EXAMPLES

Case 1: Panfacial injury and delayed (3 weeks) reconstruction following crush injury from a 300 lb crab pot while fishing in the Bering Strait (Figs. 1.19.14 and 1.19.15).

Case 2: Panfacial injury and reconstruction in a 5-year-old girl resulting from a motor vehicle collision. Pediatric panfacial injuries, like all facial fractures in the growing craniofacial skeleton, require appreciation of deciduous/mixed dentition, accelerated healing times, differences in facial proportions, growth centers of the face, and psychosocial issues specific to children (Figs. 1.19.16 and 1.19.17).

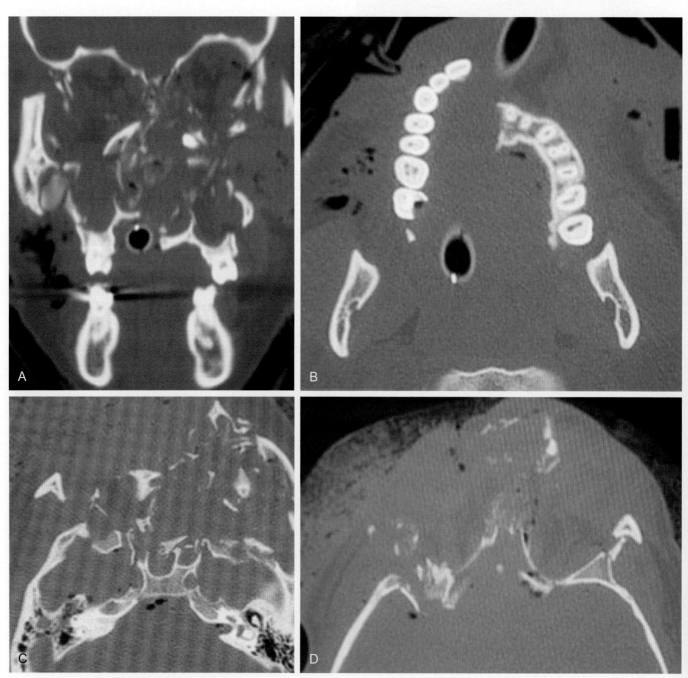

Fig. 1.19.14 *Case 1:* Preoperative imaging demonstrating extensive panfacial fractures of all facial thirds.

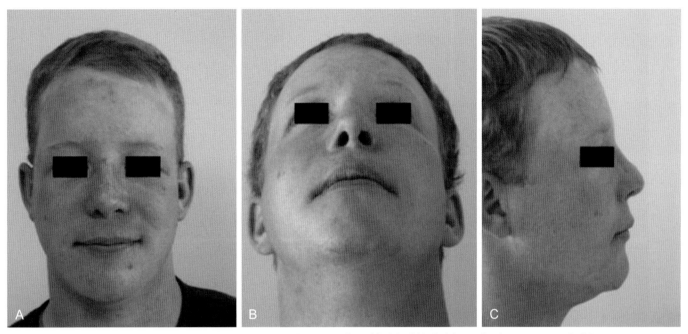

Fig. 1.19.15 *Case 1:* Postoperative result with restoration of facial width, height, projection, transverse facial curve, and globe position.

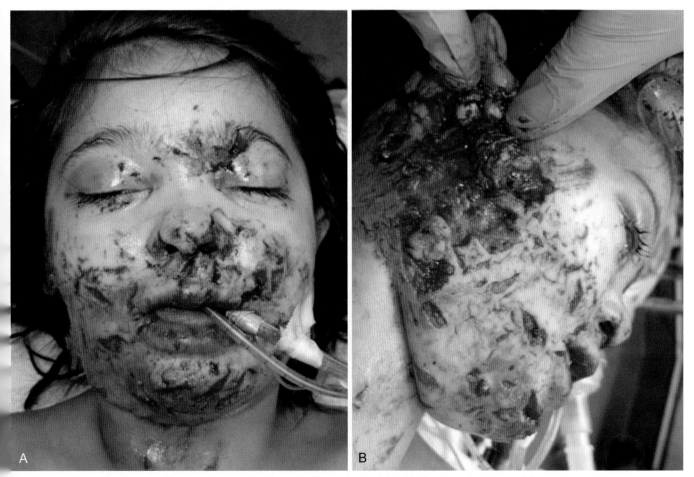

Fig. 1.19.16 *Case 2:* Preoperative images illustrating facial widening, lengthening, and loss of nasal projection.

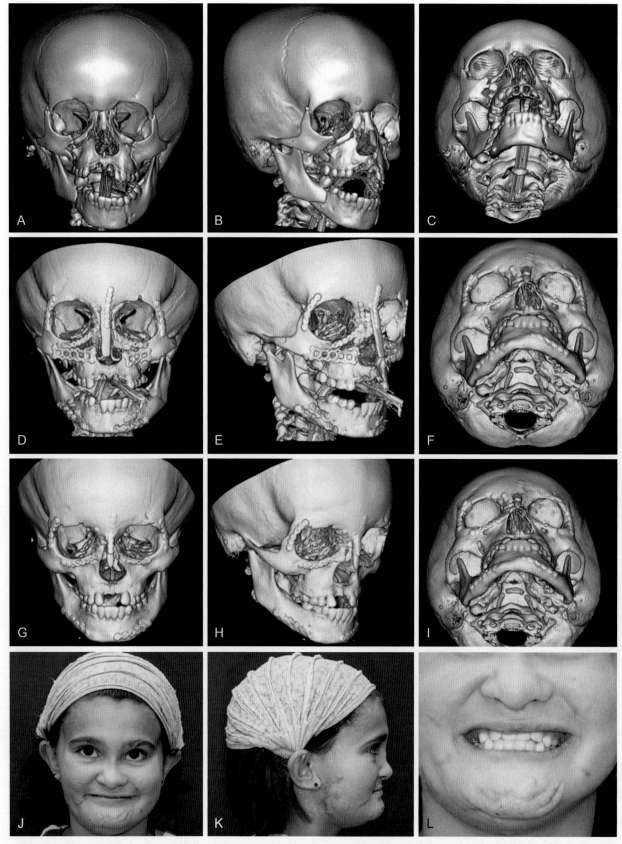

Fig. 1.19.17 *Case 2:* (A–C) Preoperative CT imaging demonstrating bilateral ZMC, NOE, orbital, Le Fort, and mandible fractures with facial flattening, widening, and bigonial splaying. (D–F) Immediate postoperative CT scan following fracture reduction and fixation with cantilever bone grafting to narrow facial width, improve facial projection and restore occlusion. (G–I) Two-year postoperative CT scan demonstrating stability of reconstruction with some cantilever bone graft resorption. (J–L) Two-year postoperative photographs.

EXPERT COMMENTARY

No injury of the face is more challenging nor more urgently in need of treatment than the panfacial injury. The bony buttresses of the face are crushed to various extents, and the soft tissue is suffused with hematoma. Contracture of the soft tissue begins immediately and forms an internal pattern of scar tissue in the shape of the unreduced bone fragments. This irreversible soft tissue deformity is reversed by early or immediate open reduction of the bone with the soft tissue anatomically replaced at its usual locations onto the craniofacial skeleton. [1–4] Curiously the reduction is easiest when the patient is freshly injured.

Various schemes for the sequencing of the steps in reduction of the bone have been proffered, with each of us having our favorite.[17] Conceptually, I like addressing the increased facial width in each anatomical area first, which reciprocally establishes facial projection. Then last in each anatomical area, the facial height is simply adjusted. While I prefer (in the absence of acute neurosurgical needs) beginning in the split palate, then arch bars, with transfer of that width to the horizontal mandible. The mandible for me is first linked with interfragment wires, which provide temporary stability in the horizontal and vertical mandible. Rigid fixation then establishes mandibular position, working on subtle adjustments and alignment to achieved a perfect fit, making sure that the mandible segments are not lingually rotated (I use the technique of Ellis, placing compressing fingers on the condyle and angle, while another operator looks for the anterior "gap" in the front cortex of the mandible when the segments are correctly rotated) and one must be sure that the true length of the ramus and condyle unit are restored. The frontal bone frontal bar reassembly is preceded by defunctionalizing and obliterating or cranializing the frontal sinus, then replacing frontal bone pieces, then reducing the nasoethmoid. The nasoethmoid is actually better visualized without the nose bones and before the frontal bone reassembly, correcting its width by a true transnasal canthopexy behind and above the lacrimal fossa. The zygomas are brought to fit the medially correctly positioned NOE segments,

preventing excess facial width by making sure the zygomatic arch is flat, and if it is, the orbital process of the zygoma is aligned with the greater wing of the sphenoid. Beware the fractured anterior lip of the greater wing of the sphenoid, which can create a false impression of alignment in the lateral orbit when displacement is present.

The facial halves are then linked at the Le Fort I level, correcting facial length by buttress alignment or by viewing old pictures of upper lip-incisor tooth position. Bone grafts restore eye position, and the height, contour, and length of the nose.

Soft tissue must then be replaced onto the reassembled facial skeleton by closing incisions in the temporal aponeurosis, the temporal aponeurosis over the frontal process of the zygoma, the gingival–buccal sulcus, the muscular layers of the mandible, and at the medial and lateral canthal attachments following careful repositioning. While it is a formidable undertaking to complete the repair of an acute panfacial injury, nowhere in facial injury treatment are the results more gratifying or the needs more urgent in restoring the original facial appearance, which must be verified at the time of reconstruction from old pictures obtained from license wallet photographs or the family.

References

1. Manson PN. *Dimensional Analysis of the Facial Skeleton in Problems in Plastic Surgery*. Philadelphia, PA: J.B. Lippincott Co.; 1991.
2. Hendrickson M, Clark N, Manson P. Sagittal fractures of the maxilla: classification and treatment. *Plast Reconst Surg*. 1998;101:319–332.
3. Manson P, Clark N. Sequencing treatment of segmental fractures. *Plast Reconstr Surg*. 1999;103:1287–1306.
4. Clark N, Robertson B, Slezak S, et al. Subunit principles in midface fractures: the importance of sagittal buttresses, soft tissue reductions and sequencing treatment of segmental fractures. *Plast Reconstr Surg*. 1999;103:1287–1306.

REFERENCES

1. Follmar KE, Debruijn M, Baccarani A, et al. Concomitant injuries in patients with panfacial fractures. *J Trauma*. 2007;63(4):831–835.
2. Mundinger GS, Bellamy JL, Miller DT, et al. Defining population-specific craniofacial fracture patterns and resource use in geriatric patients. *Plast Reconstr Surg*. 2016;137(2):386e–393e.
3. Girotto JA, Mackenzie E, Fowler C, et al. Long-term physical impairment and functional outcomes after complex facial fractures. *Plast Reconstr Surg*. 2001;108(2):312–327.
4. Markowitz BL, Manson PN. Panfacial fractures: organization of treatment. *Clin Plast Surg*. 1989;16(1):105–114.
5. Manson PN, Markowitz B, Mirvis S, et al. Toward CT-based facial fracture treatment. *Plast Reconstr Surg*. 1990;85(2):202–212, discussion 213–214.
6. Hopper RA, Salemy S, Sze RW. Diagnosis of midface fractures with CT: what the surgeon needs to know. *Radiographics*. 2006;26(3):783–793.
7. Bellamy JL, Mundinger GS, Flores JM, et al. Facial fractures of the upper craniofacial skeleton predict mortality and occult intracranial injury after blunt trauma. *J Craniofac Surg*. 2013;24(6):1922–1926.
8. Vaca EE, Mundinger GS, Kelamis JA, et al. Facial fractures with concomitant open globe injury. *Plast Reconstr Surg*. 2013;131(6):1317–1328.
9. Mithani SK, St Hilaire H, Brooke BS, et al. Predictable patterns of intracranial and cervical spine injury in craniomaxillofacial trauma: analysis of 4786 patients. *Plast Reconstr Surg*. 2009;123(4):1293–1301.
10. Mundinger GS, Rodriguez ED, Manson PN. Craniofacial trauma. In: Zins JE, Gordon CR, eds. *Handbook of Craniomaxillofacial Surgery*. River Edge, NJ: 2014.
11. Rodriguez ED, Mundinger GS. Evaluation and treatment of common facial injuries. In: Fischer JE, Jones DB, Pomposelli FB, eds. *Fischer's Mastery of Surgery*. 6th ed. Philadelphia, PA: Lippincott Williams & Wilkins; 2011.
12. Ho K, Hutter JJ, Eskridge J, et al. The management of life-threatening haemorrhage following blunt facial trauma. *J Plast Reconstr Aesthet Surg*. 2006;59(12):1257–1262.
13. Mundinger GS, Dorafshar AH, Gilson MM, et al. Analysis of radiographically confirmed blunt-mechanism facial fractures. *J Craniofac Surg*. 2014;25(1):321–327.
14. Hoelzle F, Klein M, Schwerdtner O, et al. Intraoperative computed tomography with the mobile CT Tomoscan M during surgical treatment of orbital fractures. *Int J Oral Maxillofac Surg*. 2001;30(1):26–31.
15. Curtis W, Horswell BB. Panfacial fractures: an approach to management. *Oral Maxillofac Surg Clin North Am*. 2013;25(4):649–660.
16. Gruss JS. Complex craniomaxillofacial trauma: evolving concepts in management. A trauma unit's experience – 1989 Fraser B. Gurd lecture. *J Trauma*. 1990;30(4):377–383.
17. Manson PN, Clark N, Robertson B, et al. Subunit principles in midface fractures: the importance of sagittal buttresses, soft-tissue reductions, and sequencing treatment of segmental fractures. *Plast Reconstr Surg*. 1999;103(4):1287–1306, quiz 1307.
18. Rodriguez ED, Stanwix MG, Nam AJ, et al. Twenty-six-year experience treating frontal sinus fractures: a novel algorithm based on anatomical fracture pattern and failure of conventional techniques. *Plast Reconstr Surg*. 2008;122(6):1850–1866.
19. Stanley RB. Management of severe frontobasilar skull fractures. *Otolaryngol Clin North Am*. 1991;24(1):139–150.
20. Gruss JS, Van Wyck L, Phillips JH, Antonyshyn O. The importance of the zygomatic arch in complex midfacial fracture repair and correction of posttraumatic orbitozygomatic deformities. *Plast Reconstr Surg*. 1990;85(6):878–890.

21. Stanley RB. The zygomatic arch as a guide to reconstruction of comminuted malar fractures. *Arch Otolaryngol Head Neck Surg.* 1989;115(12):1459–1462.

22. Gruss JS. Naso-ethmoid-orbital fractures: classification and role of primary bone grafting. *Plast Reconstr Surg.* 1985;75(3):303–317.

23. Markowitz BL, Manson PN, Sargent L, et al. Management of the medial canthal tendon in nasoethmoid orbital fractures: the importance of the central fragment in classification and treatment. *Plast Reconstr Surg.* 1991;87(5):843–853.

24. Sargent LA. Nasoethmoid orbital fractures: diagnosis and treatment. *Plast Reconstr Surg.* 2007;120(7 suppl 2):16S–31S.

25. Phillips JH, Gruss JS, Wells MD, Chollet A. Periosteal suspension of the lower eyelid and cheek following subciliary exposure of facial fractures. *Plast Reconstr Surg.* 1991;88(1):145–148.

26. Mundinger GS, Borsuk DE, Okhah Z, et al. Antibiotics and facial fractures: evidence-based recommendations compared with experience-based practice. *Craniomaxillofac Trauma Reconstr.* 2015;8(1):64–78.

27. Rodriguez ED, Bluebond-Langner R, Park JE, Manson PN. Preservation of contour in periorbital and midfacial craniofacial microsurgery: reconstruction of the soft-tissue elements and skeletal buttresses. *Plast Reconstr Surg.* 2008;121(5):1738–1747.

Characteristics of Ballistic and Blast Injuries

David B. Powers, Eduardo D. Rodriguez

INTRODUCTION

Ballistic injury patterns to the craniomaxillofacial region present a unique, and challenging, dilemma for the facial trauma surgeon. The tissue disruption associated with ballistic injury to the head and neck region can be daunting, and the identification of normal anatomic planes, potentially lost within bleeding, destroyed soft and hard tissues, can challenge the skills of even the most experienced facial trauma specialist. While classically considered to be under the purview of the military trauma surgeon, ballistic and blast injuries are routinely treated by the civilian surgeon due to the incidence of intentional and unintentional firearm injuries and industrial accidents. Unfortunately, as evidenced by the recent surge of terrorist attacks in locales such as Paris, France and Orlando, Florida, the civilian craniomaxillofacial trauma surgeon must have not only a working knowledge of the management of ballistic wounds to the craniofacial region, but also an understanding of the staging and timing of treatment in these injuries. A basic understanding of the definitions and characteristic clinical findings of ballistic and blast wounds should be an important tool in the armamentarium of the practicing craniomaxillofacial trauma surgeon.

BACKGROUND

Any introduction to the study of ballistic injuries should provide a review of commonly used terms. Box 1.20.1 provides the necessary background information to recognize the terminology associated with ballistics, and how those components correlate to an understanding of ballistic injuries:

As historical concepts of ballistics teach that impact kinetic energy is equal to one half the mass of the projectile times velocity squared ($KE = \frac{1}{2} MV^2$), one would wrongly assume caliber (size) of the projectile and velocity are the sole components of injury calculation. Actually, the increased energy transmitted from a high-velocity projectile does not necessarily translate to increased wounding capacity, as will be noted throughout the remainder of this chapter, and the physical properties of the projectile, and its fate upon striking the victim, are more important than the caliber. Caliber alone has no alteration to the surgical treatment of the injury, and primarily serves to satisfy the curiosity of the attending medical staff. By understanding the basic mechanical properties of the projectile expelled towards the target, the correlation of velocity and subsequent energy transfer, and the anatomical properties of the head and neck, the craniomaxillofacial trauma surgeon will have a better understanding of the consequences of ballistic injury to the facial skeleton (see Box 1.20.2).

Yaw, precession, and nutation are frequently referenced when initially studying ballistics. Yaw and precession decrease as the distance of the bullet from the barrel increases, and along with nutation, are terms generally associated with shooting from a distance, as seen in military grade artillery weaponry (Fig. 1.20.1). Illustrative examples of yaw are exaggerated in excess of 30 degrees for graphic representation, while in actuality the degree of yaw is generally less than 1–2 degrees, affording tight control of the projectile in flight and allowing the projectile to hit what the firearm is aimed towards. Should the yaw be as exaggerated as seen in most artistic renderings, the projectile would be uncontrollable due to tumbling along the path of fire. A clear clinical example of the effects of yaw and precession is the fact that when examined on a shooting range, projectile holes in targets are consistently circular in nature, indicating the spherical shape of the projectile, not a ragged opening consistent with *"tumbling"* or excessive yaw. Of interest, projectiles *do* tumble within the body of the target causing increased damage after striking hard tissue, or with deformation of the projectile. While these terms have practical applications in weaponry, the clinical significance of these items in craniomaxillofacial ballistic trauma is negligible at best.

The Magnus and Coriolis Effects are also frequently referenced in the discussion of ballistics, but again are isolated to the military applications of projectile flight, as well as the recreational aspects of long-range firing for hunting or competitive shooting. As the overwhelming majority of ballistic injuries to the head and neck region occur within relatively short distances, well within the effective range of the weapon and projectiles, these definitions and concepts have minimal to no correlation to the remainder of this chapter, or for the surgical management of these ballistic injuries.

COMPONENTS OF BALLISTIC MISSILES

As previously described, the cartridge or round describes a unit of firearm ammunition. Each round consists of the following components (Fig. 1.20.2A–B):
- Projectile
- Casing
- Propellant
- Primer

The components of a round provide a basic understanding of the principles of firearm injury. The projectile is the portion of the bullet that is expelled and strikes the target. The compositional makeup of the projectile (soft lead, hollow point, full copper covering, or multiple pellets as seen in shotguns) has a direct correlation on the wounding potential of the weapon. As a projectile deforms after striking the victim, either as a result of metallurgic composition during manufacturing, or as a direct consequence of striking the underlying bone, the energy transfer to the victim, and potential injury to associated tissues, is increased (Fig. 1.20.2C). As noted earlier, the actual projectiles expelled by firearms are limited in type only by the imagination of the manufacturers and firearm enthusiast. The casing is the container packaging the projectile, propellant (gunpowder or cordite) and primer as a single

BOX 1.20.1   Terminology of Ballistics

Components of Ammunition

Cartridge/Round	A unit of firearm ammunition
Projectile	The component of the round that is expelled towards the target, sometimes referred to as the "bullet"
Magnum	A cartridge loaded with either a greater volume or more powerful propellant than the original cartridge design, imparting greater velocity to the projectile

Components of Weapon

Rifling	Helical grooves in the barrel of a weapon, which imparts spin along the long axis of the projectile
Caliber	The internal diameter of the barrel of a weapon, usually measured in millimeters or fractions of an inch
Gauge/Bore	The total number of round lead balls that would fill the diameter of the barrel and weigh 1 pound

Associated Terms Seen in Ballistic Literature

Yaw	Movement along the longitudinal access of the projectile
Precession	Rotation of the projectile around the center of mass
Nutation	Small circular movement along the projectile tip
Magnus Effect	Lateral crosswind effect of a spinning projectile in flight
Coriolis Effect	Spherical shape and rotational properties of the Earth, and its orbit, as it applies to the projectile

BOX 1.20.2   Factors Affecting Energy Transfer Between a Projectile and Body Tissue

Velocity
Profile
Shape
Stability
Fragmentation
Expansion
Secondary impact

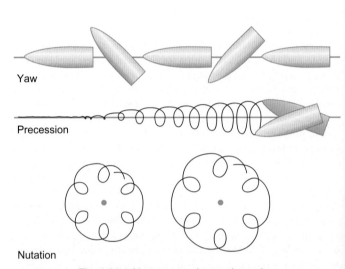

Yaw

Precession

Nutation

Fig. 1.20.1 Yaw, precession, and nutation.

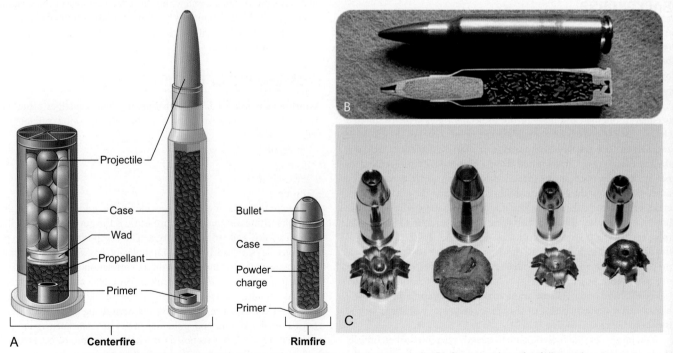

Projectile

Case

Wad

Propellant

Primer

Centerfire

Bullet

Case

Powder charge

Primer

Rimfire

A

B

C

Fig. 1.20.2 (A) Cross-sectional analysis of a cartridge and shotgun shell. (B) Cross-section of a full metal jacketed rifle cartridge. (C) Photograph of the projectile changes associated with hollow-point ammunition after they strike resistance (i.e., tissue) in flight

unit for placement into the firing mechanism of the weapon. The propellant, such as gunpowder or cordite, is the accelerant that actually allows for expulsion of the projectile from the weapon. The more propellant in a cartridge, as is seen in Magnum and rifle rounds, the greater velocity the projectile exhibits. Wadding, or *wads*, are generally plastic frameworks with a paper or felt insert that hold the various pellets (projectiles) together in relation to the propellant, allowing for accurate and safe release of all the projectiles simultaneously from the barrel in scattershot and shotgun cartridges. Without the presence of wadding, the gas produced by the propellant would push through the pellets, and not propel them as a unit. The primer is the only portion of the bullet with an explosive charge. As the primer is struck by the firing pin of the weapon, the explosive charge is activated, igniting the propellant and sending the projectile on its flight. Some cartridges are referred to as *rimfire* as the priming mechanism is contained within the rim of the base rather than a separate primer in the center of the base. Generally, rimfire cartridges are less powerful and cannot be reloaded, while centerfire cartridges can have the primer replaced and reloaded with another projectile.

Rifles, handguns, and machine guns have rifled barrels – essentially, spiral grooves cut into the length of the interior of the bore of the barrel. The grooves impart spin upon the projectile, stabilizing it in flight and allowing the projectile to travel in a controlled manner to the target. The grooves are separated by segments of metal, called lands, which project into the middle of the barrel. The diameter of the barrel measured between the lands represents the caliber of the projectile. Caliber specifications based on nomenclature used in the United States can be difficult to comprehend, and utterly confusing to the healthcare team. The .30-06 and the Winchester .308 cartridges are both loaded with bullets that have a diameter of .308 inches. The "06" in this term describes the year, 1906, when the cartridge was introduced to the market. The term "grains" originally was applied to black powder charges and refers to the weight of the powder in the cartridge, not the number of granules contained in the cartridge case. A .30-30 cartridge has a .308 inch diameter bullet propelled by 30 grains of smokeless powder. As newer forms of gunpowder were developed, this powder charge was no longer used, but the terminology persists to this day. Additional misperceptions regarding caliber exist because the North Atlantic Treaty Organization (NATO) and United States military projectiles are described using the metric system (7.62 mm or 9 mm rounds), while United States civilian firearm munitions are generally referred to in measurements relating to inches (.357 or .38). Unfortunately, no uniform mechanism exists for the description of firearm cartridges and manufacturers continue to inundate the market with further descriptions to add to the confusion, such as velocity, country of manufacture, number of grains of propellant, year of manufacture, etc. (Fig. 1.20.3). As noted earlier, the question regarding caliber is commonly asked in the management of ballistic injury. In reality, caliber has minimal practical impact on the care of the patient as the surgical management of a wound caused by a .357 projectile is no different from a wound caused by a 9 mm round, and should be directed to the specific anatomical anomaly created by the projectile not the weapon used. Experienced surgical providers cannot accurately determine the caliber of a weapon by visual examination of the wound alone, and would never alter the required treatment based on the diameter of the projectile.

Handguns are handheld firearms, with a barrel length generally 10½ inches or less, which usually fire projectiles of a lower velocity and caliber. Handgun injuries generally have a tendency to "push-away," or stretch soft tissues, including vessels or nerves as opposed to avulsive loss. The characteristic low-velocity wound has a small rounded, or slightly ragged entrance wound, causing fragmentation of teeth and bony comminution, often exhibiting no exit wound (Figs. 1.20.4A–C).

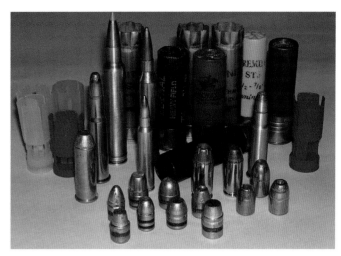

Fig. 1.20.3 Photograph of the tremendous variety of caliber, projectile composition or construction, and variable volumes of propellant and casings available for the modern firearm. (From Powers DB, Delo RI. Maxillofacial ballistic and missile injuries. In Fonseca RJ, Walker RV, Betts NJ, et al., editors. Oral and maxillofacial trauma, 4th ed. St. Louis, MO; 2012.)

If an exit wound does occur, it is generally slit-shaped or stellate. Rifles are long guns with barrel lengths generally more than 24 inches. At distance, rifle wounds create a low-energy transfer similar to those seen with handguns. At close range the wounding characteristics are different due to the increased potential injury associated with velocity and high-energy transfer (Figs. 1.20.4D–H). The presence of an exit wound is usually found, which may be stellate and larger than the entry wound. The existence of avulsive soft/hard tissue wounds and significant fragmentation of the bone can be characteristic findings of rifle wounds. A shotgun is a long gun that may fire a single pellet, or numerous pellets, at a relatively low velocity. The gauge of the shotgun is classified as the number of lead balls/pellets placed together equaling the interior diameter of the barrel, which would weigh one pound. For contact with close range injuries, the effect of the gas that is discharged under pressure into the wound also needs to be considered. This scenario is extremely important in shotgun and improvised explosive blast wounds due to the higher degree of contamination and presence of propelled gas and shock waves. Powder gases are expelled from the muzzle of the weapon after combustion of the gunpowder and follow the projectile out of the barrel. When the muzzle of the weapon is in contact with the target, this can be an additional source of tissue displacement, injury, and thermal burning.

Shotgun pellet injuries essentially depend completely on the distance the weapon is from the target at the time of discharge. Sherman and Parrish devised a classification system to describe shotgun wounds in relation to the distance from the target. Type I injury occurs from a distance longer than 7 yards; Type II injury is sustained when the discharge is within 3–7 yards; Type III injury is within 3 yards. Type III injuries usually sustain dramatic soft and hard tissue injuries and avulsion of tissue, whereas Type I injuries may be minimal (Figs. 1.20.5A–D). Because victims often have difficulty in determining how far away the shotgun was at the time of discharge, Glezer and colleagues revised this classification system and directed their attention to the size of the pellet scatter. Type I injuries occur when pellet scatter is within an area of 25 cm²; Type II injuries are within 10 cm² to 25 cm²; Type III injuries have pellet scatter less than 10 cm². Although the Glezer classification originally was developed for abdominal injuries, the information is transferable to other areas of the body, and determinations of tissue

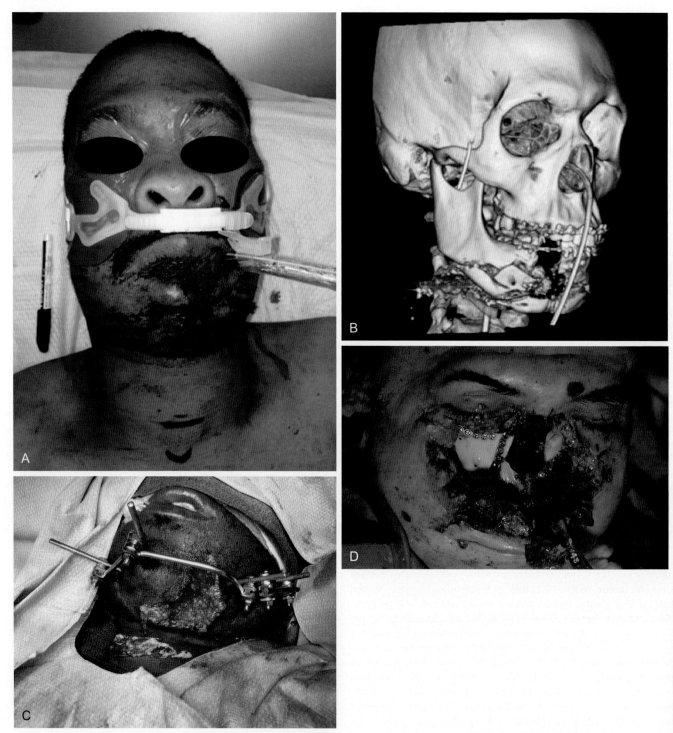

Fig. 1.20.4 (A) Characteristic clinical appearance of low-energy/low-velocity gunshot wound to the anterior mandible. No exit wound was detected. (B) 3-Dimensional reconstruction of computed tomography scan indicating the degree of comminution associated with this gunshot wound. 3-D reconstructions provide superior visualization, and localization, of anatomic variants in the management of ballistic injuries to the craniomaxillofacial unit. (C) Application of a modern external fixator for the management of a low-energy/low-velocity gunshot wound to the mandible. (D) High-energy/high-velocity rifle wound to the anterior maxilla with complete avulsion of the nasal complex. Note the significant difference in the wounding characteristics of the high-energy weapon, as the patient was shot in the face at a distance by an assailant with a rifle. Reconstruction shows utilization of calvarial bone to reconstruct the vertical pillars of support for the maxilla.

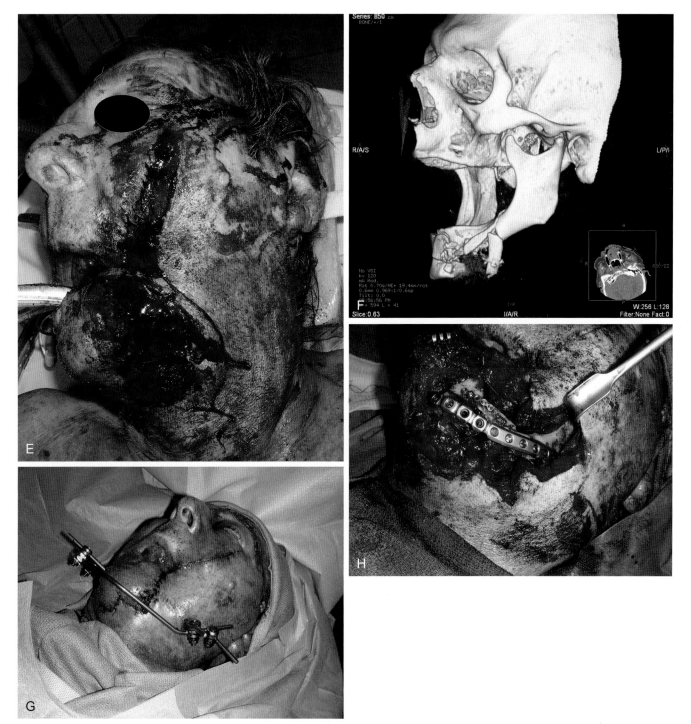

Fig. 1.20.4, cont'd (E) High-energy gunshot wound to the anterior mandible. Note the presence of soft tissue disruption as the projectile exited the patient's mouth and then tracked along the soft tissues of his anterior maxilla. (F) 3-Dimensional reconstruction of computed tomography scan indicating the degree of comminution and avulsive bone loss associated with this gunshot wound. (G) Initial stabilization of the patient was accomplished with an external fixator. (H) Definitive reconstruction with open reduction and internal fixation with a reconstruction plate. (Panel (D) from Powers DB, Delo RI. Maxillofacial ballistic and missile injuries. In: Fonseca RJ, Walker RV, Betts NJ, et al., editors. Oral and maxillofacial trauma, 4th ed. St. Louis, MO; 2012. Panels (E–H) from Powers DB, Delo RI. Characteristics of ballistic and blast injuries. Atlas Oral Maxillofac Surg Clin North Am 2013; 21;15–24.)

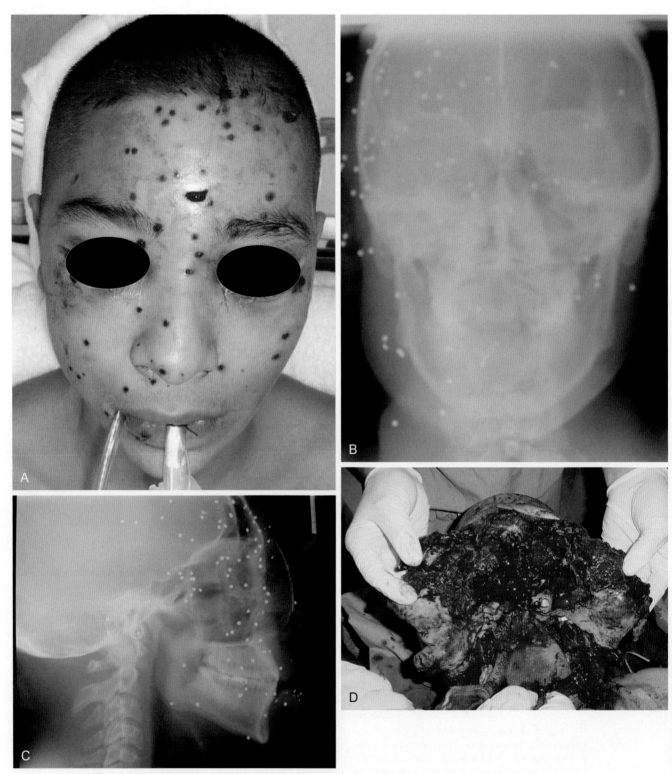

Fig. 1.20.5 (A) Characteristic facial appearance of a patient sustaining a shotgun wound from a distance (Sherman and Parrish – Class I *or* Glezer – Class I). Note the presence of multiple punctate entry wounds, but no significant disruption of the facial features. (B–C) Classic radiographic appearance of a patient sustaining a shotgun wound from a distance (Sherman and Parrish – Class I *or* Glezer – Class I). Note the presence of multiple shotgun pellets on the radiographs. (D) Self-inflicted shotgun wound in a suicide attempt. Note significant hard and soft tissue disruption and avulsion (Sherman and Parrish – Class III *or* Glezer – Class III) (Panels (A) and (D) from Powers DB, Delo RI. Maxillofacial ballistic and missile injuries. In: Fonseca RJ, Walker RV, Betts NJ, et al., editors. Oral and maxillofacial trauma, 4th ed. St. Louis, MO; 2012. Panels (B–C) from Powers DB, Delo RI. Characteristics of ballistic and blast injuries. Atlas Oral Maxillofac Surg Clin North Am 2013; 21: 15-24.)

injury can be correlated directly to the size of the pellet scatter. Intuitively, the closer the shotgun is to the patient, the more dramatic the hard and soft tissue damage. For rifles and handguns, the practical clinical difference in whether the weapon was 10 feet, 100 feet, or 1000 feet away from the patient otherwise has no bearing on surgical and medical treatment.

COMPONENTS OF IMPROVISED EXPLOSIVE DEVICES

The recent conflicts in the Middle East have introduced a "new" mechanism for delivery of craniomaxillofacial missile projectiles resulting in gruesome and avulsive craniomaxillofacial injuries – the improvised explosive device (IED). While not a new entity, as the concept of IEDs has been deployed by guerrilla forces since World War II, the description and media interest in the IED warrants a brief discussion of its characteristic properties. Explosives are broadly classified as low-order explosives (LE – such as pipe bombs, gunpowder or petroleum-based bombs) or high-order explosives (HE – such as TNT, C4, Semtex). Additionally, explosives are categorized as manufactured, which implies military-grade mass production and quality control, or improvised. An IED is a bomb fabricated in an "*improvised*" manner designed to destroy or incapacitate military personnel or civilians. The bomb itself may be a conventional military grade weapon, or an assortment of explosive components such as gasoline, or agricultural fertilizer as seen in the Oklahoma City bombing of 1995. An IED has five components (Fig. 1.20.6):

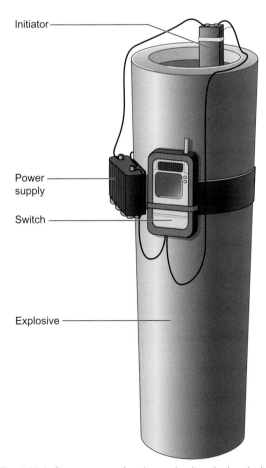

Fig. 1.20.6 Components of an improvised explosive device.

- Switch (activator)
- Initiator (fuse)
- Container (body)
- Charge (explosive)
- Power source (battery)

Antipersonnel IEDs typically contain shrapnel-generating components such as nails, ball-bearings, metal fragments, wood or glass. The victim may first sustain a burn injury from ignited explosives. Blunt and penetrating injury from contact by exploded fragments will further injure the patient. These fragments will be propelled at high- or ultra-high velocity and therefore cause ultra-high kinetic energy injuries. Direct shrapnel injury is only a single element to be considered, as detonation of any powerful explosive generates a blast wave of high pressure that spreads out from the point of explosion and travels hundreds of yards in all directions. The relative proximity the victim is to the site of the explosion, the greater the exposure to the shock wave energy. The initial shock wave of very high over-pressurization, which is referred to as the *primary*, or "*blast wave,*" is unique to the HE and is followed closely by a "*secondary wind,*" a huge volume of displaced air flooding back into the area, again under pressure. It is these sudden and extreme differences in pressures, and associated dispersal of secondary projectiles, which can lead to significant neurological, skeletal or soft tissue injury (Fig. 1.20.7, Tables 1.20.1 and 1.20.2).

THE PRINCIPLES OF VELOCITY

All else being equal, velocity has the largest impact on kinetic energy. However, velocity cannot be examined in a vacuum, as at suboptimal levels expanding projectiles do not expand, and at excessive velocity projectiles lose their stability in flight. The terms "high velocity" and "low velocity" as they relate to projectiles can also be somewhat misleading. Consensus between United States and European research does not occur in the literature, with varying definitions correlating to where the study was performed (Tables 1.20.3–1.20.5). The US literature designates high velocity as being between 2000 and 3000 feet/second (610–914 meters/second), whereas studies from the United Kingdom designate the line between low- and high-velocity projectiles as being 1100 feet/second (335 meters/second), which is the speed of sound in air. The earliest recognized entry of high-velocity projectiles having an association with increased wounding potential occurred during the Vietnam War. In 1967, Rich reported in the *Journal of the American Medical Association* that bullets fired from the M16 rifle inflicted tremendous tissue destruction and injuries upon enemy combatants. The muzzle velocity of the projectile shot from the M16 was 3100 feet/second. When coupled with erroneous information published by Rybeck in 1974 and in the 1975 edition of the *Emergency War Surgery* manual regarding the size of the temporary cavity caused by the missile, this information led to the common misperception that high-velocity projectiles caused more significant injuries. Part of the confusion regarding the wounding potential of high-velocity projectiles is caused by misinterpretation of ballistic gelatin model studies. Ballistic gelatin is 10%–20% gelatin refrigerated to 4–10°C and is used as the tissue model for ballistic studies. The wound profile diagrams included in this chapter and others represent the findings of these studies. The validity of the ballistic gelatin model has been confirmed by comparison with human autopsies, although there is confusion in correlating these studies to living patients, because the human body is much more resistant to deformation than gelatin. The effects of skin resistance, clothing, and opposition to separation of the fascial planes cannot be replicated in gelatin. Harvey evaluated the two types of pressure waves produced by penetrating objects in 1947: the sonic pressure wave and the temporary cavity. The first wave is the sonic pressure wave, sometimes referred to as the "*shock wave,*"

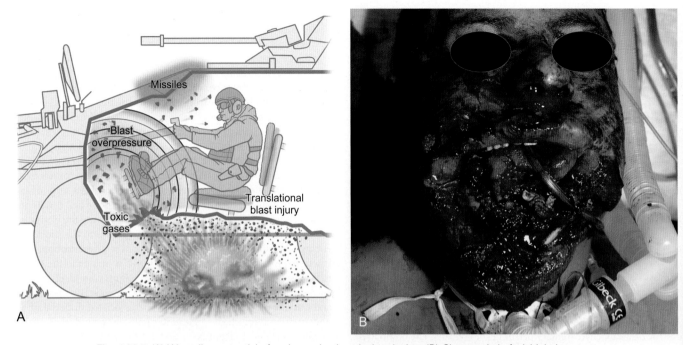

Fig. 1.20.7 (A) Wounding potential of an improvised explosive device. (B) Characteristic facial injuries sustained by an improvised explosive device. (Panel (A) from: Emergency War Surgery Course, Washington DC, United States Government; 2009.)

TABLE 1.20.1	**Mechanisms of Blast Injury**		
Category	**Characteristics**	**Body Part Affected**	**Types of Injuries**
Primary	Unique to high-order explosives (HE), resulting from impact of the overpressurization wave with body surfaces	Gas filled structures are most susceptible (lungs, middle ear and GI tract)	Pulmonary barotrauma (*blast lung*) Tympanic membrane rupture Abdominal hemorrhage and perforation Globe rupture Traumatic brain injury (*TBI*)
Secondary	Results from flying debris and bomb fragments	Any	Penetrating ballistic injury due to shrapnel or fragmentation Blunt injuries Globe penetration (can be occult)
Tertiary	Results from individuals being thrown by the blast wind	Any	Fractures Traumatic amputation Open/closed TBI
Quaternary	All blast/explosion-related injuries/illnesses/diseases not related to other mechanisms (includes exacerbations or complications associated with existing diseases)	Any	Burns Crush injuries Open/closed TBI Asthma/chronic obstructive pulmonary disease/angina/hypertension/hyperglycemia

and it relates to the sound of the projectile striking the target. This wave transmits at the speed of sound (i.e., approximately 4750 feet/second [1450 meters/second]) and is traveling considerably faster than the projectile entering the target. No temporary cavity is formed with the sonic pressure wave, and in that regard it is analogous to the lithotripsy devices used for renal calculi destruction, with corresponding minimal risks for tissue injury. Although American and Swedish researchers have tried to disprove Harvey's conclusions, no definitive evidence suggests that his findings are in error, and additional studies by French and American researchers support the original findings of 1947.

The secondary pressure wave, referred to as the temporary cavity, is formed when the penetrating projectile strikes tissue and the wave radiates laterally away from the permanent cavity of the projectile path. After being struck by the projectile, the ballistic gelatin/tissue displays an obvious temporary cavity, which potentially injures tissues such as muscle, vessels, and organs. The clinical significance of this cavity is variable with no real consensus in the literature, and the temporary cavity caused by the M16 in animal laboratory models is much smaller than the approximate 18 cm temporary cavity seen in ballistic gelatin. Dog models indicated that acute tissue injury secondary to temporary cavity formation sustained with high-velocity projectile strikes were no more than 5 cm and were able to resolve within 72 hours. The United States military conducted extensive research into the wounding patterns of projectiles, and the results are summarized in Figs. 1.20.8A–C.

TABLE 1.20.2   Overview of IED/Blast-Related Injuries to the Craniomaxillofacial Region

System	Injury or Condition
Auditory	Tympanic membrane rupture Ossicular disruption Cochlear damage Foreign body entrapment
Eye/orbit/face	Perforated/penetrated globe Foreign body entrapment Air embolism Fractures Thermal injury Soft tissue disruption
Respiratory	*Blast lung* – direct consequence of the HE overpressurization wave. The most common fatal primary blast injury among initial survivors Hemothorax Aspiration pneumonitis Airway thermal injury Pulmonary contusion/hemorrhage
CNS injury	Open/closed traumatic brain injury Cerebrovascular accident Spinal cord injury Air embolism-induced injuries

The unique anatomic differences of the craniomaxillofacial skeleton, a relatively thin soft tissue layer overlying a dense foundation of bone, mitigate some of the expected responses of the temporary tissue stretch as the overall thickness of the soft tissue envelope is generally less than the required total distance needing to be traveled prior to exhibiting secondary cavitation. While sequential soft tissue necrosis and small-vessel damage can occur, it is much more likely to be in response to the exaggerated permanent cavity of the projectile, which is greatly enhanced after striking the underlying facial skeleton. The key point of understanding in the management of ballistic injuries is that the permanent cavity, which involves all of the tissues that are pushed aside or destroyed during the flight of the projectile, is the location of the extent of the initial, or immediate, damage. A projectile striking bone may cause fragmentation of the bullet and/or native bone, forming numerous secondary missiles, each capable of producing additional wounds, dramatically increasing the size of the permanent cavity (Fig. 1.20.9). The size and shape of the permanent cavity are determined by the density and anatomical characteristics of the tissue lying in the projectile's path, the velocity of the projectile, the shape/characteristics of the projectile, and likely most importantly the degree of deformation of the missile as it travels through the tissues.

CHARACTERISTICS OF BALLISTIC INJURIES

Gunshot injuries have been categorized in the literature as penetrating, perforating, or avulsive. Penetrating wounds are caused by the projectile striking the victim but not exiting the body. The perforating injuries have entrance and exit wounds, classically described as being without

TABLE 1.20.3   Ballistic Table for Common Handgun Cartridges

Cartridge	Velocity (fps) – Muzzle	Velocity (fps) – 100 yd	Energy (fpe) – Muzzle	Energy (fpe) – 100 yd
.25	900	742	63	43
.32	1000	834	133	96
.38	800	735	199	168
9 mm	975	899	310	264
.357 Magnum	1500	1153	624	298
.44 Magnum	1500	1196	999	635
.45	970	860	386	304
.50 Magnum	1700	1289	2246	1291

TABLE 1.20.4   Ballistic Table for Common Rifle/Machine Gun Cartridges

Cartridge	Velocity (fps) – Muzzle	Velocity (fps) – 100 yd	Energy (fpe) – Muzzle	Energy (fpe) – 100 yd
.22 Hornet	3070	2246	732	392
.243	3010	2744	1911	1588
.270	3060	2851	2702	2345
.30 – 30	2390	1959	1902	1278
.30 – 06	2960	2750	3209	2769
5.56 mm (NATO)	2910	2675	1410	1192
7.62 mm (AK 47)	2360	2060	1521	1159
9 mm Parabellum (Uzi)	1060	946	338	268
.50 BMG Sniper	2820	2732	13421	12428

TABLE 1.20.5   Ballistic Table for Common Shotgun Slugs

Cartridge (2.75 in Shell)	Velocity (fps) – Muzzle	Velocity (fps) – 100 yd	Energy (fpe) – Muzzle	Energy (fpe) – 100 yd
12 gauge (1 oz slug)	1560	977	2364	927
16 gauge (0.9 oz slug)	1590	975	2320	875
20 gauge (0.87 oz slug)	1590	975	2080	780

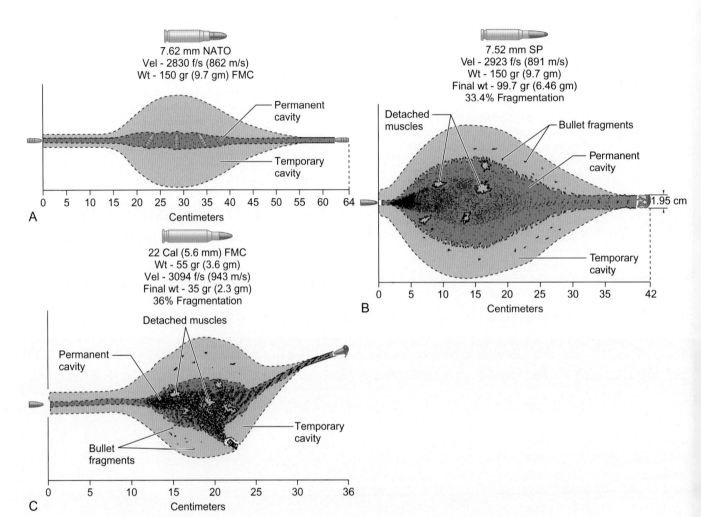

Fig. 1.20.8 (A) Ballistic representation of NATO 7.62 mm full metal case (FMC) round fired from an M16 rifle. Observe the relatively consistent permanent cavity and laterally radiating temporary cavity, which begins to develop at approximately 20 cm into the tissue as the projectile begins to tumble. This chart represents the projectile not striking any hard structures causing deformation or alteration in trajectory. The anatomical characteristics of the head and neck do not have over 20 cm of soft tissue present prior to encountering the bony skeleton, which would have a clinical significance in regards to the temporary cavity should the projectile be of a trajectory to encounter only soft tissue and miss the underlying facial bones. (B) Ballistic representation of a 7.52 mm soft point (SP) round striking muscle and bone. Note as the projectile strikes the underlying structures, there is a tremendous increase in the permanent cavity, as well as the temporary cavity, as the projectile deforms and fragments due to the soft tip construction. This deformation in the structural characteristic of the projectile, and associated increase in the permanent and temporary cavities, greatly enhances the wounding potential of this round. (C) Ballistic representation of a 22 caliber (5.6 mm) full metal case round striking bone and muscle. Note as the relatively small caliber projectile strikes the underlying structures there is a tremendous increase in the permanent cavity and associated temporary cavity as the projectile deforms and continues on a new trajectory. This representation illustrates the wounding potential of a smaller caliber weapon should the projectile actually strike the target and engage in energy transfer to the tissues. A troy grain is equivalent to the abbreviation "gr" while a gram is equivalent to the abbreviation "gm". (From Emergency War Surgery, 3rd ed. Washington DC: United States Government Printing Office; 2004.)

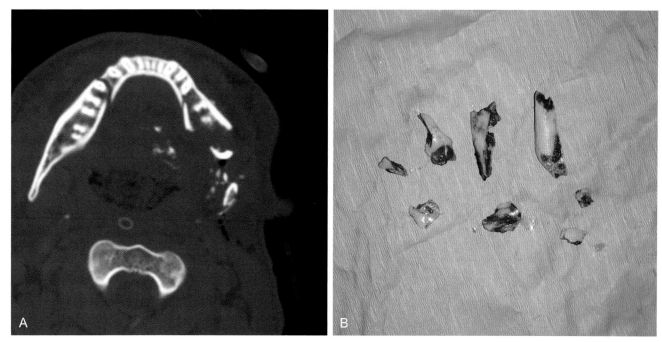

Fig. 1.20.9 Example of a projectile striking the mandible, causing fragmentation of the bone with the formation of numerous secondary projectiles, which enlarged the size of the permanent cavity.

appreciable tissue loss. Avulsive injuries have entrance and exit wounds, generally presenting with an acute loss of tissue associated with the passage of the projectile out of the victim. The type of firearm used has implications in the wounding potential of the projectile. As referenced earlier in this chapter, traditional concepts of ballistics teach that impact kinetic energy is equal to one-half the mass of the projectile times velocity squared ($KE = \frac{1}{2} MV^2$), the increased energy transmitted from a high-velocity projectile does not necessarily translate to increased wounding capacity. Cunningham and others suggest modifications need be used to correct the kinetic energy estimate of wounding potential for the type of tissue being struck by the projectile. Cunningham's belief was softer tissues, such as brain and muscle, should be associated with a lower exponent of injury (0.5) than harder tissues, such as bone, which would have a higher exponent (2.5) and therefore higher likelihood of permanent injury. The corrected formula for estimating wounding capacity by kinetic energy should be $KE = \frac{1}{2} MV^{0.5}$ to $KE = \frac{1}{2} MV^{2.5}$.

The soft tissue injuries inherent in ballistic trauma may exhibit avulsive loss, sequential necrosis over days to weeks, and compromised vascularity negating, or delaying, potential microvascular or pedicled soft tissue reconstruction. Due to the frequent occurrence of comminuted bony fractures, the necessity for open reduction of the hard tissue injuries further complicates the soft tissue healing response. A compromised soft tissue bed can lead to necrosis of free-floating bone fragments, avascular necrosis of the underlying facial skeleton, devitalization of stabilized fracture segments, and development of soft tissue infection or osteomyelitis resulting in increased tissue loss and scarring of the facial composite. Hard tissue loss, including both bone and teeth, presents the unique challenges of reconstruction including reconstitution of the masticatory complex to support the oral intake of nutrition, reestablishment of the normal anterior–posterior projection and angular shape of the facial skeleton, maintenance of lip competence and control

of salivation. Beyond the anatomical concerns of reconstruction, the presence of specialized vascular and neurosensory components in the maxillofacial region, including the great vessels of the neck, the various branches of the cranial nerves compromising both motor and sensory functions such as sight, smell, hearing, and taste, only serve to further complicate the potential for catastrophic injury and life-long deformity that ballistic injuries cause to the craniomaxillofacial region.

CONCLUSION

Ballistic injury wounds are formed by variable interrelated factors such as the nature of the tissue, the compositional makeup of the bullet, distance to the target, and the velocity, shape and mass of the projectile. This complex arrangement, with the ultimate outcome dependent upon each other, make the prediction of wounding potential difficult to assess. As the facial features are the component of the body most involved in a patient's personality and interaction with society, preservation of form, cosmesis and functional outcome should remain the primary goals in the management of ballistic injury. A logical, sequential analysis of the injury patterns to the facial complex is an absolutely necessary component for the treatment of craniomaxillofacial ballistic injuries. Fortunately, these skill sets should be well honed in all craniomaxillofacial surgeons through their exposure to generalized trauma, orthognathic, oncologic and cosmetic surgery patients. Identification of injured tissues, understanding the functional limitations of these injuries, and preservation of both hard and soft tissues minimizing the need for tissue replacement are paramount. By obtaining an understanding of the mechanism of the injury received, appropriate timing and selection of surgical treatment options can be performed minding the caveat of Dr. Paul Manson, "You never get a second chance to do a good primary reconstruction."

KEY POINTS

- The permanent cavity is the site of initial permanent tissue destruction.
- Deformation of the projectile after impacting hard tissues causes an increase in the size of the permanent cavity.
- After striking bone, fragmentation of the projectile and/or bone can result in the formation of numerous secondary projectiles, each producing additional wounding potential, enlarging the size of the permanent cavity.
- The ultimate fate and compositional makeup of the projectile is more important than its velocity or caliber.

- Soft tissue injuries inherent in ballistic trauma may exhibit avulsive loss, sequential necrosis over days to weeks, and compromised vascularity negating/delaying potential microvascular or pedicled soft tissue reconstruction.
- Projectiles do not "tumble" in flight, but do tumble within the target after striking hard tissue.
- Penetration of the skin can occur by projectiles traveling as slow as 148–197 feet per second.

EXPERT COMMENTARY

This chapter is one of the best discussions of the subject of ballistics physics and management, and the material for a solid basis for caring for these challenging patients with overlying lacerations. My own algorithm for managing these patients is that for small caliber gunshot wounds, I manage them as facial fractures overlying lacerations, closing the wound and ORIF of the fractures. When the damage is more extensive, i.e., close-range shotgun wounds, there is often missing soft tissue and missing bone.

There are four areas to consider (and frequently, the patterns can be defined) and care rendered to three separate areas:

1. In the area of soft tissue that is injured but present, exposure of the fractures is performed being careful to plan incisions differently as required to preserve soft tissue vascularity.
2. In the area of missing soft tissue, skin to mucosa closure needs to be accomplished, or some maneuver to preserve soft tissue length.
3. In the area where fractures of the bone are present, but there is damaged or intact soft tissue, the bone is repaired in the standard fashion with rigid fixation, designing exposures so as not to devascularize injured soft tissue.

BIBLIOGRAPHY

Barach E, Tomlanovich M, Nowak R. Ballistics: a pathophysiologic examination of the wounding mechanisms of firearms. Part I. *J Trauma.* 1986;26:225.

Barnes FC. *Cartridges of the World: A Complete and Illustrated Reference for Over 1500 Cartridges.* 12th ed. Iola, WI: F+W Media Inc.; 2009.

Clark N, Birely B, Manson PN, et al. High-energy ballistic and avulsive facial injuries: classification, patterns, and an algorithm for primary reconstruction. *Plast Reconstr Surg.* 1996;98(4):583–601.

Cunningham LL, Haug RH, Ford J. Firearm injuries to the maxillofacial region: an overview of current thoughts regarding demographics, pathophysiology and management. *J Oral Maxillofac Surg.* 2003;61:932–942.

Di Maio VJM. *Gunshot Wounds: Practical Aspects of Firearms, Ballistics, and Forensic Techniques.* 2nd ed. Washington, DC: CRC Press; 1999:16–27.

National Center for Injury Prevention and Control, Centers for Disease Control and Prevention. Explosions and blast injuries: a primer for clinicians. http://www.bt.cdc.gov/masscasualties/explosions.asp. Accessed September, 2012.

Fackler ML, Bellamy RF, Malinowski JA. The wound profile: illustration of the missile–tissue interaction. *J Trauma.* 1988;28:S21.

Fackler ML. Civilian gunshot wounds and ballistics: dispelling the myths. *Emerg Med Clin North Am.* 1998;16:17–28.

Fackler ML. Gunshot wound review. *Ann Emerg Med.* 1996;28:194–203.

Fackler ML. The wound and the human body: damage pattern correlation. *Wound Ballist Rev.* 1994;1:12–19.

Glezer JA, Minard G, Croce MA, et al. Shotgun wounds to the abdomen. *Am Surg.* 1993;59:129.

Harvey EN, Korr IM, Oster G, et al. Secondary damage in wounding due to pressure changes accompanying the passage of high velocity missiles. *Surgery.* 1947;21:218–239.

Ordog GJ, Balasubramanian S, Wasserberger J, et al. Extremity gunshot wounds. I. Identification and treatment of patients at high risk of vascular injury. *J Trauma.* 1994;36:358–368.

Ordog GJ, Wasserberger J, Balasubramanium S. Wound ballistics: theory and practice. *Ann Emerg Med.* 1985;13:1113.

Powers DB, Will MJ, Bourgeois SL, Hatt HD. Maxillofacial trauma treatment protocol. *Oral Maxillofac Surg Clin North Am.* 2005;17:341–355.

Rich NM, Johnson EV, Dimond FC Jr. Wounding power of missiles used in the Republic of Vietnam. *JAMA.* 1967;199:157–161.

Robertson BC, Manson PN. High-energy ballistic and avulsive injuries: a management protocol for the next millennium. *Surg Clin North Am.* 1999;79(6):1489–1502.

Rybeck B. Missile wounding and hemodynamic effects of energy absorption. *Acta Chir Scand.* 1974;450(suppl):5–32.

Sherman RT, Parrish RA. Management of shotgun injuries: a review of 152 cases. *J Trauma.* 1963;3:76.

Suneson A, Hansson HA, Lycke E, et al. Pressure wave injuries to rat dorsal root ganglion cells in culture caused by high-energy projectiles. *J Trauma.* 1989;29:10–18.

Suneson A, Hansson HA, Seeman T. Central and peripheral nervous system damage following high-energy missile wounds in the thigh. *J Trauma.* 1988;28(suppl 1):S197–S203.

Suneson A, Hansson HA, Seeman T. Pressure wave injuries to the nervous system caused by high-energy missile extremity impact. I. Local and distant effects on the peripheral nervous system: a light and electron microscopic study on pigs. *J Trauma.* 1990;30:281–294.

Tan YH, Zhou SX, Liu IQ, et al. Small-vessel pathology and anastomosis following maxillofacial firearm wounds: an experimental study. *J Oral Maxillofac Surg.* 1991;49(4):348–352.

United States Government Printing Office. *Emergency War Surgery.* 3rd United States revision. Washington, DC: United States Government Printing Office; 2004.

Ziervogel JF. A study of the muscle damage caused by the 7.62 NATO rifle. *Acta Chir Scand Suppl.* 1979;489:131.

Geriatric and Edentulous Maxillary and Mandibular Fractures

George M. Kushner, Robert L. Flint

Through medical advances, the world's population is living longer and the geriatric age group is increasing. Edentulism is often associated with the geriatric population. Edentulism is defined as the condition of being without natural teeth.[1] The edentulous population statistics are difficult to interpret fully and are related to multiple factors, including socioeconomic status. The rate of edentulism appears to be declining in the United States, however there are regions with high rates of edentulism, sometimes greater than 20% of the population. There is an estimated 12.2 million edentulous population in the United States in the 2009–2012 survey.[2]

The edentulous population is subject to the same mechanisms of trauma as the rest of the population. Motor vehicle collisions, assaults, and falls account for the majority of maxillofacial trauma seen in the geriatric population.[3]

DIAGNOSIS

A thorough physical exam should be performed on all maxillofacial trauma patients. Indicators of bony trauma and fracture are similar between edentulous and dentate patients.

1. Facial deformity
2. Ecchymosis
3. Mobility of segments and pain
4. V3 paresthesia in the mandible
5. V2 paresthesia in the maxilla
6. Malocclusion if dentures are in place

See Figs. 1.21.1 and 1.21.2.

If maxillofacial trauma is suspected, radiographs will most likely be performed. Plain films of the maxillofacial region such as the mandible series, Waters view and submental vertex view are almost always now being replaced by the computed tomography (CT) scan. CT scans of the maxillofacial region give much better detail in a 3-dimensional aspect to assist the provider in diagnosing the injury and formulating a treatment plan. Occasionally, patients seen in the outpatient office will have an orthopantomogram (panorex) as a screening film for mandibular trauma. The orthopantomogram should have another radiograph in a second plane such as an AP film or CT scan to fully assess the injury. A CT scan is the optimal study to assess maxillary and upper face trauma. Additionally, the CT scan can be carried through the skull to assess bony and soft tissue injuries to the central nervous system and cervical spine (Figs. 1.21.3–1.21.6).

The basis for treatment of maxillofacial trauma for hundreds of years has been to "put the teeth together and the bones will follow." This is the rationale for the classic closed reduction of mandible and maxillary fractures with intermaxillary fixation. The teeth will heal in the correct occlusion and the bony fractures will remodel over time to correct any residual bony deformity. Edentulous patients by definition do not have any natural teeth which causes a problem with the basics of treatment.

There are multiple options to treat edentulous fractures of the jaws. One option is to maintain a dental soft diet. This option is best for minimally displaced fractures or a patient who is medically unfit for surgery. There is the obvious potential for the patient to go on to a nonunion or malunion, both of which would be considered complications in the management of the patient. The atrophic edentulous mandible fracture patient has a high complication rate of nonunion at approximately 20%.[4]

MANDIBLE FRACTURES

Historically, edentulous mandible fractures were treated by closed reduction. This required altering the patient's denture and fixating the dental prostheses to the patient's jaws and using postoperative maxillomandibular fixation (MMF). Alternatively, dental splints could be fabricated and secured to the patient and postoperative maxillomandibular fixation could be used. The dental splints could be one- or two-piece constructs. The one-piece constructed dental prosthesis is known as the Gunning splint. Treating edentulous mandible fractures with dental prostheses required additional knowledge not available to all surgeons managing facial fractures. A dental laboratory facility needed to be available in order to fabricate the acrylic prostheses after dental models had been obtained. This could be cumbersome, time-consuming and delay patient care. Additionally, the patient's postoperative course was very difficult because of the dental appliances fixated to their jaws and the postoperative MMF. External fixators have also been used to stabilize edentulous mandible fractures as there are no teeth present. Precise anatomical reduction is often difficult with external fixators, especially in the atrophic mandible fracture with reduced bone stock. Management of edentulous mandible fractures by closed reduction techniques was difficult for the patient and had a high complication rate of nonunion (Figs. 1.21.7–1.21.11).

Open reduction techniques then evolved in management of edentulous mandible fractures. Osteosynthesis was accomplished using stainless steel wire, K wires, and finally miniplates. Often, postoperative MMF was still required as the fixation was not strong enough to withstand the forces of mastication or the pull of muscles attached to the mandible. The open reduction techniques using wire, K wires, and miniplates still had an unacceptably high complication rate.

Contemporary management of edentulous mandible fractures is best accomplished with open reduction and internal fixation of the fracture with a stable plate, usually a locking reconstruction plate. This permits anatomical reduction of the fracture with fixation that can withstand the forces of mastication and no postoperative MMF. The treatment does not require use of dental prostheses, dental consultation or dental laboratory use and is well tolerated by the patient as there is no postoperative MMF. Patients can enjoy the immediate function of chewing and speaking normally. This treatment of edentulous mandible

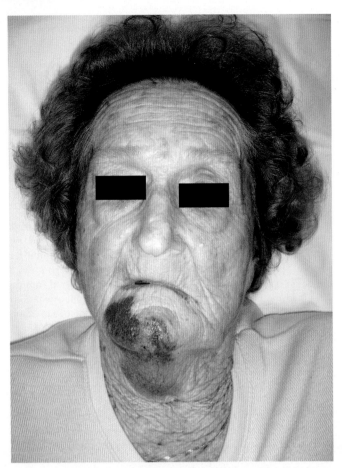

Fig. 1.21.1 Facial ecchymosis and deformity.

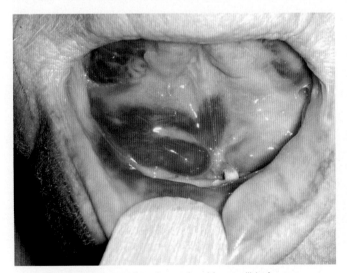

Fig. 1.21.2 Intraoral ecchymosis with mandible fracture.

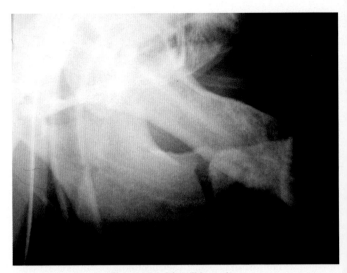

Fig. 1.21.3 Mandible series.

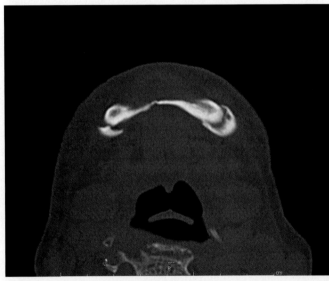

Fig. 1.21.4 Axial CT scan.

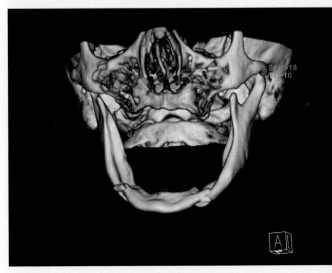

Fig. 1.21.5 3D CT scan.

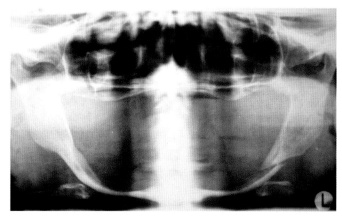

Fig. 1.21.6 Panorex of atrophic edentulous fracture.

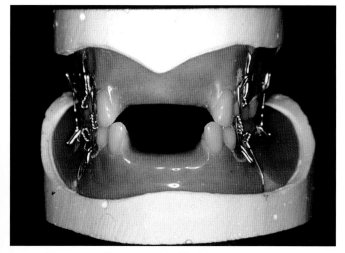

Fig. 1.21.7 Modified denture.

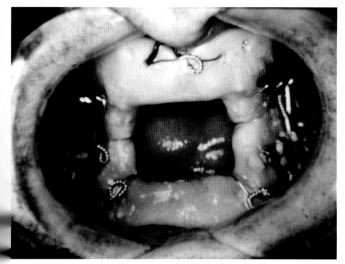

Fig. 1.21.8 Gunning splint.

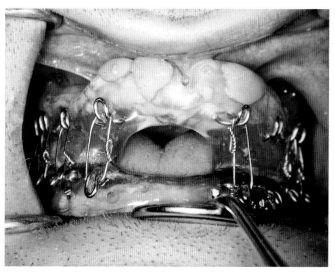

Fig. 1.21.9 Modified Gunning splint.

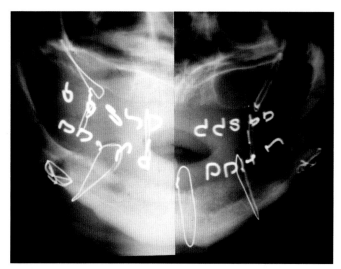

Fig. 1.21.10 Radiograph of modified Gunning splint.

fractures follows the recommendations of the AO/ASIF, a group of surgeons committed to advancing the care of musculoskeletal injuries, and their principles have been employed successfully all over the world[5,6] (Figs. 1.21.12 and 1.21.13)

The principles of the AO/ASIF group are well accepted and used all over the world. Treatment of edentulous mandible fractures is best accomplished using load-bearing osteosynthesis. Another name for this type of fixation is stabilization by splinting. This requires the plate to withstand the forces of mastication and allow immediate function for the patient. Typically, this requires a reconstruction plate with at least three screws on either side of the fracture. Locking reconstruction plates have been shown to provide adequate stability and have the benefit of a lower incidence of screw loosening.[5,6]

The open reduction and internal fixation of edentulous mandible fractures can be accomplished via a transoral approach. However, the transoral approach is quite difficult and requires multiple sets of trained hands to assist the surgeon. In the severely atrophic mandible the inferior alveolar nerve and inferior alveolar artery can sit on the crest of the ridge of the mandibular bone because of previous bone absorption and are at risk for damage with intraoral incisions. We have found the extraoral approach permits excellent access to align the fractures and place the reconstruction plates, which often are large. The extraoral approach is our preferred method to treat the edentulous mandible fracture patient. Transcutaneous incisions allow adequate access to place longer reconstruction plates. These patients often have neck skin creases which mask the scar of an extraoral incision to heal with an excellent cosmetic result.[4] Often, temporary stabilization with smaller plates of

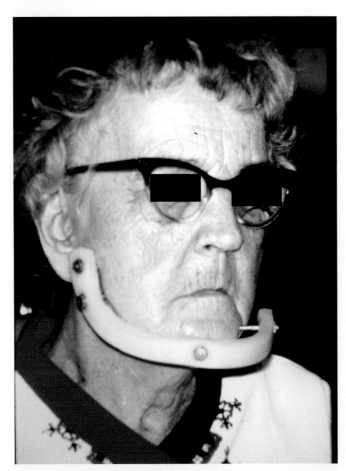

Fig. **1.21.11** External fixator.

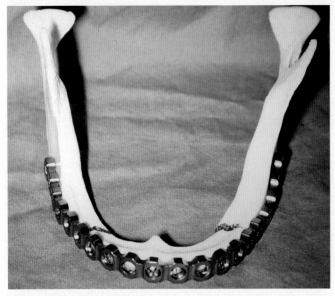

Fig. **1.21.12** Atrophic edentulous bone model with reconstruction plate.

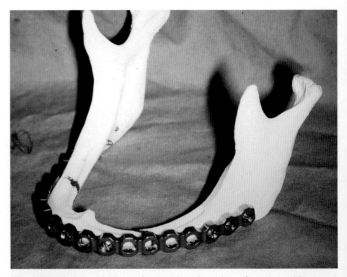

Fig. **1.21.13** Lateral view of atrophic edentulous fracture with reconstruction plate.

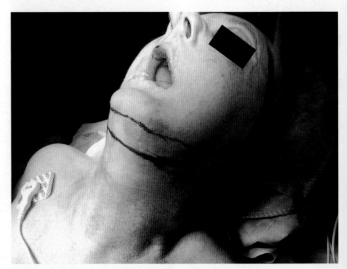

Fig. **1.21.14** Extraoral approach to atrophic edentulous mandible fracture.

edentulous mandible fractures is helpful as there are no teeth to provide occlusion. These smaller plates provide temporary fracture reduction and stabilization while the reconstruction plate is being bent and applied to the mandible. Bending templates are used to assist the surgeon in appropriate contouring of the reconstruction plate. The reconstruction plate is placed at the inferior border of the mandible to avoid damage

to the inferior alveolar nerve. The temporary plates are removed after the reconstruction plate is in place with all screws applied. The principle of at least 3–4 screws on either side of the fracture provides adequate stability for immediate function. Often, the edentulous mandible fractures bilaterally or in more than one place due to the weak nature of the bone, especially in atrophic mandibles.[7] The reconstruction plate is often taller than the native mandible in cases of severe mandibular atrophy. The bilateral edentulous mandible fracture often requires a single long reconstruction plate adapted from angle to angle to fulfill the requirements for stable fixation. The bone at the fracture sites of atrophic edentulous mandible sites is very often of poor quality. There is dense cortical bone with very little cancellous bone or marrow. Surgeons will often overgraft the fracture with autogenous cancellous bone at the fracture sites after the plate has been applied to augment healing at the fracture site. Additionally mandibular bone height can also be gained with this technique.. Many of these patients are poor surgical candidates for multiple general anesthetics so the open reduction, fixation, and autogenous grafting are performed as a single procedure under anesthetic[8,9] (Figs. 1.21.14–1.21.24).

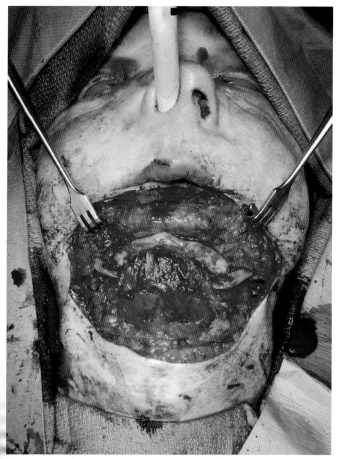

Fig. 1.21.15 Extraoral approach visualizing atrophic edentulous mandible fracture.

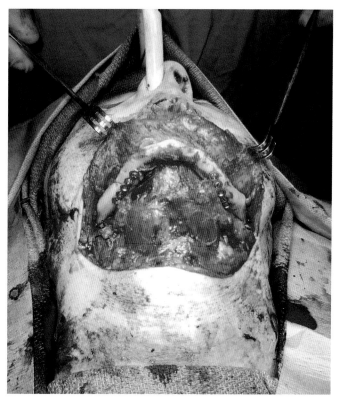

Fig. 1.21.17 Temporary miniplate fixation to simplify mandible fracture.

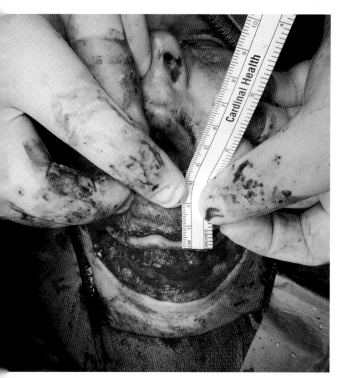

Fig. 1.21.16 Bone height in atrophic edentulous mandible fracture.

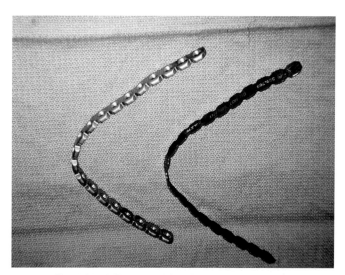

Fig. 1.21.18 Reconstruction plate bent to template.

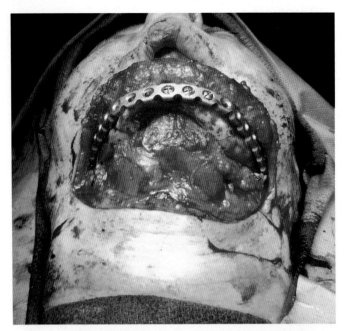

Fig. 1.21.19 Reconstruction plate in place.

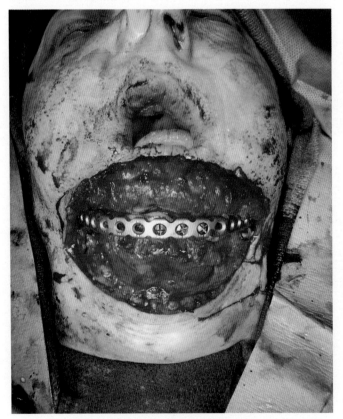

Fig. 1.21.20 Reconstruction plate in place.

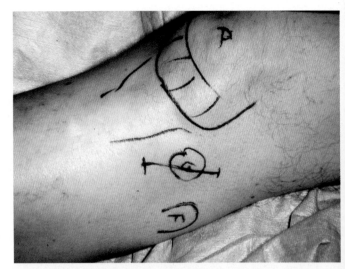

Fig. 1.21.21 Autogenous tibia bone graft harvest site.

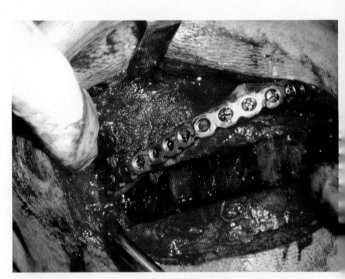

Fig. 1.21.22 Autogenous bone graft to fracture site.

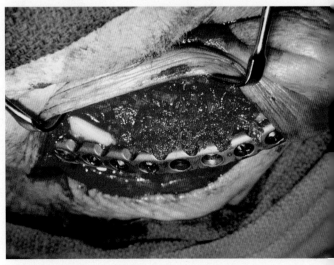

Fig. 1.21.23 Autogenous graft to fracture site to aid healing.

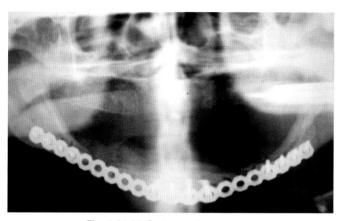

Fig. 1.21.24 Postoperative panorex.

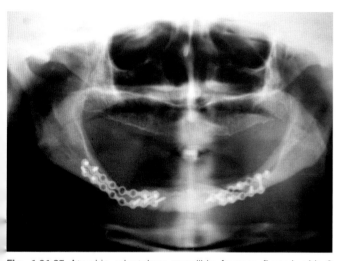

Fig. 1.21.25 Atrophic edentulous mandible fracture fixated with 2 miniplates.

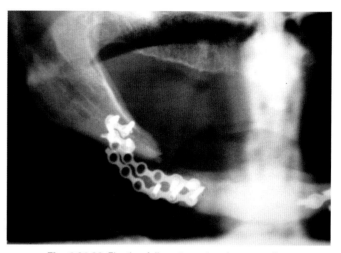

Fig. 1.21.26 Fixation failure 3 weeks after operation.

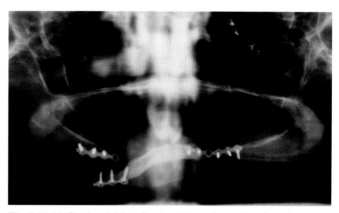

Fig. 1.21.27 Single miniplate fixation failure of atrophic edentulous mandible fracture.

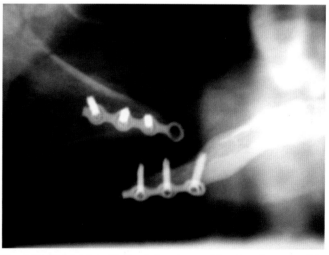

Fig. 1.21.28 Miniplate fixation failure in atrophic edentulous mandible fracture.

Following the principles of the AO/ASIF for treating edentulous mandible fractures with "load bearing" osteosynthesis, the patient has the tremendous benefit of immediate function and no MMF. Often the edentulous mandible fracture patients are elderly, frail, and have limited reserve. MMF creates respiratory pulmonary difficulties and hampers normal dietary intake. The ability to breathe unobstructed and have fairly normal eating capabilities can be a life-saving benefit for these patients.

It may being tempting to treat the small, atrophic mandible with small miniplates. This technique is certainly easier to perform. However, treatment of atrophic edentulous mandible fractures with miniplates is fraught with disaster. The treatment of these fractures with miniplates often results in fixation failure and additional surgery. Surgeons would be wise to remember the advice "the smaller the bone … the bigger the plate" when treating atrophic edentulous mandible fractures[10-12] (Figs. 1.21.25–1.21.28).

COMPLICATIONS

Complications were common in edentulous mandible fractures managed with closed reduction or wire osteosynthesis techniques and postoperative MMF. Prolonged periods of MMF were seen, ranging from 6 to 12 weeks, to enable the fractured mandible to heal. The patient often had difficulty in maintaining adequate nutrition during these long periods of MMF fixation. Patients were often elderly and infirm and experienced respiratory pulmonary complications during the long period of MMF. Nonunions and malunions were common and seen in up to 20% of the patients. Malunion of fractures with subsequent deformities were also frequently seen.

With use of load-bearing osteosynthesis (reconstruction plates) in the management of edentulous mandible fractures, the incidence of nonunion and malunion has decreased. There is no postoperative MMF, which has been a tremendous benefit for the patient. Oral intake and pulmonary toilet are greatly improved when compared to the use of postoperative MMF fixation. Plate exposure occasionally occurs in the mandible, especially when a hard acrylic denture is placed on the mandibular ridge. Consideration should be given to a permanent soft liner in the denture or denture fabrication by an experienced dentist who can monitor the denture fit and avoid excess pressure on mucosa under the denture. Secondarily, dental implants can be used to assist in the dental rehabilitation of these patients. The dental implants can provide increased stability of a dental prosthesis in the atrophic mandible with reduced bone stock. After treatment of the edentulous mandible fracture it is very common for the existing dentures to fit poorly and require fabrication of new dentures or rebasing/modification of the existing dentures to insure an appropriate fit.

MAXILLARY FRACTURES

The geriatric patient is occasionally involved with midface trauma. The most common mechanism of injury is falling, but also includes motor vehicle collisions, assaults, and unfortunately, elder abuse. Medical advances have increased the numbers of the elderly population and therefore the number of geriatric fractures is increasing.[13] Fractures of the midface are diagnosed by clinical and radiographic exam similar to the mandible fracture patient. The CT scan is the gold standard for diagnosing midface fractures. The Le Fort classification of midface fracture patterns is applicable to the edentulous maxilla. Clinically, pure Le Fort classifications are seen infrequently. More commonly a combination of classic Le Fort patterns are seen together. Midface fractures in the elderly tend to be minimally displaced and some do not require surgical intervention. However, displaced and mobile fractures which are symptomatic should be treated by classic techniques of open reduction, plate fixation, and where indicated, immediate bone grafting[3] (Figs. 1.21.29–1.21.32).

Le Fort fractures of the edentulous maxilla were historically treated with closed reduction by wiring the patient's denture in place and using MMF. Additionally, Gunning splints were fabricated and used similar to treatment of mandibular fractures. Wire fixation and suspension wires were used historically as "open reduction" techniques but generally required postoperative MMF.[14,15] They frequently compressed the face, shortening and retruding the facial profiles. External fixators and head frames were also used but often lacked the precise anatomical reduction needed for optimal postoperative results. These techniques have fortunately been abandoned and are mentioned only for historical purposes. Modern operative treatment of midface fracture management involve use of miniplates along the facial buttresses to restore the height, width, and projection of the face in conjunction with anatomic reduction of the fractures and immediate postoperative function and no MMF. Bone grafts may augment the volume of the atrophic midface bone, which is usually deficient.

The midface fractures are approached primarily with a maxillary vestibular incision, possibly in conjunction with a variety of transcutaneous approaches, depending on the fracture pattern. Using a maxillary vestibular approach, the surgeon can identify the zygomatic buttress, the nasomaxillary buttress, the orbital rim and infraorbital nerve. The bony buttresses can be reduced anatomically and fixated with miniplates. The four main buttresses of the maxilla are the two zygomatic and two nasomaxillary buttresses. These bony buttresses have the best quantity and quality of bone to align and stabilize the midface fractures.[5,6] In the edentulous maxilla, there is often bony atrophy or poor quality and

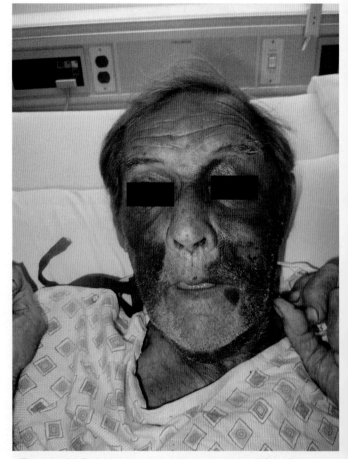

Fig. 1.21.29 Facial edema and ecchymosis with midface fractures.

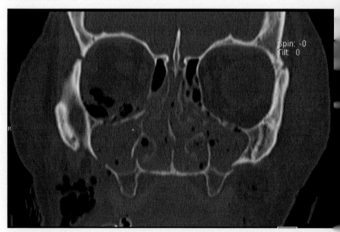

Fig. 1.21.30 Coronal CT scan showing fractures of edentulous midface.

quantity of bone. Occasionally, one or more buttresses are severely comminuted and cannot be plated. The bite force in the edentulous patient is greatly reduced and the surgeon must decide if plating the existing buttresses will give adequate stability to allow for healing. Alternatively, comminuted maxillary buttresses can be stabilized with a strut bone graft acting as the plate to span the comminuted area with screws in stable bone where available.[16] Contemporary management o

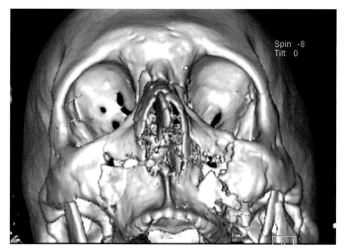

Fig. 1.21.31 3D CT scan reconstruction showing midface fractures.

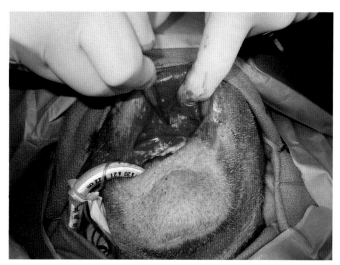

Fig. 1.21.33 Maxillary vestibular approach to midface fractures.

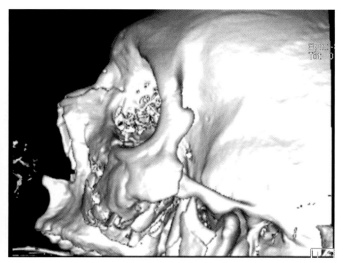

Fig. 1.21.32 Lateral view of 3D CT scan showing midface fractures.

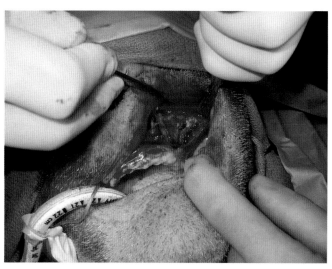

Fig. 1.21.34 Anatomic reduction and fixation of left midface fractures.

edentulous midface fractures does not require postoperative MMF. The patient has immediate function which facilitates eating, drinking, oral hygiene and ease of breathing during the convalescent period (Figs. 1.21.33–1.21.42).

COMPLICATIONS

Complications in management of the edentulous maxillary fractures are also seen. Minor jaw position discrepancies (malunions) can be treated with fabrication of a new denture which can camouflage the discrepancy in acrylic. Nonunions can result in chronic mobility of the maxilla. The reduced bone stock of the atrophic maxilla occasionally has difficulty in obtaining union. Depending on the patient's symptoms and desires, the nonunion may require anything from no treatment to additional surgery to apply new hardware and bone graft to the affected bony buttresses. Midface plates often interfere with the denture flange and require removal after adequate healing and bony union since stable bone is found only in the lower aspect of the maxillary alveolar ridge.

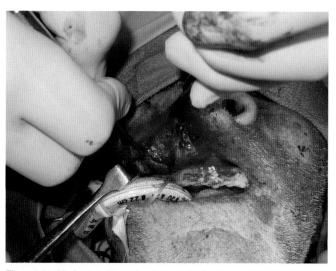

Fig. 1.21.35 Anatomic reduction and fixation of right midface fractures.

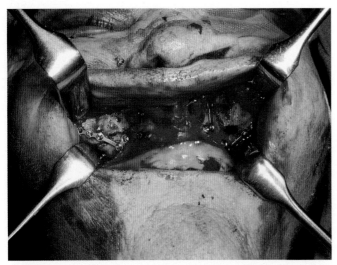

Fig. 1.21.36 Postoperative view of treated midface fractures.

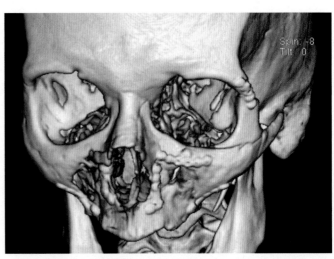

Fig. 1.21.39 Postoperative 3D CT scan showing good reduction.

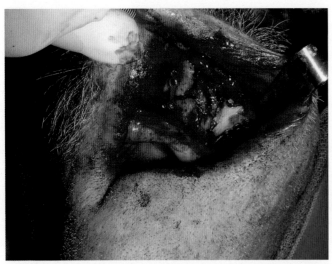

Fig. 1.21.37 Maxillary vestibular approach to comminuted left midface fractures.

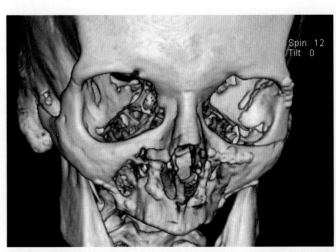

Fig. 1.21.40 Postoperative 3D CT scan of edentulous midface fractures.

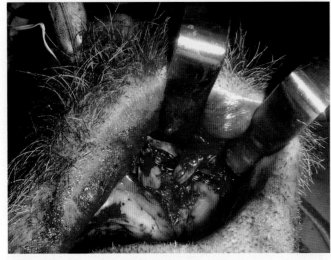

Fig. 1.21.38 Maxillary vestibular approach to midface fractures demonstrating plating of the orbital rim.

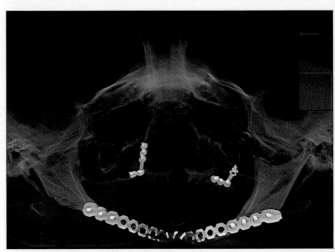

Fig. 1.21.41 Postoperative imaging of edentulous maxillary and mandibular fractures.

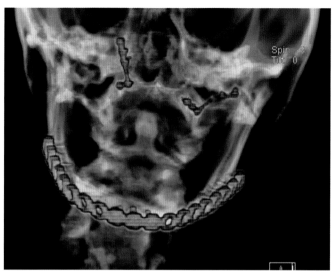

Fig. 1.21.42 Postoperative 3D CT scan of edentulous maxillary and mandibular fractures.

EXPERT COMMENTARY

The classic descriptions of edentulous mandibular and maxillary fracture treatment are a relic of the past, and should be replaced by well-thought-out plans of open reduction, secure plate fixation and bone grafting. A way to confirm good positioning of the mandible and maxilla is required in edentulous fracture treatment [1–4].

For the edentulous mandible whose height exceeds 20–25 mm, varied types of plate fixation are stable because there is sufficient bone stock to serve as a "buttress" to small plates. The bone stock is sufficient to predict good healing. Intermediate heights of the mandible demonstrate progressively worse healing, and a height of 15 mm predicts the need for larger plates to overcome the strong pull of the mandibular musculature which acts to depress the anterior mandibular segment and open and disrupt the fracture. Small, short plates simply cannot resist or counteract these forces, the screws pull out of the bone, and the disrupted plates are ineffective in preventing displacement.

Fractures of the edentulous mandible which are less than 10 mm in height display most of the complications and are prone to nonunion because of poor bone quality. A large reconstruction plate with locked screws, and at least four sites of fixation in reasonable bone away from the fracture site are recommended. Extraoral approaches are preferred, and the author prefers cancellous bone grafting to augment the poor bone quality where feasible. Plates frequently require removal for dentures to be accommodated or "fit" and further sulcus correction/revision may have to be accomplished.

The edentulous maxilla is not well understood or described in terms of its fracture treatment. Its operative treatment is frequently minimized, allowing it to heal in a displaced position, frequently retrodisplaced, with a tilt anteriorly and posteriorly, inferiorly displaced posteriorly and superiorly displaced anteriorly and frequently tilted from side to side. While the displacements may be able to be partially corrected by new denture reconstruction (which is the classic treatment in the literature), one has to honestly ask whether this is the best treatment, or merely the easiest treatment. Also, the elderly are frequently poorer risks healthwise, and multiple injuries and poorer prognosis may complicate treatment decisions about this component of the injury.

Frequently the anterior maxilla is displaced into the nasal airway anteriorly. Looking into the nose, the inferior part of the nasal airway is constricted by the displaced maxilla. The only way to prevent these maxillary deformities is an open reduction with immediate bone grafting to supplement the atrophic walls and struts of the maxilla, and essentially the process is the same as one would pursue in treating a dentulous maxilla, first achieving alignment properly with the mandible, then fixing it and supplementing atrophic areas where healing in the buttresses would not be acceptable with bone grafts, which also help by augmenting the volume of the atrophic skeleton. In this way, the patient can benefit from the exposure and fixation required with an improved bone structure correcting the appearance and strengthening the quality of the repair.

The critical step is positioning the maxilla to the mandible, the same as in dentulous Le Fort fracture treatment. Without this, the maxilla is invariably positioned too posteriorly, and even lining up the pieces of the maxilla does not correct the posterior displacement of the entire maxilla, as aligning the surface of the anterior walls of the maxilla does not prevent the displacement of the entire structure, which is *only* prevented by alignment to a properly positioned mandible, the same as in dentulous Le Fort fracture treatment. So the critical step is at the operation to open the fractures, and physically relate the maxilla's position to that of a properly positioned mandible by using dentures or splints to achieve the temporary alignment while fixation is completed. Bone grafts may then be used to augment fixation, and to provide better contour to the atrophic bone. The temporary fixation of the mandible to the maxilla may be released postoperatively, but may benefit from elastic traction in the same manner that dentulous fractures are managed.

Admittedly, this takes the treatment of the edentulous fracture out of the reconstructive domain, and takes it to the preventive, restorative or aesthetic areas, but then is this not a desirable outcome of a more comprehensive treatment of a challenging problem?

References

1. Francel T, Birely B, Ringleman P, Manson PN. The fate of plates and screws after facial fracture reconstruction. *Plast Reconstr Surg.* 1992;90:505–573.
2. Evans G, Clark N, Manson PN, Leipinger L. The role of mini- and micro-plate fixation in significant fractures of the midface and mandible. *Ann Plast Surg.* 1995;34: 453–456.
3. Manson P, Clark N, Robertson B, Crawly W. Comprehensive management of panfacial fractures. *J Craniomaxillofac Trauma.* 1995;11:43–56.
4. Crawley W, Clark N, Azman P, Manson P. The edentulous LeFort fracture. *J Craniofac Surg.* 1997;8:298–308.

Evidence-based medicine (EBM) content available in Appendix 1 (online only)

REFERENCES

1. *Mosby Medical Dictionary*. 9th ed. Philadelphia, PA: Elsevier; 2009.
2. Slade GD, Akinkugbe AA, Sanders AE. Projections of U.S. edentulism prevalence following 5 decades of decline. *J Dent Res*. 2014;93(10):959–965.
3. Zelken J, Khalifian S, Mundinger G, et al. Defining predictable patterns of craniomaxillofacial injury in the elderly: analysis of 1,047 patients. *J Oral Maxillofac Surg*. 2014;72:352–361.
4. Pereira FL, Gealh WC, Barbosa CE, et al. Different surgical approaches for multiple fractured atrophic edentulous mandibles. *Craniomaxillofac Trauma Reconstr*. 2011;4(1):19–24.
5. Prein J, ed. *Manual of Internal Fixation in the Craniofacial Skeleton*. Berlin: Springer Verlag; 1998.
6. Ehrenfeld M, Manson P, Prein J, eds. *Principles of Internal Fixation of the Craniomaxillofacial Skeleton, Trauma and Orthognathic Surgery*. Stuttgart: Georg Thieme; 2012.
7. Franciosi E, Mazzaro E, Larranaga J, et al. Treatment of edentulous mandible fractures with rigid fixation: case series and literature review. *Craniomaxillofac Trauma Reconstr*. 2014;7(1):35–42.
8. Tiwana PS, Abraham MS, Kushner GM, Alpert B. Management of atrophic mandible fractures: the case for primary reconstruction with immediate bone grafting. *J Oral Maxillofac Surg*. 2009;67(4):882–887.
9. Ellis E, Price C. Treatment protocol for fractures of the atrophic mandible. *J Oral Maxillofac Surg*. 2008;66(3):421–435.
10. Santos GS, de Assis Costa MD, de Oliveira Costa C, et al. Failure of miniplate osteosynthesis for the management of atrophic mandible fracture. *J Craniofac Surg*. 2013;24(4):415–418.
11. Madsen M, Kushner G, Alpert B. Failed fixation in atrophic mandibular fractures: the case against miniplates. *Craniomaxillofac Trauma Reconstr*. 2011;4(3):145–150.
12. Chee NS, Park SJ, Son MH, et al. Surgical management of edentulous atrophic mandible fractures in the elderly. *Maxillofac Plast Reconstr Surg*. 2014;36(5):207–213.
13. Yakamoto K, Matsusue Y, Murakami K, et al. Maxillofacial fractures in older patients. *J Oral Surg*. 2011;69(8):2204–2210.
14. Farmand M, Baumann A. The treatment of the fractured edentulous maxilla. *J Craniomaxillofac Surg*. 1992;20(8):341–344.
15. Crawley WA, Azman P, Clark N, et al. The edentulous LeFort fracture. *J Craniofac Surg*. 1997;8(4):298–307.
16. Gruss JS, Mackinnon SE. Complex maxillary fractures: role of buttress reconstruction and immediate bone grafts. *Plast Reconstr Surg*. 1986;78(1):9–22.

2.1

Pediatric Skull Fractures

Matthew R. Louis, Jeffrey G. Trost Jr., Larry H. Hollier

BACKGROUND

Skull fractures are a common injury in the pediatric population and are often associated with significant morbidity and mortality. A strong foundational knowledge of pediatric skull fractures is essential for appropriate treatment and prevention of long-term complications. Although most skull fractures can be treated with conservative management, timely identification of more severe injuries can be life-saving. The surgeon should be comfortable identifying various fracture patterns and initiating appropriate management for each.

EPIDEMIOLOGY

Head trauma is the leading cause of traumatic death in children.[1] It is estimated that more than 600,000 children visit the emergency room each year for blunt head trauma. Of these, 1%–3% will die as a result of intracranial injuries.[1-3] In the outpatient setting, 2%–20% of children presenting with head trauma will have a skull fracture.[4]

Falls are the most common mechanism of head injury in children, especially under the age of 2, and comprise 35%–54% of cases.[2,3] Sports-related injuries, peaking between ages 13 to 15 years old, represent another common mechanism of skull fracture and contribute 29% of cases.[2] These patients typically have favorable outcomes and lower rates of mortality. Baseball and softball are the most frequently implicated sports, with the most common mechanism being direct contact between ball and skull. Motor vehicle accidents (MVAs) are the cause of 21%–24% of pediatric skull fractures and increase in prevalence with age.[3-4] The clinician should have a high suspicion for associated facial, cardiothoracic or cervical spine injuries as the mechanism of injury involves higher energy transfer.

PEDIATRIC SKULL AND FRACTURE ANATOMY

An understanding of the differences between the pediatric and adult skull is important in evaluating fractures and formulating the appropriate management. Thinner bones, a larger head-to-torso ratio, and developing sinuses increase a child's susceptibility to cranial injury. In addition, the retruded position of the face relative to the skull results in a higher incidence of cranial injuries in younger children.

During the first years of life, the pediatric brain and craniofacial skeleton undergo rapid development. At birth, the neurocranium is 25% of its final adult size. It grows to 75% of adult dimensions by age 2 and 95% by age 10.[3] Although the ethmoid and maxillary sinuses are present at birth, both the sphenoidal and frontal sinuses undergo aeration from childhood into puberty.[3] During this period of aeration, frontal fractures become more common. While conservative management is favored prior to frontal sinus aeration in younger patients, teenagers and adults are more often treated operatively.

The parietal bone is the most frequently fractured calvarial bone.[3] These fractures typically occur in younger children, while the incidences of frontal and temporal bone fractures increase with age. Frontal bone fractures can involve the frontal sinus, skull base, and orbit, putting patients at an increased risk for cerebrospinal fluid (CSF) leak and ocular complications. Temporal bone fractures carry the highest risk of mortality, as injury to the underlying middle meningeal artery may lead to an epidural hematoma.

Fracture patterns include linear, comminuted, depressed, open, and growing types (Figs. 2.1.1 and 2.1.2). Each type differs in its presentation and management. Linear fractures, the most common fracture pattern, characteristically arise at the point of maximum impact and spread along the involved bone without crossing suture lines. Comminuted fractures result from higher impact forces and are comprised of multiple associated linear fractures. More significant trauma can result in depressed fractures which are usually associated with underlying cerebral injury and may present as hemorrhage, posttraumatic seizures, or infection. Since open fractures produce a communication between the skull through the scalp or upper respiratory tract, there is an increased risk for central nervous system (CNS) infection. Growing skull fractures are an uncommon late complication of wide skull fractures with underlying dural tear and subsequent brain parenchymal herniation.

CLINICAL PRESENTATION

A detailed history is essential in evaluating children with head trauma. In the emergency center setting, the AMPLE mnemonic (Allergies, Medications, Past medical history, Last meal, Events surrounding injury) is a useful guide for rapid assessment. Important considerations include the presence of penetrating trauma, intentional injury, and loss of consciousness. Older children may be able to vocalize important aspects of the history, localize pain, and bring other symptoms to attention.

Physical examination begins with a primary survey of the child's airway, breathing, and circulation – the ABCs. The secondary survey should include a head-to-toe examination for soft tissue swelling, hematoma, and palpable skull step-offs, bony irregularity or crepitus. The surgeon should be aware that skull fractures are often associated with

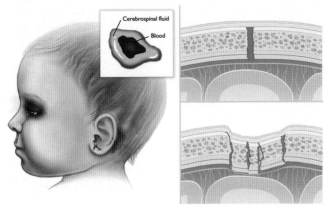

Fig. 2.1.1 Signs of various fracture types. (*Left*) Basilar skull fracture. Cutaneous findings suggestive of basilar skull fractures include raccoon's eyes, Battle's sign over the mastoid process, as well as otorrhea and rhinorrhea. The "halo sign" (inset) is considered positive when blood coalesces in the center and clear fluid (CSF) distributes around the blood. (*Top right*) Linear skull fracture. (*Bottom right*) Depressed and comminuted fracture. Findings may include palpable step-offs on physical examination. Underlying dural tears may serve as the nidus for the future development of a growing skull fracture. (Reproduced with permission from Texas Children's Hospital.)

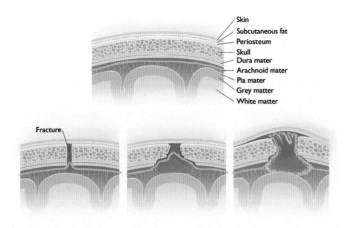

Fig. 2.1.2 Growing skull fracture. After injury and fracture, the arachnoid membrane will herniate into the fracture site and over time a leptomeningeal cyst will develop. The cyst communicates with the subarachnoid space but is contained by pia-arachnoid adhesions. As the cyst grows, it will erode away the underlying bone and begin to cause a noticeable deformity. The leptomeningeal cyst may become clinically apparent a year after the inciting injury. (Reproduced with permission from Texas Children's Hospital.)

underlying intracranial injuries. Independent predictors of intracranial injury include focal neurological deficits, seizures, and altered mental status (AMS); however, not all patients with intracranial injuries will exhibit either skull fractures or focal neurological findings upon initial examination.

Linear fractures most frequently involve the parietal bone and are associated with intracranial injury in 15%–30% of patients.[5] Examination may reveal overlying hematoma or soft tissue swelling, although these findings may require some time to develop. Subgaleal hematomas are largely predictive of underlying skull fractures in infants.[1,5,6] Linear fractures of the temporal bone should be evaluated for injury to the middle meningeal artery and subsequent development of an epidural hematoma. Occipital bone fractures may involve the underlying venous sinus and result in hematoma of the posterior fossa.

Comminuted fractures of the occipital bone suggest repeated blows against a solid surface and should raise suspicion for nonaccidental trauma. Diastatic fracture is a term used to describe fractures that traverse suture lines and manifest as widening of the involved suture. This subset of fractures is typically seen in children under the age of 3.

Depressed fractures may be appreciated as palpable step-offs at the site of injury. Of the children with depressed skull fractures, 30% have associated dural or brain injury, with risk of underlying injury directly correlated to the depth of depression.[5,7] Further complications include hemorrhage, mass effect, ectopic bone fragments, and cosmetic deformity.

Basilar skull fractures often demonstrate unique physical exam findings (Fig. 2.1.1). These include hemotympanum, CSF rhinorrhea or otorrhea, or subcutaneous bleeding over the mastoid process (Battle's sign) or orbit (raccoon eyes or spectacle hematoma). Associated cranial nerve injuries may manifest as hearing loss, facial paralysis, anosmia, vertigo, or tinnitus.[8] Half of these children experience resolution of their deficits while the other half exhibit residual deficiencies.[8] CSF leak is a major complication. Although most leaks resolve spontaneously within a week of injury, 0.7%–5.0% of cases may be complicated by meningitis.[9,10] Failure of a CSF leak to resolve may necessitate placement of a spinal drain or open repair.

Open fractures result in a communication between the skull and outside environment. A scalp laceration overlying the site of fracture is highly suggestive of an open fracture. Otorrhea, rhinorrhea, or frank CSF present in the wound suggest an underlying dural injury. In cases where bleeding may mask the presence of CSF, a "halo test" can be performed. The patient's dressings can be examined for a lighter ring or "halo" of CSF fluid around blood (Fig. 2.1.1). These patients must be closely monitored for the development of CSF infection.

Dural tears that fail to heal properly may give rise to a "growing skull fracture." This type of fracture manifests as a slow-growing subcutaneous mass at the fracture site typically detected within the first year after injury (Fig. 2.1.2). Etiologies of this mass include brain herniation, development of a leptomeningeal cyst, or dilation of the ventricles.[11–15] These fractures are rare and occur mainly in children under 3 who have had suture diastasis, or widening of the skull sutures, greater than 3–4 mm. In one study of 592 consecutive pediatric head injuries, the incidence of growing skull fractures was 1.2%.[16] The most common sites of growing skull fractures are parietal and frontoparietal.[17]

RADIOLOGICAL EVALUATION

Computed tomography (CT) is the imaging modality of choice to assess skull fractures and intracranial injury. Although all children with presumed head trauma should be considered for CT, imaging is required for patients with AMS, focal neurological deficits, seizures, or a palpable depression.[1] CT should be strongly considered in the case of loss of consciousness, vomiting, headache, drowsiness, amnesia, or when the etiology of trauma is unknown. A low threshold for imaging is employed for infants, as intracranial injuries in this age group may result from minor trauma and manifest with subtle signs and symptoms. The PECARN Pediatric Head Injury/Trauma Algorithm can be used to guide the decision of whether or not to utilize CT imaging.

Skull radiographs are no longer routinely used as meta-analyses have found plain radiographs are neither sensitive nor specific in diagnosing the intracranial injury.[18] Although ultrasonography is becoming increasingly popular in the emergency setting, this technique is operator-dependent and requires advanced training.[19] As technology advances, ultrasound may prove useful in cases when CT is not immediately available.

SURGICAL INDICATIONS

In the majority of cases, skull fractures can be managed without surgery.[18] Predictors of operative intervention include increasing age, being hit in the head by an object, presence of a hematoma, and involvement of the frontal bone.[3,18] Patients over 1 year of age with linear fractures, resulting bone gaps fewer than 3 mm, and no evidence of acute mental status changes can be safely sent home with close follow-up within 2 days.[19] Caregivers should be instructed to closely observe the child for 24 hours after the injury and awaken the child at night to confirm neurological stability. Infants should be evaluated for a potential growing skull fracture 1–2 months after the initial injury.

Surgery is typically reserved for severely comminuted or depressed fractures. Indications for emergent intervention include underlying mass shift, hematoma, or evidence of a dural tear with pneumocephalus. In the case of depressed skull fractures, the degree of depression is correlated with prognosis. As depression depth increases, so does the likelihood of dural tears and cortical lacerations. A nonoperative approach can be pursued in pediatric patients with simple, mildly depressed skull fractures without underlying intracranial hematoma. A cutoff of 5 or 10 mm of depression is often used in deciding to pursue surgical elevation.[7,20]

SURGICAL TECHNIQUES

Surgical management of skull fractures includes repair of underlying dural injury, anatomical reduction, and fixation. For optimal results, primary reconstruction of depressed fractures, particularly open injuries, should take place within 6 hours of injury.[21] Due to their great potential for bone remodeling, pediatric skull fractures are generally more forgiving in achieving anatomical reduction. Surgical reconstruction includes rigid fixation across the fracture with nonresorbable or resorbable plates, while small comminuted bone fragments are often amenable to semirigid fixation with wires or sutures.

If a dural tear is suspected, a CSF leak can be sought intraoperatively. Dural tears can often be repaired directly with water-tight suturing. Larger defects can be closed using a dural graft material that may be synthetic or autogenous. Vascularized flaps can also be used to isolate the intracranial space in the event an anterior skull base fracture predisposes the patient to infection.

Titanium has long been favored in craniofacial surgery for its resistance to corrosion, light weight, strength, and biocompatibility.[21] Disadvantages include its permanence and the potential need for future removal. Although some suggest plate removal after the bone has healed, small titanium plates are not routinely removed at this author's institution unless indicated by infection, hardware failure, visibility, soft tissue thinning prominence or exposure. If removal is planned, this should occur no later than 12–16 weeks after the initial fixation. Delayed removal may result in a very difficult surgery since the titanium plates may become incorporated into newly developed bone.[22]

Resorbable plates are typically composed of a polymer of polylactic and polyglycolic acids. These plates retain their strength for the duration of fracture healing before resorbing by hydrolysis. Resorption typically occurs by 1 year postimplantation, making them ideal for the pediatric population. The safety profile of resorbable plates is comparable to that of metal plates, with postoperative infection encountered in 0.4% of patients and 0.3% requiring reoperation due to device failure. At 3 month follow-up, foreign body reactions were experienced in 0.7% of patients and were clinically recognized as scalp swelling or cyst formation. There are currently no randomized controlled trials that compare titanium and resorbable plates for treatment of skull fractures.[23]

Semirigid fixation with wire or suture can achieve adequate remodeling of small comminuted fragments. Wire, however, may later become painful or palpable and require removal. To overcome this potential complication, semirigid fixation with PDS suture is preferred.

POSTOPERATIVE COURSE

Common post-surgical complications include wound infection, the need for revision, poor cosmesis, CSF leak, and pain at the hardware site. Persistent bleeding in the form of intracranial hematoma and venous sinus thrombosis are less likely, but possible. Signs of increased intracranial pressure include persistent neurological deficits, headache, or vomiting.

Antibiotic use often depends on the mechanism of injury, risk of exposure, and the presence of a CSF leak suggesting communication between the environment with the brain. Antibiotic selection is individualized depending on exposure profiles but often includes broad spectrum coverage. Prophylactic antiepileptic drugs are commonly employed in patients who have sustained depressed skull fractures. However, in patients with Glasgow Coma Score (GCS) over 8, prophylactic phenytoin is not indicated and has not been shown to decrease seizure rates in these children.[24]

ILLUSTRATIVE CASE EXAMPLES

Case 1

A 4-year-old girl was ejected from a car following a high-speed motor vehicle accident. Upon arrival in the emergency room she was unconscious with an extensive scalp laceration. CT showed a large, mildly displaced fracture of the frontal bone, a diastatic fracture of the left squamosal suture, and a non-displaced fracture of the left parietal bone (Fig. 2.1.3). There was no significant intracranial hemorrhage or mass effect.

Although large in size, minimal displacement and a lack of underlying hematoma or mass effect allowed this fracture to be managed without surgical reconstruction or fixation. After thorough irrigation and closure of her scalp laceration, the patient was closely monitored for a temporal lobe contusion and concern for elevated ICP with a monitor.

Case 2

A 6-year-old boy suffered a head injury after being kicked by a horse. He presented with a large, contaminated laceration over the left parietal bone, a subgaleal hematoma, and clear rhinorrhea. CT showed a comminuted left parietal fracture extending to the left squamosal suture. A depression of about 3 mm was noted (Fig. 2.1.4). No parenchymal hemorrhage or mass effect was observed.

Given the contamination of the wound, the patient was brought to the operating room for irrigation and closure. Upon wound exploration, no CSF leak was readily identified. Given the minimal amount of depression (less than 5 mm), the depressed bone fragment was left alone to heal without elevation and fixation. Given the potential severity of microbial exposure and concern for CSF leak, broad-spectrum antibiotic therapy was continued throughout hospitalization.

Case 3

A 10-year-old boy presented to the emergency room after suffering a blunt force trauma by a baseball bat. Upon arrival, the patient was sleepy, concerning for post-ictal state. Examination showed a scalp laceration down to bone and a palpable bony step-off. CT revealed a depressed comminuted skull fracture of the left parietal bone (Fig. 2.1.5A). Given the degree of depression, the patient was brought to the

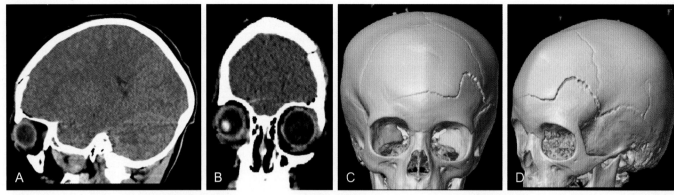

Fig. 2.1.3 Linear skull fracture. Although large, this linear, non-displaced fracture did not require fixation for proper healing to occur.

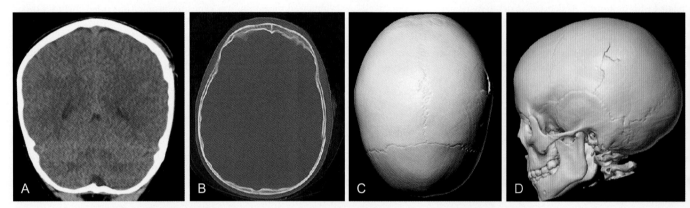

Fig. 2.1.4 Minimally depressed skull fracture. Surgical elevation of the depressed bone was not required in this patient with a depression of 3 mm.

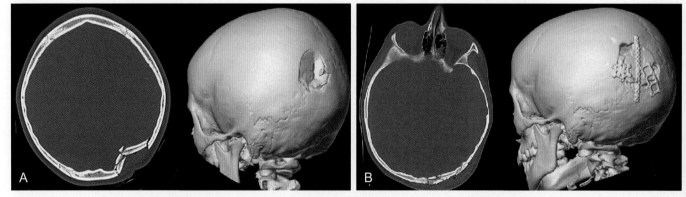

Fig. 2.1.5 Largely depressed skull fracture. (A) Preoperative CT images of a depressed skull fracture are shown. The patient underwent surgery for a depression greater than 1 cm and for repair of CSF leak. (B) Postoperative scans showing reconstructed skulls with titanium plating system.

operating room for elevation of the skull fracture and repair of any underlying dural injury.

In the operating room, the patient's laceration was continued superiorly and inferiorly to expose an adequate area of bone. Bur holes were placed superior and inferior to the depressed fragments. Bone flap elevation revealed an underlying dural laceration. An anteriorly based pericranial flap was raised to facilitate closure of the dural laceration in a watertight manner. The comminuted fracture was then repaired off-table with titanium plates and secured into the craniotomy site (Fig. 2.1.5B). The patient received three doses of perioperative antibiotics followed by a 5-day course of clindamycin.

Case 4

A 15-month-old boy presented to the emergency room after a fall and subsequent posturing. On arrival the patient demonstrated anisocoria and a GCS of 3. CT demonstrated a small, minimally displaced fracture of the inferior right parietal bone with a large underlying epidural hematoma with significant mass effect (Fig. 2.1.6). The patient was brought to the operating room emergently for evacuation of the hematoma.

A bone flap was elevated over the hematoma, and the clot was evacuated by suction and irrigation. A bleeding epidural vessel, likely an

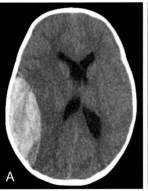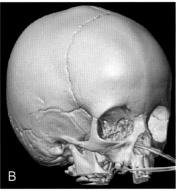

Fig. 2.1.6 Linear skull fracture with underlying hematoma. Alone, this small linear fracture would not necessitate surgical intervention. However, hematoma and mass effect required emergent craniotomy and surgical evacuation.

injured branch of the middle meningeal artery, was noted at the inferior aspect of exposure and controlled with cautery. After irrigation, epidural tacking holes were placed centrally and around the edges of the craniotomy. The bone flap was inset with titanium plates and screws, and the tack-up sutures secured. In the postoperative period, both antibiotics and antiepileptics were employed as prophylaxis.

COMPLICATIONS

Acute Complications

The most concerning acute complications include meningitis or encephalitis. To prevent infection patients with open skull fracture should receive prophylactic antistaphylococcal antibiotics and appropriate vaccination against tetanus.[25] Empiric coverage for nosocomial Gram-negative rods and staphylococcus is also commonly employed in patients with basilar skull fracture; however, prophylactic antibiotics have not been shown to decrease the risk of meningitis in these patients.[26,27] Patients with CSF leak for greater than 7 days are at substantially increased risk for meningitis, regardless of antibiotic use.

Long-Term Complications

Development of a growing skull fracture is a rare but serious long-term complication following pediatric skull trauma. Other terms used to describe this type of fracture include leptomeningeal cyst, subdural hygroma, traumatic meningocele, and cerebrocranial erosion. Growing skull fractures have been poorly studied but are believed to occur in 0.6–1.6% of patients who have sustained severe head trauma in the first year of life.[12] For a growing skull fracture to occur, the resulting defect must be wide (greater than 3–4 mm) with an associated unrepaired dural tear. The brain parenchyma deep to the fracture site herniates through the torn dura and its pulsations erode the overlying bone. The herniating brain is often revascularized by the scalp vessels, further complicating management.[13–15]

Clinically, growing skull fractures are appreciated as cranial asymmetry or a slowly growing lesion within the injury site. Although growing skull fractures are most commonly recognized within a year of a skull fracture, some may present later with neurologic sequelae including headache or delayed seizures.[15] Seizures eventually affect 34% of children with growing skull fractures.[12]

Treatment is best directed toward identification and prevention. One author has suggested extensive exploration of wide skull fractures to search for a dural tear. Dural repair should be pursued once the patient is stable and cerebral edema has abated.[15] If growing skull

fractures are discovered later, the clinician should look for signs of increased intracranial pressure. If present, a shunt is warranted. The dural defect needs to be closed, often with graft material, and cranioplasty may be required for skeletal reconstruction.[13]

Permanent fixation devices should not be placed across suture lines to allow for cranial vault growth with aging.

CONCLUSION

A knowledge of the pediatric skull and fracture anatomy is essential to timely and appropriate management of cranial fractures. Although the majority of patients can be managed nonoperatively, significantly depressed or comminuted fractures should undergo operative treatment and reconstruction. Rigid fixation can be accomplished with either titanium or resorbable plating, depending on surgeon preference and patient factors. Complications include infection, neurological deficits, or seizures. Large fractures with significant diastasis or depression should be explored to correct fracture displacement dural injury. All fractures should receive late follow-up X-rays to identify the occasional patient with a "growing skull fracture."

EXPERT COMMENTARY

Since trauma is a leading cause of death and disability in children, and since injuries of the skull and face frequently coexist, the proper management of skull injuries in children is a routine part of the management of the injured child.

Frequently the skull serves as a donor site for bone grafts, which may be utilized as the child grows older. Good management of pediatric trauma must include that of the skull, as injuries of the skull and face are frequently combined, and comprehensive management requires attention to the entire injury with the brain injury, and here the aesthetics, the function and the appearance are all combined as multiple important priorities. The principles of both operative and nonoperative management of the pediatric skull injury are outlined, and this chapter is a nice companion to Chapter 3.2 by Liang, Vercler and Buchman on pediatric skull reconstruction.

REFERENCES

1. Quayle KS, Jaffe DM, Kuppermann N, et al. Diagnostic testing for acute head injury in children: when are head computed tomography and skull radiographs indicated? *Pediatrics*. 1997;99(5):E11.
2. Kraus JF, Fife D, Cox P, et al. Incidence, severity, and external causes of pediatric brain injury. *Am J Dis Child. 1960*. 1986;140(7):687–693.
3. Adetayo OA, Naran S, Bonfield CM, et al. Pediatric cranial vault fractures: analysis of demographics, injury patterns, and factors predictive of mortality. *J Craniofac Surg*. 2015;26(6):1840–1846.
4. Gallagher SS, Finison K, Guyer B, Goodenough S. The incidence of injuries among 87,000 Massachusetts children and adolescents: results of the 1980-81 Statewide Childhood Injury Prevention Program Surveillance System. *Am J Public Health*. 1984;74(12):1340–1347.
5. Schutzman SA, Greenes DS. Pediatric minor head trauma. *Ann Emerg Med*. 2001;37(1):65–74.
6. Greenes DS, Schutzman SA. Clinical significance of scalp abnormalities in asymptomatic head-injured infants. *Pediatr Emerg Care*. 2001;17(2):88–92.
7. Erşahin Y, Mutluer S, Mirzai H, Palali I. Pediatric depressed skull fractures: analysis of 530 cases. *Childs Nerv Syst*. 1996;12(6):323–331.
8. Kitchens JL, Groff DB, Nagaraj HS, Fallat ME. Basilar skull fractures in childhood with cranial nerve involvement. *J Pediatr Surg*. 1991;26(8):992–994.

9. Kadish HA, Schunk JE. Pediatric basilar skull fracture: do children with normal neurologic findings and no intracranial injury require hospitalization? *Ann Emerg Med.* 1995;26(1):37–41.

10. Baltas I, Tsoulfa S, Sakellariou P, et al. Posttraumatic meningitis: bacteriology, hydrocephalus, and outcome. *Neurosurgery.* 1994;35(3):422-426-427.

11. Naim-Ur-Rahman, Jamjoom Z, Jamjoom A, Murshid WR. Growing skull fractures: classification and management. *Br J Neurosurg.* 1994;8(6):667–679.

12. Pezzotta S, Silvani V, Gaetani P, et al. Growing skull fractures of childhood. Case report and review of 132 cases. *J Neurosurg Sci.* 1985;29(2):129–135.

13. Zemann W, Metzler P, Jacobsen C, et al. Growing skull fractures after craniosynostosis repair: risk factors and treatment algorithm. *J Craniofac Surg.* 2012;23(5):1292–1295.

14. Muhonen MG, Piper JG, Menezes AH. Pathogenesis and treatment of growing skull fractures. *Surg Neurol.* 1995;43(4):367-372-373.

15. Sanford RA. Prevention of growing skull fractures: report of 2 cases. *J Neurosurg Pediatr.* 2010;5(2):213–218.

16. Rinehart GC, Pittman T. Growing skull fractures: strategies for repair and reconstruction. *J Craniofac Surg.* 1998;9(1):65–72.

17. Gupta SK, Reddy NM, Khosla VK, et al. Growing skull fractures: a clinical study of 41 patients. *Acta Neurochir (Wien).* 1997;139(10):928–932.

18. Bonfield CM, Naran S, Adetayo OA, et al. Pediatric skull fractures: the need for surgical intervention, characteristics, complications, and outcomes. *J Neurosurg Pediatr.* 2014;14(2):205–211.

19. Mannix R, Monuteaux MC, Schutzman SA, et al. Isolated skull fractures: trends in management in US pediatric emergency departments. *Ann Emerg Med.* 2013;62(4):327–331.

20. van den Heever CM, van der Merwe DJ. Management of depressed skull fractures. Selective conservative management of nonmissile injuries. *J Neurosurg.* 1989;71(2):186–190.

21. Marbacher S, Andres RH, Fathi A-R, Fandino J. Primary reconstruction of open depressed skull fractures with titanium mesh. *J Craniofac Surg.* 2008;19(2):490–495.

22. Siy RW, Brown RH, Koshy JC, et al. General management considerations in pediatric facial fractures. *J Craniofac Surg.* 2011;22(4):1190–1195.

23. Dorri M, Nasser M, Oliver R Resorbable versus titanium plates for facial fractures. In: Cochrane Database of Systematic Reviews [Internet]. 2009. Available from: http://onlinelibrary.wiley.com.ezproxyhost.library.tmc.edu/doi/10.1002/14651858.CD007158.pub2/abstract.

24. Lewis RJ, Yee L, Inkelis SH, Gilmore D. Clinical predictors of post-traumatic seizures in children with head trauma. *Ann Emerg Med.* 1993;22(7):1114–1118.

25. Rabinowitz RP, Caplan ES. Management of infections in the trauma patient. *Surg Clin North Am.* 1999;79(6):1373–1383, x.

26. Villalobos T, Arango C, Kubilis P, Rathore M. Antibiotic prophylaxis after basilar skull fractures: a meta-analysis. *Clin Infect Dis.* 1998;27(2):364–369.

27. Ratilal BO, Costa J, Pappamikail L, Sampaio C Antibiotic prophylaxis for preventing meningitis in patients with basilar skull fractures. In: The Cochrane Collaboration, editor. Cochrane Database of Systematic Reviews [Internet]. Available from: http://doi.wiley.com/10.1002/14651858.CD004884.pub4.

Superior Pediatric Orbital and Frontal Skull Fractures

Devin O'Brien-Coon, Richard J. Redett

BACKGROUND AND INCIDENCE

Within the pediatric age group, orbital fractures are among the most common facial fractures.[1,2] Although pediatric craniofacial trauma remains relatively uncommon when compared to the adult population, it continues to cause significant morbidity and mortality.[3] Orbital trauma can be caused by a range of mechanisms from low energy falls to high energy trauma caused by motor vehicles or sporting injuries. While orbital floor fractures are a common occurrence in both children and adults, orbital roof fractures are found disproportionately more often in children.

It is well described in the literature that the relative frequency of orbital floor to roof fractures is dependent on age. The fracture patterns of the orbit are affected by the differing craniofacial shape among children by age.[4] After birth the cranium grows faster than the face, reaching 80% of its final size by the age of 2 years. Brain and ocular growth are nearly complete by age 7 years; however, facial growth then continues well into the teenage years, eventually resulting in a final cranium:facial ratio of 2:1.[4] Orbital roof fractures occur primarily in younger children, and are associated with high-energy mechanisms and less commonly need surgical intervention.[4] On the other hand, orbital floor fractures occur more commonly after the age of 7 years as a consequence of the proportionally larger cranium and the lack of maxillary sinus pneumatization in younger children. In contrast, due to the lack of frontal sinus pneumatization in these young children, impact to the superior aspect of the orbital rim cannot be dissipated by the frontal sinus, and is thus transmitted through to the orbital roof.[5] However, as the frontal sinus pneumatizes into the superior orbital rim as the child becomes older, it serves as a buffer to shield the direct transmission of energy from the superior orbital rim into the orbital roof, and the incidence of orbital roof fractures decreases.[4]

SURGICAL ANATOMY

The orbital roof is formed almost completely by the frontal bone, though it extends laterally to the greater wing of the sphenoid and zygoma. The lesser wing of the sphenoid forms the most posteromedial portion of the orbital roof as it extends upwards to the superior orbital fissure and optic canal.[6] Medially, the orbital roof extends to the orbital plate of the ethmoid, posterior lacrimal crest, and the frontal process of the maxilla. The orbital roof is thin with comparable structure to the orbital floor and serves to separate the brain and anterior cranial fossa from the orbit and ocular structures. The anteromedial portion of the orbital roof borders the frontal sinus in children in whom it is developed,

separating the orbit from the frontal sinus and communication with the nasal cavity.[7]

CLINICAL PRESENTATION

Examination of patients with upper third facial fractures begins with a complete craniomaxillofacial trauma history and physical. Younger children may be more difficult to examine and indirect measures must sometimes be resorted to, particularly for extraocular movement evaluation and visual acuity examination.

For frontal bone fractures, examination of the skull contour for irregularity should be performed. Any evidence of CSF leak should be noted, through the nose, ear or from lacerations. Overlying lacerations are relatively common and can sometimes be used as access approaches for limited surgical repair. For orbital roof fractures, evidence of vertical dystopia or proptosis should be looked for, as well as visual acuity and full range or limitation extraocular movements. Evidence of an afferent pupillary defect (Marcus Gunn pupil) is also a highly concerning sign. At our institution, in addition to the surgical team survey most patients with orbital fractures receive comprehensive ocular examination by the ophthalmology service.

RADIOLOGICAL EVALUATION

In most centers, plain skull films have largely been supplanted by computed tomography (CT) with multiplanar reconstruction (MPR). Evaluations of axial, sagittal, and coronal views are all valuable given the complex frontal/orbital anatomy and significant symptomatology that can be caused by relatively small bone fragments. Three-dimensional reconstructions can sometimes offer added value, particularly to contextualize the significance of skull fractures to overall cranial contour.

Radiation dose from imaging is an important consideration, especially in younger children. Our radiology department, as a tertiary care center performing a significant number of pediatric head/face CTs, has developed special scanning protocols to offer lower dose scans of the head and face in children (e.g., angling cuts away from the brain, taking slightly thicker cuts in less essential areas, etc.) while still maintaining quality. Unnecessary scans should be avoided and, when scans are indicated, dose should be minimized to the extent possible.

In patients with developed frontal sinuses, evaluation of the integrity of the anterior and posterior tables should be performed, as well as the status of the nasofrontal duct. Orbital fractures should be carefully examined to identify both the integrity of the orbital contents and the position of any dislodged bony fragments that may lead to ophthalmic symptoms.

SURGICAL INDICATIONS

Indications for surgery in these fractures are undoubtedly the most controversial aspect of their management. Consideration must be given to the overall status of the patient, possibility of future growth, alterations, and risk of long-term complications. Concomitant neurosurgical pathology and need for neurosurgical intervention are often an important adjunctive consideration.

Orbital Roof Fractures

In our review of 159 pediatric patients with orbital roof fractures, we found that most can be managed nonoperatively.[8] Only 14 (9%) of the patients who sustained orbital roof fractures required surgical management. In four of these patients only the orbital floor was repaired. Three patients were treated for isolated orbital roof fractures (with a mean fracture size in these cases of 3.9 cm^2). One of these patients received an orbitotomy with fragment reduction only while the other two patients underwent craniotomies with open reduction and internal fixation (ORIF) and pericranial flaps.

Seven patients presented with both frontal bone and orbital roof fractures. Three of these patients had the orbital roof directly addressed via craniotomy and wiring or plating and/or onlay alloplastic implant (SynPor). Three patients underwent frontal bone ORIF. One patient underwent frontal sinus obliteration.

In our cohort, most orbital roof fractures were noncomminuted and were treated nonoperatively. Management of operative orbital roof fractures will be dictated by the concomitant frontal bone or neurosurgical injuries. If a craniotomy is already necessary, it is a relatively straightforward decision to reduce and repair the roof or place an implant or split cranial bone graft, external to the roof defect. Similarly, in older children who have involvement of the frontal sinus that necessitates intervention, treatment should first address reconstruction of the orbital rim and the frontal sinus, including the possible need for obliteration or cranialization (see below).[9] In our experience isolated roof fractures <2 cm^2 are unlikely to develop orbital encephalocele or leptomeningeal cysts.

Our analysis strongly supports the management concept that displacement direction in orbital roof fractures is significant, with inferiorly displaced "blow-in" fractures representing a substantially worse prognostic sign than superior displacement.[8] Despite representing nearly half of fractures, none of the 10 patients who had operative roof repair had superior displacement. The magnitude of displacement was also predictive of need for surgery but only for fractures displaced inferiorly, lending further support to this concept. Two patients who had superiorly displaced roof fractures did have ORIF of the orbital floor performed but nothing done to their orbital roof fractures, suggesting that the "blow-out" mechanism can lead to simultaneous roof-floor fracture but rarely causes roof fractures that need repair. All other patients requiring surgery had significant inferior displacement of the roof bone fragments.

Direct comparison of "defect size" with roof fractures can be misleading as a concept because a 2 cm^2 defect in an infant is far different proportionally than the same area in a teenager. However, it does seem likely that there is a size below which herniation of the leptomeninges will not occur and thus fracture size should be a consideration in repair. We followed long-term outcomes on 9 patients with sub-2 cm^2 defects and 14 patients with sub-4 cm^2 defects, and none of these patients developed late complications. We therefore believe that roof fractures that measure less than 2 cm^2 in size and do not have a significant frontal bone component are unlikely to develop encephalocele and can be regarded with less concern. Fig. 2.2.1 represents our overall algorithm for management of pediatric orbital roof fractures. In the absence of

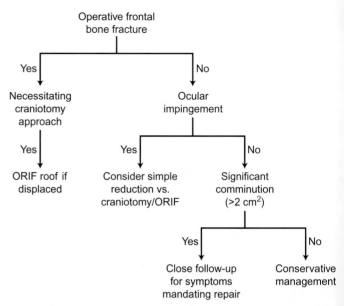

Fig. 2.2.1 Algorithm for management of orbital roof fractures in children. (From Coon D, Yuan N, Jones D, et al. Defining pediatric orbital roof fractures: patterns, sequelae, and indications for operation. Plast Reconstr Surg 2014;134:442e–448e.)

any symptoms or concomitant injuries, we generally recommend close follow-up rather than prophylactic intervention even in larger defects.

Frontal Bone Fractures

In a review of 897 pediatric skull fractures, frontal bone fractures were the most commonly in need of repair, though only about 16% of patients needed surgery.[10] In their series, the authors reported one late case of a growing frontal bone fracture in an 8-year-old boy whose fracture had not been treated.

Surgical decision making in these fractures must necessarily be bifurcated into two cohorts: children with developed frontal sinuses and those without. The latter case is more straightforward: the primary indications for surgical repair are depression or displacement of the frontal bone fragment (which will lead to a contour depression) or underlying dural injury, after which the bone can be fixed into place using the surgeon's preferred method of osteosynthesis.

Management is more complex in children with pneumatized frontal sinuses, especially those with rudimentary but not fully formed sinuses. Even in adults, indications for cranialization versus obliteration versus observation can be controversial. There is even less evidence to base intervention upon in children. Vu et al. reviewed a series of 39 pediatric patients with frontal sinus fractures.[11] For the management of posterior table injuries, they distinguished between nasofrontal outflow tract injury and persistent CSF leakage. The latter was generally treated first by observation, followed by cranialization if it did not resolve. However, they proposed that nasofrontal outflow tract (NFOT) obstruction requiring intervention should be treated by obliteration. In contrast, Whatley presented a series of pediatric frontal sinus fractures where cranialization was the procedure of choice for both CSF leakage and NFOT obstruction.[12]

Given the residual potential for skull growth and the many decades of anticipated future life for problems resulting from microscopic mucosal remnants after obliteration to arise, we generally favor cranialization over obliteration. Intervention is recommended in the presence of a persistent CSF leak or imaging evidence that the sinus function is unlikely to be adequate (e.g., comminution of the posterior wall or obstruction of the nasofrontal duct). Isolated anterior wall fractures can generally be managed in a similar fashion to frontal bone fractures as discussed above.

SURGICAL TECHNIQUES
ORIF Orbital Roof
The surgical technique used to repair orbital roof fractures is determined by the degree of comminution and the presence of concomitant neurosurgical injuries. Inferiorly displaced fractures with a mild degree of comminution can sometimes be managed through existing lacerations or an orbitotomy with direct reduction of the bone fragment. More comminuted fractures or those requiring a frontal craniotomy for a neurosurgical injury are best managed by intracranial elevation of the bone fragments followed by placement of an autologous onlay bone graft or alloplastic implant. Our preferred method is to reduce any displaced bone fragments and place a thin piece of alloplast (Synpor, 0.85 mm) on the orbital roof. A small pericranial flap is used to cover the cranial side of the implant. We prefer to use alloplast as in our experience autologous bone graft will frequently resorb.

ORIF Frontal Bone
Isolated, depressed frontal bone fractures or those associated with a dural tear and CSF leak will sometimes require repair using open reduction and internal fixation (Fig. 2.2.2). Depressed fractures that do not require neurosurgical intervention can be managed through forehead lacerations if present or a coronal scalp incision. We usually use

resorbable fixation if possible because of concerns of passive intracranial force transmission of titanium osteosynthesis plates and screws in the growing skull. A craniotomy may be required for severely depressed fractures or those associated with persistent CSF leak requiring dural repair.

Cranialization
Extensive fractures involving the anterior and posterior tables and/or nasofrontal duct of the frontal sinus can be treated by frontal sinus cranialization. To accomplish cranialization, the disrupted posterior wall of the frontal sinus is removed, the sinus mucosa in remaining walls is burred away, and the nasofrontal duct is tightly obliterated with bone graft to block communication of the aerodigestive tract and intracranial space. The entire sinus is then covered with a vascularized pericranial flap and the brain and dura are permitted to rest against the repaired anterior wall and sinus floor. It is important to make sure all of the mucosa or the sinus and the proximal portion of the frontal duct is thoroughly surface burred to prevent late mucocele formation.

Bone Graft vs. Mesh, Fixation Method (Including Resorbable vs. Permanent)
A comparative analysis of autogenous bone graft vs. alloplast does not exist, and the choice of implant ultimately lies with the surgeon. The implants most often employed in children include porous polyethylene and autogenous bone graft, including split cranial bone graft and iliac crest. A well-developed diploic space is required to harvest split cranial

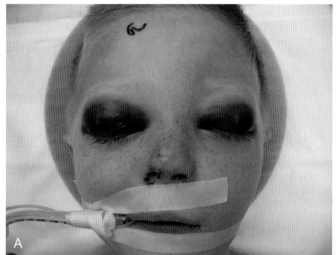
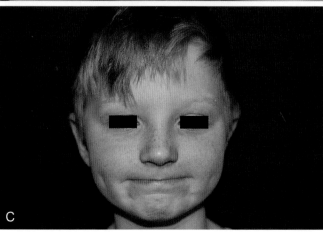
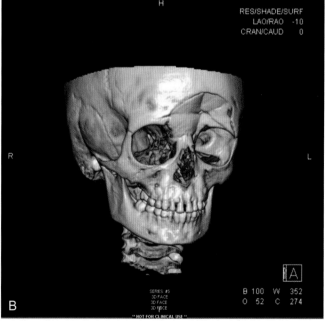

Fig. 2.2.2 A case example of a 6-year-old boy who presented after being struck in the forehead with a golf club (A). CT scan demonstrated a depressed frontal bone fracture (B). He underwent open reduction and internal fixation through a coronal approach which restored frontal contour without long-term complications (C).

bone graft. This method is less feasible in children younger than the age of 5 years although recent reports suggest split cranial bone graft can be harvested in children less than 3 years of age.[13] Split cranial bone graft can be used to reconstruct skull and orbital roof defects.

ACUTE COMPLICATIONS

Optic Nerve Injury/Orbital Apex Syndrome

The optic nerve (CN II) travels through the optic canal, emerging through the optic foramen. Fractures that propagate posteriorly through the orbital roof or sphenoid can in principle go to the optic canal with the potential for nerve injury or bony compression. This is an extremely rare complication, as compared to the comparatively more common situation of traumatic optic neuropathy caused by direct globe injury or traction. Unexpected deterioration in visual acuity or development of an afferent pupillary defect should merit consideration of immediate ophthalmologic consultation, steroids, and potential optic nerve decompression.

Cerebrospinal Fluid (CSF) Leak

CSF leaks through the nose are more common with frontal bone fractures than orbital roof fractures and are suggestive of an underlying dural tear. Most will stop with conservative treatment; persistent leaks are typically managed in conjunction with neurosurgery via cranialization as discussed above. Antibiotic coverage during the period of CSF leakage continues to be a topic without a clear consensus.

LONG-TERM COMPLICATIONS

Encephalocele/Leptomeningeal Cyst/Growing Skull Fracture

Encephalocele is a rare but feared late complication after orbital roof fractures. Typically limited to case reports, incidence rates are hard to estimate. In our series of 149 patients, we did not see any cases. Menkü reported two cases of late growing skull fractures with underlying encephalocele,[14] while Suri et al. reported two more cases, with both of these presenting as exophthalmos from expansion of the dura through the orbital defect.[15] While the enlargement of the anterior cranial fossa caused by inferior displacement of the orbital roof appears to be a key aspect of encephalocele formation (by creating potential space for brain expansion), it alone is probably not sufficient to cause a growing fracture. Havlik proposes that a combination of a dural injury with an expanding intracranial process (i.e., brain growth) is also required to provoke development of an encephalocele into a bone space resulting from a fracture.[16] Any patient presenting with pulsatile exophthalmos should raise suspicion for an underlying encephalocele and this diagnosis should be ruled out.

Much of the evidence supporting the proposed mechanism and management of these pathologies in the anterior skull base and orbital roof is extrapolated from the substantially more common scenario of growing fractures in the external skull.[17] Growing fractures of the frontal bone are much more common than the orbit, with the parietal bone being an even more common site.[18,19] From a review of the 132 cases reported in the literature, it is clear that age is the strongest risk factor, with babies at vastly disproportionate risk (which is unsurprising given their more rapid rate of skull growth).[19]

Growth Impairment

Much concern around surgical intervention in the pediatric population revolves around the possibility of impairment of further growth, however there is relatively little evidence for these fractures to support whether or not surgery affects long-term growth. These concerns have also often underlain the move to resorbable fixation from surgeons who choose to use these devices.

Mucocele

Prevention of late mucocele or pyomucocele is one of the driving forces behind management of frontal sinus injuries. Because the indolent period may be years or decades prior to presentation, the small series in the literature of pediatric frontal sinus fractures rarely include these cases. There have been isolated case reports of pediatric mucocele after both craniofacial surgery (orbital box osteotomies)[20] and frontal sinus fractures.[21] At our center, presentation of this rare complication in a patient still in the pediatric age range would be managed similarly to an adult.

EXPERT COMMENTARY

Pediatric orbital trauma is traditionally considered to involve the lower and medial orbit and zygoma.

The large size of the frontal cranium early in life predisposes to trauma to the orbital roof and frontal skull; there is an absence in the literature of good descriptions, treatment and follow-up in the literature of these upper orbital injuries. The difficulty of following children through growth contributes to the lack of data. While many authors describe the "spontaneous correction with growth" of pediatric fractures before age 5, I have usually pursued anatomical correction; there is an orbital roof deformity which follows more subtle but displaced frontal bone fractures and those of the accompanying roof which magnifies with growth, and is challenging to correct. I often, when seeing these unusual cases, think of how straightforward it would have been to pursue correction at the time of the injury.

Here, O'Brien-Coon and Redett have produced one of the best categorized descriptions of fractures of this area, and they outline their recommendations for diagnosis and treatment in each specific anatomical area and for each age group. Their outline of "what to do and when" is one based upon much case study, and the extensive experience in a major pediatric trauma center.

REFERENCES

1. Grunwaldt L, Smith DM, Zuckerbraun NS, et al. Pediatric facial fractures: demographics, injury patterns, and associated injuries in 772 consecutive patients. *Plast Reconstr Surg.* 2011;128:1263–1271.
2. Chapman VM, Fenton LZ, Gao D, et al. Facial fractures in children: unique patterns of injury observed by computed tomography. *J Comput Assist Tomogr.* 2009;33:70–72.
3. Bank DE, Carolan PL. Cerebral abscess formation following ocular trauma: a hazard associated with common wooden toys. *Pediatr Emerg Care.* 1993;9:285–288.
4. Koltai PJ, Amjad I, Meyer D, et al. Orbital fractures in children. *Arch Otolaryngol Head Neck Surg.* 1995;121:1375–1379.
5. Messinger A, Radkowski MA, Greenwald MJ, et al. Orbital roof fractures in the pediatric population. *Plast Reconstr Surg.* 1989;84:213–216, discussion 217–218.
6. Conforti PJ, Haug RH, Likavec M. Management of closed head injury in the patient with maxillofacial trauma. *J Oral Maxillofac Surg.* 1993;51:298–303.
7. Haug RH. Management of the trochlea of the superior oblique muscle in the repair of orbital roof trauma. *J Oral Maxillofac Surg.* 2000;58:602–606.
8. Coon D, Yuan N, Jones D, et al. Defining pediatric orbital roof fractures: patterns, sequelae, and indications for operation. *Plast Reconstr Surg.* 2014;134:442e–448e.
9. Haug RH, Likavec MJ. Frontal sinus reconstruction. *Atlas Oral Maxillofac Surg Clin North Am.* 1994;2:65–83.

10. Bonfield CM, Naran S, Adetayo OA, et al. Pediatric skull fractures: the need for surgical intervention, characteristics, complications, and outcomes. *J Neurosurg Pediatr*. 2014;14:205–211.

11. Vu AT, Patel PA, Chen W, et al. Pediatric frontal sinus fractures: outcomes and treatment algorithm. *J Craniofac Surg*. 2015;26:776–781.

12. Whatley WS, Allison DW, Chandra RK, et al. Frontal sinus fractures in children. *Laryngoscope*. 2005;115:1741–1745.

13. Vercler CJ, Sugg KB, Buchman SR. Split cranial bone grafting in children younger than 3 years old: debunking a surgical myth. *Plast Reconstr Surg*. 2014;133:822e–827e.

14. Menku A, Koc RK, Tucer B, et al. Growing skull fracture of the orbital roof: report of two cases and review of the literature. *Neurosurg Rev*. 2004;27:133–136.

15. Suri A, Mahapatra AK. Growing fractures of the orbital roof. A report of two cases and a review. *Pediatr Neurosurg*. 2002;36:96–100.

16. Havlik RJ, Sutton LN, Bartlett SP. Growing skull fractures and their craniofacial equivalents. *J Craniofac Surg*. 1995;6:103–110, discussion 111–102.

17. Rinehart GC, Pittman T. Growing skull fractures: strategies for repair and reconstruction. *J Craniofac Surg*. 1998;9:65–72.

18. While B, Saha K, Radford R, et al. A reliable surgical technique for the management of growing fractures of the frontal bone involving the orbit. *Orbit*. 2013;32:166–170.

19. Pezzotta S, Silvani V, Gaetani P, et al. Growing skull fractures of childhood. Case report and review of 132 cases. *J Neurosurg Sci*. 1985;29:129–135.

20. Tatla T, East C, Marucci DD, et al. Frontoethmoidal mucocele following pediatric craniofacial surgery. *J Craniofac Surg*. 2014;25:2008–2012.

21. Smoot EC III, Bowen DG, Lappert P, et al. Delayed development of an ectopic frontal sinus mucocele after pediatric cranial trauma. *J Craniofac Surg*. 1995;6:327–331.

Pediatric Orbital Fractures

Jonathan Y. Lee, Jesse A. Goldstein, Joseph E. Losee

BACKGROUND

Pediatric orbital fractures differ from the adult population in terms of presentation, management, and complications. The craniofacial skeleton undergoes significant anatomical and physiological changes from birth into adulthood; therefore, the fracture patterns in the pediatric population present differently, influencing diagnosis and management. The understanding of these injuries is evolving and controversial in some aspects: particularly the decision to operate and the timing of the operation. In pediatrics, fracture repair must be weighed against the potential skeletal growth disruption resulting from surgery versus preventing globe malposition and motility complications. The objective of this chapter is to highlight the pertinent differences in anatomy, presentation, and management, as well as clinical outcomes of pediatric orbital fractures.

SURGICAL ANATOMY

In the infant, the cranium is relatively large compared to the face, with an estimated ratio of 8:1. As the skeleton matures, facial growth predominates resulting in an adult cranium to facial ratio of 2.5:1. During major trauma, craniofacial fractures (i.e., orbital roof) are more likely than maxillofacial fractures (i.e., orbital floor) in early life due to a more prominent cranium and developing sinuses (Fig. 2.3.1).[1–3]

Seven bones articulate to form the orbit: frontal, maxillary, zygomatic, palatine, ethmoid, lacrimal, and sphenoid. Three of the four orbital walls – roof, floor, and medial wall – are adjacent to a sinus.[4] In the setting of trauma, the sinuses help dissipate the force transmitted to the facial skeleton and brain.

The sinuses begin to separate from the nasal cavity in utero, and begin to pneumatize and expand after birth.[5] The maxillary sinuses are the first to develop, but in a biphasic pattern, with a delay between 7 and 12 years of age. During this period of mixed dentition, the cuspid teeth are unerupted in the maxilla, directly below the orbital floor. The halt in pneumatization results in increased bone stock beneath the orbital floor, helping the floor resist fracture. As the permanent dentition erupts, maxillary sinus growth continues, reaching adult size by age 16.

The ethmoid sinuses grow from birth to age 12, from anterior to posterior. As they expand, the medial orbital wall becomes progressively thinner and more susceptible to fracture. At adulthood, the medial wall is named the lamina papyracea or "paper wall."

The frontal sinuses pneumatize and enlarge, typically starting at age 7, completing growth in adulthood.[6] Prior to their development, traumatic forces placed on the superior orbital rim are not dissipated through the frontal sinus but rather, transmitted to the roof, causing either roof fractures or cranial fractures extending into the orbit. Posnick et al. reported a relatively high incidence of pediatric orbital roof fractures,

representing 18% of orbital fractures in their cohort.[2] Losee et al. reported an even higher incidence, at 33.3%.[7] Lastly, orbital floor fractures become more common than orbital roof fractures with increasing age, following the timeline of maxillary sinus pneumatization.[2,8,9]

There are also physiological differences in the craniofacial tissues that help the pediatric skeleton resist fracture.[10] Pediatric bones have a higher proportion of cancellous bone, which has less stiffness than cortical bone. The stiffness of a material is inversely related to its elasticity – the material's ability to deform with force. Cancellous bone can therefore better conform to traumatic forces, resulting in higher incidence of "greenstick" fractures or minimal to no displacement. The metabolic turnover of the pediatric skeleton is also significantly greater. Clinically, this means that the healing and remodelling potential of the pediatric skeleton is superior, supporting nonoperative management.

Increased elasticity of the periorbital soft tissue also helps avoid operative management in many cases. The periosteal lining, supporting check ligaments, and suspensory ligaments of the orbital cavity, can also help resist deformation, even in the setting of fracture.[5,7] The elastic soft tissue may act to splint fractures or, in the setting of a blow-out fracture, prevent orbital malposition (Fig. 2.3.2). Increased skeletal elasticity also means that a more significant amount of force is required to cause pediatric fractures. This, in addition to rudimentary sinuses, leads to more transmitted force to the neurocranium. Losee et al. found that 43.4% of pediatric orbital fractures were associated with neurosurgical injuries.[7]

Pediatric facial fractures are relatively uncommon due to the aforementioned bone elasticity, cancellous composition, and higher cranium-to-face ratio. Within pediatric facial fractures, orbital fractures have a wide reported incidence, ranging from 3% to 45% of all facial fractures. Grunwaldt et al. demonstrated that the orbital fracture was the most common facial fracture (Fig. 2.3.3) in all age groups (0–5 years, 6–12 years, 13–18 years).[11] This differs from prior work evaluating the epidemiology of pediatric facial fractures.[10,12,13] However, Grunwaldt et al. utilized emergency department-based assessment at a level one trauma children's hospital, eliminating an inherent selection bias of individual surgeons, consulting department, and hospital admissions.[11]

CLASSIFICATION

Orbital fractures can be isolated to the orbital walls or they can extend into adjacent structures. To guide management based on the presenting pattern, Losee et al. described a pediatric orbital fracture classification system based on three presenting patterns: pure orbital fractures, craniofacial fractures, and orbital fractures associated with common fracture patterns (Table 2.3.1).[7]

Pure orbital fractures (Type 1) describe fractures limited to the orbit without extension into adjacent structures, and can be subdivided into five subcategories: floor, medial wall, combined medial wall and floor,

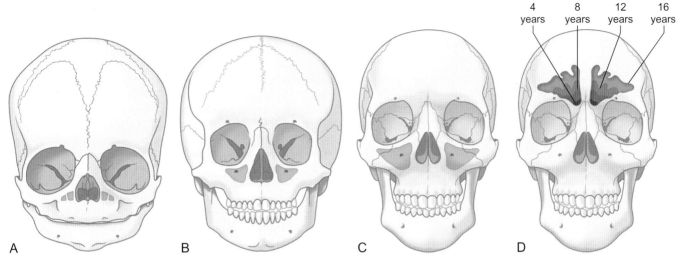

4 years 8 years 12 years 16 years

A B C D

Fig. 2.3.1 Craniofacial development. Cranium to face ratio at birth (A) is 8:1 and evolves to 2.5:1 at adulthood (C). Maxillary sinus (green) progressive pneumatization at birth (A), at 5 years of age (B), and at adulthood (C). Frontal sinus (D) pneumatization. (Adapted from Oppenheimer AJ, Monson LA, Buchman SR. Pediatric orbital fractures. Craniomaxillofac Trauma Reconstr 2013;6:9–20 and Golden BA, Jaskolka MS, Vescan A, et al. Evaluation and management of frontal sinus injuries. In: Fonseca RJ, Walker RV, Barber HD, editors. Oral and maxillofacial trauma, 4th ed. St. Louis, MO: Elsevier Saunders; 2013. p.470–490.)

TABLE 2.3.1	**Pediatric Orbital Fracture Classification**
Type 1	Pure orbital fractures
1a	Floor fractures
1b	Medial wall fractures
1c	Roof fractures
1d	Lateral wall fractures
1e	Combined floor and medial wall fractures
Type 2	Craniofacial fractures
2a	Growing skull fractures
Type 3	Orbital fractures associated with common fracture patterns
3a	Fractures of the floor and inferior orbital rim
3b	Zygomaticomaxillary fractures
3c	Naso-orbito-ethmoid fractures
3d	Other fracture patterns

Adapted from Losee JE, Afifi A, Jiang S, et al. Pediatric orbital fractures: classification, management, and early follow-up. Plast Reconstr Surg 2008;122:886–897.

superior roof, and lateral wall. Type 1 fractures are commonly referred to as "blow-out" or "blow-in" fractures but without involvement of the orbital rim. The orbital floor is the most common wall involved.

Craniofacial fractures (Type 2) describe fractures of the skull that extend into the orbital roof. This type of fracture is commonly seen in younger pediatric patients, often with neurological injury.[11] The orientation also tends to be obliquely positioned, traveling from the frontal bone or temporal bone crossing diagonally through the orbital roof and extending to the orbital apex or sphenoid wings. Growing skull fractures are a unique complication of Type 2 fractures, which involve bony and dural disruption in the setting of surface tension on the dura, which most commonly arises from the growing brain. As the dural and bony defects enlarge, there is herniation of the leptomeninges, causing pulsatile proptosis, vertical orbital dystopia, and perhaps vision loss.[14]

Common pattern fractures (Type 3) are orbital fractures that occur in the setting of a well-described facial fracture pattern. This group can

be further separated into four subcategories: impure blow-out fractures involving the orbital rim, zygomaticomaxillary complex fractures, naso-orbito-ethmoid fractures, and other fracture patterns such as Le Fort II and III fractures. The orbital fractures in this group tend to be more displaced, and the associated fractures often carry indications for operative management.

CLINICAL PRESENTATION

Obtaining an adequate history and physical examination in the pediatric patient can be difficult due to the uncooperative nature of this patient population. Furthermore, the clinical presentation of orbital fractures in children is often different from the adult due to many of the anatomical and physiological differences described earlier. Therefore, there should be a low threshold for obtaining radiographic imaging when neurological injury or fracture is suspected.

While comminuted "blow-out" fractures are commonly seen in adults, linear, minimally displaced fractures occur more commonly in the pediatric orbit.[15] The elasticity of the pediatric orbital bone is the key difference, resulting in a unique clinical presentation: trapdoor fractures. The trapdoor pattern describes the entrapment of orbital tissue, the most concerning of which are extraocular muscles, in a linear orbital wall fracture that is usually minimally or non-displaced (Fig. 2.3.4). When force is placed on the orbit, the intraorbital pressure increases and creates a fracture of the orbital wall. Periorbital tissue is then pushed into the open fracture. In the adult, the fracture remains open and displaced, resulting in the classic "blow-out" presentation characterized by enophthalmos and/or hypoglobus. In the pediatric patient, however, the bone fracture is incomplete, and the partially fractured bone will rapidly recoil back to the original position trapping the periorbital tissue and leading to possible strangulation. Furthermore, children presenting with radiographic "blow out" fractures often times do not present with globe malposition as do their adult counterparts (Fig. 2.3.5). The periosteum and supporting soft tissue may remain intact, maintaining orbital volume despite a large displaced wall fracture.[10]

Subconjunctival hemorrhage in the setting of orbital trauma is always a sign of possible orbital fracture. However, the absence of this finding

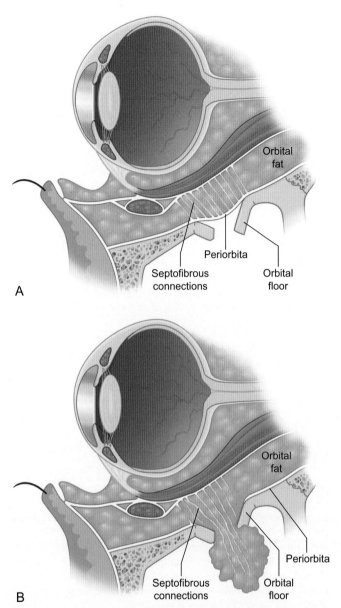

Fig. 2.3.2 Schematic isolated orbital floor blow-out fracture. (A) Pediatric orbit with intact periosteum and ligamentous support. (B) Adult orbit with composite injury and periorbital herniation into fracture. (Adapted from Losee JE, Afifi A, Jiang S, et al. Pediatric orbital fractures: classification, management, and early follow-up. Plast Reconstr Surg 2008;122:886–897.)

in the pediatric patient does not rule out a diagnosis of an entrapped orbital wall fracture. This presentation was termed "white-eyed blow-out" fracture by Jordan et al. in 1998.[16] The conjunctiva may appear normal, but the entrapped periorbital tissue will result in severe gaze restriction. Radiographically, a fracture may not be significantly displaced, but periorbital tissue may often be identified in the adjacent sinus.

Entrapment of the extraocular muscles can result in the oculocardiac reflex, describing the clinical constellation of bradycardia, nausea, and syncope.[17] Aschner first described this phenomenon in 1908 with a decrease in heart rate when applying pressure to the globe.[18] In addition to muscle entrapment, other triggering stimuli including ocular pain, increased intraocular pressure, and globe injury. Patients demonstrating signs of the oculocardiac reflex need urgent treatment, ophthalmic consultation, and forced duction assessment.

Given the elasticity and the robust nature of the pediatric facial skeleton and soft-tissue, higher traumatic forces are needed to cause facial fractures. Therefore, pediatric patients with facial fractures frequently have other associated injuries. Losee et al. found that 60% of children presenting with an orbital fracture had a nonfacial laceration, 12.6% had an ocular injury, 43.4% had a neurosurgical injury, and 20% had a significant injury beyond their head and neck. Pediatric facial fractures with more severe injuries to the regions of the head and chest are associated with a higher mortality.[7] The high incidence of associated injuries in pediatric orbital fractures reinforces the importance of a thorough primary and secondary traumatic survey and a multidisciplinary approach to assessment and management.

RADIOGRAPHIC EVALUATION

In the pediatric population, there should be a low threshold for obtaining imaging because it is often necessary to adequately diagnose an orbital fracture. High resolution, noncontrast computed tomography (CT) is the gold standard modality to assess the orbit. The image slice should be axial with thin cuts, ranging from 1.0 mm to 2.0 mm; coronal and sagittal views should be reconstructed. This form of traditional CT has limitations due to increased scan times and radiation dosage. Helical orbital CT may be a good alternative with scan times as short as 18 seconds while producing high-resolution images with reduced motion artifact.[19] Magnetic resonance imaging (MRI) with a microscopy orbital coil is superior to CT in visualizing entrapment of soft tissue while reducing radiation exposure. However, CT remains more sensitive in detecting smaller fractures and fractures towards the orbital apex.[20,21] Ultrasound (US) has also been used to detect infraorbital rim and orbital floor fractures with sensitivity and specificity similar to CT.[22] However, US evaluation is subject to interrater reliability discrepancies and is less familiar to many surgeons.[23]

SURGICAL INDICATIONS

The management of pediatric orbital fractures needs to be balanced between the benefits of anatomic restoration and the potential complications from surgery. There is a clear rationale for either operative or nonoperative management. Patients presenting with acute enophthalmos, acute vertical orbital dystopia, or clinical entrapment of an extraocular muscle have strong indications for prompt operative management. However, management should not be dictated by CT findings alone regardless of the size of the fracture. Patients with a radiographically nondisplaced or minimally displaced orbital fracture, and even those with significantly displaced Type 1 fractures, without any associated clinical findings, may safely avoid operative management.[7,24,25] In the setting of a moderate to large Type 1 orbital wall defect, with no acute enophthalmos, vertical orbital dystopia, or muscle entrapment, the patient benefits from time to allow for resolution of swelling and serial examinations by the plastic surgeon and ophthalmologist (Video 2.3.1).

In the adult, large orbital wall defects are generally accepted as an indication for reduction and internal fixation in order to prevent the high likelihood of globe malposition.[7,26,27] Enophthalmos occurs as a result from a discrepancy between the bony orbital volume and the orbital soft tissue content, resulting from herniation of orbital soft tissues into the surrounding sinuses, fat necrosis, retrobulbar soft tissue cicatricial contraction, entrapment of tissue holding the globe in a recessed position, or enlargement of the orbital cavity. According to CT evaluation of the facial skeleton, an increase of orbital volume of as little as 5% may lead to enophthalmos.[28,29] Fractures involving 50% of an orbital wall or defects greater than 2–3 cm² have become generally accepted indications of operative management.[30,31] However, these

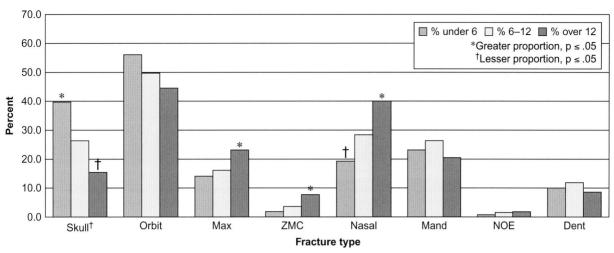

Fig. 2.3.3 Percent incidence of facial fracture stratified by age (*max*, maxillary; *ZMC*, zygomaticomaxillary; *mand*, mandible; *NOE*, naso-orbito-ethmoid; *dent*, dentoalveolar). (Adapted from Grunwaldt L, Smith DM, Zuckerbraun NS, et al. Pediatric facial fractures: Demographics, injury patterns, and associated injuries in 772 consecutive patients. Plast Reconstr Surg 2011;128:1263–1271.)

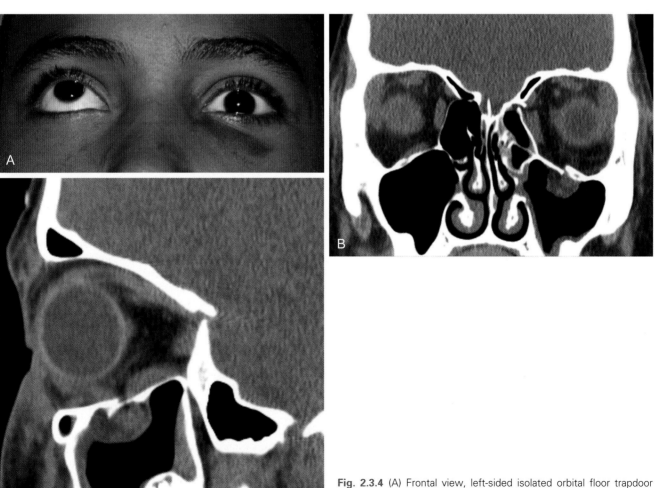

Fig. 2.3.4 (A) Frontal view, left-sided isolated orbital floor trapdoor fracture with severe restriction of upward gaze. Computed tomography coronal view (B) and sagittal view (C) demonstrate entrapment of the inferior rectus muscle.

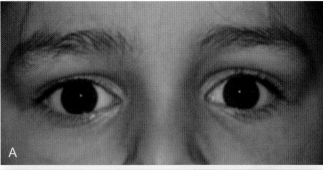

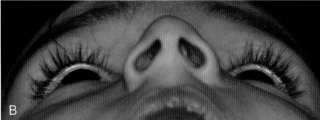

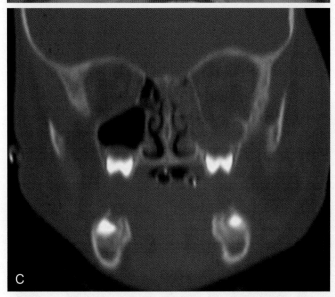

Fig. 2.3.5 (A) Frontal view, left-sided isolated orbital floor blow-out fracture. No surgery performed. (B) Worm's-eye view demonstrating minimal perceivable enophthalmos. (C) Coronal computed tomographic scan demonstrating left-sided orbital floor fracture affecting 46% area.

radiographic indications are based upon studies in the adult population, which may not be as applicable to pediatric patients.

Losee et al. demonstrates that, despite nonoperative management, no pediatric patients with orbital fractures developed functionally significant enophthalmos, regardless of the size of their Type 1 orbital fracture.[7] This may be a result of the elasticity of pediatric bone and the associated ligaments and periosteum, which can resist deformation of the fractured orbital wall. The size of the fracture alone may not be an adequate indicator for surgery in the pediatric population; however, these patients still need close follow-up for persistent/developing diplopia and globe malposition.

Conversely, Broyles et al. conclude that operative intervention in large orbital wall fractures may prevent the development of enophthalmos in the pediatric orbit.[26] In their retrospective cohort study of 76 orbital fractures, 33% underwent surgical reconstruction. In their study,

surgery did not improve visual outcomes, but the risk of developing enophthalmos was significantly reduced in the operative group. A critical defect size could not be determined.

Similarly, Coon et al. found it important to consider large orbital fractures as an indicator for early operative management to prevent globe malposition in pediatric patients.[27] They highlight the displaced two-wall fracture with concomitant displacement of the medial transition zone between the medial orbital wall and the orbital floor. Although radiographically these fractures may seem minimally displaced, the large nature of the fragment can result in significant orbital volume expansion. Yet, radiographic orbital volume expansion may not correlate with enophthalmos in pediatric patients.

Clinical findings of enophthalmos, vertical orbital dystopia, continued diplopia on central gaze, and extraocular muscle entrapment are generally accepted indications for operative repair; however, surgical timing can vary.[32] Timing to treatment can be divided into urgent (within 24 hours), early (24–96 hours), or late (greater than 96 hours).[33] Trapdoor fractures directly involving extraocular muscles have historically been an indication for urgent to early surgical management. Patients presenting with muscle entrapment in the setting of oculocardiac reflex demonstrate prompt resolution of pain, nausea, and vomiting after surgical repair.[34] Furthermore, repair of the fracture within a week of injury in patients with severe limitation of movement resulted in more rapid improvement of globe motility and diplopia. Gerbino et al. demonstrate that diplopia in the setting of a trapdoor fracture resolved in 91.7% of patients treated within 24 hours, 62.5% treated at 24–96 hours, and 0% treated more than 96 hours after trauma.[33] The pathophysiology of long-term extraocular muscle dysfunction resulting from entrapment is unclear; however, ischemia and fibrosis is likely involved, causing cicatricial changes and impaired function.[35]

SURGICAL TECHNIQUE

The orbital floor is accessed through the lower eyelid. The transconjunctival approach describes a posterior lamella incision with a dissection plane that is either preseptal or retroseptal. The transcutaneous approach describes an anterior lamella incision that can either be subciliary, subtarsal, or transjugal. For isolated orbital floor fractures, the authors routinely perform a transconjunctival, retroseptal approach with lateral canthotomy if needed. This approach is most likely to avoid injury to the middle and anterior lamellae, and with canthoplasty, will minimize risk of lower lid malposition.

If needed, a lateral canthotomy with cantholysis is first performed. The lower lid is retracted inferiorly and the inferior orbital rim can be easily palpated through the palpebral conjunctiva. A transconjunctival incision is made down through the periosteum. The periosteum of the orbital floor, medial, and lateral orbital wall can be elevated to expose the full extent of the orbital wall fracture and to reduce any entrapped or herniated periorbital tissue. For further exposure of the medial orbit, the incision can be extended into the transcaruncular approach. Orbital fractures associated with zygomaticomaxillary fractures can be approached with a subciliary incision, extended laterally into a "crow's foot" crease lateral to the lateral canthus. Appropriate resuspension of the soft tissue will prevent lower lid malposition.

Once the periorbital tissue has been reduced, the fracture is reconstructed. The authors advocate using either autologous calvarial bone grafts or resorbable mesh in pediatric patients. The implant is shaped to account for the slight concavity of the normal orbital floor. Positioning and shape of the implant should take into consideration the superior slant of the orbital floor as it reaches the orbital apex posteriorly. The shape of the floor in the area of fracture is reproduced by contouring the material. After satisfactory contouring and positioning of the implant, it can be secured to the rim or internal orbit with a low profile 4–5 mm screw to ensure position.

Before closure is performed, forced duction testing is performed to ensure there is no entrapment of periorbital tissue. A canthopexy is performed using a 5-0 PDS suture where required. Three to four buried, interrupted 6-0 fast absorbing gut sutures can be used to reapproximate the conjunctiva. Clinical assessment of globe position is critically assessed, while standing at the head of the patient and retracting the upper lids. Following reduction and repair, the globe should appear slightly over-corrected with mild exophthalmos. However, globe position must be perfectly aligned and symmetric with the unaffected globe in the vertical plane: hyper- or hypoglobus will not "get better" with time. Lastly, a Frost suture may be placed at the level of the lateral limbus.

Pediatric patients with severely comminuted, multiwall fractures, bilateral orbital fractures, and/or significantly displaced associated fractures can benefit from utilizing intraoperative CT scans, virtual surgical planning with 3D models, and precontoured templates/implants to reduce operative time and facilitate successful repair, particularly when surgeons have less experience in these more complex injuries.

POSTOPERATIVE COURSE

In the immediate postoperative period, the surgical team confirms vision in the operated eye; swelling impacts the extent of this exam. Postoperative care after orbital reconstruction aims to monitor/prevent infection, promote periocular soft tissue healing, and survey for intraorbital hypertension. These approaches are not often standardized and individual variations lack strong clinical evidence of success.

Antibiotic prophylaxis in the postoperative period remains controversial. The concern is that the fracture is in direct communication with a sinus, potentially leading to orbital cellulitis or implant infection.[36] Nevertheless, prolonged postoperative antibiotics are not routinely used, and the incidence of infection after surgical repair is not well characterized. Wladis et al. report a cohort of 153 patients treated for an orbital floor fracture with an alloplastic implant without postoperative antibiotics – none of the patients developed orbital cellulitis or implant infection.[37] Although postoperative antibiotics may not be necessary, standard preoperative antibiotic prophylaxis is encouraged because orbital cellulitis can result in catastrophic complications including vision loss, intracranial abscess, cavernous sinus thrombosis, and death.

Sinus precautions are often recommended in the setting of orbital trauma and operative repair in order to prevent colonized air being forced into the orbit, negative pressure drawing intraorbital contents into the sinus, or implant malposition. Precautions include no nose blowing, no sucking, no pushing/lifting heavy objects, and open-mouthed sneezing. Several case studies have shown intraorbital emphysema associated with orbital cellulitis and orbital fractures occurring with sudden sinus pressure changes.[38–40] However, the role of sinus precautions in the postoperative care of orbital fractures is not well studied.

The rationale for the use of steroids is to reduce periorbital swelling; however, there are concerns for delayed healing, infection, and adrenal insufficiency. Flood et al. demonstrated that methylprednisolone given preoperatively followed by three postoperative doses significantly improved eye-opening compared to placebo, allowing for better globe assessment.[41] Thoren et al. showed that the rate of delayed healing and infection in patients treated with open repair of facial fractures receiving perioperative steroids was 6.0%, while in patients not receiving steroids it was 2.8%.[42] The difference was not significantly different, although there is a trend towards increased surgical site complications with steroid use, especially when there was an intraoral incision. Although perioperative steroids may reduce periorbital swelling after surgical repair,

caution should be taken in the setting of concomitant fractures requiring an additional intraoral approach.

Frost sutures are frequently used in the postoperative period to minimize lower eyelid malposition and chemosis. The Frost suture acts to suspend the lower-lid tarsal plate to the brow thereby preventing cicatricial retraction and soft tissue malposition. Since the first description in 1934,[43] there has been little evidence on the efficacy of the Frost suture in preventing lower lid malposition. Furthermore, the duration of Frost suture use is highly variable among surgeons, although initially described for 4 days. A retrospective review comparing patients receiving Frost suture versus no suture was performed in a cohort of 96 patients.[44] There was no significant difference in the incidence of postoperative lower lid malposition between using the Frost suture or not. The Frost suture may, however, interfere with thorough globe examination and vision testing in the postoperative course and causes discomfort for the patient, which can be significant in the pediatric population.

ACUTE COMPLICATIONS

Complications following orbital reconstruction include infection, injury to periorbital and ocular structures, vision loss from malignant intraocular hypertension or optic nerve injury, altered globe motility, and malposition of the globe, implant, or lower eyelid. These complications can either be a result from the initial traumatic injury, or can be iatrogenic. Therefore, thorough examination is required both pre- and postoperatively.

Persistent diplopia is the most commonly reported complication after surgical repair of the orbital floor in children. This may be due to the higher prevalence of the trapdoor fracture pattern in the pediatric population leading to extraocular muscle injury, fibrosis, and long-term dismotility. Additionally, higher rates of misdiagnosis of muscle entrapment can delay treatment that further contributes to persistent dysfunction.[45] Given the plasticity of the neurovisual system in children, long-term diplopia may sometimes resolve without intervention.[46] However, treating persistent diplopia and strabismus can be challenging, involving specialized glasses and/or re-balancing the extraocular muscles, and should generally not be considered until 6 months have elapsed.

Globe injury can occur in up to 30% of orbital trauma; therefore, all pediatric patients with orbital fractures should have an evaluation by an ophthalmologist where possible. Injury can range from corneal abrasions to globe rupture, resulting in blindness.[12] Other causes of traumatic visual changes and blindness can occur from retinal injury, hyphema, ocular vessel thrombosis, and direct injury to the optic nerve. Management of the neurovisual axis takes priority in orbital trauma, and timing for orbital reconstruction should be coordinated with the ophthalmology consultant. Postoperatively, blindness is most often a result of increased pressure at the orbital apex; however, this occurs rarely.[47] A retrobulbar hemorrhage is the most common cause of a postoperative orbital apex syndrome and initially presents with proptosis, significant pain, and decreased vision. This requires prompt consideration for steroids, surgical decompression with canthotomy and exploration, and possibly optic nerve decompression. Thankfully, this is a very unusual phenomenon in orbital trauma because the periorbital and bony orbit has been "released" by the inciting trauma.

LONG-TERM COMPLICATIONS

Caution should be advised when considering a nonabsorbable (titanium mesh, porous polyethylene, silicone) alloplastic implant for reconstruction in the pediatric orbit. Extrusion or malposition can occur as the orbit grows. The long-term risk of infection is also a consideration. Autogenous bone grafts have been the gold standard material for orbital reconstruction in children because they incorporate with the surrounding bone, revascularize, and have minimal fibrous reaction to the soft tissue;[48] however, resorbable plates and screws have been gaining popularity.[49] Several investigators have demonstrated intermediate and long-term success with using resorbable materials in orbital floor reconstruction in the pediatric and adult population with minimal globe malposition.[50,51] Localized inflammation along the infraorbital rim seems to be the only significant adverse event, and is likely implant-dependent, and if significant may contribute to lid reactions/ectropion. Nonetheless, investigators such as Hollier et al. caution against resorbable mesh due to concerns for globe malposition over time as the plate dissolves, since the current resorbable plates lose the majority of their tensile strength at 2 months.[51]

Persistent enophthalmos occurs from inadequate correction of increased orbital volume.[52] Enophthalmos should be accurately and objectively measured using a Hertel exophthalmometer; however, cooperation in children is limited.[53] Alternatively, enophthalmos can be followed using serial worm's eye photography, positioning the tip of the nose between the eyebrows of the patient to ensure the proper visual angle.

Lower lid malposition ranging from scleral show to ectropion is frequently reported after orbital reconstruction, at least on a temporary basis. Disruption and cicatricial changes in the anterior and middle lamellae have been sited as the primary pathophysiology.[54,55] Ridgway et al. demonstrated that the risk of ectropion was highest with a subciliary incision, and the risk of entropion was highest with a transconjunctival incision, and risk of hypertrophic scarring was highest with a subtarsal incision.[56] Utilizing canthopexy/canthoplasty in patients with significant laxity of the lower lid, prominent globes, or poor lower lid tone can help prevent malposition. Frost sutures may have benefit; however, little evidence supports significant prevention. Conservative scar massage is used initially for early postoperative lower lid malposition. Persistent malposition may require release of anterior lamellar scarring with full-thickness skin grafting and/or lower lid tightening with canthopexy/canthoplasty.[57]

CONCLUSIONS

The changing anatomy and physiology of the pediatric craniofacial skeleton give unique characteristics to the pattern, clinical presentations, and clinical outcomes of pediatric orbital fractures. Therefore, the management of these fractures should be performed differently from adult patients. For children with type 1 orbital fractures, the size of the defect on CT scan should not solely drive the decision to operate – independent of physical exam findings. A more conservative approach to operative management should be pursued when signs of muscle entrapment, acute enophthalmos, or hypoglobus are not present. Careful clinical and radiographic evaluations of the pediatric orbit with an interdisciplinary approach are strongly advised to help deliver the optimal treatment plan to balance clinical outcomes and support the developing craniofacial skeleton.

EXPERT COMMENTARY

This chapter, one of the most comprehensive on the subject, is a product of the extensive experience of the senior author. The views expressed are traditionally focused, and the classification system and advice presented are the product of much thought and reflection. While I have a slightly more forward posture toward surgery in equivocal cases, the sound advice of the authors can certainly serve as a basis for good practice. While I have not experienced

EXPERT COMMENTARY—cont'd

the long-term problems with alloplastic implants which are smooth on one surface and textured on the other, certainly bone grafts are the traditional recommendation in children, particularly with more extensive injuries.

While the adaptive potential of growth in children has never been conclusively proven to correct residual deformity, certainly the normal appearance of the child may often mask slight bone or eye malposition. I would emphasize early correction of the incarcerated muscle as leading to improved outcomes, and alternately conservative management of minimally or nondisplaced fractures.

REFERENCES

1. Kaban LB, Mulliken JB, Murray JE. Facial fractures in children: an analysis of 122 fractures in 109 patients. *Plast Reconstr Surg.* 1977;59:15–20.
2. Posnick JC, Wells M, Pron GE. Pediatric facial fractures: evolving patterns of treatment. *J Oral Maxillofac Surg.* 1993;51:836–844, discussion 844–5.
3. Rowe NL. Fractures of the facial skeleton in children. *J Oral Surg.* 1968;26:505–515.
4. Turvey TA, Golden BA. Orbital anatomy for the surgeon. *Oral Maxillofac Surg Clin North Am.* 2012;24:525–536.
5. Oppenheimer AJ, Monson LA, Buchman SR. Pediatric orbital fractures. *Craniomaxillofac Trauma Reconstr.* 2013;6:9–20.
6. Golden BA, Jaskolka MS, Vescan A, et al. Evaluation and management of frontal sinus injuries. In: Fonseca RJ, Walker RV, Barber HD, et al, eds. *Oral and Maxillofacial Trauma.* 4th ed. St. Louis: Elsevier Saunders; 2013:470–490.
7. Losee JE, Afifi A, Jiang S, et al. Pediatric orbital fractures: classification, management, and early follow-up. *Plast Reconstr Surg.* 2008;122:886–897.
8. Escaravage GK Jr, Dutton JJ. Age-related changes in the pediatric human orbit on CT. *Ophthal Plast Reconstr Surg.* 2013;29:150–156.
9. Hatton MP, Watkins LM, Rubin PA. Orbital fractures in children. *Ophthal Plast Reconstr Surg.* 2001;17:174–179.
10. McGraw BL, Cole RR. Pediatric maxillofacial trauma. Age-related variations in injury. *Arch Otolaryngol Head Neck Surg.* 1990;116:41–45.
11. Grunwaldt L, Smith DM, Zuckerbraun NS, et al. Pediatric facial fractures: demographics, injury patterns, and associated injuries in 772 consecutive patients. *Plast Reconstr Surg.* 2011;128:1263–1271.
12. Imahara SD, Hopper RA, Wang J, et al. Patterns and outcomes of pediatric facial fractures in the United States: a survey of the National Trauma Data Bank. *J Am Coll Surg.* 2008;207:710–716.
13. Vyas RM, Dickinson BP, Wasson KL, et al. Pediatric facial fractures: current national incidence, distribution, and health care resource use. *J Craniofac Surg.* 2008;19:339–349, discussion 350.
14. Muhonen MG, Piper JG, Menezes AH. Pathogenesis and treatment of growing skull fractures. *Surg Neurol.* 1995;43:367–372, discussion 372–3.
15. Kwon JH, Moon JH, Kwon MS, et al. The differences of blowout fracture of the inferior orbital wall between children and adults. *Arch Otolaryngol Head Neck Surg.* 2005;131:723–727.
16. Jordan DR, Allen LH, White J, et al. Intervention within days for some orbital floor fractures: the white-eyed blowout. *Ophthal Plast Reconstr Surg.* 1998;14:379–390.
17. Cohen SM, Garrett CG. Pediatric orbital floor fractures: nausea/vomiting as signs of entrapment. *Otolaryngol Head Neck Surg.* 2003;129:43–47.
18. Aschner B. Ueber einen bisher noch nicht heschriebenen reflex vom auge auf kreislauf und atmung: Verschwinden des Radialispulses bei Druck auf das Auge. *Wien Klin Wochenschr.* 1908;21:1529–1530.
19. Lakits A, Prokesch R, Scholda C, et al. Orbital helical computed tomography in the diagnosis and management of eye trauma. *Ophthalmology.* 1999;106:2330–2335.
20. Freund M, Hahnel S, Sartor K. The value of magnetic resonance imaging in the diagnosis of orbital floor fractures. *Eur Radiol.* 2002;12:1127–1133.
21. Kolk A, Stimmer H, Klopfer M, et al. High resolution magnetic resonance imaging with an orbital coil as an alternative to computed tomography

scan as the primary imaging modality of pediatric orbital fractures. *J Oral Maxillofac Surg.* 2009;67:348–356.

22. Jank S, Emshoff R, Etzelsdorfer M, et al. Ultrasound versus computed tomography in the imaging of orbital floor fractures. *J Oral Maxillofac Surg.* 2004;62:150–154.

23. Jank S, Deibl M, Strobl H, et al. Interrater reliability of sonographic examinations of orbital fractures. *Eur J Radiol.* 2005;54:344–351.

24. Bansagi ZC, Meyer DR. Internal orbital fractures in the pediatric age group: characterization and management. *Ophthalmology.* 2000;107:829–836.

25. Burnstine MA. Clinical recommendations for repair of orbital facial fractures. *Curr Opin Ophthalmol.* 2003;14:236–240.

26. Broyles JM, Jones D, Bellamy J, et al. Pediatric orbital floor fractures: outcome analysis of 72 children with orbital floor fractures. *Plast Reconstr Surg.* 2015;136:822–828.

27. Coon D, Kosztowski M, Mahoney NR, et al. Principles for management of orbital fractures in the pediatric population: a cohort study of 150 patients. *Plast Reconstr Surg.* 2016;137:1234–1240.

28. Dolynchuk KN, Tadjalli HE, Manson PN. Orbital volumetric analysis: clinical application in orbitozygomatic complex injuries. *J Craniomaxillofac Trauma.* 1996;2:56–63, discussion 64.

29. Manson PN, Grivas A, Rosenbaum A, et al. Studies on enophthalmos: II. The measurement of orbital injuries and their treatment by quantitative computed tomography. *Plast Reconstr Surg.* 1986;77:203–214.

30. Bite U, Jackson IT, Forbes GS, et al. Orbital volume measurements in enophthalmos using three-dimensional CT imaging. *Plast Reconstr Surg.* 1985;75:502–508.

31. Parsons GS, Mathog RH. Orbital wall and volume relationships. *Arch Otolaryngol Head Neck Surg.* 1988;114:743–747.

32. Hawes MJ, Dortzbach RK. Surgery on orbital floor fractures. Influence of time of repair and fracture size. *Ophthalmology.* 1983;90:1066–1070.

33. Gerbino G, Roccia F, Bianchi FA, et al. Surgical management of orbital trapdoor fracture in a pediatric population. *J Oral Maxillofac Surg.* 2010;68:1310–1316.

34. Egbert JE, May K, Kersten RC, et al. Pediatric orbital floor fracture: direct extraocular muscle involvement. *Ophthalmology.* 2000;107:1875–1879.

35. Smith B, Lisman RD, Simonton J, et al. Volkmann's contracture of the extraocular muscles following blowout fracture. *Plast Reconstr Surg.* 1984;74:200–216.

36. Westfall CT, Shore JW. Isolated fractures of the orbital floor: risk of infection and the role of antibiotic prophylaxis. *Ophthalmic Surg.* 1991;22:409–411.

37. Wladis EJ. Are post-operative oral antibiotics required after orbital floor fracture repair? *Orbit.* 2013;32:30–32.

38. Hwang K, Kim HJ. Medial orbital wall fracture caused by forceful nose blowing. *J Craniofac Surg.* 2014;25:720–721.

39. Rahmel BB, Scott CR, Lynham AJ. Comminuted orbital blowout fracture after vigorous nose blowing that required repair. *Br J Oral Maxillofac Surg.* 2010;48:e21–e22.

40. Watanabe T, Kawano T, Kodama S, et al. Orbital blowout fracture caused by nose blowing. *Ear Nose Throat J.* 2012;91:24–25.

41. Flood TR, McManners J, el Attar A, et al. Randomized prospective study of the influence of steroids on postoperative eye-opening after exploration of the orbital floor. *Br J Oral Maxillofac Surg.* 1999;37:312–315.

42. Thoren H, Snall J, Kormi E, et al. Does perioperative glucocorticosteroid treatment correlate with disturbance in surgical wound healing after treatment of facial fractures? A retrospective study. *J Oral Maxillofac Surg.* 2009;67:1884–1888.

43. Frost A. Supporting suture in ptosis operations. *Am J Ophthalmol.* 1934;17:633.

44. Bartsich S, Yao CA. Is Frosting effective? The role of retention sutures in posttraumatic orbital reconstruction surgery. *J Plast Reconstr Aesthet Surg.* 2015;68:1683–1686.

45. Gerber B, Kiwanuka P, Dhariwal D. Orbital fractures in children: a review of outcomes. *Br J Oral Maxillofac Surg.* 2013;51:789–793.

46. Cope MR, Moos KF, Speculand B. Does diplopia persist after blow-out fractures of the orbital floor in children? *Br J Oral Maxillofac Surg.* 1999;37:46–51.

47. Girotto JA, Gamble WB, Robertson B, et al. Blindness after reduction of facial fractures. *Plast Reconstr Surg.* 1998;102:1821–1834.

48. Wolfe SA, Ghurani R, Podda S, et al. An examination of posttraumatic, postsurgical orbital deformities: conclusions drawn for improvement of primary treatment. *Plast Reconstr Surg.* 2008;122:1870–1881.

49. Avashia YJ, Sastry A, Fan KL, et al. Materials used for reconstruction after orbital floor fracture. *J Craniofac Surg.* 2012;23:1991–1997.

50. Eppley BL. Use of resorbable plates and screws in pediatric facial fractures. *J Oral Maxillofac Surg.* 2005;63:385–391.

51. Hollier LH, Rogers N, Berzin E, et al. Resorbable mesh in the treatment of orbital floor fractures. *J Craniofac Surg.* 2001;12:242–246.

52. Kawamoto HK Jr. Late posttraumatic enophthalmos: a correctable deformity? *Plast Reconstr Surg.* 1982;69:423–432.

53. Grant MP, Iliff NT, Manson PN. Strategies for the treatment of enophthalmos. *Clin Plast Surg.* 1997;24:539–550.

54. Lorenz HP, Longaker MT, Kawamoto HK Jr. Primary and secondary orbit surgery: the transconjunctival approach. *Plast Reconstr Surg.* 1999;103:1124–1128.

55. Rohrich RJ, Janis JE, Adams WP Jr. Subciliary versus subtarsal approaches to orbitozygomatic fractures. *Plast Reconstr Surg.* 2003;111:1708–1714.

56. Ridgway EB, Chen C, Colakoglu S, et al. The incidence of lower eyelid malposition after facial fracture repair: a retrospective study and meta-analysis comparing subtarsal, subciliary, and transconjunctival incisions. *Plast Reconstr Surg.* 2009;124:1578–1586.

57. Yaremchuk MJ. Changing concepts in the management of secondary orbital deformities. *Clin Plast Surg.* 1992;19:113–124.

2.4

Pediatric Midface Fractures

Elizabeth Zellner, Christopher R. Forrest

BACKGROUND

The management of pediatric facial fractures presents some unique and specific opportunities that differ from those in the adult world. It is important to recognize that children are not small adults, and when possible, treatment should be conservative. There is no single approach to the management of midface fractures in children and care must be individualized. The dimensions of age and growth can add to the complexity of their management.

The midface region traditionally involves the maxilla although the contents of this chapter will touch on regions of the orbital–zygomatic complex and nasal–orbital zone. Skeletal maturity is considered to be the age of transition to adulthood (14–16 years in females; 18–20 years in males) but it is useful to conceptualize pediatric facial trauma by the stage of dentition (primary, mixed and permanent).

Pediatric facial fractures occur with much less frequency and severity and make up between 1% and 15% of all facial fractures series.[1–3] They are less common in very young children below the age of 5, representing less than 1% of all facial fractures.[1,4,5] As children mature and start to move with increasing velocity, fracture incidence increases, representing nearly adult levels in the late teenage years. Of midfacial fractures, nasal and dentoalveolar fractures are quite common, with zygomaticomaxillary complex (ZMC) and maxillary fractures less frequently represented.[6,7] When maxillary fractures do occur in young children, traditional pure Le Fort patterns are varied. Oblique fracture patterns involving the orbits and piriform aperture are more likely to occur.[2] Nasal bone fractures and dentoalveolar fractures represent the most common facial fractures in the pediatric population.[7–9] With increasing age, eruption of dentition and growth of the lower face and sinuses, there is a transition to more typical adult fracture patterns.

Pediatric facial fractures occur primarily as the result of motor vehicle collisions (MVC), falls and sports-related injuries.[2,10–13] While changing traffic laws and safety standards (e.g. increased use of air bags, car seats, and seat belts) over the years have led to fewer MVCs, compliance varies dramatically, and up to 70% of children with MVC-related facial fractures were unrestrained at the time of injury.[14]

Lower-velocity injuries such as falls are more common in younger children, while teenagers and young adults are more likely to suffer traffic accidents and sports-related trauma. Violent altercations are much less common causes of craniofacial trauma in children compared to adults, although this also increases with age.[5] Child abuse as a cause of isolated maxillofacial trauma is quite rare.[4]

Like most traumatic injuries, incidence peaks in the warmer months, attributed to more outdoor physical activity.[13] Facial fractures are more common in boys, though this varies greatly in reports from 1.1:1 to 8.5:1 depending on the publication.[4,13] This difference is less notable in younger age groups.[15]

SURGICAL ANATOMY

Children have a lower blood volume with overall higher cardiac output and smaller airway volume. This puts them at increased risk of complications from blood loss and airway obstruction compared to adults. As a result, the principles of initial trauma management regarding volume resuscitation and securing the airway are especially relevant in treating pediatric trauma patients. Fractures of the midface and mandible are associated with higher velocity impact and are more likely to be associated with other systemic injuries than isolated nasal or orbital fractures.[13]

The target zone for facial trauma in the pediatric population changes with age. At birth, the cranial vault/orbital region makes up roughly an 8:1 ratio compared with the facial region that halves to 4:1 by 4 years of age and then gradually decreases to around 2.5:1 at skeletal maturity (Fig. 2.4.1).[16] As the facial bones are smaller in size and more retruded relative to the overlying skull at younger ages, this provides relative protection to the midface. Therefore, younger patients, especially under the age of 5, have a predilection for cranio-orbital injuries (Fig. 2.4.2). As the face grows, the prominent areas (nose, zygoma, mandible) become more frequently involved and prone to injury.[15]

Facial fractures in children are often less displaced than those of adults and greenstick fractures are common given their more flexible bones with more mobility at suture lines and less bone mineralization. The bone exhibits a higher cancellous-to-cortical bone ratio, and without the development of the air-filled paranasal sinuses which affect the compliance of the craniofacial skeleton.[16] At birth, the maxillary sinus is present but very small, enlarging gradually downward as the permanent dentition erupts, to fill the area previously occupied by the tooth buds. As such, it does not reach its adult size until eruption of the third molars.[6] Ethmoid air cells are also usually present at birth, slowly expand and are the first sinuses fully developed, which occurs around puberty (Fig. 2.4.2). The sphenoid sinus first appears around age 2 and continues to enlarge until skeletal maturity, with some further septation into adulthood.[17] The frontal sinus first appears at age 5 and continues to expand into late teen years. Increased soft tissue padding, thicker fat pads, and the strong, developing tooth buds within the maxilla and mandible also provide increased resistance to complete fractures (Fig. 2.4.3).[3,4,13,18] While these factors act to provide protection for the pediatric skeleton, a higher impact force per unit area is required for the facial bones to fracture in children compared with their adult counterparts and as such, there may be a higher incidence of associated injuries

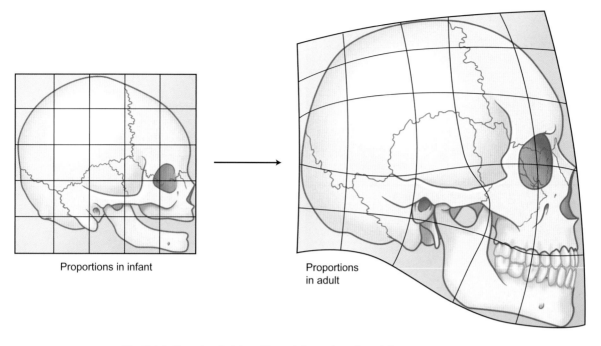

Proportions in infant

Proportions in adult

Fig. 2.4.1 Changing facial profile and dimensions from infancy to teen years.

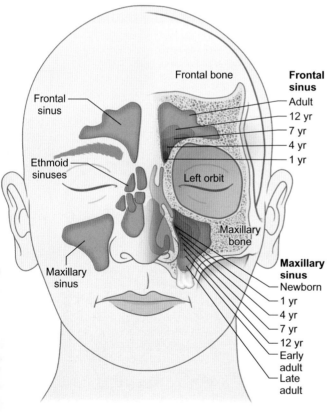

Frontal bone

Frontal sinus

Frontal sinus

Frontal sinus
- Adult
- 12 yr
- 7 yr
- 4 yr
- 1 yr

Ethmoid sinuses

Left orbit

Maxillary bone

Maxillary sinus

Maxillary sinus
- Newborn
- 1 yr
- 4 yr
- 7 yr
- 12 yr
- Early adult
- Late adult

Fig. 2.4.2 Development of the sinuses in the facial skeleton.

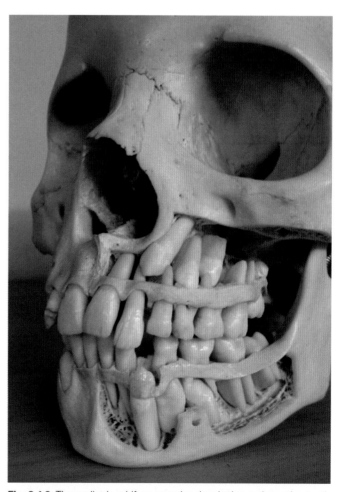

Fig. 2.4.3 The pediatric midface contains developing and erupting teeth which contribute to the strength of the maxilla. The transition into adult dentition and the development of the maxillary sinuses results in the predisposition for standard Le Fort fractures instead of dentoalveolar fractures.

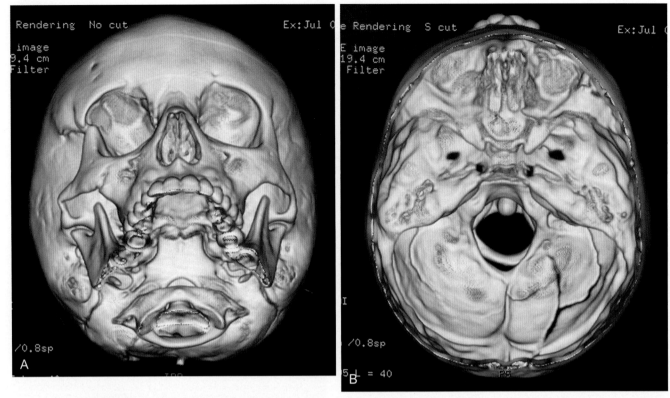

Fig. 2.4.4 An example of the unique nature of the elastic compliant pediatric craniofacial skeleton which can result in greenstick fractures and discontinuity between fracture zones in a 7-year-old female following an equestrian injury. A blow-in fracture of the right ZMC is associated with basal skull fractures extending into the right posterior fossa and occiput (A–B).

The unique nature of the elastic compliant pediatric craniofacial skeleton can result in greenstick fractures and discontinuity between fracture zones (Fig. 2.4.4).

CLINICAL PRESENTATION

Pediatric midfacial fractures tend to occur as the result of significant trauma and usually warrant the assessment of a trauma team. A history of the injury and details of the velocity involved will give the treating physician clues as to the potential extent of the injury. Information about the use of seatbelts, helmets, height of falls, loss of consciousness, and preexisting conditions are standard elicited history. Features of the child may make obtaining a detailed history and the presence of symptoms (pain, loss of sensation, malocclusion, visual disturbances) problematic and an index of suspicion may help direct clinical investigation. It is often useful to obtain an orthodontic history given the frequency of orthodontic appliance use in children and young adults. Premorbid scans, impressions, and models may give useful information regarding the state of the preinjury dentition and occlusion.

Physical examination is focused on the zone of trauma. Overlying lacerations, ecchymosis and soft tissue disruption may give clues as to directed injuries. Due to the lack of pneumatization of the sinuses and strength from unerupted tooth buds, forces applied to the midface are transferred to the dentoalveolar complex resulting in tooth avulsion and fractures. Dentoalveolar fractures are the commonest form of pediatric midface fractures and occasionally may be associated with midface gingival degloving (Fig. 2.4.5). An understanding of the patterns of tooth eruption will be useful in assessing children between ages 6 to 12 in mixed dentition (Fig. 2.4.6).

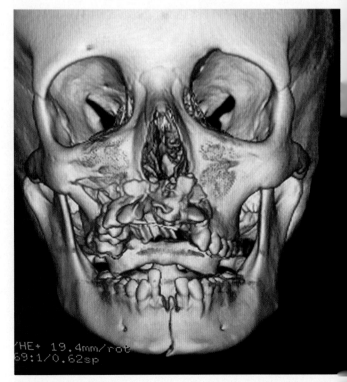

Fig. 2.4.5 Dentoalveolar fractures of the maxilla in association with a mandibular fracture in a 16-year-old female. CT (A) and panorex are useful to assess the extent of the injuries and determine the presence of tooth fractures.

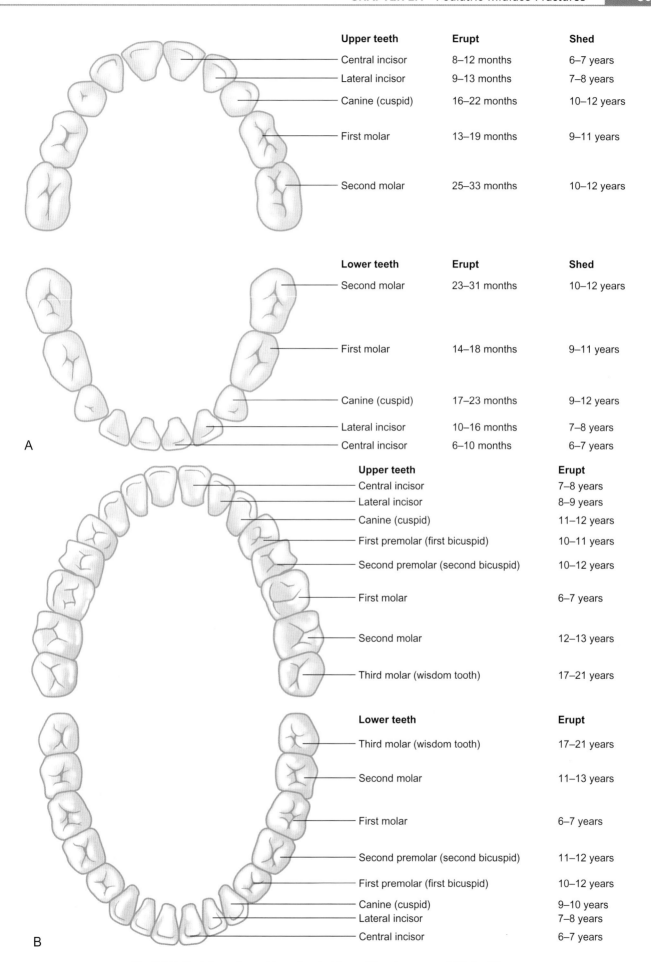

Upper teeth	Erupt	Shed
Central incisor	8–12 months	6–7 years
Lateral incisor	9–13 months	7–8 years
Canine (cuspid)	16–22 months	10–12 years
First molar	13–19 months	9–11 years
Second molar	25–33 months	10–12 years

Lower teeth	Erupt	Shed
Second molar	23–31 months	10–12 years
First molar	14–18 months	9–11 years
Canine (cuspid)	17–23 months	9–12 years
Lateral incisor	10–16 months	7–8 years
Central incisor	6–10 months	6–7 years

A

Upper teeth	Erupt
Central incisor	7–8 years
Lateral incisor	8–9 years
Canine (cuspid)	11–12 years
First premolar (first bicuspid)	10–11 years
Second premolar (second bicuspid)	10–12 years
First molar	6–7 years
Second molar	12–13 years
Third molar (wisdom tooth)	17–21 years

Lower teeth	Erupt
Third molar (wisdom tooth)	17–21 years
Second molar	11–13 years
First molar	6–7 years
Second premolar (second bicuspid)	11–12 years
First premolar (first bicuspid)	10–12 years
Canine (cuspid)	9–10 years
Lateral incisor	7–8 years
Central incisor	6–7 years

B

Fig. 2.4.6 Dental eruption patterns for deciduous (A) and permanent (B) dentition.

Systematic assessment of the integrity of the craniofacial skeleton will involve inspection for obvious asymmetries and deviations, palpation for areas of tenderness, bony steps and disruptions, and manipulation for midface instability and mobility. A careful dental examination to assess for malocclusion, mobile, lost or devitalized teeth is important. The possibility of aspirated teeth may warrant a chest X-ray.

Orbital examination is always mandated with potential midface fractures. Periorbital ecchymosis, subconjunctival hemorrhage, visual acuity, extraocular mobility, telecanthus, enophthalmos and facial sensation should be assessed. All suspected orbital injuries should have a formal ophthalmological consultation when possible. The forced duction test should be performed in any patient that cannot supply a satisfactory voluntary examination but is not tolerated in the awake child and should be done under anesthesia in order to prevent a false-positive result. A delay in diagnosis and treatment of these injuries can have significant consequences on the patient's long-term outcome.[19]

Midface fractures are rare in children. When present, due to the high velocities involved, associated systemic injuries may be seen in up to 88% of patients.[4] As such, a thorough trauma and possible neurosurgical evaluation should be performed for all patients with substantial facial fractures.

RADIOLOGICAL EVALUATION

Plain films of the craniofacial skeleton, especially the midface, are of no use in the assessment of facial trauma in the pediatric population.[11,20] Developing sinuses and tooth buds may obscure already overlapping planes. Computed tomography (CT) scans are necessary in order to accurately diagnose pediatric facial trauma.[4,11,13] Fine facial cuts are necessary to adequately define facial fractures, and 3D reconstructions can be extremely useful in planning surgical intervention and teaching trainees.[21] Cone beam CT scans and orthopantomograms (panoramic radiographs or panorex) are also useful to assess for dental injuries.

CLASSIFICATION

Pediatric midfacial fractures are classified anatomically and will vary according to the age of the patient. The velocity of the injury will give clues to the types of fractures seen. The orbitozygomatic and nasal regions are susceptible to lower velocity trauma than the midface maxillary complex. The degree of displacement and comminution will be used to classify these fractures. Naso-orbito-ethmoid fractures are quite rare in young children due to the flatter nasal dorsum but may be classified according to the degree of comminution of the segments containing the medial canthal ligament (Type I: large fragment; Type II: small fragment; Type III: canthal avulsion). The typical Le Fort fracture classification may be applied but usually does not occur until teen years when the maxillary sinuses have aerated and the teeth erupted. Dentoalveolar fractures are much more common in the pediatric population. Midface fractures in the pediatric age group follow oblique and unpredictable lines extending often into the cranial base and frontal areas.[22] The palatal suture does not fuse until teen years and midline palatal fractures may be more commonly seen in children.

SURGICAL INDICATIONS

The indications for open reduction and rigid fixation of facial fractures in the pediatric population are more conservative than those in adults, especially in very young children. With higher metabolic activity, osteogenic potential and bone healing, children will heal more rapidly than adults, and have the added element of facial growth that may be negatively impacted by surgical intervention and periosteal stripping.[12,18]

Indications for surgical intervention in the midface region are both functional and aesthetic. The maxilla provides the centerpiece of the face, and the vertical and horizontal buttresses of the midface must be intact to establish appropriate facial height and width. Fracture displacement, malocclusion, severe comminution, associated soft tissue injuries and lacerations, large orbital wall defects with the potential for late enophthalmos and disruption of the medial canthal complex in NOE fractures are indications for surgical intervention in pediatric midface fractures.

Often, the compliance of the pediatric facial skeleton results in less displacement in young patients than their adult counterparts and can be treated with observation or closed reduction aided by splinting or limited MMF. General principles dictate that non- or minimally displaced fractures of the midface can be treated with observation, generally combined with a soft diet for 2–3 weeks for comfort. Displaced fractures, on the other hand, may require either closed or open reduction and fixation. If surgical intervention is necessary, quick healing times implicitly require more rapid intervention. Additionally, children require shorter periods of bony immobilization in order to heal: 2–3 weeks versus 4–6 weeks in adults.

MAXILLOMANDIBULAR FIXATION

Maxillomandibular fixation (MMF) in children with deciduous or mixed dentition can prove challenging (Fig. 2.4.7). The conical shape of the primary teeth and partially erupted permanent teeth may be difficult to adequately fixate with interdental wires and arch bars.[1] Likewise, use of MMF screw fixation may be limited given the various permanent tooth buds present in both the maxilla and mandible. In very young children, temporary suspension wiring around the zygomatic arch or piriform aperture to the arch bar may be necessary for fixation. Fortunately, major midface fractures affecting occlusion and mandibular fractures are more common in patients with more mature dentition, such as adolescents and teenagers.

Prior to the 1960s, closed reduction with MMF was utilized for nearly all pediatric fractures. Open reduction and internal fixation (ORIF) transitioned slowly to open reduction with wires and now has become accepted for displaced fractures given technical improvements in plating technology. However, the permanent placement of hardware in growing children raises important questions in terms of cost, iatrogenic trauma to erupting tooth buds, migration of plates and effects on bony growth. Animal studies have shown slight adverse effects on growth, but no similar effects have been proven in humans.[23] Resorbable plates may have some efficacy in pediatric fractures under the age of 10 years where a permanent implant is not desired, but do not have

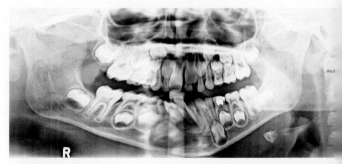

Fig. 2.4.7 Examples of panorex X-rays in mixed dentition. Note the presence of exfoliating teeth and short tooth roots in mixed dentition making the application of arch bars problematic. Pyriform aperture and zygomatic wires may be combined with circum-mandibular wires to overcome this issue.

the shear strength of metal miniplates, and as such are not used in load-bearing bone.[24] In general, our treatment philosophy involves consideration of hardware removal in the pediatric midface 6 months following repair in order to prevent theoretical concerns of retained hardware (bone stress shielding, bony overgrowth, dental concerns) in later years.

SURGICAL TECHNIQUES

Nasal Bone Fractures

Nasal bone fractures are the most common facial fractures in children. Despite this, they are often overlooked as immediate swelling and difficult compliance with intranasal exam may mask the fracture displacement. Diagnosis is made by clinical examination. Unless an NOE fracture is suspected, CT imaging is not necessary. As in adults, septal hematomas must be drained immediately to avoid septal cartilage necrosis and/or infection with potential nasal deformity (saddle nose). This is especially important in children, as a saddle nose deformity may also be associated with long-term facial growth restriction.[25]

Displaced nasal bone fractures should be reduced within a week following injury if possible (Fig. 2.4.8).[12,25] Ideally this should be done in the operating room with a secure airway, and should not be attempted in the emergency department where significant epistaxis could be life-threatening. Once reduced with a Goldman elevator or Asch forceps, intranasal packing or splints for 2–4 days are helpful to maintain the reduction and to assist with hemostasis. External splinting for 7–14 days is also crucial to guide healing, but may be difficult to maintain in noncompliant younger patients. Septoplasty in the case of septal fractures is a controversial topic, and if attempted, should take care to avoid the growth center at the nasal spine of the maxilla.[25] It is important to note that some nasal deformity may persist despite closed reduction. In the case of residual deformity outside the acute traumatic period, definitive rhinoplasty is usually deferred until skeletal maturity if possible in order to preserve nasal growth.

Naso-Orbito-Ethmoid Fractures

Naso-orbito-ethmoid (NOE) fractures are rare in younger children, and generally are related to high-impact trauma (Fig. 2.4.9). This area of the face can be difficult to access through camouflaged incisions, and treatment should be conservative if little to no displacement is observed. NOE fractures are classified by the Markowitz and Manson classification depending on the degree of comminution and whether or not the medial canthal tendon is avulsed which helps determine treatment.[26] The patient should be assessed for telecanthus upon initial presentation, and an intercanthal distance greater than 30–35 mm warrants evaluation of the medial canthal tendon bearing bone fragment for fracture or displacement. For simple displaced fractures with large fragments, the nasal portion may be reducible with a closed approach combined with external splinting or possibly through a buccal sulcus vestibular incision. For comminuted or complete fractures, a full coronal incision combined with buccal sulcus and transconjunctival/subciliary incisions for complete exposure may be necessary (Fig. 2.4.10). We do not advocate use of an "open sky" or extended glabellar approach over the nasal bones, as the scarring is frequently problematic and the visualization more limited. Transnasal wiring or suturing may be necessary in cases of avulsed medial canthal tendons to address the resulting telecanthus.

Dentoalveolar Fractures

Isolated dentoalveolar fractures are most commonly associated with low-impact injuries such as falls and sports-related accidents, and are often non-displaced.[6] Dental injuries such as fractured, displaced or missing teeth accompany the underlying skeletal injury, and alveolar fractures can be present in approximately 5% of dental trauma patients.[27] Nondisplaced fractures can be treated with a soft diet and appropriate dental care to avoid aspiration of loose or broken teeth with restoration of any permanent dentition as soon as possible. In the case of mobile or displaced fractures, surgery may be necessary to reduce the fragments (Fig. 2.4.11). For fixation, dental colleagues may be helpful in providing intraoral splints to stabilize the fracture in the desired position. Plating the maxilla itself is challenging in terms of tooth roots and unerupted tooth buds in younger children. Splinting or possibly MMF should be considered when possible to avoid damage to the developing maxilla.

Zygomatic Complex Fractures

Nondisplaced, asymptomatic zygomatic complex fractures can be treated with observation. It is important to evaluate thoroughly for sensory deficits, enophthalmos (which may evolve over time), entrapment, diplopia, and facial asymmetry. In symptomatic cases or aesthetic facial

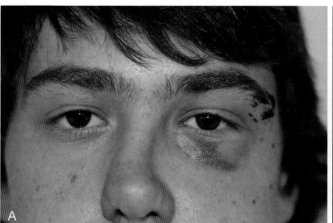
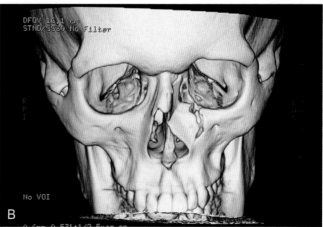

Fig. 2.4.8 A 14-year-old male with a nasal fracture following a low-velocity bicycle accident (A). Deviation of the nose is a clinical sign. A CT demonstrates a segmental fracture of the left inferior orbital rim (B). Radiographic imaging is not required to make the diagnosis of nasal fractures. The patient underwent a closed reduction of the fracture.

changes, open reduction and internal fixation may be indicated. A "trapdoor" entrapment of the extraocular musculature is a fracture mostly unique to children and is considered a surgical urgent consideration (Fig. 2.4.12). Classically a linear fracture of the orbital floor is seen with a double-density of herniated tissue into the maxillary sinus in association with entrapment of the inferior rectus muscle. It should be decompressed as soon as possible to avoid permanent damage to the muscle and periorbital fat. Other indications for ORIF should be performed when suitable, but within 3–7 days of the accident.[19]

Zygomatic complex fractures, previously misidentified as tripod fractures, are in fact tetrapod injuries, disrupting the intersections of the zygoma with the frontal bone, temporal bone, maxilla and sphenoid bone (Fig. 2.4.13). All of these attachments must be positioned to complete reduction of the fracture fragments. One key is approximating the lateral orbital wall as a point of reference. Historically, a Gilles closed approach through the temporal region and reduction with an instrument placed below the deep temporal fascia was performed but is not advised due to the lack of stable support and high incidence of repeat displacement. For displaced zygomatic complex fractures, access is always obtained through an upper buccal incision to visualize and fixate the zygomaticomaxillary buttress. The lateral orbital wall and zygomaticofrontal suture are approached through a blepharoplasty-type incision

in the upper lid crease. When indicated (entrapment, large orbital floor defects, enophthalmos), the orbital floor and rim can be approached via transconjunctival approach but routinely, this access point is not used. Reduction may be facilitated by placing a wire through the zygomaticofrontal suture allowing alignment of the lateral orbital wall and then placement of the first point of fixation along the lateral zygomaticomaxillary buttress. The wire may be replaced with a small fixation plate. Reduction is checked and the prominence of the malar eminence is compared with the opposite side. Two-point fixation is usually adequate in the majority of cases. If there is severe comminution, addition of a plate along the inferior orbital rim may be required. In very young children with unerupted permanent dentition, care should be taken before placing screws into developing tooth buds. In general, titanium fixation plates are used due to their zygomaticofrontal suture stability and routinely removed 6 months later.

Isolated fractures of the zygomatic arch may require closed reduction if they result in impingement on the mandibular coronoid, limiting mouth opening or closing or if the width of the face is altered or disrupted. The only direct approach to the zygomatic arch is through a coronal incision, but this is always excessive for an isolated arch fracture. Often, if reduction is required, this can be performed transorally through

Text continued on p. 317

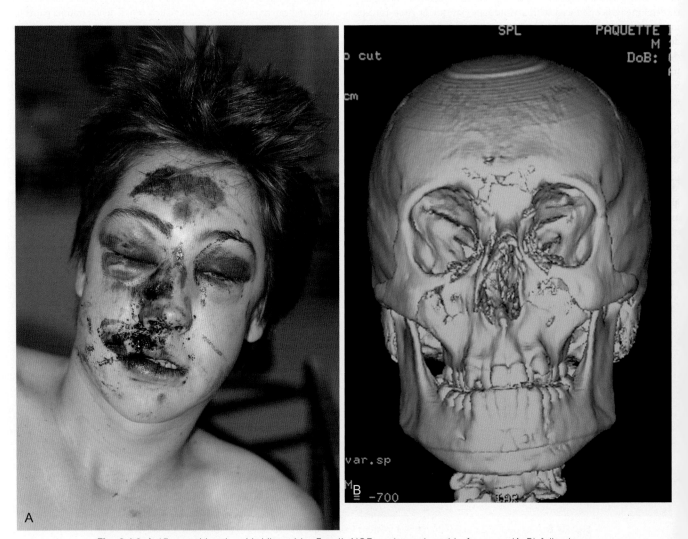

A

Fig. 2.4.9 A 15-year-old male with bilateral Le Fort II, NOE, and anterior table fractures (A–B) following a bicycle fall. The bone fragments of the NOE component are large enough (Type I) and not severely comminuted or displaced (C–D).

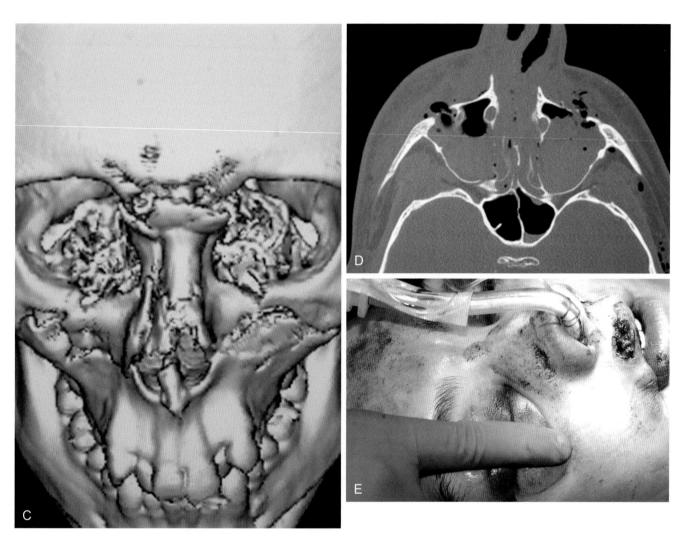

Fig. 2.4.9, cont'd Clinical examination demonstrates midface instability. The bowstring test by pulling the medial canthus laterally and seeing the webbing at the site of the medial canthus indicates that the canthus is attached to the bone (E). Treatment of this injury pattern consisted of a reduction of the maxillary component of the fracture by placing the teeth into MMF followed by stabilization of the lateral maxillary buttresses with rigid internal fixation and a closed reduction of the NOE component and splint application. It would have been inappropriate to rely on MMF alone as a treatment option for this patient as lack of stabilization would have resulted in midface lengthening and extrusion due to mandibular pull.

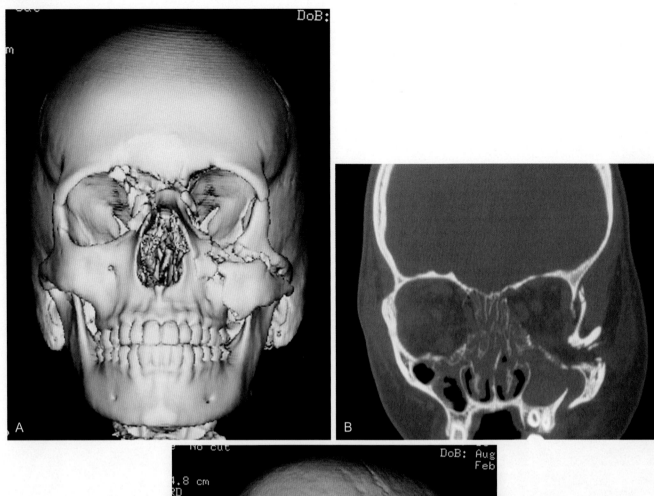

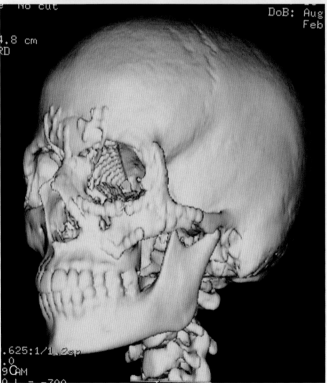

Fig. 2.4.10 A 15-year-old female with a severely comminuted Type III NOE fracture in association with a fracture of the left ZMC (A). Coronal view shows comminution of the medial orbital walls and floors bilaterally (B). Postoperative CT scans demonstrate restoration of orbital integrity with medial wall and orbital titanium mesh plates and reduction/internal fixation of the NOE component with transnasal wires to restore the position of the medial canthal tendons (C). Reduction and fixation of the left ZMC was performed to restore midface width and zygomatic projection.

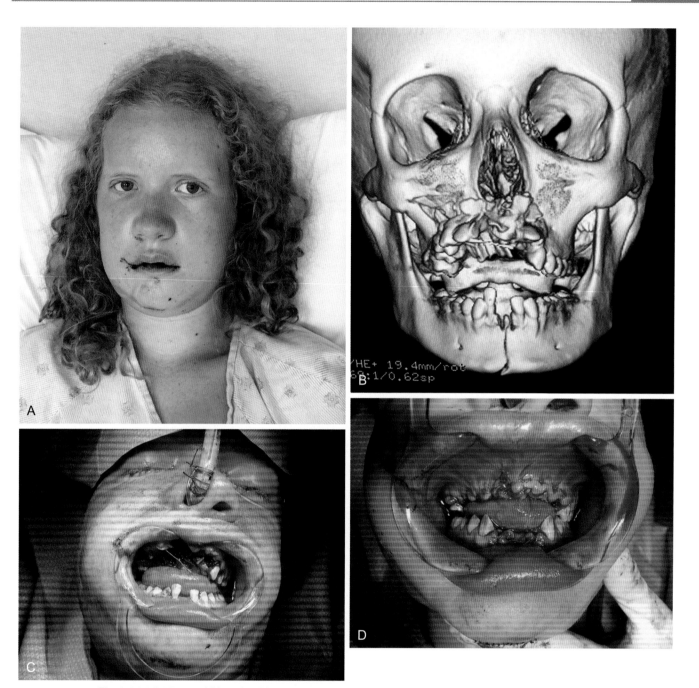

Fig. 2.4.11 A 15-year-old female with a severe maxillary dentoalveolar fractures, multiple dental losses, and midline mandibular fracture following a boating accident (A–C). A lingual arch wire is present (C) following pretrauma orthodontic treatment. All devitalized and loose teeth are removed and soft tissue is repaired (D).

Continued

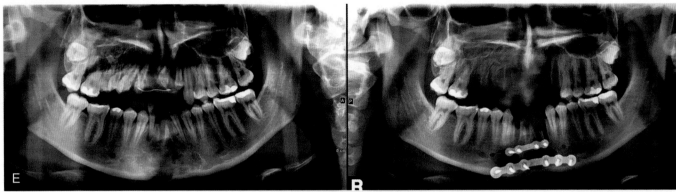

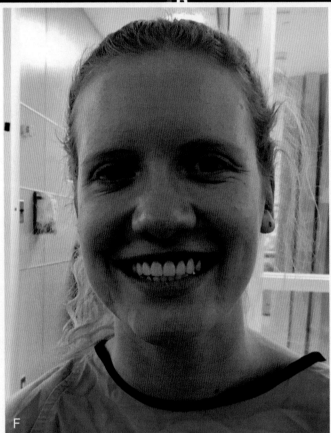

Fig. 2.4.11, cont'd Pre- and postoperative panorex X-rays show the extent of the injury (E). Patient is seen 6 months post injury for removal of her mandibular plate (F). She has been fitted with dentures in anticipation of osseointegrated dental implants.

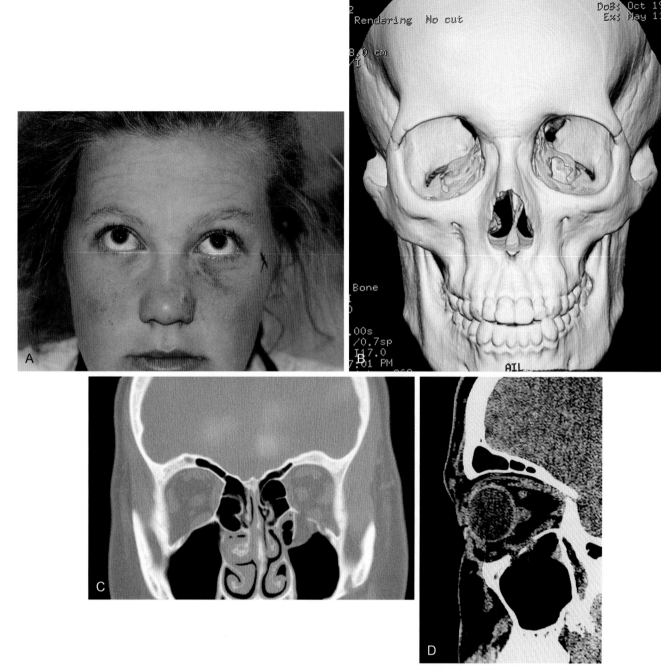

Fig. 2.4.12 A 14-year-old female presents with a left orbital floor trapdoor fracture with mechanical limitation of superior gaze in association with nausea and vomiting (A). CT images show a defect of the left orbital floor (B–C). Oblique sagittal views show the minimal displacement of the fracture and entrapment of the inferior rectus muscle (D). Immediate surgical exploration and release of the inferior rectus relieved the vagal symptoms and restored range of motion of the globe.

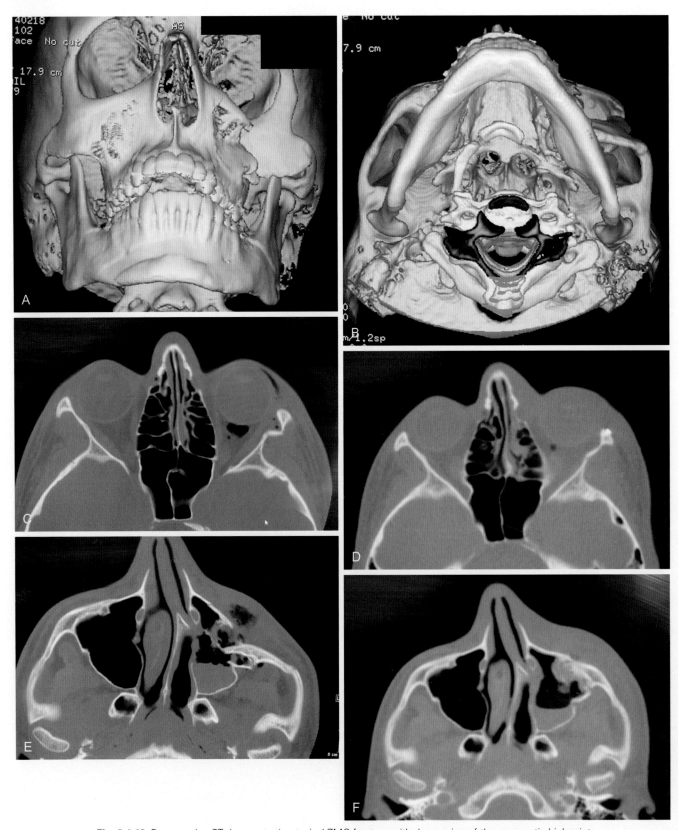

Fig. 2.4.13 Preoperative CT demonstrating typical ZMC fracture with depression of the zygomatic highpoint (A) and widening of the arch (B). For a displaced ZMC fracture to occur, fracture lines run through the zygo-maticofrontal suture, sphenoid–zygomatic attachments, lateral maxillary buttress, inferior orbital rim, and the zygomatic arch. Reduction of the ZMC fracture relies on alignment of the lateral orbital wall as noted on the prereduction and postreduction CT images (C–D). Fixation of the zygomatic arch is rarely necessary unless there is comminution of the lateral orbital wall preventing its use to reduce the ZMC. The arch tends to restore its anatomic position when the body is reduced and fixed (E–F).

a buccal sulcus incision with direct access under the zygomatic arch. An elevator can then be used to reduce the fracture, with no fixation necessary. Alternately, a Gillies approach, through the hair-bearing temporal scalp just superior and anterior to the upper helix, can be used. This dissection continues through the temporoparietal fascia and the deep layer of the deep temporal fascia and an instrument is passed just superficial to the temporalis muscle in order to spare the facial nerve. In this plane, an elevator then reduces the fracture similarly to the transoral approach with no fixation.

Le Fort/Maxillary Fractures

As mentioned previously, true Le Fort fracture patterns are rare in children, especially before the age of 10, who demonstrate oblique fracture patterns (Fig. 2.4.14).[2] The maxilla in conjunction with the zygomatic complex establishes midface facial height and width and is a centerpiece of the craniofacial skeleton. In the case of a nondisplaced fracture, this can be treated with soft diet and conservative management. Anterior wall maxillary fractures are not uncommon and rarely require treatment. Displaced midface fractures require basic principles of reducing the fracture by restoring premorbid occlusion and maintaining the reduction with MMF for 3 weeks (Fig. 2.4.15). In cases where there is comminution and instability, a standard open reduction through upper buccal sulcus incisions and fixation of the maxilla along the four anterior buttresses works well. In cases where segmental fracture of the maxilla exists, or a midpalatal split has occurred, restoration of the maxillary

arch is performed and then the maxilla may be fixed to the upper facial buttresses. Use of a dental splint in these cases will help maintain the integrity of the reduction at the dental level. Younger patients may sometimes be better treated with MMF given the developing tooth buds although the difficulties of this have been mentioned.[3] Over the age of 12, ORIF via a buccal sulcus incision may be a more palatable option, with less risk of tooth bud injury. Occlusion should be confirmed intraoperatively, as inadequate reduction may result in malocclusion or an open-bite.

POSTOPERATIVE COURSE

As mentioned above, children do not require as prolonged immobilization of fractures as do adults due to their increased osteoblastic potential and rapid healing. There is no consensus about the use of prolonged antibiotics following surgery. Activity is curtailed until bone healing has occurred (around 3 weeks). Nasal splints are worn for a week postoperatively. MMF need only be applied for 2–3 weeks with the relatively longer treatment times reserved for older children. Elevating the patient's head of bed both in the hospital and home setting for the first 5–7 days can significantly reduce swelling and hasten healing time. Ice, if tolerated by the child, is most useful within the first 24–48 hours after injury or surgical intervention.

Postoperative care of midface fractures includes adequate dental hygiene and oral mouthwashes. A soft "no-chew" diet may be employed

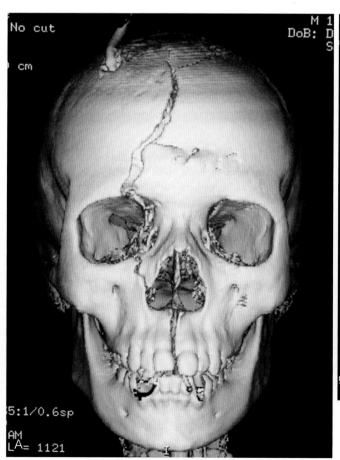
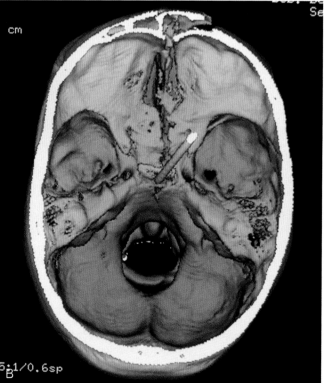

Fig. 2.4.14 Oblique and unique midfacial fracture in a 14-year-old male who landed on his head during a bicycle fall. The CT demonstrates a vertical split through the midface extending into the right orbit and craniofrontal region (A–B). Fractures occurred across the skull base into the pituitary fossa. An extraventricular drain is present. The patient died several days post injury due to a carotid artery dissection.

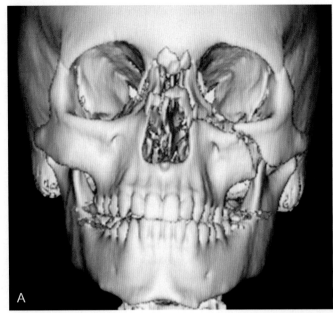
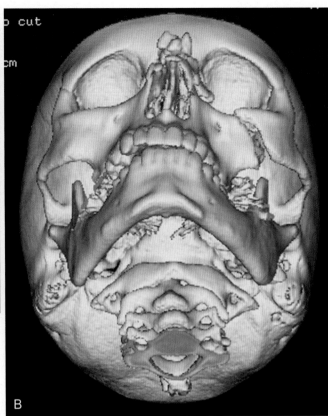

Fig. 2.4.15 An example of a right Le Fort III and left Le Fort II fracture in a 14-year-old male (A). Due to the increased compliance of the young craniofacial skeleton, the right-sided fracture has impacted and a shift of the occlusion with resultant cross-bite has occurred (B). At the time of surgery 10 days post injury, disimpaction of the right side was not easily performed due to advanced healing of the bone. As such, a Le Fort I osteotomy was performed on the right side in order to mobilize and reduce the maxilla prior to rigid fixation.

during the healing phase for the purpose of comfort and ease. A consultation with a dietician is advantageous when the patient is in MMF. Patients are discharged home with wire-cutters and instructions. Scar management techniques (massage, use of sunscreen, silicone gel) are employed when soft tissue injuries require management.

Acute Complications

Complications may be related to the injury or occur as the result of surgical treatment. General complications in the immediate posttrauma/postoperative period relate to the zone of injury and include bleeding, swelling, scars, airway issues, pain, and infection. Site-specific issues include failure of adequate reduction, persistent nasal deviation, and airway obstruction postnasal bone fracture. Following a reduction, nasal packs and/or septal splints may prevent nasal synechiae and maintain the position of the septum. It is important to use prophylactic antibiotics to prevent toxic shock syndrome when prolonged nasal packs are maintained. Any fractures involving the orbit (ZMC, NOE) may incur visual symptoms (blindness, extraocular muscle dysfunction, and diplopia) necessitating postoperative visual assessments. Midface and maxillary fractures may have airway compromise, nutritional issues, sinusitis, and rarely, life-threatening delayed hemorrhage following treatment. Delayed hemorrhage occurring around 7–10 days post injury can be seen. The history of a "sentinel" bleed in these cases should be taken seriously. Dental injuries should be managed in a timely fashion to prevent late onset infection. In patients managed with MMF, it is mandatory to have wire-cutters with the patient at all times in case of

emergency. Iatrogenic complications such as dental injury, scars due to exposure, failure to properly reduce the fracture and damage to soft tissues (e.g. extraocular muscles) may also occur. Complications related to surgical treatment may include poorly positioned incisions with resultant visible scars, inadequately reduced bone fragments with application of rigid fixation resulting in malunion and inadequate fixation (Figs. 2.4.16 and 2.4.17).

Long-Term Complications

Long-term complications will depend on the location of the injury. Growth abnormalities are possible with all forms of midface trauma but fortunately tend to be rare. Care should be taken to not upset future growth centers or overly expanding suture lines with permanent fixation if surgical intervention is required. While titanium fixation is well tolerated by the bony facial skeleton, with time, it will become overgrown and enveloped by bone. Occasionally loose hardware will necessitate removal following bone healing.

Despite undergoing a closed reduction, there is the possibility of a late and permanent nasal deformity following a nasal bone fracture and parents should be warned about the potential need for a corrective septorhinoplasty at skeletal maturity.[7,11,25] NOE fractures can be complicated by similar deformity and possible telecanthus (Fig. 2.4.18), which can be addressed with canthopexy outside the acute perioperative period.

Zygomatic and maxillary fractures involving the orbit can be complicated by persistent diplopia, late enophthalmos and cicatricial ectropion or entropion. Late enophthalmos may occur as swelling around the

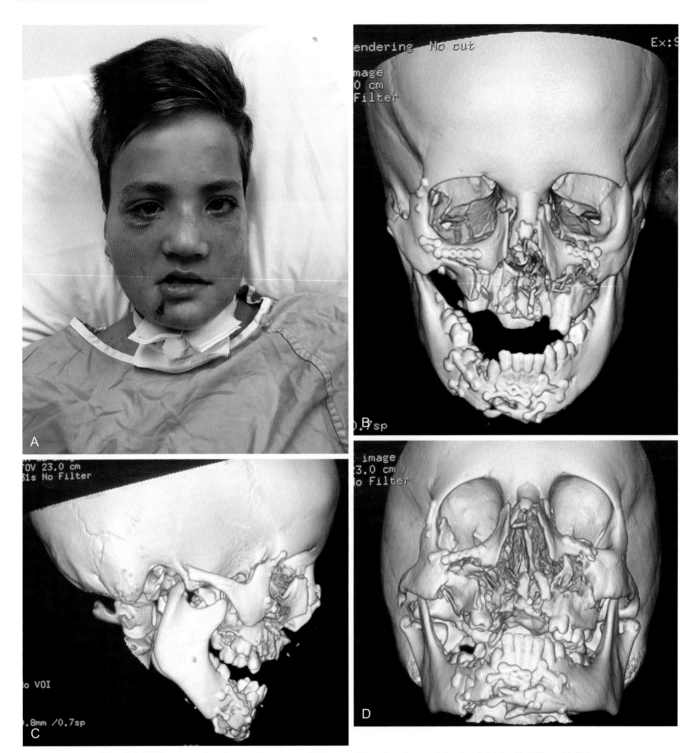

Fig. 2.4.16 An example of a poorly managed 11-year-old male who sustained a right Le Fort III and left Le Fort II fracture with comminuted central mandibular fractures in addition to significant dentoalveolar fractures presenting 3 weeks post injury after surgery at an out-of-country institution (A). A tracheostomy has been established to manage the airway. In general, this is unusual in the management of panfacial fractures. Surgical exposure of the inferior orbital rims has been performed through bilateral lower eyelid incisions (A). These have been placed nonanatomically. CT scans post reduction show the extensive loss of dentition and bone in the maxilla (B–C). A critical error has been made in not adequately reducing the right ZMC, which has sheared off at the base of the zygomatic arch and posteriorly displaced. This has resulted in nonanatomic fixation of the ZMC with lateral displacement, increased right orbital volume, and lateral displacement of the right nasal bone complex and medial canthus. The maxillary fracture has been ignored with no stabilization. Internal fixation of the mandibular fracture has been performed without adequate reduction, using inadequate unstable miniplate fixation placed with screws entering into the tooth roots (D–E).

Continued

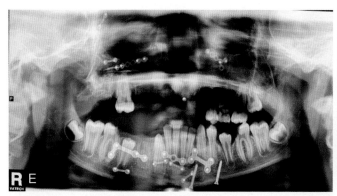
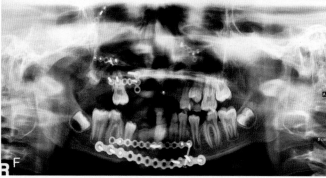

Fig. 2.4.16, cont'd The patient subsequently underwent removal of mandibular fixation, removal of devital-ized teeth, bony reduction using the remaining maxillary dentition, and stabilization using a titanium plate that provides support and stability (F). The displaced right ZMC fracture was reduced and plated.

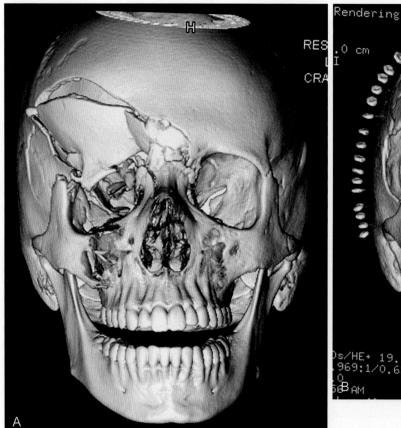
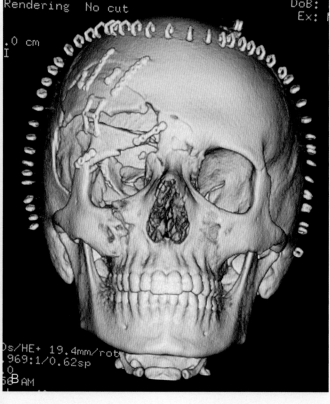

Fig. 2.4.17 An example of a poorly managed right compound fronto-orbital fracture involving the right ZMC in a 16-year-old female 2 weeks following an ATV accident. Preoperative CT scans demonstrate comminuted fractures of the right frontotemporal region, anterior table of the frontal sinus and right ZMC (A). The patient underwent open reduction through an anterior hairline incision. In general, a bicoronal incision would place the scar back in the hairline as unsightly hairline scars are difficult to manage. Nonanatomic reduction of the right supraorbital rim in a depressed position has narrowed the vertical height of the right orbit and has resulted in posttrauma inferior displacement of the right ZMC, a step-off along the inferior orbital rim with widening of the transverse facial dimension with segmental bone defects of the frontal and temporal region (B). The orbital roof fracture was ignored in the original surgery. CT scans demonstrate the results following a re-repair with open reduction of the right ZMC using the lateral maxillary buttress and inferior orbital rim as landmarks due to the comminuted nature of the lateral orbital wall (C).

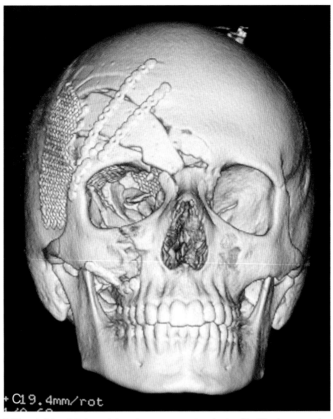

Fig. 2.4.17, cont'd The right orbital roof has been reconstructed with titanium mesh plates. A sheet of titanium mesh was used to replace missing bone in the temporoparietal region (C).

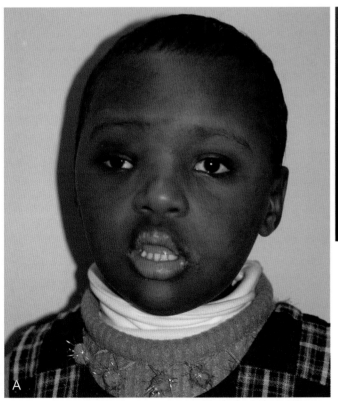

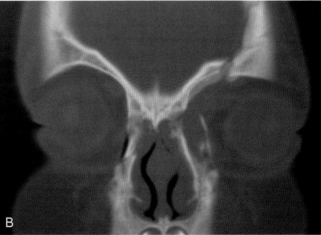

Fig. 2.4.18 An example of a posttraumatic right telecanthus occurring following a displaced unrecognized unilateral NOE fracture in a 6-year-old female (A). CT scan demonstrates the displaced segment that contains the medial canthal ligament in addition to an orbital roof fracture (B). Treatment will involve a transnasal canthopexy and restoration of the anatomic location of the medial canthus.

orbit subsides if the bony orbital volume has not been appropriately restored, and necessitates close follow-up of patients, especially those treated conservatively.

With some cases of maxillary trauma and pterygoid disjunction, malocclusion can occur following intervention. However, given the adaptive nature of the developing dentition, this is quite rare.[28] Depending on the age of the patient, either orthodontic or formal orthognathic surgical interventions may be necessary to address this. Dental rehabilitation following the loss of teeth may take the form of a dental plate but definitive tooth replacement with osseointegrated implants is generally deferred until skeletal maturity.

CONCLUSION

Children with facial trauma present specific challenges and the basic principles of adult-based management may have to be modified when dealing with the pediatric craniofacial region. Appropriate and accurate diagnosis requires a careful clinical examination supplemented with the application of CT scans. A high index of suspicion should be present when high-velocity trauma has occurred and concomitant injuries (C-spine and intracranial) must be excluded.

In general, in the treatment of the pediatric patient who has sustained facial trauma, consideration should be given to a conservative approach whenever possible. Fortunately, children seem to have a unique resilience and remodeling potential that allows a good recovery from significant facial trauma but the possibility that growth impairment may occur should be discussed with parents. As such, it is suggested that children be followed until skeletal maturity has been reached to confirm long-term stable outcomes.

EXPERT COMMENTARY

The authors present a good and classic discussion of the treatment of midface fractures in children. I agree with the authors that minimally displaced fractures often do not need any treatment except observation for displacement. I have generally approached displaced fractures with open reductions, trying to be as conservative as possible in terms of doing the least number of approaches that I need to align and stabilize the fracture.

I would emphasize that the needs of confirming "alignment" are often greater than the needs of providing "fixation" in terms of the number of exposures for a particular fracture. Considering that the ZF suture plate is often both palpable and visible, and frequently requires removal, some might consider using a wire alone at this site for stabilization, as recommended by Kawamoto. I prefer using shallow screws when overdeveloping teeth or when tooth injury is likely, and I have not noticed a significant incidence of remote tooth problems, but I did not go looking for them either.

Frequently, the patients disappear, as the families of patients with children are notoriously mobile, and do not return for plate removal, and so one wonders whether plate retention really contributes to significant noticeable deformity; admittedly, the follow-up is challenging. The authors' experience, however – one of the most extensive in the world – must be respected, particularly their warning that the mixed dentition patients experience the most post-fracture growth issues requiring repeat osteotomy. Finally, judicious use of incomplete exposures may significantly minimize scarring and more extensive use of fixation materials which may contribute to late growth problems. We know that growth problems are the injury, the exposure, the fixation and the healing, and any complications, so that the etiology is multifactorial, and the fixation equipment is only one factor [1].

Reference
1. Wong L, Richtsmeier JT, Manson PN. Craniofacial growth following rigid fixation: suture excision, miniplating, microplating. *J Craniofac Surg*. 1993;4:234–245.

REFERENCES

1. Rowe NL. Fractures of the facial skeleton in children. *J Oral Surg.* 1968;26(8):505–515.
2. Naran S, MacIsaac Z, Katzel E, et al. Pediatric craniofacial fractures. *J Craniofac Surg.* 2016;27(6):1535–1538.
3. Roeder RA, Thaller S. Unique Features of the pediatric craniofacial anatomy. *J Craniofac Surg.* 2011;22(2):392–394.
4. McGraw BL, Cole RR. Pediatric maxillofacial trauma: age-related variations in injury. *Arch Otolaryngol Head Neck Surg.* 1990;116(1):41–45.
5. Adekeye EO. Pediatric fractures of the facial skeleton: a survey of 85 cases from Kaduna, Nigeria. *J Oral Surg.* 1980;38(5):355–358.
6. Iizuka T, Thoren H, Annino D, et al. Midfacial fractures in pediatric patients. *Arch Otolaryngol Head Neck Surg.* 1995;121:1366–1371.
7. Kaban LB, Mulliken JB, Murray JE. Facial fractures in children. *Plast Reconstr Surg.* 1977;59(1):15–20.
8. Anderson PJ. Fractures of the facial skeleton in children. *Injury.* 1995;26(1):47–50.
9. Thaller SR, Huang V. Midfacial fractures in the pediatric population. *Ann Plast Surg.* 1992;29(4):348–352.
10. Haug RH, Foss J. Maxillofacial injuries in the pediatric patient. *Oral Surg Oral Med Oral Pathol Oral Radiol Endod.* 2000;90(2):126–134.
11. Zimmermann CE, Troulis MJ, Kaban LB. Pediatric facial fractures: recent advances in prevention, diagnosis and management. *Int J Oral Maxillofac Surg.* 2005;34(8):823–833.
12. Kaban L. Oral and maxillofacial surgery. In: Kaban L, ed. *Pediatric Oral and Maxillofacial Surgery*. Philadelphia: WB Saunders; 1990:209–232.
13. Posnick JC, Wells M, Pron GE. Pediatric facial fractures: evolving patterns of treatment. *J Oral Maxillofac Surg.* 1993;51(8):836–844.
14. Murphy RX, Birmingham KL, Okunski WJ, et al. Influence of restraining devices on patterns of pediatric facial trauma in motor vehicle collisions. *Plast Reconstr Surg.* 2001;107(1):34–37.
15. Hoppe IC, Kordahi AM, Paik AM, et al. Age and sex-related differences in 431 pediatric facial fractures at a level 1 trauma center. *J Craniomaxillofac Surg.* 2014;42(7):1408–1411.
16. Maisel H. Postnatal growth and anatomy of the face. In: Mathog RH, ed. *Maxillofacial Trauma*. Baltimore, MD: Williams & Wilkins; 1984:21–38.
17. Spaeth J, Krügelstein U, Schlöndorff G. The paranasal sinuses in CT-imaging: development from birth to age 25. *Int J Pediatr Otorhinolaryngol.* 1997;39(1):25–40.
18. Maniglia AJ, Kline SN. Maxillofacial trauma in the pediatric age group. *Otolaryngol Clin North Am.* 1983;16(3):717.
19. Neinstein RM, Phillips JH, Forrest CR. Pediatric orbital floor trapdoor fractures: outcomes and CT-based morphologic assessment of the inferior rectus muscle. *J Plast Reconstr Aesthet Surg.* 2012;65(7):869–874.
20. Holland AJ, Broome C, Steinberg A, et al. Facial fractures in children. *Pediatr Emerg Care.* 2001;17(3):157–160.
21. Hopper RA, Salemy S, Sze RW. Diagnosis of midface fractures with CT: what the surgeon needs to know. *Radiographics.* 2006;26(3):783–793.
22. Moore M, David D, Cooter R. Oblique craniofacial fractures in children. *J Craniofac Surg.* 1990;1(1):4–7.
23. Polley J, Figueroa A, Hung K. Effect of rigid microfixation on the craniomaxillofacial skeleton. *J Craniofac Surg.* 1995;6(2):132–138.
24. Eppley BL. Use of resorbable plates and screws in pediatric facial fractures. *J Oral Maxillofac Surg.* 2005;63(3):385–391.
25. Desrosiers AE, Thaller SR. Pediatric nasal fractures. *J Craniofac Surg.* 2011;22(4):1327–1329.
26. Markowitz BL, Manson PN, Sargent L, et al. Management of the medial canthal tendon in nasoethmoid orbital fractures: the importance of the central fragment in classification and treatment. *Plast Reconstr Surg.* 1991;87(5):843–853.
27. Perez R, Berkowitz R, McIlveen L, et al. Dental trauma in children: a survey. *Endod Dent Traumatol.* 1991;7:212–213.
28. Gussack G, Luterman A, Powell R, et al. Pediatric maxillofacial trauma: unique features in diagnosis and treatment. *Laryngoscope.* 1987;97(8):925–930.

Pediatric Mandible Fractures

Lewis C. Jones, Robert L. Flint

BACKGROUND

The topic of pediatric mandible fractures covers a wide range of patients with multiple clinical variables. Patients can range from a neonate with a mandible fracture stemming from birth trauma to an 18-year-old with full permanent dentition and multiple fractures. Because of this range of differences, the "pediatric" population in regards to mandible fractures can be further divided into the following:

Neonate/infants – 0 to 1 year of age (developing/unerupted dentition)
Toddlers – 1 to 3 years of age (erupting primary dentition)
Children – 4 to 12 years of age (primary and mixed dentition)
Adolescents – 12 to 18 years of age

Fractures of the mandible can be characterized as favorable or unfavorable, or according to site; however, the crucial information in pediatric mandible fractures is the stage of the dentition. Whether the patient has primary, mixed or permanent dentition can drastically affect the overall treatment plan. The pediatric mandible is the storage warehouse for the developing teeth. Developing tooth buds that exist in the growing patient will add complexity to a case, as the routine methods to control occlusion (intermaxillary fixation) and apply fixation can prove to be difficult, or even impossible. Unfortunately, pediatric mandible fractures are a common problem.

The incidence of pediatric mandible fractures, as demonstrated in Imahara's review of the National Trauma Data Bank from 2001 to 2005, is not insignificant. Imahara found that of 12,739 pediatric patients diagnosed with facial fractures, the most common fracture was that of the mandible (32.7%).[1] A recent review of the Healthcare Cost and Utilization Project's National Emergency Department Sample demonstrated mandible fractures (defined as fractures in patients 18 years of age and younger) to have a 4:1 male to female ratio and an overall mean age of 14 years. The major etiologies of mandible fractures in this study included falls (17%), motor vehicle collisions (13%), and assault (8%). The mechanism of trauma varies according to age, with the leading cause in both females and males in patients under 12 years of age being falls, while male and older adolescent (≥12 years) patient populations had assault as their leading cause of mandible fracture.[2]

The site of fracture also varies according to age. Owusu and colleagues reviewed more than 1200 mandible fractures in pediatric patients, revealing that the most commonly fractured anatomic sites of the mandible varied depending on age.[2] This is likely a result of two factors: first, the developing dentition, which would provoke changes in the mandible's weak points as teeth develop and erupt, and second, the change in the mechanisms based on the common activities specific to each age group. Young patients (≤12 years of age) most commonly fractured the condyle (27.9%) while older patients' most common site of fracture was the angle (17.6%).[2] Several additional studies have demonstrated that while many pediatric mandibular condylar fractures will

occur in isolation, up to 20% will present with bilateral condylar fractures.[3–5] Mandible fractures also occur with concomitant injuries in regions other than the face in 11%–65% of trauma patients.[6,7] Forces that are significant to fracture a pediatric mandible have a high likelihood of concomitant injury. Injuries associated with mandible fractures include other facial fractures (13%), facial soft tissue injury (34%), C-spine (0.9%–4.4%), neurocranial (8.5%–34%), extremity (9.1%–16.4%), chest (1.8%), and abdominal injuries (1.6%).[2,6,7] Concomitant injuries vary based on the mechanism of injury. While ER visits involving facial fractures are relatively uncommon (0.03%),[2] all surgeons are mandatory reporters of suspected child abuse—any suspicion of the mechanism/injury should provoke notification through the proper channels for investigation and any necessary intervention.

EMBRYOLOGY AND GROWTH OF THE MANDIBLE

The mandible develops by intramembranous ossification and is derived from the first branchial cleft with contributions from the proximal portion of Meckel's cartilage. By the sixth week of embryologic development, the bilateral mandibular processes have fused to form a fibrous symphysis. The mandible is then the second site (after the clavicle) to undergo ossification.[8,9] Ossification continues throughout the first year of life.

The growth of the mandible is a complex, multifactorial process. Its growth is influenced by the growth of the alveolar process, the developing dentition, the associated muscular processes, and the mandibular condyle. Disruptions in growth (either due to congenital factors or due to trauma) can lead to abnormal development, with significant cosmetic and functional consequences, including asymmetries and malocclusions (Fig. 2.5.1).

The importance of the relationship of the developing dentition to alveolar growth cannot be overstressed. In patients with congenitally missing dentition (such as ectodermal dysplasia), the alveolar process is undeveloped. The growth of the alveolar process mirrors the eruption sequence. After tooth eruption, the mechanical forces of mastication and parafunctional habits exert forces on the alveolar bone that will also influence development and maintenance of bone. While this complex process has not been fully elucidated, it is imperative that the surgeon understands the interactive role the developing dentition plays in alveolar bone development and does everything possible to minimize disruption during the treatment of mandible fractures.

The position of the mental foramen changes relative to the mandibular body throughout mandibular growth. At age 3 it lies between the deciduous canine and first molar and is near the inferior border. By age 6, the mental foramen is posterior and superior in its relative position, eventually residing inferior to the first or second premolar and is no longer near the inferior border, but is often equidistant between the inferior and superior aspect of the mandibular body.[10]

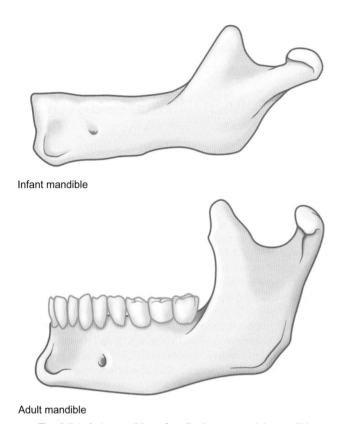

Infant mandible

Adult mandible

Fig. 2.5.1 Artist rendition of pediatric versus adult mandible.

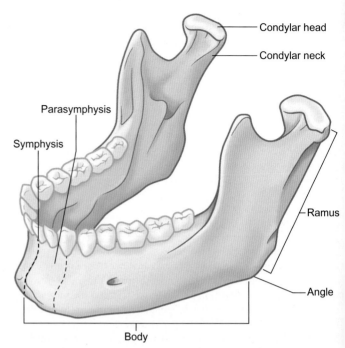

Fig. 2.5.2 Artist rendition of anatomic regions of the mandible.

The muscles of mastication play a role in the development of both the coronoid process and mandibular angle (which grow by periosteal apposition). However, disruption of these regions with fractures rarely impacts the overall growth of the mandible.

The mandibular growth derived from the condylar process is complex and fracture of this region can impede growth and result in asymmetry and malocclusion.[10] While other growth mechanisms exist within the mandible, the condyle is a major contributing source of both vertical and horizontal growth of the mandible. The growth of the condylar process is linked to the presence of secondary cartilage in this location.[11] The direction of this growth of the condyle is influenced by the mandibular posture, condyle/fossa relationship, and a multitude of mechanical factors.[12] Fractures of the condyle can have a significant impact on normal mandibular growth/development and will be discussed later in this chapter.

ANATOMY OF THE MANDIBLE

The bony mandible is comprised of the following anatomic subunits: the condyle, condylar neck, ramus, angle, body, and symphysis. Use of these terms in describing the injury is paramount in helping a practitioner understand the problem at hand – as fractures of the mandible are treated differently based on the age of the patient and the anatomic subunit involved (Fig. 2.5.2).

The third division of the trigeminal nerve (cranial nerve V) provides sensory innervation to the mandible after exiting the foramen ovale. This nerve also provides innervation to the muscles of mastication (masseter, temporalis, and medial/lateral pterygoid muscles). The major arterial supply to the mandible is the inferior alveolar artery (a branch of the internal maxillary artery). The associated inferior alveolar vein completes the neurovascular bundle that enters at the mandibular

foramen proximally and divides at the first molar region into an incisive branch that continues anteriorly within the mandible and a mental branch that exits at the mental foramen. The orientation of the neurovascular bundle is that the vein (or veins) reside superior to the nerve, and the artery is located lingual to the nerve.[13]

The mandible is a bone suspended in space by its musculature. The paired muscles that help with mastication are the medial and lateral pterygoids, masseter, temporalis, with some contribution from the digastric muscles. The medial aspect of the mandibular body is the site of attachment for the mylohyoid and the anterior lingual aspect provides the site of attachment for the digastric, the genioglossus, and geniohyoid muscles. The mandible is also the site of attachment for the paired muscles of the mentalis (anteriorly) and buccinator (superiorly at the posterior body), as well as the platysma (along the inferior border).

This complex musculoskeletal unit provides the ability for basic life functions such as speech and mastication. An injury to the mandible can lead to compromise, and its proper repair is necessary in reestablishing both form and function.

STAGES OF DENTITION

Understanding the dentition and its stages is crucial in the treatment of pediatric mandible fractures. In general, pediatric mandible fractures can be divided into three simple groups: primary dentition, mixed dentition, and permanent dentition stages. The dentition phase, as well as the condition of the dentition, will significantly affect the treatment plan for mandible fractures.

The tooth buds for the primary teeth are present in utero with the dental lamina from which they develop present as early as 12 weeks in utero.[14] The first teeth to erupt are most often the lower central incisors at 6–10 months of age. The primary dentition is comprised of 20 teeth that most often erupt prior to age 3 (Fig. 2.5.3). Primary teeth have crowns that are more bulbous than their permanent counterparts, and have roots with increased divergence, which allows space for the development of permanent tooth buds inferiorly. The roots of primary teeth will resorb as the permanent teeth develop and begin to erupt, ending

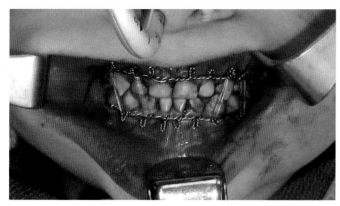

Fig. 2.5.3 Primary dentition in a 4-year-old patient with Risdon cables in place.

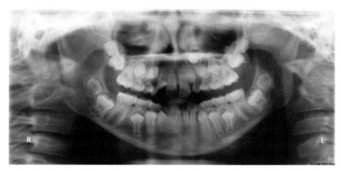

Fig. 2.5.4 Mixed dentition: panoramic image of mixed dentition (age 11) – note the eruption of permanent first molars and incisors. The developing canines and premolars (and second and third molars) have yet to erupt.

with the exfoliation of the primary teeth. Primary teeth should have some spacing between all of the teeth, although spacing between the primary teeth will close with the eruption of the first permanent molar, which ushers in the beginning of the mixed dentition phase.[15]

The mixed dentition phase begins around age 6 and extends until approximately age 12 when the final primary tooth exfoliates (Fig. 2.5.4). The mixed dentition presents significant challenges in establishing the maxillomandibular relationship due to unerupted or partially erupted permanent teeth, loose deciduous teeth that have not exfoliated, and discrepancy in crown size of the newly erupted permanent dentition adjacent to smaller, retained primary teeth. These challenges can impede the placement of secure maxillomandibular fixation (MMF) for both closed and open procedures to correct alignment of a mandible fracture. Similarly to the primary dentition phase, existing unerupted tooth buds within the mandible can present challenges when open reduction/rigid fixation is required.

Following the exfoliation of the final primary tooth, the dentition is considered to be in the permanent dentition phase (Fig. 2.5.5). It is at this point that the methods of treatment for a mandible fracture begin to mirror the treatments rendered in the adult population. The fracture patterns of the mandible also resemble that of the adult population.

FRACTURE PATTERNS IN PEDIATRIC POPULATIONS

Fracture patterns in pediatric populations vary based on the stage of the dentition of the patient as both the activities a child/youth/adolescent

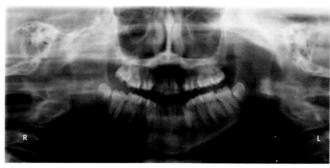

Fig. 2.5.5 Early permanent dentition (age 13) with developing third molars.

is involved in and the weak points of the mandible vary with age. In various studies evaluating the distribution of mandible fractures in pediatric patients, the condylar (condylar neck or condylar head) region is consistently the most frequently fractured structure (7%–45%), the parasymphysis is the second most frequently injured (20%–32%), the percentage of angle fractures ranges from 4.4% to 45%, with an increased incidence during the teenage years, coinciding with third molar development. Siegel et al. demonstrated that children in mixed dentition aged 7–12 have increased risk of mandibular body fractures (20%) compared to younger children aged birth to 6 (4.4%) or those aged 13–18 years (9.7%). Patients often presented with multiple fractures (28%–59%).[7,16,17]

EVALUATION

Evaluation of the mandible during the secondary trauma survey (following ATLS protocol) should replicate the exam in an adult patient – however, it will often require patience and ingenuity. A thorough evaluation of the mandible will include examination of the temporomandibular joints, bony continuity at the posterior/inferior border, dentition, occlusion, and the associated soft tissue.

The temporomandibular joint (TMJ) should be assessed for appropriate range of motion, tenderness overlying the joint, pop/click/crepitus, and deviation on opening. From the TMJ region, the practitioner should palpate for bony steps or irregular surface along the posterior border of the ramus and inferior border of the body and symphysis region, also noting any discrete regions of tenderness. The dentition should be inspected for loose or missing teeth as well as "steps" in the occlusal plane. The occlusion with the maxillary dentition (if intact) should be evaluated for a stable/repeatable occlusion, as alterations in occlusion can be indicative of fracture or TMJ hemarthrosis/edema. The overlying attached and unattached gingival tissues require inspection for lacerations and bleeding, which often harbor fragments of traumatized dentition (or entire teeth).

Imaging of the mandible for suspected fractures/injury is best performed with a combination of images.[18] Imaging of the mandible can be accomplished with a single panoramic image (Fig. 2.5.6). This single image allows visualization of the mandible and dentition in its entirety on a single image with minimal radiation exposure. Unfortunately, young patients may not be tall enough or remain motionless long enough for this image to be obtained, and many emergency rooms and trauma centers are not equipped to provide this image as it is most often employed in a dental setting. AP and lateral mandible films can be helpful in augmenting the panoramic image (Fig. 2.5.7). They may be used alone to demonstrate fractures, but can be difficult to interpret if the practitioner is not accustomed to viewing these images and non-displaced fractures or greenstick fractures (more common

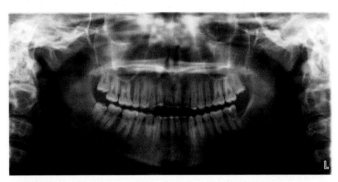

Fig. 2.5.6 Fracture from between teeth 22 and 23 extending to symphysis detected on panoramic radiograph (age 18).

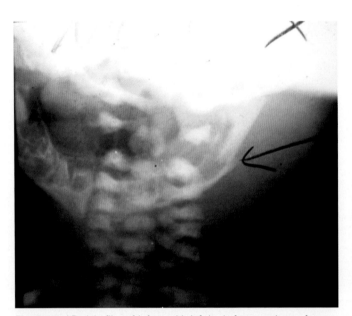

Fig. 2.5.7 AP plain film of infant with left body fracture due to forceps delivery.

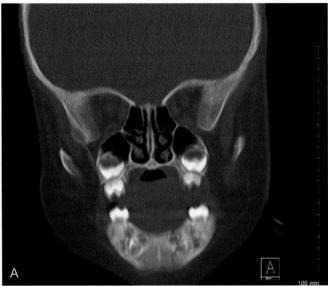

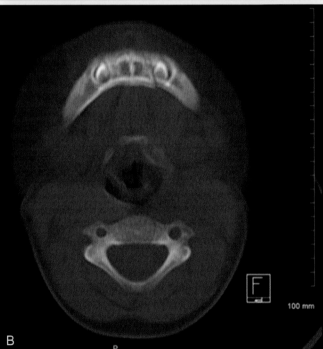

Fig. 2.5.8 Coronal CT of 2-year-old male with left parasymphysis fracture (ATV accident) – coronal (A) and axial (B) views.

in pediatric populations) can be missed. For all of the above reasons, further characterization of mandible fractures is most often provided by a non-contrast computerized tomogram (CT) of the mandible (Fig. 2.5.8). Appropriate imaging ensures extension of the area imaged from the glenoid fossa to the inferior border of the mandible. Finally, surgeons who have cone beam technology available to them can utilize this method of imaging to decrease radiation dose, while still affording axial, coronal and sagittal slices for three-dimensional evaluation of the injury, but like a panoramic image they require a patient to remain motionless in an upright position for the period of time it takes to obtain the image.

TREATMENT

The treatments described below are directed toward the growing patient, and for the purposes of this chapter, treatments for patients where growth cessation has already occurred are not discussed – as these patients should be treated consistent with "adult" modalities. The major "take-home" point from any chapter on pediatric fractures should be the role for conservative therapy, which often occupies a much larger spectrum than in the adult population. This is due to the pediatric

patient's ability to heal more rapidly, as well as avoidance of potential complications associated with open management of a growing/developing bony structure. The discussion of management is divided into anatomic regions and includes fractures of the condylar/subcondylar region, angle, and the body/symphyseal region.

Fractures of the Condyle/Subcondylar Region

Condylar fractures in pediatric patients are almost always managed closed; these patients have proven regenerative/healing potential and the risk of growth disturbance usually precludes open treatment.[19] The indications for open treatment of condylar fractures, introduced by Zide,[20] also apply to pediatric patients as there are few scenarios outside of these in which the benefits of an open procedure would outweigh

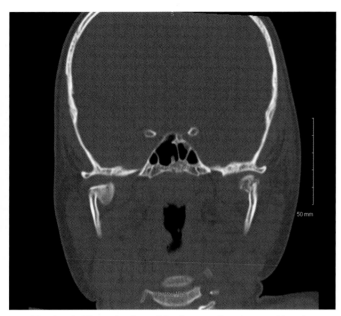

Fig. 2.5.9 Bilateral subcondylar fracture in a 9-year-old male.

the risks. These indications, as outlined in the 1983 paper, include the following scenarios:
1. Displacement of the condyle into the middle cranial fossa or external auditory canal
2. Lateral extracapsular dislocation.
3. Contaminated open joint wound.
4. Inability to obtain adequate occlusion.

It should be noted that in pediatric patients, there may exist a much more loose definition of what defines adequate occlusion. In the primary and mixed dentition phase, the developing dentition can often compensate for discrepancies introduced by a condylar fracture. In situations where occlusion is difficult to determine, a set of dental models can often prove useful as it can allow the practitioner to evaluate the occlusion with some manipulation of the models and thus help determine the necessity for opening a condylar fracture. When in doubt, it is prudent to err on the side of conservative treatment. In general, conservative therapy is preferred for treating pediatric condylar fractures – even in bilateral cases (Fig. 2.5.9). Several practitioners have demonstrated good results in published reports.[21,22] Conservative therapy for condylar and subcondylar fractures includes a soft diet and antiinflammatory medications. The soft diet should be adhered to for 4–6 weeks and the antiinflammatory medications should be prescribed for the first 5–7 days in patients where contraindications do not exist. Both unilateral and bilateral fracture patients require close observation for persistent decreased range of motion that may indicate a patient on the path to ankylosis. Early referral to a physical therapist to increase range of motion is advised. Patients are also observed for development of growth disturbances with resultant asymmetry (Figs. 2.5.10A–D). The traumatized condyle may cease to grow while the unaffected condyle continues to grow normally resulting in obvious asymmetry with a compensatory occlusal cant. Appropriate follow-up and early referral to an orthodontist for evaluation and intervention is paramount (Fig. 2.5.10E).

Like condylar fractures, subcondylar fractures should also be managed conservatively. These fractures are contained within the pterygomasseteric sling and as such will most often heal without complication. The healing of a subcondylar fracture is facilitated by light function with Risdon cables and elastics in primary and mixed dentition, and

Erich arch bars with elastics in the growing patient with permanent dentition (Figs. 2.5.11 and 2.5.12).

In all cases, it is important to maintain long-term follow-up to observe the developing mandible after a fracture of the condyle. Fractures in young patients can take years to manifest the developing asymmetry.

Angle Fractures

Fractures of the mandibular angle increase with the development of the third molar – thus inducing a weak point at the angle of the mandible.[23–26] As such, only 4% of mandible fractures in children <12 years of age were angle fractures, versus almost 18% of patients over age 12 who presented with mandibular angle fractures.[2] These fractures can be treated with MMF as described above with the use of Risdon cables or Erich arch bars and wire MMF for a period of 2–3 weeks followed by elastics for an additional 2–4 weeks depending on the patient's age and severity of the fracture. Open reduction and internal fixation of angle fractures can be addressed with the use of 3D or "ladder" plates, a single superior lateral border plate, a plate on the external oblique ridge ("Champy technique"), or with an inferior border plate[27] (Fig. 2.5.13). Several circumstances will impact the decision-making process regarding the technique to be employed, such as the nature of the fracture, the presence or absence of a third molar, and the need for extraction of the third molar (if present) at the time of fixation.

Fractures of the Mandibular Body/Symphysis

Fractures of the body and symphysis region (dentate portion) of the mandible should be assessed for mobility. If no mobility is noted and imaging is consistent with a greenstick fracture (which is common in pediatric populations), then soft diet and follow-up are recommended. Minimal mobility or displacement may be amenable to Risdon cables/arch bar placement with a short (2–3 week) period of MMF followed by elastics for an additional 2–4 weeks depending upon the severity of the fracture. The severity of the fracture is based upon bony displacement and subsequent occlusal stability. Alternatively, a lingual splint can be used to stabilize the fracture with the aid of circumdental wires (Fig. 2.5.14). However, this usually necessitates multiple trips to the operating room for impressions, followed by pouring of dental stone models and fabrication of a lingual splint, which is then wired into place. This laborious process is generally avoided as a technique. Fractures of the body which are oblique in nature may be amenable to circumdental wiring, which is another effective technique that is rarely employed (Fig. 2.5.15).

Grossly displaced fractures often require open reduction and internal fixation. Resorbable plates are not FDA-approved for use in mandible fractures, but have been utilized with some success.[28] If used, they may require placement of two plates and therefore placement of the second, more superior plate can cause damage to developing tooth buds in primary and mixed dentition patients. A single mandibular miniplate at the inferior border with the use of a superior "tension band" of a Risdon cable or Erich arch bar is often sufficient and minimizes injury to tooth buds and/or the inferior alveolar nerve (Figs. 2.5.16 and 2.5.17). The plate can be removed after adequate healing has taken place. This can usually be accomplished in conjunction with removal of the arch bars/wires at 6–8 weeks after injury.

Conservative, nonoperative management of the pediatric mandible fracture is often the preferred method of treatment. Open treatment of the symphysis, body, or ramus is typically indicated when there is significant skeletal displacement resulting in malocclusion, limited range of motion, inhibition of proper function, and/or the possibility of airway compromise. Rarely, if ever, is open treatment performed for a pediatric

Text continued on p. 332

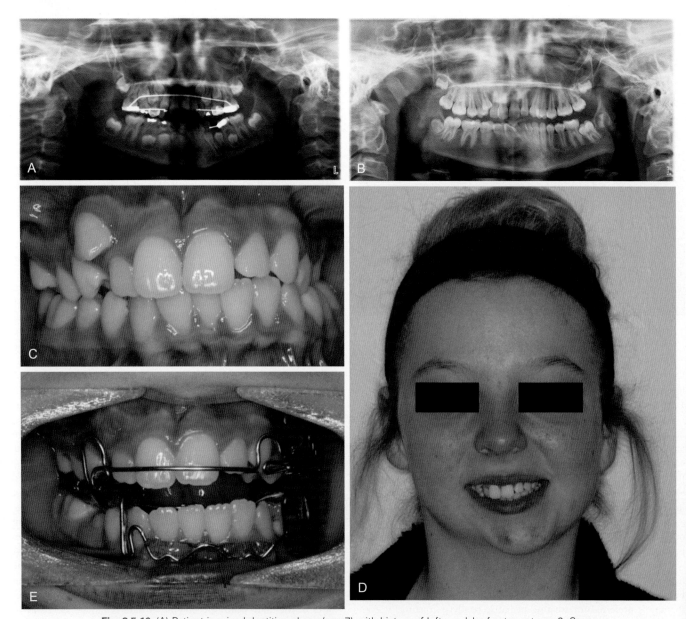

Fig. 2.5.10 (A) Patient in mixed dentition phase (age 7) with history of left condylar fracture at age 2. Some mild to moderate asymmetry can be seen at the inferior border of the mandible. (B) Same patient at age 13 with worsening asymmetry due to condylar fracture at age 2. (C) Intraoral view exhibiting occlusal cant and mandibular asymmetry with left posterior crossbite present. Severe dental midline discrepancy also exists. (D) Anteroposterior facial view of patient at age 13 with noted asymmetry. Note the significant chin point deviation toward the affected left side and the dental midline discrepancy is also present. (E) Patient with orthodontic appliance in place. This appliance is fabricated and worn in order to help inhibit right maxillary tooth eruption and promote continued eruption of that on the left. This will help prevent development of a compensatory maxillary occlusal cant.

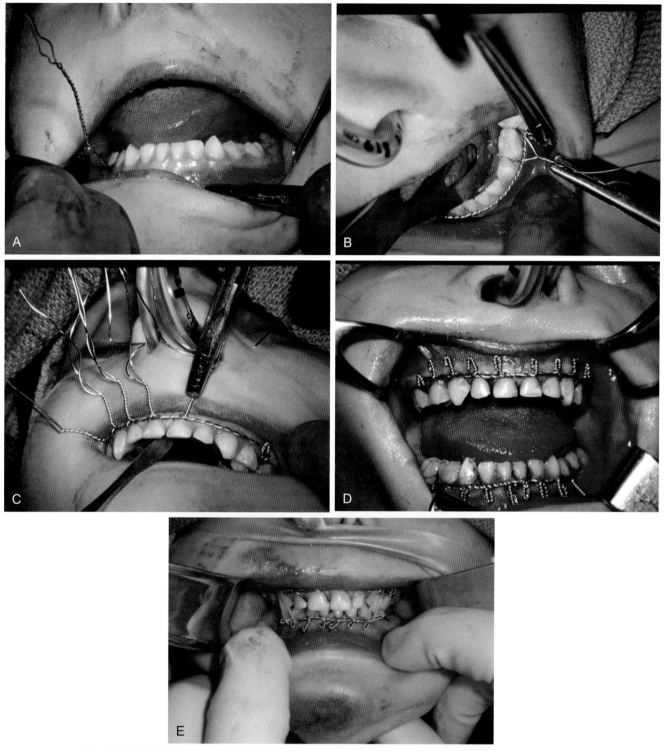

Fig. 2.5.11 (A) Risdon cables are placed by first placing a circumdental wire around a stable molar. The wire is then twisted to the length appropriate to reach the contralateral molar and a loop can be placed around this molar as well. (B) Circumdental wires are then placed around each tooth in the arch, securing it to the initial cable. (C) This is done in the maxilla and mandible both in order to obtain maxillomandibular fixation. (D) The final product should appear similar to this – with rosettes placed to avoid additional trauma to adjacent soft tissues. (E) Elastics can then be placed bilaterally for elastic MMF to allow for light function through the convalescent period.

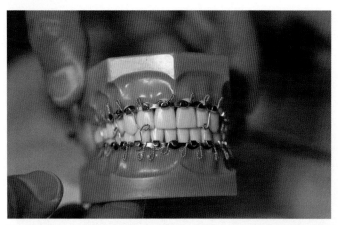

Fig. 2.5.12 Erich arch bars are applied similarly to Risdon cables. Note that Erich arch bars are more able to maintain stability with wire MMF compared with Risdon cables.

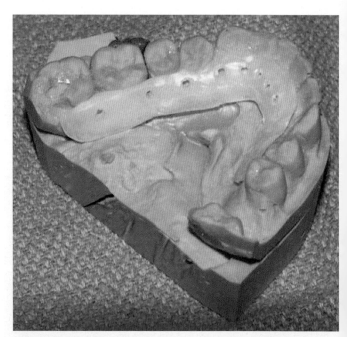

Fig. 2.5.14 Lingual splint fabricated from acrylic for stabilization of left mandibular body fracture. Note the holes placed for stabilization with circumdental wires.

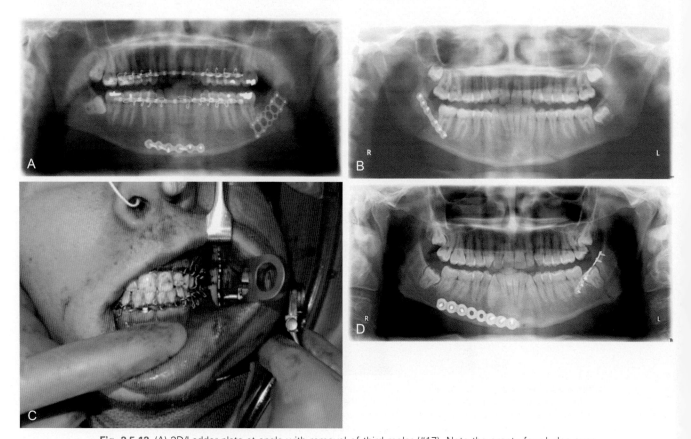

Fig. 2.5.13 (A) 3D/Ladder plate at angle with removal of third molar (#17). Note the empty four holes over the region of fracture. The screws at the angle are monocortical. Note that arch bars remain in place and single mandibular reconstruction plate was used for the symphysis fracture. (B) Superior lateral border plate can be used for fixation of an angle fracture. This is a 14-year-old female with angle fracture. Tooth #32 was removed due to displacement and six-hole monocortical plate was placed with three screws on each side of the fracture. (C) One disadvantage of a 3D or a superior border plate is the necessity for a transbuccal trocar for placement of proximal screws. Several types of transbuccal retractors exist for use with the trocar. Pictured below is the blade cheek retractor (KLS Martin). (D) Champy plate at left angle fracture with third molar remaining in place. Rigid fixation achieved at contralateral fracture with reconstruction plate at inferior border. This plate can most often be placed with a transoral approach.

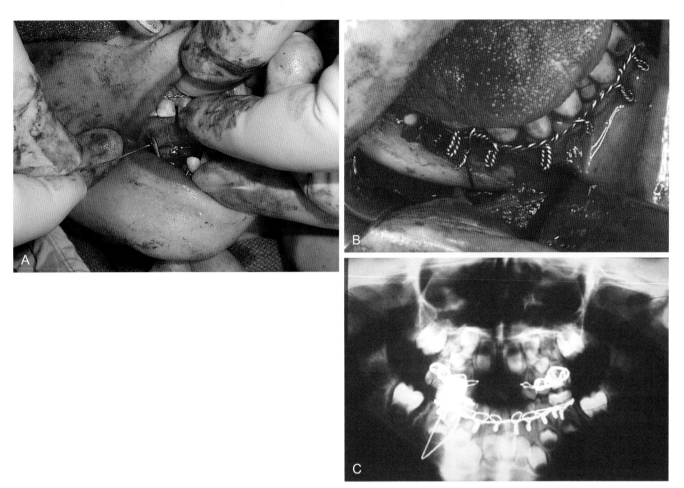

Fig. 2.5.15 Placement of circum-mandibular wire is accomplished with the aid of an awl which is passed first on the lingual aspect (A), the wire is secured through the hole on the awl and then brought inferiorly (taking care not to exit the skin) and reintroduced at the buccal aspect. The fracture is then reduced by twisting the wire into place (B). (C) Panoramic image after placement of the circum-mandibular wire pictured in (B).

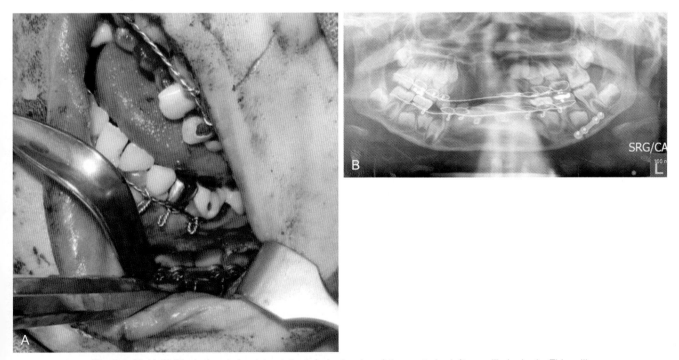

Fig. 2.5.16 (A,B) Single four-hole plate at the inferior border of the posterior left mandibular body. This will ideally be below the developing tooth buds. As evidenced on the panoramic image, the plate appears to be placed at the inferior aspect of the developing #20 follicle.

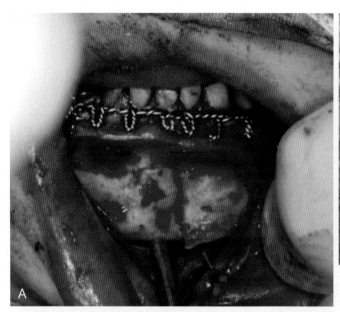
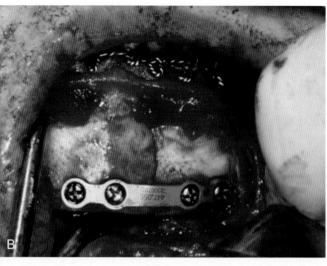

Fig. 2.5.17 (A,B) Fracture of the parasymphysis region with developing tooth buds in place. A single inferior border four-hole plate was placed for stabilization.

condyle fracture unless the condyle is displaced into the middle cranial fossa.

Treatment of the Associated Dentition

Tooth buds that are displaced and in the line of fracture preventing reduction should be replaced within the alveolus, where possible. If preventing fracture reduction, the tooth bud should be removed – with clear communication to the patient's dentist/pedodontist for space maintenance, where appropriate. Avulsed primary teeth should *never* be replaced. Primary teeth loose enough to present an aspiration risk should be removed. Permanent teeth that have been avulsed or luxated should be reimplanted, reduced, and splinted/stabilized appropriately and referred to a dentist/endodontist for vitality testing to determine the necessity of root canal therapy.

MAJOR COMPLICATIONS AND MANAGEMENT

Ankylosis

This is a complication that is often described but seldom seen in the pediatric patient. Trauma to the TMJ region that results in fracture of the condyle or high subcondylar region can lead to bone formation in and around the condylar head/glenoid fossa. Inadequate reduction of mandible fractures can lead to fixation with resultant mandibular widening and a condyle that functions lateral to the glenoid fossa. These scenarios can result in bony ankylosis, which is a difficult problem to successfully treat. Treatment of ankylosis may involve resection of the bony ankylosis followed by reconstruction with a costochondral graft or distraction osteogenesis. Growth of the costochondral graft is quite variable and requires a delay in initiation of physical therapy for 10–14 days following reconstruction (while distraction patients can begin immediately). Preventing reankylosis is best accomplished by adequate bony resection combined with postoperative physical therapy, which is crucial in preventing reankylosis (Fig. 2.5.18). This therefore requires the surgery to be performed in an age-appropriate patient who can participate in postoperative physical therapy.[29] The techniques in pediatric bony ankylosis release and reconstruction have been well described by Kaban et al.[30]

Growth Disturbance

Thankfully, like bony ankylosis, growth disturbance following trauma to the mandible is an uncommon complication (Figs. 2.5.10A–D). One retrospective study evaluating adverse outcomes in pediatric populations noted that 2 of 57 patients (3.5%) with isolated mandible fractures exhibited post-injury mandibular hypoplasia.[31] Pediatric mandible fractures, especially those in the condylar/subcondylar region, should be followed as they continue to grow to evaluate for disturbance in growth. This is most often noted as chin point deviation and dental midline discrepancies. A panoramic radiograph (orthopantomogram) will confirm clinical suspicion for hypoplasia of the mandible following trauma. Treatment will be dependent upon age and severity of the asymmetry – most often, surgical correction will include orthodontics in conjunction with orthognathic surgery. According to a single center, retrospective study at the Hospital for Sick Children (Toronto, Canada) of 88 patients with mandible fractures, the children most likely to require orthognathic surgery after mandible fracture were those between ages 4 and 7 (22%) and 8 and 11 (17%). As expected, these growth disturbances most often resulted from condylar trauma.[29]

Internal fixation hardware in the pediatric mandible fracture, although controversial as to its impact on skeletal growth, can easily be removed at the time of MMF hardware removal. Since bony healing is so rapid in the pediatric population, a short course of 6–8 weeks is often all that is necessary for internal fixation. Removal at that time will reduce bony overgrowth of the hardware, which may make plate removal more difficult at a later date, and will also alleviate the concern for growth restriction.

Malunion/Malocclusion

Typically, pediatric patients that develop or have persistent malocclusion following a fracture with or without operative intervention are observed without further operative intervention until growth is completed. Referral to an orthodontist with a combined approach for correction is often the best solution. Some minor malocclusions can be amenable to orthodontic correction alone, while other more severe presentations will require a combined effort to correct the underlying problem (Figs 2.5.19 and 2.5.20).

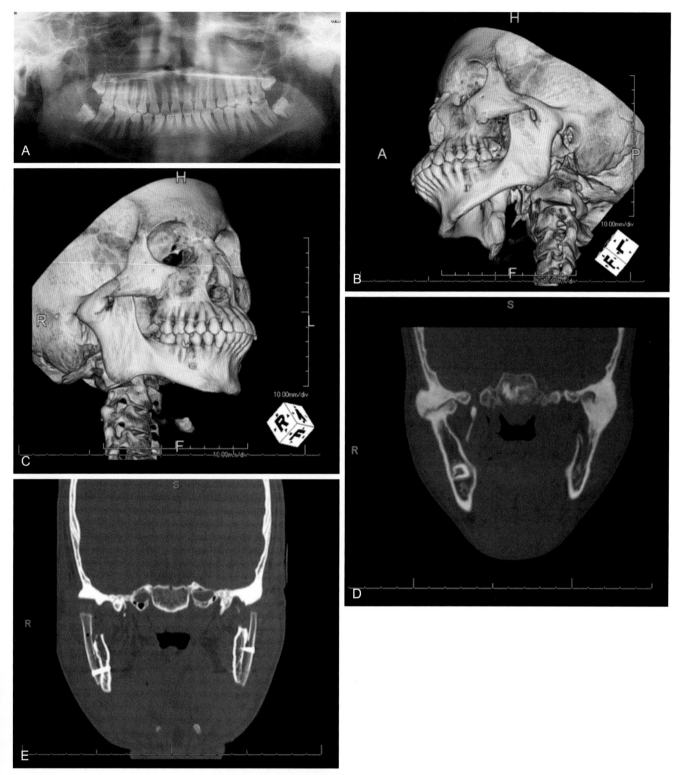

Fig. 2.5.18 (A) Panoramic image of 16-year-old male with bilateral ankylosis from untreated condylar fractures from a fall at a young age. (B–C) Three-dimensional renderings of CT scan demonstrating ankylosis. (D) Coronal slice of CT of same patient. (E) Coronal image with costochondral grafts in place. (Photos courtesy of Drs. Waite and Louis, Univeristy of Alabama at Birmingham.)

CONCLUSION

The evaluation, diagnosis, and treatment of mandible fractures in the pediatric trauma patient differs from that of an adult. It requires a complete knowledge of the growth and development of the dentition, and the mandible and its subunits. The surgeon should also comprehend tooth development and the difficulties that are often encountered in the mixed dentition stage. The application of all of this information, along with understanding of the various techniques available for fracture management, is integrated to make the final recommendation regarding treatment in an effort to avoid both short- and long-term complications.

EXPERT COMMENTARY

This chapter contains much valuable classification and thought organization, including a comprehensive description of "ages" of mandibular growth and development, organized to guide treatment considerations. Development and anatomical regions are further used to guide surgery/treatment planning in the regions, and growth considerations are well managed.

The long-term follow-up of pediatric patients is notoriously difficult, however the authors do as good a job with this as anyone I have read, and offer a reliable guide to the practice of pediatric mandibular trauma.

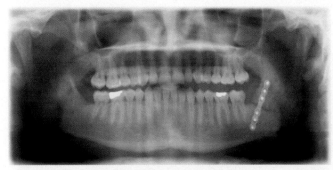

Fig. 2.5.19 This 19-year-old patient was referred by his orthodontist after he had previously undergone ORIF of his angle fracture 3 months prior to referral. He exhibited a posterior open-bite from inadequate reduction at the time of surgery. Note the difference in interocclusal distance with increase on right compared with left.

REFERENCES

1. Imahara SD, Hopper RA, Wang J, et al. Patterns and outcomes of pediatric facial fractures in the United States: a survey of the National Trauma Data Bank. *J Am Coll Surg.* 2008;207(5):710–716.
2. Owusu JA, Bellile E, Moyer JS, Sidman JD. Patterns of pediatric mandible fractures in the United States. *JAMA Facial Plast Surg.* 2016;18(1):37–41.
3. Wolfswinkel EM, Weathers WM, Wirthlin JO, et al. Management of pediatric mandible fractures. *Otolaryngol Clin North Am.* 2013;46(5):791–806.
4. Goth S, Sawatari Y, Peleg M. Management of pediatric mandible fractures. *J Craniofac Surg.* 2012;23(1):47–56.
5. Smartt JM Jr, Low DW, Bartlett SP. The pediatric mandible: II. Management of traumatic injury or fracture. *Plast Reconstr Surg.* 2005;116(2):28e–41e.
6. Thoren H, Schaller B, Suominen AL, Lindqvist C. Occurrence and severity of concomitant injuries in other areas than the face in children with mandibular and midfacial fractures. *J Oral Maxillofac Surg.* 2012;70(1):92–96.
7. Glazer M, Joshua BZ, Woldenberg Y, Bodner L. Mandibular fractures in children: analysis of 61 cases and review of the literature. *Int J Pediatr Otorhinolaryngol.* 2011;75(1):62–64.
8. Zohrabian VM, Poon CS, Abrahams JJ. Embryology and anatomy of the jaw and dentition. *Semin Ultrasound CT MR.* 2015;36(5):397–406.
9. Dixon A. Prenatal development of the facial skeleton. In: Dixon A, Hoyte D, Ronning O, eds. *Fundamentals of Craniofacial Growth.* New York: CRC Press; 1997.
10. Smartt JM Jr, Low DW, Bartlett SP. The pediatric mandible: I. A primer on growth and development. *Plast Reconstr Surg.* 2005;116(1):14e–23e.
11. Enlow DH, Hans MG. *Essentials of Facial Growth.* Philadelphia, PA: Saunders; 1996. xiv, 303 p. p.
12. Kantomaa T, Rönning O. Growth mechanisms of the mandible. In: Dixon A, Hoyte D, Ronning O, eds. *Fundamentals of Craniofacial Growth.* New York: CRC Press; 1997.
13. Pogrel MA, Dorfman D, Fallah H. The anatomic structure of the inferior alveolar neurovascular bundle in the third molar region. *J Oral Maxillofac Surg.* 2009;67(11):2452–2454.
14. Tinanoff N. Development and developmental anomalies of the teeth. In: Kliegman R, ed. *Nelson Textbook of Pediatrics.* 20th ed. Philadelphia, PA: Saunders; 2016:1768–1769.
15. Bruun R. Vasudavan S. Dental occlusion and its management. In: Rudolph CD, Rudolph AM, Lister GE, et al, eds. *Rudolph's Pediatrics.* 22nd ed. New York, NY: McGraw-Hill; 2011; ch. 376.
16. Smith DM, Bykowski MR, Cray JJ, et al. 215 mandible fractures in 120 children: demographics, treatment, outcomes, and early growth data. *Plast Reconstr Surg.* 2013;131(6):1348–1358.

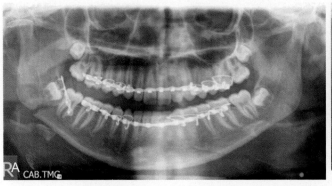
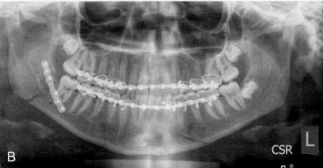

Fig. 2.5.20 (A) 14-year-old female with angle fracture with third molar (#32) that impeded adequate fracture reduction with a Champy technique. Again, note the increased interocclusal distance on right compared with left. (B) This patient returned to the OR on postop day 1, the plate was removed, the third molar extracted, and a superior border plate placed for reduction. Adequate occlusion achieved with small gap at inferior border.

17. Siegel MB, Wetmore RF, Potsic WP, et al. Mandibular fractures in the pediatric patient. *Arch Otolaryngol Head Neck Surg.* 1991;117(5):533–536.
18. Reiner SA, Schwartz DL, Clark KF, Markowitz NR. Accurate radiographic evaluation of mandible fractures. *Arch Otolaryngol Head Neck Surg.* 1989;115(Sept):1083–1085.
19. Chrcanovic BR. Open versus closed reduction: mandibular condylar fractures in children. *Oral Maxillofac Surg.* 2012;16(3):245–255.
20. Zide MF, Kent JN. Indications for open reduction of mandibular condyle fractures. *J Oral Maxillofac Surg.* 1983;41(2):89–98.
21. Zhou HH, Han J, Li ZB. Conservative treatment of bilateral condylar fractures in children: case report and review of the literature. *Int J Pediatr Otorhinolaryngol.* 2014;78(9):1557–1562.
22. Ghasemzadeh A, Mundinger GS, Swanson EW, et al. Treatment of pediatric condylar fractures: a 20-year experience. *Plast Reconstr Surg.* 2015;136(6):1279–1288.
23. Gaddipati R, Ramisetty S, Vura N, et al. Impacted mandibular third molars and their influence on mandibular angle and condyle fractures – a retrospective study. *J Craniomaxillofac Surg.* 2014;42(7):1102–1105.
24. Naghipur S, Shah A, Elgazzar RF. Does the presence or position of lower third molars alter the risk of mandibular angle or condylar fractures? *J Oral Maxillofac Surg.* 2014;72(9):1766–1772.
25. Antic S, Saveljic I, Nikolic D, et al. Does the presence of an unerupted lower third molar influence the risk of mandibular angle and condylar fractures? *Int J Oral Maxillofac Surg.* 2016;45(5):588–592.
26. Tiwari A, Lata J, Mishra M. Influence of the impacted mandibular third molars on fractures of the mandibular angle and condyle – a prospective clinical study. *J Oral Biol Craniofac Res.* 2016;6(3):227–230.
27. Al-Moraissi EA, Ellis E 3rd. What method for management of unilateral mandibular angle fractures has the lowest rate of postoperative complications? A systematic review and meta-analysis. *J Oral Maxillofac Surg.* 2014;72(11):2197–2211.
28. Eppley BL. Use of resorbable plates and screws in pediatric facial fractures. *J Oral Maxillofac Surg.* 2005;63(3):385–391.
29. Wheeler J, Phillips J. Pediatric facial fractures and potential long-term growth disturbances. *Craniomaxillofac Trauma Reconstr.* 2011;4(1):43–52.
30. Kaban LB, Bouchard C, Troulis MJ. A protocol for management of temporomandibular joint ankylosis in children. *J Oral Maxillofac Surg.* 2009;67(9):1966–1978.
31. Rottgers SA, Decesare G, Chao M, et al. Outcomes in pediatric facial fractures: early follow-up in 177 children and classification scheme. *J Craniofac Surg.* 2011;22(4):1260–1265.

3.1

Reconstruction of Full-Thickness Frontocranial Defects

S. Anthony Wolfe, Mark W. Stalder

BACKGROUND

Paul Manson, Bill Crawley, and Jack Hoopes in 1986 published a paper entitled "Frontal cranioplasty: risk factors and choice of cranial vault reconstructive material."[1] In that paper they examined their series of 42 cranioplasties, 25 of which were treated with methylmethacrylate (MMA), and 17 with autogenous bone. Both groups had about 60% preexisting infections.

In the MMA group, there were no infections, and in the autogenous bone group there were four infections (23%). One would draw the conclusion from their data that an acrylic cranioplasty would be the treatment of choice.

I [S.A.W] was asked to write the commentary for their paper, and I said that my experience with 73 autogenous cranioplasties differed from theirs: there were no infections. I had no experience with MMA to compare, since I did not use alloplastic materials, but still felt that autogenous bone grafts were the material of choice.

As of 2017, our series of autogenous cranioplasties had grown to 176, including 72 preexisting defects, and 104 "primary cranioplasties" wherein a large parietal bone flap was removed, split through the diploic space, and half replaced as a cranioplasty, and the other to serve as a large autogenous bone graft. In 23 cases, split rib was used, in 6 cases iliac bone, and the remainder were split calvarial. In this entire series, there have been no infections, and no complications associated with the harvesting of the bone grafts.

Since our series extends over a time period of 42 years (1975–2017), I think we can confidently support the assertion made in 1986 that autogenous bone grafts are indeed the material of choice, the "gold standard."

Hydroxyapatite/Methylmethacrylate

Methylmethacrylate is an alloplastic substance that has long been used to reconstruct small to moderate cranial defects. It is mixed prior to use to form a moldable putty, and has a substantial exothermic reaction while hardening which must be taken into account when applying the material to tissue *in situ*. It has substantial tensile strength and compression resistance, is cheap, and relatively easy to use. However, as a foreign substance, it provides a nidus for infection, and even those surgeons with extensive experience using MMA for cranioplasty procedures recommend against its use in proximity to the frontal sinus due to unacceptably high risk for infection.[2]

Hydroxyapatite is an inorganic phosphate-based compound that forms a hard cement after it is cured, similar in that with regard to MMA. This material, too, has limitations with regard to the size of the defect it is reliably able to reconstruct. It demonstrates superior osseointegration relative to MMA, a minimal inflammatory response, as well as some degree of osseoconduction that would theoretically mitigate some of the infection risk associated with alloplastic materials.[3,4] A distinct advantage is that there is no associated exothermic reaction, and associated risk of thermal damage to surrounding tissue. However, as with MMA, there is compelling evidence that hydroxyapatite should never be used in close proximity to the frontal sinus due to significantly increased risks of bacterial seeding and subsequent infection.[5]

In 2003 Moriera-Gonzalez et al. conducted a large study analyzing the clinical outcomes in long-term follow-up between autogenous bone, methylmethacrylate, and hydroxyapatite. Infection and implant exposure were the most common complications seen in those patients treated with methylmethacrylate and hydroxyapatite, and occurred in 13.3% and 22.4% of these cases respectively. In comparison, the rate of infection and exposure seen with autologous bone was significantly lower at 7.1% and 1.3% respectively.[6]

Titanium Mesh

Titanium is a commonly used material in the fixation of bony fractures and reconstructions, and is reasonably well tolerated by the body. Typically, for cranioplasty procedures, it is used in the form of a moldable mesh, which can be cut, bent, and fitted to cover the relevant defect. In this form it has been used successfully (particularly in conjunction with free tissue transfer for improved soft tissue coverage) for reconstruction of large frontocranial defects.[7,8] It is, however, still a foreign substance, and thus prone to the complications inherent to such materials. Infection risk remains higher than that of autogenous bone, there is an ever-present risk of attenuation of the overlying native soft tissue envelope (especially in large reconstructions), and when used in context of irradiated tissue the results will be predictable and poor.

Polyetheretherketone (PEEK)

Polyetheretherketone (PEEK) is biocompatible, inert, and reported to have similar mechanical properties to bone. Importantly, it can be formed to precisely fit frontocranial defects preoperatively based off 3-dimensional CT scans. For these reasons PEEK has been growing in popularity based on the arguments that these implants save operative time, prevent donor site morbidity, and result in improved aesthetic outcomes. While early results seem to indicate better outcomes relative to other alloplastic materials, clinical series are limited in scope (between 5 and 38 patients), and follow-up times are probably inadequate at this point (from 6 to 24 months) to provide an accurate representation of the potential for long-term success.[9–13] There does appear to be an implant failure rate of up to 27% reported with PEEK, typically due to exposure and/or infection.[9,10,12,14] A few direct comparison studies with PEEK cranioplasties have suggested a lower complication rate relative to autogenous bone, however these were small series with short follow-up times, and this was clearly not consistent with our experience.[15]

Autogenous Nonvascularized Bone

Through our experience over the past 41 years, autogenous bone grafts are generally the most appropriate material with which to reconstruct the frontocranial region. Grafts can be readily harvested from split calvarium, split rib, or iliac crest cortical bone. The ability of these grafts to revascularize and consolidate after reconstruction allows them to become resistant to infection over the long term. While other published experiences vary in their quality and results, we have experienced zero graft failures as a result of infection or extrusion. The notion is commonly put forth that these nonvascularized grafts are prone to significant resorption, but again, this has not been the case in our experience.

The most comprehensive recent investigation to date regarding the use of autogenous bone for cranioplasties was published by Fearon et al.[16] Their 14-year series of 96 patients had zero incidences of postoperative infections resulting in loss of the cranioplasty graft, all of which were performed with split calvarium. Only one patient experienced clinically significant graft resorption that required operative revision. Additionally, their extensive review of the literature concluded that alloplastic cranioplasty grafts demonstrated a nearly fivefold higher infection rate relative to autogenous bone grafts. They also noted that should infection occur with an autogenous graft, it can often be treated with drainage alone, as opposed to the near universal need to remove an alloplastic implant under similar circumstances.

Free Tissue Transfer

Rodriguez, and a number of other craniofacial microsurgeons, have used the fibula extensively to reconstruct limited frontal and zygomatic defects (the scapula has been used to a lesser degree as well), but there is no vascularized bone flap that can be used for the repair of a large defect. The latissimus flap is an excellent option to provide well-vascularized muscle capable of nourishing free bone grafts for reconstructing larger bony defects, and several fasciocutaneous perforator flaps have been used in this regard with good success as well. For patients with suspect soft tissue coverage, particularly the irradiated, free flaps must be used preliminarily in order to prepare the recipient site for the bone graft.[7,8] This can also be performed concomitantly with a bone graft dependent upon the specific clinical scenario, however we have preferred to stage these procedures in order to allow the sometimes very significant swelling of the free flap to resolve prior to placement of the graft.

CASE EXAMPLES

Case 1

Just before his first birthday this boy was bitten by a Boxer dog and sustained a loss of most of his right parietal bone, dura, and a good bit of parietal lobe (Fig. 3.1.1). Excellent neurosurgical care debrided nonvital brain and repaired the dura with an artificial dural substitute. Because of the lack of native dura, spontaneous regeneration of the bone was unlikely. Three months later, at 14 months of age, a switch cranioplasty was performed, taking the entire left parietal bone to replace what was missing on the right. This left the left side devoid of bone, but with healthy dura and pericranium. Several fragments of his skull, which had been saved and frozen from the original operation, along with a large segment of rBMP-2 impregnated in collagen sponge, were placed between the dura and the pericranium. At 2 years of age the boy had an intact skull and only a mild left hemiplegia.

Case 2

This 19-year-old male lost control of his bicycle on a wet bridge and was run over by a truck (Fig. 3.1.2). After debridement of his compound right fronto-orbital defect, along with complete removal of the remnants of his frontal sinus (proper neurosurgical treatment), he was left with the defect shown, which was easily repaired with split calvarial bone from adjacent parietal bone.

Case 3

This 22-year-old man suffered a comminuted displaced but not compound frontal fracture in an automobile accident. A dural repair was

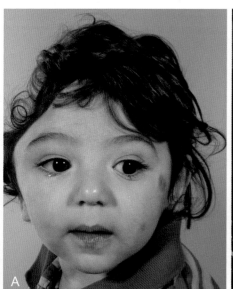
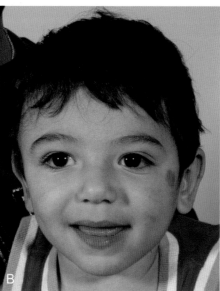

Fig. 3.1.1 One-year-old boy attacked by a dog, suffering severe trauma of his right parietal bone, dura, and parietal lobe pictured after initial treatment by the neurosurgical team (A). (C–E) The cranial defect was reconstructed in a delayed fashion using autogenous contralateral parietal bone in a switch cranioplasty technique. The donor site was supported by healthy osteogenic dura and preserved pericranium, and bone was regenerated with the assistance of bone morphogenic protein. Less than one year later (B) he had an intact skull.   *Continued*

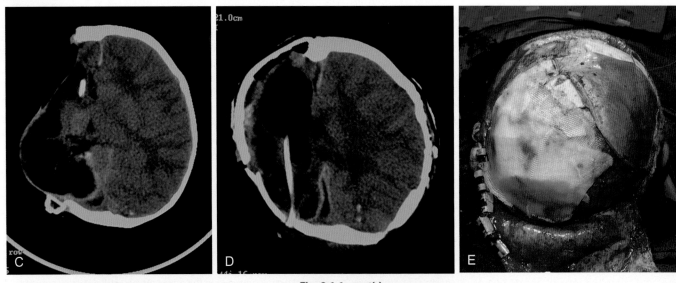

Fig. 3.1.1, cont'd

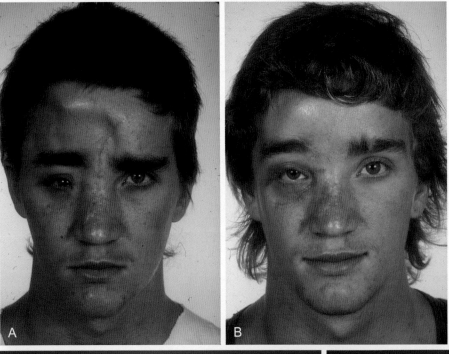

Fig. 3.1.2 Nineteen-year-old male involved in bicycle versus motor vehicle accident resulting in a right fronto-orbital defect. (A,C) Before and (B,D) after reconstruction.

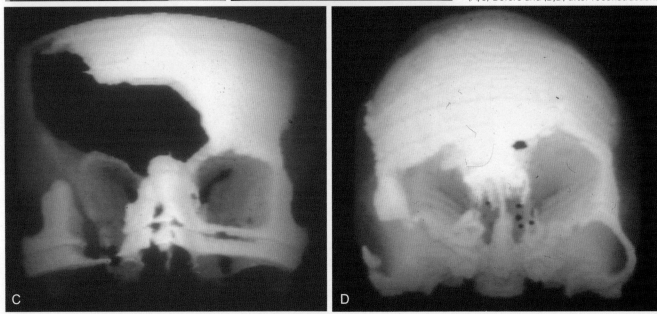

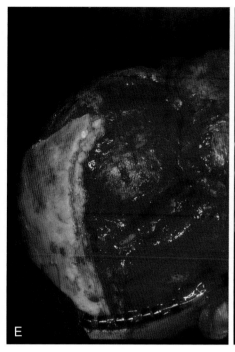
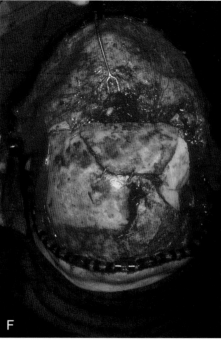

Fig. 3.1.2, cont'd (E–F) He was initially treated with cranialization of the frontal sinus, and then the bony defect was reconstructed using autogenous split calvarial graft in a delayed manner.

performed along with reduction of the fractures. The neurosurgeon felt that due to brain swelling, he could not dissect the anterior cranial base and cranialize the frontal sinus.

Initially his wounds healed well, but after about 6 months small abscesses began to crop up along his coronal suture line. These were drained and he was treated with antibiotics, but the process continued to smolder on over the next year. Finally, the coronal incision was opened and the frontal bone was found floating on a bed of epidural purulence, and was removed. After a wait of 6 months, a successful cranioplasty was performed using split rib (Fig. 3.1.3).

Case 4

Female patient involved in a remote motor vehicle collision in which she suffered fronto-orbital trauma, and lost her left eye. She arrived in our office with a moderately enophthalmic prosthesis on the left, and significant hypoglobus and proptosis of her right eye (Fig. 3.1.4). A CT scan revealed a mucocele extending from her frontal sinus into her right orbit, resulting in the ocular malposition. She underwent exploration of bilateral orbits, and the mucocele was exenterated. Cancellous iliac bone graft was used to pack and obliterate the frontal sinus along with BMP (due to the large size of the sinus), and cortical graft was used to reconstruct the outer table of the sinus and the roof of the orbit on the right side.

Case 5

Male patient involved in a pedestrian versus automobile accident. He suffered multiple facial fractures, including involvement of the frontal sinus. He was treated at a different facility with open reduction and internal fixation through the frontal laceration. Ultimately he developed a draining osteocutaneous fistula at the site of original injury (Fig. 3.1.5). We performed exploration, debridement, and removal of hardware and methylmethacrylate from the infected area, in addition to obliteration of the frontal sinus. This resulted in a supraorbital defect. The sinus cavity was packed with cancellous iliac bone, and the outer table of the frontal bone was reconstructed with a cortical iliac bone graft.

Case 6

Male patient involved in a remote motorcycle accident in India in which he suffered extensive frontocranial trauma. When seen in our clinic he had a 15 x 10 cm bony defect in the left temporoparietal calvarium, as well as a malpositioned zygoma and exotropia on the left side (Fig. 3.1.6). He underwent reconstruction of the bony defect using split rib grafts fixated with surgical wires. BMP was placed into the periosteal sleeves from which the ribs were harvested.

Case 7

Male patient who sustained a gunshot wound, with loss of his left eye, left frontal bone, and part of his frontal lobe (Fig. 3.1.7). Split calvarial bone graft was harvested from the ipsilateral side, and contoured to fit the frontal bone defect. He also received an ocular prosthesis, and lower lid canthopexy in order to improve the appearance of the injured periorbital soft tissue.

CONCLUSIONS

The following are some of the lessons learned and important takeaways from over 40 years of experience performing autogenous frontocranial reconstruction:

Ease of usage. It is certainly easier to place a prefabricated alloplastic implant than to harvest autogenous bone, shape it, and fix it to rigidly span the defect. The solution to this is for surgeons to develop the skills necessary to harvest rib, cranial bone, and iliac bone. Paul Tessier won the James Barrett Brown award for the second time for his 2005 Supplement to *Plastic and Reconstructive Surgery* on the tools and techniques of harvesting autogenous bone.[17] Using the techniques described in this monograph, we had no complications associated with the harvesting of bone.

Infection and extrusion. Once primary healing has taken place, an autogenous cranioplasty becomes vascularized and fully integrated, and has no chance of developing a late infection. In contrast, late infection is the primary reason for failure of alloplastic cranioplasty implants. Additionally, autogenous bone will not cause atrophy of

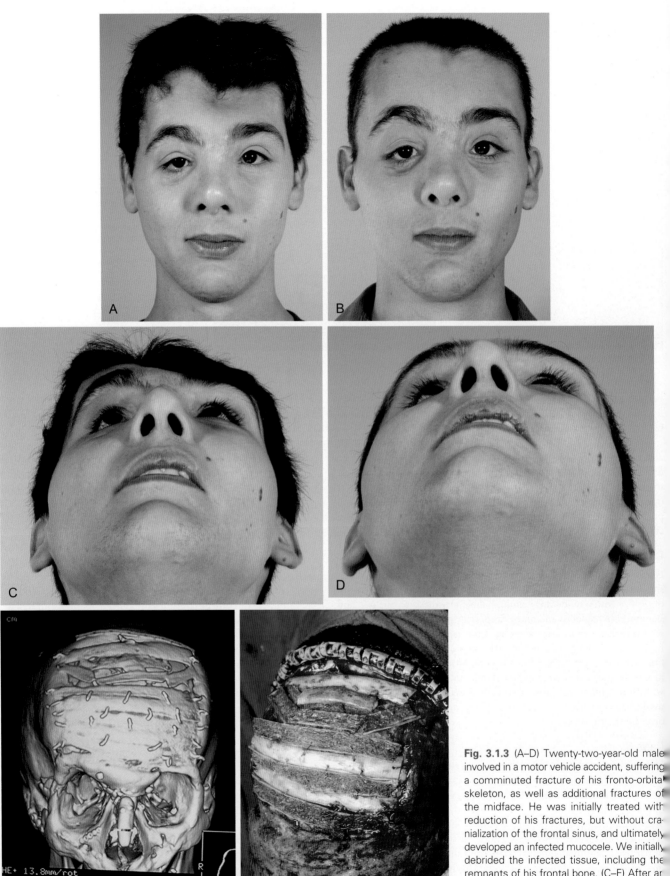

Fig. 3.1.3 (A–D) Twenty-two-year-old male involved in a motor vehicle accident, suffering a comminuted fracture of his fronto-orbital skeleton, as well as additional fractures of the midface. He was initially treated with reduction of his fractures, but without cranialization of the frontal sinus, and ultimately developed an infected mucocele. We initially debrided the infected tissue, including the remnants of his frontal bone. (C–F) After an additional 6 months' delay, we performed a split-rib reconstruction of the bony defect and restored near premorbid contour.

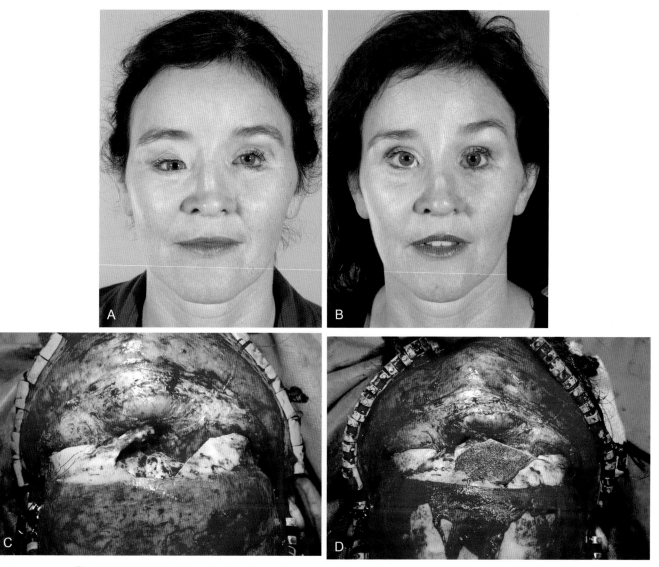

Fig. 3.1.4 Middle-aged female remotely involved in a motor vehicle collision, suffering severe fronto-orbital trauma and loss of her left eye. On presentation to our practice (A) she had a mucocele extending into her right orbit. (C–D) She was treated with exenteration of the mucocele and obliteration of the frontal sinus with cancellous iliac bone graft and bone morphogenic protein. A cortical iliac bone graft was used to reconstruct the outer table and roof of the right orbit. Postoperatively (B) she demonstrated improved frontal contour and position of the right globe.

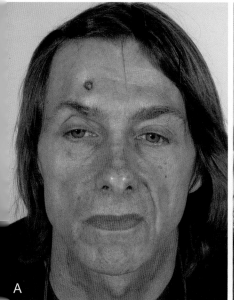
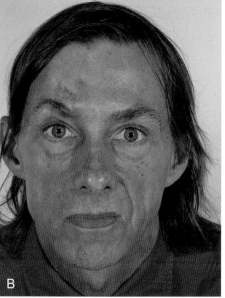

Fig. 3.1.5 Middle-aged male patient involved in pedestrian versus motor vehicle accident, suffering fracture of the frontal bone involving the sinus. He was initially treated elsewhere with internal fixation and methylmethacrylate reconstruction of the frontal bone. He presented to our practice with a draining fistula (A). We debrided the infected alloplastic materials, obliterated the frontal sinus with iliac cancellous bone graft (C), and reconstructed the supraorbital region with cortical iliac bone graft (D). Postoperatively (B) he has good fronto-orbital contour, and has been relieved of the chronic infection.   *Continued*

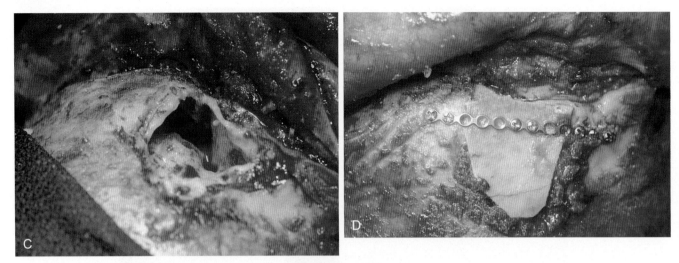

Fig. 3.1.5, cont'd

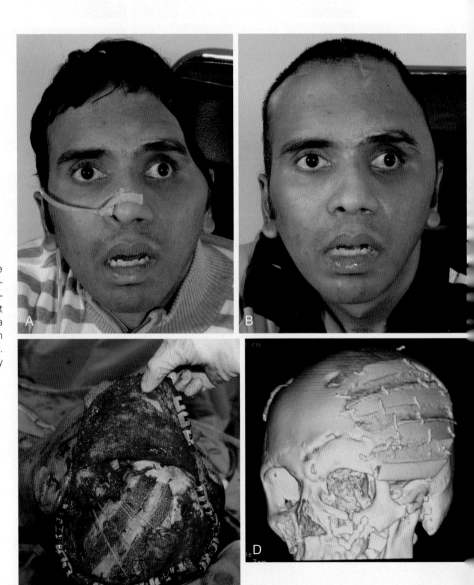

Fig. 3.1.6 Male patient involved in remote motorcycle accident, suffering extensive frontocranial injuries. On presentation to our practice he had a large bony defect in the left temoporoparietal calvarium, resulting in a severe aesthetic deformity (A). Reconstruction was accomplished using split rib grafts (C–D). Postoperatively the patient had significantly improved cranial contour (B).

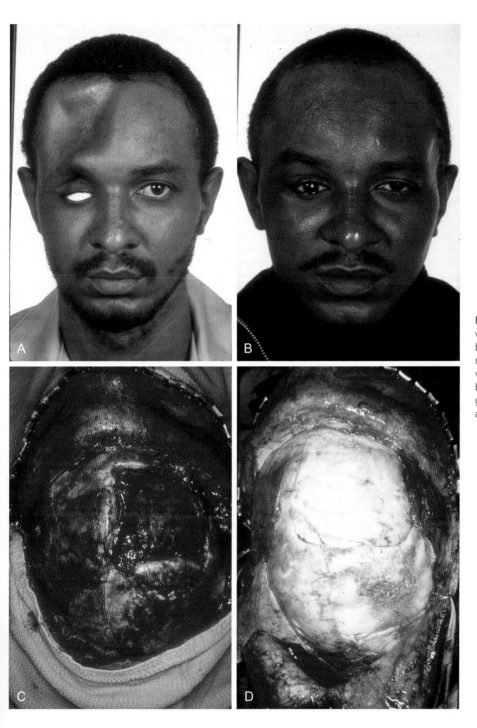

Fig. 3.1.7 Male patient who suffered a gunshot wound, with loss of his left eye, left frontal bone, and part of his frontal lobe (A). Delayed reconstruction was undertaken using split calvarial bone graft from the ipsilateral parietal bone (C–D). Postoperatively he benefitted from greatly improved frontal contour (B), as well as an ocular prosthesis.

the overlying soft tissue, which is too frequently the case with large alloplastic implants, ultimately resulting in extrusion and failure of the reconstruction.

Resorption. This is the complication most commonly reported in association with nonvascularized autogenous bone cranioplasties, with rates of resorption varying wildly among available studies, anywhere from 2% to 32% in adults, and 20% to 81.8% in pediatric patients.[6,18–24] If the bone graft is placed properly – with good contact with adjacent bone and rigid fixation – then no significant resorption will be noted. These outcomes are most certainly due to aberrant variations in surgical technique, disparate determinations of the severity and clinical relevance of resorption, and vast differences in postoperative follow-up times.

Management of the frontal sinus. In all cases where there is a full-thickness frontocranial defect with exposure of the frontal sinus, the sinus should be completely cranialized, i.e. removed down to the base of the skull where the duct passes into the nose. The ducts should be plugged with pericranial graft and a small calvarial bone graft.

Free tissue transfer. When planning the reconstruction of any frontocranial defect, the quality of the overlying soft tissue must be taken into consideration, and must provide adequate vascularized coverage for placement of underlying bone grafts, or certainly any alloplastic materials that would be considered. Transfer of free muscle or fasciocutaneous flaps is commonly required in the event of radiation-damaged tissue, and may be needed in other circumstances of severely scarred, atrophied, or otherwise absent soft tissue.

EXPERT COMMENTARY

The authors make a compelling argument for the use of autogenous bone in frontal cranial reconstruction, and back it up with their series and that of Fearon (2017) [1] . Their technical skill makes the procedure seem straightforward, efficacious, and safe.

To begin, the paper we published in 1986 [2] had two groups of patients: one, patients who were deemed safe for alloplastic cranioplasty (safe frontal and ethmoid sinuses and nose, and good soft tissue and bone partition between the nose and sinuses and the intracranial cavity); and two, patients who were of higher risk and therefore bone was used because it was logically felt to be safer in higher-risk environments. Therefore, in the bone group, there was a higher risk of infection as they were selected, and not randomized.

I do not personally believe there is substantial difference in any of the alloplastic materials except for two things: one, titanium mesh alone seems to have less infectious problems than any of the other materials for some reason (I do note that secondary traumatic injury to mesh alone has resulted in inbending of the mesh, as it is not substantial enough to withstand point trauma); two, the use of hydroxyapatite is plagued by infections, as it somehow attracts *Staphylococcus epidermidis* organisms and then drains until removed. The other problem with hydroxyapatite is that it fragments, and is not good protection [3–4].

In my experience, nothing is stronger than methylmethacrylate cured on metallic mesh so that it resists splintering with secondary trauma, and it is certainly stronger than any of the other alloplastics. Bone partially takes, is revascularized *only* at its periphery, and often has contour defects and holes noticeable at the time of secondary reconstruction.

The main problem with autogenous bone is that it is prone to variable resorption and irregularity; no study has ever tested its strength following its "take," which always involved partial resorption. No one who has done large numbers of repeat craniofacial operations would deny that one can sometimes see partially resorbed bone with "holes" and thin bone of unpredictable protective strength. No studies exist that quantify the strength of bone cranioplasty, assess their relative rates of bone resorption, and their final (20-year) contour results. Bone is never completely revascularized, but only its outer surface is penetrated for a short distance by vessels, which makes it resist infection. The same is true in porous artificial materials, where penetration of 100–200 micrometers of the surface by vessels resists infection.

While I agree that thinning of skin can occasionally be observed over alloplastic cranioplasty, most of these issues are thin areas of scalp which were potential problems before the cranioplasty. The demanding aesthetics of the frontal region argue for artificial material being the most predictable aesthetic result, whose long-term durability is sufficient most times for the life of the patient.

What we now see in all types of cranioplasty, regrettably, is less skilled surgeons using expensive preformed implants; their lack of experience is generating frequent complications giving cranioplasty a poor reputation. In neurosurgery, it is considered a "minor" procedure, and assigned to the most junior residents who work alone with understandable results. Individuals like Chad Gordon, working with neurosurgeons consistently on a cranioplasty and scalp reconstruction service, have dramatically improved the results of cranioplasty and made scalp safe for artificial materials.

References

1. Fearon JA, Griner D, Ditthakasem K, Herbert M. Autogenous bone reconstruction of large secondary skull defects. *Plast Reconstr Surg.* 2017;139(2):427–438.
2. Manson PN, Crawley WA, Hoopes JE. Frontal cranioplasty: risk factors and choice of cranial vault reconstructive material. *Plast Reconstr Surg.* 1986;76:888–904.
3. Matic D, Manson P. Biomechanical analysis of hydroxyapatite cement cranioplasty. *J Craniofac Surg.* 2004;15(3):415–422.
4. Reddy S, Khalifian S, Flores J, et al. Clinical outcomes in cranioplasty: risk factors and choice of reconstructive material. *Plast Reconstr Surg.* 2014;133(4):864–873.

REFERENCES

1. Manson PN, Crawley WA, Hoopes JE. Frontal cranioplasty: risk factors and choice of cranial vault reconstructive material. *Plast Reconstr Surg.* 1986;77:888–904.
2. Marchac D, Greensmith A. Long-term experience with methylmethacrylate cranioplasty in craniofacial surgery. *J Plast Reconstr Aesthet Surg.* 2008;61:744–752.
3. Eppley BL, Holier L, Stal S. Hydroxyapatite cranioplasty: 2. Clinical experience with a new quick-setting material. *J Craniofac Surg.* 2003;14(2):209–214.
4. Matic DB, Manson PM. Biomechanical analysis of hydroxyapatite cement cranioplasty. *J Craniofac Surg.* 2004;15(3):415–423.
5. Wong RK, Gandolfi BM, St. Hilaire H, et al. Complications of hydroxyapatite bone cement in secondary pediatric craniofacial reconstruction. *J Craniofac Surg.* 2011;22(1):247–251.
6. Moreira-Gonzalez A, Jackson IT, Miyawaki T, et al. Clinical outcome in cranioplasty: critical review in long term follow up. *J Craniomaxillofac Surg.* 2003;14:144–153.
7. St. Hilaire H, Mithani SK, Taylor J, et al. Restoring the failed cranioplasty: nonanatomical titanium mesh with perforator flap. *Plast Reconstr Surg.* 2009;123(6):1813–1817.
8. Fisher M, Dorafshar A, Bojovic B, et al. The evolution of critical concepts in aesthetic microsurgical reconstruction. *Plast Reconstr Surg.* 2012;130(2):389–398.
9. O'Reilly EB, Barnett S, Madden C, et al. Computed-tomography modeled polyether ether ketone (PEEK) implants in revision cranioplasty. *J Plast Reconstr Aesthet Surg.* 2015;68:329–338.
10. Thien A, King NKK, Ang BT, et al. Comparison of polyetheretherketone and titanium cranioplasty after decompressive craniectomy. *World Neurosurg.* 2015;83(2):176–180.
11. Rammos CK, Cayci C, Castro-Garcia JA, et al. Patient-specific polyetheretherketone implants for repair of craniofacial defects. *J Craniofac Surg.* 2015;26(3):631–633.
12. Jonkergouw J, van de Vijfeijken SECM, Nout E, et al. Outcome in patient-specific PEEK cranioplasty; a two-center cohort study of 40 implants. *J Craniomaxillofac Surg.* 2016;44:1266–1272.
13. Jalbert F, Boetto S, Nadon F, et al. One-step primary reconstruction for complex craniofacial resection with PEEK custom-made implants. *J Craniomaxillofac Surg.* 2014;42:141–148.
14. Mundinger GS, Latham K, Friedrich J, et al. Management of the repeatedly failed cranioplasty following large postdecompressive craniectomy: establishing the efficacy of staged free latissimus dorsi transfer/tissue expansion/custom polyetheretherketone implant reconstruction. *J Craniofac Surg.* 2016;27(8):1971–1977.
15. Gilardino MS, Karunanayake M, Al-Humsi T, et al. A comparison and cost analysis of cranioplasty techniques: autologous bone versus custom computer-generated implants. *J Craniofac Surg.* 2015;26(1):113–117.
16. Fearon JA, Griner D, Ditthakasem K, Herbert M. Autogenous bone reconstruction of large secondary skull defects. *Plast Reconstr Surg.* 2017;139(2):427–438.
17. Tessier P, Kawamoto H, Matthews D, et al. Autogenous bone grafts and bone substitutes-tools and techniques: I. A 20,000-case experience in maxillofacial and craniofacial surgery. *Plast Reconstr Surg.* 2005;116(5 suppl):6S–24S, discussion 92S–94S.
18. Grant GA, Jolley M, Ellenbogen RG, et al. Failure of autologous bone-assisted cranioplasty following decompressive craniectomy in children and adolescents. *J Neurosurg.* 2004;100(2 supplPediatrics):163–168.
19. Iwama T, Yamada J, Imai S, et al. The use of frozen autogenous bone flaps in delayed cranioplasty revisited. *Neurosurgery.* 2003;52:591–596, discussion 595–596.

20. Pochon JP, Kloti J. Cranioplasty for acquired skull defects in children – a comparison between autologous material and methylmethacrylate 1974–1990. *Eur J Pediatr Surg.* 1991;1:199–201.
21. Bobinski L, Koskinen LO, Lindvall P. Complications following cranioplasty using autologous bone or polymethylmethacrylate – retrospective experience from a single center. *Clin Neurol Neurosurg.* 2013;115:1788–1791.
22. Schoekler B, Trummer M. Prediction parameters of bone flap resorption following cranioplasty with autologous bone. *Clin Neurol Neurosurg.* 2014;120:64–67.
23. Schuss P, Vatter H, Oszvald A, et al. Bone flap resorption: risk factors for the development of a long-term complication following cranioplasty after decompressive craniectomy. *J Neurotrauma.* 2013;30:91–95.
24. Bowers CA, Riva-Cambrin J, Hertzler DA 2nd, Walker ML. Risk factors and rates of bone flap resorption in pediatric patients after decompressive craniectomy for traumatic brain injury. *J Neurosurg Pediatr.* 2013;11:526–532.

Pediatric Cranial Reconstruction

Fan Liang, Christian J. Vercler, Steven R. Buchman

BACKGROUND

Pediatric head trauma is a major source of morbidity, resulting in 600,000 emergency room visits annually within the United States.[1,2] Between 10% and 30% of head traumas are associated with calvarial fractures,[1,3] and of those greater than 50% have neurological injury.[4] While the overall mortality rate from cranial fractures is low (2.9%), cranial trauma still accounts for 7000 deaths per year in the United States.[3] The most frequently cited causes for calvarial fractures that require operative treatment include objects hitting the head (48.2%), followed by falls (13.8%), and motor vehicle collisions (MVC) (10.3%).[1,3,5] There are clear sex- and age-associated trends: boys have twice as many calvarial fractures as girls and young children (<5 years) are injured predominantly by falls while older children are more likely to sustain head trauma from collisions and sports.[1,3]

Among children less than one year of age, nonaccidental head trauma (NAHT) is the leading cause of death.[6] Estimates of the prevalence of NAHT are almost certainly underreported, with studies showing anywhere from 24 to 47 cases per 100,000 children less than a year old.[7–10] Children suffering from NAHT are predominantly male (61%), less than 6 months of age (55%), and African American (47%).[10] Infants and toddlers with a history of abuse frequently will have long-standing neurological compromise that extends into adulthood.[11] Despite significant effort on the part of practitioners to diagnose NAHT, one study showed that one-third of all cases of abuse go unrecognized.[12] Of the children who belong to the unrecognized NAHT group, four out of five deaths can be prevented by earlier diagnosis of abuse.[12] Children that are discharged with a missed diagnosis of NAHT frequently sustain further abuse, leading to rehospitalization or death.[12] Abuse is missed more frequently in white children than minorities, in two-parent vs. single-parent families, and in children presenting before the age of 6 months, likely secondary to evaluation bias on the part of practitioners.[12]

Diagnosis of nonaccidental head trauma is particularly difficult because the symptoms are nonspecific (vomiting, fever, irritability), the patients are preverbal, and the history surrounding the trauma can be misleading.[13] Furthermore, a false-positive diagnosis of child abuse can cause significant grievance to the family and child and result in dissolution of the practitioner–patient relationship. Several studies have attempted to isolate findings to differentiate nonaccidental from accidental head trauma. A systematic review on clinical and radiographic characteristics associated with pediatric head trauma found that children with NAHT had increased rates of cerebral ischemia, skull fractures, subdural hematoma, retinal hemorrhage, rib and long bone fractures, seizures, apnea at time of presentation, and inadequate or inconsistent histories.[13] Despite these findings, the authors acknowledge the overall nonspecificity of presenting symptoms and history and recommend a holistic and discerning approach to evaluating all cases of pediatric trauma. All patients should be evaluated for bruises on the head and face when they present with nonspecific symptoms such as vomiting, fever, and irritability. Dedicated pediatric radiologists are also better able to discover radiographic evidence of skeletal trauma than nonspecialized practitioners.[12]

Nonoperative management is typically advocated whenever possible for calvarial fractures in children, given the cranium's increased capacity for remodeling and healing at this age.[14,15] A large retrospective review of 897 children at a Level I trauma center noted that the overwhelming majority of patients with acute skull fractures were managed nonoperatively (86.1%).[1] Of the patients who did undergo operative intervention, more than half did so to address underlying traumatic brain injury. Only 6.5% of all pediatric skull fracture patients had surgical intervention to address the fracture in isolation; the children who underwent surgery did so primarily for depressed or open skull fractures, as well as for frontal sinus fractures or injuries with intracerebral processes.[1]

While there is copious data on management of acute head trauma in adults and children, there is less consensus on management principles for delayed calvarial reconstruction in the pediatric population. Long-term outcomes in managing rare complications such as growing skull fractures or follow-up for nonautologous cranioplasty is lacking. Here we seek to consolidate the evidence supporting indications for pediatric reconstruction, and offer the authors' management principles in dealing with complex defects.

CLINICAL PRESENTATION

Pediatric calvarial fractures are classified by pattern (linear or comminuted, depressed or nondepressed, open or closed), and location (flat bone or skull base). Ninety percent of all pediatric skull fractures are linear, and approximately 15%–30% of these are associated with intracranial injuries.[16–19] Linear skull fractures frequently advance to, but do not violate, suture lines. Most children with linear skull fractures will have overlying subgaleal hematomas (Fig. 3.2.1). Comminuted fractures are a constellation of linear fractures. When found within the occipital or basilar regions, these are particularly concerning for repetitive or NAHT.

Lacerations with associated skull depressions warrant surgical exploration for foreign bodies, cerebrospinal leak, and injury to the dura or underlying brain parenchyma. Depressed skull fractures are commonly associated with intracranial injury (30%) and have an increased incidence of posttraumatic seizure and infection.[18,20] Some children with depressed skull fractures will present with a palpable bony step-off or bony defect. Depressed skull fractures are clinically significant when displacement of the inner table is greater than one thickness of the bone; 33% of these will have dural lacerations. In the newborn or very young infant, depressed skull fractures are frequently referred to as ping-pong fractures, and can be managed nonoperatively with an obstetrical vacuum extractor.[21] All depressed skull fractures, basilar skull fractures, linear skull fractures with greater than 3 mm diastasis, and fractures with intracranial injury, warrant evaluation by a pediatric neurosurgeon.

Several studies have attempted to risk stratify children who sustain head trauma into those who require hospitalization for observation or further radiological workup. Patients with a normal neurological

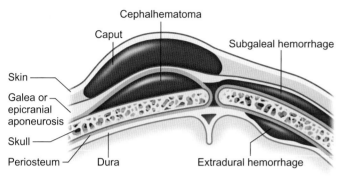

Fig. 3.2.1 Cephalhematomas are seen frequently with birth trauma and do not cross suture lines. The majority of subgaleal hematomas (90%) result from vacuum-assisted delivery and rupture of the emissary veins. Subgaleal hematomas can also be seen, however, in head trauma with associated skull fracture or intracranial hemorrhage and does cross suture lines. The growth of the hematoma can be insidious and lead to hemorrhagic shock. (From http://www.childneurologyfoundation.org/wp-content/uploads/2015/08/GillesFigure4.jpg.)

exam in the setting of head trauma have less than a 5% chance of intracranial injury.[22] Of those, only 1% require neurosurgical intervention.[23] Current guidelines stipulate that children with an isolated, narrow (<3 mm diastasis) linear skull fracture and no focal neurological findings can be discharged without hospitalization.[22,24] Follow-up studies have shown that this subset of patients is at low risk for complications, but national practices have yet to adopt the recommendations for direct discharge from the emergency room, resulting in avoidable healthcare expenditures.[19–21,24,25] After discharge, the patient should be monitored at home for the first 24 hours following injury, and be assessed overnight for signs of vomiting or decreased arousal. Any neurological symptoms such as increased somnolence, seizure, persistent nausea or vomiting, coordination difficulties, confusion, or visual disturbance, warrants a repeat workup. A recent algorithm published by Blackwood and colleagues for evaluation and management of blunt head trauma (excluding NAHT) is depicted in Fig. 3.2.2.[22]

In infants, growing skull fractures (GSF), leptomeningeal cysts, or posttraumatic cephaloceles are a group of rare but serious complications that result from traumatic head injury with associated dural tears. Half of all cases are seen in children less than 12 months of age, and 90% of cases are found in children less than 3 years of age. Diagnosis of GSF is frequently missed as it is frequently seen in linear fractures in a closed head injury, and symptoms may present in a delayed fashion. Swelling, cephalhematoma or bony depressions at the site of the defect are also commonly noted.[26] The challenge arises in risk stratifying patients with high probability of developing GSF or leptomeningeal cysts, prior to irreversible brain damage. Clinical presentation of GSF is varied;

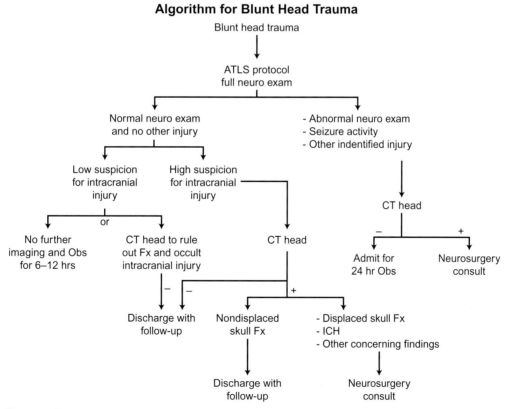

Algorithm for Blunt Head Trauma

Fig. 3.2.2 Management algorithm for simple, isolated skull fractures. Children with depressed skull fractures, penetrating head trauma, basilar skull fractures, polytrauma, pneumocephalus, neurological deficits on examination, and those suspected of sustaining NAHT are excluded from this algorithm. Neurological exam was considered normal if there were no witnessed seizures and no localizable neurological deficits. (Reproduced from Blackwood BP, Bean JF, Sadecki-Lund C, et al. Observation for isolated traumatic skull fractures in the pediatric population: unnecessary and costly. J Pediatr Surg 2016;51(4):654–658.)

children can be asymptomatic or profoundly impaired with spasticity, seizures, hemiparesis, or visual disturbances.[26]

Current guidelines for early diagnosis of GSF include the following parameters: (1) age <5 years with cephalohematoma; (2) bony diastasis greater than 4 mm; (3) underlying parenchymal injury; and (4) contrast MRI demonstrating dural tear and brain herniation.[26,27] Definitive treatment relies on a successful duraplasty and cranioplasty, performed within a month of trauma to mitigate the effects on underlying brain parenchyma.[27] Strict follow-up in patients who are managed conservatively is paramount, with care taken to document new neurological symptoms or an expanding scalp mass.

Neuroimaging

All pediatric patients with major head trauma require evaluation with a head computed tomography (CT) scan. For children with minor head trauma, current recommendations for ordering a head CT are based off of the Pediatric Emergency Care Research Network (PECARN) guidelines.[28] The PECARN flow-chart is derived from a validated study that identifies children at very low risk of traumatic brain injury using clinical examination findings and Glasgow Coma Scores (Fig. 3.2.3).[28]

In brief, for children younger than 2 years of age, CT radiographs are not indicated if the child has normal mental status, no scalp hematoma, no loss of consciousness (LOC), no palpable skull fractures, has

normal behavior, and has a nonsevere mechanism of injury. For children aged 2 years or older, CTs are not indicated for children demonstrating normal mental status, no LOC, no vomiting, nonsevere mechanism of injury, no symptoms of basilar skull fracture, and no headache.[28]

Plain radiographs are not recommended as a screening tool when head trauma is suspected because of their limitations in assessing intracranial injuries. Orman and colleagues demonstrated that 3D reconstruction of CT images increased the sensitivity of diagnosing linear skull fractures in children across age groups.[29] In addition, 3D-reconstructed images also increase the specificity of fracture diagnosis in children under 2 years of age, and where the fracture site is located close to a suture line.[29] For children with suspected basilar skull fractures, a temporal bone CT without contrast with thin sections along the axial and coronal axes is helpful in providing a more nuanced understanding of involved structures.

The role of ultrasound is limited for the same reasons as that for plain radiographs. Namely, while it possesses good sensitivity (88%) and specificity (97%) for fractures diagnosis, it is less reliable in assessing intracranial pathology. Moreover, the technique is highly operator-dependent, and is unreliable in evaluating fractures of the orbital roof. The one area where ultrasound is effective is for screening patients for dural tears as seen with growing skull fractures or leptomeningeal cysts. The dura can be visualized as a bright linear structure through the

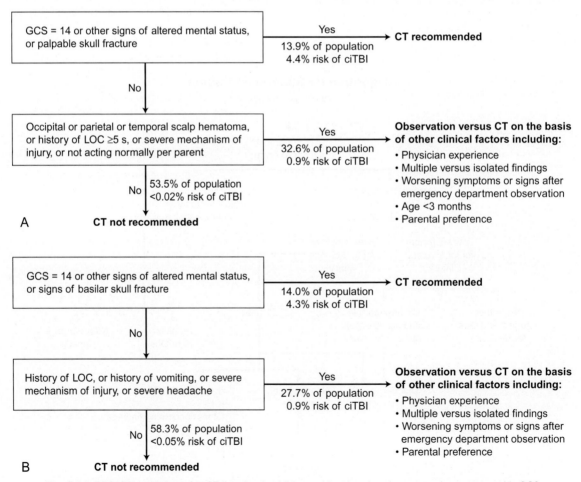

Fig. 3.2.3 PECARN guidelines for CT imaging in children with minor head trauma who present with GCS scores of 14–15. The treatment algorithm is slightly different for patients younger than 2 years of age (A), and those who are 2 and older (B). ciTBI, clinically important traumatic brain injury; GCS, Glasgow Coma Score; LOC, loss of consciousness. (Reproduced from Kuppermann N, Holmes JF, Dayan PS, et al. Identification of children at very low risk of clinically-important brain injuries after head trauma: a prospective cohort study. Lancet 2009;374(9696):1160–1170.)

acoustic window at the fracture site. The absence of a bright signal from the dura is indicative of a dural tear; either CSF or brain parenchyma fills the diastatic space.[30]

For patients presenting for delayed calvarial reconstruction, CT with 3D reconstruction is helpful for evaluating the size, dimensions, and topography of the defect. Furthermore, patient-specific 3D-printed implants can be generated from the posttraumatic CT films and aid in allogeneic reconstruction techniques.

Indications for Repair

Several developmental and anatomical differences exist between pediatric patients and adults with respect to skull fractures. At birth, the skull is only 25% of its final size. By age 2, it has reached 75% of its adult size, and by age 10, 95%.[31,32] The ratio in height between the cranium and midface diminishes as the child grows, owing to the preferential enlargement of the facial skeleton (Fig. 3.2.4). At birth, the height discrepancy between the cranium and face is 8:1, decreasing to 4:1 at age 5, and 2:1 by adulthood.[32] As such, within the 0–5-year age range, skull and orbital fractures are more common, while midface and mandibular fractures are more common in the 6–16-year-old age group.[31,33] Retrospective reviews of facial trauma within the maxillofacial and neurosurgical literature demonstrate that decreasing age is an independent predictor for need of surgical intervention, due to several factors, including a protected environment, greater elasticity of immature bone, and the low ratio of midface to neurocranium height.[3,32]

Infants and very young children have a higher remodeling capacity compared to young adults, and thus, nonoperative management has frequently been recommended for acute skull fractures in the young.[14,15] In infants younger than one year, the osteogenic effects of dura compensate for small bony defects.[34] However, conservative management must be weighed against anticipated cranial vault growth and expansion, which places the child at risk for unique complications.[1] For example, fractures of the anterior cranial fossa can impact orbital growth, and structures of the upper face can be distorted by growth restriction or trauma to the calvarium, orbit, and frontal sinus.[1]

The remodeling potential of pediatric calvarial bone is supported by case reports of complete resolution of anterior table contour deformities in the absence of operative management. In cases of isolated anterior table fractures without involvement of the posterior table or the nasofrontal outflow tract (NFOT), watchful waiting has resulted in spontaneous remodeling and resolution of minor contour depressions.[35]

Growing Skull Fractures

Growing skull fractures, or leptomeningeal cysts, are frequently cited as a potential long-term complication of untreated linear skull fractures. The actual incidence of fracture extension is very rare, with reported rates ranging from 0.05% to 1.6%, and found almost exclusively in patients under the age of 3 years.[36] Bonfield and colleagues reviewed 897 patients with skull fractures at a Level I trauma center and found that only 0.1% of patients with initial conservative treatment of a linear, frontal bone fracture (with orbital extension) developed a growing skull fracture that required delayed operative reconstruction.[1] Growing skull fractures require an inciting dural injury. After the initial injury, herniation of intracranial tissues through the osteodural defect precludes apposition of dural tissues and healing. The defect ultimately enlarges as the child grows and can result in glial changes to the underlying brain parenchyma.[27]

Most growing skull fractures are diagnosed within a year of the initial injury and present with localized swelling or pulsatile exophthalmos. On occasion, patients can have a delayed presentation, with neurologic symptoms such as headache, seizure, or other focal neurologic deficits that prompt further workup.[37–39] Given the low incidence of late complications, current guidelines recommend close follow-up of all linear fractures with a diastasis greater than 4 mm, and early exploration only in cases with evidence of brain herniation on MRI.[36,40] Liu et al. propose surgical exploration in all children with a linear fracture and MRI-proven brain herniation as close to the time of initial injury as possible, in an attempt to stymie progressive neurologic deficits.[26] All children under 2 years of age with isolated skull fractures should be followed up 1–2 months after injury to assess for pulsatile swelling or a localized scalp defect raising concern for a growing skull fracture.[41]

Definitive treatment for growing skull fracture requires resection of the leptomeningeal cyst and nonviable brain parenchyma, a watertight duraplasty, and cranioplasty.[26] In patients with associated hydrocephalus, a ventriculoperitoneal shunt may be placed. Liu et al. recommend autologous dural reconstruction using pericranium and fascia lata, given the lower complication rates as compared to artificial dural substitutes.[26]

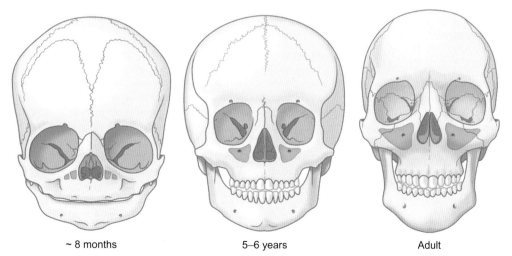

~ 8 months   5–6 years   Adult

Fig. 3.2.4 Postnatal growth of the craniofacial skeleton. Note the changes in ratio between the neurocranium and viscerocranium from infancy to skeletal maturity. The shaded area in green reflects the growth and aeration of the maxillary sinuses. (Reproduced from Ali Baba Attaie, Mairaj K Ahmed, Ferro's fundamentals of maxillofacial surgery. 2nd ed. Berlin: Springer; 2015. p.57.)

In instances of early diagnosis and repair, the bony margins along the fracture site are healthy and well vascularized. Significant cranioplasty can be avoided as long as the bone along the fracture site is well reapproximated. In patients with late presentation and diagnosis, long-term changes to the bone and dura result in a larger defect that may require significant cranioplasty and staged reconstruction. The neurological sequelae from late stage growing skull fracture are also less likely to be reversible than if the fracture were treated at an earlier point.[26]

PEDIATRIC CRANIOPLASTY – SURGICAL TECHNIQUES

Calvarial cranioplasty on a growing skeleton presents unique challenges in the pediatric population. The timing of repair and choice of reconstructive technique are still frequently debated, without a clear consensus except in select situations. The fundamental principle of "replace like with like" is particularly relevant in this population, making autologous reconstruction the gold standard. Some surgeons find alloplastic options necessary, which includes ceramics, metals, hyaluronic acid, or a combination. The authors prefer the utilization of autogenous bone graft when at all possible as the pernicious sequelae of alloplastic material can arise at any point with complications that can potentially last a lifetime. The common indications for cranioplasties include repair after decompressive craniectomy (36%), bone flap infection following previous neurosurgical intervention (18%), osteomyelitis (14%), traumatic bone loss (14%), congenital calvarial dysmorphology (9%), or growing skull fractures (9%).[42] Goals of repair include improved cosmesis and restoration of a protective encasement of the brain. In some instances, reconstructive cranioplasty can also provide the added benefits of improved cerebral blood flow, improved cerebrospinal fluid dynamics, and resolution of the syndrome of the trephined.[43,44]

In the acute setting, the timing of reconstruction is dictated by the clinical condition of the patient. Extensive cranioplasty is generally not attempted until the patient is hemodynamically stable, free from infection, and has normalized intracranial pressures (3–6 months).[45,46] Piedra and colleagues advocate for early repair (less than 6 weeks) following decompressive cranioplasties using autologous bone grafting.[47] However, several other groups saw no clear difference in timing of repair.[46,48,49] In infants younger than 12 months of age, a switch cranioplasty can be performed. Native calvarium is taken from the unaffected side and used to reconstruct the defect. The donor site then regenerates by harnessing the osteogenic potential of dura.

Autologous Reconstruction

Autologous reconstruction provides a restorative option that can grow with the patient. Once fully integrated and vascularized, bone grafts pose minimal infectious risk. However, autologous methods are often erroneously thought to be constrained by availability of donor tissue when the closure of large defects can actually be enhanced by utilizing advanced harvesting techniques.[42,46] The most commonly used autologous tissues for cranioplasty are calvarial bone, hip, and rib.

In adults, replacement of the bone "flap"* following decompressive craniotomies is generally regarded as the most expedient method to restore contour and provide protection of the brain. In children, bone resorption following delayed replantation of autologous bone flaps can

---

*Neurosurgical literature will frequently refer to the bone removed during a decompressive craniotomy as a bone flap, despite its lack of vascularity. For purposes of consistency, plastic surgeons frequently adopt the nomenclature of their neurosurgical colleagues and use "bone flap" in lieu of the more precise terminology, "bone graft."

be significant, and on occasion compromises the longevity of the repair.[46,49,50] Grant and colleagues found that 50% of children who had delayed bone flap replacement following decompressive craniectomy required reoperation due to bone resorption, compared to 6.5%–26% in adults.[46,51] Other groups reported similar rates of reoperation due to either resorption or infection, and found an inverse correlation between age at time of repair and risk of resorption.[52]

At the time of replacement, maximizing apposition of the bone flap edges within the craniotomy defect will promote greater osteointegration. Rigid fixation of the nonvascularized autologous bone graft also minimizes graft resorption and is shown to facilitate osteoconduction.[46,53] Indeed, the high rate of bone resorption described in the neurosurgical literature is likely to be largely a function of poor bone to bone apposition and inadequate rigid fixation at the time of surgery.[46,53]

Rates of resorption correlate to the size of the cranial defect; defects greater than 75 cm^2 have a failure rate greater than 60%, whereas smaller defects have a negligible failure rate.[46] Bone flaps are preserved following craniotomy via subcutaneous storage or cryopreservation. Bone flaps can be stored in an abdominal pocket, anterolateral thigh, or under the scalp where their osteocytes can be nourished by the surrounding blood supply.[51] At our institution, bone flaps that are set aside for delayed reconstruction are predominantly cryopreserved. However, if there is a possibility that the patient will move or be transferred to a separate institution, the flaps are embedded within the abdomen to ensure transport with the patient.

Subcutaneous storage can reduce the degree of bone devitalization as well as infection, but can be uncomfortable for children, and require creation of a second surgical site.[54,55] Cryopreserved bone flaps are associated with high rates of bone resorption (up to 50%), which in turn, can lead to increased rates of infection and cosmetic deformity from inadequate bone stock.[46,56,57] Alternative methods of sterilization such as autoclaving and irradiation have also been proposed, but are associated with equal or higher rates of bone devitalization and are thought to suffer from the destruction of bone healing factors such as BMP.[58,59] Ultimately, large, long-term comparative studies in adults evaluating the efficacy and morbidity of subcutaneous bone flap storage versus cryopreservation indicate similar outcomes between the two methods.[49] Within the pediatric literature, however, there is suggestion that increased devitalization of bone is seen with cryopreserved bone flaps, though the data is limited and more extensive studies are needed prior to drawing a definitive conclusion.[45]

Despite the limitations and high resorption rates, the pediatric neurosurgical community still recommends delayed primary reconstruction with bone flaps. In the event of bone resorption, a delay of at least one year is recommended before attempting another repair to maximize the opportunity for spontaneous ossification.[46] At our institution, the authors replace the bone flap in the immediate phase, insofar as the patient is stable and brain swelling has resolved. In instances requiring significant bone grafting or delayed reconstruction (i.e., where the original bone flap was lost or resorbed), the reconstruction is delayed months to years to allow for maximal spontaneous ossification and fibrosis around the defect. Between the ages of 6 and 8, we acquire a CT scan to evaluate the diploic space prior to proceeding with a large split calvarial graft cranioplasty.

In children with full-thickness calvarial defects from trauma or infection, split calvarial bone grafts, particulate calvarial grafts, and split rib grafts are commonly used in repair.[60,61] Cranial bone has a lower rate of resorption than grafts harvested from elsewhere along the body, as it is denser.[42,62–64] Split and particulate grafts demonstrate lower levels of resorption and infection as compared to bone flaps.[65] The traditional assumption that calvarial splitting is unreliable in children under 5 has largely been debunked. Vercler, Buchman, and colleagues demonstrate use of split bone grafts in children as young as 3 months applied to a range of calvarial defects.[66] Bone is harvested as a full-thickness segment, and split between the inner and outer cortices through the diploic space. For large reconstructions requiring bone grafting, the procedure is delayed until the child is between 6 and 8 years of age, at which point a CT scan is obtained to ensure adequate development of the diploic space for bone splitting. One cortex is used to repair the donor site while the second cortex is used for repair of the defect[67] (Fig. 3.2.5) (Video 3.2.1).

The use of particulate bone grafting is also advocated by some groups given its ease of harvest and minimal donor site morbidity. However, it is of limited utility in more extensive reconstruction as it lacks independent structural integrity and relies instead on underlying dura, alloplastic scaffolding, or bone for support.[34,62,68,69] In our practice, we have found that for easy and rapid generation of particulate bone, a Hudson brace or hand-held bone shaver (MX Grafter, Salvin Dental Specialties) can provide copious amounts of cortical bone with minimal donor site morbidity (Fig. 3.2.6).

Rib grafts have been successfully used in cranioplasty, but demonstrate greater resorption than split calvarial grafts.[70] Donor site complications such as chest wall deformity, postoperative pain, and pneumothorax

limit the use of rib graft when other options exist.[70] Combinations of donor sites can also be utilized to assure an autogenous reconstruction with results that can last, without complications, for a lifetime.

Postoperative antibiotics are used for 10 days following any bone grafting procedure, to mitigate bone resorption from infection. Patients are monitored overnight in all cranioplasty cases with dural exposure and discharged the following day. Skin sutures or staples are removed on postoperative days 10–14 when the patient returns for follow-up evaluation.

Acute complications include hematoma, wound dehiscence, and surgical site infection, but are rare. Hematoma formation is precluded by meticulous hemostasis at the time of closure and placement of a snug circumferential head wrap. In our practice, the placement of a drain depends on the degree of exposure, undermining, and scalp mobilization. Infectious complications usually warrant a return to the operating room for washout. If the infection is localized and draining, children can be observed on antibiotics insofar as the patient is clinically stable. Local wound care with frequent follow-up can lead to resolution of infection and healing by secondary intention.

Long-term complications include scar alopecia, scar widening, bone graft resorption, bone graft migration, and infrequently, temporalis

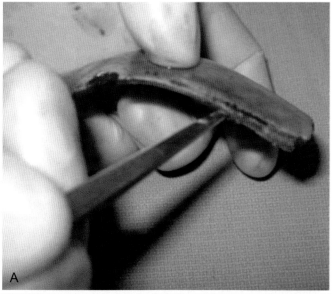
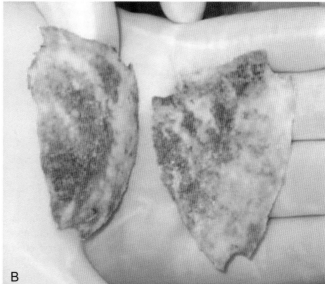
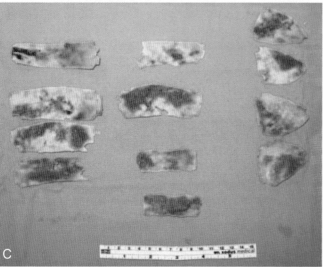

Fig. 3.2.5 (A) The first step in splitting cranial bone is to gain access to the diploic space. This is accomplished by inserting a 2 mm straight osteotome between the inner and outer cortices along the cut bone edge. (B) A complete split of the frontal bone in an 8-month-old patient. (C) Splitting cranial bone essentially doubles the amount of rigid bone available for reshaping the calvaria. (Reproduced with permission from Christian Vercler.)

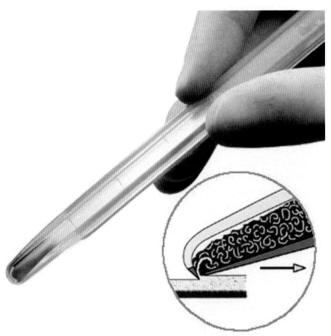

Fig. 3.2.6 The MX Grafter can be used for quick and easy harvesting of bone shavings through a small scalp incision. (From http://www.salvin.com/bone-grafting/MX-Grafter.html.)

muscle hypertrophy. In our clinical practice, the severity of bony resorption is low as we use almost exclusively autologous reconstruction, and few patients (<5%) require secondary reconstruction with additional bone grafting or fat transfer for contour deformities. Large full-thickness calvarial defects that reappear from resorption of bone graft can be treated with additional bone grafting and pericranial flaps in a secondary procedure. For patients who have a donor site defect from areas of split thickness bone harvest, we advocate the use of protective headgear in contact sports, as the structural integrity at the donor site is diminished in these cases.

Again, a significant advantage in using autologous tissue in pediatric calvarial reconstruction is the excellent long-term aesthetic and functional outcomes and low complication rates. We rarely observe bone graft extrusion or rejection when a purely autologous reconstruction is undertaken. In cases where alloplastic materials are used in conjunction with bone grafts, infection of mesh or other hardware can spread to contiguous bone grafts and bony particulates. On surgical reexploration, these areas of bone will exhibit advanced resorption and poor integration.

Alloplastic Reconstruction

There is still much controversy surrounding the use of alloplastic materials in the pediatric population. The most commonly used biomaterials include ceramics, polyethene, polyetheretherketone (PEEK), and titanium.[42,71,72] Concerns surrounding biomaterials include infection, tissue reaction, and material breakdown.[42] In the pediatric population, a growing skull presents added challenges, such as restriction of normal growth, implant extrusion or migration, inadequate cosmesis and the need for implant replacement for the enlarging skeleton.[73] The authors find little use for alloplastic materials in pediatric cranioplasty. Insidious side effects often ignored when placing allograft under the scalp and forehead are the associated gradual thinning of the overlying skin. Breakdown of the thin skin spontaneously or secondary to minor trauma can occur many years after the reconstruction and require extensive,

complex, and disfiguring operations that often require staging in order to restore soft tissue cover and the reconstruction of the cranial defect after alloplastic removal.

However, some studies have shown reliable outcomes with titanium cranioplasties. Williams et al. report successful reconstruction with titanium mesh in patients under 18, without need for revision or implant removal at 4-year follow-up.[42] Technically, titanium plates can be difficult to contour to a child's skull shape, and also induces artifact during CT follow-up.[46] Other groups have reported good outcomes with beta-tricalcium phosphate bone graft substitute, in defects less than 40 cm^2.[74] However, long-term data for most alloplastic materials is unavailable, which is of particular concern given the necessary longevity of such implanted materials.

Temporal Hollowing

Temporal hollowing following cranioplasty is not an uncommon long-term complication. At our institution, we have extensive experience using temporalis turnover flaps for recapitulation of normal temporal fossa anatomy in the craniosynostosis population (Fig. 3.2.7). A similar procedure is performed to augment areas of soft tissue deficiency in patients with sequelae from calvarial trauma.

After infiltrating the subcutaneous tissues with 1:200,000 epinephrine, the cranial flaps are elevated in the supraperiosteal plane with care to preserve the integrity of the temporalis muscle and overlying deep temporal fascia. The temporalis muscle is then elevated in a subperiosteal plane from its origin to the superior temporal line, avoiding the external auditory canal (Fig. 3.2.7A). The muscle is dissected down to the level of the zygomatic arch and mobilized anteriorly, medially, and inferiorly to maximize the arc of rotation for an advancement temporalis flap that can be utilized to reconstruct the temporal fossa (Fig. 3.2.7B). The temporalis muscle is mobilized and secured with 0 Vicryl suture to position it in an area of depression. On occasion, it can be folded on itself to double the projected thickness along the region. Augmentation with split bone grafts is frequently employed to bolster the muscle from below, and give additional projection along areas of deficiency. Leftover bone dust and pericranium are used to smooth irregular areas and optimize the desired final contour.[75]

In patients with damaged and atrophied temporalis muscles, augmentation of the temporal region can be accomplished with either bone grafts or fat transfer. We routinely harvest split bone from the nondominant hemisphere using a combination of straight and curved osteotomes at the time of primary reconstruction.

On occasion (<1%), children with temporal augmentation using a temporalis turnover flap will develop muscle hypertrophy, manifesting as bulges along the temporal region. These cases have been noted primarily following adolescence in patients who demonstrate excessive mastication (e.g. gum chewing) or trauma. Botox and kenalog injections into the temporalis are attempted first before reoperation and excision of excess temporalis tissue.

EXPERT COMMENTARY

This chapter on pediatric cranial reconstruction, which includes a second discussion of the importance of pediatric cranial injuries, is carefully written and meticulously researched. Its detail and extensive references provide the best concise description of the issues of which I am aware. The authors emphasize the importance of autogenous reconstruction, and outline the ways that this can be accomplished, and provide the opinion that split skull cranioplasties may be done far younger than traditionally considered. The authors' emphasis on using autogenous materials is echoed by many experts who deal with the pediatric population.

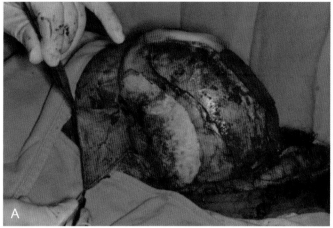
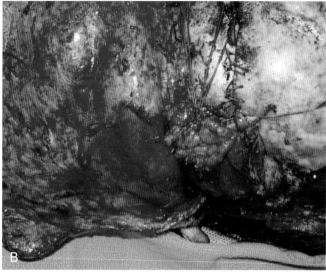

Fig. 3.2.7 (A) Temporalis muscle elevated from the temporal fossa, without violation into the body of the muscle, thus retaining its blood supply. (B) Temporalis flap advanced and folded on itself along the area of greatest bony concavity for soft tissue augmentation. Bone dust can be placed over the muscle to increase projection. Split bone graft can be used as either overlay or underlay relative to the muscle to also provide additional support. (Courtesy Steven Buchman.)

REFERENCES

1. Bonfield CM, Naran S, Adetayo OA, et al. Pediatric skull fractures: the need for surgical intervention, characteristics, complications, and outcomes. *J Neurosurg Pediatr.* 2014;14(2):205–211.
2. Schneier AJ, Shields BJ, Hostetler SG, et al. Incidence of pediatric traumatic brain injury and associated hospital resource utilization in the United States. *Pediatrics.* 2006;118(2):483–492.
3. Adetayo OA, Naran S, Bonfield CM, et al. Pediatric cranial vault fractures: analysis of demographics, injury patterns, and factors predictive of mortality. *J Craniofac Surg.* 2015;26(6):1840–1846.
4. Grunwaldt L, Smith DM, Zuckerbraun NS, et al. Pediatric facial fractures. *Plast Reconstr Surg.* 2011;128(6):1263–1271.
5. Sherick DG, Buchman SR, Patel PP. Pediatric facial fractures: a demographic analysis outside an urban environment. *Ann Plast Surg.* 1997;38(6):578–584, discussion584–585.
6. Duhaime AC, Christian CW, Rorke LB, Zimmerman RA. Nonaccidental head injury in infants – the "shaken-baby syndrome. *N Engl J Med.* 1998;338(25):1822–1829.
7. Barlow KM, Minns RA. Annual incidence of shaken impact syndrome in young children. *Lancet.* 2000;356(9241):1571–1572.
8. Minns RA, Jones PA, Mok JY-Q. Incidence and demography of non-accidental head injury in southeast Scotland from a national database. *Am J Prev Med.* 2008;34(4 suppl):S126–S133.
9. Keenan HT, Runyan DK, Marshall SW, et al. A population-based comparison of clinical and outcome characteristics of young children with serious inflicted and noninflicted traumatic brain injury. *Pediatrics.* 2004;114(3):633–639.
10. Boop S, Axente M, Weatherford B, Klimo P. Abusive head trauma: an epidemiological and cost analysis. *J Neurosurg Pediatr.* 2016;18(5):542–549.
11. Hadley MN, Sonntag VK, Rekate HL, Murphy A. The infant whiplash-shake injury syndrome: a clinical and pathological study. *Neurosurgery.* 1989;24(4):536–540.
12. Jenny C, Hymel KP, Ritzen A, et al. Analysis of missed cases of abusive head trauma. *JAMA.* 1999;281(7):621–626.
13. Piteau SJ, Ward MGK, Barrowman NJ, Plint AC. Clinical and radiographic characteristics associated with abusive and nonabusive head trauma: a systematic review. *Pediatrics.* 2012;130(2):315–323.
14. Hung K-L, Liao H-T, Huang J-S. Rational management of simple depressed skull fractures in infants. *J Neurosurg Pediatr.* 2005;103(1):69–72.
15. van den Heever CM, van der Merwe DJ. Management of depressed skull fractures. Journal of neurosurgery. *J Neurosurg.* 1989;71(2):186–190.
16. Greenes DS, Schutzman SA. Infants With isolated skull fracture: What are their clinical characteristics, and do they require hospitalization? *Ann Emerg Med.* 1997;30(3):253–259.
17. Thompson JB, Mason TH, Haines GL, Cassidy RJ. Surgical management of diastatic linear skull fractures in infants. *J Neurosurg.* 1973;39(4):493–497.
18. Muhonen MG, Piper JG, Menezes AH. Pathogenesis and treatment of growing skull fractures. *Surg Neurol.* 1995;43(4):367–373.
19. Hassan SF, Cohn SM, Admire J, et al. Natural history and clinical implications of nondepressed skull fracture in young children. *J Trauma Acute Care Surg.* 2014;77(1):166–169.
20. Mannix R, Monuteaux MC, Schutzman SA, et al. Isolated skull fractures: trends in management in US pediatric emergency departments. *Ann Emerg Med.* 2013;62(4):327–331.
21. Metzger RR, Smith J, Wells M, et al. Impact of newly adopted guidelines for management of children with isolated skull fracture. *J Pediatr Surg.* 2014;49(12):1856–1860.
22. Blackwood BP, Bean JF, Sadecki-Lund C, et al. Observation for isolated traumatic skull fractures in the pediatric population: unnecessary and costly. *J Pediatr Surg.* 2016;51(4):654–658.
23. Schunk JE, Rodgerson JD, Woodward GA. The utility of head computed tomographic scanning in pediatric patients with normal neurologic examination in the emergency department. *Pediatr Emerg Care.* 1996;12(3):160–165.
24. Rollins MD, Barnhart DC, Greenberg RA, et al. Neurologically intact children with an isolated skull fracture may be safely discharged after brief observation. *J Pediatr Surg.* 2011;46(7):1342–1346.
25. Reid SR, Liu M, Ortega HW. Nondepressed linear skull fractures in children younger than 2 years: Is computed tomography always necessary? *Clin Pediatr (Phila).* 2012;51(8):745–749.
26. Liu X-S, You C, Lu M, Liu J-G. Growing skull fracture stages and treatment strategy. *J Neurosurg Pediatr.* 2012;9(6):670–675.
27. Singh I, Rohilla S, Siddiqui SA, Kumar P. Growing skull fractures: guidelines for early diagnosis and surgical management. *Childs Nerv Syst.* 2016;32(6):1117–1122.
28. Kuppermann N, Holmes JF, Dayan PS, et al. Identification of children at very low risk of clinically-important brain injuries after head trauma: a prospective cohort study. *Lancet.* 2009;374(9696):1160–1170.

29. Orman G, Wagner MW, Seeburg D, et al. Pediatric skull fracture diagnosis: Should 3D CT reconstructions be added as routine imaging? *J Neurosurg Pediatr*. 2015;16(4):426–431.

30. Décarie JC, Mercier C. The role of ultrasonography in imaging of paediatric head trauma. *Childs Nerv Syst*. 1999;15(11–12):740–742.

31. Haug RH, Foss J. Maxillofacial injuries in the pediatric patient. *Oral Surg Oral Med Oral Pathol Oral Radiol Endod*. 2000;90(2):126–134.

32. Singh DJ, Bartlett SP. Pediatric craniofacial fractures: long-term consequences. *Clin Plast Surg*. 2004;31(3):499–518–vii.

33. Iizuka T, Thorén H, Annino DJ, et al. Midfacial fractures in pediatric patients. Frequency, characteristics, and causes. *Arch Otolaryngol Head Neck Surg*. 1995;121(12):1366–1371.

34. Fu KJ, Barr RM, Kerr ML, et al. An outcomes comparison between autologous and alloplastic cranioplasty in the pediatric population. *J Craniofac Surg*. 2016;27(3):593–597.

35. Macisaac ZM, Naran S, Losee JE. Pediatric frontal sinus fracture conservative care: complete remodeling with growth and development. *J Craniofac Surg*. 2013;24(5):1838–1840.

36. Ersahin Y, Gülmen V, Palali I, Mutluer S. Growing skull fractures (craniocerebral erosion). *Neurosurg Rev*. 2000;23(3):139–144.

37. Schutzman SA, Greenes DS. Pediatric minor head trauma. *Ann Emerg Med*. 2001;37(1):65–74.

38. Kutlay M, Demircan N, Akin ON, Basekim C. Untreated growing cranial fractures detected in late stage. *Neurosurgery*. 1998;43(1):72–76.

39. Vignes J-R, Jeelani NUO, Jeelani A, et al. Growing skull fracture after minor closed-head injury. *J Pediatr*. 2007;151(3):316–318.

40. Sanford RA. Prevention of growing skull fractures: report of 2 cases. *J Neurosurg Pediatr*. 2010;5(2):213–218.

41. Naim-Ur-Rahman, Jamjoom Z, Jamjoom A, Murshid WR. Growing skull fractures: classification and management. *Br J Neurosurg*. 1994;8(6):667–679.

42. Williams L, Fan K, Bentley R. Titanium cranioplasty in children and adolescents. *J Craniomaxillofac Surg*. 2016;44(7):789–794.

43. Fodstad H, Love JA, Ekstedt J, et al. Effect of cranioplasty on cerebrospinal fluid hydrodynamics in patients with the syndrome of the trephined. *Acta Neurochir (Wien)*. 1984;70(1–2):21–30.

44. Suzuki N, Suzuki S, Iwabuchi T. Neurological improvement after cranioplasty. Analysis by dynamic CT scan. *Acta Neurochir (Wien)*. 1993;122(1–2):49–53.

45. Lam S, Kuether J, Fong A, Reid R. Cranioplasty for large-sized calvarial defects in the pediatric population: a review. *Craniomaxillofac Trauma Reconstr*. 2015;8(2):159–170.

46. Grant GA, Jolley M, Ellenbogen RG, et al. Failure of autologous bone – assisted cranioplasty following decompressive craniectomy in children and adolescents. *J Neurosurg Pediatr*. 2004;100(2):163–168.

47. Piedra MP, Thompson EM, Selden NR, et al. Optimal timing of autologous cranioplasty after decompressive craniectomy in children. *J Neurosurg Pediatr*. 2012;10(4):268–272.

48. Bowers CA, McMullin JH, Brimley C, et al. Minimizing bone gaps when using custom pediatric cranial implants is associated with implant success. *J Neurosurg Pediatr*. 2015;16(4):439–444.

49. Yadla S, Campbell PG, Chitale R, et al. Effect of early surgery, material, and method of flap preservation on cranioplasty infections: a systematic review. *Neurosurgery*. 2011;68(4):1124–1129.

50. Bowers CA, Riva-Cambrin J, Hertzler DA II, Walker ML. Risk factors and rates of bone flap resorption in pediatric patients after decompressive craniectomy for traumatic brain injury. *J Neurosurg Pediatr*. 2013;11(5):526–532.

51. Matsuno A, Tanaka H, Iwamuro H, et al. Analyses of the factors influencing bone graft infection after delayed cranioplasty. *Acta Neurochir (Wien)*. 2006;148(5):535–540.

52. Martin KD, Franz B, Kirsch M, et al. Autologous bone flap cranioplasty following decompressive craniectomy is combined with a high complication rate in pediatric traumatic brain injury patients. *Acta Neurochir (Wien)*. 2014;156(4):813–824.

53. Citardi MJ, Friedman CD. Nonvascularized autogenous bone grafts for craniofacial skeletal augmentation and replacement. *Otolaryngol Clin North Am*. 1994;27(5):891–910.

54. Yap C, Macarthur DC, Hope DT. "Mind the gap": resorption of a bone flap stored subcutaneously for 6 months. *Br J Neurosurg*. 2009;16(5):523–524.

55. Bhaskar IP, Inglis TJJ, Lee GYF. Clinical, radiological, and microbiological profile of patients with autogenous cranioplasty infections. *World Neurosurg*. 2014;82(3–4):e531–e534.

56. Baldo S, Tacconi L. Effectiveness and safety of subcutaneous abdominal preservation of autologous bone flap after decompressive craniectomy: a prospective pilot study. *World Neurosurg*. 2010;73(5):552–556.

57. Oppenheimer AJ, Mesa J, Buchman SR. Current and emerging basic science concepts in bone biology. *J Craniofac Surg*. 2012;23(1):30–36.

58. Mracek J, Hommerova J, Mork J, et al. Complications of cranioplasty using a bone flap sterilised by autoclaving following decompressive craniectomy. *Acta Neurochir (Wien)*. 2015;157(3):501–506.

59. Osawa M, Hara H, Ichinose Y, et al. Cranioplasty with a frozen and autoclaved bone flap. *Acta Neurochir (Wien)*. 1990;102(1–2):38–41.

60. Tessier P, Kawamoto H, Matthews D, et al. Autogenous bone grafts and bone substitutes: tools and techniques. I. A 20,000-case experience in maxillofacial and craniofacial surgery. *Plast Reconstr Surg*. 2005;116(suppl): 6S–24S.

61. Jackson IT, Helden G, Marx R. Skull bone grafts in maxillofacial and craniofacial surgery. *J Oral Maxillofac Surg*. 1986;44(12):949–955.

62. Rogers GF, Greene AK. Autogenous bone graft. *J Craniofac Surg*. 2012;23(1):323–327.

63. Rosenthal AH, Buchman SR. Volume maintenance of inlay bone grafts in the craniofacial skeleton. *Plast Reconstr Surg*. 2003;112(3):802–811.

64. Ozaki W, Buchman SR. Volume maintenance of onlay bone grafts in the craniofacial skeleton: micro-architecture versus embryologic origin. *Plast Reconstr Surg*. 1998;102(2):291–299.

65. Frodel JL, Marentette LJ, Quatela VC, Weinstein GS. Calvarial bone graft harvest: techniques, considerations, and morbidity. *Arch Otolaryngol Head Neck Surg*. 1993;119(1):17–23.

66. Vercler CJ, Sugg KB, Buchman SR. Split cranial bone grafting in children younger than 3 years old: debunking a surgical myth. *Plast Reconstr Surg*. 2014;133(6):822e–827e.

67. Jaskolka MS, Olavarria G. Reconstruction of skull defects. *Atlas Oral Maxillofac Surg Clin North Am*. 2010;18(2):139–149.

68. Chao MT, Jiang S, Smith D, et al. Demineralized bone matrix and resorbable mesh bilaminate cranioplasty: a novel method for reconstruction of large-scale defects in the pediatric calvaria. *Plast Reconstr Surg*. 2009;123(3):976–982.

69. Beederman M, Alkureishi LWT, Lam S, et al. Exchange hybrid cranioplasty using particulate bone graft and demineralized bone matrix. *J Craniofac Surg*. 2014;25(2):451–454.

70. Blair GAS, Gordon DS, Simpson DA. Cranioplasty in children. *Childs Brain*. 1980;6(2):82–91.

71. Cho YR, Gosain AK. Biomaterials in craniofacial reconstruction. *Clin Plast Surg*. 2004;31(3):377–385.

72. Hanasono MM, Goel N, DeMonte F. Calvarial reconstruction with polyetheretherketone implants. *Ann Plast Surg*. 2009;62(6):653–655.

73. Lin AY, Kinsella CR Jr, Rottgers SA, et al. Custom porous polyethylene implants for large-scale pediatric skull reconstruction. *J Craniofac Surg*. 2012;23(1):67–70.

74. Biskup NI, Singh DJ, Beals S, et al. Pediatric cranial vault defects: early experience with beta-tricalcium phosphate bone graft substitute. *J Craniofac Surg*. 2010;21(2):358–362.

75. Mesa JM, Fang F, Muraszko KM, Buchman SR. Reconstruction of unicoronal plagiocephaly with a hypercorrection surgical technique. *Neurosurg Focus*. 2011;31(2):E4.

Secondary Reconstruction of Facial Soft Tissue Injury and Defects

Christian Petropolis, Jeffrey Fialkov

Despite the craniofacial surgeon's best efforts to minimize soft tissue disruption, secondary scarring and deformity are not infrequent following the treatment of facial injuries.[1,2] These deformities may arise as a consequence of the trauma itself or may be an iatrogenic consequence of the exposure and soft tissue disruption required for facial fracture fixation.[3] Such scarring and deformity are both functionally and psychologically disturbing to the patient and often need to be addressed surgically.[4] This is especially true in the head and neck region, where anatomical distortions measured in millimeters can be visible at conversation distance. The purpose of this chapter is to describe these deformities, how to avoid them through modified surgical approaches, and the techniques used for correcting them secondarily.

BACKGROUND AND ETIOLOGY

Prevention of secondary deformity is the primary long-term goal of treating acute facial injuries. However, as outlined in the previous chapter on primary repair of soft tissue injuries, the need for secondary revision is often unavoidable. When the zone of injury is extensive, healing and soft tissue viability become unpredictable, limiting the reconstructive options available in the acute period. In addition, patients may be too unstable to receive an optimal primary reconstruction. In these cases in which the patient requires stabilization first and foremost, the immediate surgical goal is confined to soft tissue closure and coverage of vital structures and bone.

Soft tissue disruption is often associated with underlying skeletal injury in need of open reduction and internal fixation. The surgical approaches to the craniofacial skeleton required for fixation carry with them a predictable risk of iatrogenic secondary deformity.[3] Ptosis of soft tissues, transection or disinsertion of muscles, atrophy of fat pads, alopecia, and nerve damage are just some of the postoperative complications attributed to craniofacial exposures. These complications arise from the required soft tissue dissection, subperiosteal degloving, and subsequent scarring.

With the advent of plate and screw osteosynthetic systems for the craniofacial skeleton, internal fixation of facial fractures followed the principles of extensive fracture exposure in order to maximize rigidity and minimize interfragmentary movement. This principle was followed even in cases of low energy trauma with simple fracture patterns and in spite of a lack of understanding of the physiological loading of the craniofacial skeleton.[5–7] Over time it has become clear that the complications arising from the soft tissue disruption and biological compromise inherent in this aggressive approach offset the benefits of rigid fixation.[8–10] This has lead to the paradigm for facial fracture stabilization changing over the last few decades, with a shift from stabilization by maximal rigidity to stabilization using the minimum stiffness required to achieve bone healing, consequently better preserving biology, which in turn has led to a reduction in complication rates.[11,12]

This approach is also less likely to disrupt soft tissue support structures and hence result in less secondary soft tissue deformity. As an example, lower eyelid incisions, a significant source of secondary soft tissue deformity, can often be avoided in the fixation of low-energy zygoma fractures not requiring orbital floor exploration. Mechanical stabilization of these fractures can effectively be achieved with fixation at the zygomatic–frontal fracture and/or at the zygomatic–maxillary buttress.[7,12–14] Furthermore, the inferior orbital rim fracture site can be readily visualized from the upper buccal sulcus incision (Fig. 3.3.1), precluding the need for the lower lid exposure for the purposes of ensuring an adequate reduction in cases where orbital floor exploration is not necessary.[7]

Complications can also arise from the fixation hardware itself, with visibility and prominence, loosening, pain and infection being common reasons for secondary removal.[15,16] Complete mitigation of hardware-related complications is impossible, which again emphasizes the need to achieve stable bony fixation with the least amount of hardware possible.

INITIAL ASSESSMENT

History and Physical Examination

Comprehensive assessment should begin with a history documenting details of the initial injury and primary treatment. The timeline of secondary interventions, both surgical and nonsurgical, should also be documented. The patient's chief concerns need to be thoroughly explored and placed in order of priority. Risk factors for poor soft tissue healing such as diabetes, smoking, use of glucocorticoid steroids, and personal or family history of keloid scarring need to be identified.[17]

Examination should assess for facial asymmetries, tissue deficiencies, and distortion of key structures and landmarks. Both static and dynamic asymmetries should be assessed along with function of all divisions of the facial nerve. If bilateral injuries are present, the use of preinjury photographs will assist in this process. The quality of the soft tissues should then be assessed noting all scars and their characteristics including pigmentation, vascularity, pliability, and height.[18] For each soft tissue deformity an attempt should be made to determine the underlying cause. This can be as simple as the incorrect alignment of key landmarks during the primary repair, or in complex cases, a combination of malalignment, abnormal scarring, tissue deficiency, and bony malunion. The contribution of each of these factors to the deformity must be carefully considered to appropriately plan for stepwise correction. Assessment of the underlying facial skeleton should determine if accurate reconstruction has been achieved, and if not which areas are malunited, deficient or unstable. Temporal and cheek contour deformities are then examined in relation to the facial skeleton. The mobility of displaced soft tissues should be assessed to determine if they are fixed or passively correctable.

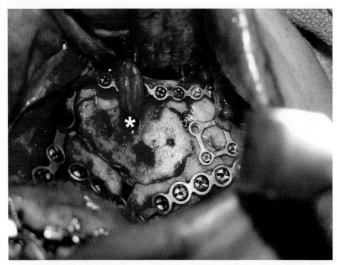

Fig. 3.3.1 Exposure and fixation of the infraorbital rim through an upper buccal sulcus approach. The nerve and infraorbital foramen are marked by the asterisk (*).

A cranial nerve examination should be performed with particular attention to the facial and trigeminal nerves. The power of each muscle group and the presence of synkinesis should be noted along with any functional issues such as corneal exposure, nasal airway obstruction, and oral incompetence. Dysaesthesias and painful neuromas can result from damage to any of the trigeminal nerve branches. The most common cause of posttraumatic trigeminal nerve injury is compression followed by partial nerve laceration and, infrequently, complete laceration.[19] Operative decompression and neurolysis at the foramen or fracture site is effective in most compressive injuries. Complete lacerations require microsurgical repair, and may require autologous nerve grafting if the repair is delayed.

Finally, a set of standard facial photographs should be obtained for documentation and operative planning.[20] Three-dimensional (3D) facial scanning technology is also becoming more accessible for use in preoperative planning and documentation. These techniques have the advantage of allowing computer-based simulation of corrective procedures and development of 3D templates to aid in soft tissue reconstruction.[21–23]

Fig. 3.3.2 demonstrates a case of posttraumatic dysaesthesia of the supraorbital nerve following laceration and fracturing of the supraorbital rim. Laceration of the nerve went unrecognized during primary soft tissue repair and open reduction internal fixation. Secondary exploration was carried out revealing the nerves' discontinuity and direct microsurgical repair was performed with eventual resolution of symptoms.

Radiographic Examination

In evaluating significant secondary soft tissue deformities, computed tomography (CT) examination should be routinely performed to assess the adequacy of skeletal reconstruction, including symmetry and position of key segments.[24,25] High resolution images are useful for preoperative planning of skeletal corrective procedures, including osteotomies, bone grafting, and customized implants. Soft tissues can also be assessed through CT providing information on their quantity, quality, and location relative to bony structures. Axial images best demonstrate the soft tissues of the midface and their relation to the infraorbital rim. Coronal slices are best for evaluation of the temporalis muscle and overlying fat pad.[3]

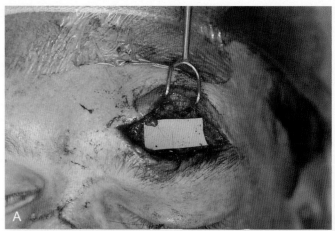

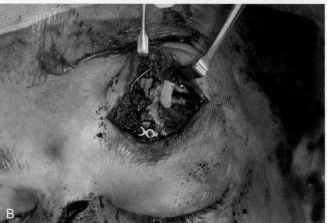

Fig. 3.3.2 Patient presenting with painful neuroma following laceration and fracturing of the supraorbital rim. Exploration revealed complete discontinuity of the supraorbital nerve which was repaired with direct neurorrhaphy.

PRINCIPLES OF SECONDARY SOFT TISSUE CORRECTION

Sequence of Revision

A specific sequence of reconstruction provides optimal correction of posttraumatic facial soft tissue deformities. Skeletal deformities are corrected first, as an accurately reconstructed facial skeleton is required for the correct repositioning or reconstruction of soft tissues. Defects and contour irregularities of the facial skeleton should be corrected with bone graft, free tissue transfer or alloplastic implants depending on the clinical situation. Grossly malpositioned bony segments should be osteotomized and repositioned.

With skeletal correction complete, the deformity and deficiency of the soft tissues can be appropriately addressed. Soft tissues should be fully freed from any points of adhesion to allow for tension-free resuspension. Bone suture anchors are useful for fixation of soft tissues. Key soft tissue landmarks such as the canthi and oral commissures are carefully repositioned with anchoring of ligamentous attachments to bone, and resuspension of muscles.

Finally, residual soft tissue deficiencies are corrected with submuscular or subcutaneous volume augmentation.

Fig. 3.3.3 demonstrates a patient following a motor vehicle collision resulting in a compound skull fracture and loss of the right zygomatic arch. Initial treatment of the patient's skeletal defects was limited due to their critical condition and severe neurotrauma. Following the acute

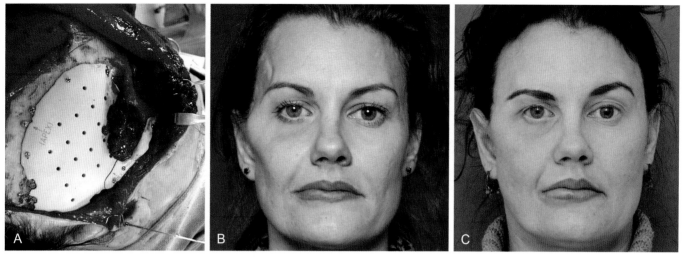

Fig. 3.3.3 (A) Custom PEEK implant for secondary correction of cranial and zygomatic defect. (B) Residual temporal hollowing was present following implant placement. (C) Final result was obtained after structural fat grafting.

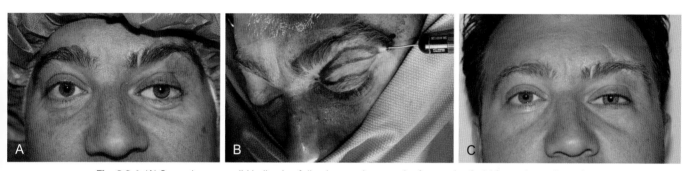

Fig. 3.3.4 (A) Secondary upper lid hollowing following previous repair of extensive facial fracturing and enucleation of the left globe. (B) Structural fat grafting of the deformity with slight overcorrection. (C) Final result.

phase, staged secondary reconstruction was planned. First, a custom made PEEK implant to address the cranial and zygomatic defects was designed based on CT imaging. Following skeletal correction, the true soft tissue deficit in the temporal fossa became apparent and could be appropriately addressed. Serial fat grafting was then employed to complete the soft tissue reconstruction.

SOFT TISSUE CONTOUR AUGMENTATION

Corrective techniques for soft tissue contour deformities include autologous fat grafting, synthetic fillers, alloplastic implants, and occasionally free tissue transfer. Selecting the appropriate technique requires consideration of amount of volume loss, quality of the overlying skin and soft tissues as well as the defect location. Small volume deficiencies are readily corrected using autologous fat grafting, while moderate-sized defects may require serial grafting. Hyaluronic acid-based synthetic fillers can be useful for small volume soft tissue augmentation, however the temporary nature of these products makes them less ideal in this patient population.

Fat Grafting

Although initially described over 100 years ago it was not until the 1990s that the modern technique for fat grafting became well accepted.[26] Fat grafting has now become a common procedure within the armamentarium of most reconstructive surgeons. Although there is much

debate over the technical aspects of graft harvest, preparation, and injection, evidence is largely lacking to endorse one protocol over another.[27] Our current practice follows the principles of structural fat grafting described by Coleman.[28,29]

1. Gentle handling of fat to prevent damage to its delicate structure of parcels.
2. Limited centrifugation to refine and concentrate the fat, removing non-viable components.
3. Small volume injection of fat aliquots.

As seen in Fig. 3.3.4, our usual donor sites are the distal thigh/medial knee or the abdomen accessed through a stab incision made within the umbilicus, leaving an inconspicuous scar. The location of harvest has not been proven to affect overall graft take and so can be adjusted based on availability of adipose tissue and patient preference.[30] Harvesting of fat using both syringe suction and pump aspiration have been shown to yield equivalent graft take, and so the choice is based on surgeon preference and availability of equipment.[31] Our preference is to use syringe suction because of the small volumes required for facial augmentation, its simplicity, and low cost. Harvest sites are infiltrated with 1% lidocaine with 1:200,000 epinephrine diluted in normal saline (generally 1:5). Once harvested, the fat is centrifuged for 3 minutes at 3000 rotations per minute. The aqueous layer is then drained from the syringe and the oil is decanted. Further oil can be wicked from the fat using gauze. The prepared fat is then transferred into one milliliter (mL) syringes for injection.

If performed with the patient awake, such as in the case of small defects, injection sites are sparingly infiltrated with local anesthetic containing epinephrine, and stab incisions are made in inconspicuous locations such as within the hairline, natural creases or existing scars. Each pass of the cannula should deposit a small parcel of fat into a tunnel surrounded by vascular tissue. Multiple tunnels are created with successive passes and no more than 0.1 mL of fat deposited per pass as the cannula is withdrawn.[28] Larger deposits per pass are thought to inhibit graft take and lead to fat necrosis and oil cyst formation. Depth of injection can be varied depending on the desired effect. Augmentation of depressed scars is accomplished through superficial injection into a subdermal plane. An intermediate subcutaneous plane is injected for augmentation of soft tissue volume. A deep plane of injection adjacent to the periosteum will affect the draping of soft tissues over the bony skeleton.

With proper technique, long-term graft take is reported up to 60%.[27] Optimal correction in one sitting is difficult because of the variability in rates of graft take, and patients should be informed about the possibility of multiple grafting sessions. The most common complication following fat grafting is visible irregularities, which can occur due to superficial placement of graft or fat necrosis and oil cyst formation.[28] Fat embolism is a known but very rare complication following vascular cannulation. Use of blunt injection cannulas and epinephrine solution at the injection site help to mitigate this risk.[32]

Fig. 3.3.4 demonstrates a patient with significant facial deformity following repair of extensive midfacial fracturing. Staged secondary reconstruction began with osteotomy and repositioning of the malunited zygoma and enucleation of the left globe with eventual prosthetic placement. A lateral canthoplasty was then performed to correct the canthal dystopia and ectropion. With the skeletal and periorbital structures accurately repositioned, fat grafting to the left upper lid hollowing was undertaken. Superficial injection of graft was avoided to prevent contour irregularities in the thin eyelid skin. A slight overcorrection was obtained immediately following grafting, leading to a satisfactory postoperative result.

TEMPORAL CONTOUR DEFORMITY

The temporal fossa is filled by the temporalis muscle and superficial temporal fat pad creating a smooth convex contour from the insertion of the temporalis fascia on the superior temporal line to the zygomatic arch. Concavity in the temporal region presents with prominence of the lateral orbital rim and zygomatic arch. This can result from either soft tissue volume loss or expansion of the skeletal boundaries of the temporal fossa. Lateral displacement of the zygomatic arch or rotation of the zygoma leads to increased depth of the temporal fossa with resulting contour deformity. Soft tissue volume loss in the temporal fossa can result from atrophy or displacement of the temporalis muscle or temporal fat pads. The deformity is most commonly associated with coronal flap exposure of the lateral orbital rim and zygomatic arch.[3] MRI and cadaver studies have demonstrated that atrophy or prolapse of the superficial temporal fat pad is the primary cause of the contour deformity following this approach and failure to close the periosteum over the zygomaticofrontal suture (orbital periosteum and temporalis fascia).[33,34] Dissection within the superficial fat pad may result in ischemic injury to the fat with subsequent atrophy, or dehiscence of supporting ligaments causing inferior displacement of the fat pad.

Direct injury to the temporalis muscle from trauma or surgical access can also result in tissue loss, atrophy or ptosis. In traumatic injuries repair and resuspension of the muscle should be performed as best as possible with priority placed on filling the anterior portion of the temporal fossa adjacent to the lateral orbital rim and zygomatic

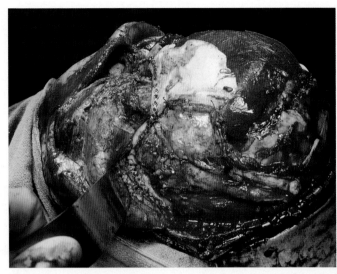

Fig. 3.3.5 Devastating craniofacial trauma with open skull fracture and partial loss of the temporalis muscle. The remaining temporalis was elevated to access and fixate the associated skull base fractures. The temporalis was preferentially resuspended to the lateral orbital rim and frontal bone to prevent visible hollowing in the non-hair-bearing region.

arch (Fig. 3.3.5). Resuspension is facilitated through use of drill holes, suture anchors or fixation to fracture plates. If elevation of the temporalis muscle is required for surgical access to the lateral skull base, a cuff of muscle and fascia at the superior temporal line should be left to facilitate accurate resuspension.

The patient's fracture type and overall injury severity can also influence postoperative rates of temporal hollowing.[35,36] Higher energy injuries are more difficult to accurately reconstruct, and have more direct soft tissue injury. Polytrauma patients are also at risk of significant decreases in body mass index, which increases their risk of temporal hollowing.[36]

Prevention of temporal contour deformity focuses on avoiding disruption of the superficial temporal fat pad during coronal flap elevation. Direct damage to the fat pad, its vascular supply and dehiscence of its suspensory fibers are all proposed mechanisms for the development of hollowing. Our preferred method and the most common variation of the coronal approach passes through the anterior layer of the deep temporalis muscle fascia 2–3 cm above the zygomatic arch. Dissection then continues on the undersurface of the superficial fascia leaving the underlying fat pad undisturbed. This theoretically allows for simultaneous protection of the fat pad and temporal branch of the facial nerve which is closely associated with the periosteum of the zygomatic arch.[37,38] Use of marking sutures on both sides of the cut temporal fascia allows for accurate reapproximation during closure. Some authors bypass dissection of the superficial temporal fat pad entirely by dissecting above the temporalis fascia until the superior posterior edge or the zygomatic arch can then be directly accessed. The reported rates of both facial nerve injury and temporal hollowing are low with this approach.[36,39] However, in the setting of severe trauma it may be difficult to perform this approach safely given the displacement of bony landmarks and the disruption of soft tissue planes. Another approach transects the temporalis fascia above the superficial temporal fat pad and continues the dissecting on the undersurface of the deep layer of the temporalis fascia. This supratemporalis approach bypasses the fat pad entirely and also preserves the blood supply from the middle temporal artery.[40] There are currently no large randomized trials showing definitive benefit to one approach over another.

Several treatments have been described for correction of established temporal hollowing, with the goal of treatment being to address any underlying bony abnormality and deficiencies of the soft tissues. Prior to the popularization of structural fat grafting, soft tissue augmentation was achieved with many different alloplastic materials including hydroxyapatite, porous high-density polyethylene, and methylmethacrylate.[41–44] These firm, adynamic materials were most often placed in a submuscular plane to mask their borders and prevent palpability. Unfortunately dissection of the temporalis muscle could itself lead to further soft tissue atrophy. Subcutaneous placement was performed in patients where the temporalis muscle was missing or deficient, and although this filled the soft tissue defect, it resulted in an unnatural appearance.[44] Custom temporal implants theoretically offer a technologically superior means of mirroring the unaffected side following traumatic injuries of the temporal region, however the limitations of using alloplastic materials still apply. The thin traumatized soft tissues present in these cases do little to hide visible irregularities and shadow lines that occur even with the best implant-based reconstruction. When an implant is required, such as for cranial reconstruction, secondary use of structural fat grafting offers an excellent means of "fine tuning" the reconstruction. Fig. 3.3.6 demonstrates a case of posttraumatic temporal hollowing with temporal bone resorption and soft tissue atrophy following a decompressive craniectomy. A custom PEEK implant was first placed to reconstruct the defect in the temporal bone and correct the bony deficiency. Serial fat grafting was then used to complete the reconstruction, providing excellent symmetry and masking of the implant.

For patients without skeletal defects our current practice for correction of temporal hollowing is primarily through structural fat grafting. Depending on the degree of deformity one or more sessions may be required to achieve full correction. The success of this technique in head and neck reconstruction has been well documented.[45–47] Dermal fat grafting has also been successfully described for temporal soft tissue augmentation, with the authors claiming lasting correction in a one-stage procedure.[48] Unlike implant-based reconstructions, fat grafting can provide a softer, less artificial appearance and feel. It also

mitigates the risk of implant-related complications such as infection and extrusion.

CHEEK PTOSIS

Ptosis of cheek tissues is a well-known complication following subperiosteal degloving of the midfacial skeleton.[9] The anterior surface of the maxilla and zygoma are the origin of attachment for the muscles of the upper lip, as well as the suspensory ligaments supporting the midface soft tissue.[49,50] Release of these periosteal attachments therefore results in descent of the midface and cheek soft tissues. This retinacular support system starts at the periosteum and forms an arborized pattern as it connects to the superficial musculoaponeurotic system (SMAS) before finally inserting into the dermis. A histological depiction of this is shown in Fig. 3.3.7.

Disruption of this retinacular support network results in the appearance of premature facial aging. This may occur as a consequence of a direct traumatic injury, or as a result of operative midfacial soft tissue degloving. The characteristics of this deformity are malar volume loss, skeletonization of the lid–cheek junction with ptosis of the malar fat pad, and fullness of the nasolabial fold due to descent of the soft tissues.[9] Midface ptosis also increases the downward pull on the eyelid increasing the risk of ectropion and scleral show following lower lid approaches.[51] This malar volume loss occurs despite adequate bony reconstruction and was initially thought to be due to soft tissue atrophy secondary to the trauma.[9,50] Without correction, the descended periosteum heals to the anterior maxillary wall in its new descended position.

Prevention of the deformity is always preferred to secondary correction. Phillips et al. described a technique for prevention of cheek ptosis following a subciliary approach in which the descended periosteum is identified and resuspended to the inferior orbital rim prior to closure. This can be done either through drill holes in the orbital rim, suture anchors or around existing hardware applied for fixation of the rim. A heavy absorbable or permanent suture is used for resuspension of the tissues.[9] Correcting the position of the ptotic cheek tissues prevents

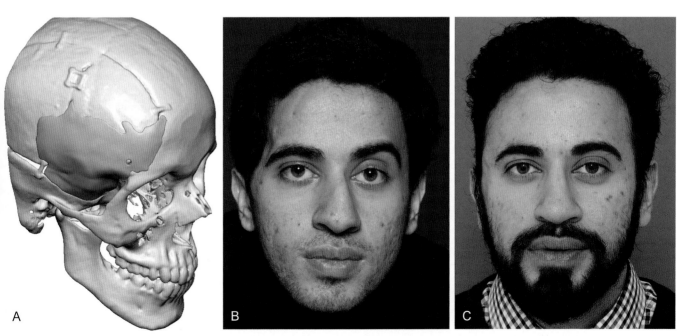

Fig. 3.3.6 (A) Posttraumatic temporal hollowing with underlying temporal bone resorption and soft tissue atrophy following a decompressive craniectomy. (B) Design of custom PEEK implant. (C) One year postoperative result following serial fat grafting.

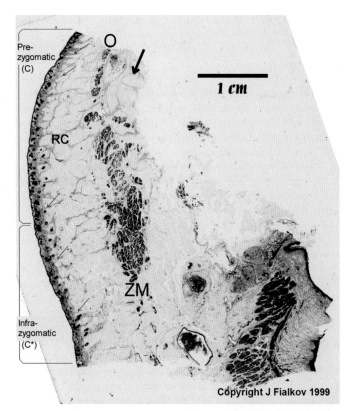

Fig. 3.3.7 A histological cross-section of the midface soft tissues showing the arborized retinacular support system (*arrows*) traveling through the SMAS to insert onto the dermis. (Copyright J Fialkov, 1999.)

TABLE 3.3.1   Ptosis Procedure and Levator Resection in Relation to Amount of Ptosis and Levator Function

Amount of Ptosis	Levator Excursion	Levator Resection
Mild (1–2 mm)	Excellent (> 10 mm)	Levator resection or Müllerectomy
Mild (1–2 mm)	Good (8–10 mm)	10–13 mm
Moderate (3–4 mm)	Fair (5–7 mm)	14–20 mm
Severe (> 4 mm)	Poor (1–4 mm)	21–26 mm
Severe (> 4 mm)	None	Frontalis sling

From Finsterer J. Ptosis: causes, presentation, and management. Aesth Plast Surg 2003;27:193–204.

secondary pull on the lower lid which can lead to ectropion and scleral show. The suture purchase on the cheek tissues should include enough of the deep periosteal layer to ensure transmission of the suspensory force through the retinacular network to the skin.

Established ptosis of cheek tissues is a reconstructive challenge due to retraction and scarring of the descended periosteum and shortened mimetic muscles. Success in correction is dependent on the degree to which the scarred soft tissues can be mobilized and repositioned. The surgical approach to the infraorbital rim used during the initial procedure should be determined and again implemented so as to not introduce any additional scarring in the lid. Once the infraorbital rim has been exposed, the maxilla and zygoma are degloved over their anterior surface. Full mobility of the cheek tissues is only achieved when the scarred contracted periosteum is sharply released. This release should be performed well inferior to the infraorbital nerve. The superior edge of the periosteum is grasped and placed on vertical traction ensuring there is full mobility of the cheek tissues. The mobilized periosteum is then secured with a heavy permanent suture to the infraorbital rim through drill holes, with suture anchors or around existing hardware.[3]

PERIORBITAL DEFORMITY

Background

Periorbital soft tissue deformities are commonly seen following facial trauma and fracture repair. Asymmetry and disproportion of the palpebral aperture is closely related to the underlying bony orbital anatomy onto which the ligamentous attachments insert. Changes to the insertions of the canthal tendons greatly affect the appearance of the upper and lower lid, making identification of naso-orbito-ethmoid (NOE)

and zygoma malunions essential to appropriate treatment of canthal dystopias. Globe projection must also be considered as it directly affects upper and lower lid position and palpebral aperture height.

Prevention as always is the most effective treatment. Accurate primary reconstruction of the bony orbit sets the position of the canthal tendons and globe projection. Canthoplasty should be employed in the setting of tendon avulsion with reinsertion to bone. Traumatic disinsertion of the levator superioris should be repaired to the tarsal plate. The secondary treatment of canthal dystopia and lower lid malposition will be covered in another chapter.

Upper Lid Ptosis

The levator palpebrae superioris takes its origin from the lesser wing of the sphenoid just superior to the annulus of Zinn. Its average muscle length is 36 mm with the muscle transitioning to its aponeurosis at Whitnall's ligament. The aponeurosis is 14–20 mm in length with insertion onto the anterior tarsus and overlying orbicularis and skin which varies with ethnicity. Innervation is through the oculomotor nerve. The levator palpebrae along with Müller's muscle are responsible for upper lid elevation.[52–55]

Traumatic upper lid ptosis can be due to lid avulsion, muscle contusion, orbital roof fracture, foreign body impingement, secondary scarring and neurogenic causes. The cause of the ptosis may also be multifactorial making careful examination essential to obtain the correct diagnosis. Ptosis following blunt trauma will usually be transient and with time full recovery should be expected. Small lacerations with accurate primary repair will also usually result in good levator function.[56] Avulsive injuries are far more unpredictable and permanent ptosis can result even with appropriate primary repair.[57] Neurogenic causes include isolated third nerve palsy, superior orbital fissure syndrome and more central lesions due to traumatic brain injury.[58,59] If a neurogenic component to the patient's ptosis is suspected, treatment should be delayed 6–12 months to allow for recovery prior to surgical correction.[56,60]

Examination should include the degree of ptosis and levator excursion as well as a complete cranial nerve examination. The presence of a Bell's phenomenon is important to note, especially if a static ptosis correction is being considered. The degree of ptosis is measured as the distance of the lid margin from the upper limbus and is divided into mild (1–2 mm), moderate (3–4 mm) and severe (>4 mm).[55] Levator excursion should be similarly determined (Table 3.3.1).[60] When considering the options for ptosis correction, these measurements play an important role in determining the choice of operation and the amount of levator advancement required (Table 3.3.1).

Cases of mild ptosis can be corrected with a external levator resection and advancement, or Müllerectomy. For patients with severe ptosis with maintained levator excursion, levator advancement is the procedure of choice. Severe ptosis with absent levator function will usually require a frontalis sling procedure. Secondary correction of severe injuries should be delayed until the scar has remodeled 6–12 months post injury.[55,56]

NASAL DEFORMITIES

Secondary reconstruction of posttraumatic nasal defects is challenging due to the complex multilamellar structure of the nose and its roles as a key aesthetic and functional unit of the face. All secondary defects should be assessed for deficiencies in lining, structure and cutaneous coverage. Defining the cutaneous defect by affected nasal subunits as described by Burget and Menick is particularly important in planning effective reconstructive strategies. The nasal subunits include the tip, soft triangles, alae, sidewalls, and dorsal subunits.[61] The underlying principle of nasal subunit reconstruction dictates that defects greater than 50% of a given subunit are best treated with excision of the remaining tissue and reconstruction of the entire subunit. This ensures that subunits or defined surfaces are reconstructed with similar homogenous tissues, while scars are hidden along boundaries or junctions of anatomical units, corresponding to natural planar and reflected light transitions. However, considerable judgment is required here in traumatic facial injuries as youthful patients have poorer results than older patients with this approach. In the case of secondary reconstruction residual portions of subunits that are to be replaced may be used as part of the reconstruction, as turnover lining flaps for example, rather than disposing of them.

The case depicted in Fig. 3.3.8 demonstrates these principles. The initial trauma occurred during a fall from height resulting in multiple facial lacerations and avulsion of his nasal tip and columella. Initial treatment was layered primary closure. Several months following the injury the patient presented with greater than 60% loss of the tip with complete loss of the columella and caudal septum as well as some medial alar loss. The residual tip skin was used as a turnover flap to reconstruct the lining. The tip and right soft triangle subunit were then resurfaced with a folded three-stage forehead flap. Restructuring of the underlying cartilage was completed at the second stage. Our preferred cartilage source is rib cartilage autograft from the sixth–seventh rib synchondrosis, or rib allograft in older individuals with calcified cartilage.[62] Grafts are placed to recreate both the caudal and dorsal septal supports followed by nonanatomic grafting under the reconstructed tip and ala to support the soft tissue and prevent contraction and distortion during healing.

Although small, an isolated defect to the soft triangle as seen in Fig. 3.3.9 can be significantly disfiguring. Recreation of the thin, defined structure of the nasal rim with both lining and coverage is challenging. The helical rim bears a striking resemblance to the alar rim and can be used as a composite graft for defects under 1 cm². To aid in graft take the composite area containing cartilage and lining should be minimized to the rim itself. Turnover flaps from the residual subunit or scar, delayed and then turned over, can be used to supply a vascularized recipient bed of additional lining to improve composite graft take. Larger defects involving two or more subunits are best reconstructed with

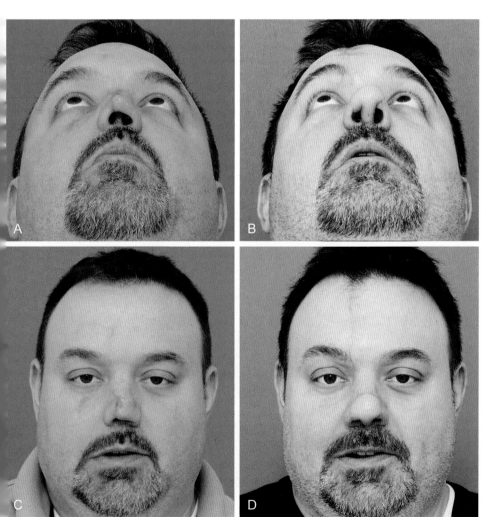

Fig. 3.3.8 (A and C) Secondary nasal deformity following avulsion of the nasal tip and columella initially treated with primary closure. (B and D) Early postoperative result following a three-stage forehead flap with rib cartilage grafts and lining turnover flap from the remaining tip subunit.

folded forehead flaps. Helical rim free flaps are useful for the largest defects containing alar, soft triangle, and columellar subunits.[63]

BROW PTOSIS

The brow is a dynamic structure, the position of which is determined by the balance of several forces. The pull of the frontalis is opposed by the corrugator, procerus, orbicularis oculi and depressor supercilii muscles. Gravity also contributes to downward pull on the brow.[64]

Traumatic ptosis of the brow is usually secondary to either injury to the upper temporal branch of the facial nerve, or direct trauma to the frontalis muscle resulting in dysfunction. Injury to the temporal branch is also a known complication of the coronal approach for access to the upper craniofacial skeleton.

Correction of brow ptosis has been described through several approaches, including open and endoscopic. Open approaches include the direct brow lift, midforehead, pretrichial, coronal, and blepharoplasty. The direct and midforehead lifts allow for greater elevation per amount of tissue resected, with the tradeoff being visible scarring. The coronal and pretrichial approaches hide visible scars, while greatly increasing the required dissection. Although the endoscopic approach limits scarring, it may not provide as durable a result.[65]

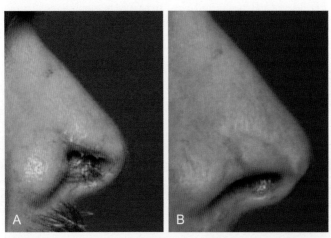

Fig. 3.3.9 (A) Dog bite injury to the nose resulting in an isolated right soft triangle defect. (B) Result following composite graft from the ascending helical rim.

Our preferred approach for brow elevation is through a coronal approach. Preoperatively the desired amount of elevation is determined. The forehead is raised in a subgaleal plane, with a transition to the subpericranial plane at the level of the brow pads (Fig. 3.3.10). The inferior edge of the pericranium with incorporated brow pad can then be elevated and fixated to superior pericranium as required to correct the ptotic brow. The elevation of the pericranium is overcorrected by 2–3 mm. Fixation is accomplished with a non-absorbable braided suture, one placed at the brow apex and one just medial to this. Redundant skin is resected carefully to ensure a tension-free closure. If inadequate correction or relapse of the brow ptosis occurs a secondary direct brow lift is performed.

SCAR REVISION

Cutaneous and soft tissue craniofacial injuries far outnumber cases of skeletal trauma, with scarring being the unfortunate outcome. Achieving an aesthetically pleasing scar without secondary revision should be the goal of primary repair and the techniques to optimize primary soft tissue repair are covered in another chapter. Poor quality scarring cannot always be avoided with the complex process of wound healing and remodeling creating unpredictability even when appropriate techniques are employed. Unaesthetic scars include widened atrophic scars as well as prominent hypertrophic and keloid scars. Scar visibility can also be due to poor positioning across aesthetic units or running perpendicular to relaxed skin tension lines.

Although elimination of scars is impossible, conversion of an unfavorable scar to a more favorable scar can be facilitated by employing both surgical and nonsurgical interventions. Conservative treatment should first be attempted in most situations, with the rare exception being scar contracture resulting in significant functional impairment, such as corneal exposure.

Early use of topical therapies has undergone significant investigation in the recent past. Most agree that a slightly moist warm environment facilitates early wound healing through enhanced reepithelization.[66] Use of occlusive or semiocclusive dressings can facilitate this, however there is a risk of maceration and increased bacterial load in exudative wounds. Use of vitamin E (alpha-tocopherol) has been proposed as an early prophylactic scar treatment because of its antiinflammatory effect with inhibition of fibroblast and collagen production.[67] Multiple studies have been published showing mixed results, with some evidence showing worse healing and skin irritation to the surrounding area.[68,69] Without

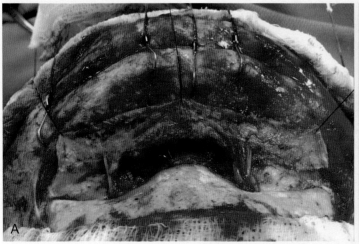
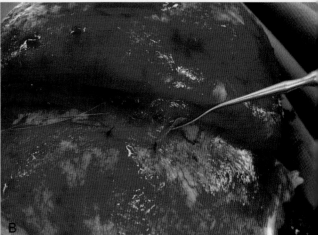

Fig. 3.3.10 (A) Technique for correction of brow ptosis with elevation of the brow pad in the subperiosteal plane. (B) Elevation and fixation of the brow pad to the superior periosteum using nonabsorbable sutures.

the existence of strong evidence, the use of topical vitamin E is not recommended.

Silicone sheeting has been used since the early 1980s for treatment of hypertrophic and keloid scarring.[70] The mechanism of action is felt to be increased hydration and temperature relating to the occlusive nature of silicone.[71] This may result in decreased fibroblast proliferation and modulation of collagen remodeling. Although silicone sheeting is one of the few conservative measures with evidence for its use, the quality of the evidence is low and the reported benefit is small.[72] Despite this, the low cost and simplicity of silicone sheeting makes it a first line treatment for hypertrophic scars and as prophylactic treatment for scars in patients at higher risk. Silicone along with pressure can be used in conjunction and is facilitated with the use of a custom mask. With the exception of facial burn scars, prolonged use of a mask is not usually tolerated and rarely employed.

Corticosteroid injections are another intervention for treatment of hypertrophic and keloid scarring. They act to decrease fibroblast activity while also promoting collagen breakdown. Injections are usually every 4–6 weeks and serial injection may be required over several months. Triamcinolone 40 mg/mL is typically diluted into a small volume of local anesthetic to decrease the pain of injection. Care should be taken to inject only into the scar tissue to avoid atrophy of the subcutaneous tissue and surrounding skin. Other complications can include hypopigmentation and the development of telangiectasias. Although there is a lack of high-level evidence demonstrating benefit, corticosteroids are still widely used as a first-line treatment.[71]

RESURFACING TECHNIQUES

Resurfacing of Scarred Tissues

Laser treatments that are used to improve scar appearance can employ both ablative and nonablative lasers. Lasers work through the principle of selective photothermolysis which allows for controlled damage to tissues while minimizing damage to surrounding structures. Nonablative lasers such as the ND-YAG selectively cause injury to the dermal and subdermal collagen structures without loss of the epithelium. This results in collagen remodeling with a shorter recovery, however the amount of remodeling is more modest than that which is achieved with ablative lasers.[73] Patients with hypertrophic scars may benefit from treatment with pulsed dye lasers that target oxyhemoglobin. Multiple studies have shown significant improvement to erythema, scar height, skin surface texture, and pruritus.[74] This effect is most pronounced in immature hypertrophic scars still in the remodeling phase of wound healing. Treatments are usually performed every 6–8 weeks as required.

Ablative CO_2 and Er-YAG lasers act by removing the epidermis and variable amount of superficial (papillary) dermis with each pass. The remaining reticular dermis and adnexal structures regenerate collagen and the overlying epidermis. The creation of a superficial wound which must heal and prolonged erythema are disadvantages of ablative lasers. To overcome these disadvantages, fractional versions of ablative lasers were developed. Instead of uniformly ablating an area of skin, fractional lasers create microperforations with intervening areas of intact skin. Epithelization from these intact areas allows for faster healing and decreased side effects.[73] Care should be taken when resurfacing patients with higher Fitzpatrick skin types (IV and V) because of this risk of hyperpigmentation or hypopigmentation. For at-risk patients there is some evidence for the use of topical corticosteroids during the healing phase. Direct sun avoidance should also be employed to prevent melanocyte stimulation. Topical hydroquinone is the usual treatment for established hyperpigmentation.[75] Reactivation of herpes simplex is another serious complication of skin resurfacing techniques. Treatment is contraindicated in patients with an active infection. Patients with a

known history should be treated prophylactically with aciclovir. Treatment should begin 1 day prior to, and 5–10 days post procedure.[73]

Dermabrasion is another method of skin resurfacing resulting in controlled abrasion of the epidermis and superficial dermis. The technique employs a rotary handpiece such as wire brush or diamond fraise. This is a technique requiring skilled clinical judgment on the part of the operator to determine the depth of abrasion. Regeneration of the remodeled dermis and epidermis results in improvement in scar quality. Postoperatively, skin returns to a normal appearance at approximately 1 month. Similar to laser ablation techniques prolonged erythema and pigmentation changes can complicate the recovery.

TRAUMATIC TATTOOING

Traumatic tattooing occurs when foreign body particulate matter becomes embedded into the dermis. Prevention is critical and careful cleansing and debridement should be performed on initial treatment of abrasive or explosive wounds. The Versajet hydrosurgery system has been successfully used for this purpose, and may facilitate the process by providing a finely tunable debridement.[76] Failure to remove these particles results in an irregularly distributed blue to black tattooing, with color depending on particle depth. Treatment of established traumatic tattooing is very difficult. Q-switch lasers are commonly employed and use high-energy nanosecond bursts to break apart embedded particulate matter. Treatments can be repeated every 4–6 weeks as required.[77] The larger particle size seen in these patients makes the tattoos difficult to fully eliminate. Skin resurfacing with ablative lasers can be attempted and may help eliminate larger particles. Caution must be taken when using lasers to treat tattoos caused by embedded gunpowder or explosive material as there is a risk of ignition.[78] Overall treatment yields moderate improvement, and the patient should be guided on realistic expectations prior to initiating treatment.

EXCISIONAL TECHNIQUES

Scars that cross aesthetic units or run perpendicular to relaxed skin tension lines are often more noticeable even if they do not have hypertrophic features. Several techniques exist to camouflage these unaesthetic scars through excision, redirection, and relocation. Ideally scars should fall at the junction of the facial subunits or parallel to the relaxed skin tension lines (RSTL). This not only decreases visibility but also tension across the wound, optimizing scar healing.

For small scars simple elliptical excision can be enough to revise and redirect the scar parallel to the RSTL. In larger scars it can be advantageous to break up the scar into shorter nonlinear segments. These shorter segments tend to be better camouflaged compared to a long linear segment. Multiple techniques exist and can follow a regular pattern, such as the W-plasty, or an irregular pattern, such as geometric broken line techniques. Templates can be made or acquired to facilitate planning of these excision techniques.

The Z-plasty technique can serve multiple purposes including redirection, lengthening, and effacement when there is webbing of the scar. Most commonly the triangular flaps are designed with limbs of equal length with angles of 60 degrees. Increasing the angle will increase the gain in scar length, however flap transposition becomes more difficult and may create standing cones. Smaller angles transpose easily but are less robust and do not create much lengthening.[79]

TISSUE EXPANSION

Tissue expansion is a powerful tool that allows for reconstruction with local and regional tissue when redundant tissues are not available. This method provides the best match for color and texture compared to the native tissues. In the case of defects involving the scalp it also allows for reconstruction of hair-bearing tissues. The molecular mechanisms of tissue expansion are complex and involve multiple intracellular and extracellular pathways. The mechanical strain results in increases in growth factors as well as activation of intracellular pathways, the outcome being cellular growth and creation of new tissue.[80]

The physiological response of expansion varies by tissue type. In the skin the epidermis thickens while the dermis thins. Following expansion these changes typically reverse over several months in the epidermis and over 2 years in the dermis. Adipose tissue undergoes permanent atrophy during expansion ranging from 30% to 50%. Muscle similarly undergoes atrophy during expansion, however function is usually maintained. An additional benefit of tissue expansion is the resulting angiogenesis, with formation of a highly vascularized capsule. Flaps raised with this intact capsule are far more robust than comparable local and regional flaps. Expansion of hair-bearing scalp effectively produces new hair-bearing tissue. In this process hair follicles are not generated but rather the existing follicles are shared over a larger area. An area of scalp can be expanded to twice its original size before an appreciable thinning of the hair occurs.[81]

Expansion can be done intraoperatively with immediate inflation and stretching of tissues leading to a modest gain in size. More commonly though, expansion is done in a staged fashion with use of an implanted expansion device. These devices typically feature an integrated or separate injection port, although self-expanding implants employing osmotic fluid shifts also exist. Expanders come in a variety of shapes with rectangular, round, and crescentic being commonly used. Size selection is usually based on the amount of advancement required, which can be roughly correlated to the expander circumference minus the base width of the expander. Initially the expander should be inflated enough to fill the deadspace without putting undue tension on the surgical closure. Expansion is usually carried out over several weeks with injection intervals of 1 or 2 weeks. The endpoint for injection at each expansion session is determined by both patient comfort and perfusion of the overlying skin.

Complications of expansion include implant exposure, infection, deflation, and underlying bone resorption. If premature exposure does occur then consideration should be given to either expander deflation to allow for closure and attempted salvage, or expander removal and transposition of the flap as much as possible.

Fig. 3.3.11 depicts a secondary brow and forehead deformity resulting from an avulsion injury which was primarily treated with split-thickness skin grafting. Goals of reconstruction were removal of all grafted skin, release of the contracted brow and upper lid, and eventual brow reconstruction. Tissue expansion of the remaining ipsilateral forehead was undertaken with an expander placed in a submuscular

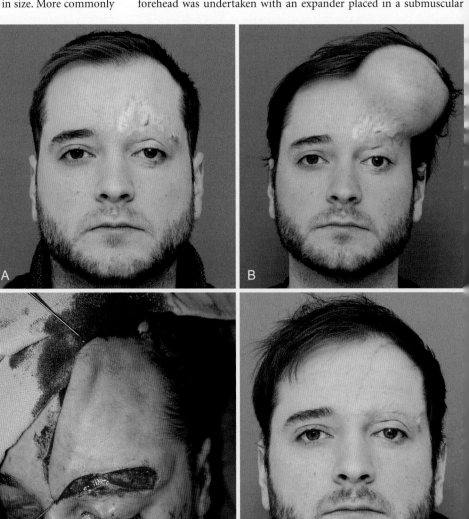

Fig. 3.3.11 (A) Avulsion injury of the left brow and forehead following treatment with split-thickness skin grafting. (B) Expansion of the remaining ipsilateral forehead. (C) Excision of the grafted area with rotation of the expanded tissue. (D) Early postoperative result.

plane. Following several weeks of inflation the expander was removed and reconstruction was completed with rotation of the expanded tissue. Note that despite the initial expansion of the hair-bearing scalp there is no distortion of the hairline. Subsequent eyebrow reconstruction is planned with hair transplantation.

EXPERT COMMENTARY

This chapter (a companion to the chapter on primary soft tissue injury treatment) is a subject few have written about, and what is written is often not good advice, in my opinion. The use/effectiveness of Z-plasties, for instance, is not something that can be trusted to improve the appearance of scars, and some of these techniques merely turn the scar into something with a more curious shape and configuration.

What can be said, however, is well said here, and reconstruction should be aimed at improving scars and replacing missing tissue and augmenting what is there by techniques of fat grafting.

The effects of fat grafting on scars are still being evaluated, however newer techniques still promise more hope. The main point is that proper initial management can prevent/minimize soft tissue injury, and the use of carefully chosen incisions, can camouflage the results of exposure techniques.

Soft tissue injury, and the use of carefully chosen incisions, can camouflage the results of exposure techniques [1–2].

The principles of cutaneous replacement which have been employed in more major cancer defects may also have use in trauma, and the principles are good basic information to consider. Children and young adults differ in their healing from the cancer population, however, and their different healing patterns and differences in scar formation must be learned.

The seasoned advice from two long-established practitioners who have devoted their careers to trauma is an excellent starting point for our own journey toward better results.

References

1. Manson P. Reconstruction of traumatic cutaneous facial defects. *Oper Tech Plast Reconstr Surg*. 1998;5(4):368–379.
2. Manson PN. Facial Injuries. In: McCarthy JG, ed. *Plastic Surgery*. Vol. 2. The Face, Part I. Philadelphia, PA: Saunders; 1990:867–1142.

REFERENCES

1. Hutchison IL, Magennis P, Shepherd JP, et al. The BAOMS United Kingdom survey of facial injuries. Part 1: aetiology and the association with alcohol consumption. *Br J Oral Maxillofac Surg*. 1998;36:3–13.
2. Ong TK, Dudley M. Craniofacial trauma presenting at an adult accident and emergency department with an emphasis on soft tissue injuries. *Injury*. 1999;30:357–363.
3. Antonyshyn OM. Soft tissue deformity after craniofacial fracture repair: analysis and treatment. *J Craniomaxillofac Trauma*. 1999;5(3):19–29, discussion 30–31.
4. Brown BC, McKenna SP, Siddhi K, et al. The hidden cost of skin scars: quality of life after skin scarring. *J Plast Reconstr Aesthet Surg*. 2008;61(9):1049–1058.
5. Gruss JS, Mackinnon SE. Complex maxillary fractures: role of buttress reconstruction and immediate bone grafts. *Plast Reconstr Surg*. 1986;78(1):9–22.
6. Manson PN, Crawley WA, Yaremchuk MJ, et al. Midface fractures: advantages of immediate extended open reduction and bone grafting. *Plast Reconstr Surg*. 1985;76(1):1–12.
7. Pakdel A, Whyne C, Fialkov JA. Structural biomechanics of the craniomaxillofacial skeleton under maximal masticatory loading: inferences and critical analysis based on a validated computational model. *J Plast Reconstr Aesthet Surg*. 2017;70(6):842–850.
8. Lacey M, Antonyshyn O, MacGregor JH. Temporal contour deformity after coronal flap elevation: an anatomical study. *J Craniofac Surg*. 1994;5(4):223–227.
9. Phillips JH, Gruss JS, Wells MD, et al. Periosteal suspension of the lower eyelid and cheek following subciliary exposure of facial fractures. *Plast Reconstr Surg*. 1991;88(1):145–148.
10. Ridgway EB, Chen C, Colakoglu S, et al. The incidence of lower eyelid malposition after facial fracture repair: a retrospective study and meta-analysis comparing subtarsal, subciliary, and transconjunctival incisions. *Plast Reconstr Surg*. 2009;124(5):1578–1586.
11. Regev E, Shiff JS, Kiss A, et al. Internal fixation of mandibular angle fractures: a meta-analysis. *Plast Reconstr Surg*. 2010;125(6): 1753–1760.
12. Ellis E 3rd, Perez D. An algorithm for the treatment of isolated zygomatico-orbital fractures. *J Oral Maxillofac Surg*. 2014;72(10):1975–1983.
13. Ellis E 3rd, Kittidumkerng W. Analysis of treatment for isolated zygomaticomaxillary complex fractures. *J Oral Maxillofac Surg*. 1996;54(4):386–400, discussion 400–401.
14. Kim ST, Go DH, Jung JH, et al. Comparison of 1-point fixation with 2-point fixation in treating tripod fractures of the zygoma. *J Oral Maxillofac Surg*. 2011;69(11):2848–2852.
15. Orringer JS, Barcelona V, Buchman SR. Reasons for removal of rigid internal fixation devices in craniofacial surgery. *J Craniofac Surg*. 1998;9(1):40–44.
16. Francel TJ, Birely BC, Ringelman PR, et al. The fate of plates and screws after facial fracture reconstruction. *Plast Reconstr Surg*. 1992;90(4):568–573.
17. Guo S, DiPietro LA. Factors affecting wound healing. *J Dent Res*. 2010;89(3):219–229.
18. Sullivan T, Smith J, Kermode J, et al. Rating the burn scar. *J Burn Care Rehabil*. 1990;11(3):256–260.
19. Bagheri SC, Meyer RA, Khan HA, et al. Microsurgical repair of peripheral trigeminal nerve injuries from maxillofacial trauma. *J Oral Maxillofac Surg*. 2009;67(9):1791–1799.
20. Ettorre G, Weber M, Schaaf H, et al. Standards for digital photography in cranio-maxillo-facial surgery - Part I: basic views and guidelines. *J Craniomaxillofac Surg*. 2006;34(2):65–73.
21. Sultan B, Byrne PJ. Custom-made, 3D, intraoperative surgical guides for nasal reconstruction. *Facial Plast Surg Clin North Am*. 2011;19(4):647–653, viii–ix.
22. Lekakis G, Claes P, Hamilton GS 3rd, et al. Three-dimensional surface imaging and the continuous evolution of preoperative and postoperative assessment in rhinoplasty. *Facial Plast Surg*. 2016;32(1):88–94.
23. Hontscharuk R, Fialkov JA, Binhammer PA, et al. Primary orbital fracture repair: development and validation of tools for morphologic and functional analysis. *J Craniofac Surg*. 2012;23(4):1044–1049.
24. Mayer JS, Wainwright DJ, Yeakley JW, et al. The role of three-dimensional computed tomography in the management of maxillofacial trauma. *J Trauma*. 1988;28(7):1043–1053.
25. Fox LA, Vannier MW, West OC, et al. Diagnostic performance of CT, MPR and 3DCT imaging in maxillofacial trauma. *Comput Med Imaging Graph*. 1995;19(5):385–395.
26. Mazzola RF, Mazzola IC. History of fat grafting: from ram fat to stem cells. *Clin Plast Surg*. 2015;42(2):147–153.
27. Sinno S, Wilson S, Brownstone N, et al. Current thoughts on fat grafting: using the evidence to determine fact or fiction. *Plast Reconstr Surg*. 2016;137(3):818–824.
28. Coleman SR, Katzel EB. Fat grafting for facial filling and regeneration. *Clin Plast Surg*. 2015;42(3):289–300, vii.
29. Coleman SR. Structural fat grafting. *Aesthet Surg J*. 1998;18(5):386–388.
30. Small K, Choi M, Petruolo O, et al. Is there an ideal donor site of fat for secondary breast reconstruction? *Aesthet Surg J*. 2014;34:545–550.
31. Smith P, Adams WP Jr, Lipschitz AH, et al. Autologous human fat grafting: effect of harvesting and preparation techniques on adipocyte graft survival. *Plast Reconstr Surg*. 2006;117:1836–1844.
32. Lazzeri D, Agostini T, Figus M, et al. Blindness following cosmetic injections of the face. *Plast Reconstr Surg*. 2012;129:995–1012.
33. Lacey M, Antonyshyn O, MacGregor JH. Temporal contour deformity after coronal flap elevation: an anatomical study. *J Craniofac Surg*. 1994;5(4):223–227.

34. Kim S, Matic DB. The anatomy of temporal hollowing: the superficial temporal fat pad. *J Craniofac Surg.* 2005;16(5):760–763.
35. Guo J, Tian W, Long J, et al. A retrospective study of traumatic temporal hollowing and treatment with titanium mesh. *Ann Plast Surg.* 2012;68(3):279–285.
36. Matic DB, Kim S. Temporal hollowing following coronal incision: a prospective, randomized, controlled trial. *Plast Reconstr Surg.* 2008;121(6):379e–385e.
37. Tzafetta K, Terzis JK. Essays on the facial nerve: part I. Microanatomy. *Plast Reconstr Surg.* 2010;125(3):879–889.
38. Roostaeian J, Rohrich RJ, Stuzin JM. Anatomical considerations to prevent facial nerve injury. *Plast Reconstr Surg.* 2015;135(5):1318–1327.
39. Baek RM, Heo CY, Lee SW. Temporal dissection technique that prevents temporal hollowing in coronal approach. *J Craniofac Surg.* 2009;20(3):748–751.
40. Luo W, Wang L, Jing W. A new coronal scalp technique to treat craniofacial fracture: the supratemporalis approach. *Oral Surg Oral Med Oral Pathol Oral Radiol.* 2012;113(2):177–182.
41. Cheung LK, Samman N, Tideman H. The use of mouldable acrylic for restoration of the temporalis flap donor site. *J Craniomaxillofac Surg.* 1994;22:335.
42. Gosain AK. Hydroxyapatite cement paste cranioplasty for the treatment of temporal hollowing after cranial vault remodeling in a growing child. *J Craniofac Surg.* 1997;8:506.
43. Burstein FD, Cohen SR, Hudgins R, et al. The use of porous granular hydroxyapatite in secondary orbitocranial reconstruction. *Plast Reconstr Surg.* 1997;100:869.
44. Lacey M, Antonyshyn O. Use of porous high-density polyethylene implants in temporal contour reconstruction. *J Craniofac Surg.* 1993;4:74.
45. Reiche-Fischel O, Wolford LM, Pitta M. Facial contour reconstruction using an autologous free fat graft: a case report with 18-year follow-up. *J Oral Maxillofac Surg.* 2000;58:103.
46. Clauser LC, Tieghi R, Galiè M, et al. Structural fat grafting: facial volumetric restoration in complex reconstructive surgery. *J Craniofac Surg.* 2011;22(5):1695–1701.
47. Francesco A, Matteo B, Nicola B, et al. The role of fat grafting in the treatment of posttraumatic maxillofacial deformities. *Craniomaxillofac Trauma Reconstr.* 2013;6(2):121–126.
48. McNichols CH, Hatef DA, Cole P, et al. Contemporary techniques for the correction of temporal hollowing: augmentation temporoplasty with the classic dermal fat graft. *J Craniofac Surg.* 2012;23(3):e234–e238.
49. Wong CH, Mendelson B. Facial soft-tissue spaces and retaining ligaments of the midcheek: defining the premaxillary space. *Plast Reconstr Surg.* 2013;132(1):49–56.
50. Moss CJ, Mendelson BC, Taylor GI. Surgical anatomy of the ligamentous attachments in the temple and periorbital regions. *Plast Reconstr Surg.* 2000;105(4):1475–1490, discussion 1491–1498.
51. Yaremchuk MJ, Kim WK. Soft-tissue alterations associated with acute, extended open reduction and internal fixation or orbital fractures. *J Craniofac Surg.* 1992;3(3):134–140.
52. Ng SK, Chan W, Marcet MM, et al. Levator palpebrae superioris: an anatomical update. *Orbit.* 2013;32(1):76–84.
53. Ezra DG, Beaconsfield M, Collin R. Surgical anatomy of the upper eyelid: old controversies, new concepts. Expert Rev Ophthalmol. 4(1):47.
54. Dutton JJ, Frueh BR. Eyelid anatomy and physiology with reference to blepharoptosis. In: Cohen AJ, Weinberg DA, eds. *Evaluation and Management of Blepharoptosis.* Berlin: Springer Business + Media; 2011:13–26.
55. Finsterer J. Ptosis: causes, presentation, and management. *Aesth Plast Surg.* 2003;27:193–204.
56. Boyle NS, Chang EL. Traumatic blepharoptosis. In: Cohen AJ, Weinberg DA, eds. *Evaluation and Management of Blepharoptosis.* Berlin: Springer Business + Media; 2011:129–140.
57. Berke RN. Surgical treatment of traumatic blepharoptosis. *Am J Ophthalmol.* 1971;72:691–698.
58. Kim YJ, Choi WKJ. Delayed superior orbital fissure syndrome after reconstruction of blowout fracture. *J Craniofac Surg.* 2016;27(1):e8–e10.
59. Li G, Zhang Y, Zhu X, et al. Transient traumatic isolated neurogenic ptosis after a mild head trauma: a case report. *BMC Ophthalmol.* 2015;15:161.
60. Satchi K, Kumar A, McNab AA. Isolated traumatic neurogenic ptosis with delayed recovery. *Ophthal Plast Reconstr Surg.* 2014;30(1):57–59.
61. Burget GC, Menick FJ. The subunit principle in nasal reconstruction. *Plast Reconstr Surg.* 1985;76(2):239–247.
62. Teshima TL, Cheng H, Pakdel A, et al. Transverse slicing of the sixth–seventh costal cartilaginous junction: a novel technique to prevent warping in nasal surgery. *J Craniofac Surg.* 2016;27(1):e50–e55.
63. Pribaz JJ, Falco N. Nasal reconstruction with auricular microvascular transplant. *Ann Plast Surg.* 1993;31(4):289–297.
64. Ducic Y, Adelson R. Use of the endoscopic forehead-lift to improve brow position in persistent facial paralysis. *Arch Facial Plast Surg.* 2005;7:51–54.
65. Bastidas N, Zide B. Suspension of the brow in facial paralysis and frontalis loss. *Plast Reconstr Surg.* 2010;126(2):486–488.
66. Winter GD. Formation of the scab and the rate of epithelisation of superficial wounds in the skin of the young domestic pig. *Nature.* 1962;193:293–294.
67. Ehrlich HP, Tarver H, Hunt TK. Inhibitory effects of vitamin E on collagen synthesis and wound repair. *Ann Surg.* 1972;175(2):235–240.
68. Baumann LS, Spencer J. The effects of topical vitamin E on the cosmetic appearance of scars. *Dermatol Surg.* 1999;25(4):311–315.
69. Zampieri N, Suin V, Burro R. A prospective study in children: pre- and post-surgery use of vitamin E in surgical incisions. *J Plast Reconstr Aesthet Surg.* 2009;63(9):1474–1478.
70. Perkins K, Davey RB, Wallis KA. Silicone gel: a new treatment for burn scars and contractures. *Burns.* 1983;9(3):201–204.
71. Mustoe TA, Cooter RD, Gold MH. International clinical recommendations on scar management. *Plast Reconstr Surg.* 2002;110(2):560–571.
72. O'Brien L, Jones DJ. Silicone gel sheeting for preventing and treating hypertrophic and keloid scars. *Cochrane Database Syst Rev.* 2013;(9):CD003826.
73. Alexiades-Armenakas MR, Dover JS, Arndt KA. The spectrum of laser skin resurfacing: nonablative, fractional, and ablative laser resurfacing. *J Am Acad Dermatol.* 2008;58(5):719–737, quiz 738–740.
74. Alster TS, Williams CM. Treatment of keloid sternotomy scars with 585 nm ashlamp-pumped pulsed-dye laser. *Lancet.* 1995;345:1198–1200.
75. Goldman MP. The use of hydroquinone with facial laser resurfacing. *J Cutan Laser Ther.* 2000;2(2):73–77.
76. Vrints I, Den Hondt M, Van Brussel M, et al. Immediate debridement of road rash injuries with Versajet® hydrosurgery: traumatic tattoo prevention? *Aesthetic Plast Surg.* 2014;38(2):467–470.
77. Seitz AT, Grunewald S, Wagner JA. Fractional CO_2 laser is as effective as Q-switched ruby laser for the initial treatment of a traumatic tattoo. *J Cosmet Laser Ther.* 2014;16(6):303–305.
78. Taylor C. Laser ignition of traumatically embedded firework debris. *Lasers Surg Med.* 1998;22(3):157–158.
79. Thomas JR, Prendiville S. Update in scar revision. *Facial Plast Surg Clin North Am.* 2002;10(1):103–111.
80. Takei T, Mills I, Arai K, et al. Molecular basis for tissue expansion: clinical implications for the surgeon. *Plast Reconstr Surg.* 1998;102(1):247–258.
81. Buchanan PJ, Kung TA, Cederna PS. Evidence-based medicine: Wound closure. *Plast Reconstr Surg.* 2014;134(6):1391–1404.

Ocular Considerations: Ectropion, Entropion, Blink, Ptosis, Epiphora

Shannath Merbs, Sarah DeParis

BACKGROUND

Approximately 2.4 million eye injuries occur each year.[1] Ocular and periocular trauma can occur by a variety of mechanisms, some of the most common including assault and blunt trauma, motor vehicle collisions, gunshot, fireworks, and falls.[2] The cumulative lifetime prevalence of eye injuries in the United States is approximately 1400 per 100,000 population.[2,3] In one study, medical treatment was not sought for 18% of these injuries.[4] Acute management of traumatic injury necessitates immediate evaluation by an ophthalmologist, as vision loss is a serious risk, and more than half of those with eyelid injury have underlying globe injury.[5] However, in one study 60% of injured eyes showed improvement in visual acuity after treatment.[2]

The United States Eye Injury Registry estimates that periocular injuries occur in 5% of all serious injuries, with 80% affecting the canalicular structures and 70% affecting the eyelids.[5] As discussed in Chapter 1.9, eyelid lacerations must be repaired to properly align the eyelid structures and avoid the later development of an eyelid notch. Eyelid lacerations, including the canaliculi, require repair and stenting of the canaliculi to prevent future epiphora.

Even if visual function is preserved following an acute periocular injury, scarring can occur, which can further threaten vision years later. Ectropion, entropion, eyelid retraction, ptosis and epiphora can occur months to years following trauma, and may have functional and visual consequences necessitating secondary reconstruction.

SURGICAL ANATOMY

Eyelid and Soft Tissue Anatomy

Knowledge of the normal anatomy of the eyelids is vital to identifying and repairing conditions such as entropion that may interfere with their function.

The peak of the upper eyelid slope is at the medial edge of the pupil. The lateral canthus lies slightly higher than the medial canthus. The palpebral fissure, or vertical distance between the upper and lower eyelid margins is normally about 9 mm. The eyelid height may be measured by the marginal reflex distance 1 (MRD1) and marginal reflex distance 2 (MRD2). The MRD1 is the distance from the pupillary light reflex to the upper eyelid margin, and is normally approximately 4 mm. The MRD2 is the distance from the light reflex to the lower eyelid margin and is typically about 5 mm. The lower eyelid margin normally rests at the inferior junction between the cornea and sclera, the inferior limbus. Lower eyelid retraction is present if the eyelid margin falls below this, and can be quantified by measuring the inferior scleral show, or millimeters of sclera visible between the inferior limbus and the lower eyelid margin.

The eyelids are anchored to the orbital bones by the medial and lateral canthal tendons. The lateral canthus is typically a few millimeters higher than the medial canthus, creating a slight downward slope of the palpebral fissure from the lateral to the medial aspect. The medial canthal tendon divides into anterior and posterior limbs, which attach at the anterior and posterior lacrimal crests, respectively, surrounding the lacrimal sac. The lateral canthal tendon is divided into superior and inferior limbs, which join and attach together at Whitnall's tubercle on the lateral orbital rim.

Beneath the upper and lower eyelid skin lies the orbicularis muscle, which is responsible for eyelid closure and is innervated by the seventh cranial nerve. The pretarsal portion of the orbicularis overlies the tarsal plate, the preseptal portion overlies the septum, and the orbital portion overlies the orbital rim.

The tarsal plate is located posterior to the orbicularis and is made of fibrous tissue. In the upper eyelid, the tarsal plate extends approximately 10 mm above the upper eyelid margin. Posterior to the tarsal plate is the conjunctiva, which contains goblet cells that supply the mucin layer of the tear film.

The two main retractors of the upper eyelid are the levator palpebrae superioris and Müller's muscle. The levator is the primary retractor of the upper eyelid and is innervated by the superior division of the third cranial nerve. Müller's muscle is innervated by sympathetic fibers and extends from the superior border of the tarsus to Whitnall's ligament. Superior to the tarsal plate, the orbital septum, the boundary between the eyelid and orbit, lies posterior to the orbicularis, overlying the preaponeurotic fat. The levator aponeurosis lies posterior to the preaponeurotic fat and anterior to Müller's muscle and conjunctiva.

In the lower eyelid, the orbicularis lies posterior to the skin. The tarsal plate extends 4–6 mm from the lower eyelid margin posterior to the orbicularis, and is lined posteriorly by the conjunctiva. The lower eyelid retractors, or the capsulopalpebral fascia, attach to the inferior aspect of the tarsal plate and are analogous to the function of the levator muscle in the upper eyelid.

The anterior lamella of the eyelids consists of the skin and orbicularis muscle. The posterior lamella includes the tarsal plate and conjunctiva. The gray line, visible at the eyelid margin, marks the boundary between the anterior and posterior lamellae and is a useful anatomical landmark during eyelid surgery.

Lacrimal System Anatomy

The lacrimal system includes the tear film of the eye and the tear drainage system. The tear film is made up of three layers. The most anterior layer is the oil layer, produced by the meibomian glands and glands of Zeis, and functions to prevent evaporation of the tear film. The middle layer is the aqueous layer, produced by the lacrimal gland and accessory glands of Wolfring and Krause. The mucous layer is the most posterior layer, produced by the goblet cells of the conjunctiva.

The openings to the lacrimal drainage system are the superior and inferior puncta, located medially in the upper and lower eyelid, respectively. Tears travel through the puncta into the superior and inferior canaliculi, which join to form the common canaliculus. The common canaliculus enters the lacrimal sac via the valve of Rosenmuller.

The lacrimal sac lies in the lacrimal fossa, bounded by the anterior and posterior lacrimal crests. The anterior portion of the fossa is made up of a portion of the maxillary bone, and the posterior portion of the fossa is composed of the much thinner lacrimal bone. The blinking action of the eyelids acts as a pump to fill and empty the lacrimal sac. This pumping function is compromised in patients with facial nerve palsy, which is in part responsible for tearing in those patients. The lacrimal sac drains into the nasolacrimal duct, which is lined by mucosa and enters the nose through the valve of Hasner beneath the inferior turbinate in the inferior meatus. Dacryocystorhinostomy surgery bypasses obstruction in the nasolacrimal duct by creating a new orifice into the nose at the level of the lacrimal sac.

CLINICAL ASSESSMENT

History

A thorough history is necessary to guide clinical and surgical decision-making. The mechanism of injury and amount of time elapsed are important elements of the history. Past imaging, if available, should be reviewed. The history of present illness should elicit the patient's primary complaints and allows the surgeon to determine if functional impairment is present. Ocular surface irritation, discomfort, and dryness are common complaints with ectropion, entropion, and eyelid retraction. Corneal epithelial defects or ulcerations may cause significant pain and erythema of the eye. Prior canalicular laceration or fracture through the nasolacrimal duct may result in significant epiphora, which can impair function. Traumatic seventh nerve palsy may result in poor orbicularis function and impairment of the eyelid blink and closure, which can result in ocular surface exposure and desiccation, creating significant discomfort for the patient. Ptosis, which can occur secondary to trauma, can obstruct the superior and temporal visual fields, interfering with visual function. In each case, the surgeon and patient must weigh the risks of surgery against the degree of functional impairment that is present.

Examination

Dilated fundus examination should be performed at the time of initial injury, as there is significant correlation between periocular and concurrent intraocular injuries. Visual acuity, confrontational visual fields, pupils, and ocular motility should be assessed in all patients with a history of trauma. If possible, slit lamp examination should be performed, and should include evaluation of all anterior ocular structures. Careful attention should be paid to the eyelids. MRD1 and MRD2 should be assessed. The patient should be asked to close their eyes gently to assess for lagophthalmos (Fig. 3.4.1). Hertel exophthalmometry can be helpful in the setting of orbital fractures to assess for enophthalmos.

ENTROPION

Entropion, or posterior rotation of the eyelid margin, with or without trichiasis, may occur after trauma. Although there are several types of entropion, cicatricial entropion is often present in the setting of prior trauma, where scarring and contracture of the posterior lamella rotates the eyelid margin inward. The palpebral conjunctiva of both the upper and lower eyelids should be evaluated, and careful eversion of the upper eyelid should be performed. Scarring of the conjunctiva and posteriorly displaced meibomian gland orifices are suggestive of cicatricial entropion. There may also be concurrent horizontal laxity of the eyelid,

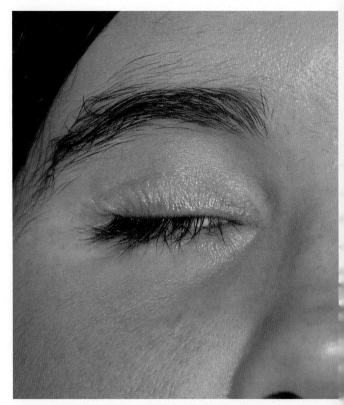

Fig. 3.4.1 Lagophthalmos. Upper eyelid scarring causing limitation of the right upper eyelid excursion and resulting in the abnormal ability to see the sclera of the eye nasally with the individual's eye closed.

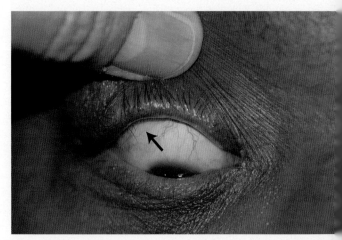

Fig. 3.4.2 Trichiasis. Abnormal lashes growing towards the eye (*arrow*)

which should be evaluated by performing snap-back testing, or pulling the lower eyelid away from the globe and assessing how quickly it snaps back into place. Trichiasis (Fig. 3.4.2) may be present with or without corresponding corneal surface breakdown due to mechanical trauma from eyelashes. Fluorescein staining should be performed if indicated to determine whether the corneal epithelium is intact. In the most severe cases, a corneal epithelial defect may become superinfected to become a corneal ulcer. Corneal ulceration typically appears as focal corneal opacification with overlying epithelial defect, and if present should be urgently evaluated by an ophthalmologist.

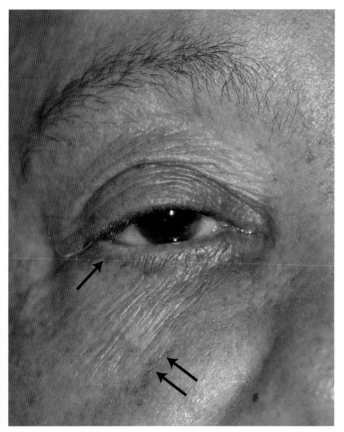

Fig. 3.4.3 Ectropion. Turning outward of the lateral aspect of the lower eyelid (*arrow*) resulting in the ability to see the inflamed tarsal conjunctiva. Note the vertical tension lines in the skin (*double arrow*).

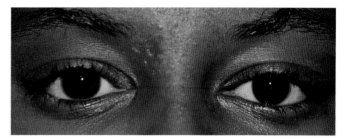

Fig. 3.4.4 Dye disappearance test. Elevated tear meniscus and retention of the fluorescein dye on the right side secondary to tear outflow obstruction.

PTOSIS

Traumatic ptosis can occur due to dehiscence or laceration of the levator tendon or muscle, or by injury to the branch of the superior division of the third cranial nerve supplying the levator palpebrae superioris. In the case of nerve injury, this may recover spontaneously as late as 6 months after injury, and a trial of observation is warranted prior to surgical intervention.

The eyelid height and contour should be assessed and compared with the contralateral side. Eyelid height may be quantified using the MRD1. Levator function should be quantified by asking the patient to look down, and then look up while the examiner prevents the use of the frontalis muscle of the forehead with their hand. The excursion of the upper eyelid margin from downgaze to upgaze is the levator function measurement in millimeters. Lagophthalmos should be assessed as well by asking the patient to gently close their eyes. This may be relevant when considering ptosis repair, as if significant lagophthalmos is present, aggressive lifting of the eyelid may be contraindicated due to the risk of corneal exposure.

ECTROPION

Cicatricial ectropion can also occur after past trauma due to scarring of the anterior lamella, leading to anterior rotation of the eyelid margin (Fig. 3.4.3). The eyelid skin and margin should be assessed for tautness and evidence of scarring. The eyelid should be assessed for horizontal laxity with the snap-back technique. The corneal surface should be examined and fluorescein staining should be performed if indicated. Eyelid retraction may also be present, and the amount of inferior scleral show (the distance from the inferior corneoscleral limbus to the lower eyelid margin) and lagophthalmos should be quantified. In severe cases, exposure of the inferior cornea can cause corneal epithelial breakdown.

BLINK

In the case of facial nerve palsy from trauma, the patient's eyelid closure and blink may be affected. The blink should be observed, and may be noted to be hypometric. The patient should be asked to gently close their eyes, mimicking sleep, to assess for lagophthalmos. If present, this should be measured. Lower eyelid retraction may be present, which can be quantified by measuring the amount of inferior scleral show and the MRD2. Again, the corneal surface should be evaluated and fluorescein staining performed. A normal corneal epithelium will appear smooth with an even tear film overlying. In exposure keratopathy, punctate epithelial erosions may indicate ocular surface dryness, and appear as faint individual dots of staining on fluorescein testing. In the case of severe exposure keratopathy, the cornea may be thinned. A corneal ulcer may also occur in this instance due to superinfection.

EPIPHORA

With a complaint of epiphora, the height and quality of the lacrimal lake should be assessed. In patients with nasolacrimal duct obstruction, the tear lake will be elevated. The puncta should be examined and assessed for patency, stenosis, and punctal ectropion. A dye disappearance test (Fig. 3.4.4) may show a delay of fluorescein disappearance from the eye compared to the contralateral side. Irrigation of the tear system should be performed to determine if a nasolacrimal duct obstruction is present.

Ancillary Testing

Humphrey visual field testing can be considered in patients with complaints of visual loss or with visual field defects on confrontational testing. In patients with epiphora, perform irrigation testing of the tear drainage system and note as to whether there is recovery of fluid in the patient's throat. The amount of reflux should be quantified, and it should be noted whether reflux occurs through the opposite or same punctum. With nasolacrimal duct obstruction and a history of trauma, computed tomography (CT) imaging of the orbital and facial structures should be considered as this can guide surgical planning. Ptosis visual field testing is useful and may be required by insurance companies for approval of ptosis repair. It can be performed with the upper eyelid in its natural state and then with the eyelid manually elevated with tape to determine if reversible obstruction of the superior visual field is present.

Surgical Indications

The patient's complaints, degree of functional impairment, and examination findings should be assessed as a whole to determine if surgical intervention is indicated. If there is significant functional impairment, aesthetic impairment, or risk to the health of the eye, and examination findings that explain the patient's complaints, surgery may be considered.

SURGICAL TECHNIQUES

Cicatricial Ectropion Repair

Cicatricial ectropion results from horizontal laxity and a shortage of anterior lamella due to scarring. Therefore, repair of cicatricial ectropion typically requires a full-thickness skin graft. This can be harvested from the upper eyelid in a fashion similar to a blepharoplasty, or can be taken from the preauricular, postauricular or supraclavicular skin. Eyelid skin is preferable as it is closest in thickness and pigmentation and lacks hair follicles. The skin graft should be combined with a horizontal tightening procedure such as a wedge excision, lateral tarsal strip, or lateral canthoplasty to elevate the eyelid.[6]

Wedge Excision

A subciliary incision is initiated with a #15 blade at the lateral canthus and continued with sharp iris scissors. A traction suture is placed inferior to the lid margin through the orbicularis to provide exposure. Submuscular dissection is performed across the length of the incision (Fig. 3.4.5A). Thickened conjunctiva should be removed and the bare tarsus allowed to reepithelize. A full-thickness base-up wedge is excised with iris scissors from the tarsus at the location of the worst ectropion (Fig. 3.4.5B). The tarsus is re-approximated with 6-0 polyglactin sutures (Fig. 3.4.5C). Eyelid margin sutures are then placed with 8-0 silk at the gray line and the lash line, taking care to ensure good alignment and eversion of the wound edges to prevent development of a notch.

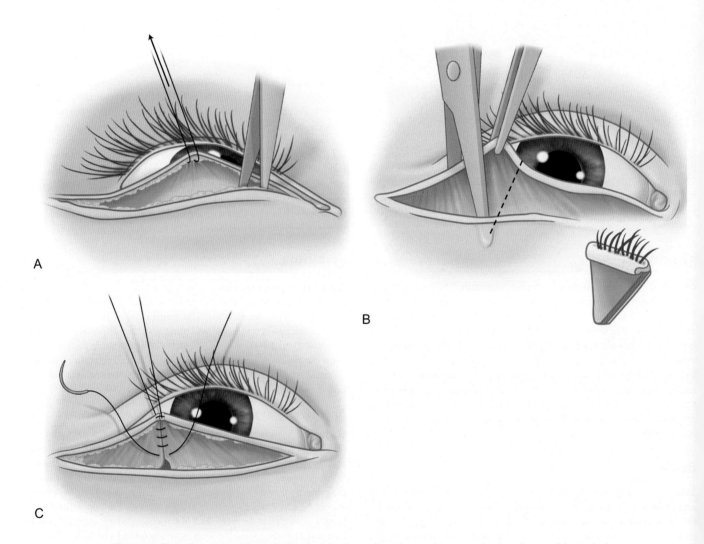

Fig. 3.4.5 Ectropion repair. (A) A subciliary incision is made and a traction suture is placed to provide vertical tension to the lower eyelid. A skin/muscle flap is raised by dissecting between the orbicularis and orbital septum allowing the eyelid to be raised. Thickened, inflamed conjunctiva should be removed to allow the freed eyelid to become apposed to the eye. The bare tarsus will reepithelize. (B) A full-thickness, base-up triangular resection of the tarsus is performed at the location of the worst ectropion, which is often nasal because the lateral canthal ligament helps to stabilize the lateral aspect of the lower eyelid. (C) The tarsus is reapproximated with partial-thickness 6-0 polyglactin sutures. The eyelid margin and subciliary incision are then closed. (From Iliff NT, Merbs SL. Ectropion. In: Gottsch JD, Stark WJ, Goldberg MF, editors. Rob & Smith's operative surgery: Ophthalmic surgery. 5th ed. London: Arnold; 1999. (A) p.20, Figure 2; (B) p.20, Figure 3; (C) p.21, Figure 4.)

Lateral Tarsal Strip

A lateral canthotomy and cantholysis is performed (Fig. 3.4.6A). The anterior lamella and eyelashes are removed from the tarsal strip. The conjunctiva is ablated with bipolar cautery or debrided with a #15 blade. Both arms of a double-armed 4-0 polyester suture are then passed from the posterior to anterior surface of the tarsal strip (Fig. 3.4.6B). Each arm is then passed through the inner aspect of the periosteum of the lateral orbital rim. The suture is tied with appropriate tension, and a 6-0 polyglactin suture is then used to reform the lateral canthal angle (Fig. 3.4.6C).

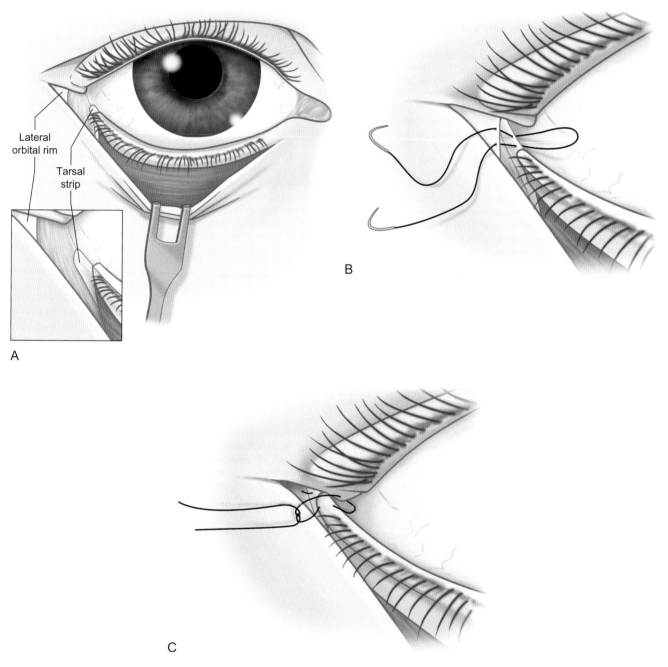

Fig. 3.4.6 Tarsal strip procedure. (A) A subciliary incision is made across the length of the eyelid and is extended into a lateral canthal incision for about 1 cm. A 3–4 mm tarsal strip is created by removing the skin, orbicularis, and eyelashes. The conjunctiva on the strip is either ablated with cautery or removed with a blade. (B) Both arms of a double-armed 4-0 polyester suture are then passed from the posterior to anterior surface of the tarsal strip, and then each arm is passed, posterior to anterior, through the periosteum of the inner aspect of the lateral orbital rim. (C) The lateral canthal angle is reformed with a 6-0 polyglactan suture with the knot buried laterally. (From Iliff NT, Merbs SL. Entropion. In: Gottsch JD, Stark WJ, Goldberg MF, editors. Rob & Smith's operative surgery: Ophthalmic surgery. 5th ed. London: Arnold; 1999. (A) p.14, Figure 1; (B) p.14, Figure 2a; (C) p.14, Figure 2b.)

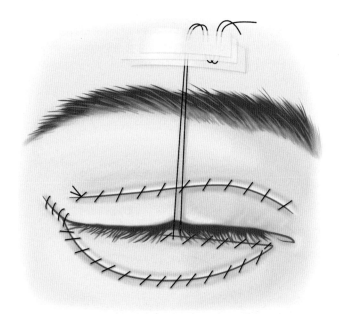

Fig. 3.4.7 Skin graft. After a subciliary incision and dissection of a skin/muscle flap to release the anterior tension on the eyelid margin, the skin deficit is measured and the skin obtained from a blepharoplasty incision. The skin is trimmed of its subcutaneous tissue and secured in place, and the donor site closed, with a running 8-0 nylon sutures. A traction suture placed anterior to the margin is taped above the brow to stretch the recipient bed, which should be dry. A bolster is not needed; a patch overnight is sufficient. (From Iliff NT, Merbs SL. Ectropion. In: Gottsch JD, Stark WJ, Goldberg MF, editors. Rob & Smith's operative surgery: Ophthalmic surgery. 5th ed. London: Arnold; 1999. (A) p.24, Figure 14.)

Full-Thickness Skin Graft

The skin graft is first harvested. In the upper eyelid, markings are made as for a blepharoplasty in the upper eyelid crease of the appropriate dimensions, ensuring that enough anterior lamella is preserved to allow complete eyelid closure. The incision is made with a #15 blade and the graft harvested and thinned with iris scissors. Careful hemostasis with bipolar cautery is important throughout. The graft is then positioned into the lower eyelid defect and secured with 8-0 nylon sutures in a running fashion. The eye can be closed by a Frost traction suture, which can be left in place while the eye is patched for 3 days (Fig. 3.4.7). 6-0 Nylon suture is passed through the lower eyelid margin at the gray line, out through skin, and back in through skin and exiting at the gray line. The suture ends are secured to the forehead with a liquid adhesive and Steri-Strips.

Cicatricial Entropion Repair

Repair of cicatricial entropion requires release of the conjunctival scarring by tarsotomy and placement of rotational sutures. A mucous membrane graft may be used to extend the posterior lamellar surface. Eyelid laxity or dehiscence of the retractors may be present concurrently. If the eyelid can be retracted from the globe by more than 3–4 mm, horizontal tightening (such as lateral tarsal strip, see above) should be performed in conjunction with tarsotomy and eyelid margin rotation. If there is evidence of the entire tarsal plate rotating inward due to dehiscence of the retractors, they should be reinserted.[7]

Tarsotomy and Eyelid Margin Rotation

An incision is made through conjunctiva and tarsus just inferior where the anatomical posterior edge of the eyelid margin would be (Fig. 3.4.8A). The location of the meibomian glands can be used to guide the location

of the incision. Both arms of a double-armed 7-0 chromic gut suture are passed through the posterior edge of the wound, full thickness through the eyelid, exiting at the lash line, and are tied, creating eversion of the lid margin and a resulting conjunctival defect (Fig. 3.4.8B). This is repeated in several locations along the length of the eyelid.

A mucous membrane graft is then harvested from the buccal mucosa (Fig. 3.4.8C). The area is marked to match the size of the conjunctival defect. A #15 blade is used to incise at the marks, and the graft is harvested with iris scissors. After hemostasis is achieved, the mucosal donor site is then reapproximated with 5-0 chromic gut sutures or left to heal by secondary intent. The gloves and instruments should then be changed prior to continuing with the procedure. The graft is placed in antibiotic solution, thinned, and placed in the conjunctival defect. It is secured with running 7-0 chromic gut suture with the knots on the skin to avoid a corneal abrasion.

Reinsertion of Eyelid Retractors

A subciliary incision is initiated with a #15 blade at the lateral canthus and continued with sharp iris scissors. A traction suture is placed inferior to the lid margin through the orbicularis to provide exposure. Sharp iris scissors are used to dissect through orbicularis to the inferior border of tarsus. Dissection is carried further inferiorly through the septum until orbital fat is encountered. The retractors are identified lying just posterior to the orbital fat and inferior to the tarsus (Fig. 3.4.9). Interrupted passes of 6-0 polyglactin suture are then used to reattach the retractors to the inferior aspect of the tarsal plate.

Eyelid Retraction Repair

Acellular porcine dermal matrix may be used as a lower eyelid spacer to bolster the eyelid height in the case of lower lid retraction. This can be done in combination with a tightening procedure if laxity is present.

A subciliary incision is started with a #15 blade at the lateral canthus and continued with sharp iris scissors. A traction suture is placed inferior to the lid margin through the orbicularis to provide exposure. Subcutaneous dissection is performed across the length of the incision. The orbicularis is then entered with sharp iris scissors and elevated separately from the cutaneous flap. An acellular porcine dermal matrix implant (such as ENDURAGen, Stryker, Kalamazoo, MI) is cut to size and placed deep to the preorbital orbicularis inferior to the tarsal plate (Fig. 3.4.10). It is secured with interrupted passes of 6-0 polyglactin to the inferior aspect of the tarsal plate. The biplanar flap is then advanced, with the muscular portion overlying the implant, and the cutaneous portion over the pretarsal orbicularis.

Dacryocystorhinostomy

Dacryocystorhinostomy (DCR) is indicated in patients with significant epiphora and complete or near-complete nasolacrimal duct obstruction as diagnosed by punctal irrigation.[8]

The incision site is marked along the anterior lacrimal crest within the eyelid skin crease. The incision is made with a #15 blade down to the orbital rim through skin, orbicularis, and periosteum. Skin rakes are used for retraction. A Freer elevator is used to elevate the periosteum and carry dissection into the lacrimal sac fossa (Fig. 3.4.11A). The medial wall of the lacrimal sac fossa is then removed with a sphenoid bone punch (Fig. 3.4.11B). A Surgitron radiofrequency dissector is then used to make a vertical incision in the lacrimal sac and a corresponding vertical incision in the nasal mucosa (Fig. 3.4.11C). A groove director is placed in the nose to the level of the ostium. A bicanalicular silicone stent is threaded through the canaliculi and into the nose within the groove director (Fig. 3.4.11D). The two ends are tied with 6-0 silk suture within the ostium to prevent prolapse and trimmed to appropriate length. A 12-French rubber catheter is threaded over the silicone tube

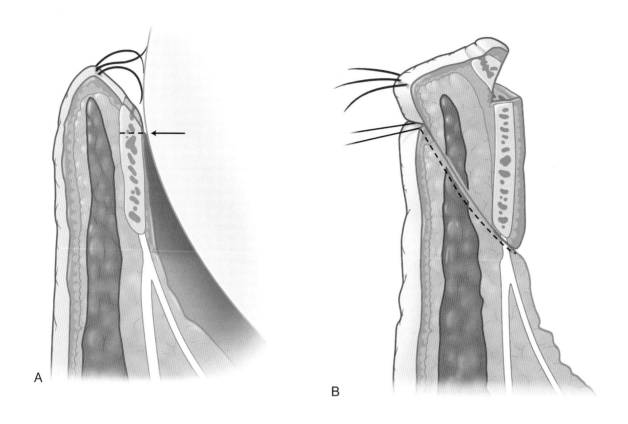

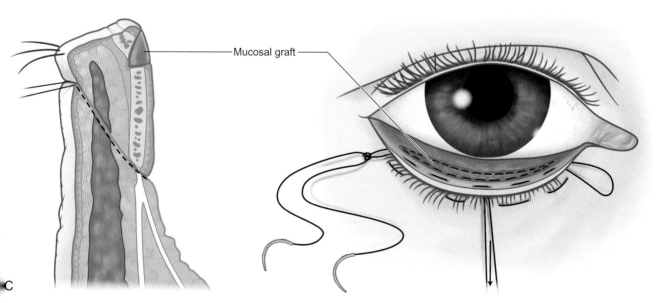

Fig. 3.4.8 Cicatricial entropion repair. (A) A horizontal incision is made through the conjunctiva and tarsus, posterior to the meibomian glands, at a point corresponding to the normal posterior eyelid margin. (B) Mattress sutures, using a double-armed 5-0 chromic suture, are placed from the bottom of the tarsus to the lash line. When these sutures are tied, the lashes rotate anteriorly and the posterior incision is widened. Typically three sutures are required to rotate the entire margin. (C) The posterior lamellar deficit, demonstrated by the gap in the incision, is filled with a mucous membrane graft obtained from the mouth. The graft is sutured in place with a running 7-0 chromic suture with knots on the skin to minimize the chance of corneal abrasion. (From Iliff NT, Merbs SL. Entropion. In: Gottsch JD, Stark WJ, Goldberg MF, editors. Rob & Smith's operative surgery: Ophthalmic surgery. 5th ed. London: Arnold; 1999. (A) p.16, Figure 5; (B) p.16, Figure 6; (C) p.17, Figure 7.)

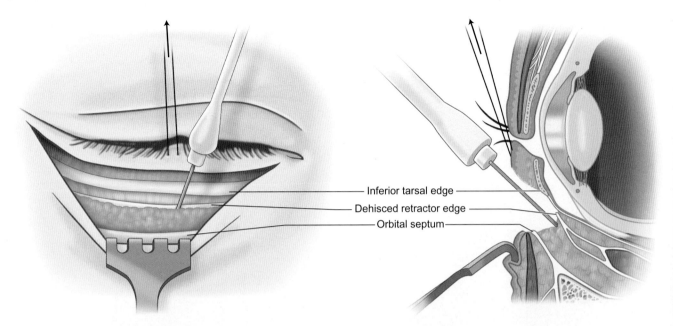

Inferior tarsal edge
Dehisced retractor edge
Orbital septum

Fig. 3.4.9 Reinsertion of eyelid retractors. Dissection is performed from a subciliary incision to expose the inferior edge of the lower tarsus. Inferior to this, the orbital septum is identified and opened. The lower eyelid retractors are just posterior to the orbital fat. They can be grasped and pulled forward, unlike the orbital septum, which is firmly attached to the orbital rim. The retractors are reapproximated to the inferior edge of the lower tarsus with interrupted 6-0 polyglactin sutures with care not to cause lower eyelid retraction. (From Iliff NT, Merbs SL. Entropion. In: Gottsch JD, Stark WJ, Goldberg MF, editors. Rob & Smith's operative surgery: Ophthalmic surgery. 5th ed. London: Arnold; 1999. p.13, Figure 3.)

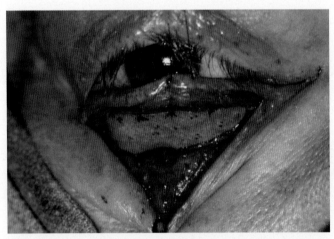

Fig. 3.4.10 Lower eyelid retraction repair. After the lower eyelid retractors have been released from the inferior border of the lower tarsus, a mid-lamellar spacer is placed to support the retracted lower eyelid. An acellular porcine dermal matrix implant, placed deep to the preorbital orbicularis and inferior to the tarsal plate, is secured with interrupted 6-0 polyglactin sutures to tarsus.

and sutured to the fundus of the lacrimal sac with a 4-0 chromic gut suture (Fig. 3.4.11E). The opposite end of the catheter is secured to the nasal vestibule with a 5-0 Prolene suture, and the tubes are trimmed. The incision is closed with a running 8-0 nylon suture.

Ptosis Repair

Ptosis repair by external levator advancement should be performed in the operating room under monitored anesthesia care. As the patient's

cooperation is required for portions of the procedure, excessive sedation should be avoided.

The upper eyelid crease incision is marked, and three additional markings placed at the midpoint of the pupil, medial limbus, and lateral limbus. The eyelid crease incision is made with a #15 blade. Sharp iris scissors are used to carry the dissection posteriorly through orbicularis and then superiorly until the orbital fat is visible posterior to the orbital septum (Fig. 3.4.12A). The orbital septum is opened where the preaponeurotic fat lies between the orbital septum and levator tendon (Fig. 3.4.12B). The levator tendon is identified and dissected free anteriorly and posteriorly from the surrounding tissues (Fig. 3.4.12C). Hemostasis is achieved with bipolar cautery, taking care to elevate the tissues from the ocular surface prior to cautery when working in the area of conjunctiva and Müller's muscle. The tarsal plate is dissected free from the overlying tissues. One arm of a double-armed 6-0 Surgidac suture is passed through the tarsal plate at the previously placed medial limbal mark (Fig. 3.4.12D). The tarsal plate is everted and inspected to ensure that a full-thickness pass has not been placed, as doing so can cause ocular surface irritation and abrasion. Both arms are then passed through the levator tendon and tied in a slipknot (Fig. 3.4.12D). This is repeated for the midpupillary and lateral limbal marks.

The patient is then asked to open their eyes, and the knots are adjusted so that the eyelid is at the optimal height and contour, considering symmetry as compared to the contralateral side. The patient's eyelid position should be evaluated in both the supine and sitting positions. The sutures are then cut and tied permanently, and the skin incisions closed with 8-0 nylon suture in a running fashion.[9]

POSTOPERATIVE CONSIDERATIONS

Following eyelid surgery, steroid–antibiotic ointment should be applied to the surgical sites for 7–14 days after surgery to aid in healing and

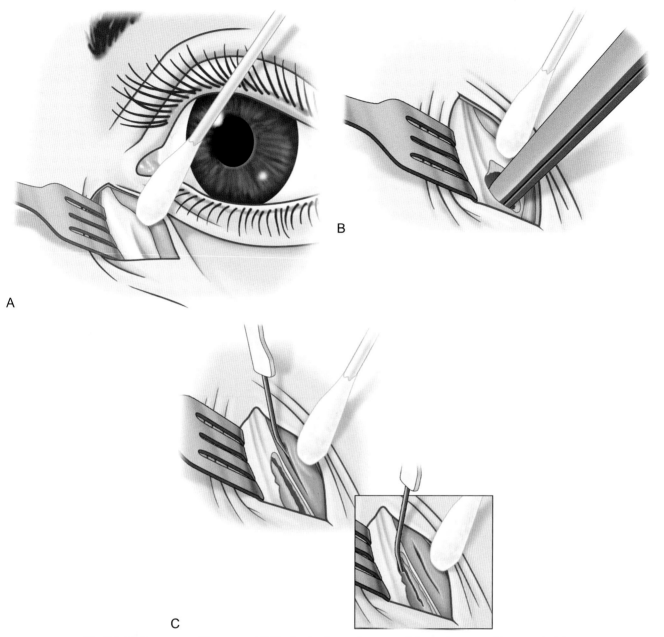

Fig. 3.4.11 Dacryocystorhinostomy. (A) The lacrimal crest is exposed from a lower eyelid crease incision. The sac is being retracted with a cotton tip applicator. (B) The bone separating the lacrimal sac fossa from the nose is removed with a sphenoid bone punch. (C) The lacrimal sac and nasal mucosa are opened with corresponding vertical incisions using a blade or radiofrequency dissector.   *Continued*

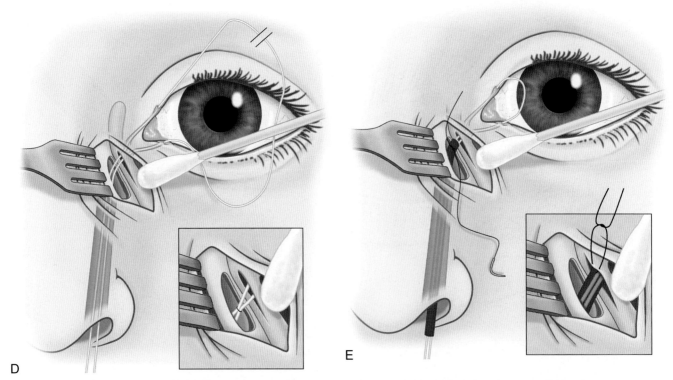

Fig. 3.4.11, cont'd (D) Silicone tubes are placed through the puncta and canaliculi, into the sac, and through the corresponding incisions, into the nose. The tubes are tied together with a 6-0 silk suture so that they cannot prolapse. (E) As an alternative to sewing flaps together to form the dacryocystorhinostomy ostium, a 12-French red rubber catheter is threaded over the silicone tubes and secured to the fundus of the lacrimal sac with an absorbable 4-0 chromic suture, thereby approximating the edges of the flap without sutures. (From Iliff NT, Merbs SL. Dacryocystorhinostomy. In: Gottsch JD, Stark WJ, Goldberg MF, editors. Rob & Smith's operative surgery: Ophthalmic surgery. 5th ed. London: Arnold; 1999. (A) p.54, Figure 2; (B) p.55, Figure 3; (C) p.55, Figure 4; (D) p. 56, Figure 5; (E) p.56, Figure 6.)

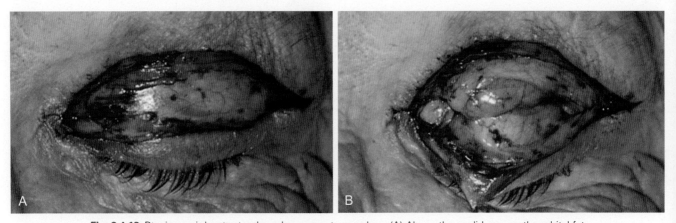

Fig. 3.4.12 Ptosis repair levator tendon advancement procedure. (A) Above the eyelid crease, the orbital fat is visible though the orbital septum, which is still intact. (B) The septum is opened above where the septum fuses with the levator tendon and where preaponeurotic orbital fat is between the septum and tendon.

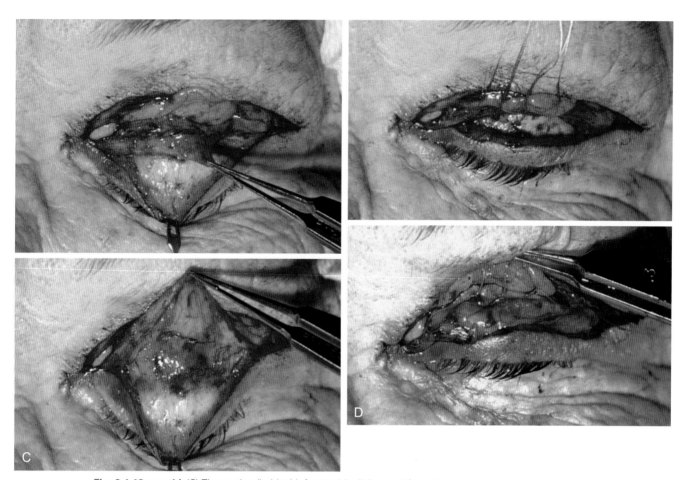

Fig. 3.4.12, cont'd (C) The tendon (held with forceps) is disinserted from its tarsal attachment and dissected anteriorly and posteriorly from surrounding tissues. (D) Double armed 6-0 polyester sutures are first placed partial thickness through the tarsus (*above*) and then full-thickness through the tendon and tied in slip knots (*below*) so the height of the eyelid can be assessed when the eyes are opened and the tension adjusted.

prevent infection. The authors prefer more frequent applications of ointment (twice to four times daily) in the case of skin grafts. A monocular occlusive dressing is often placed, and can be left in place for 1–3 days after surgery. If such a dressing is placed, ophthalmic ointment should be placed in the eye and eyelid closure under the patch should be ensured. If a Frost suture is performed, this can be taken down by the patient upon removal of the patch. The patient is instructed to cut one of the arms of the suture just below the Steri-Strips. When they remove the Steri-Strips from the forehead, the suture will be pulled free from the eyelid. Application of ice 20 minutes per hour can be helpful to reduce edema in the first 48 hours after surgery, however this should be avoided if a skin graft is present.

If an implant such as porcine dermis is used, a short course of oral antibiotics may be considered. If there is poor closure of the eyelids, frequent lubrication with over-the-counter artificial tears and ointment should be used in addition to any postoperative medications prescribed. Occasionally, with poor closure of the eyelids resulting from facial nerve palsy or expected postoperative periocular edema, a temporary tarsorrhaphy may be considered in the postoperative period to prevent ocular surface exposure and keratopathy.

LONG-TERM COMPLICATIONS

In patients with a history of periocular trauma, a thorough discussion of the risks of surgery should be held as a part of the informed consent process. Due to the altered anatomy and significant scarring that may often be present, surgery may carry a higher risk of failure than in a patient with no history of prior trauma. The risk of recurrence or worsening of eyelid malposition after surgery should be discussed.

EXPERT COMMENTARY

This well-written chapter serves as brief instruction to an exceedingly complex discipline which has become a specialty in itself, Oculoplastic Surgery. The chapter is meant to educate the facial surgeon about the importance of examination of the eye and orbit, to acquaint them with basic surgical techniques and management skills, and should serve to alert the practitioner as to when such expert consultation is warranted and will contribute to improved patient outcomes.

In my career, I have learned as much from excellent oculoplastic colleagues as I have from anyone, and I have spent many enjoyable hours examining patients together, sharing reconstructive surgery procedures, and benefitting from close associative follow-up. Many of the contributions we have made to the care of patients with orbital injuries would not have occurred in the absence of these relationships, studying patient's problems carefully and their outcomes.

I would strongly recommend that those who want to be proficient in facial reconstruction in the periorbital area develop a strong relationship with an oculoplastic colleague, see patients together, operate together, manage problems together, and discuss better ways to perfect operations, manage/avoid problems, and to better care for patients. Nonophthalmologist practitioners can benefit from the expertise and insight of oculoplastic surgeons in the challenging problems we face about the orbit. Together, the best results and patient care can be achieved.

REFERENCES

1. Centers for Disease Control and Prevention Morbidity and Mortality Weekly Report. 2013; http://www.cdc.gov/mmwr/preview/mmwrhtml/mm6218a9.htm.
2. Kuhn F, Morris R, Witherspoon CD, Mann L. Epidemiology of blinding trauma in the United States Eye Injury Registry. *Ophthalmic Epidemiol.* 2006;13(3):209–216.
3. May DR, Kuhn FP, Morris RE, et al. The epidemiology of serious eye injuries from the United States Eye Injury Registry. *Graefes Arch Clin Exp Ophthalmol.* 2000;238(2):153–157.
4. Katz J, Tielsch JM. Lifetime prevalence of ocular injuries from the Baltimore Eye Survey. *Arch Ophthalmol.* 1993;111(11):1564–1568.
5. Murchison AP, Bilyk JR. Management of eyelid injuries. *Facial Plast Surg.* 2010;26(6):464–481.
6. Iliff NT, Merbs SL. Ectropion. In: Gottsch JD, Stark WJ, Goldberg MF, eds. *Rob & Smith's Operative Surgery: Ophthalmic Surgery.* 5th ed. London: Arnold; 1999:19–25.
7. Iliff NT, Merbs SL. Entropion. In: Gottsch JD, Stark WJ, Goldberg MF, eds. *Rob & Smith's Operative Surgery: Ophthalmic Surgery.* 5th ed. London: Arnold; 1999:13–18.
8. Iliff NT, Merbs SL. DCR. In: Gottsch JD, Stark WJ, Goldberg MF, eds. *Rob & Smith's Operative Surgery: Ophthalmic Surgery.* 5th ed. London: Arnold; 1999:53–57.
9. Iliff NT, Merbs SL. Ptosis. In: Gottsch JD, Stark WJ, Goldberg MF, eds. *Rob & Smith's Operative Surgery: Ophthalmic Surgery.* 5th ed. London: Arnold; 1999:26–38.

Secondary Nasoethmoid Fracture Repair

Kristopher M. Day, Larry Sargent

BACKGROUND

High-energy midfacial trauma commonly results in naso-orbito-ethmoid (NOE) fractures, which present some of the greatest diagnostic and therapeutic challenges in facial trauma reconstruction.[1–7] Fractures of the nasoethmoid region are defined as a midface fracture resulting in lateral displacement of the medial canthal-bearing segment of the medial orbital wall.[8] These fractures may be isolated but frequently occur as part of more extensive "panfacial" fractures.[7–9] The degree of comminution is proportional to the amount of trauma to the nasoethmoid skeleton, which also determines the degree of difficulty for reduction and primary repair.[4,5] Nasoethmoid injuries are often misdiagnosed and inadequately treated because of the complex anatomy and technical challenges associated with this region. Failed management of nasoethmoid fractures in the primary setting can result in functional and cosmetic deformities that are difficult to correct secondarily. The pitfalls leading to secondary deformities are summarized in Box 3.5.1.

While nasoethmoid fracture management presents a challenge to even experienced surgeons, the best treatment of secondary nasoethmoid deformity remains its avoidance by the early diagnosis and appropriate treatment of the primary injury.[10–12] Soft tissue swelling may obscure the severity of nasoethmoid fractures, so a high degree of suspicion is required to diagnose their initial presentation.[9] The missed diagnosis and failed surgical treatment of nasoethmoid fractures can be best avoided with detailed knowledge of the surgical anatomy of this region, a thorough understand of the clinical presentation and management of such fractures, and a high degree of clinical suspicion.[1,3,4] Once diagnosed, the treatment of nasoethmoid fractures remains one of the most difficult surgical repairs in facial trauma. It therefore remains somewhat common that patients present in a delayed fashion for both primary repair and secondary surgical revision (Fig. 3.5.1).

The treatment of secondary nasoethmoid fractures is more complicated and often results in inferior outcomes compared to optimal primary management.[12] Posttraumatic tissue scarring and contour irregularities add complexity to delayed repair. The surgeon must widely expose the deformity, recreate the injury with selective osteotomies, and then reduce the tissue to its premorbid state with rigid bony fixation and soft tissue stabilization. The possibility of lost bone stock due to resorption of comminuted fragments increases the need for autogenous bone grafts, but this is rarely needed in the medial orbital wall. Soft tissue scarring and contracture result in the loss of elasticity and limit redraping the soft tissues with an optimal recreation of the subtle soft tissue contours that distinguish the nasoethmoid region. This chapter presents the senior author's approach to secondary nasoethmoid fracture repair, including case examples that illustrate the surgical management of these complex deformities (Fig. 3.5.2).

SURGICAL ANATOMY

Nasoethmoid Region (Fig. 3.5.3)

The nasoethmoid skeleton consists of the confluence of orbital, nasal, maxillary, and cranial bones.[4,13,14] Multiple facial buttresses support the nasoethmoid region, including the frontal process of the maxilla vertically and the supraorbital and infraorbital rims horizontally. Together these buttresses create a relatively stable anterior framework. Weakness exists posteriorly in the form of the thinner lacrimal and ethmoid bones of the internal medial orbital walls, which are prone to blow-out fracture and comminution. The inadequate reduction of displaced medial orbital rim and wall fragments results in a loss of definition of the naso-orbital valley. This may require wide scar release during delayed or revision surgery while taking care to avoid iatrogenic injury to the medial canthal tendon. Soft tissue buttressing may then be required for recontouring in secondary nasoethmoid fracture repair[9,11] (Fig. 3.5.4).

Interorbital Space

Between the two medial orbital walls and below the floor of the anterior cranial fossa lies the interorbital space, which consists of two ethmoidal labyrinths divided by the perpendicular plate of the ethmoid and nasal septum.[1–7] Anterior to this region are the nasal bones, and care must be taken to avoid confusing fractures of these bones with those of the nasoethmoid region.[8] The cribriform plate is found in the posterior roof of the interorbital space, which explains the occasional occurrence of persistent cerebrospinal fluid rhinorrhea or dysosmia with delayed nasoethmoid fractures. The interorbital space is both vulnerable to fracture from central midface trauma and adds complexity to the accurate diagnosis of nasoethmoid fractures, which may contribute to delays in presentation.

Medial Canthal Tendon and Central Bone Fragment (Fig. 3.5.5)

The single most important region of the medial orbital rim to optimal surgical repair of complex nasoethmoid fractures in both the acute and delayed setting is the "central bone fragment," into which the medial canthal tendon inserts.[2,3,14–18] There are three limbs of the medial canthal tendon. The anterior limb is distributed over the frontal process of the maxilla onto the posterolateral nasal bones. The superior limb inserts at the junction of the frontal process of the maxilla and the internal angular process of the frontal bone. The thin posterior portion inserts behind the lacrimal sac into the posterior portion of the lacrimal fossa. Nasoethmoid orbital fracture lines may extend through the frontal process of the maxilla, the medial orbital wall, inferior orbital rim, and lateral nasal bones, resulting in a mobile central medial orbital rim fragment.[15–21] This can result in a mobile canthal-bearing segment, which can compromise the integrity of eyelid support ligaments and the contour of the palpebral fissure. The degree of displacement is often proportional to the extent of comminution, which varies greatly between injuries. An intimate knowledge of these anatomical relationships is essential to appropriately manage secondary nasoethmoid fractures, whose pre-morbid anatomy must be reapproximated despite being altered at the time of presentation (Fig. 3.5.6).

BOX 3.5.1 Typical Reasons for Failed Management of Primary Nasoethmoid Orbital Fracture

Missed diagnosis
Inadequate operative exposure
Poor reduction and stabilization of bone fragments
Reduction plating placement in the medical canthal region
Undetected loss of normal nasal contours
Missed orbital defects
Failure to adequately reduce soft tissues in the naso-orbital valley

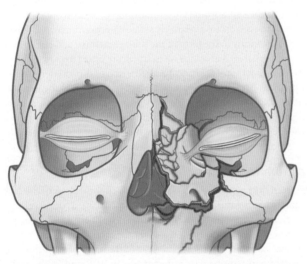

Fig. 3.5.1 Secondary nasoethmoid fractures of variable grade and complexity. Bone and soft tissue deformities can be unilateral or bilateral. Bone fragments may be displaced, partially resorbed, and encased by scar tissue. (Courtesy Caleb M. Steffen, MD; Chattanooga, TN.)

CLINICAL PRESENTATION

Patient History

The delayed presentation of nasoethmoid fractures may occur after missed diagnosis or inadequate treatment of an acute injury, so the presentation may share certain elements of the original trauma setting with some important distinctions. The astute clinician should be mindful

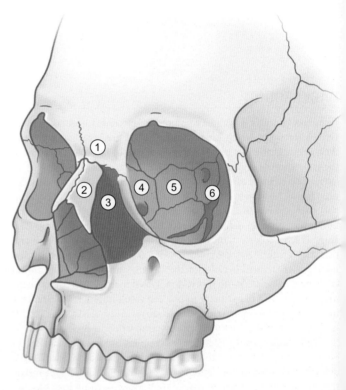

Fig. 3.5.3 Nasoethmoid region osseous components: (1) nasal process of frontal bone; (2) nasal bones; (3) nasal process of maxilla; (4) lacrimal bone; (5) lamina papyracea; (6) lesser wing of sphenoid bone. The key central bone fragment is shaded. (Reproduced with permission from Resident Manual of Trauma to the Face, Head, and Neck. A publication of the American Academy of Otolaryngology – Head and Neck Surgery Foundation. Alexandria, VA; 2012.)

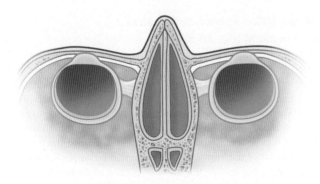
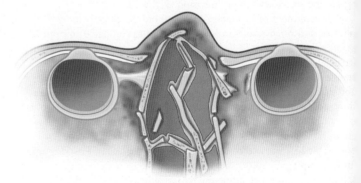

Fig. 3.5.2 Comparison of normal and traumatized nasoethmoid region anatomy. Medial orbital walls with medial canthal tendons displaced laterally. Radix of nose telescopes in. Chronic edema can be present. Collapse of the septum and vomer is frequently seen. (Courtesy Caleb M. Steffen, MD; Chattanooga, TN.)

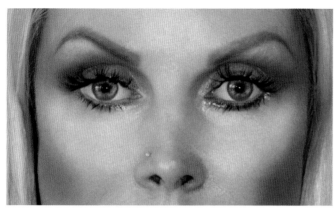

Fig. 3.5.4 Normal naso-orbital surface anatomy. The naso-orbital valley displays complex and multidimensional surface anatomy. This is distinguished by a delicate soft tissue–bony interface where millimeters can make a significant difference in appearance. (Courtesy Caleb M. Steffen, MD; Chattanooga, TN.)

BOX 3.5.2 Presentation of Secondary Nasoethmoid Fracture

General
Soft tissue scarring and contraction
Chronic central midface pain

Nasal
Widened nasal bridge
Foreshortened nose
Lack of nasal tip support or projection
Saddle nose deformity

Orbital
Traumatic telecanthus
Canthal asymmetry
Enophthalmos
Vertical orbital dystopia
Persistent diplopia
Orbital rim step-off
Grossly enlarged orbit
Strabismus
Lacrimal dysfunction

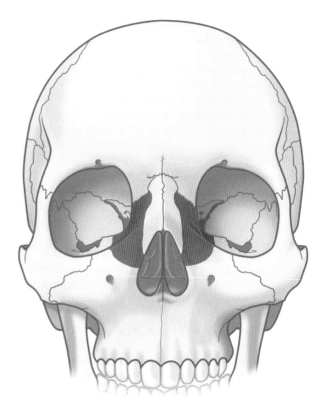

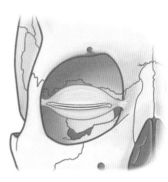

Fig. 3.5.5 The key structures of the nasoethmoid orbital fracture. Central bone fragment is shaded bilaterally. The insertion of the medial canthal tendon into this bony segment can be seen. (Courtesy Alina Sholar, MD; Austin, TX; reproduced with permission from Sargent LA. Naso-ethmoid orbital fractures: diagnosis and treatment. Plast Reconstr Surg 2007;120(7):16S-31S.)

---

of the varied manner in which delayed nasoethmoid fractures may present in order to avoid repeating its misdiagnosis or inadequate treatment. A recent history of blunt trauma to the central midface is the typical presentation of the acute nasoethmoid fracture, but initial injury sequelae may not prompt presentation for weeks to months.[9–12] Ideally, details of the original mechanism of injury and initial surgery would be obtained prior to any remote operative intervention. Without adequate primary nasoethmoid fracture repair, patients present with a variety of deformities, which are summarized in Box 3.5.2.

Physical Examination (Fig. 3.5.7)

Physical examination findings of medial orbital rim step-off, mobile medial orbital bone segments, a "telescoped" nasal radix, or telecanthus may be obscured by central midface scar tissue or chronic edema.[12–15] Common orbital findings in the representation of patients with naso-ethmoid fractures include: an asymmetric corneal light reflex, displaced and misshapen bony fragments creating step-offs, enophthalmos, or

periorbital soft tissue scarring and contracture.[1–8] Due to lost nasal and septal support, the nose may appear flat and foreshortened with a wide nasal dorsum and upturned tip. Nasal deformity as a result of healed nasal bone fractures must be distinguished from the nasoethmoid deformity. Lacrimal dysfunction from a traumatized nasolacrimal duct may manifest with epiphora. The physical exam findings may reflect displaced bone fragments[17–21] (Fig. 3.5.8).

RADIOLOGICAL EVALUATION

A high-quality CT scan with no more than 1.5 mm thickness axial and coronal cuts confirms the diagnosis of secondary nasoethmoid fracture.[22] Two-dimensional axial and coronal images provide a blueprint for the surgical plan, including planning the incision, use of bone grafts, location of osteotomies, and avoidance of adjacent structures. After

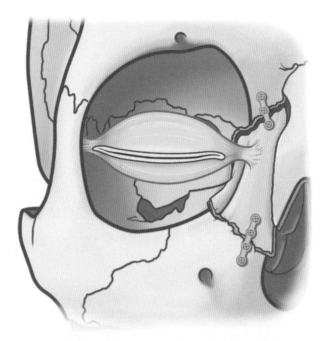

cross-sectional imaging has been evaluated, three-dimensional reconstructions may be utilized to refine and improve the assessment. Care should be taken not to rely on 3-dimensional reconstructions in isolation to avoid underestimation of the details of the fracture. The surgeon should be mindful that abnormal bony and soft tissue densities from scarring or edema may be present and obfuscate anatomic boundaries in secondary nasoethmoid fractures. This may complicate the determination of the fracture pattern, degree of comminution, and displacement, which must be considered in the development of an adaptable surgical plan.

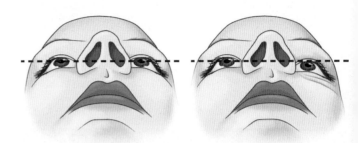

Fig. 3.5.6 Displaced nasoethmoid fracture plated in nonanatomical position. Persistent abnormalities can be caused by inadequate reduction of the primary defect, as shown in this medial bone fragment malpositioning. (Courtesy Alina Sholar, MD; Austin, TX; reproduced with permission from Sargent LA. Nasoethmoid orbital fractures: diagnosis and treatment. Plast Reconstr Surg 2007;120(7):16S-31S.)

Fig. 3.5.7 Submental view assessment of enophthalmos. (Reproduced with permission from Edward Ellis III, Marcelo Figari, Gregorio Sánchez Aniceto, Kazuo Shimozato, Daniel Buchbinder, editors. AO Surgery Reference: Craniomaxillofacial Section. https://www2.aofoundation.org/wps/portal/surgery?showPage=diagnosis&bone=CMF&segment=Overview.)

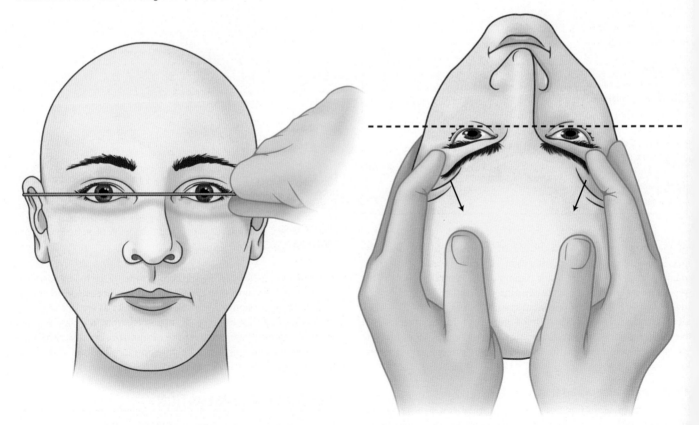

Fig. 3.5.8 Examination for orbital dystopia. (Reproduced with permission Edward Ellis III, Marcelo Figari, Gregorio Sánchez Aniceto, Kazuo Shimozato, Daniel Buchbinder, editors. AO Surgery Reference: Craniomaxillofacial Section. https://www2.aofoundation.org/wps/portal/surgery?showPage=diagnosis&bone=CMF&segment=Overview.)

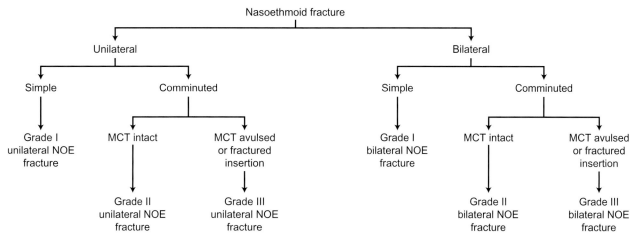

Fig. 3.5.9 Classification of nasoethmoid fractures. *NOE = nasoethmoid; MCT = medial canthal tendon. (Courtesy of Kristopher M. Day, MD; Chattanooga, TN.)

CLASSIFICATION (FIG. 3.5.9)

Secondary nasoethmoid fracture classification mirrors that of acute fractures and is useful in formulating a treatment plan. Many alternative systems exist in the literature, but basic distinctions begin with categorizing the fracture(s) as unilateral or bilateral and simple or comminuted. A straightforward classification system previously described by the author is based on the degree of comminution of the medial orbital bone fragment and integrity of the medial canthal tendon.[15–18,22,23] Type I fractures are characterized as large medial orbital rim fragments bearing an intact medial canthal tendon. Type II fractures feature comminuted central bone fragments without extension under the canthal insertion site. The medial canthus is thereby attached to a relatively large piece of intact medial orbital rim. Type III fractures display severe comminution with fracture lines extending under the medial canthal tendon insertion site. The medial canthal tendon is either avulsed or attached to small, nonusable bone fragments. Asymmetry usually exists with higher-grade injuries on one side and lower-grade or absent fractures on the other. The treatment plan is primarily dictated by the higher-grade injury, but an individualized surgical plan for each side is essential (Fig. 3.5.10).

SURGICAL INDICATIONS

Individualized Operative Planning

Once secondary nasoethmoid deformities have been detected, an individualized treatment plan must be made to address each patient's specific problem while omitting unnecessary surgical interventions.[24] For example, inadequate nasal projection may require cantilever bone grafting, while a foreshortened nose may call for lengthening of the nasal lining, and each of these conditions may or may not be accompanied by an overlying soft tissue derangement that may require its own specific intervention.[25,26] Enophthalmos requires orbital reconstruction, while a blunted canthal region may require medial canthopexy.[15,16,26–29] Increased interorbital distance often requires medial orbital osteotomy prior to repositioning of bone fragments, perhaps even with slight overcorrection to compensate for expansion due to scarring.[23,27,28] The role of the nasoethmoid region in determining orbital relationships cannot be overestimated.[13] Whether due to displacement of the medial orbit or medial canthal tendon or due to an abnormal relationship between orbits from inadequate bony or soft tissue reduction, special attention must be paid to orbital symmetry during secondary nasoethmoid reconstruction.[30]

Traumatic Telecanthus

The assessment and measurement of traumatic telecanthus is a skill that must be honed to ensure the accurate treatment of secondary nasoethmoid fractures.[15–18,23,27,30,31] Telecanthus refers to an abnormally increased distance between the medial canthi and differs from orbital hypertelorism, which refers instead to an increased interpupillary distance or bony interorbital distance (dacryon to dacryon). Calipers may be used to measure intercanthal and interpupillary distances, which average 30–31 mm and 60–62 mm in a typical adult, respectively.[13–18] Telecanthus becomes noticeable at varying distances, since the interpretation is relative to other facial structures, but distances greater than 40 mm are typically an indication for operative intervention.

Enophthalmos

Subtle variations in the degree of ocular projection may go unnoticed and do not require intervention when asymptomatic.[31] Enophthalmos becomes noticeable when greater than 3–4 mm, which indicates the possibility of improvement by surgical management.[27–31] Enophthalmos is measured from the lateral orbital rim to the anterior border of the cornea with a Hertel exophthalmometer. If the lateral orbital rim is also malpositioned, then a Naugle exophthalmometer may be used, which uses reference points above and below the superior and inferior orbital rims, respectively.[27,28,31]

The preoperative consultation should include a discussion of reasonable expectations for outcome. Photographs predating the original injury may help guide the reconstruction, although they must be viewed in the context of the delayed nasoethmoid repair setting. An anticipation of a restored perfect premorbid appearance must be tempered to the actual goals of symmetry, correction of any obvious deformity, and relief of the patient's symptoms.

Virtual Surgical Planning

Three-dimensional computerized planning may be employed in the virtual environment or physical models may be generated for operative planning and visualization prior to repair of secondary nasoethmoid fractures. However, unlike other secondary craniomaxillofacial deformities, which might feature larger bony structures amenable to individualized custom implant reconstruction or custom cutting guides, the fine

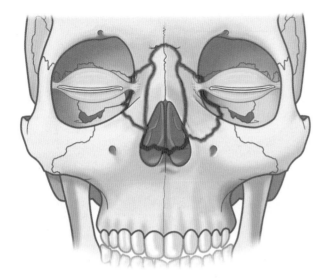

Grade I, noncomminuted, tendon intact

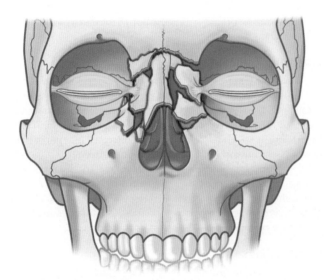

Grade II, comminuted, tendon intact

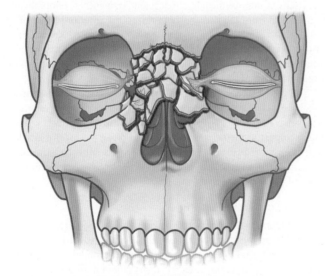

Grade III, comminuted, tendon detached

Fig. 3.5.10 Nasoethmoid fracture grading system. In descending order: (1) Grade I noncomminuted, tendon intact; (2) grade II comminuted, tendon intact; (3) grade III comminuted, tendon detached. (Courtesy Alina Sholar, MD; Austin, TX; reproduced with permission from Sargent LA. nasoethmoid orbital fractures: diagnosis and treatment. Plast Reconstr Surg 2007;120(7):16S-31S.)

BOX 3.5.3   Components of Customized Surgical Plan

Medial canthal position and symmetry
Soft tissue contour of medial canthal area/naso-orbital valley
Nasal contour, including dorsal contour and tip projection
Bilateral globe position and symmetry

---

anatomy of the nasoethmoid region requires meticulous repair of native tissue. Therefore, the benefit of virtual planning is largely for the surgeon's preoperative visualization of the intended reconstruction. However, 3D models are beneficial in analyzing the displaced or deformed medial orbital wall segments as well as planning osteotomies.

SURGICAL TECHNIQUES (FIG. 3.5.11)

In determining the operative approach it is important to analyze, if possible, the initial injury fracture pattern and the reason for loss of preinjury appearance. The areas to be assessed to establish a customized treatment plan are summarized in Box 3.5.3.[24] Once each of these areas is adequately assessed, then a customized treatment plan can be made to address the abnormal areas in an attempt to reconstruct this deformity back to "normal." The most common type of secondary nasoethmoid deformity is widened and asymmetric medical canthal tendon positions, with thickened, scarred medial canthal region soft tissue and loss of naso-orbital valley contour with a widened nasal dorsum, lack of nasal projection, and foreshortened nose with upturned tip.[12,14,17,25,27] Varying degrees of orbital malposition are typically present (Fig. 3.5.12).

A successful operative plan must include treatment of each of these deformities. In the senior author's 35-year experience in treating over 500 nasoethmoid fractures, the key steps in creating a successful treatment plan are:

1. *Adequate surgical exposure*: usually a coronal incision combined with other local incisions (eyelid and gingival buccal sulcus) are required.

   Once the operative plan is formulated, then it is the technical execution of the procedure that determines the quality of the results. A complex bilateral nasoethmoid fracture that is healed in a displaced position requires recreating the initial injury by doing multiple osteotomies. Exposure is the key to being able to do these types of osteotomies in an appropriate fashion. It can be approached through a coronal incision combined with eyelid incisions or upper buccal sulcus incisions; however, local incisions are an alternative option. This would involve a short vertical midline incision in the radix glabellar area of about 1.5–2 cm, or the horizontal limb alone of the converse "open sky" incision.

   For the inexperienced surgeon, the midline glabella/nasal incision allows excellent exposure with good visualization of the anatomy as well as your reduction. Doing this through a coronal incision without a midline nasal incision requires more experience and the exposure is more difficult. The midline nasal excision exposes the nasal bone, the subciliary incision exposes the medial inferior orbital rim and internal orbit. The upper sulcus incision exposes the piri-form area, distal nasal bones, and the medial maxilla and inferior orbital rim. Through these incisions and exposure, the planned osteotomies or recreation of the fracture can be done. It is helpful to do an osteotomy on the nasal bones to temporarily either dislocate or remove these so you can expose the medial orbital walls from the nasal side, effectively from within the nose.

2. *Re-securing the medial canthal tendon insertion with 3-0 wire*: Rarely is the canthal tendon avulsed from the "central bone fragment" unless there is an overlying laceration or it has been avulsed during exposure of the medial orbital wall (Fig. 3.5.13).

Osteotomies are then made with a small osteotome at the superior medial orbital rim and inferior lower rim to create a canthal bearing medial orbital wall "central" segment that can then be mobilized. This is the key segment, which contains the medial canthal tendon insertion. The tendon is carefully dissected out in all of these cases. A small transverse incision about 3–4 mm is made over the tendon in the skin at the corner of the medial eyelid commissure. The tendon is dissected out, and then a 3-0 surgical steel suture with an FS-2 curved needle is used to pass through the tendon twice in a tendon stitch-type fashion. The two ends of the wires are then threaded through the wound into the nasal side via the midline nasal incision. Two drill holes are made into the medial orbital wall near the canthal insertion. The two ends of the 3-0 wire are passed through that so that the tendon can be reinforced or, if necessary, reinserted into the medial orbital wall and secured down with this wire. These two drill holes must be adjacent to the tendon insertion.

3. *Custom bone osteotomies, as needed, to reposition the central medial bone fragment*: Over-reduction is usually required. One wire can resecure the medial canthal tendon and central medial orbital wall bone fragment. Treating the opposite side in an identical fashion and twisting these two wires together insures symmetry (Figs. 3.5.14 and 3.5.15).

Once these two wires are twisted, then it not only secures the tendon down to the medial orbital wall but it then controls the medial orbital wall and tendon with one twisted wire. The identical procedure is done on the opposite side so that the medial orbital segments can then be mobilized and the two wires twisted together,

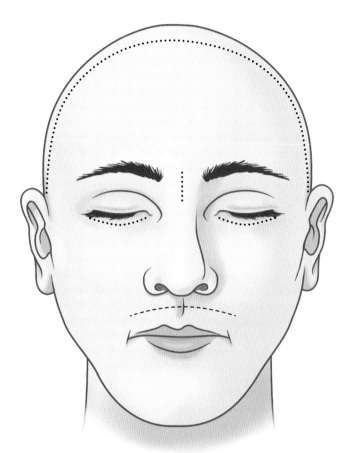

Fig. 3.5.11 Surgical approaches to nasoethmoid fracture repair. Various incisions used to provide exposure of nasoethmoid orbit complex. Existing lacerations frequently are present and used in conjunction with the incisions. (Courtesy Alina Sholar, MD; Austin, TX; reproduced with permission from Sargent LA. Nasoethmoid orbital fractures: diagnosis and treatment. Plast Reconstr Surg 2007;120(7):16S-31S.)

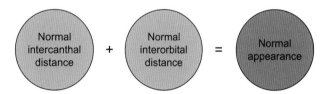

Fig. 3.5.12 Relationship of intercanthal and interorbital distances to normal appearance. The achievement of normal intercanthal and interorbital distances is not equivalent to the achievement of a normal appearance. Both premorbid intercanthal and interorbital distances may be reestablished with an abnormal appearance, which is also a function of soft tissue reduction and contour in the medial canthal area. (Courtesy of Kristopher M. Day, MD; Chattanooga, TN.)

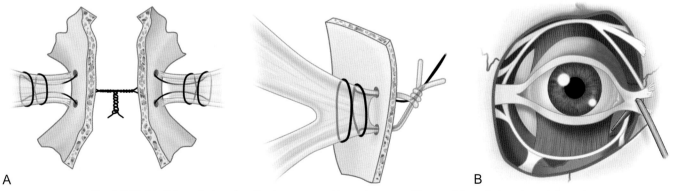

A   B

Fig. 3.5.13 Medial canthal tendon fixation to central bone fragment. The medial canthal tendon reinforced and further secured to the central bone fragment (A) and anchored in anatomical position (B) with transnasal wires. (Courtesy of Caleb M. Steffen, MD.)

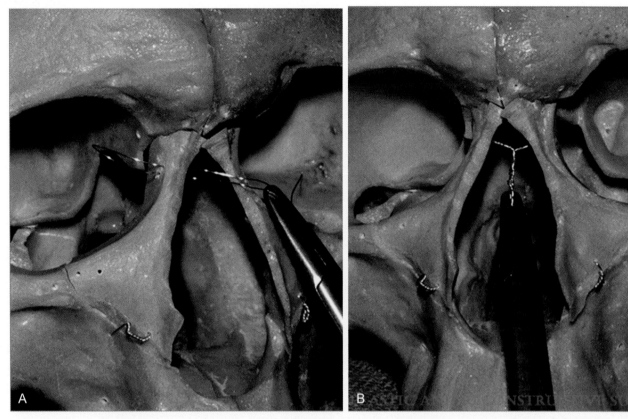

Fig. 3.5.14 Anatomy of transnasal wiring. Transnasal wires are secured within the interorbital space (A) with sufficient tension (B) to correct any lateral displacement of the central bone fragments. (Courtesy Larry A. Sargent, MD; Salt Lake City, UT; reproduced with permission from Sargent LA. Nasoethmoid orbital fractures: diagnosis and treatment. Plast Reconstr Surg 2007;120(7):16S-31S.)

bringing them together in a very symmetric transverse fashion so that you have good symmetry of the medial orbital wall segments as well as the tendon insertion. Slight overcorrection of these medial orbital wall segments is always accomplished as well as securing this segment to the nasofrontal area with wires or very small plates.[15,16,22,27] At no time is any plate placed in the medial canthal area as this causes thickening and loss of contour of this delicate area.

4. *Extensive thinning of thickened, scarred soft tissue anterior and lateral to medial canthal tendon is mandatory to re-establish a normal contour in this area.*

Once the two medial orbital wall segments are stabilized so that they control the medial canthal tendon insertion, then the next step is perhaps as important as the medial orbital wall reduction. One of the most difficult parts of this procedure is being able to restore soft tissue contour. A great deal of attention and time must be devoted to thinning the soft tissue as needed and to securing the soft tissue that has been abnormally positioned from the displaced fracture and then further elevated and distorted from the dissection required to do the osteotomies. Without attention to this important step, good results cannot be routinely obtained. In fact, the soft tissue deformity alone may mimic the entire appearance of the poorly repaired bone/soft tissue of the original deformity.

This is soft tissue fixation anterior to the tendon down to the naso-orbital valley. Thinning of the soft tissue anterior to around the tendon insertion is almost always needed in secondary nasoethmoid reconstruction. This area has usually become thickened with loss of contour. Small tenotomy scissors are used to trim this tissue down to a thin skin flap resecting the periosteum and scar tissue and then dermal pexy sutures are used to provide a progressive

tension type of fixation of the soft tissue creating the normal contour of the naso-orbital valley. This is key to reestablish a normal contour of the medial canthal area and to avoid thickened epicanthal folds with loss of definition of the medial canthal insertion. The appropriate height of this area is determined by the nasal reconstruction. It may be that there has been some foreshortening of the nose from the secondary deformity, and a calvarial bone graft is frequently used to provide a good contour to the dorsum, support to the middle and distal third of the nose where there has been a significant septal injury.[24,25] This creates height which then allows a more normal definition of the intercanthal contour. Dorsal and caudal bone grafts may be required, and the residual septum may have to be relocated to insert on the anterior nasal spine.

5. *Soft tissue reduction and fixation using dermal pexy sutures of the medial orbital region to recreate the naso-orbital valley contour.*

Dermal pexy sutures using 4-0 PDS or 3-0 wire suture to the dermis are used to secure the skin down to the sidewalls of the nasal bones to give a good contour and prevent any thickening and hematoma formation. At the end, this area should have a very "pinched" appearance to end up with a normal contour 6–8 weeks postoperatively.

6. *Reconstruction of the nose with calvarial bone graft is almost always needed. This graft is contoured, shaped, and rigidly fixed to re-establish nasal length and projection* (Fig. 3.5.16).

7. *Soft tissue compression bolsters of the medial canthal area that are secured with two transnasal pull-out wires are used to prevent hematoma and swelling of the soft tissue of the medial canthal area and naso-orbital valley preserve the right-angle between the nose and the maxilla. This can also serve as a secure nasal splint for the nasal bones if left in place 10–14 days* (Fig. 3.5.17).

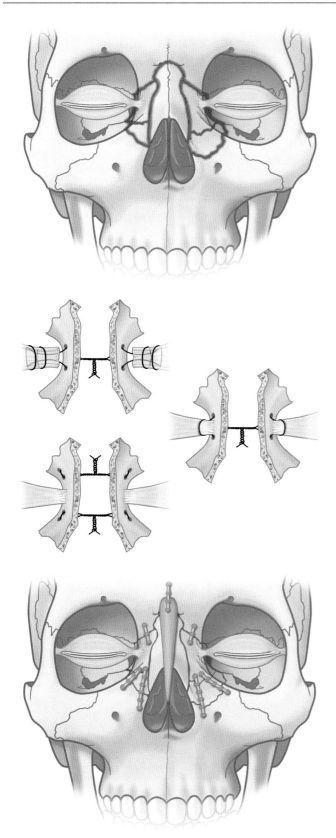

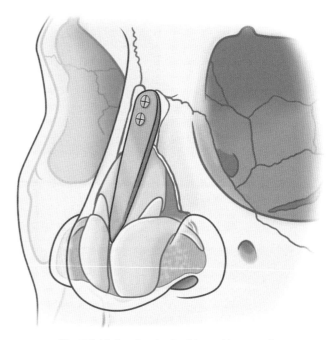

Fig. 3.5.16 Cantilevel calvarial nasal bone graft.

The final step is adding a soft tissue bolster that is made of lead padded with orthopedic felt and wrapped with Xeroform. These are placed by passing a 22-gauge spinal needle through the tendon insertion area through an osteotomy site and out the opposite side in a symmetric fashion. A 28-gauge wire is then passed through this and then the distal wire is passed flush to the maxilla just beneath the end of the nasal bones over the piriform aperture. With these two wires in place, drill holes are placed in the lead plates, wires passed through orthopedic felt, and then twisted down so there is a compression of the soft tissue that results in further contouring of this soft tissue to the nose in the medial canthal area and lateral nose. This also serves as a secure nasal bone splint in addition to its more important role of providing soft tissue compression and molding in the medial canthal area and lateral nose.

8. *Titanium mesh to repair internal orbital defects and reestablish normal orbital volume and globe position* (Figs. 3.5.18 and 3.5.19).

Lag screws, or fine plates, are used to secure the bone graft and segments of the medial orbital wall to the nasal frontal area as long as the plates do not come anywhere near the medial canthal region, as this distorts and thickens the contour. Internal orbital defects are repaired with orbital mesh as needed.[31–37] The key components of secondary nasoethmoid fracture repair technique are summarized in Box 3.5.4, with illustrated case examples in Figs. 3.5.20–3.5.25.

Text continued on p. 393

Fig. 3.5.15 Relationship of medial canthal tendon fixation to transnasal wiring. Dissection of the medial orbital bone segment may be best approached from the nasal side. Osteotomy and temporary dislocation of the nasal bone segments may be needed. (Courtesy Alina Sholar, MD; Austin, TX; reproduced with permission from Sargent LA. Naso-ethmoid orbital fractures: diagnosis and treatment. Plast Reconstr Surg 2007;120(7):16S-31S.)

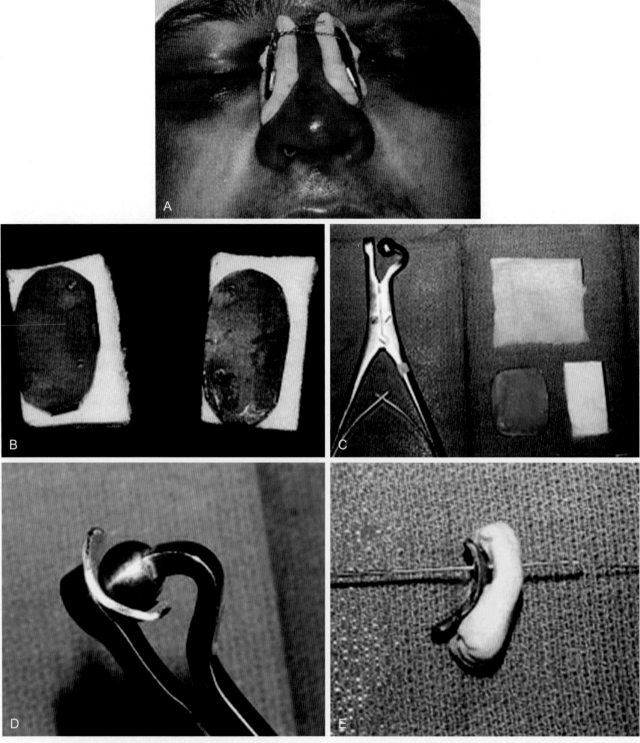

Fig. 3.5.17 Soft tissue buttress. Soft tissue bolsters reinforce the soft tissue (A) over the canthopexies as well as the multiple dermal pexies. Lead plates with orthopedic padding (B–C) may be contoured (D) to the convexity of the naso-orbital valley and combined with transnasal wire (E) for reinforcement of the soft tissue reduction. This provides essential soft tissue compression, which achieves optimal contour and hematoma prevention. (Courtesy Larry A. Sargent, MD; Salt Lake City, UT; reproduced with permission from Sargent LA. Nasoethmoid orbital fractures: diagnosis and treatment. Plast Reconstr Surg 2007;120(7):16S-31S.)

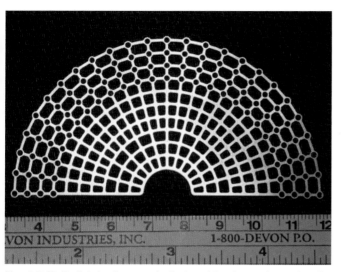

Fig. 3.5.18 Radial titanium mesh designed by the senior author for internal orbital defect reconstruction. The radial contour mimics native conical orbital shape and may be easily customized. (Courtesy Larry A. Sargent, MD; Salt Lake City, UT; reproduced with permission from Sargent LA. Nasoethmoid orbital fractures: diagnosis and treatment. Plast Reconstr Surg 2007;120(7):16S-31S, 2007.)

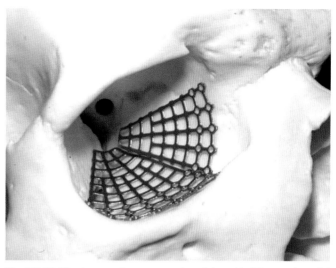

Fig. 3.5.19 Titanium mesh reconstruction of the orbital floor and medial orbital wall. These pieces of radial mesh have been cut to the appropriate size and contoured to each orbital wall defect individually. (Courtesy Larry A. Sargent, MD; Salt Lake City, UT; reproduced with permission from Sargent LA. Nasoethmoid orbital fractures: diagnosis and treatment. Plast Reconstr Surg 2007;120(7):16S-31S.)

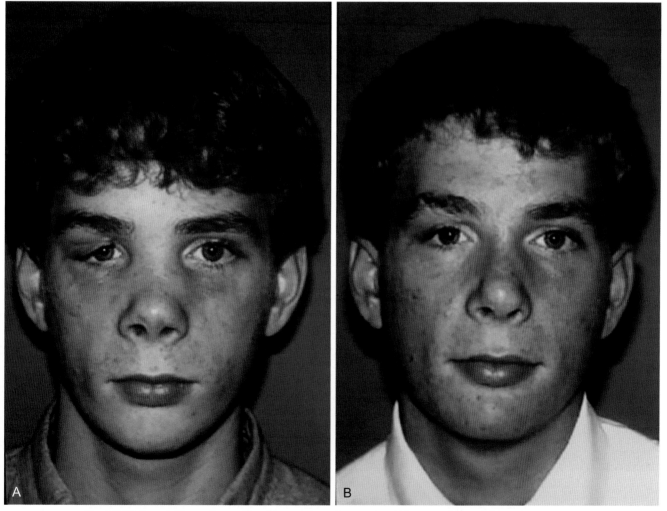

Fig. 3.5.20 Case 1: The patient suffered a comminuted nasoethmoid fracture after an ATV rollover accident. He underwent repair by attempted open reduction and internal fixation at an outside institution that resulted in secondary deformities. He presented to the senior author with a healed nasoethmoid fracture exhibiting traumatic telecanthus, nasal foreshortening, and a widened dorsal nasal bridge resulting in decreased projection and loss of nasal contour (A). This patient underwent customized osteotomies to recreate the nasoethmoid fractures, repeat open reduction and internal fixation of fractures, transnasal wiring, and soft tissue pexies and bolsters. A cantilevel bone graft was used to reconstruct the nose, restoring projection and contour (B).

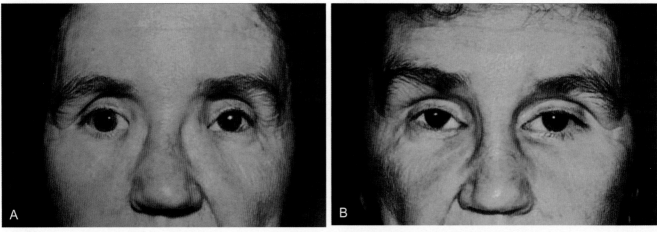

Fig. 3.5.21 Case 2: This elderly woman sustained a comminuted bilateral nasoethmoid fracture after a motor vehicle collision. She presented to the senior author with residual deformities after an unsuccessful attempt at repair. She has traumatic telecanthus due to laterally displaced medial orbital wall segment, asymmetric globe positions with bilateral enophthalmos. She has a displaced widened nasal dorsal contour (A). The patient underwent bilateral medial orbital wall osteotomies with repositioning, transnasal wiring/medial canthopexies, soft tissue thinning and reduction using dermal pexies and soft tissue compression bolsters. The internal orbits were reconstructed with radial titanium mesh and the nose was reconstructed with a cantilever calvarial bone graft (B).

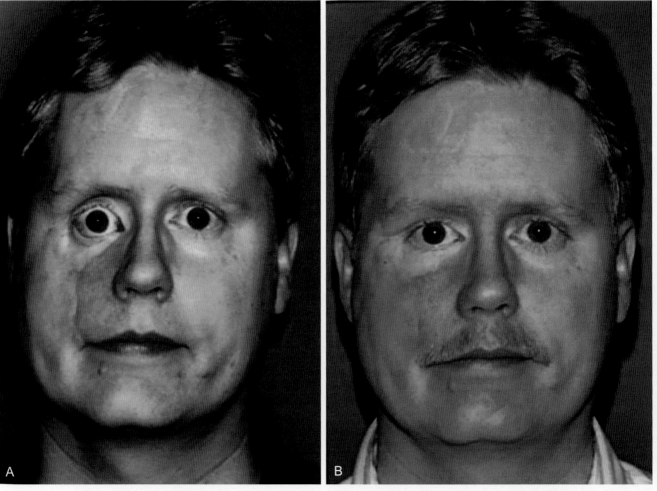

Fig. 3.5.22 Case 3: This patient sustained a complex crushing left-sided facial fracture including a left uni-lateral nasoethmoid injury from being side-swiped by a subway train. He presented to the senior author secondarily with a displaced left unilateral nasoethmoid segment, severe displacement of the right zygoma/maxilla with vertical orbital dystopia and enophthalmos. He additionally had excessive scarring of the right cheek and eyelid with an ectropion (A). He underwent osteotomy of the left medial orbital wall segment and repositioning with transnasal canthopexy and osteotomy and repositioning of the right zygoma with calvarial bone grafting of defects. Internal orbit reconstruction with titanium mesh was required to correct globe position. Extensive release of eyelid and cheek soft tissue with resuspension and fixation was performed. Suspension of soft tissue with fixation to bone was key in repositioning and maintaining eyelid position (B).

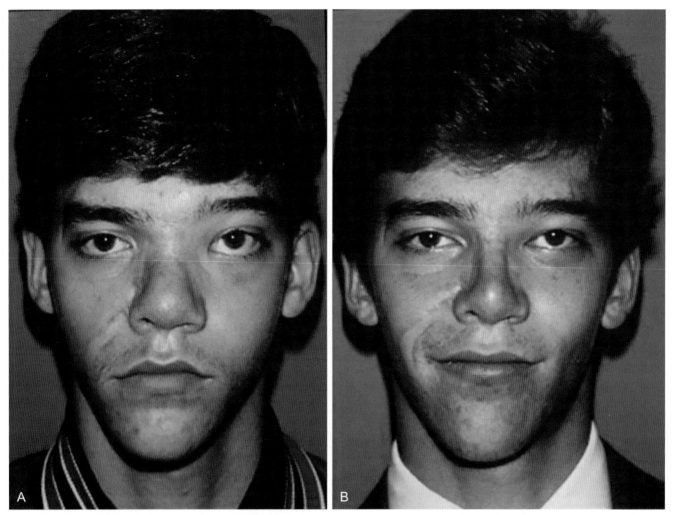

Fig. 3.5.23 Case 4: This patient presented after attempted open reduction and internal fixation of a comminuted bilateral nasoethmoid fracture following a motor vehicle accident. He shows significant asymmetric traumatic telecanthus with loss of the naso-orbital valley, especially on the left. He has blunted contour to the medial eyelid commissures and widened dorsal nasal bridge with thickened soft tissue (A). This was corrected with medial orbital wall osteotomies that were reduced, transnasal canthopexies, extensive soft tissue thinning with reduction and fixation using dermal pexies. A cantilever calvarial bone graft was used to restore nasal height and contour (B).

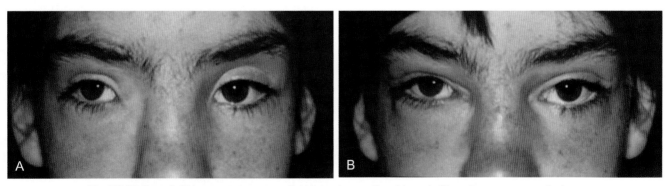

Fig. 3.5.24 Case 5: This was an unsuccessful bilateral nasoethmoid repair. There is more severe displacement of right medial orbital wall segment than left (A). The patient underwent bilateral medial orbital wall osteotomies with over-reduction and transnasal canthopexies as described. Soft tissue contouring was performed with reduction and stabilization using dermal pexies and compression bolsters (B).

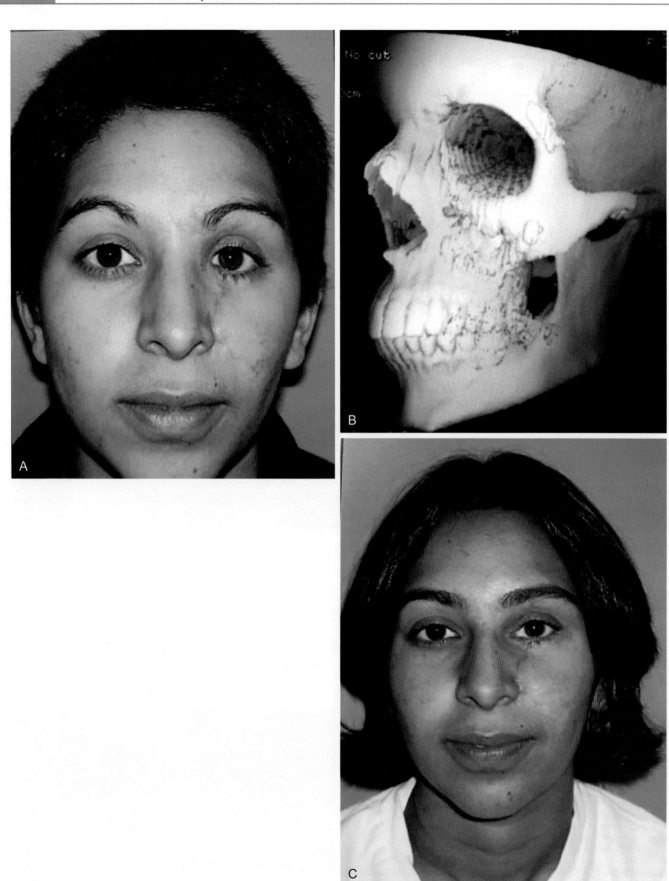

Fig. 3.5.25 Case 6: This patient had her left zygomatic fracture reduced and stabilized but the left nasoethmoid fracture was missed. This resulted in a deformity of the left medial canthal area as well as an enophthalmos (A–B). Repositioning of the left medial orbital wall segment with a left transnasal canthopexy and soft tissue contouring and reduction was performed. The internal orbit was reconstructed with radial titanium mesh to correct the enophthalmos. As in all the other cases, detailed attention to soft tissue fixation in the medial canthal area with dermal pexies and compression bolsters was done (B).

POSTOPERATIVE COURSE

The postoperative management after secondary nasoethmoid repair requires assessing the stability and skin circulation under the soft tissue bolsters, evaluation of the integrity of the soft tissue envelope, and management of soft tissue swelling. The soft tissue buttress is maintained until outpatient follow-up, or approximately 1–2 weeks, to optimize soft tissue positioning and molding during the initial remodeling phase. Antibiotic therapy may be administered, especially if there is concurrent sinus involvement or gross contamination. The routine use of prophylactic antibiotics, however, is not supported by the literature for isolated secondary nasoethmoid fracture repair.

COMPLICATIONS

Acute Complications

Hematoma is a potential complication of the immediate postoperative period. The scarred nature of tissue undergoing revision surgery predisposes it to ongoing bleeding, and every effort should be made intraoperatively to attain meticulous hemostasis. The tension of the soft tissue buttress is a balance between insufficient, which risks hematoma formation, and inadequate tissue contouring, and excessive pressure that may precipitate skin necrosis. Judicious soft tissue buttress pressure should be applied, considering the risk of inducing soft tissue ischemia while compressing the tissues enough to attain desired anatomic contours. If tissue compromise is detected, these buttresses should be loosened and repositioned to avoid further injury.

Long-Term Complications

Chronic soft tissue edema and swelling occurs not uncommonly after revision nasoethmoid fracture repair. The central midface has suffered significant trauma following secondary nasoethmoid surgery and is prone to scarring, swelling, and contracture. The avoidance of unnecessary soft tissue trauma during dissection is therefore of paramount importance. Careful handling of the soft tissue envelope and prudent reapproximation provides the best opportunity for an anatomic revision.

The most technically demanding aspect of both acute and delayed nasoethmoid fractures with medial canthal tendon involvement is precise tendon reinsertion. Placement of wires anterior to tendon insertion may lead to splaying of the central bone fragment, which can result in persistent telecanthus. Transnasal wires must therefore be carefully positioned superior and posterior to the medial canthal tendon insertion (Surgical Techniques steps 2 and 3 above). The soft tissue techniques in the medial canthal area described are the key to improving your results in secondary nasoethmoid reconstruction. If medial canthal tendons are not reinforced or securely fixed to the medial orbital wall central segment, then stretching or lateral drift can take place with resultant telecanthus.

The soft tissue of the naso-orbital valley may be altered by chronic edema, scarring, or previous hematoma that must be managed with judicious debridement and thinning. Failure to reduce abnormal tissue bulk during repair of delayed nasoethmoid fractures may result in blunted naso-orbital valley contour which mimics the original deformity. The primary mechanism to reestablish the contour of the naso-orbital valley is soft tissue periosteal resection molding and fixation.

CONCLUSION

Avoidance of delayed nasoethmoid deformities by optimal primary management remains the best treatment of secondary nasoethmoid orbital fractures, which present one of the most challenging scenarios in maxillofacial trauma reconstruction. Patients may present with a variety of orbital, nasal, and lacrimal signs and symptoms of inadequate primary repair. Keys to the repair of secondary nasoethmoid fractures include: careful anchoring of the medial canthal tendon to the central bone fragment, meticulous debulking and redraping of the soft tissue of the naso-orbital valley, accurate transnasal wire and soft tissue buttress placement, and reconstruction of nasal and internal orbital deformities.

EXPERT COMMENTARY

Long the most difficult primary fracture and what was once thought to be an impossible secondary correction, this chapter on the secondary nasoethmoid deformity, whose senior author, Larry Sargent, has obtained the best primary and secondary results in nasoethmoid fracture treatment, carefully and in much detail lays out the sequence and steps in secondary reconstruction. More emphasis is placed on the soft tissue than on the bone, clearly indicating the importance of thickened, malpositioned, and contracted soft tissue in the secondary correction. Positioning the medial canthal ligament while augmenting the nasal dorsum are opposing actions, but they must be combined in order to achieve good results. The steps in soft tissue remodeling necessary in the secondary management are clearly outlined, and the use of wires rather than plates in the sidewall of the nose and anterior to the medial canthal ligament is stated but deserves further emphasis here, as their use creates additional thickness and deformity. Bolsters and special sutures help to mold, reposition, and remodel the soft tissue, preventing hematoma and soft tissue contracture. The thinness, delicacy, and angles of the covering soft tissue must be realized and recreated; the soft tissue, thickened and suffused with scar tissue from resolved hematoma, must be thinned to the limits of its circulation, and then repositioned and held in position by soft tissue fixation until the initial healing has been completed. In no previous publication is the important management of the soft tissue emphasized and so clearly described – the careful descriptions given here make us all think that we are capable of managing this recalcitrant secondary deformity. One should read Sargent's chapter on hypertelorism [1], in which one can see how his experience with nasoethmoidal fracture treatment has molded his craniofacial surgical career, and again his results are the best that have been achieved in these congenital deformities.

References

1. Sargent LA. Orbital hypertelorism. In: Prein J, Ehrenfeld M, Futran N, Hanson PN, eds. *AOCMF Manual of Advanced Techniques in Surgery of the Craniofacial Skeleton.* New York: Thieme; 2012.

REFERENCES

1. Gruss JS. Fronto-naso-orbital trauma. *Clin Plast Surg.* 1982;9:577.
2. Hoffmann JF. Naso-orbital-ethmoid complex fracture management. *Facial Plast Surg.* 1998;14(1):67–76.
3. Leipziger LS, Manson PN. Nasoethmoid orbital fractures. Current concepts and management principles. *Clin Plast Surg.* 1992;19:167.
4. Morrison AD, Gregoire CE. Management of fractures of the nasofrontal complex. *Oral Maxillofac Surg Clin North Am.* 2013;25(4):637–648.
5. Papadopoulos H, Salib NK. Management of naso-orbital-ethmoidal fractures. *Oral Maxillofac Surg Clin North Am.* 2009;21(2):221–225, vi.
6. Paskert JP, Manson PN, Kiff NT. Nasoethmoidal and orbital fractures. *Clin Plast Surg.* 1988;15:209.
7. Pawar SS, Rhee JS. Frontal sinus and naso-orbital-ethmoid fractures. *JAMA Facial Plast Surg.* 2014;16(4):284–289.
8. Manson PN. Facial injuries. In: McCarthy J, ed. *Plastic Surgery.* Philadelphia: Saunders; 1990:867–1141.
9. Sargent LA. Acute management of nasoethmoid orbital fractures. *Oper Tech Plast Reconstr Surg.* 1998;5:213.

10. Rosenberger E, Kriet JD, Humphrey C. Management of nasoethmoid fractures. *Curr Opin Otolaryngol Head Neck Surg.* 2013;21(4):410–416.

11. Sargent LA. Nasoethmoid orbital fractures. *Problems Plast Reconstr Surg.* 1991;1:426.

12. Wolff J, Sándor GK, Pyysalo M, et al. Late reconstruction of orbital and naso-orbital deformities. *Oral Maxillofac Surg Clin North Am.* 2013;25(4):683–695.

13. Farkas LG, Ross RB, Posnick JC, Indech GD. Orbital measurements in 63 hyperteloric patients. Differences between the anthropometric and cephalometric findings. *J Craniomaxillofac Surg.* 1989;17(6):249–254.

14. Fedok FG. Comprehensive management of nasoethmoid-orbital injuries. *J Craniomaxillofac Trauma.* 1995;1(4):36–48.

15. Converse JM, Smith B. Naso-orbital fractures and traumatic deformities of the medial canthus. *Plast Reconstr Surg.* 1966;38:147.

16. Markowitz BL, Manson PN, Sargent LA, et al. Management of the medial canthal tendon in nasoethmoid orbital fractures: the importance of the central fragment in classification and treatment. *Plast Reconstr Surg.* 1991;87:843.

17. Sargent LA, Rogers GF. Nasoethmoid orbital fractures: diagnosis and management. *J Craniomaxillofac Trauma.* 1999;5:19.

18. Sargent LA. Nasoethmoid orbital fractures: diagnosis and treatment. *Plast Reconstr Surg.* 2007;120(7):16S–31S.

19. Merville LC, Real JP. Fronto-orbito-nasal dislocations: initial total reconstruction. *Scand J Plast Reconstr Surg.* 1981;15:287.

20. Paskert JP, Manson PN. The bimanual examination for assessing instability in naso-orbitoethmoid injuries. *Plast Reconstr Surg.* 1989;83:165.

21. Manson PN, Markowitz B, Mirvis S, et al. Toward CT-based facial fracture treatment. *Plast Reconstr Surg.* 1990;85:202.

22. Gruss JS. Naso-ethmoid-orbital fractures: classification and role of primary bone grafting. *Plast Reconstr Surg.* 1985;75:303.

23. Ellis E 3rd. Sequencing treatment for naso-orbito-ethmoid fractures. *J Oral Maxillofac Surg.* 1993;51(5):543–558.

24. Vora NM, Fedok FG. Management of the central nasal support complex in naso-orbital ethmoid fractures. *Facial Plast Surg.* 2000;16(2):181–191.

25. Craft P, Sargent LA. Membranous bone healing and techniques in calvarial bone grafting. *Clin Plast Surg.* 1989;16:11.

26. Elbarbary AS, Ali A. Medial canthopexy of old unrepaired naso-orbito-ethmoidal (NOE) traumatic telecanthus. *J Craniomaxillofac Surg.* 2014;42(2):106–112.

27. Clauser L, Galiè M, Pagliaro F, Tieghi R. Posttraumatic enophthalmos: etiology, principles of reconstruction, and correction. *J Craniofac Surg.* 2008;19(2):351–359.

28. Roncević R, Stajcić Z. Surgical treatment of posttraumatic enophthalmos: a study of 72 patients. *Ann Plast Surg.* 1994;32(3):288–294.

29. Hammer B, Prein J. Correction of post-traumatic orbital deformities: operative techniques and review of 26 patients. *J Craniomaxillofac Surg.* 1995;23(2):81–90.

30. Priel A, Leelapatranurak K, Oh SR, et al. Medial canthal degloving injuries: the triad of telecanthus, ptosis, and lacrimal trauma. *Plast Reconstr Surg.* 2011;128(4):300e–305e.

31. Koo L, Hatton MP, Rubin PA. When is enophthalmos "significant"? *Ophthal Plast Reconstr Surg.* 2006;22(4):274–277.

32. Gear AJ, Lokeh A, Aldridge JH, et al. Safety of titanium mesh for orbital reconstruction. *Ann Plast Surg.* 2002;48(1):1–9.

33. Sargent LA. Safety of titanium mesh for orbital reconstruction (Discussion). *Ann Plast Surg.* 2002;48:7.

34. Sargent LA, Fulks KD. Reconstruction of internal orbital fractures with vitallium mesh. *Plast Reconstr Surg.* 1991;88:31.

35. Sargent LA. Reconstruction of internal orbit fractures with internal mesh. *Plast Reconstr Surg.* 1992;89:1177.

36. Sargent LA, Kennedy JW. Long-term evaluation of metallic mesh in acute internal orbital reconstruction. *Plast Surg Forum.* 1996;19:63.

37. Sargent LA. Orbital floor repair with titanium mesh screen (Discussion). *J Craniomaxillofac Trauma.* 1999;5:17.

Posttraumatic Nasal Deformities

Dane J. Genther, Ira D. Papel

BACKGROUND

Nasal bone fractures are the most common type of facial fracture, and the third most common fracture of the human skeleton. Nasal trauma is often the result of motor vehicle collisions, sports-related injuries, altercations, and falls. The annual incidence has been estimated to be 53/100,000 in the United States, with the incidence of post-traumatic nasal deformity ranging from 14% to 50% if such fractures are left untreated.[1] Immediate fracture reduction in the acute setting can reduce the incidence of posttraumatic nasal deformity, but does not eliminate the risk entirely.

Nasal deformity following trauma is one of the most common reasons that patients seek evaluation by a rhinoplasty surgeon. Depending on the type of deformity, concerns may be aesthetic, functional, or a combination of the two. Surgical correction of the complex acquired deformities that occur after trauma requires a keen understanding of nasal anatomy and physiology and honed skills of nasal analysis and physical examination. Two of the most challenging problems to address are crooked nose and saddle nose deformities. These deformities often result in both cosmetic irregularities and nasal obstruction, which should be addressed simultaneously as a unified problem.

SURGICAL ANATOMY

Normal Nasal Anatomy

When discussing nasal anatomy (Fig. 3.6.1), the nose is typically divided into thirds. The upper third consists of the paired nasal bones and bony septum. The nasal bones articulate with the frontal bones superiorly, frontal processes of the maxilla laterally, perpendicular plate of the ethmoid medially, and upper lateral cartilages inferiorly. The nasal bones are thickest superiorly and become thinner inferiorly.[2]

The middle third of the nose is composed of the upper lateral cartilages and the dorsal cartilaginous nasal septum. The upper lateral cartilages are fused with the nasal bones superiorly, dorsal cartilaginous septum medially, and lower lateral cartilages inferiorly. Externally, the shape of the middle vault plays a critical role in shaping the nasal dorsal aesthetic lines. Endonasally, the middle vault defines the internal nasal valve, which represents the narrowest portion of the nasal airway and the site of highest airflow resistance. The internal nasal valve is formed by the caudal edge of the upper lateral cartilage laterally, cartilaginous nasal septum medially, and head of the inferior turbinate posteriorly.

The lower third of the nose comprises the paired lower lateral cartilages, caudal septum, and bony nasal spine. Attachments of the lower lateral cartilages to the upper lateral cartilages in the scroll region and to the caudal septum and the strength of the lower lateral cartilages themselves are major determinants of tip support.[3] Additionally, the position of the caudal septum relative to the nasal spine and the shape of the caudal septum itself play a key role in determining the shape and position of the lower third of the nose.

Crooked Nose

Asymmetry of the upper third of the nose results from fractures of the nasal bones with or without fracture of the bony septum. As deflections of the bony pyramid can be highly variable, it is important to determine the site of nasal bone fractures, contour of the nasal bones, and involvement of the bony septum. In simple cases, a single nasal bone is displaced medially by direct trauma. However, bilateral nasal bone fractures with involvement of the bony septum and subsequent deviation to one side is often the case.

Fractures of the bony pyramid are often accompanied by deviation of the middle third of the nose. Deviation to one side as a result of fractures of the bony pyramid often cause deviation of the cartilaginous septum to the same side superiorly, resulting in a "C-shaped" deformity (Fig. 3.6.2). However, deformity of the middle vault can be seen without abnormality of the bony pyramid. Isolated cartilaginous septal involvement will result in deviation inferior to the nasal bones. If trauma results in disruption of the attachments of the upper lateral cartilage to the dorsal septum or caudal nasal bone, depression of the middle vault on that side will occur over time. If the attachments of upper lateral cartilages to the nasal bones in the keystone area are disrupted bilaterally, the upper lateral cartilages may become depressed over time, resulting in external visibility of the caudal aspect of the nasal bones (inverted-V deformity or saddle nose).

Post-traumatic deformity of the lower third of the nose often results from caudal septal fracture with subsequent deviation of the nasal tip to one side. Additionally, traumatic displacement of the caudal septum from the nasal spine results in potentially more severe tip deviation. An "S-shaped" deformity results from tip deviation to one side with contralateral deviation of the nasal bones and can result in significant cosmetic irregularity and nasal obstruction (Fig. 3.6.3). This scenario is often associated with a high septal deviation, which can be challenging to repair.

Saddle Nose

Saddle nose deformity results from the loss of integrity of the cartilaginous septum and results in loss of dorsal height and a scooped-out appearance (Fig. 3.6.4). Following trauma, a saddle nose may develop from an untreated septal hematoma leading to infection and subsequent necrosis of the cartilaginous septum or from direct fracture of the septum. Various features may accompany the loss of dorsal height and include shortened vertical length, loss of tip support, tip overrotation, and columellar retrusion. The appearance and symptoms may be mild with a minimal supratip depression and slight widening of the nose to severe with complete loss of cartilaginous septal support, flattening of the nose, and nasal obstruction.[4]

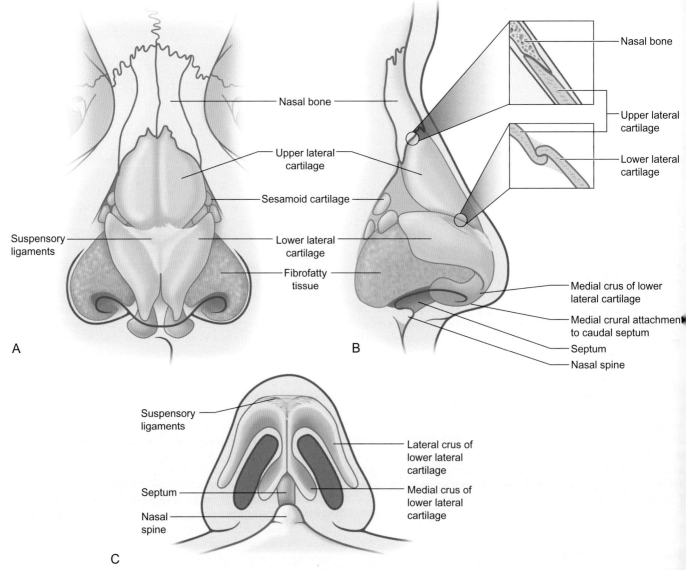

Fig. 3.6.1 Nasal anatomy: (A) frontal view; (B) profile view; (C) base view. (From Papel ID, et al., editors. Facial plastic and reconstructive surgery. New York: Thieme; 2016. p. 446)

CLINICAL PRESENTATION

History

A comprehensive history should include details of the timing and mechanism of injury and determination of the magnitude and vector of the traumatic force. High-velocity trauma resulting from motor vehicle collisions or similar mechanisms often causes significant comminution and septal injury, whereas low-velocity trauma resulting from personal assault and sports-related injuries often leads to less comminution and nasal deviation to one side.[2] Cosmetic deformity and changes in breathing resulting from the injury must be evaluated in the context of preexisting aesthetic abnormalities and nasal obstruction. Preinjury photographs are helpful in establishing a baseline. The patient's concerns regarding the appearance of the nose and patency of the nasal airway must be elicited to clearly establish goals of treatment.

Physical Examination

Determination of the anatomical cause of external deviation of the nose following trauma requires careful nasal analysis. In all cases, external

examination should be accompanied by thorough endonasal examination. Determination of the nature and severity of nasal obstruction or subjective changes in nasal breathing are vital.

On inspection of the frontal view, symmetry and width of each third should be evaluated to elucidate any abnormalities of the bony pyramid, middle vault, and nasal tip. The brow–nasal tip aesthetic lines as determined by shadowing and transitions from the medial orbital rims, nasal root, middle vault, and nasal tip should be symmetric and smooth. On the lateral view, projection of the radix, bony dorsum, cartilaginous dorsum, and tip should be evaluated. The profile should be smooth with adequate relative projection at each level and appropriate rotation of the nasal tip. On the base view, columellar position and orientation, tip projection, and nostril symmetry should be evaluated. Any asymmetries or deviations should be noted and further evaluated.

Following inspection, careful palpation is required. Palpation of the nasal bones may reveal subtle bony step-offs or depressions even if not visible on inspection. Middle vault palpation may reveal loss of support or deficiency of the cartilaginous septum, separation of the cephalic

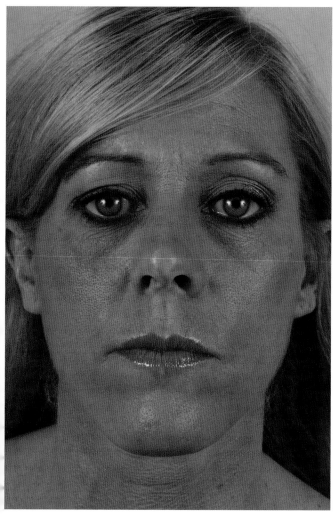

Fig. 3.6.2 C-shaped posttraumatic nasal deformity.

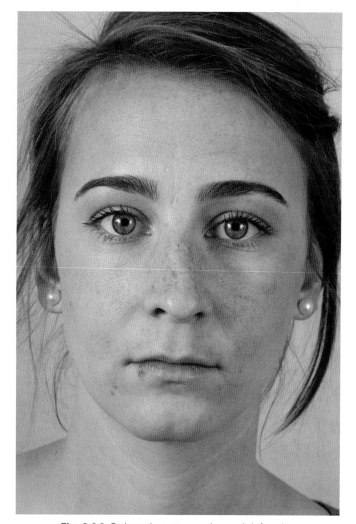

Fig. 3.6.3 S-shaped posttraumatic nasal deformity.

edge of the upper lateral cartilages from the nasal bones, or asymmetric recoil, position, or strength of the upper lateral cartilages themselves. Downward and lateral pressure on the nasal tip can provide information on tip support and status of the relationship between the caudal septum and lower lateral cartilages.

Endonasal and airway evaluation should include examination of the entirety of the nasal septum and static and dynamic evaluation of the external and internal nasal valves. Examination should be performed first without the use of topical decongestant and then performed a second time following adequate decongestion with a topical agent, such as oxymetazoline. Initially, the external nasal valves, which are formed by the columella, nasal floor, and nasal alar rim, should be evaluated for integrity. Movement and collapse at the level of the external valve should be evaluated during restful breathing and forced nasal inspiration. Function of the dilator naris muscle, which dilates the nasal vestibule, should also be evaluated. The internal nasal valves are then inspected using a nasal speculum for an appropriate valve angle of 10–15 degrees and stability during comfortable breathing and forced inspiration. A modified Cottle maneuver can then be performed to further evaluate support at the external and internal nasal valves (Fig. 3.6.5). During the maneuver, a ring curette or other narrow instrument is used to support and/or elevate the lateral nasal wall at the level of the internal and external nasal valves to see if this prevents collapse and improves subjective breathing. An improvement with this maneuver

may indicate amenability to surgical correction at the corresponding location. Following valve examination, a nasal speculum allows direct inspection of the anterior septum and potentially the posterior septum. If visualization of the posterior septum is difficult, a 0- or 30-degree endoscope can aid in septal examination. Any deviations or evidence of mucosal lacerations, which may indicate the site of septal fracture, should be noted. Additionally, the size and position of the inferior turbinates should be inspected as they can have a profound impact on patency of the nasal airway.

Photographic Documentation

High-quality photographic documentation should be performed for all patients seen for functional or cosmetic rhinoplasty consultation. Photographs are invaluable for preoperative surgical planning and patient discussion, intraoperative reference, and postoperative comparison. Standard photographic views for rhinoplasty surgery photos include frontal, base, "skyline," bilateral oblique, and bilateral profile views (Fig. 3.6.6). The "skyline" view of the dorsum is particularly valuable for visualizing the alignment of all three portions of the nose. A digital single-lens-reflex camera with a resolution of at least 1.5 megapixels is recommended. A camera lens with a focal length of 90–105 mm with macro capability is needed to minimize distortion and provide an adequate depth of field for the entire face to be in focus. Ideal lighting should be provided by two lights of equal intensity positioned at 45

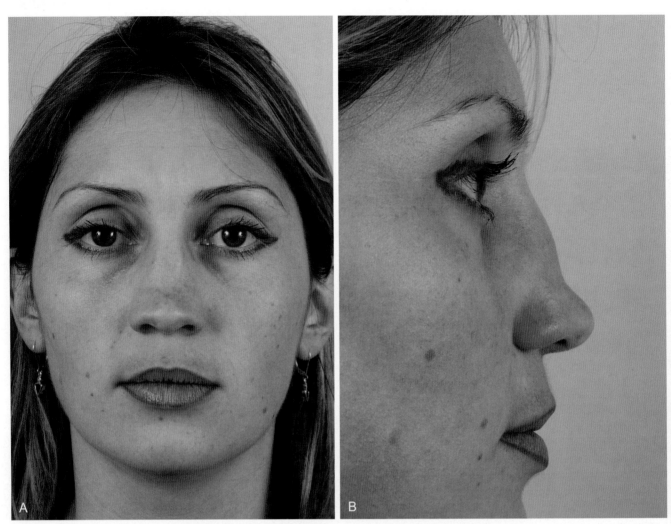

Fig. 3.6.4 Posttraumatic saddle nose: (A) frontal view; (B) profile view.

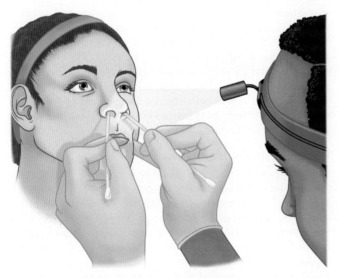

Fig. 3.6.5 Modified Cottle maneuver to evaluate for nasal valve compromise. (From Papel ID, et al., editors. Facial plastic and reconstructive surgery. New York: Thieme; 2016. p. 393.)

degrees from the subject–camera axis to prevent shadowing and uneven lighting. A plain background devoid of shiny material or creases should be used. In terms of color, an electrochromic blue background is preferred for facial medical photography. A distance of 12–18 inches between the subject and background should be maintained to minimize shadowing by the subject on the background.[5]

Radiological Evaluation

Computed tomography (CT; Fig. 3.6.7) may be useful in the acute setting to evaluate the nature and severity of facial fractures following severe trauma, but the majority of patients who subsequently follow up for correction of posttraumatic nasal deformity do not require imaging. However, if concomitant bony facial injuries are suspected, such as an untreated naso-orbital-ethmoid complex fracture, a CT scan can be considered. Plain radiographs taken at the time of trauma may provide information on the nature of nasal injury (Fig. 3.6.8), but are often of limited value in the acute setting or upon planning for corrective surgery.

SURGICAL TECHNIQUES

Approach

The choice of surgical approach depends upon the type and complexity of the deformity to be addressed and experience of the surgeon. A

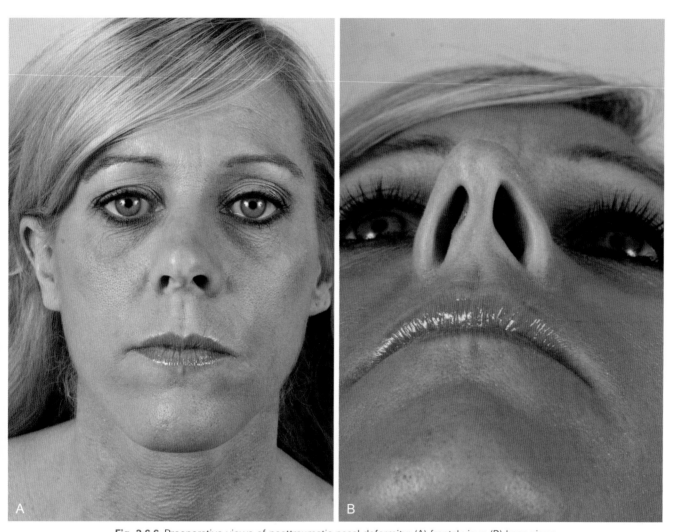

Fig. 3.6.6 Preoperative views of posttraumatic nasal deformity: (A) frontal view; (B) base view;

Continued

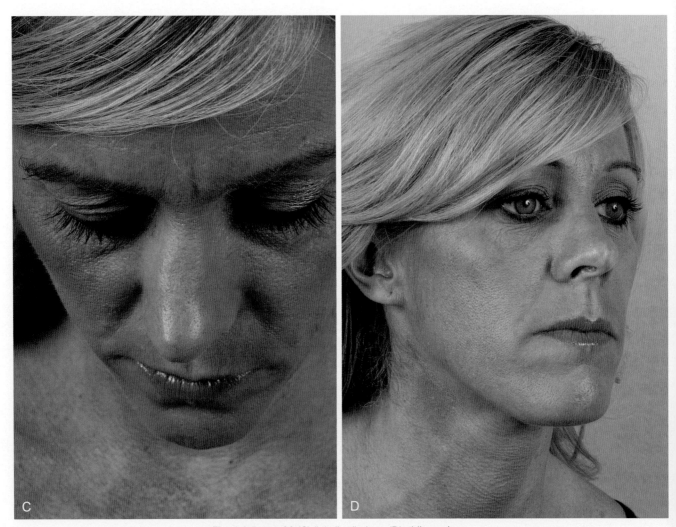

Fig. 3.6.6, cont'd (C) "skyline" view; (D) oblique view;

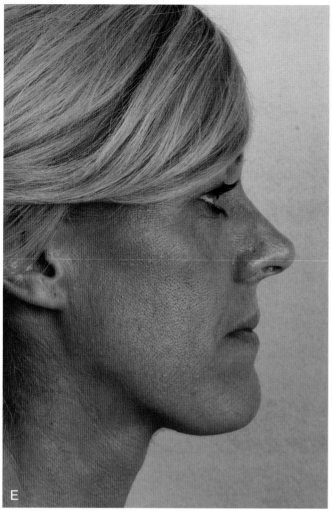

Fig. 3.6.6, cont'd (E) profile view.

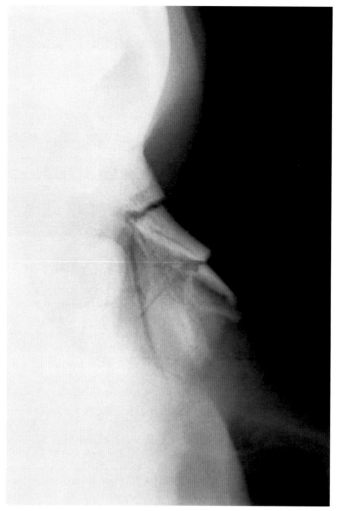

Fig. 3.6.8 Plain radiograph showing nasal bone fractures, lateral view.

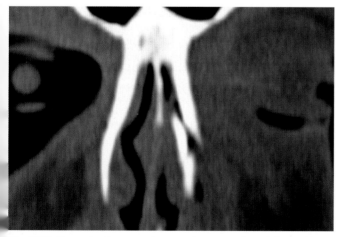

Fig. 3.6.7 Computed tomography scan demonstrating a left nasal bone fracture, coronal view.

endonasal approach may be preferred in patients requiring modest profile reduction, conservative tip management, or other minor modifications. Advantages of the endonasal approach include less tissue dissection, less postoperative edema, and more rapid postoperative healing; however, by its very nature the endonasal approach affords inferior visualization compared to the external or open approach. Indications for an open rhinoplasty approach include asymmetric nasal tip or middle vault, saddle nose deformity, and other complex nasal deformities requiring significant grafting or modification. Advantages of the open approach include excellent exposure allowing for precise tissue manipulation, suturing, and grafting. Disadvantages include an external transcolumellar incision, greater field of dissection that may disrupt some of the inherent nasal support mechanisms, and greater postoperative edema.[6] In general, procedures that do not involve complex tip changes or grafting can be performed with endonasal approaches. When middle vault grafting or tip changes are necessary, an open approach offers distinct advantages.

Graft Material

Surgical correction of nasal deformities often requires the use of grafting material. Autologous cartilage is the gold standard in rhinoplasty due to its effectiveness, similar biomechanical characteristics to the native nasal framework, and long-term safety profile. The primary

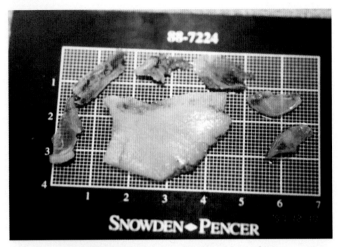

Fig. 3.6.9 Septal cartilage for potential grafting.

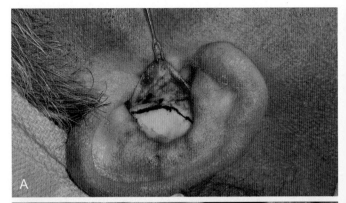

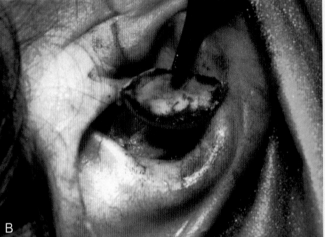

Fig. 3.6.10 (A) Exposure of conchal cartilage via an anterior approach. (B) Harvested conchal cartilage.

sources for autologous cartilage grafts include septal, auricular, and costal cartilage. Septal cartilage is the preferred material for most rhinoplasty surgeons and is typically available in adequate quantity and quality unless the patient has a history of severe septal trauma or previous septoplasty (Fig. 3.6.9). It can be easily harvested from the same surgical site through an endonasal or open approach, is generally straight, and provides strong structural support. It is highly versatile and typical uses include dorsal onlay, columellar strut, caudal septal extension, lateral crural strut, alar batten, alar rim, spreader, and tip grafts. Auricular cartilage is the second most commonly used graft in nasal surgery. It is more pliable and less rigid than septal cartilage, making it less ideal for (but not precluding) structural grafting, and is an excellent choice for most nonstructural applications when septal cartilage is inadequate or unavailable. A significant amount of the conchal bowl can be harvested en bloc without cosmetic deformity through an anterior or posterior approach with minimal donor site morbidity (Fig. 3.6.10). When a significant amount of grafting material is required or when septal and auricular cartilage are unavailable or inadequate, costal cartilage can be harvested. Costal cartilage is strong, abundant, durable, and pliable and can be easily sliced, carved, and fashioned into essentially any graft. It is particularly useful when significant dorsal grafting or restoration of nasal structural integrity is required (Fig. 3.6.11). Postoperative pain can be significant in some patients and there exists a risk of pneumothorax, although this risk is minimal if performed by an experienced surgeon. Crushed cartilage is an attractive option to conceal contour deformities and soften transition zones. Septal cartilage works best in this regard and can be lightly crushed without significant cellular loss. Diced cartilage wrapped in oxidized regenerated cellulose (Surgicel, Johnson & Johnson Medical, New Brunswick, NJ) or autologous fascia (typically the superficial layer of the deep temporal fascia) has been popularized in recent years and is an excellent tool to augment the dorsum and other areas of the nose while providing a smooth contour that is free of palpable edges.[7]

Additional sources of graft material include autologous bone, most often harvested from the bony septum or calvarium, although other sources are available. Split calvarial bone can provide significant structural support for nasal reconstruction (Fig. 3.6.12); however, its stiffness lends itself to an unnatural feel and visible or palpable edges if not properly camouflaged or fashioned. Homologous grafts are also an option if autologous sources are unavailable or the morbidity associated with harvest is undesirable. Irradiated rib cartilage is a reasonable alternative to autologous rib and can be used in the same way, albeit with a potentially greater risk of resorption and infection. Acellular dermal

matrix (AlloDerm, LifeCell Corporation, Palo Alto, CA) can be used for nonstructural augmentation or camouflaging of contour deformities; however, it is subject to potentially high rates of resorption and postoperative removal can be difficult if revision is required. Additionally, various alloplastic implants are available, including silicone, expanded polytetrafluoroethylene (e-PTFE; Gore-Tex, W. L. Gore & Associates, Flagstaff, AZ), and porous high-density polyethylene (pHDPE; Medpor, Stryker, Kalamazoo, MI). While these implants have the attractive qualities of an essentially infinite supply and avoidance of the need for a second surgical site for harvest, they confer additional risks not seen with autologous implants, including higher rates of extrusion and infection (among others), and should be used only in select circumstances and with the appropriate level of caution and consideration.[7]

Crooked Nose
Upper Third
Closed reduction. If identified early, nasal bone deviations following trauma can be treated with closed reduction (Fig. 3.6.13). In order for closed reduction to be successful, this technique must be performed before bony union has occurred. This time point varies from person to person, but within 2 weeks can be used as a general guideline. Unless reduction can be performed within hours after the initial injury, closed reduction should be delayed several days to allow resolution of edema, which can impede mobilization of the nasal bones. Additionally, because closed reduction is less precise than open reduction, residual deformity following this procedure is not uncommon.

Osteotomies. If correction of nasal bony deviation is to be attempted after bony union has occurred, an open reduction technique with the

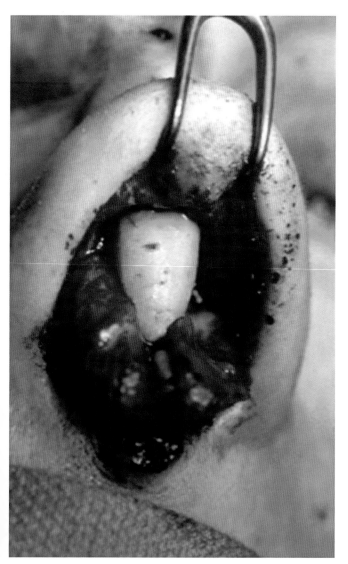

Fig. 3.6.11 Costal cartilage graft for dorsal nasal reconstruction.

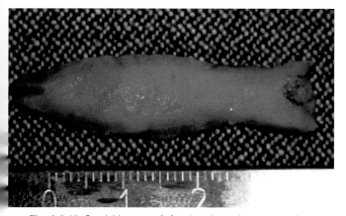

Fig. 3.6.12 Cranial bone graft for dorsal nasal reconstruction.

use of osteotomies will be required. In general, waiting at least 6 weeks after the fracture has occurred to utilize osteotomies is recommended, as this will allow the bony unions to be more stable and will make the osteotomies more predictable. Osteotomies are created through the use of various osteotomes tapped carefully by a mallet to create a controlled

fracture resulting in mobile bony segments that can be reduced to a more favorable anatomic position. These maneuvers, while called "open," rely on tactile discrimination rather than direct visualization. Importantly, if a dorsal hump reduction is to be performed, this should be done prior to any osteotomies.

Medial osteotomies are typically performed first, unless there is a significant open roof created by removal of a dorsal hump or if the nasal bones are thin. A 2–3 mm straight, unguarded osteotome is placed at the rhinion near the junction of the nasal bones and bony septum. The osteotomy is advanced cephalad, fading 15–20 degrees laterally toward the head of the eyebrow (Fig. 3.6.14).[2,8] These osteotomies allow for a predictable site of back fracture in association with lateral osteotomies.

Lateral osteotomies are then performed beginning with the side opposite the deviation. A high–low–high technique allows for reshaping of the nasal bones without narrowing the airway (Fig. 3.6.15). A 3–4 mm, curved, guarded osteotome is used, with the curve allowing for easier establishment of the high–low–high fracture pattern and the guard reducing the risk of injury to the nasal skin.[2] For access, an intranasal stab incision is made just above the anterior insertion of the inferior turbinate, approximately 3–4 mm above the base of the pyriform aperture. The osteotomy then proceeds toward the cephalad aspect of the medial osteotomy and is halted inferior to the medial canthus, often where the lateral nasal bones meet the frontal process.[2,8]

In some cases, medial and lateral osteotomies alone may be insufficient to restore nasal symmetry. Significant convexity or concavity of the nasal bones themselves can be corrected with the addition of intermediate osteotomies, which should be performed prior to the lateral osteotomies and parallel their course.[8] Transcutaneous perforated osteotomies with a sharp 2 mm osteotome is the preferred method (Fig. 3.6.16). This is often a unilateral maneuver.

Bony septal deviation. If a bony septal deviation is present that is not corrected after osteotomies and repositioning of the bony pyramid have been performed, closed reduction can be attempted with septum-straightening forceps or a blunt instrument such as a Boise elevator to manually fracture the bony septum toward the midline. These closed reduction techniques are less precise and may not result in stable reduction. In many cases, direct visualization through a formal septoplasty with specific attention paid to the deviated bony portion may be required.[8]

Camouflage grafts. Precisely placed grafts can be used to camouflage contour irregularities following reduction of bony abnormalities. Autologous crushed or diced cartilage or fascia can be effective at reducing visibility and palpability of bony edges or small depressions. Subperiosteal placement decreases the chance of graft migration and has the theoretic advantages of improved camouflaging. Grafts can be placed supraperiosteally but this increases the risk of migration and may appear more prominent, especially in patients with thin nasal skin.[2]

Middle Third

Middle third deviations may be corrected by reduction of the bony pyramid due to the attachments between the nasal bones and upper lateral cartilages. However, if the middle vault does not return to the midline following reduction of the bony pyramid or if deviation of the middle vault occurred in the absence of bony pyramid abnormalities, the middle third deviation is likely the result of dorsal septal deviation.

Septoplasty. Because of the firm fibrous attachments between the upper lateral cartilages and dorsal cartilaginous septum, dorsal septal deviations often manifest as external nasal asymmetry. Complex septal deviations resulting in nasal asymmetry are best approached through an open rhinoplasty approach, which affords direct visualization and

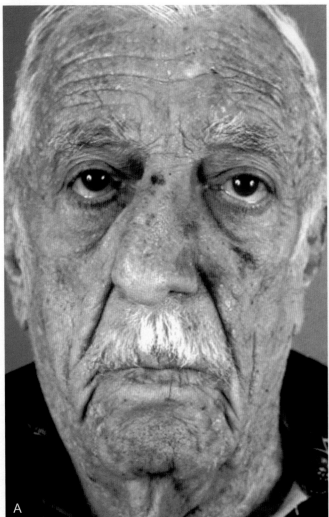
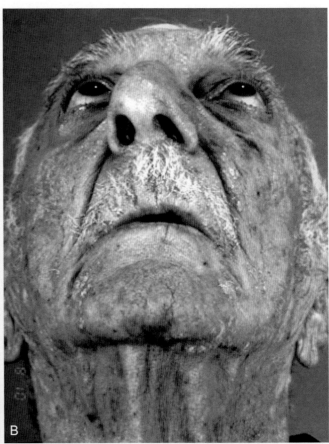

Fig. 3.6.13 Acute nasal fracture: (A) frontal view; (B) base view.

wide exposure of the dorsal septum and its attachment to the upper lateral cartilages. To visualize the entire septum and reestablish its relationship with the upper lateral cartilages, the fibrous attachments are sharply separated from the dorsal septum and mucoperichondrial flaps are elevated. Septal cross-hatching or shaving may help to restore symmetry if the asymmetry is primarily due to intrinsic deviation of the septal cartilage. In the case of direct septal fracture, the fracture can be reduced and secured in the midline. However, the majority of cases require structural grafting in the form of spreader grafts to restore septal straightness and integrity. In the most severe cases, extracorporeal septoplasty, during which the entire septum is explanted, reconstructed *ex vivo*, reimplanted, and secured, may be required.

    Spreader grafts. Spreader grafts are an indispensable tool in management of dorsal septal deviation and internal nasal valve compromise that often accompanies it. The dimensions of each graft depend upon the intended function and specific anatomy but typically range from 6 mm to 12 mm in length, 3 mm to 5 mm in height, and 2 mm to 4 mm in thickness.[8] Unilateral, bilateral symmetric, or bilateral asymmetric grafts can be used as necessary depending on the specific deformity. Each spreader graft is placed between the dorsal septum and ipsilateral upper lateral cartilage (Fig. 3.6.17) and secured using horizontal mattress sutures placed through and through the spreader graft, septum, upper lateral cartilages, and any additional spreader grafts previously

placed (Fig. 3.6.18). If the goal is simply to straighten the nose with a mild-to-moderate dorsal septal deviation, a single spreader graft may be placed on the concave side. For more severe deviations, bilateral spreader grafts are used. Occasionally, double or asymmetric spreaders can be used to restore symmetry and establish appropriate width to the middle vault. Even in the absence of a septal deviation, depression or pinching at the level of the middle third can be treated with a unilateral or bilateral spreader graft.[9]

    Camouflage grafts. Following establishing septal straightness and adequate securing of the upper lateral cartilages and any spreader grafts to the septum itself, any residual depression or contour deformity can be addressed with camouflage grafts. Autologous crushed or diced cartilage or fascia work well in this capacity. Care should be taken to not inappropriately widen the middle vault by overzealous grafting.

Lower Third

    Caudal septal deformity. Caudal septal deformity results in twisting of the lower third of the nose and nasal obstruction. The caudal septum starts at the anterior septal angle near the nasal tip and continues to the posterior septal angle at its junction with the nasal spine. Deviation or displacement anywhere along this path results in deformity and/or nasal obstruction at the level of the lower third of the nose. Various techniques exist to address deformities in this area.

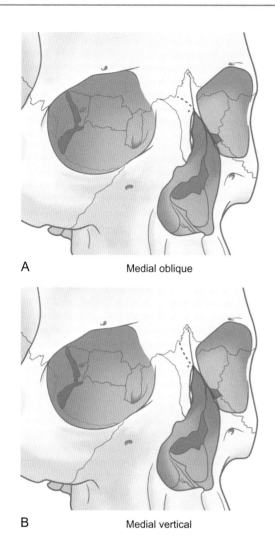

A Medial oblique

B Medial vertical

Fig. 3.6.14 Placement of medial osteotomies. (A) Oblique course to assist with control of back-fracture in conjunction with a lateral osteotomy to treat a deviated nose or to close an open roof deformity. (B) Vertical course to widen a narrow bony vault. (From Papel ID, et al., editors. Facial plastic and reconstructive surgery. New York: Thieme; 2016. p. 443.)

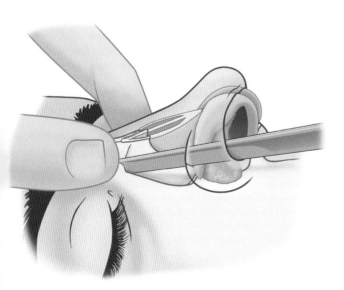

Fig. 3.6.15 Illustration of lateral high–low–high osteotomy.

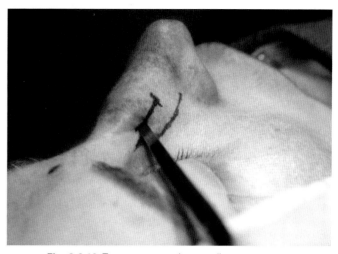

Fig. 3.6.16 Transcutaneous intermediate osteotomy.

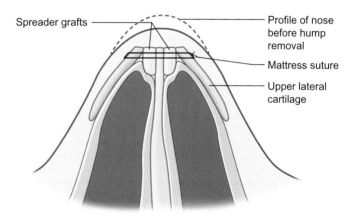

Fig. 3.6.17 Illustration of extramucosal placement of spreader grafts. (From Papel ID, et al., editors. Facial plastic and reconstructive surgery. New York: Thieme; 2016. p. 449.)

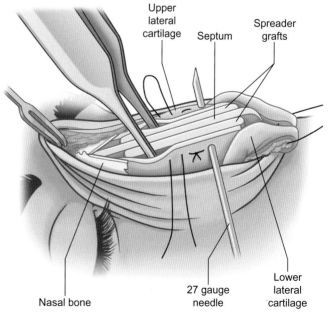

Fig. 3.6.18 Placement of spreader grafts to stabilize middle vault.

If the septum is displaced from the nasal spine at the posterior septal angle (Fig. 3.6.19), caudal repositioning may restore symmetry and alleviate nasal obstruction. After exposure of the septum through a septoplasty approach, the septum at the posterior septal angle is trimmed, shifted back over the nasal spine in the midline, and sutured to the nasal spine using a nonabsorbable suture. Alternatively, the septum can be repositioned to the other side of the nasal spine, with or without trimming at the posterior septal angle, and sutured into place, as long as this results in symmetry and patency at the nasal vestibule. In this case, the nasal spine acts as a "doorstop" to keep the septum from returning to its previous position and may be particularly useful if the nasal spine is off midline.[10]

If the caudal septum is mild-to-moderately deviated, conservative maneuvers may serve to straighten it. Scoring of the cartilage through a series of incomplete incisions on the concave side or careful morselization will alleviate the warped memory of the caudal strut. Suture techniques may also be considered to further stabilize the septum in a more vertical position. Following scoring, 2–4 horizontal mattress sutures are placed through the cartilage using nonabsorbable sutures, similar to Mustarde sutures used to correct prominent ears.[10]

If more severe deviation is present or significant septal repositioning is performed, more substantive techniques may be required to maintain long-term integrity of the reconstruction with regard to prevention of recurrence of the deviation and loss of tip support. Spreader grafts, which are a long-recognized method of widening the internal nasal valve angle, can be extended beyond the caudal border of the upper lateral cartilages to stabilize the caudal septum and improve tip support. These extended spreaders can be unilateral or bilateral depending on the need of middle vault treatment and desired degree of stabilization of the caudal septum. Cartilage can be used in many cases, but if extra stabilization is required, bony grafts from the perpendicular plate of the ethmoid bone can be used. Holes for suture stabilization of the bony graft can be made with a small drill bit or 18-gauge needle, through

which horizontal mattress sutures are used to secure it to the caudal septum. Stabilization can also be accomplished with the tongue-in-groove technique, in which the septum is stabilized in a groove between the medial crura of the lower lateral cartilages. A caudal septal extension graft can also be used to stabilize and maintain a vertical position of the caudal septum. In this technique, a cartilage or bony graft is secured to the caudal aspect of the septum and secured with at least two horizontal mattress sutures. If necessary, the overlapping edges of the cartilage can be beveled to prevent nasal obstruction that may otherwise occur from widening of this area. A slight curve of the graft can be used to the surgeon's advantage to counteract the inherent curvature of the deviated septum. The medial crura are then sutured to the extension graft, and the graft may be further secured to the nasal spine. This is a particularly versatile graft that can be shaped to affect changes in nasal projection, nasal rotation, nasolabial angle, and columellar show.[8,10]

The most severe deviations may require replacement of the caudal septum. This technique requires an open approach with separation of the nasal cartilages from the septum, wide elevation of mucoperichondrial flaps, and excision of the offending portion of the septum. This portion is then replaced with a straight and stable graft that is sutured to the remaining septum and nasal spine. A straight portion of the remaining septum, double-layer auricular cartilage, or costal cartilage can be used in this regard. If inadequate stabilization is achieved with suturing alone, extended spreader grafts or a thin semi-rigid material, such as polydioxane (PDS; Ethicon Inc., Somerville, NJ) flexible plate, can be used to secure the graft into place.[8,10] If severe caudal septal deviation is accompanied by significant deformity of the dorsal cartilaginous septum, a subtotal or total extracorporeal septoplasty may be required. In this more extreme case, the entire septum is removed after wide exposure, reconstructed, replaced, and secured to remnant cartilage or nasal bones and nasal spine. Polydioxanone plate works well to serve as a scaffold for the multiple pieces of cartilage that are often required.

Tip modification. Following treatment of the caudal septum, tip modification may be required. This can be accomplished via tip grafts, such as cap or shield grafts, or suture techniques. Additionally, ensuring a stable relationship of the lower lateral cartilages is paramount. Interdomal, intradomal, and spanning sutures can be used to restore the lower lateral cartilages to their preinjury position and create symmetry of the nasal tip.

Saddle Nose

Following trauma, untreated septal hematoma with subsequent abscess formation may result in resorption of septal cartilage and consequent "saddling." In minor cases, septal support is only partially comprised resulting in a cosmetic deformity; however, in more severe cases, loss of all septal support with significant dorsal depression, loss of tip support and nasal obstruction ensue.

In mild cases, dorsal onlay grafting with carved or diced cartilage wrapped in fascia (Fig. 3.6.20) can improve cosmetic appearance. If internal nasal valve compromise is also present, spreader grafts can be used to widen the internal nasal valve angle and also provide additional septal support. When septal support is severely compromised, reconstruction of the dorsal–caudal L-strut may be required. While septal and auricular cartilage sutured together can be used in some cases if these cartilages are available in adequate amounts, costal cartilage is ideal due to its strength and availability in large quantity. It is imperative that the costal cartilage used for the L-strut is straight and should be obtained from a concentrically carved portion of the rib to prevent warping. Alternatively, split calvarial bone can be harvested and used for this purpose, but proper fashioning can be difficult, postoperative visibility and palpability of the rigid framework is difficult to avoid and the risk of resorption is higher.[8] Once the dorsal strut is carved

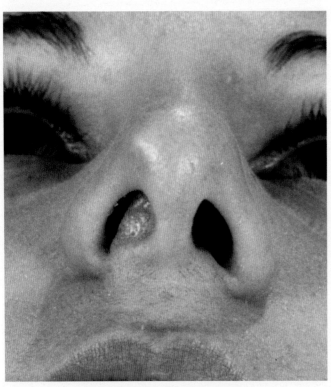

Fig. 3.6.19 Caudal septal deviation.

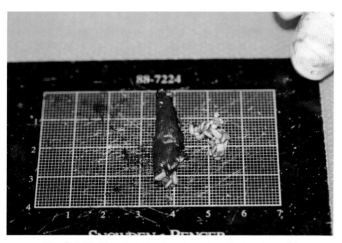

Fig. 3.6.20 Diced cartilage and temporalis fascia graft.

to achieve adequate dorsal projection and length, it is placed into a tight subperiosteal pocket over the nasal bones and may be further secured using a temporary transcutaneous retention suture. The columellar strut portion of the "L" is fashioned to achieve appropriate tip projection and support, columellar show, and nasolabial angle. It is secured to the nasal spine and adjacent soft tissues, and then secured to the caudal edge of the dorsal graft, resulting in a stable L-strut.[4,8] Following this, the upper lateral and lower lateral cartilages are suspended from the new construct and additional grafting is applied to restore patency of the nasal airway and recontour any depressions or deformities.

CASE EXAMPLES

Case 1

A middle-aged female presented 1 week after a nasal fracture resulting from a fall. Preoperative nasal analysis demonstrated leftward deviation of the nasal bones and dorsal septum, resulting in a reverse "C-shaped" deformity (Fig. 3.6.21A–D). Given the severity of her injury and the desire for immediate surgical correction, she was taken to the

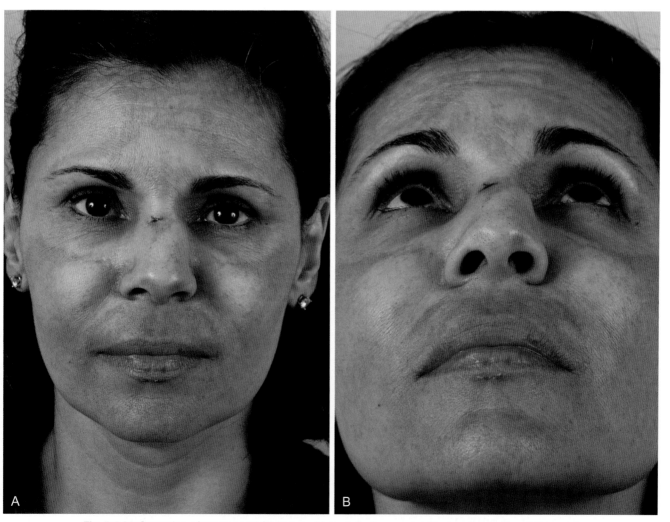

A   B

Fig. 3.6.21 Correction of acute nasal fracture and lateral displacement with closed reduction of the nasal bones and septoplasty via an endonasal approach. (A–D) Preoperative views. (E–H) Postoperative views at one year. *Continued*

operating room to undergo closed reduction of her nasal bone fractures and septoplasty via a hemitransfixion incision. Evaluation one year after surgery demonstrated a straight nasal dorsum and septum (Fig. 3.6.21E–H).

Case 2

A 40-year-old male presented years after multiple nasal fractures resulting in an obvious posttraumatic nasal deformity with nasal obstruction. Preoperative analysis demonstrated leftward deviation of the nasal bones, bilateral narrowing of the middle vault (right greater than left),

prominent dorsal hump, rightward tip deviation, bilateral external nasal valve compromise (left greater than right), and bilateral internal nasal valve compromise (right greater than left) (Fig. 3.6.22A–D). He was taken to the operating room and underwent dorsal hump reduction, lateral and intermediate osteotomies, septoplasty, bilateral spreader graft placement, and bilateral alar strut graft placement via an open approach. Evaluation one year after surgery demonstrated a straight dorsal contour, symmetry of the nasal tip, and improved stability of the external and internal nasal valves (Fig. 3.6.22.E–H).

Text continued on p. 414

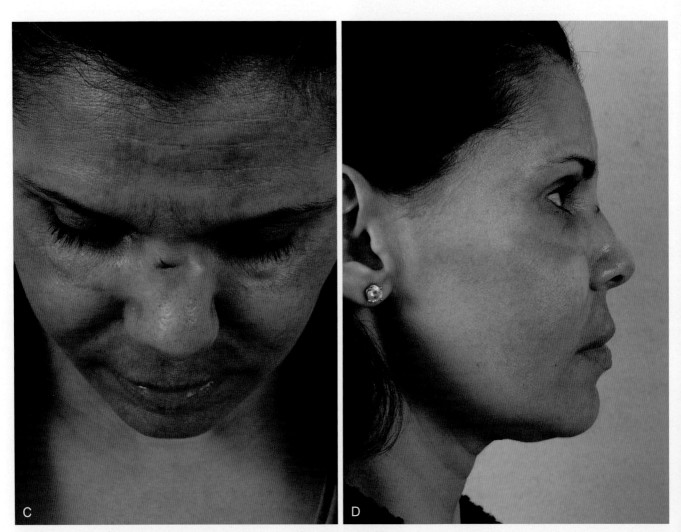

Fig. 3.6.21, cont'd

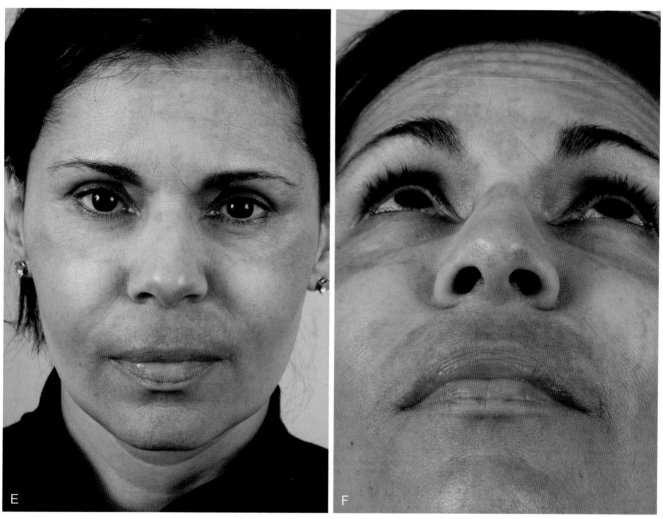

Fig. 3.6.21, cont'd

Continued

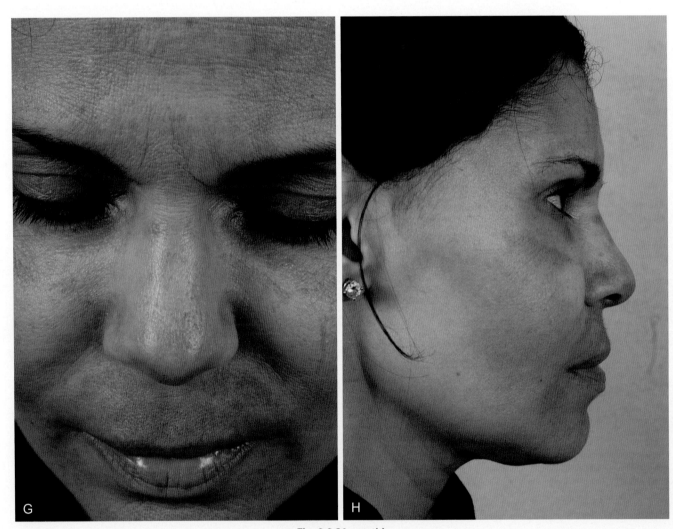

Fig. 3.6.21, cont'd

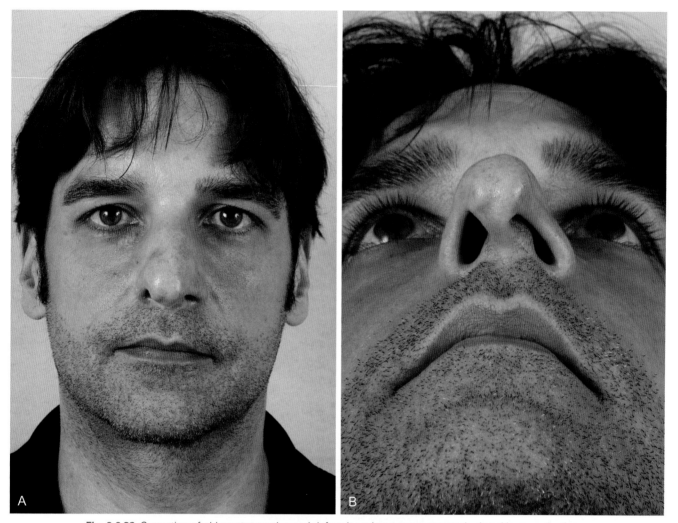

Fig. 3.6.22 Correction of old posttraumatic nasal deformity using an open approach, dorsal hump reduction, lateral and intermediate osteotomies, septoplasty, bilateral spreader graft placement, and bilateral alar strut graft placement. (A–D) Preoperative views. (E–H) Postoperative views at one year.   *Continued*

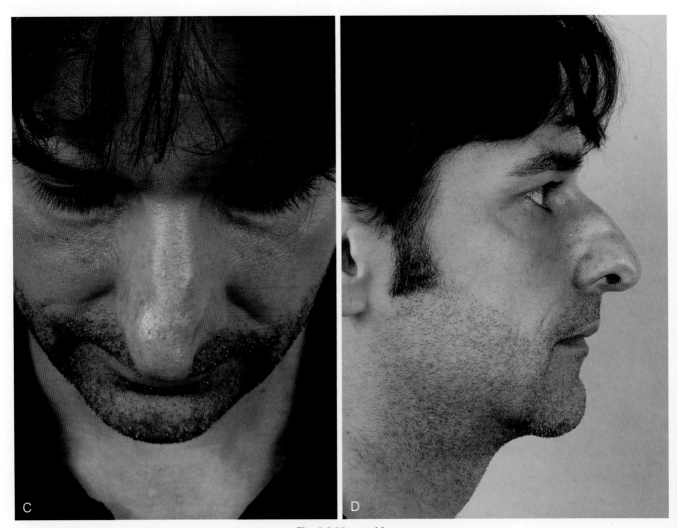

Fig. 3.6.22, cont'd

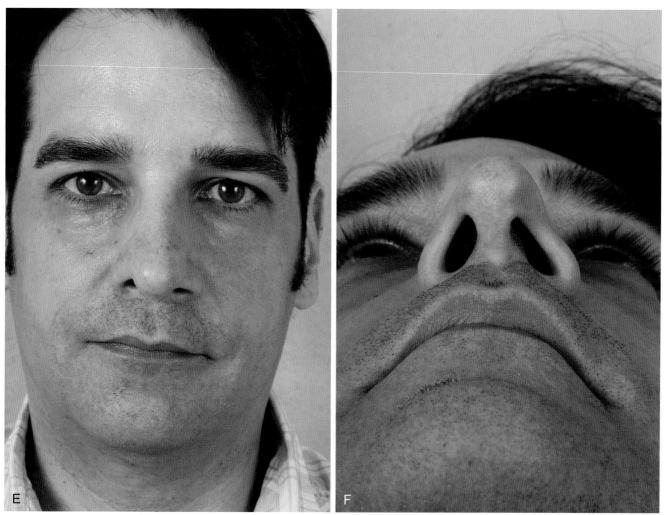

Fig. 3.6.22, cont'd   *Continued*

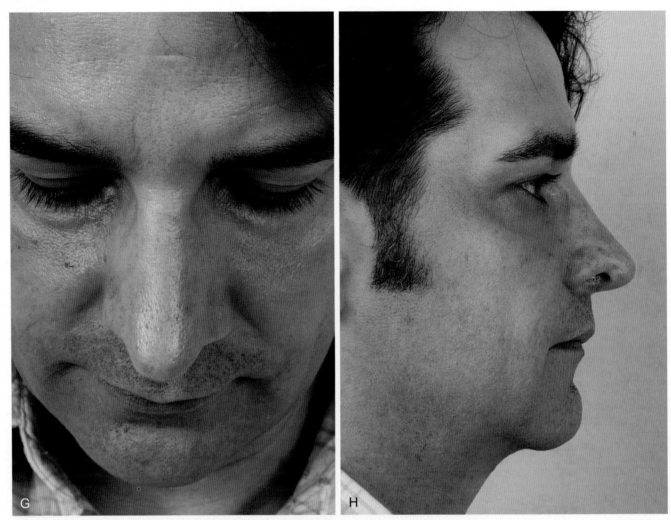

Fig. 3.6.22, cont'd

POSTOPERATIVE COURSE

Postoperative Edema

Following rhinoplasty, edema persists for up to a year in primary cases and up to 2 years in revision cases. Various techniques have been employed to manage postoperative edema. Exacerbated swelling can occur particularly in patients with thick skin, and the dead space under the soft tissue envelope has been speculated to contribute to chronic edema. Postrhinoplasty taping is a widely employed method to reduce postoperative edema and has been shown to reduce swelling, with particular utility in thick-skinned patients and for reducing supratip fullness.[11] Postrhinoplasty tape is typically left in place for 1–4 weeks and can be reapplied by the patient at home as needed according to surgeon preference. Edema can also affect adjacent soft tissue, especially the eyelids, and the administration of perioperative corticosteroids has been shown to reduce edema as well as bruising in the upper and lower eyelids. An intravenous dose of corticosteroids is typically administered prior to surgery, and oral corticosteroids may be prescribed for up to 3 days postoperatively with significant reduction in edema and ecchymosis; however, beyond 3 days postrhinoplasty, no additional benefit has been shown.[12]

Antibiotic Prophylaxis

Typical antibiotic regimens (according to surgeon preference) include no antibiotics, a single dose of intravenous antibiotics at induction of anesthesia, and up to 7 days of postoperative oral antibiotics; however, multiple studies have shown that antibiotic prophylaxis is not associated with a decreased infection rate in most patients. Complications related to antibiotic use were significantly higher in patients who received a 7-day postoperative course of oral antibiotics compared to a single perioperative dose in one study. Another study showed a decreased infection rate with antibiotic prophylaxis only if surgery lasted longer than 3 hours or if the American Society of Anesthesiologists score was 3 or higher.[13] Antibiotics should be considered in patients who receive alloplastic grafts, such as silicone, since these represent a foreign body. Additional considerations include revision surgery or the use of multiple autologous grafts. Overall, there is no consensus as to what antibiotic should be used, but typical choices for intravenous antibiotics include cefazolin, ampicillin-clavulanic acid, clindamycin, or sulfamethoxazole/trimethoprim and for oral antibiotics include cephalexin, amoxicillin-clavulanic acid, clindamycin, or sulfamethoxazole/trimethoprim. There is no evidence for the use of antibiotics that specifically target methicillin-resistant *Staphylococcus aureus* (MRSA) for patients undergoing outpatient rhinoplasty unless there is a clear history of MRSA-related infections.[12]

Nasal Stabilization

If osteotomies or manipulation of the bony pyramid are performed, an external nasal cast should be applied for approximately 1 week. If a simple septoplasty is performed, the septum can be approximated by septal quilting sutures, internal nasal splints, or nasal packing. Quilting sutures have been shown to be associated with less patient discomfort without a difference in postoperative complications related to the septum, suggesting that quilting sutures may be superior to and obviate the need for more uncomfortable nasal packing or splints.[13] However, if a complex septal reconstruction is performed, nasal splints can be used to stabilize the reconstruction in the midline and may be indicated in such a case. If splints or packing are used, antistaphylococcal antibiotics should be administered while these foreign bodies are in place.[13] In our experience, the use of nasal packing is almost never indicated.

Nasal Exercises

In patients with persistent nasal bone deviation after osteotomies and following external cast removal, surgeon- and patient-directed nasal exercises can be undertaken. These exercises consist of application of direct pressure to the edge of the bone that has shifted for approximately 1 minute up to 20 times per day. These can be particularly effective in treating minor deviations of the bone. If shifting of a dorsal onlay graft has occurred, direct pressure can be similarly applied to move this graft back to the midline (Fig. 3.6.23). These exercises can also be performed to correct minor contour irregularities due to edema in a specific location. These exercises are particularly useful in the first 2 weeks following rhinoplasty.

COMPLICATIONS

Acute Complications

Acute complications following rhinoplasty include graft displacement, bleeding, and infection. Early after surgery, graft displacement typically manifests as shifting of onlay grafts. Within the first few postoperative weeks, repositioning exercises may help to restore these grafts to their ideal location. Bleeding typically occurs in the perioperative period out

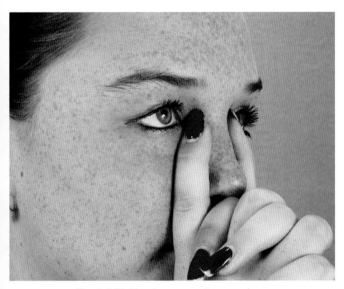
Fig. 3.6.23 Nasal compression exercises.

to approximately 2 weeks and is one of the most common complications. Bleeding resulting from incision lines or traumatized mucosa can typically be managed with conservative measures such as direct pressure and topical vasoconstriction. More severe bleeding may require nasal packing with either a compressive or hemostatic agent. Additionally, intravenous desmopressin can be considered as an adjunctive treatment in patients with refractory bleeding requiring bedside intervention. Major or refractory bleeding warrants a return trip to the operating room for exploration and control of epistaxis.[12]

Infection is uncommon following rhinoplasty and typically manifests as cellulitis with erythema, induration, and tenderness. If identified early, frank purulence or abscess formation is often not present. Management involves oral antibiotics and topical intranasal bacitracin or mupirocin ointment. Rarely, severe infections may require admission to the hospital for intravenous antibiotics. The infection risk depends in part upon the nature of the operation (primary versus revision) and the type of graft(s) used. In primary rhinoplasty with only autologous grafting, infection risk is far less than 1%, but this risk may be higher in revision surgery. Alloplastic grafting materials are associated with a significantly higher risk of infection in both primary and revision nasal surgery. If alloplast is used, minor infections can be treated with antibiotics, but severe infections may warrant implant removal.[7]

Long-Term Complications

Complications that occur after the acute postoperative phase include prolonged edema, persistent or iatrogenic nasal deformity, and nasal airway obstruction. Edema typically resolves over several months following rhinoplasty surgery and may be present for up to a year following an open approach with wide dissection or even longer in revision cases, despite the use of rhinoplasty tape and steroids in the perioperative period to reduce the amount of initial swelling. While the bulk of the postoperative edema resolves within the first 6–8 weeks after surgery, some degree of edema should be expected for several months, and patients must be counseled that the edema may take up to one year or longer to fully resolve. In the case of exuberant or asymmetric edema, particularly in the tip or supratip areas, conservative localized steroid injection can help to speed resolution. Steroid injection should not start before 6–8 weeks following surgery, and serial injections should be spaced out at least 6 weeks apart. Care must be taken while injecting to avoid significant dermal atrophy or hypopigmentation of the surrounding skin.

Poor cosmetic outcomes, which may be related to undercorrection of the initial deformity or iatrogenic changes, should be addressed on a case-by-case basis. Patient satisfaction strongly influences the decision to intervene following a non-ideal outcome following rhinoplasty surgery. Contour deformities or visible bony or cartilaginous edges can typically be treated with in-office procedures with local anesthesia. Options for conservative intervention include injection of temporary fillers (such as hyaluronic acid), rasping of bony edges, or shaving of cartilage grafts. However, more prominent abnormalities or those that are particularly troubling to the patient may require more extensive revision surgery. Additionally, persistent or new nasal obstruction after rhinoplasty must be addressed. Minor nasal obstruction resulting from a slightly narrowed nasal airway or persistent edema may improve with topical corticosteroid therapy. However, significant nasal obstruction may require surgical revision. Minor interventions can be undertaken as early as 3–6 months after surgery, but revision requiring extensive surgery should be delayed until at least 6–12 months to allow for resolution of edema, evolution of any graft resorption, scar maturation, and completion of the healing process.

The use of alloplastic implants imparts additional risks of delayed infection and implant extrusion that are not seen with autologous

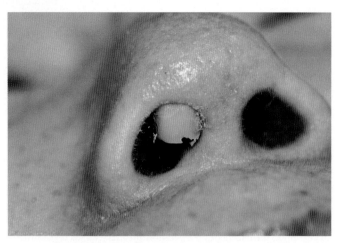

Fig. 3.6.24 Intranasal extrusion of silicone implant.

cartilage grafts. Infection may occur months or even decades after rhinoplasty surgery when alloplastic grafts such as silicone, Gore-Tex, or Medpor are used. The infections may be minor requiring oral antibiotic treatment and close follow-up, but severe infections or those that fail to resolve with antibiotic treatment require implant removal, which can be complicated by fibrovascular ingrowth and tissue incorporation. Additionally, implants have a risk of extrusion that may occur up to decades after surgery (Fig. 3.6.24). Extrusion may occur intranasally or through the nasal skin and often requires implant removal and revision of the previous reconstructive efforts.

CONCLUSION

Posttraumatic nasal deformity is a complex problem that requires astute preoperative assessment and nasal analysis. A keen knowledge of the normal nasal anatomy and physiology is required to recognize abnormalities and to develop a treatment plan for each individual patient that appropriately addresses both cosmetic and functional concerns. The intraoperative techniques and maneuvers are many and vary according to the problem at hand. Following surgical treatment, an understanding of the postoperative healing process will help to increase patient understanding and satisfaction during recovery.

The chapter is filled with experience-derived templates for analysis and planning treatment. This helpful chapter should make the interested reader want to invest in more voluminous and sophisticated literature, which, when supplemented by the good rhinoplasty courses available which stress anatomy, technique, and surgical performance, create continuous improvement in outcomes in this challenging field.

REFERENCES

1. Basheeth N, Donnelly M, David S, Munish S. Acute nasal fracture management: a prospective study and literature review. *Laryngoscope.* 2015;125:2677–2684.
2. Chua DY, Park SS. Posttraumatic nasal deformities: correcting the crooked and saddle nose. *Facial Plast Surg.* 2015;31:259–269.
3. Schinkel ML, Nayak LM. Nasal tip modifications. *Oral Maxillofac Surg Clin North Am.* 2012;24:67–74.
4. Daniel RK, Brenner KA. Saddle nose deformity: a new classification and treatment. *Facial Plast Surg Clin North Am.* 2006;14:301–312.
5. Swamy RS, Most SP. Pre- and postoperative portrait photography: standardized photos for various procedures. *Facial Plast Surg Clin North Am.* 2010;18:245–252.
6. Cafferty A, Becker DG. Open and closed rhinoplasty. *Clin Plast Surg.* 2016;43:17–27.
7. Genther DJ, Papel ID. Surgical nasal implants: indications and risks. *Facial Plast Surg.* 2016;32:488–499.
8. Kim DW, Toriumi DM. Management of posttraumatic nasal deformities: the crooked nose and the saddle nose. *Facial Plast Surg Clin North Am.* 2004;12:111–132.
9. Kim L, Papel ID. Spreader grafts in functional rhinoplasty. *Facial Plast Surg.* 2016;32:29–35.
10. Haack J, Papel ID. Caudal septal deviation. *Otolaryngol Clin North Am.* 2009;42:427–436.
11. Ozucer B, Yildirim YS, Veyseller B, et al. Effect of postrhinoplasty taping on postoperative edema and nasal draping: a randomized clinical trial. *JAMA Facial Plast Surg.* 2016;18:157–163.
12. Beck DO, Kenkel JM. Evidence-based medicine: rhinoplasty. *Plast Reconstr Surg.* 2014;134:1356–1371.
13. Han JK, Stringer SP, Rosenfeld RM, et al. Clinical consensus statement: septoplasty with or without inferior turbinate reduction. *Otolaryngol Head Neck Surg.* 2015;153:708–720.

Secondary Orbital Reconstruction

Bartlomiej Kachniarz, Michael Grant, Amir H. Dorafshar

BACKGROUND

Persistent enophthalmos and diplopia following primary orbital reconstruction lead to unsatisfactory aesthetic and functional outcomes, respectively. Diplopia after surgical repair of orbital fractures has been reported in 8%–52% of patients, while clinically significant enophthalmos has been reported in 27%.[1–3] Large combined medial wall and orbital floor fractures tend to carry a higher risk of enophthalmos, particularly if the fracture compromised the inferonasal bony strut support. Secondary orbital reconstruction has traditionally been seen as extremely challenging, and keys to success are careful preoperative planning, appropriate imaging and identifying which patients are most likely to benefit from surgical treatment.[4]

Changes in orbital volume as small as 2.1–2.3 mL have been shown to result in clinically significant globe malposition.[5,6] Suboptimal reduction of orbital fractures in the acute setting results in increased orbital volume and in both secondary enophthalmos and diplopia. Symptoms may present in a delayed fashion, as a poorly fixed implant becomes displaced or changes in orbital anatomy after trauma are not considered properly. For instance, if the posterior bony orbit remodels following trauma, the retrobulbar volume may increase; the orbital fat is frequently repositioned posteriorly, further compromising support of the globe.[7] Such anatomic reasons for globe malposition tend not to improve, and frequently worsen, over time following inadequate primary reconstruction.

Persistent diplopia following orbital fracture repair may be broadly categorized into either restrictive or paralytic etiologies. Poor primary reduction may lead to increased orbital volume and muscle impingement. Developing adhesions surrounding the implant and implant displacement may also restrict muscle movement. Such anatomic causes of symptoms result in restrictive strabismus and most often improve with revision surgery. Conversely, paralytic diplopia secondary to neuromuscular injury will not benefit from reoperation, although symptoms tend to improve over time with conservative management which depends upon nerve regeneration.

CLINICAL PRESENTATION

Patient history and physical examination should include all details relevant to any orbital trauma patient. Specific details pertinent in secondary reconstruction include a thorough understanding of prior reconstructive procedures, and a timeline of presentation of symptoms. Operative reports should be obtained if possible, detailing surgical approaches, incision choice, and implant type. An understanding of how symptoms have been changing over time may lend clues to the etiology. Diplopia that has been improving very slowly suggests neurogenic causes; new onset symptoms that have worsened since primary repair are more suggestive of a restrictive process.

Compared to patients with acute orbital trauma, those who have undergone prior repair warrant a more thorough eye examination. Patients should be referred for strabismus evaluation by an extraocular muscle specialist. A detailed extraocular motion exam may help differentiate between restrictive and paralytic symptoms, as the latter is unlikely to improve with repeat surgery. Additionally, accurate measurements of the relative position of orbital rims, lateral, and medial canthi, and pupils should be taken. An exophthalmometer may be used to measure globe position relative to the lateral orbital rim, or the ear canal if necessary (Fig. 3.7.1).

RADIOLOGICAL EVALUATION

Recent computed tomography imaging should be available as part of any secondary reconstruction evaluation. As in acute trauma, thin-cut computed tomography (CT) imaging of the face is the gold standard for evaluating the bony orbit. In patients with contraindications to CT imaging, MRI has been used to assess orbital volume and anatomy.[5] Repeat imaging should be compared to prior studies and focus on identifying abnormalities amenable to surgical revision. Orbital volume should be assessed and compared to the contralateral uninjured side if possible. Any implant displacement or impingement, herniation of orbital contents, or muscle entrapment should be noted.

SURGICAL INDICATIONS

Persistent symptoms, including diplopia, enophthalmos, or disfigurement, attributable to an anatomical surgically correctable defect generally warrant repair. Most surgeons consider enophthalmos greater than 2 mm as clinically significant and an indication for surgery.[8] An observer will generally not notice globe asymmetry of 1–2 mm.[9] Restrictive diplopia caused by muscle impingement, or enophthalmos in the setting of orbital content herniation or implant displacement are likewise reasons for reoperation. Care must be taken to rule out paralytic diplopia unlikely to improve with surgery.

Another consideration in planning revision orbital surgery is that of best timing. Postponing nonemergent reoperation for several months affords tissue time to heal and symptoms to stabilize. On the other hand, waiting more than one year after initial repair may result in significant bone remodeling and scarring that could complicate reoperation.[10] Many surgeons choose to wait 3–6 months before undertaking any elective orbital revision.[11] Acute symptoms suggestive of nerve or

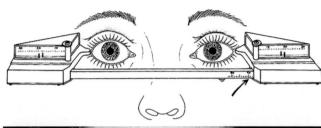

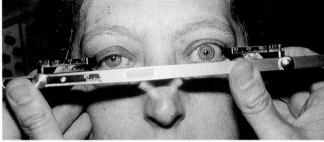

Fig. 3.7.1 Hertel exophthalmometer. (From Cockerham KP, Chan SS. Thyroid eye disease. Neurol Clin 2010;28(3):729–755.)

muscle impingement, implant displacement, or orbital compartment syndrome warrant immediate intervention, as they would following primary injury.

SURGICAL TECHNIQUES

Surgical approaches used in primary orbital reconstruction apply in secondary procedures. Transconjunctival, subciliary, or transcutaneous incisions may all be used; scarring and aberrant anatomy may make reoperation more challenging, but the surgical approach may be chosen independently of that used in primary repair. Some surgeons have even employed endoscopic approaches, although success is highly dependent on experience in endoscopic surgery.[12] Most importantly, the techniques employed in revision orbital reconstruction should be tailored to the specific preoperative diagnosis and mechanism behind symptoms. All prior orbital implants should be removed, and replaced with pre-planned devices. Care must be taken as radiolucent implants may be difficult to visualize on preoperative imaging and intraoperatively. Retained implant material should be suspected if a prefabricated implant or virtual planning results do not correspond to intraoperative findings. Some surgeons avoid placement of radiolucent orbital implants partly because of challenges during any revision procedures.

Computer-assisted surgical (CAS) planning is essential for precise secondary orbital reconstruction.[13] Recent axial orbital CT scan data should be available for virtual planning. Software mirrors the intricate orbital wall anatomy of the uninjured side onto the symptomatic orbit. Any deficits and asymmetries may readily be seen by superimposing the contralateral template. Although preformed implants are generally not recommended in secondary reconstruction, virtual planning software may aid in planning cuts and position of fixation screws if necessary. Use of CAS has been shown to improve accuracy of bony reconstruction and reduce the need for bony revision surgery.[14,15]

Patient-specific implant fabrication has advanced greatly in recent years and is imperative in secondary orbital reconstruction[16] (Fig. 3.7.2). Accurate restoration of the intricate anatomy of the orbital walls is critical to success, but is greatly complicated by prior attempts at repair and delayed timeframe. Further, the non-emergent nature of the surgery affords time for careful implant design (Fig. 3.7.3). Many surgeons exclusively employ custom implants in cases of secondary reconstruction. The technology has been reported to achieve orbital volumes comparable to the contralateral side with favorable long-term outcomes.[17] Notably, intraoperative overcorrection of enophthalmos by an average 2.7 mm is necessary for satisfactory results.[18]

Intraoperative navigation has likewise proven invaluable in secondary orbital surgery.[17] The anatomy is frequently distorted and tissue-scarred; presence of misplaced old implants may further complicate the surgical approach. Intraoperative CT imaging and navigation not only aids in safe access to the bony orbit, but ensures ideal reduction and implant placement. One study noted that intraoperative imaging led to repositioning of the implant in 25% of cases.[19] When only postoperative imaging is used, patients return to the operating room only in cases of severe misplacement or impingement, as greater error in positioning is ultimately accepted.

POSTOPERATIVE COURSE

Postoperative care following secondary orbital reconstruction largely mirrors that following primary repair. Immediate postoperative forced duction testing and computed tomography imaging is used to assess implant placement and muscle entrapment. Patients are monitored postoperatively for development of compressive symptoms, which would warrant emergent decompression. Frequent light perception checks are employed to assess optic nerve function. Temporary suture tarsorrhaphy and lubricating eye drops may be used to reduce the risk of exposure keratitis. Head of bed elevation and ice applications may help with swelling and likewise reduce the risk of lagophthalmos in the immediate postoperative period. Antibiotics are generally not indicated beyond the perioperative period. Patients should be discharged on nose blowing precautions and instructed to avoid heavy lifting and strenuous exercise for 2 weeks.

COMPLICATIONS

Patients should be forewarned and monitored for development of all acute complications pertinent in primary orbital repair. Patients should likewise be cautioned of the possibility of persistent symptoms. Secondary orbital reconstruction has traditionally been viewed as extremely challenging, resulting in higher rates of complications.[4] That said, at least some degree of improvement in diplopia has been noted in 56%–100% of patients following revision orbital surgery.[20–22] Nearly all patients have reported some improvement in enophthalmos and hypoglobus. Patient selection is key to success in secondary orbital reconstruction. Patients with restrictive diplopia or enophthalmos attributable to an anatomic defect are most likely to improve with surgery. A careful preoperative evaluation, including referral for a strabismus examination, is imperative for diagnosis. Computer-assisted surgical planning, custom implant prefabrication, and intraoperative navigation are emerging technologies that have helped surgeons achieve consistent outcomes in cases of complex revision orbital reconstruction.

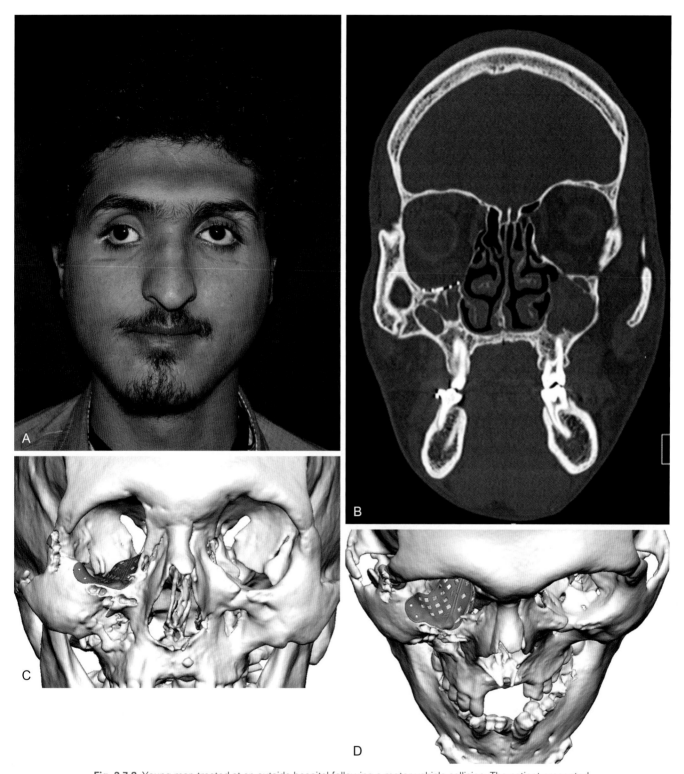

Fig. 3.7.2 Young man treated at an outside hospital following a motor vehicle collision. The patient presented with no light perception and enophthalmos in the right eye. (A–B) Preoperative clinical and coronal CT images demonstrating enophthalmos secondary to poor primary reduction leading to increased orbital volume. (C–D) Virtual surgical planning software was used to design a custom implant to reconstruct the orbital floor.

Continued

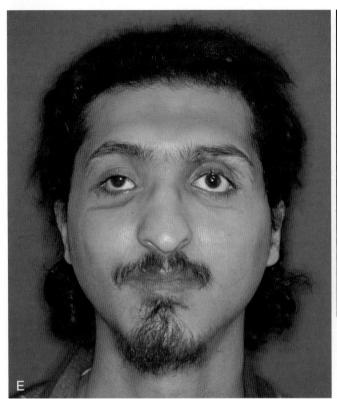

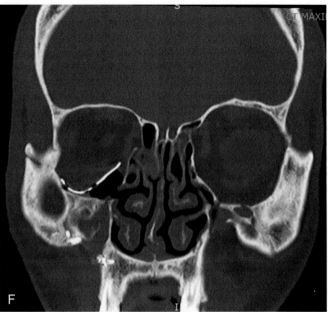

Fig. 3.7.2, cont'd (E–F) Postoperative clinical and coronal CT images demonstrating improvement in enophthalmos. The patient is pending right lower eyelid reposition. (Courtesy Drs. Amir H. Dorafshar and Michael Grant.)

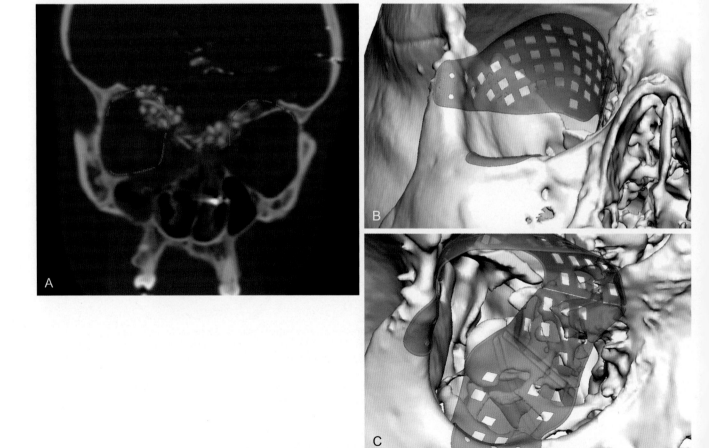

Fig. 3.7.3 Use of virtual planning software for complex orbital reconstruction following ballistic injury. (A) Ideal orbital contour designed via mirroring of uninjured side. (B) Design of complex orbital roof. (C) Orbital floor implants. (Courtesy Drs. Amir H. Dorafshar and Michael Grant.)

EXPERT COMMENTARY

Secondary orbital reconstruction ranks with secondary nasoethmoidal orbital fracture correction as one of the most demanding and challenging facial injuries. The problem is generally soft tissue and bone combined, and the injuries are usually fixed by scar tissue, which makes any correction difficult, challenging, and hazardous. One must begin with old pictures, and a history of the previous injury and each of its previous treatments including CTs, operative results, and photographic results.

Original and subsequent CT scans are reviewed, and a good present CT scan is essential, preferably with 3D rendering. One looks at the patient, feels and examines the soft tissue and feels the globe and rims of the orbit, measuring the pupil to midline nasal distance, and the rim positions. If the contralateral orbit is uninjured, it forms a reasonable template for reconstruction, but the pictures preinjury should be reviewed to note differences in the prominence of the globes, level of the eyes and the pupils, and differences in the position of the globe on the other side. Usually, one side of the face is longer than the other, and one globe more prominent than the other, and the globe is higher on the side of the larger hemiface. The dimensions of both orbital rims are measured, and compared. The parts of the orbit on the injured side which were fractured are noted, and their relative displacement recorded. The amount of enophthalmos is measured and noted and if the rim is out of position, this will affect the relative measurements of globe position, which are based on rim anatomy.

The amount of double vision is measured in each field of gaze, as is the visual acuity and the excursion of the globe in each direction, noting limitation and double vision. Formal visual fields measuring extraocular muscle functions are a good idea when there is diplopia. Postoperatively, diplopia may be improved, the same or worse following secondary reconstruction.

Old incisions are noted, including their problems of tissue thinning or thickening, an estimation of what previous incisions have done to disorganize the lid tissue, presence of lid/periorbital lacerations, lid margin issues, lid flexibility and position, ectropion and disorders of "blink" and ocular lubrication. The incisions are planned for complete exposure of all of the problems, and the choice must include consideration of fixing previous incisional problems. After fixing the bony problems, the soft tissue must be repaired, reorganized, and repositioned by reorganization and repair and then fixation to the reconstructed facial skeleton.

A plan for getting each of the rim segments into proper position is developed for the naso-ethmoid, zygoma/inferior rim and supraorbital sections of the orbital rim. A plan is made for repositioning each segment, and for the exposure to do so, and for confirming the correct position of the repositioned segment with measurements, intraoperative positioning guides, and/or intraoperative CT. Once the orbital rim is correctly positioned, and its new dimensions compared and confirmed with the contralateral side, the four parts of the internal orbit may be serially reconstructed, one at a time in the same manner as that for primary fracture treatment. The subtle internal curves of the internal orbit must be reconstructed, as they provide the shape and volume correction for the soft tissue, and thus control the postoperative appearance.

Having reconstructed the internal walls of the orbit, one proceeds with the replacement, reorganization, and fixation of the soft tissue onto the reconstructed craniofacial skeleton. Marking the layers of the incisions as they are disassembled assists in their proper repair and assembly by layered closure/fixation of the incisions at the proper position to the bone.

REFERENCES

1. Biesman BS, Hornblass A, Lisman R, Kazlas M. Diplopia after surgical repair of orbital floor fractures. *Ophthal Plast Reconstr Surg.* 1996;12(1):16, discussion 17.
2. Brucoli M, Arcuri F, Cavenaghi R, Benech A. Analysis of complications after surgical repair of orbital fractures. *J Craniofac Surg.* 2011;22(4):1387–1390.
3. Hossal BM, Beatty RL. Diplopia and enophthalmos after surgical repair of blowout fracture. *Orbit.* 2002;21(1):27–33.
4. Converse JM, Smith B, Obear MF, Wood-Smith D. Orbital blowout fractures: a ten-year survey. *Plast Reconstr Surg.* 1967;39(1):20–36.
5. Kolk A, Pautke C, Schott V, et al. Secondary post-traumatic enophthalmos: high-resolution magnetic resonance imaging compared with multislice computed tomography in postoperative orbital volume measurement. *J Oral Maxillofac Surg.* 2007;65(10):1926–1934.
6. Ahn HB, Ryu WY, Yoo KW, et al. Prediction of enophthalmos by computer-based volume measurement of orbital fractures in a Korean population. *Ophthal Plast Reconstr Surg.* 2008;24(1):36–39.
7. Kellman RM, Bersani T. Delayed and secondary repair of posttraumatic enophthalmos and orbital deformities. *Facial Plast Surg Clin North Am.* 2002;10(3):311–323.
8. Nkenke E, Vairaktaris E, Spitzer M, et al. Secondary reconstruction of posttraumatic enophthalmos: prefabricated implants vs titanium mesh. *Arch Facial Plast Surg.* 2011;13(4):271.
9. Koo L, Hatton MP, Rubin PAD. When is enophthalmos "significant"? *Ophthal Plast Reconstr Surg.* 2006;22(4):274–277.
10. Gruss JS. Craniofacial osteotomies and rigid fixation in the correction of post-traumatic craniofacial deformities. *Scand J Plast Reconstr Surg Hand Surg Suppl.* 1995;27:83–95.
11. Imola MJ, Ducic Y, Adelson RT. The secondary correction of post-traumatic craniofacial deformities. *Otolaryngol Head Neck Surg.* 2008;139(5):654–660.
12. Park J, Kim J, Lee J, et al. Secondary reconstruction of residual enophthalmos using an endoscope and considering the orbital floor and medial wall slope. *J Craniofac Surg.* 2016;27(4):992–995.
13. Bittermann G, Metzger MC, Schlager S, et al. Orbital reconstruction: prefabricated implants, data transfer, and revision surgery. *Facial Plast Surg.* 2014;30(5):554–560.
14. Lauer G, Pradel W, Schneider M, Eckelt U. Efficacy of computer-assisted surgery in secondary orbital reconstruction. *J Craniomaxillofac Surg.* 2006;34(5):299–305.
15. Zimmerer RM, Ellis E 3rd, Aniceto GS, et al. A prospective multicenter study to compare the precision of posttraumatic internal orbital reconstruction with standard preformed and individualized orbital implants. *J Craniomaxillofac Surg.* 2016;44(9):1485–1497.
16. Zhang Y, He Y, Zhang ZY, An JG. Evaluation of the application of computer-aided shape-adapted fabricated titanium mesh for mirroring-reconstructing orbital walls in cases of late post-traumatic enophthalmos. *J Oral Maxillofac Surg.* 2010;68(9):2070–2075.
17. Rana M, Chui CHK, Wagner M, et al. Increasing the accuracy of orbital reconstruction with selective laser-melted patient-specific implants combined with intraoperative navigation. *J Oral Maxillofac Surg.* 2015;73(6):1113–1118.
18. Gellrich N, Schramm A, Hammer B, et al. Computer-assisted secondary reconstruction of unilateral posttraumatic orbital deformity. *Plast Reconstr Surg.* 2002;110(6):1417–1429.
19. Schmelzeisen R, Gellrich NC, Schoen R, et al. Navigation-aided reconstruction of medial orbital wall and floor contour in cranio-maxillofacial reconstruction. *Injury.* 2004;35(10):955–962.
20. Hammer B, Prein J. Correction of post-traumatic orbital deformities: operative techniques and review of 26 patients. *J Craniomaxillofac Surg.* 1995;23(2):81–90.
21. Freihofer HPM. Effectiveness of secondary post-traumatic periorbital reconstruction. *J Craniomaxillofac Surg.* 1995;23(3):143–150.
22. Kim JS, Lee BW, Scawn RL, et al. Secondary orbital reconstruction in patients with prior orbital fracture repair. *Ophthalmic Plast Reconstr Surg.* 2016;32(6):447–451.

Secondary Midfacial Reconstruction

Likith Reddy, Tyler Wildey, Andrew M. Read-Fuller

BACKGROUND

Secondary deformities resulting from complications in treating craniofacial injuries, specifically the midface, occur even when treated by experienced surgeons. Following proper surgical principles and recognizing the potential functional and aesthetic sequelae limits many complications. Ideal primary reconstruction is not always achieved. Displaced or missing bony segments result in an inadequate infrastructure, which interferes with the balance of the associated soft tissues. Lack of underlying support leads to loss of proper soft tissue dimensions and results in further reconstructive difficulty. The main focus of this chapter is the assessment of secondary deformities of the midface, specifically maxillary, zygomatic, and naso-orbito-ethmoid (NOE) fractures, and techniques for restoring both form and function are reviewed. Return of symmetry and function are the fundamental bases for reconstruction. An organized evaluation of facial structures including orbital position, bizygomatic width, and occlusion are crucial. The surgeon's goal when addressing the midface is restoration of appropriate facial height, width, and projection (Fig. 3.8.1).

There are multiple reasons for requiring a secondary correction. These include poor reduction, inadequate stabilization, and delayed treatment or nontreatment. When insufficient closed reduction or fixation means are applied, loss of skeletal and soft tissue support occurs. It is also important to understand that the first operation provides the best opportunity for a good outcome. Primary restoration of proper skeletal framework and immediate placement of grafts in areas of bone loss provides the necessary structure needed to maintain soft tissue contour. This reduces the severity of complications requiring secondary management. Operative correction of established traumatic deformities with associated soft tissue changes and permanent disfigurement poses a formidable challenge. The important aspects in reconstruction are a detailed assessment of the patient including a thorough history and physical examination, and adequate imaging studies, such as a computed tomography (CT) scan. The early correction of midface fractures yields better facial form than the treatment of established deformities. Beyond one year, the timing of repair of these defects has less influence on eventual esthetic and functional outcome.

In order to plan for secondary revision, sufficient assessment of the bone and soft tissues must be achieved. Minor distortions may be managed by more conservative options, whereas gross deformities will likely require aggressive treatment such as osteotomy and repositioning. Therefore, proper presurgical evaluation is the most important initial step when addressing secondary deformity. For this chapter, we will categorize the correction of secondary defects based on the initial fracture such as the central midface and medial canthal deformity associated with NOE fractures, orbitozygomaticomaxillary complex (OZMC) fractures and Le Fort fractures.

The functional deficits due to midfacial deformities can be grouped into ophthalmological, sinonasal, and masticatory issues. The most common ophthalmological deficit is diplopia and this is due to globe malpositioning and from adaptive changes within the extraocular muscles. The inferior rectus and superior oblique muscles are frequently involved with posttraumatic and postsurgical scarring. The secondary correction typically involves creation of stable and anatomical orbital architecture followed by delayed extraocular muscle surgery. Secondary repositioning of periorbital bony segments may further exacerbate diplopia.

Functional problems of the sinonasal system include obstruction of the nasal airway and paranasal sinuses. Septorhinoplasty and endoscopic sinus procedures can be performed at a later time. The masticatory dysfunction is primarily due to malocclusion. This will be discussed further in the section on Le Fort fractures.

CENTRAL MIDFACE AND MEDIAL CANTHAL DEFORMITY

The central midface consists of the paired nasal bones that form the nasal sidewalls and medial orbital rims conjointly. This region is common to NOE fracture, Le Fort II and III fractures. If uncorrected or inadequately treated, the secondary deformity is extremely difficult to correct. The pivotal structure that is present in this region is the medial canthal tendon. This tendon supports the canthus, enables proper apposition between the eyelid and the globe, and includes the lacrimal canaliculi. In order to have acceptable functional and esthetic outcomes, the surgeon must restore nasal projection, intercanthal width, orbital volume, and a functional lacrimal system.

The majority of late complications resulting from inadequate management of medial canthal tendons are cosmetic in nature. Late deformities include a shortened palpebral fissure, telecanthus, enophthalmos, ocular dystopia, and a shortened nose with saddle deformity of the nasal dorsum.[1] The main components involved in NOE deformities are the medial canthal area, the nose, and the medial internal orbit. There is often significant scar contracture and soft tissue thickening[2] (Fig. 3.8.2).

The secondary correction of the medial canthal tendon-bearing fragment in the central midface is managed similarly for NOE fracture and comminuted Le Fort II and Le Fort III fractures. In this chapter we will briefly discuss the management of the deformity surrounding the medial canthus. NOE fractures are discussed in detail in other chapters.

Medial Canthal Correction

Telecanthus can be corrected by re-osteotomy and repositioning medially of the old fracture site containing the medial canthal attachment. The transnasal wire when placed anterior to the medial canthal attachment

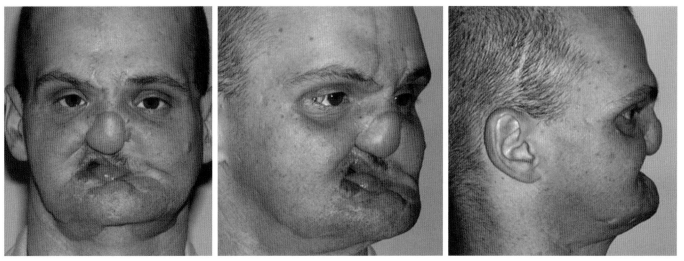

Fig. 3.8.1 Secondary midface deformity due to comminuted Le Fort III fracture demonstrating inadequate canthal correction and shortened midface.

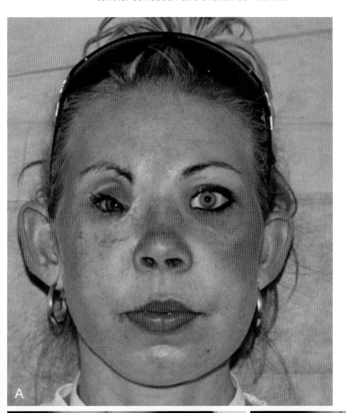

Fig. 3.8.2 (A) Primary management of medical canthal tendon. (B) Soft tissue changes due to untreated NOE fracture.

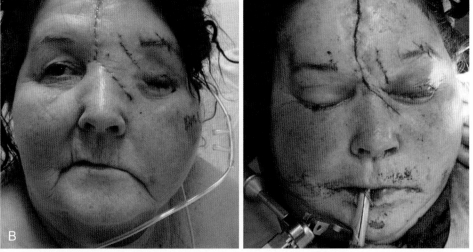

will widen the posterior portion of the segment and thus laterally displace the medial canthal tendon.[3] If one canthus is superior to the other, the inferior canthus should be elevated to achieve symmetry.[4]

If the medial canthal tendon is detached during previously operated NOE fracture, Le Fort II or Le Fort III, the medial canthal tendon itself must be found and engaged with a wire. In this situation, a small incision can be used directly over the tendon area in the skin to locate and secure the medial canthal tendon. Engaging the tendon alone tends to produce a "bow-string" appearance and also has the propensity to drift laterally over time. When absent or deficient bone is present, a calvarial graft can be placed and then the transnasal wire can be pulled through the graft and secured with a transnasal wire or perhaps a mini bone anchor.[5–7]

Medial canthal tissue thickening due to hematoma formation and scarring can be encountered if the medial canthal tendon is not addressed previously.[7] The oblique transnasal wiring technique with Y–V epicanthoplasty incision is adequate and would assist in minimizing unsightly scar formation (Fig. 3.8.3A–B). Masking of telecanthus can be done by dorsal nasal augmentation to increase the nasal profile and decrease the appearance of telecanthus. This technique will also lengthen the nose and raise the radix.[8]

Medial Wall Osteotomy

When the medial canthal tendon is displaced laterally with the bony medial orbital wall, either due to NOE or Le Fort III fracture with comminution, this results in medial orbital wall hypertelorism. Poor frontonasal angle and poor nasal projection combined with associated telecanthus or traumatic orbital hypertelorism compound the severity of the apparent deformity making the patient look worse (Fig. 3.8.4A–C).

ZYGOMA FRACTURES SECONDARY DEFORMITY

The zygomatic bone is an anatomical structure that determines the outer shape of the midface. It constitutes the lateral two-thirds of the orbital floor and lateral wall. Secondary deformities can occur due to delay in diagnosis, inability to correct in an appropriate time period or poor reduction of the zygoma. The majority of unfavorable outcomes relate to improper orientation of the zygomatic complex in three dimensions, which leads to failure to restore the facial dimensions and contour. The most common complications relate to poor cosmetic results, abnormalities in globe position, and malpositioned lateral canthus position. The common abnormal globe position is enophthalmos and inferior

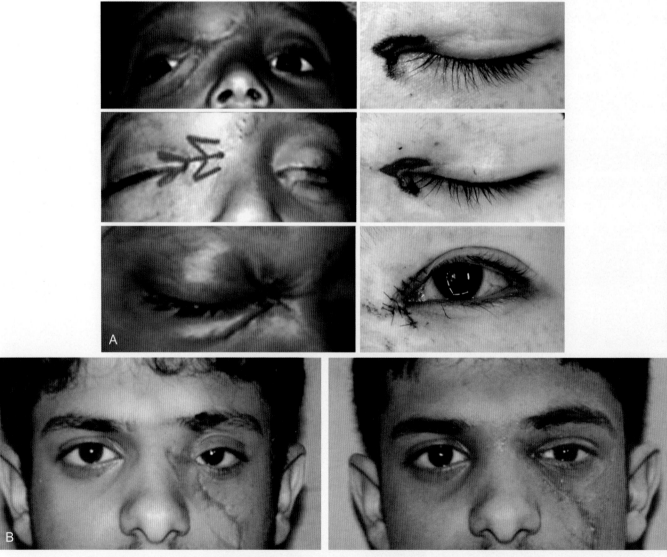

Fig. 3.8.3 (A) Y–V variations of medial epicanthoplasty. (B) Y–V epicanthoplasty 4-month postoperative result.

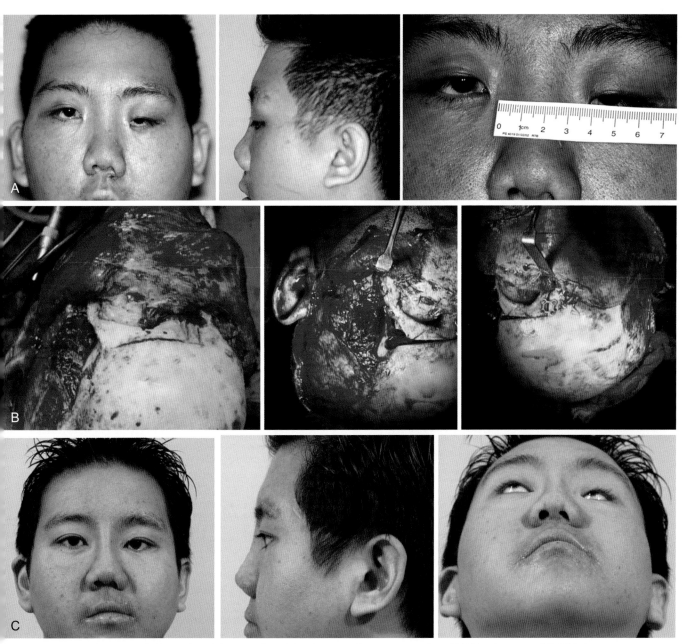

Fig. 3.8.4 (A) Secondary deformity of midface due to inadequate correction of NOE and zygoma. (B) Orbital osteotomy with medialization and superior positioning. (C) Six-month postoperative results demonstrating improvement of the central midface.

displacement. This is due to persistently increased orbital volume and inadequate correction of internal orbital defects. The meridian of the globe is at the lateral rim. A small external rotation of the lateral orbital wall often results in an increased intraorbital volume. Late enophthalmos may also result from scarring or atrophy of orbital soft tissues despite attempts at adequate reconstruction. Successful reconstruction of zygoma fractures is dependent on the correction of midface height, width, and projection. Recent emphasis is placed on the zygomaticomaxillary buttress (as opposed to the zygomaticofrontal region), not only because it is typically the mobile area but also because of its importance in restoring facial height.[9]

As malar projection decreases, facial width tends to increase. Restoring facial balance thus requires understanding ideal zygomatic positioning and returning displaced segments to these dimensions. Complications

of zygomatic fractures include poor 3-dimensional reduction resulting in residual cosmetic deformities and an increase in orbital volume with subsequent enophthalmos or dystopia.[10]

A displaced zygoma typically results in facial widening and inadequate malar projection. Severe cases will likely require osteotomy and repositioning as well as bone grafting to achieve proper aesthetic balance (Fig. 3.8.5).

ZMC Secondary Correction

The goals of secondary surgical correction are the same as primary treatment. The surgical treatment of ZMC fractures is organized into two goals: (1) restoration of facial projection and facial symmetry and (2) restoration of orbital volume, globe position, and shape of the affected palpebral fissure. Delayed repair of greater than 4 months after

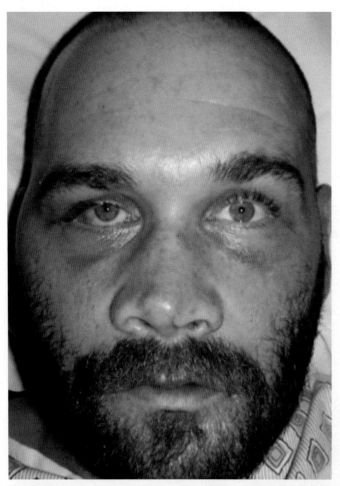

bone over time.[13] The onlay graft's site and extent of augmentation should be established preoperatively. Intraoperative judgment of the extent of necessary augmentation to achieve symmetry is extremely difficult, due to distortion of overlying soft tissues as a result of the surgical access, edema, and presence of an endotracheal tube.

In minor deformities, masking with fat injections or high-density polyethylene/silicone malar implants and soft tissue resuspension will be pursued.[14] The "ideal" characteristics of onlay grafts include the following: biocompatible, no risk of disease transmission, resistant to infection, dimensionally stable, easy to shape or mold, amenable to skeletal fixation, and long shelf-life. More recently, customized poly-etheretherketone (PEEK) implants are more frequently utilized. With the advances of 3D imaging and advancement in biocompatible allo-plastic materials, there has been a recent shift to consideration of patient-specific implants created using 3D CT scans. These implants have the distinct advantage of being tailored precisely to the exact size and contour of the defect, thus reducing intraoperative time and adjustment. Other advantages of PEEK implants include excellent chemical resistance (corrosion and acid), biocompatibility, ideal imaging properties (X-ray and CT translucency with no artifacts, and magnetic resonance imaging compatibility with no magnetic interferences), and a modulus that can be tailored by adding reinforcing fibers that enable their mechanical properties to be increased significantly (Fig. 3.8.6A–C).

Calvarial bone, bone substitutes or alloplastic implants can be used.[15] When autogenous bone grafts are used outer cortex calvarial graft from the parietal region can provide a good contour. The other alternatives for autogenous bone grafts includes the rib and iliac crest. It is essential that the grafts are stabilized to maintain the correct contours and minimize the resorption of the bone graft. Onlay grafting of the malar region can usually be carried out through a lower eyelid incision. The other access options include onlay grafting via a coronal incision, indicated when the zygoma along with the arch need to be contoured. An intraoral vestibular incision provides good access inferior and lateral to the infraorbital nerve. The placement of the bone graft at the inferior orbital rim is limited by obstruction by the infraorbital nerve when an intraoral incision is utilized.

ZMC Osteotomy

The analysis of alignment of the bony fractures at the zygomaticofrontal sutures, orbital rim, and lateral buttress of the maxilla may be lost in delayed repair due to bone remodeling. Although some secondary corrections can be made with onlay grafting alone, certain deformities can only be treated with osteotomy with or without supplemental bone grafting. Enophthalmos due to ZMC malposition is typically one of these instances. The osteotomy technique must take account of the concerns of the patient, as well as the nature and degree and extent of surgery required, potential complications, and a realistic assessment of the likely outcome. The method described for correction consists of recreating the fracture lines and reorienting the zygoma complex. The ideal access incisions include the coronal or hemicoronal flap extending to the preauricular region. This provides access to the lateral orbit, body of the zygoma and zygomatic arch. In addition, an intraoral vestibular incision corrects the zygomatic maxillary buttress region. A lower eyelid incision is required if the orbital floor needs revision. The approaches are usually determined before the surgery. A reciprocating saw is used to separate the frontozygomatic region, and then an osteotomy of the lateral orbital wall is performed. Next, a thin osteotome creates the orbital floor osteotomy followed by saw cuts through the inferior orbital rim, anterior maxilla, lateral buttress, and zygomatic arch. The location of the maxillary osteotomy can be lateral or medial to the infraorbital foramen. Before the zygoma is mobilized, the bony movements should be marked at the infraorbital rim, the zygomaticofrontal suture, and

Fig. 3.8.5 Poorly reduced zygoma demonstrating facial widening and dystopia.

injury commonly requires not only osteotomy of the segments but also bone grafting. This is due to osseous healing and bone resorption that has occurred.[11] For cases requiring refracture with osteotomies, mobilization of the ZMC can be challenging due to the scar contractures of adjacent soft tissues. In order to gain sufficient mobility, all attachments should be released, including the masseter.

Facial symmetry is achieved by restoring the 3-dimensional position of the malar prominence and orbital volume is restored by alignment of the zygoma with its internal and external articulations such as the sphenoid.[12] The secondary correction of the zygoma deformities can be done by reosteotomy, onlay grafting techniques, soft tissue fillers (autogenous fat or fillers) or a combination of techniques. The minor deformities are managed with augmentation or reduction procedures to camouflage the asymmetry. The larger corrections would typically require reosteotomy, repositioning, and supplemental bone grafting. Adjunctive soft tissue resuspension is often helpful. This can be done with lower eyelid incisions of endoscopic midface lift.

Onlay Grafting

The minor secondary deformity from zygoma malposition can be managed by onlay grafting and bony recontouring. This is especially the choice when there is good orbital volume restoration and no enophthalmos or dystopia. Due to irregular remodeling and resorption in older fractures, when repositioning segments, overcorrection as well as onlay grafting is needed. Overcorrection of the onlay graft is an important consideration because there will likely be some resorption of this

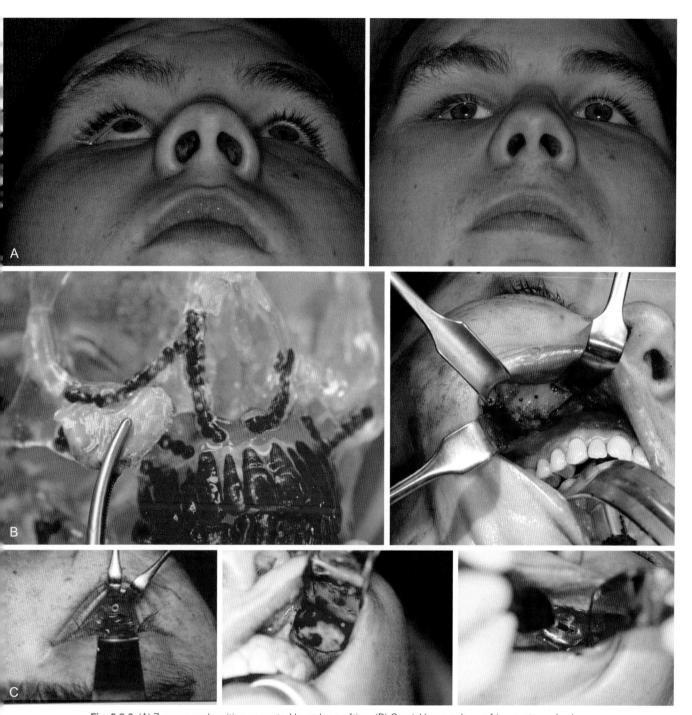

Fig. 3.8.6 (A) Zygoma malposition corrected by onlay grafting. (B) Cranial bone onlay grafting contoured using stereolithographic model. (C) Transconjunctival and intraoral approaches of onlay grafting for malar deformity.

he zygomatic arch. Posttraumatic displacement of the zygoma usually involves impaction posteriorly, inferiorly, and medially. Usually, bone removal is required at the zygomaticofrontal suture to permit superior repositioning of the zygoma, whereas advancement and lateral movement both create bony gaps. The zygoma is fixed into its new position with miniplates. Repositioning of the body of the zygoma will often produce contour deformities and steps in the zygomatic arch and the arch itself may require local osteotomies to allow it to be recontoured. Anterior, lateral, and superior movement of the osteotomized zygoma will create bony gaps and step deformities at several sites and these require bone grafting in order to insure bony union, stability, and soft tissue support and to avoid palpable bone irregularities beneath the thin periorbital skin. Gaps may occur at the infraorbital margin, orbital floor, the frontozygomatic cut, lateral orbital wall, zygomatic arch, and zygomatic buttress. In addition, the zygomatic repositioning may have created an orbit larger in volume than before and allow herniation of periorbital tissues through bony defects of the orbital walls. Considerable widening of the inferior orbital fissure may occur as a result of repositioning. This increased orbital volume predisposes enophthalmos. The inferior orbital fissure should be exposed and the infraorbital nerve

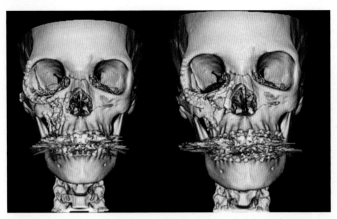

Fig. 3.8.7 CT scans of zygoma repositioning by reosteotomy along fracture lines.

and soft tissues protected. Floor reconstruction with calvarial bone grafts or a titanium plate restores orbital volume. Bone grafting is effective to treat preexisting enophthalmos and to prevent its occurrence following osteotomy. Contoured calvarial bone is used for this purpose. Calvarial bone graft exhibits considerably less tendency to resorption than the previously used rib or iliac crest bone grafts. Calvarial bone is readily available and does not require a separate incision for its harvest. Enough bone is available for the great majority of cases and the morbidity associated with its harvest is low. Once the zygoma has been completely mobilized, it can be repositioned and fixated. Fixation is typically placed at the zygomaticofrontal suture, the zygomaticomaxillary buttress, and the inferior orbital rim[16] (Fig. 3.8.7).

Use of Intraoperative Navigation

The use of navigation in management of secondary deformities of the craniofacial patient can greatly improve predictability and accuracy of the surgical outcome. The advantage is that the surgeon can instantaneously determine the position of the surgical instrument on the CT images and see, during the operation, if the reconstruction is performed according to presurgical planning.[17] Navigation systems have been shown to have an intraoperative precision of less than 2 mm.[18] Intraoperative navigation uses a facemask registration to localize anatomical points in three dimensions using LED technology. A monitor then is used to display a reconstruction of the patient's skeleton that can be viewed to assess and measure the amount of displacement and deviation from normal, especially when the opposite side remains intact. This enables the use of a "mirror image" of the unaffected side to be superimposed on the malpositioned segment to be used as a surgical guide.[19] Once the osteotomies as described above have been completed, this allows a real-time assessment of the segment repositioning and confirmation of appropriate placement (Fig. 3.8.8A–C).

To correct a right zygomatic defect, the left zygoma complex can be digitally rendered from a 3D CT reconstruction and subsequently mirrored and placed onto the right midface. The reconstituted virtual position of the zygoma serves as a template and is then used to guide intraoperative positioning of the displaced fracture.[20]

Use of Virtual Surgical Planning and Cutting Guides

The landmarks for accurate repair and the key fit of the bony fractures may be lost after initial repair via fracture remodeling and bone healing. The use of CAD/CAM technology allows the surgeon to have a 3D reconstructed image taken from the data of a CT scan, and use this information to develop a surgical plan. The surgical approach is modeled in the virtual environment and the osteotomies, repositioning, and

fixation can be virtually performed. Based on the mirroring techniques of the correct and unaffected zygoma, custom surgical cutting guides and custom bone-repositioning guides are designed.

These customized cutting guides intraoperatively provide the exact placement of the planned osteotomies and enable repositioning of the zygoma as planned preoperatively. This minimizes errors of estimation of the new position. Mirroring techniques can also be used to create custom implants, with PEEK, titanium or Medpor, to be used in reconstruction.[21]

Use of Intraoperative Imaging

The landmarks for accurate repair and the key fit of the bony fractures are lost after initial repair, fracture remodeling, and healing. The use of intraoperative imaging allows for immediate repositioning during the initial procedure if needed, thereby preventing a potential reoperation. Among the available modalities, Arcadia C-arm (GE systems) or O-arm (Medtronic) would help assess all articulation points of the zygoma, the zygomatic arch contour, and the orbital floor accurately. Other modalities have been used, such as ultrasonography and fluoroscopy, but with less accuracy than CT scans. Intraoperative spiral CT has been described for OZMC fractures, but practical limitations such as the weight and the size of the equipment significantly restrict its usage. Cone beam computed tomography (CBCT) scanners, with a size similar to a traditional C-arm, have been found to be comparable to spiral CT in terms of accuracy with the advantage of low radiation exposure. Repositioning of the zygoma and restoration of the orbital volume are extremely difficult to assess in the operating room due to the overlying soft tissue, onset of swelling, tissue dissection, etc., as described above. Intraoperative imaging typically adds time during the surgery, however it may mitigate the need for additional secondary surgeries.

LE FORT FRACTURES SECONDARY DEFORMITY

The midface connects the more stable frontal bone superiorly and the mandible inferiorly. Unfavorable outcomes in treating Le Fort fractures usually result from poor diagnosis, inadequate planning, lack of proper exposure, malreduction, and inadequate fixation. Le Fort fractures most frequently result from high-velocity blunt trauma, in particular, motor vehicle collisions. As a result, they are often associated with injuries to multiple body systems, with nearly a quarter suffering neurological injury. Bagheri found that 52% of patients with Le Fort fractures required ICU admission, with an average hospital length of stay of 9.5 days. As a result, these patients often have delayed or inadequate treatment due to the severity of their multiple injuries.

Pure Le Fort II and III fractures involve reconstruction of orbital volume and occlusion, which require very accurate reduction and fixation to prevent enophthalmos and malocclusion. Malocclusion occurs as a result of incorrect reduction and fixation during surgery. Inaccurate vertical positioning or poor seating of the condyles when applying maxillomandibular fixation produces immediate open-bite when the IMF is released as the condyles reseat themselves in the glenoid fossa. In addition, malocclusion may result from poor application of maxillomandibular fixation or failure to passively reposition the fractured maxilla because of inadequate mobility. Frequently, strong disimpaction forces or even additional osteotomies must be created to allow passive positioning of the maxilla in relation to the mandible. Because of involvement of the orbital floor and rim with Le Fort II fractures and the zygomaticomaxillary complex with Le Fort III fractures, orbital dystopia and enophthalmos are frequent delayed complications (Fig. 3.8.9).

Maxillary fractures can be confined to the maxilla alone, or may be a component of more complex fractures such as Le Fort I, II, or III

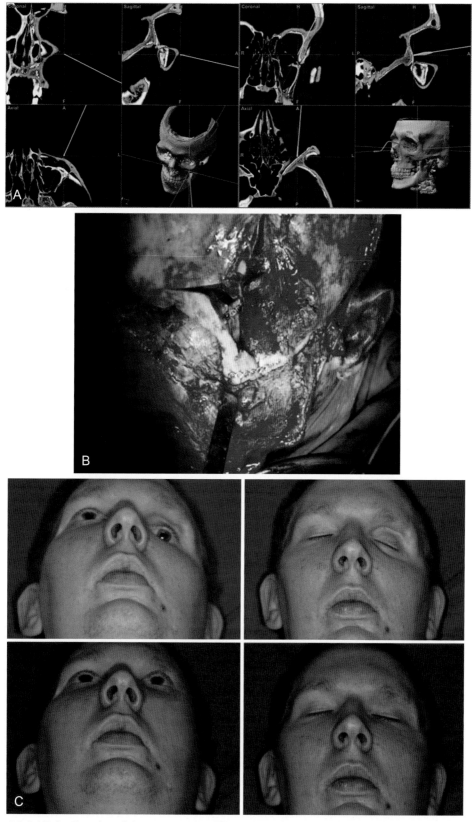

Fig. 3.8.8 (A) Confirmation of the zygoma with CT navigation. Blue is the desired position of the zygoma based on the mirroring of the intact side. (B) Repositioned zygoma. (C) Zygoma correction with osteotomy: pre- and postoperative images.

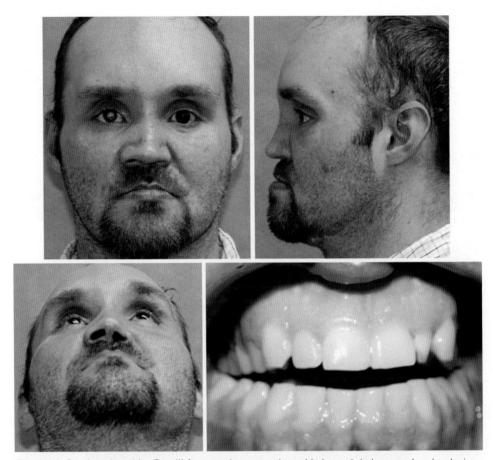

Fig. 3.8.9 Poorly reduced Le Fort III fracture demonstrating orbital enophthalmos and malocclusion.

fractures or those associated with the frontal bone and mandible. Improper or delayed treatment of these injuries can result in significant malunion and malposition. These complications result in both decreased aesthetics and function due to their direct association with the patient's occlusion. Malocclusion can be the result of inadequate fixation or more commonly from a lack of proper mobilization.[22]

The most common maxillary defects encountered after Le Fort fractures are midface retrusion, decreased midfacial height, anterior openbite, mandibular overclosure secondary to posterior displacement of the maxilla, anterior cephalad telescoping, and the inferior pull of the pterygoid musculature on the fractured pterygoid plates. Secondary malocclusion can be seen after malunion of any fracture intimately associated with the alveolar components of the maxilla. This includes isolated dentoalveolar fractures, Le Fort I, II, or III fractures, and palatal fractures. It is common to see initial bone loss or secondary bone resorption resulting in inadequate bone stock. In these cases, bone grafting will be necessary to augment these areas.[23] Deviation of the nasal septum can occur as a result of overimpaction of the maxilla, and has been shown to occur 20% of the time following Le Fort repair.[24]

Secondary Correction of Le Fort Fractures

With the introduction of CT images and incorporation of virtual surgical planning and improved fixation techniques, both primary and secondary reconstruction have greatly improved. The basic fundamentals, however, remain much the same as that stated by Tessier. If reduction cannot be entirely satisfactory, give priority to orbital function and to dental occlusion. Remodeling with bone grafts will improve contour and projection problems.[25]

Depending on the original fracture pattern, Le Fort II- or III-level osteotomies may be needed to address midface deformity. For most maxillary malocclusions, however, Le Fort I osteotomy is adequate. The technique is similar to that of the Le Fort I osteotomy performed in orthognathic surgery, which can commonly be found in the literature.[26] Because true one-piece Le Fort II and III injuries are less common, the majority of corrections can be treated by first addressing the malocclusion with a Le Fort I osteotomy. Then, the remaining components are treated with the individual techniques described in other sections of this text.[27]

In patients with orbital dystopia, enophthalmos due to Le Fort III or Le Fort II fractures would benefit from reestablishing the old orbit fractures and mobilization. More extensive osteotomies may correct the orbital rim position and the malocclusion at the same time. When the management of Le Fort II and III fractures is delayed for more than 6 months, the remodeling of the fracture edges make it difficult to anatomically estimate and reposition the components, especially at the orbital rims. Obtaining 3D preoperative stereolithographic models helps the surgeon understand the orbit position as well as the infraorbital contours. Utilizing the virtual surgical planning, the data of a CT scan will help develop a surgical plan. Based on this information, osteotomies, repositioning, and fixation can be virtually performed in a preoperative setting. From this information, customized cutting guides can be fabricated that direct exact placement of the planned osteotomies. In similar fashion, surgical occlusal guides are highly valuable in partially edentulous cases or patients with previous malocclusions.

Often, recreation of the Le Fort II or III fractures may not help obtain the desired occlusion due to remodeling and associated soft tissue changes. In such situations, the Le Fort I osteotomy should be completed at the same time. This facilitates movements of the malar and orbital components in different vectors from the occlusal plane (Fig. 3.8.10A–C).

Functional Considerations in Le Fort Fractures

The main factor when considering correction of maxillary fractures is returning the patient to pretraumatic occlusion. It can be worthwhile to attempt to obtain preinjury photos and dental records (including models when available) to aid in planning occlusion or creating surgical splints when indicated.[10] In the case of the edentulous patient, dentures may help guide the reconstruction[10] or, alternatively, the patient may simply have new dentures fabricated to match the postinjury jaw position.[27] Injury to the dentoalveolar complex is also often associated with midfacial injuries, and avulsion or fracture of the teeth may occur. In these situations, the surgeon should incorporate a general dentist or prosthodontists into the treatment team to determine the best plan for dental reconstruction, which can include dental implant placement, bone grafting, or denture fabrication.

Malocclusion that has resulted from malunion often requires osteotomies. Performing a Le Fort I osteotomy with repositioning is typically the simplest method of correction of malocclusion. Osteotomy design can also be influenced by the injury pattern and length of time elapsed since the traumatic event. Zachariades recommends a 6-month interval for performing an osteotomy at the site of the original fracture, while a 2-month period is adequate if the osteotomy is performed at an alternative location.[27] Examining the transverse dentoalveolar dimension will guide the surgeon in deciding if segmental osteotomies will be required for posterior crossbite correction (Fig. 3.8.11A–C).

Bone Grafts to the Maxilla

Secondary deformity correction may require significant bone grafting of the maxilla. Cohen and Kawamoto advocate calvarial bone grafts for replacement of the zygomaticomaxillary and nasomaxillary buttresses after mobilizing the maxilla and placing the patient into intermaxillary fixation.[28] The anterior maxilla can be reconstructed once the facial buttresses have been rebuilt. A variety of materials and methods for grafting the dentoalveolar region and interpositional bone defects created as a result of osteotomies have been described. Onlay grafting with allogenic bone[29,30] or autogenous iliac crest[30–32] are common, as are grafts from the ramus,[32,33] symphysis[33] and rib.[30] Additionally, alveolar distraction[33,34] has been similarly utilized for enhancing dentoalveolar bone volume prior to dental implant placement. Larger defects may require free tissue transfer. Interpositional grafting with block grafts has been employed,[35] particularly with larger maxillary movements that result in more extensive defects. Failure to graft these defects may result in surgical relapse and postoperative malocclusion in the long term.

CONCLUSIONS

Correction of secondary midfacial deformities is challenging. The soft tissue deformities that manifest due to scarring, malposition, and tissue loss are the limiting factors in achieving the ideal cosmetic outcome.

EXPERT COMMENTARY

Seldom is secondary midface reconstruction able to be masterfully reconstructed by a single osteotomy. In general, facial fractures are in pieces, and they heal in pieces, each demonstrating individual degrees of malalignment and each requiring separate considerations for management.

When I was young, I can recall debates over whether malaligned bones should be osteotomized or onlay grafted. In truth, they often require variations of both techniques in an attempt to restore the original shape and volume of each individual part of the facial skeleton.

So the process begins by noting the displaced pieces that make up the components of the fracture, and deciding how to get the components back into place and related to their neighbors so that a nicely shaped, properly oriented set of bone reconstructions is present.

Continued

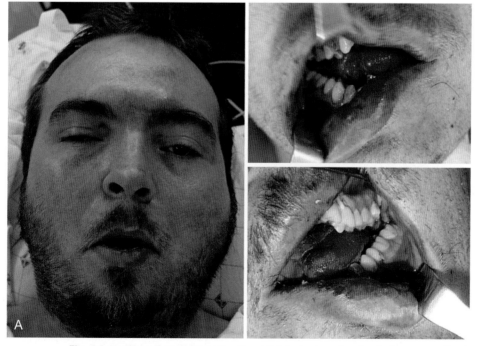

Fig. 3.8.10 (A) Le Fort III fracture with orbital dystopia and malocclusion.   *Continued*

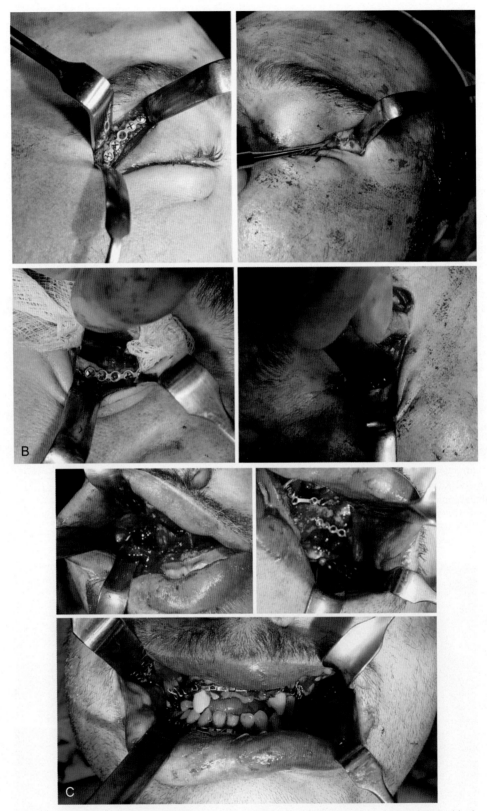

Fig. 3.8.10, cont'd (B) Fixation of remobilized midface fractures with transconjunctival and upper blepharo-plasty incisions. (C) Le Fort I osteotomy at level for correcting malocclusion; this provides different vectors of movements at Le Fort III and Le Fort I level.

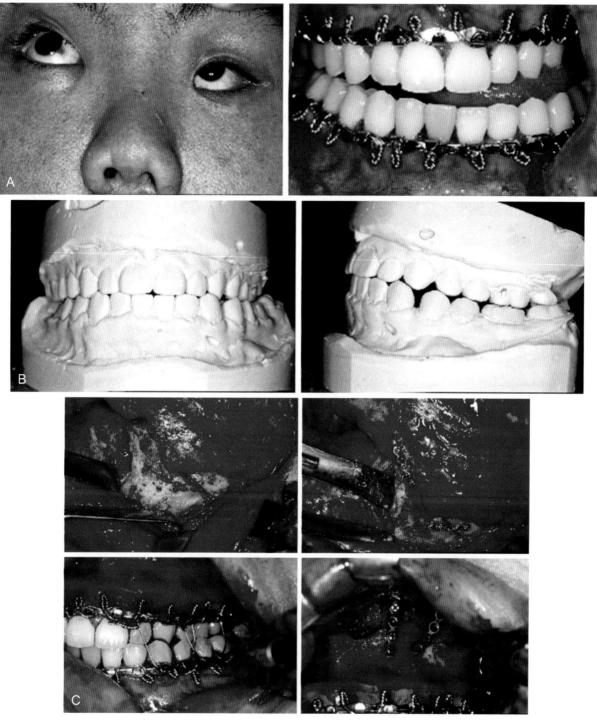

Fig. 3.8.11 Orbital dystopia and malocclusion with opposite vectors due to Le Fort III fractures. Reosteotomy at Le Fort III level alone cannot correct the deformity. (B) Dental models help understand preinjury malocclusion with the wear facets. (C) Reosteotomy of subcranial Le Fort III and Le Fort I levels for correction of orbital malposition and dental malocclusion.

REFERENCES

1. Rohrich RJ, Potter JK, Muzaffar AR, et al. Aesthetic management of the nasal component of naso-orbital ethmoid fractures. *Plast Reconstr Surg.* 2006;117(1):10e–18e.
2. Vora NM, Fedok FG. Management of the central nasal support complex in naso-orbital ethmoid fractures. *Facial Plast Surg.* 2000;16(2):181–191.
3. Herford AS, Ying T, Brown B. Outcomes of severely comminuted (Type III) nasoorbitoethmoid fractures. *J Oral Maxillofac Surg.* 2005;63:1266–1277.
4. Ellis E. Sequencing treatment for naso-orbito-ethmoid fractures. *J Oral Maxillofac Surg.* 1993;51:543–558.
5. Markowitz BL, Manson PN, Sargent L, et al. Management of the medial canthal tendon in nasoethmoid orbital fractures: the importance of the central fragment in classification and treatment. *Plast Reconstr Surg.* 1991;87(5):843–853.
6. Soodan KS, Priyadarshni P. Post trauma craniofacial deformities and treatment protocol. *J Stomat Occ Med.* 2014;7:1–5.
7. Yaremchuk MJ. Revisional surgery of nasoethmoidal orbital fractures. *Oper Tech Plast Reconstr Surg.* 1998;5(4):334–341.
8. Imola MJ, Ducic Y, Adelson RT. The secondary correction of post-traumatic craniofacial deformities. *Otolaryngol Head Neck Surg.* 2008;139(5):654–660.
9. Kochhar A, Byrne P. Surgical management of complex midfacial fractures. *Otolaryngol Clin North Am.* 2013;46(5):759–778.
10. Buehler J, Tannyhill R. Complications in the treatment of midfacial fractures. *Oral Maxillofac Surg Clin North Am.* 2003;15(2):195–212.
11. Carr RM, Mathog RH. Early and delayed repair of orbitozygomatic complex fractures. *J Oral Maxillofac Surg.* 1997;55(3):253–259.
12. Parashar A, Sharma RK. Unfavorable outcomes in maxillofacial injuries: how to avoid and manage. *Indian J Plast Surg.* 2013;46(2):221–234.
13. Perino KE, Zide MF, Kinnebrew MC. Late treatment of malunited malar fractures. *J Oral Maxillofac Surg.* 1984;42(1):20–34.
14. Mokal NJ, Desai MF. Secondary correction of posttraumatic craniofacial deformities. *J Craniofac Surg.* 2014;25(5):1658–1664.
15. Richardson D, Jones DC. Secondary osteotomies and bone grafting. In: Booth PW, ed. *Maxillofacial Trauma and Esthetic Facial Reconstruction.* Philadelphia: Saunders; 2012:443–469.
16. Longaker MT, Kawamoto HK. Evolving thoughts on correcting posttraumatic enophthalmos. *Plast Reconstr Surg.* 1998;101(4):899–906.
17. Novelli G, Tonellini G, Mazzoleni F, et al. Virtual surgery simulation in orbital wall reconstruction: integration of surgical navigation and stereolithographic models. *J Cranio-Maxillofac Surg.* 2014;42(8):2025–2034.
18. Yu H, Shen G, Wang X, Zhang S. Navigation-guided reduction and orbital floor reconstruction in the treatment of zygomatic-orbital-maxillary complex fractures. *J Oral Maxillofac Surg.* 2010;68(1):28–34.
19. Bui TG, Bell RB, Dierks EJ. Technological advances in the treatment of facial trauma. *Atlas Oral Maxillofac Surg Clin North Am.* 2012;20(1):81–94.
20. Susarla SM, Duncan K, Mahoney NR, et al. Virtual surgical planning for orbital reconstruction. *Middle East Afr J Ophthalmol.* 2015;22:442–446.
21. Lu W, Zhou H, Xiao C, et al. Late correction of orbital-zygomatic-maxillary fractures combined with orbital wall fractures. *J Craniofac Surg.* 2012;23(6):1672–1676.
22. Ellis E. Passive repositioning of maxillary fractures: an occasional impossibility without osteotomy. *J Oral Maxillofac Surg.* 2004;62(12):1477–1485.
23. Bussieres M, Tatum SA. Secondary craniofacial surgery for trauma. *Facial Plast Surg.* 2000;16(2):135–152.
24. Morgan BDG, Madan DK, Bergerot JPC. Fractures of the middle third of the face: a review of 300 cases. *Br J Plast Surg.* 1972;25:147.
25. Tessier P. Total osteotomy of the middle third of the face for faciostenosis or for sequelae of Le Fort III fractures. *Plast Reconstr Surg.* 1971;48(6):533–541.
26. Posnick JC, Le Fort I. sagittal split and genioplasty: historical perspective and step-by-step approach. In: Posnick JC, ed. *Craniofacial and Maxillofacial Surgery in Children and Young Adults.* Philadelphia, PA: Saunders; 2000:1081–1102.
27. Zachariades N, Mezitis M, Michelis A. Posttraumatic osteotomies of the jaws. *Int J Oral Maxillofac Surg.* 1993;22:328–331.
28. Cohen SR, Kawamoto HK. Analysis and results of treatment of established posttraumatic facial deformities. *Plast Reconstr Surg.* 1992;90(4):574–584.
29. Nissan J, Gross O, Mardinger O, et al. Post-traumatic implant-supported restoration of the anterior maxillary teeth using cancellous bone block allografts. *J Oral Maxillofac Surg.* 2011;69(12):e513–e518.
30. Perrott DH, Smith RA, Kaban LB. The use of fresh frozen allogeneic bone for maxillary and mandibular reconstruction. *Int J Oral Maxillofac Surg.* 1992;21:260–265.
31. Gulinelli JL, Dutra RA, Maraõ HF, et al. Maxilla reconstruction with autogenous bone block grafts: computed tomography evaluation and implant survival in a 5-year retrospective study. *Int J Oral Maxillofac Surg.* 2017;46:1045–1051.
32. Breeze J, Patel J, Dover MS, et al. Success rates and complications of autologous onlay bone grafts and sinus lifts in patients with congenital hypodontia and after trauma. *Br J Oral Maxillofac Surg.* 2017;55(8):830–833.
33. Zhao K, Wang F, Huang W, et al. Comparison of dental implant performance following vertical alveolar bone augmentation with alveolar distraction osteogenesis or autogenous onlay bone grafts: a retrospective cohort study. *J Oral Maxillofac Surg.* 2017;75(10):2099–2114.
34. Rachmiel A, Shilo D, Aizenbud D, et al. Three dimensional reconstruction of post traumatic deficient anterior maxilla. *J Oral Maxillofac Surg.* 2017;75(12):2689–2700.
35. Posnick JC, Sami A. Use of allogenic (iliac) corticocancellous graft for Le Fort I interpositional defects: technique and results. *J Oral Maxillofac Surg.* 2015;73(1):168.e1–168.e12.

Secondary Osteotomies of the Maxilla and Mandible, and Management of Occlusion

S. Anthony Wolfe, Mark W. Stalder

BACKGROUND

Unless there has been a loss of substance of portions of the maxilla and mandible, most traumatic disruptions of the maxilla and mandible are well corrected by placing the patient in the pretraumatic dental occlusion, plating the fractured segments with titanium miniplates and screws, and maintaining intermaxillary fixation where required.[1,2] In extensive maxillary fractures, autogenous bone grafting is performed to reestablish the buttresses correcting the maxillary alveolus to the base of the skull.[3,4] It is rarely indicated to do primary bone grafting of the mandible.[2] This of course presumes that the surgeon treating the jaw fractures, whether an oral surgeon or plastic surgeon, has an adequate knowledge of dental occlusion and the availability of a dental lab to fabricate splints when needed. If treated adequately, fractures of the tooth-bearing segments rarely require secondary surgery.[3]

However, when there are concomitant fractures of the facial skeleton involving the upper segments of the midface – the orbital cavities and zygomatic arches – it is not rare at all to see significant deformities requiring osteotomy and repositioning of malpositioned segments.[5] Joe Gruss has said that one of his fellows coined the wonderful acronym "OIF" for these situations – where the surgeon did open rigid fixation of the fracture, without the "R" of reduction. The reason for this is reluctance by the inexperienced surgeon to adequately expose the fracture sites through a coronal incision, and a hesitation to use autogenous bone grafts for the internal orbit and nose. This hesitation finds a comfortable option to avoid autogenous bone with the availability of a variety of alloplastic materials, so-called "bone substitutes," such as methylmethacrylate, titanium mesh, silicone, MedPore, hydroxyapatite, etc. It is best to eschew the use of *all* of these materials – there is simply no better bone substitute available than fresh autogenous bone grafts.[5,6] If there is a reluctance and hesitation to use them, then the solution is better training of surgeons in safely harvesting and using autogenous bone grafts so that they are comfortable in doing so.

Sir Harold Gillies, writing in 1920,[7] put it eloquently: "There is no royal road to the fashioning of the facial scaffold by artificial means: the surgeon must tread the hard and narrow way of pure surgery. Of the various autologous grafts available one has had enough experience to form some conclusions. It may be laid down as the guiding maxim that the replacement should be as nearly as possible in terms of the tissues lost, i.e., bone for bone, cartilage for cartilage, fat for fat, etc." In the cases that will be shown here, this advice has been followed.

PATIENT EVALUATION

Physical Examination

Upon initial presentation, a focused physical examination will identify most of the issues that will need to be addressed. Regarding bony structural deformities of the mid-face, bony step-offs and obvious facial asymmetries may be apparent if there are inadequately reduced fractures. Vertical orbital dystopia, enophthalmos, or telecanthus are findings indicative of orbital floor, zygomaticofacial, or naso-orbital-ethmoidal (NOE) fractures that will require correction.

While occlusion is frequently described using the Angle classification, this is often less important in the setting of midface trauma with occlusal deformities. Patients will often not have optimal dentition, and it is usually more beneficial to focus on determination of the patient's premorbid occlusion using the "fit" of the maxillary and mandibular teeth based on complimentary wear facets with the mandibular condyles seated in the fossa of the temporomandibular joint. There are additional findings that are relevant in diagnosing and describing occlusal deformities, and can assist in developing a surgical plan – specifically, the presence of an occlusal cant, mandibular deviation on opening, presence of an anterior open-bite, or a lateral crossbite. The presence of an obvious cant can suggest a laterally impacted or otherwise malpositioned maxillary segment, and/or nonreduced unilateral mandibular condyle fracture. Dynamic mandibular deviation or a lateral crossbite are also typically suggestive of untreated unilateral condylar pathology, while an anterior open-bite is likely due to inadequately reduced bilateral condyle fractures. Obvious step-offs in the anterior mandibular occlusion are frequently related to untreated parasymphyseal fractures.

Imaging

A maxillofacial computed tomography (CT) scan with thin cuts and 3D reconstruction is of the utmost importance to properly evaluate fractures of the craniofacial skeleton, both acutely and secondarily, and should be obtained in all cases of facial trauma. The axial, sagittal, and coronal views permit the surgeon to accurately assess bony deformities in multiple planes, and take accurate measurements that can aid in surgical planning. The reconstructed 3D image allows an excellent overview of the craniofacial skeleton that serves as a useful tool for both planning the corrective surgery, as well as for intraoperative reference. These image files can also be used for virtual surgical planning and 3D printing of osteotomy guides and occlusal splints, should the surgeon choose to pursue that option.

Plain films are of little use in these cases, as the resolution is suboptimal for accurately visualizing fractures in the context of the complex craniofacial skeleton. However, a panoramic radiograph (panorex) can be helpful specifically in the setting of dental trauma, as it does provide an accurate view of the teeth and related deformities.

CASE EXAMPLES

Case 1

This woman had a sagittal split osteotomy done elsewhere, and ended up losing full-thickness mandible from the right parasymphyseal area to the subcondylar area. She was treated with a fibular free flap extending into the glenoid fossa, another sagittal split with mandibular advancement on the left side, and a genioplasty (Figs. 3.9.1 and 3.9.2).

Case 2

This man sustained a Le Fort I fracture during the Iran/Iraq war, was taken prisoner, and the fracture went untreated. When first seen he had no nasal airway, and the maxilla was very retruded and vertically impacted (Fig. 3.9.3). The Le Fort I osteotomy performed on him was difficult since the pterygoid plates had been fractured, and it was very hard to get the maxilla adequately mobilized. This was eventually accomplished, but the usual medial and lateral buttresses were not present for rigid intersegment fixation. The one remaining maxillary tooth, a right first bisucpid, was advanced in front of the mandibular right cuspid, and a

long 2.0 mm miniplate was fixed to the infraorbital rim with several screws (through a small infraorbital incision), fixed to the edentulous alveolar ridge and palate, and extended to the mandibular symphysis where it was fixed with several long 2.0 mm screws (Fig. 3.9.4). The maxilla was lengthened vertically 21 mm; the amount of sagittal advancement was approximately the same (no cephalometric studies are available to quantitate this measurement precisely).

Large amounts of iliac bone were placed over the anterior and lateral maxilla, and the patient was maintained in intermaxillary fixation for 2 months. A stable result was obtained (Fig. 3.9.5). (Patient operated upon in Tehran, Iran, with Dr. Sayed Emami, for the Bonyad Jambazan, a Reconstructive Surgery Foundation developed in conjunction with Dr. Paul Tessier.)

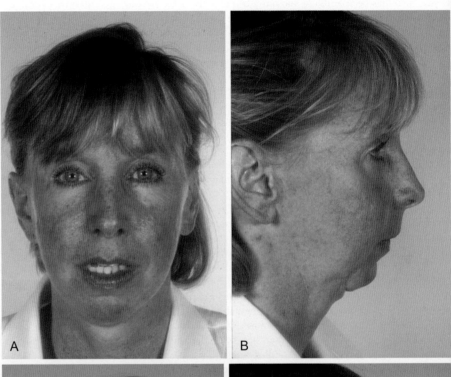

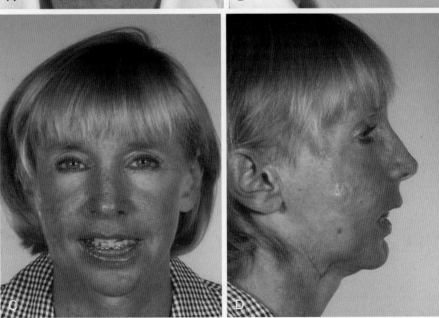

Fig. 3.9.1 Female patient who lost the right hemi-mandible secondary to a previous sagittal split osteotomy, with resulting asymmetry, malocclusion, and retrognathia (A–B). She is shown postoperatively (C–D) after reconstruction with a free fibula flap.

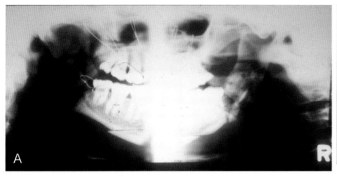
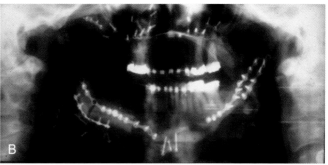

Fig. 3.9.2 Preoperative X-ray (A) demonstrating loss of much of the right hemi-mandible following sagittal split osteotomy, and postoperative X-ray (B) showing the reconstructive result after undergoing a free fibula flap for reconstruction.

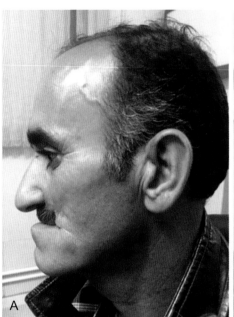
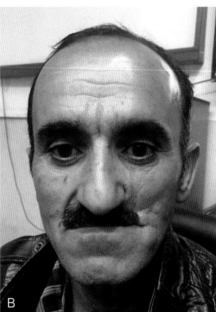

Fig. 3.9.3 Preoperative images of a patient who suffered a comminuted Le Fort I fracture, evidenced by the retruded and impacted maxillary component of the midface.

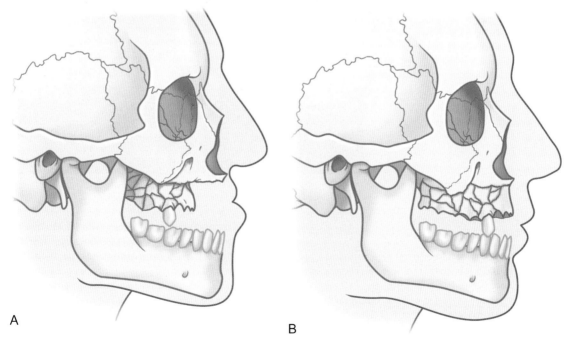

Fig. 3.9.4 Drawings of the preoperative (A) and postoperative (B) position of the involved Le Fort I segment, demonstrating the retruded post-injury position and planned position after surgery. Iliac crest bone grafts were applied in order to reinforce the damaged native bone, and vertically oriented miniplates were applied from the infraorbital rim to the mandible in order to achieve adequate fixation and immobilization (C–D).

Continued

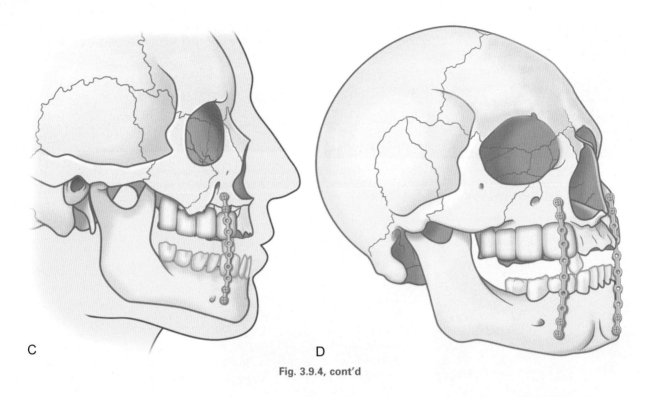

C

D

Fig. 3.9.4, cont'd

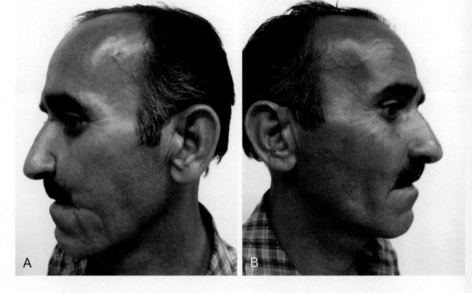

Fig. 3.9.5 Images of the patient several months following the procedure.

A

B

Case 3

Patient sustained a Le Fort I fracture and bilateral zygomatic fractures in a motor vehicle collision, and was operated on elsewhere. The zygomas were plated in an unreduced valgus position (OIF!) and he had class III malocclusion (Fig. 3.9.6). He was treated with osteotomy and varus repositioning of the zygomas, bone grafts of orbital floors, and a Le Fort I advancement.

Case 4

The patient was involved in a motor vehicle collision. She sustained a panfacial fracture: both zygomas, NOE, Le Fort I with mid-palatal split,

mandibular parasymphyseal fracture with left condyle blown into the temporal space (Fig. 3.9.7). Primary treatment involved massive primary bone grafting of maxilla, both orbits, and nose. Both iliac and calvarial grafts were used. Intermaxillary fixation was maintained for 6 weeks. A forehead flap was used for nasal reconstruction, which should have been a bit longer. The only skeletal procedure was the primary treatment. Good occlusion and mouth opening were obtained in spite of disruption of the left temporomandibular joint (Fig. 3.9.8).

Case 5

The patient was involved in a bicycle accident and was operated on elsewhere by a plastic surgeon and oral surgeon working together. The

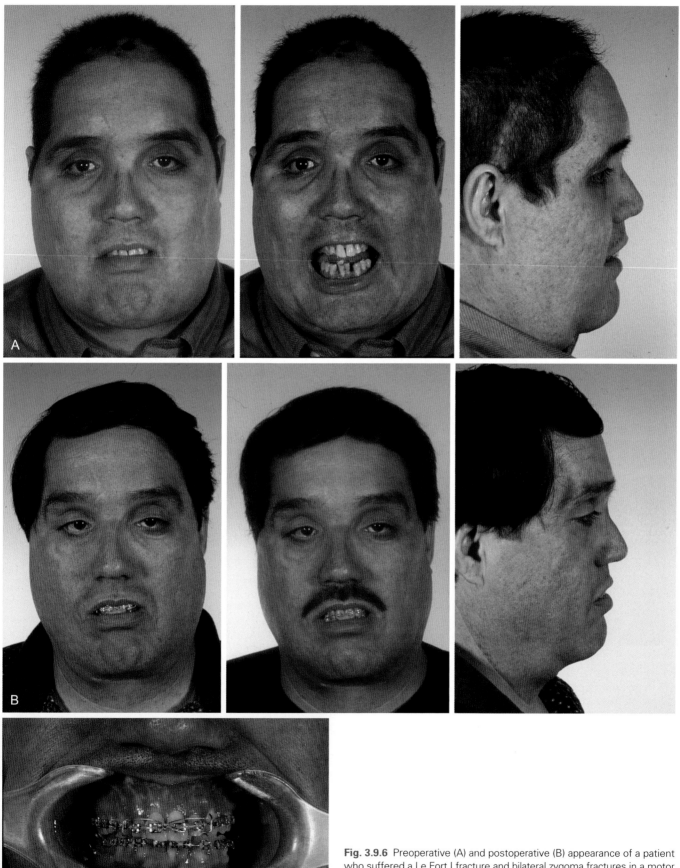

Fig. 3.9.6 Preoperative (A) and postoperative (B) appearance of a patient who suffered a Le Fort I fracture and bilateral zygoma fractures in a motor vehicle collision. He was operated on prior to his presentation to our clinic, and had malpositioned zygomas and a class III malocclusion. He underwent osteotomies and repositioning of the bilateral zygomas, Le Fort I advancement, and bilateral orbital floor bone grafting. (C) Postoperative occlusion of the patient is shown.

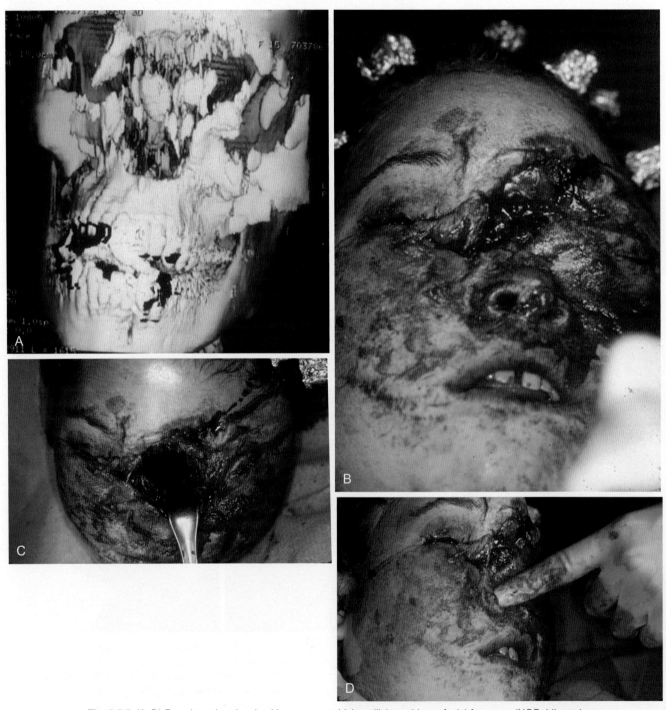

Fig. 3.9.7 (A–D) Female patient involved in a motor vehicle collision with panfacial fractures (NOE, bilateral zygomas, Le Fort I, palatal split, and mandibular fractures as evident on CT scan) and significant associated soft tissue damage and rupture of the left globe.

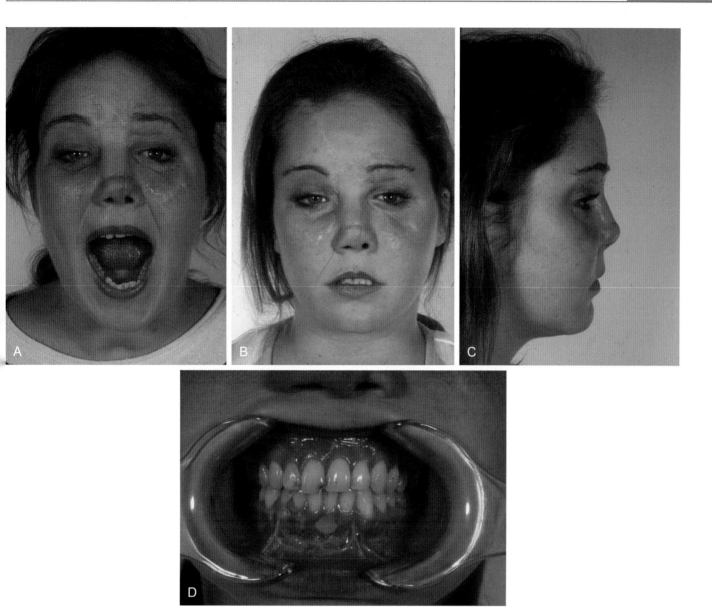

Fig. 3.9.8 (A–C) Postoperative images of a female patient who underwent primary bone grafting at time of fixation of her panfacial fractures, and maxillomandibular fixation for 6 weeks. She later underwent forehead flap reconstruction of her nasal deformity. (D) Postoperative occlusion of the patient is shown.

patient had severely displaced right zygoma and orbital floor fractures, with a right NOE component. The oral surgeon placed the patient in intermaxillary fixation. The plastic surgeon plated the zygoma in malposition, a classic OIF (Figs. 3.9.9 and 3.9.10). A coronal incision, along with proper reduction of the zygomatic and orbital fractures, and primary bone grafting of the nose and orbits should have been done, but this was beyond the plastic surgeon's comfort zone. He was referred to a colleague for secondary treatment (refracture and reposition of all malpositioned segments, bone grafting of nose and orbit, transnasal medial canthopexy), but in retrospect it would have been better for the colleague to transfer the patient for definitive primary treatment Figs. 3.9.9 and 3.9.11).

Case 6

Male patient involved in a motor vehicle collision, initially treated at a different facility where he underwent primary open fixation of his facial fractures without adequate reduction (OIF). On examination and imaging the patient had nonanatomical reduction of bilateral zygoma fractures, NOE fracture, right Le Fort II and left Le Fort III fractures, left mandibular parasymphyseal fracture, as well as bilateral telecanthus, and malposition of the left orbit and globe (Fig. 3.9.12). The patient was a Jehovah's Witness, and thus we elected to perform staged secondary reconstruction to reposition the left orbit/globe and soft tissues, and improve his occlusion to the premorbid state. Our initial procedure

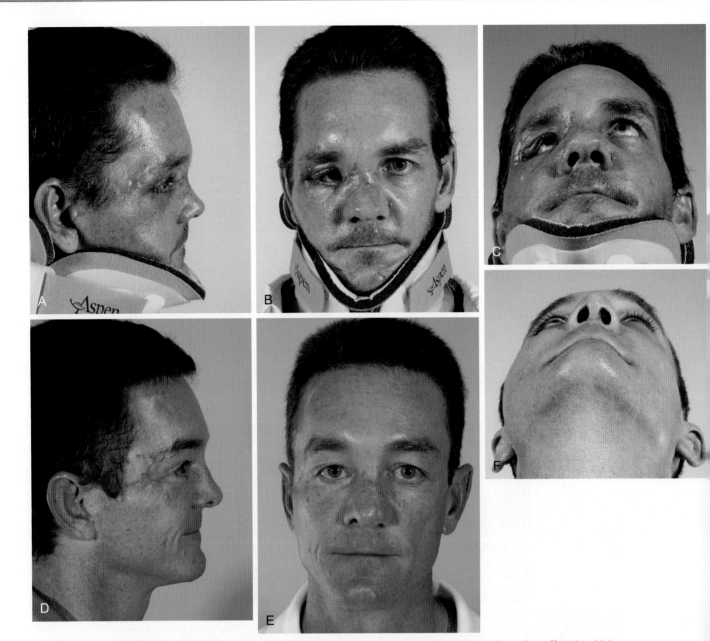

Fig. 3.9.9 (A–C) Images upon presentation (and after a primary procedure) of a patient who suffered multiple facial fractures during a bicycle accident, including displaced right zygoma, orbital floor, nasal bones, and displaced medial canthus, a classic OIF. The patient underwent secondary osteotomies and repositioning of the zygoma, along with bone grafting of the nose and orbital floor, and trans-nasal wiring. (D–F) Postoperative images.

included osteotomies of the the left zygomaticomaxillary and nasal segments, left medial orbital wall osteotomy, calvarial bone grafts to the medial orbital walls and orbital floors bilaterally, calvarial bone grafts to the nose, and bilateral medial and lateral canthopexies (Fig. 3.9.13).

At the second procedure we performed bilateral sagittal split mandibular osteotomies and Le Fort I osteotomy using preoperative facebow transfer and intermediate splints in order to accurately restore premorbid occlusion. In retrospect, we should have abandoned the intermediate splint intraoperatively and simply set his occlusion visually. The splints were ultimately incorrect, and he had an improved, though persistent, occlusal cant postoperatively (Figs. 3.9.13 and 3.9.14).

CONCLUSIONS

1. Occlusal deformities are rare in patients treated with intermaxillary fixation at primary operation. If one jaw is intact, it provides support for the fractured other. In bimaxillary fractures, one should begin with sphenoid reduction, proper zygomatic arch alignment (it should be straight), followed by maxillary reduction and buttress reconstruction, followed with relating the fractured mandible to the intact maxilla. Plating alone may not be enough: primary autogenous bone grafting should be liberally used.

2. However, upper midfacial fractures are frequently poorly treated due to lack of exposure and experience of the surgeon.

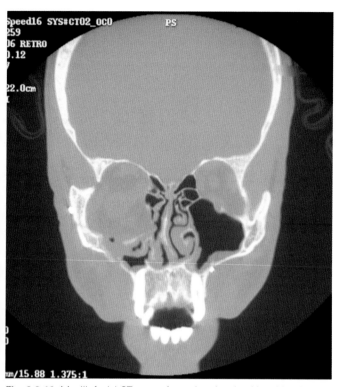

Fig. 3.9.10 Maxillofacial CT scan of a patient involved in a bicycle accident after initial OIF. Significant displacement of fractured orbital floor and zygoma fractures are evident.

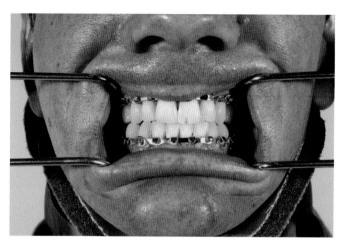

Fig. 3.9.11 Postoperative occlusion of a patient involved in a bicycle accident after undergoing secondary osteotomies and repositioning of the right zygoma, with bone grafting of the orbital floor and nasal bones.

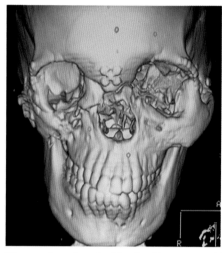

Fig. 3.9.12 CT scan of a male patient involved in a motor vehicle accident with inadequate initial reduction of numerous facial fractures, including bilateral zygoma fractures, NOE fracture, right Le Fort II and left Le Fort III fractures, and left mandibular parasymphseal fracture.

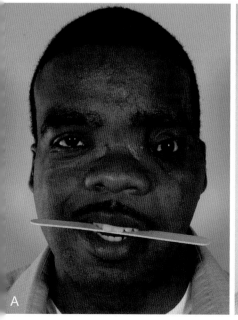
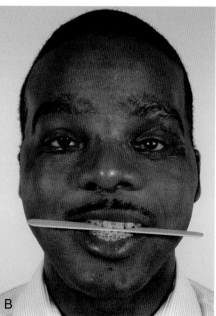

Fig. 3.9.13 Patient involved in a motor vehicle collision with extensive bony and soft tissue injuries, including bilateral zygoma fractures, NOE fracture, right Le Fort II and left Le Fort III fractures, left mandibular parasymphseal fracture, as well as bilateral telecanthus, and malposition of the left orbit and globe. He underwent primary open fixation of his fractures at a different facility without adequate reduction resulting in significant residual deformities, and malocclusion (A). He underwent secondary osteotomies of the bilateral zygomas, left medial orbital wall, nasal bones, with calvarial bone grafts to both orbits, and bilateral medial and lateral canthopexies. In a second procedure he underwent bilateral sagittal split mandibular osteotomies and Le Fort I osteotomy (B).

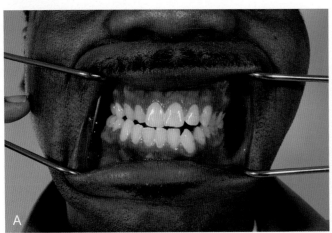 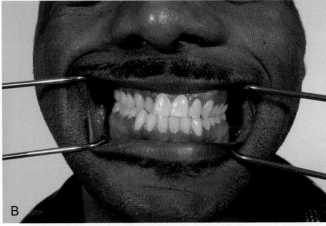

Fig. 3.9.14 Preoperative occlusion of a male patient involved in a motor vehicle collision with significant bony and soft tissue trauma and inadequate primary reconstruction (A). Postoperative occlusion after undergoing preoperative orthodontics, Le Fort I osteotomy, and bilateral sagittal split mandibular osteotomy (B).

3. An aggressive approach at the primary operation, with wide exposure, rigid fixation, and use of autogenous bone grafts without hesitation gives the best chance at an excellent result.

4. Secondary surgery with osteotomy and repositioning of malpositioned segments gives less adequate results due to soft tissue scarring and contraction. It is important to have the ability to make dental models and splints when needed. If tooth-bearing segments have been lost, more extensive reconstructive surgery with bone grafts or vascularized bone flaps may be required, along with osseointegrated implants, in order to restore proper occlusion.

EXPERT COMMENTARY

Few surgeons have had the longitudinal experience, the initial training, and subsequent relationships with Paul Tessier that Dr. Wolfe has, and few if any surgeons have had the career experience with congenital and acquired deformities and especially trauma. In particular, while most surgeons in the latter part of their careers shun trauma, Dr. Wolfe has remained involved in all aspects of craniofacial surgery including immediate and late trauma surgery. It is from this background that the present chapter on secondary maxillary and mandibular osteotomies and the management of occlusion is written.

To be able to manage secondary trauma surgery one must have managed primary trauma so well that one understands the nature of the occasional problem and its correction. Such is the teaching in this chapter, which emphasizes cases as the primary mode of teaching, which describe the use of models and occlusal analysis to plan case management. Other chapters in this text outline the principles of preoperative virtual models and surgery and

EXPERT COMMENTARY—cont'd

intraoperative imaging to guide osteotomies and reconstruction, but here reoperative surgery is still an art learned over years and practiced predominantly by the well trained. It will not be easy, in this day of shortened training and the absence of dominant role models and companions, to produce the "Tony Wolfes" of the future.

REFERENCES

1. Manson PN, Crawley WA, Yaremchuk MJ, et al. Midface fractures: advantages of immediate extended open reduction and bone grafting. *Plast Reconstr Surg.* 1986;76(1):1–10.
2. Howard P, Wolfe SA. Fractures of the mandible. *Ann Plast Surg.* 1986;17(5):391–407.
3. Gruss JS, Mackinnon SE, Kassel EE, Cooper PW. The role of primary bone grafting in complex craniomaxillofacial trauma. *Plast Reconstr Surg.* 1985;75(1):17–25.
4. Manson PN, Clark N, Robertson B, et al. Subunit principles in midface fractures: the importance of sagittal buttresses, soft-tissue reductions, and sequencing treatment of segmental fractures. *Plast Reconstr Surg.* 1999;103(4):1287–1306.
5. Gruss JS. Complex nasoethmoid-orbital and midfacial fractures: role of craniofacial surgical techniques and immediate bone grafting. *Ann Plast Surg.* 1986;17(5):377–390.
6. Wolfe SA, Ghurani R, Podda S, Ward J. An examination of posttraumatic, postsurgical orbital deformities: conclusions drawn for improvement of primary treatment. *Plast Reconstr Surg.* 2008;122(6):1870–1881.
7. Gillies HD. *Plastic Surgery of the Face: Based on Selected Cases of War Injuries of the Face.* London: Oxford University Press; 1920:12.

Secondary Traumatic TMJ Reconstruction

Zahid Afzal, Gary Warburton

BACKGROUND

The temporomandibular joint (TMJ) is a complex and unique joint unlike any other joint in the body, with both translational and rotational function, and repetitive complex movement patterns to accommodate the functions of speech, mastication, and swallowing. For these reasons, posttraumatic secondary reconstruction of this joint remains a challenging prospect for treating clinicians, and as TMJ reconstruction is performed far less commonly than other joints (knee and hip), this limits clinical experience in the field but also limits the amount of quantitative data for qualitative analysis. Following traumatic injury, it is not only the bony components of the joint, namely the mandibular fossa and condyle, but also the ligamentous and fibrocartilaginous components that may sustain injury, particularly the articular disk and the fibrocartilage joint lining. Condylar fractures account for around a quarter of all mandibular fractures highlighting the common nature of this type of injury. Potential late complications of traumatic TMJ injuries include facial asymmetry, malocclusion, growth disturbance, osteoarthritis, and ankylosis with potential functional problems.[1] There are a variety of treatment modalities to manage these problems ranging from conservative to total joint replacement surgery, which largely depends on the extent of the problem and the clinical presentation. When the mandibular condyle is extensively damaged, degenerated or lost, replacement with either autogenous graft or alloplastic implant is an acceptable approach to achieve optimal functional and symptomatic improvement.[2] The goals of TMJ reconstruction primarily are to improve mandibular form and function, to relieve pain where possible, provide cost-effective treatment and to avoid complications and morbidity. Mercuri[3] reported indications for alloplastic joint reconstruction that include ankylosis or reankylosis with severe anatomical abnormalities and failed autogenous grafts in multiply operated patients. In this chapter, we will discuss these indications further, with emphasis towards posttraumatic secondary reconstruction.

Autologous TMJ reconstruction has been described in the literature since the early 1900s and has included the use of the metatarsal graft, costochondral graft, coronoid process, scapular tip, iliac crest, sternoclavicular, deep circumflex iliac artery flap and of increasing recent use, the fibula free flap. Indeed, with improved understanding and technical abilities of the reconstructive surgeon, autologous microvascular reconstructive techniques are now widely accepted as the "gold standard" for mandibular reconstruction. In the 1970s and 1980s, alloplastic joint reconstruction resulted in significant complications associated with prostheses containing Proplast–Teflon, where fragmentation on prolonged cyclical loading often resulted in a very locally destructive foreign body giant cell reaction. The subsequent litigation and FDA recall of these devices in the United States placed progress on hold for a period until the early 1990s where newer improved devices were introduced to the market. Currently, TMJ Concepts (Ventura, CA, USA) produces

a patient-specific custom device utilizing CAD-CAM 3D technology, whereas Zimmer-Biomet Microfixation (Warsaw, IN, USA) produces both stock (in the United States) and custom devices (not available in United States). With now over 27 years of reported data, these devices have proven efficacy and safety, with outcomes similar or superior to standard orthopedic knee and hip prosthetic devices. Some common autologous and alloplastic TMJ reconstructive modalities will be discussed further in this chapter.

ANATOMY OF THE TMJ

The TMJ is a bilateral ginglymoarthrodial (hinging and sliding) synovial joint between the condylar head of the mandible and glenoid or mandibular fossa on the undersurface of the squamous part of the temporal bone, together making a craniomandibular articulation (see Fig. 3.10.1). The joint is separated into an upper and lower compartment by a fibrocartilaginous disk that is biconcave in shape against the articulating surfaces within both compartments. The bony joint surfaces are covered with the same fibrocartilage which is less susceptible to degeneration and has a greater repair ability compared to hyaline cartilage found in other synovial joints. The mandible from condyle to condyle is a continuous entity and therefore movement in either TMJ is dependent upon the other whilst the extent and direction of movement is determined by the articulating surfaces, ligaments, and local musculature.

The collateral, capsular, and temporomandibular ligaments are direct anatomic components of the TMJs whilst the sphenomandibular and stylomandibular ligaments are attached at a distance from the joints. Collectively, they provide stability and control joint movement.

The muscles of mastication are the masseter, temporalis, medial pterygoid, and lateral pterygoid. The accessory muscles of mastication include the suprahyoid (digastric, geniohyoid, mylohyoid, and stylohyoid), and infrahyoid (sternohyoid, omohyoid, sternothyroid, thyrohyoid) muscle groups. When the mouth is opened, the condylar head undergoes rotation in the lower joint compartment while an anterior gliding motion occurs in the upper compartment. The lateral pterygoid and digastric are the main muscles involved in mouth opening whilst the masseter, temporalis, and medial pterygoids are the key muscles involved in mandibular elevation and subsequent mouth closure.

POSTTRAUMATIC INDICATIONS FOR TMJ RECONSTRUCTION

The potential long-term sequelae of TMJ trauma that may require reconstruction and management are:
- Ankylosis
- Condylar malunion/malposition with malocclusion and/or facial asymmetry

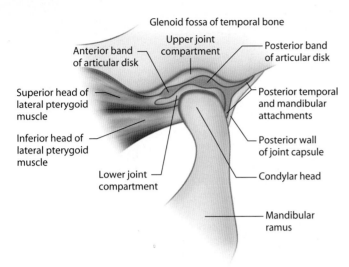

Fig. 3.10.1 Diagram showing the anatomical structure of the human temporomandibular joint. (Courtesy Dr. Zahid Afzal.)

- Degenerative joint disease
- Failed primary reconstruction (autogenous/alloplastic)

Ankylosis

Posttraumatic ankylosis of the TMJ injury is an uncommon complication of condylar injury and is of particular concern in pediatric cases where significant growth disturbances may result. This includes facial asymmetry, retrognathism, and secondary midface growth deficiency.[4,5] In the adult patient, it may present as trismus with resultant compromised mastication, speech, oral hygiene, and even psychosocial distress.[4,6] This complication usually results from comminuted intracapsular injuries, particularly when the articular disk is disrupted. It has also been suggested that concomitant anterior mandibular fractures, which allow posterior facial widening and consequent lateral displacement of fractured condyles, also increase the risk for this complication.[7,8] Treatment can depend on the severity of the condition with various treatment modalities at the clinician's disposal, including gap arthroplasty, costochondral grafting, and total joint replacement. The growing patient offers additional reconstructive challenges and often requires further corrective surgeries consequential of dynamic changes in the growing patient. Complete bony TMJ ankylosis has been typically managed with gap arthroplasty, autogenous tissue graft or alloplastic arthroplasty.[9] Autogenous grafting techniques usually require a period of immobilization postoperatively to allow adequate healing and limit the risk of graft failure resulting in mandibular functional delay. The lack of early mobilization and lack of soft tissue interface can risk reankylosis and should this occur, then total alloplastic reconstruction may be considered. In the growing patient, ankylosis of the TMJ may lead to asymmetrical mandibular growth resulting in height reduction of the affected ramus and subsequent facial asymmetry with chin deviation to the affected side, due to normal growth of the opposite side and impaired growth of the affected side. Compensatory occlusal disturbances may also occur such as overeruption and tipping of teeth to help reestablish functional occlusion. TMJ ankylosis in growing subjects has traditionally been managed by autogenous grafting, with the costochondral grafts as the most widely used method for these TMJ reconstructions.[10] The rationale for autologous grafting is to maintain growth potential[5] but growth and resorption can be unpredictable and other complications such as ankylosis have been reported.

Sawhney classified four types of pathological changes in the ankylosed TMJ.[11] Type 1 describes flattening of the condylar head with surrounding dense fibrous adhesions making movement impossible. Type 2 includes a flattened or deformed condylar head, with close proximity to the articular surfaces, and a limited bony fusion of the outer, anterior or posterior surface. Type 3 includes a bony block bridging across the ramus and the zygomatic arch, with the displaced articular head fused to the medial side of the ramus, or the presence of an atrophic condylar head. Type 4 presents as a large bony block that completely replaces the usual joint architecture.

Condylar Malunion/Malposition With Malocclusion and/or Facial Asymmetry

Loss of posterior mandibular vertical dimension due to traumatic injury can cause occlusal discrepancies as either an anterior open-bite where bilateral mandibular height is lost, or premature contact of the posterior teeth with contralateral open-bite where there is unilateral vertical height loss. Fig. 3.10.2 illustrates left condylar hypoplasia and the resultant loss of left vertical height in a young patient following an old traumatic fracture dislocation injury. In the absence of successful primary trauma reconstructive surgery or other management to help reestablish normal vertical height and correct occlusal discrepancies, then joint reconstruction (autogenous or alloplastic) or osteotomy may be considered. In the growing patient, loss of vertical height on the affected side may either be due to ankylosis and the resultant hypomobility or from direct injury to the condylar cartilaginous cap. It has been widely accepted for the growing patient where preservation of growth potential is desired, autogenous grafting such as the costochondral graft, is preferred over alloplastic TMJ reconstructive solutions. However, very good results using alloplastic devices in growing patients are emerging, with maintenance of facial symmetry in both unilateral and bilateral cases.

Degenerative Joint Disease

Traumatic injury to the TMJ, whether direct or indirect, can lead to osteoarthritic changes within the joint. Posttrauma joint effusion is well known in the orthopedic literature and has frequently been observed in posttraumatic imaging of the TMJ by magnetic resonance imaging (MRI),[12] whilst other studies have shown arthroscopic evidence of TMJ articular damage following mandibular fracture injuries.[13] The proinflammatory cytokine interleukin-6 (IL-6) has been shown to play a key role in the pathogenesis of arthritis[14] and has been found in higher concentrations in TMJs with internal derangement and osteoarthritis when compared to TMJs without joint effusion.[15] Nogami et al.[16] found a correlation between MR evidence of joint effusion and concentration of IL-6 in washed-out synovial fluid samples collected from patients with mandibular condyle fractures. TMJ arthritis is one of the most common diseases affecting this joint and has a variety of other etiologies besides trauma, including inflammatory, infectious, metabolic, degenerative osteoarthritis, and systemic arthritides. Therefore, where preexisting disease is present, then certainly a traumatic insult can exacerbate the primary disease state. Symptoms depend on disease progression but patients may typically present with constant preauricular pain, with or without radiation and crepitus. Other symptoms may include TMJ locking, clicking, popping, and mandibular deviation on opening. Although a majority of patients earlier in the disease process will respond to nonsurgical treatment modalities or limited surgical intervention, when the mandibular condyle is extensively damaged, degenerated or lost, replacement with either autogenous graft or alloplastic implant is an acceptable approach to achieve optimal functional and symptomatic improvement.[2]

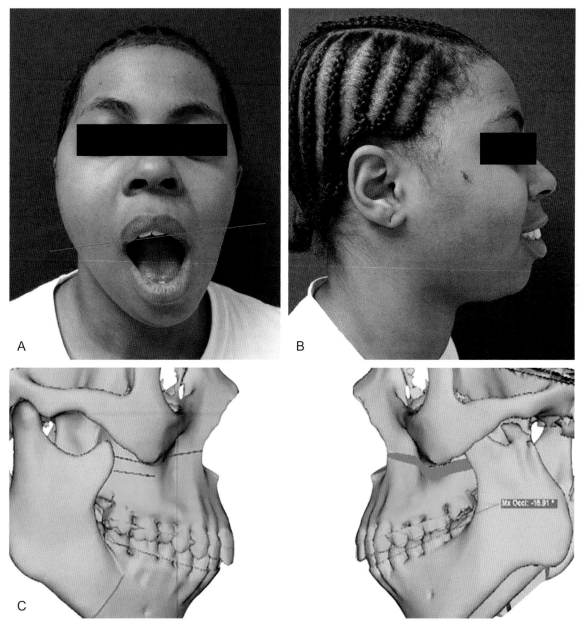

Fig. 3.10.2 Posttraumatic unilateral condylar hypoplasia, malunion with displacement in a young patient. Note chin deviation on opening to the affected side. The 3D reconstructed image (C) demonstrates the extent of left condylar hypoplasia. (Courtesy of Dr. Gary Warburton.)

AUTOGENOUS GRAFT FAILURE

The success of nonvascularized autogenous tissue reconstruction in part depends on the quality of the vascular bed at the host site, which is often compromised due to the presence of dense fibrous tissue from the trauma and also prior surgery. Marx reports that scar tissue surrounding previously operated bone averages 440 μm in thickness, however capillaries can penetrate a maximum thickness of 180–220 μm of tissue,[17] which would significantly compromise graft viability and in certain cases may explain autogenous graft failure. Auricular cartilage was once widely advocated for autogenous disk replacement, however subsequent studies have suggested it is not an ideal substitute[18] and patients treated this way primarily for posttraumatic disk replacement with subsequent graft failure, may require secondary reconstructive surgery. Patients

reconstructed with autogenous costochondral grafting normally undergo 4–6 weeks of maxillomandibular fixation following which the mandible is returned to functional activity to prevent ankylosis. However, Reitzik reported that cortex-to-cortex healing of the vertical ramus probably requires 25 weeks in humans following studies on monkeys.[19] Micromotion of these free grafts will invariably occur with early mandibular functional movement resulting in compromised graft success.[20] Furthermore, both vascularized and nonvascularized reconstructions may fail due to ankylosis, especially if there is no soft tissue interface between the condylar reconstruction and glenoid fossa of the temporal bone.

Alloplastic Joint Reconstruction Failure

Many patients who underwent TMJ reconstruction in the 1970s and 1980s with Proplast–Teflon coated alloplastic prostheses or Silastic developed foreign body giant cell reactions with subsequent osteolytic changes around the devices. The resultant bony destruction and often multiply operated surgical sites rendered the locally distorted anatomy challenging to manage. Henry and Wolford reported less success with autogenous bone and soft tissue grafts in patients who had previously had Proplast–Teflon or Silastic in place.[21] Henry and Wolford also reported in the same study that reconstruction with autogenous materials was much less predictable than with alloplastic replacement. It is therefore reasonable to consider total alloplastic TMJ reconstruction in this group of patients to achieve optimal postoperative functional value.

IMAGING OF THE TMJ

TMJ imaging of the appropriate nature and quality is fundamental for diagnostic evaluation and treatment planning in the TMJ patient. Although conventional imaging (such as panoramic radiography) is cost-effective and with lower radiation exposure compared to more advanced imaging modalities, it only provides two-dimensional detail. With superimposed regional anatomy over the region of interest, it is often necessary to take films in different planes to accomplish the detail required for diagnostic and planning purposes. For this reason, coupled with the potential for artefacts and other processing errors, conventional radiology is not the primary choice for TMJ imaging when considering secondary TMJ reconstruction where greater imaging accuracy and

detail is required. However, conventional imaging or plain film still remains a useful initial study.

Computed tomography (CT) permits detailed assessment of the TMJ, allowing views in the axial, coronal, and sagittal planes and also makes 3D volumetric reconstruction possible. CT is particularly useful in the assessment of bony structures and pathologies such as TMJ ankylosis. Indeed a "bony window" setting helps accentuate this effect, while a "soft-tissue" setting helps visualize nonosseous structures more clearly. However, despite the latter, the TMJ disk and other soft tissue structures in the region of interest are often impossible to view with CT alone. Higher radiation exposure and cost can be brought down considerably with the use of cone beam computed tomography (CBCT) technology but image artefacts from metallic objects, whether dental restorations or metallic prostheses near or in the field of interest, produce a starburst pattern of scatter. This may mask the detail required for TMJ assessment and other image modalities may be sought. Magnetic resonance imaging (MRI) is widely accepted as the study of choice to visualize the TMJ disk and ligaments,[22] adjacent soft tissues, inflammatory changes, and the presence of joint effusion. Depending on image weighting, two commonly used studies are T1 images, which are fat-enhancing and provide excellent anatomic detail such as disk position/displacement, and T2 imaging, which is used in identifying inflammatory processes and/or the presence of joint effusion in the TMJ. Open and closed views (see Fig. 3.10.3) are captured to understand changes in joint biomechanics and disk pathology. As with CT imaging, artefacts can occur with

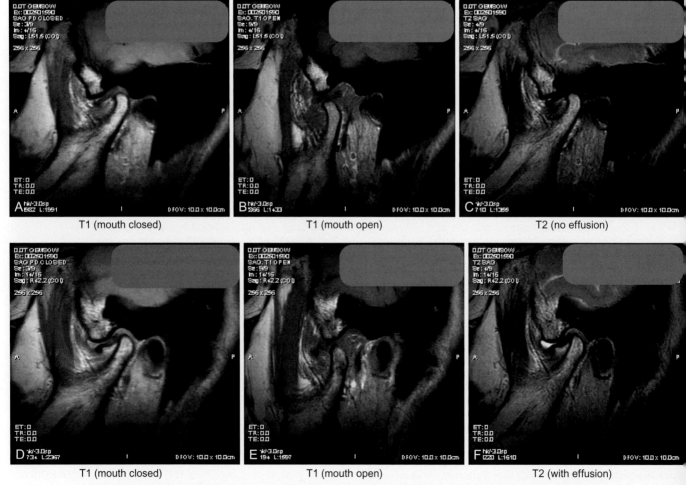

| T1 (mouth closed) | T1 (mouth open) | T2 (no effusion) |

| T1 (mouth closed) | T1 (mouth open) | T2 (with effusion) |

Fig. 3.10.3 MRI imaging showing open and closed mouth views of the TMJ for diagnostic evaluation. (Courtesy of Dr. Gary Warburton.)

metallic objects such as dental restorations. Aneurysmal brain clips or patients with indwelling cardiac pacemakers are contraindications for MRI study. Volumetric 3D reconstruction is also not easily achievable unlike with CT imaging, however Costa et al.[23] conducted a study to define the diagnostic value of a method for 3D reconstruction of MRI images for the assessment of TMJ and found the method to be a useful and an accurate tool for this purpose, particularly when focusing on internal derangement.

TMJ RECONSTRUCTIVE TECHNIQUES

Autogenous TMJ Reconstruction

In 1909 Bardenheuer first replaced the mandibular condyle with a patient's fourth metatarsal[24] and in 1920 Gillies introduced costochondral grafts (CCGs) for condylar reconstruction.[25] Autogenous grafting techniques have since continued to develop and have been of particular significance in the growing patient where preservation of growth potential has remained of primary importance. Although other grafts, for instance coronoid process, scapular tip, fibula, sternoclavicular joint and iliac crest have all been employed in TMJ reconstruction, the most widely used has been the costochondral graft, particularly in the child patient.

Costochondral Graft

In 2000, McIntosh[26] reported advantages including biological compatibility, workability, functional adaptability, minimal donor site morbidity. Kaban et al.[27] published a protocol employing CCGs for the management of TMJ ankylosis in children demonstrating excellent growth potential. However, disadvantages of costochondral grafting include donor site morbidity, fracture, ankylosis, and unpredictable growth.[28] Kaban suggested the most frequent source of failure in children treated for TMJ ankylosis has not been a lack of patient cooperation but, rather, inadequate ankylosis release. This is most commonly caused by a failure to adequately excise the ankylotic mass, resulting in failure to achieve complete, passive opening (without the need for excessive force) in the operating room.[27] In 1999 Ko et al.[29] reported a study involving 10 children all of whom underwent CCG reconstruction to manage TMJ ankylosis with a mean age of 7.4 years, two of whom had bilateral TMJ ankylosis. Ko further reported progressive deviation of the chin toward the nonaffected side in five of the children after TMJ reconstruction. The study found CCGs tended to have a more vertically directed condylar growth pattern and a more laterally positioned condyle, in the two cases with bilateral TMJ reconstruction, the CCGs grafted grew until there was a mandibular prognathism that required corrective surgery. To minimize the risk of overgrowth, it has been suggested to limit the thickness of the cartilaginous cap. In 2003, Saeed and Kent[30] conducted a retrospective review of 76 CCGs (57 patients) to determine outcome with respect to the extent of previous surgery (none, disc surgery or soft tissue graft, alloplastic disc, alloplastic joint, previous graft) and to initial and preoperative diagnosis. They concluded in patients with no previous surgery, arthritic disease or congenital deformity the costochondral graft performed well but in patients with previous alloplastic discs and/or total joints the results were less predictable. A preoperative diagnosis of ankylosis was associated with a high complication and further surgery rate suggesting caution in this group of patients.[30] CCGs can be used as an initial TMJ reconstructive approach for the adult post-traumatic patient but resorption can be problematic and for this reason, nowadays CCGs are less frequently used when compared to other autogenous options such as the fibula flap. Medra[31] reported 85 cases of CCGs for TMJ reconstruction and follow-up demonstrated resorption in 21 patients (25%), of which 10 patients showed partial resorption and 11 had complete resorption of the grafted bone.

Vascularized Fibula Free Flap

The fibula free flap (FFF) has become a widely accepted autologous reconstructive option for segmental mandibular defects after resections for cancer, benign tumors, trauma, or osteonecrosis. Advantages of this flap include the ability to repair soft-tissue composite defects, excellent bone length that can be shaped to fit the anatomical need, vascularized bone that resists resorption, suitability for dental implant placement and so allowing dental rehabilitation, and finally the ability to have a two-team approach reducing anesthesia time. Garcia et al.[32] reported six patients who underwent mandibular resection including the condyle and reconstruction using FFF where in all the cases, the fibula was placed directly into the glenoid fossa. The temporomandibular disc was preserved over the condylar end of the fibula. Panoramic radiographs were performed postoperatively to evaluate condylar position and grade of bone resorption. Five of the patients developed good function whilst one fibula ankylosed, concluding the use of the FFF directly fitted into the glenoid fossa is a reliable method in condylar reconstruction but the risk of ankylosis persists. Other options include fitting a prosthetic condyle onto the fibula to articulate against the articular eminence[33] or where the native condyle is preserved, then this can be fixated directly onto the fibula graft.[34] Figs. 3.10.4–3.10.8 illustrate secondary reconstruction of the TMJ with a fibula graft where primary reconstruction failed after many years.

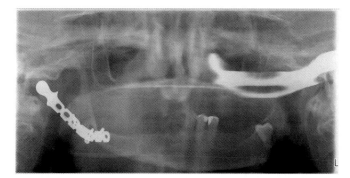

Fig. 3.10.4 Panoramic X-ray showing primary reconstructive failure with discontinuity of mandibular form. (Courtesy Dr. Gary Warburton.)

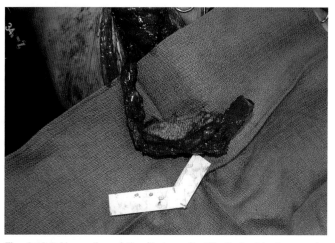

Fig. 3.10.5 Harvesting of the fibula graft still attached to its vascular supply. Note the contouring of the osseous component facilitated by the surgical template to help re-establish mandibular form. (Courtesy Dr. Gary Warburton.)

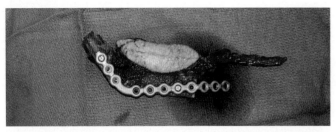

Fig. 3.10.6 The fibula microvascular free flap fixated to a reconstruction bar which is then screw fixated to the native mandible. (Courtesy Dr. Gary Warburton.)

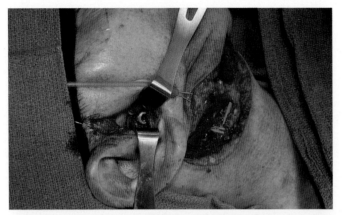

Fig. 3.10.7 Fibula graft is fixated in position with microvascular anastomosis to neck vessels for graft viability. (Courtesy Dr. Gary Warburton.)

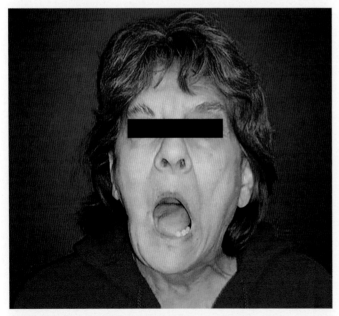

Fig. 3.10.8 Shows restored function with excellent mouth opening and improved mandibular from. (Courtesy Dr. Gary Warburton.)

Alloplastic TMJ Reconstruction

When compared to autogenous graft techniques, alloplastic joint prostheses avoid donor site morbidity, can reestablish mandibular vertical dimension reliably with joint architecture resembling more closely normal TMJ anatomy, reduce operative time, and reduce the risk of reankylosis. As the device is well adapted to the bony contours of the

recipient bone, especially in custom patient-fitted prostheses, and secured with screw fixation, immediate physiotherapy and rehabilitation is possible. In the autogenous graft, a period of around 6 weeks of MMF is required to ensure graft viability but which delays rehabilitation and joint physiotherapy. In 2002 Saeed et al.[35] reported findings comparing autogenous (CCG) reconstruction of the TMJ with alloplastic devices. In both groups of patients there was significant improvement in symptoms with a more favorable outcome in those treated by alloplastic reconstruction. Although the complication rate was similar in both groups, most of those in the alloplastic group were self-limiting whilst the autogenous group had much more serious complications such as ankylosis. The most significant disadvantage of alloplastic devices is the potential for wear debris and the associated biological responses, although there have been significant improvements, this has been a historical problem. As with all hardware, mechanical failure due to component fracture, screw loosening, and metal fatigue are other disadvantages alongside the significant cost of the device.

TMJ replacement techniques initially presented as fossa-only prostheses or only prosthetic condylar designs, but due to unacceptable bone resorption and prosthetic device failures, it was later understood that total joint replacement was necessary for more successful outcomes.[36] Our understanding of biomaterial science in the use of alloplastic TMJ materials has vastly improved and evolved since the catastrophic failures of the Proplast–Teflon (Kent/Vitek) TMJ implant several decades ago. Eventual wear of the latter implant under joint loading resulted in the release of PTFE-HA particles into surrounding tissues and bone which triggered the differentiation of monocytes into osteoclasts causing localized destruction. Metal-on-metal articulations, using cobalt-chromium-molybdenum alloys, demonstrated smaller metallic wear particles but proved to be even more problematic.[37] Today, the materials approved by the FDA for use in the manufacture of alloplastic TMJ devices are ultra-high molecular weight polyethylene (UHMWPE), cobalt–chromium alloys (Co-Cr-Mo), commercially pure titanium (cpTi), and alloyed titanium (Ti6A1V4), indeed all modern alloplastic prostheses are constructed from these materials although in varying combinations. The TMJ Concepts is a custom patient-specific total joint replacement system in which the glenoid fossa component is UHMWPE fused to an unalloyed titanium backing that is directly screwed into the zygomatic process of the temporal bone. The mandibular condyle component is made from Co-Cr-Mo and the ramus out of titanium. The Zimmer-Biomet systems glenoid fossa component is made entirely of UHMWPE and the condyle ramus component made from Co-Cr-Mo alloy and again, the glenoid fossa component is also fixed into position with titanium screws. Fig. 3.10.9 shows the custom TMJ Concepts device alongside the stock Zimmer-Biomet system. Table 3.10.1 lists the indications/contraindications for a stock device whilst Table 3.10.2 lists the advantages/disadvantages of both custom and stock TMJ Total Joint Replacement (TJR) devices.

Although TMJ implants went out of vogue following all the widely published failures of earlier devices, in the early 1990s stock or "off the shelf" devices such as the early Christensen prosthesis were being used by TMJ surgeons; however, mechanical failure, for instance metal fracture and loosening of components, remained to be addressed. In 1995 Mercuri et al.[38] published their preliminary multicenter report proving the safety and efficacy of a patient-fitted custom CAD/CAM total temporomandibular joint system (Techmedica, Camarillo, CA). Another system was developed by Biomet called the Biomet Microfixation TMJ Replacement System (Zimmer-Biomet Microfixation, Jacksonville, FL) and was granted FDA approval in 2005. The difference here was, unlike Techmedica, which only offered a custom patient-fitted device, Biomet offered both a stock and custom solution to the TMJ surgeon. For both systems, there are studies that demonstrate the efficacy and relative safety when compared to earlier generational devices. In 2007 Mercuri et al.[39]

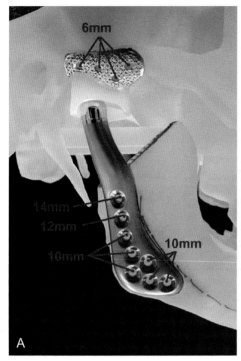
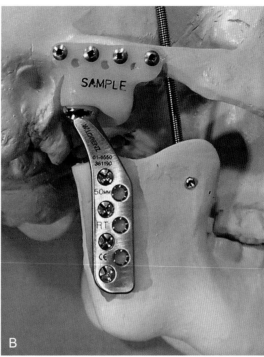

Fig. 3.10.9 (A) Patient-specific TMJ Concepts device with required screw depths and (B) an example of a Zimmer-Biomet stock device. (Courtesy Dr. Gary Warburton.)

TABLE 3.10.1 Indications and Contraindications for Alloplastic Stock TMJ Total Joint Replacement

Indications for Alloplastic Stock Joint Replacement	Contraindications to Alloplastic Stock Joint Replacement
Late-stage degenerative joint disease (osteoarthritis, rheumatoid arthritis, traumatic arthritis, etc.)	Allergy to any of the prosthetic materials
Recurrent ankylosis	Chronic infection
Irreparable condylar fracture	Systemic disease with increased susceptibility to infection
Revision procedures for failed alloplastic or autogenous reconstruction	Skeletal immaturity
Avascular necrosis	
Neoplasia requiring extensive resection	
Congenital disorders, e.g., hemifacial microsomia, Treacher Collins syndrome	

Reproduced with permission from Mercuri LG. Temporomandibular joint total joint replacement – TMJ TJR. Basle: Springer International Publishing; 2016.

TABLE 3.10.2 Advantages and Disadvantages of Stock vs. Custom Prostheses

Advantages of Stock Prostheses	Disadvantages of Stock Prostheses
Fit flexibility	Limited potential for anterior–inferior movement of mandible
Immediate availability (e.g. irreparable trauma, tumor resection)	Surgeon experience with multiple joint reconstructions required to manage variability of fit
Lower cost	

Advantages of Custom Prostheses	Disadvantages of Custom Prostheses
Patient-matched; anatomically stable	Higher cost
Addresses distorted anatomy	Potential for two-stage surgeries (e.g., removal of failed previous metallic implant)
Excessive anterior–inferior movements possible	Time for fabrication of custom implant (8–12 weeks)
	Limited flexibility (must replicate model surgery exactly)
	Potential for two-stage surgeries (e.g., removal of failed previous metallic implant)

Reproduced with permission from Mercuri LG. Temporomandibular joint total joint replacement – TMJ TJR. Basle: Springer International Publishing; 2016.

published a 14-year follow-up of assessment of the safety and effectiveness of a Patient-Fitted Total Temporomandibular Joint Reconstruction System (now, TMJ Concepts Patient-Fitted Total Temporomandibular Joint Reconstruction System, Ventura, CA; previously referred to as Techmedica, Camarillo, CA, the CAD/CAM Patient-Fitted Total Temporomandibular Joint Reconstruction System). Questionnaires were mailed to the available addresses of 193 patients who had been implanted with Techmedica/TMJ Concepts devices between 1990 and 2004. A

total of 61 surveys (31.6%) were returned properly completed. This represented 102 devices (41 bilateral, 20 unilateral), with a mean follow-up of 11.4 years. Analysis of subjective data showed a significant reduction in pain scores and an increase in mandibular function and diet consistency scores, whilst objective data showed an improvement in

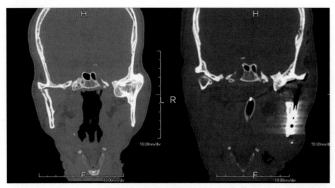

Fig. 3.10.10 CT imaging showing preoperative left TMJ ankylotic bone and postoperative imaging after alloplastic reconstruction. Note the medial proximity to the foramen ovale in both images. (Courtesy Dr. Gary Warburton.)

mandibular range of motion, 85% reported quality of life (QOL) scores that showed improvement since baseline. The study found the studied device to be safe, effective, and a reliable long-term management modality. In 2003 Wolford et al.[40] reported a prospective study evaluating 5- to 8-year subjective and objective results of 42 consecutive patients who had TMJ reconstruction using the TMJ Concepts/Techmedica custom-made total joint prosthesis. Thirty-eight of 42 patients (90%) with 69 TMJs reconstructed were included in the study and found there was statistically significant improvement in incisal opening, jaw function, and pain level. Lateral excursion movements significantly decreased whilst the occlusion remained stable in all cases. The study also found significantly better outcomes for patients with fewer previous TMJ surgeries and without exposure to Proplast–Teflon or Silastic TMJ implants. In 2012, Giannakopoulos et al.[41] reported outcomes for 442 Biomet Microfixation TMJ Replacement System TMJ TJR devices implanted in 288 patients. The study reported statistically significant improvement in pain, jaw function, and interincisal opening. Although there were complications necessitating the removal of 14 of 442 implants (3.2%), there were no device-related mechanical failures. In 2013 Lobo Leandro et al.[42] reported a 10-year follow-up of 300 patients and concluded that the reconstruction of the TMJ through the installation of the Biomet/Lorenz system prosthesis is a safe and effective option for proper reestablishment of the joint and stomatognathic system function, significant long-term improvements in mandibular range of motion are promoted and pain levels decrease.

Although evidence is emerging that both the stock and custom approaches to TMJ TJR are effective treatment modalities, in the growing patient, an autogenous joint replacement is currently preferred in the interest of preserving growth potential, and some advocate mandibular distraction osteogenesis techniques which avoid a second surgical donor site. In the multiply operated patient with significantly distorted bony architecture, a custom joint prosthesis designed with CAD/CAM technology from a 3D CT scan may be the preferred alloplastic choice to ensure a precise fit without the need for challenging surgical manipulation as would be required with a stock device.

SURGICAL TECHNIQUE (STOCK PROSTHESIS)

Figs. 3.10.10–3.10.21 illustrate a case of secondary alloplastic TMJ TJR using a Zimmer-Biomet Stock prosthesis, where unilateral complete TMJ ankylosis had occurred consequential of MMF for primary management of a traumatic condylar fracture. Preparation for surgery includes CT imaging, which can provide valuable information with regards to local structures (as shown in Fig. 3.10.10) and allows the quality of

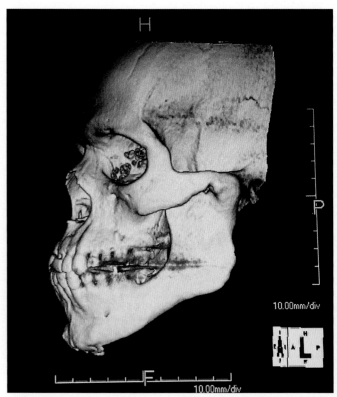

Fig. 3.10.11 3D CT reconstruction of preoperative TMJ ankylosis. (Courtesy Dr. Gary Warburton.)

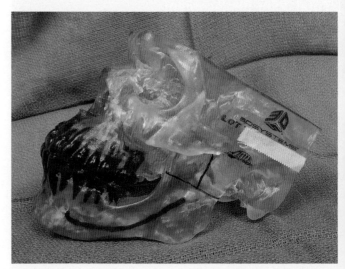

Fig. 3.10.12 Stereolithic modeling constructed from 3D CT reconstruction to facilitate surgical planning. (Courtesy Dr. Gary Warburton.)

bone to be assessed in the planning phase. The patient should understand the risks and benefits of the proposed surgery, having already undergone a detailed consent process. The patient's skin is prepped and the surgical site is isolated as shown in Fig. 3.10.13 to ensure a sterile operative field. Cefazolin and metronidazole are typically administered preincision for prophylactic coverage and vancomycin irrigation is used to clean the external ear canal. Two access incisions are required prior to any bony cuts: firstly a preauricular/endaural incision is made for access to the condyle and fossa with dissection down to the posterior

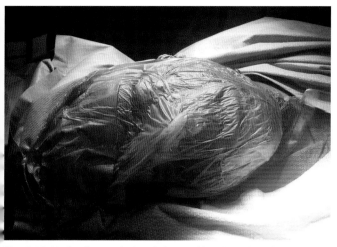

Fig. 3.10.13 Sterile surgical technique with robust isolation and skin preparation of surgical site. (Courtesy Dr. Gary Warburton.)

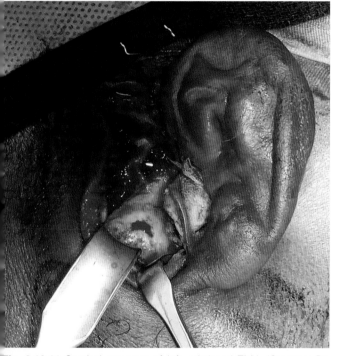

Fig. 3.10.14 Surgical exposure of left ankylosed TMJ. (Courtesy Dr. Gary Warburton.)

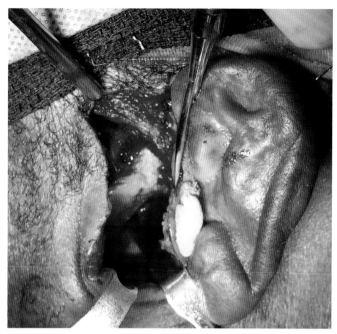

Fig. 3.10.15 Resection of ankylosed bone and establishment of sufficient space for prosthetic components. (Courtesy Dr. Gary Warburton.)

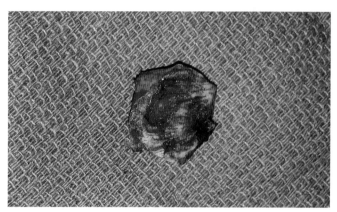

Fig. 3.10.16 Resected ankylotic condylar head. (Courtesy Dr. Gary Warburton.)

root of the zygomatic arch and then elevated in a subperiosteal plane anteriorly to expose the articular eminence, thereby avoiding branches of the facial nerve. Secondly, a retromandibular incision is made to expose the mandibular ramus through a plane of dissection in the deep cervical fascia between the parotid capsule and the sternocleidomastoid muscle towards the lower mandibular border with care to avoid the marginal mandibular branch of the facial nerve. The pterygomasseteric sling is incised and the masseter muscle is then stripped in a superior fashion until the two incisions communicate to allow proper placement of the TMJ prosthesis. Attention can now be directed to performing the condylectomy procedure and where ankylosis has occurred, resection of the ankylosed bone from the fossa is also required, as shown in Fig. 3.10.15. Special care must be taken to avoid injury to the internal maxillary artery, which runs medial to the condylar neck. The articular

eminence is then flattened to a depth determined by the fossa of the prosthesis, using a rasp with its cutting surface depth corresponding accordingly. The surgical field is then completely covered and isolated before turning attention to the oral cavity where the patient is placed in MMF prior to the condylar prosthesis placement. At this stage the range of motion is evaluated and may indicate the need for coronoidectomies. A separate intraoral instrument stand is set up for this stage of the procedure and once complete, the surgeons must change their gowns and gloves before returning to the sterile extraoral surgical field. The fossa component can now be selected using the fossa trial sizers and seated with careful angulation to help prevent the possibility of future anterior dislocation of the prosthetic condyle, achieved by slight inferior positioning of the anterior lip relative to the posterior portion. The fossa component is then secured to the zygomatic bone using 2.0 mm screws. As mentioned earlier, three sizes of the condylar component are available, namely 45 mm, 50 mm, and 55 mm. Using condylar sizers, the most appropriate size is chosen ensuring adequate condylar-fossa component contact. Utilizing both incisions, the condylar prosthesis is placed into position with the condylar head in the correct position

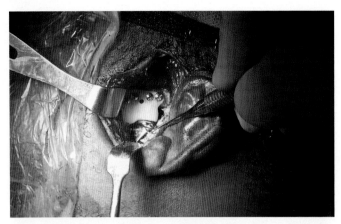

Fig. 3.10.17 Fossa and condylar prosthetic components secured into position while patient is placed in temporary MMF. (Courtesy Dr. Gary Warburton.)

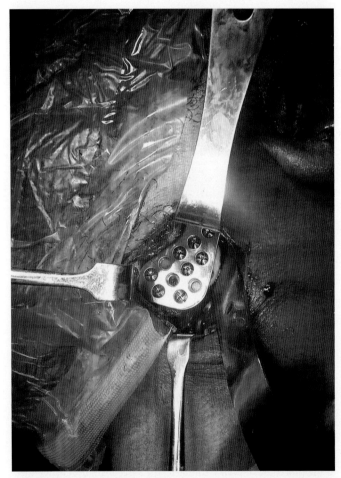

Fig. 3.10.18 Ramal aspect of condylar component screw fixed into position. (Courtesy Dr. Gary Warburton.)

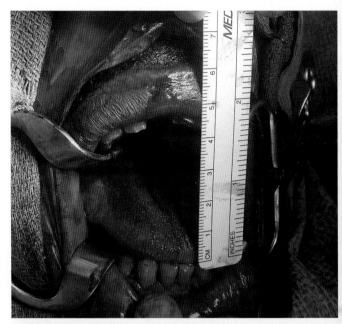

Fig. 3.10.19 Patient released from MMF demonstrating excellent immediate mouth opening. (Courtesy Dr. Gary Warburton.)

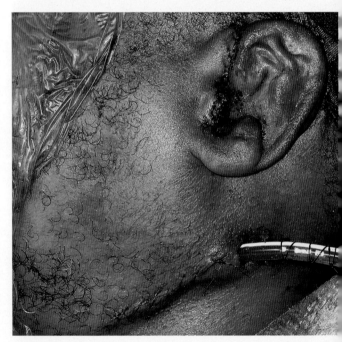

Fig. 3.10.20 Wound closure and drain placement. (Courtesy Dr. Gary Warburton.)

within the fossa component. Taking care to avoid injury to the inferior alveolar nerve, the condylar prosthesis is secured to the mandibular ramus with 2.7 mm bicortical screw fixation as shown in Figs. 3.10.17 and 3.10.18. It is recommended that the fossa and condylar prostheses are fixed provisionally with two screws in each. Before the patient can be released from MMF and mouth opening assessed, once again the extraoral surgical field is isolated in the same fashion. The expected range of mouth opening is approximately 30–35 mm but often more

than this range is achievable, as illustrated in Fig. 3.10.19. If adequate mouth opening is achieved without dislocation, then the surgeon should insert the remaining screws in both fossa and condylar components. Once satisfactory placement is achieved, the surgical site is irrigated and closure is then performed with placement of a drain to reduce the risk of hematoma, as illustrated in Fig. 3.10.20.

COMPLICATIONS

Regardless of the type of surgery performed, it is never without risks or complications and TMJ surgery is no exception. Indeed, when

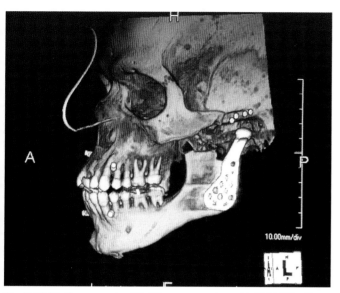

Fig. 3.10.21 Postoperative 3D CT reconstruction with TMJ TJR. (Courtesy Dr. Gary Warburton.)

considering the complex regional anatomy and functional demands on the reconstructed TMJ, complications are an understandable hazard and the TMJ surgeon should be aware of potential adverse outcomes or events and be prepared for their management. Mercuri[43] reported the most common complications resulting in adverse outcomes associated with alloplastic TMJ TJR included periprosthetic joint infection, heterotopic bone formation, dislocation, continued pain and material hypersensitivity. Some of the latter complications can also afflict autologous TMJ reconstructions such as pain and infection, but also graft failure, hyperplasia as seen with CCGs and reankylosis are all problematic.

Postoperative Infection

There are limited data on alloplastic TMJ TJR surgical site infection (SSI) rates but Mercuri and Psutka[44] in 2011 reported an infection rate of 1.51% from a retrospective study analyzing data from 2476 cases with 3368 TMJ TJRs and Speculand[45] in 2009 reported rates between 1.34% and 1.6% analyzing UK data. Infection is broadly classified as either acute, which presents less than 3 weeks, or chronic, which presents at 3 weeks or thereafter, following TMJ TJR surgery.[43] In the acute phase, fever, swelling, erythema and severe pain are typically evident whilst the chronic patient will describe progressive pain, often without fever. Although in both instances there may be purulent discharge, chronic cases may present with skin fistulae. Based on orthopedic principles, early and delayed infections that present within 2 years are regarded to have an etiological origin at the time of surgery while infections presenting beyond this period are more likely to have a hematological origin.[46] The earlier infection is identified and managed, the better the device prognostic outcome.[47] Wound cultures should be taken where possible to identify causal organisms and to initiate effective antibiotic treatment; however, broad-spectrum antibiotics should be started immediately to avoid treatment delay until culture sensitivity results are known and Infectious Disease should be consulted early in the process. Appropriate imaging will help identify drainable collections in addition to confirming device stability. In the chronic state, biofilm formation on the prosthetic surface by the offending organisms render them resistant to host defenses and systemic antimicrobial therapy. In such instances, device removal and aggressive debridement with outpatient antibiotic therapy via a PICC line for 4–6 weeks is considered the appropriate

management with replacement TMJ TJR surgery at 8–10 weeks after initial management, as proposed by Wolford and Rodrigues[47] and supported by Mercuri.[48] Prevention is of critical importance and measures to limit SSI risk should always be adopted. Preoperative optimal management of systemic disease such as diabetes mellitus, smoking cessation, optimizing nutritional status, pretreatment of existing infections, sterile operative technique with proper skin preparation and draping, avoiding device contamination and ensuring intraoperative hemostasis all help limit SSI risk.[48] Preincision prophylactic antibiotics, intraoperative soaking of device components in antibacterial solution or irrigation with antibiotic and limiting the operative time to implant the prostheses are further measures to reduce SSIs.[44]

Persistent Pain

Pain that persists beyond the acute phase despite good early postoperative pain management modalities can be challenging. Common causes such as hardware failure, screw loosening, prosthetic malposition including dislocation, infection, heterotrophic bone formation should be ruled out as potential sources. Scar tissue and even neuroma formation can be contributory and may require operative care. Better preoperative baseline pain and function tend to be good predictors of improved postoperative pain and functional outcomes,[49,50] whereas patients with preoperative anxiety and depression have poorer pain outcomes.[51] Patients with a preoperative neuropathic component to their pain or centrally mediated pain or a myofascial basis of pain are not likely to see this improve with TMJ TJR surgery and although they may experience functional improvement, they may well require specialist pain management services. Indeed, misdiagnosis of the original basis of pain is not uncommon and other etiological factors should also be considered.

Heterotopic Bone Formation

This is the aberrant bone formation in and around the soft tissue surrounding the prosthetic implanted device, which not only causes pain and limits functional motion but if allowed to progress, it bridges across the condylar and fossa components and can lead to reankylosis. To reduce the risk of heterotrophic bone formation, some advocate filling in the dead space around the device components with autologous fat graft,[52] thorough irrigation to remove bone debris and good hemostasis to avoid hematoma formation. Where imaging confirms the presence of such bone then surgical removal is necessary. In cases where there is recurrent formation leading to recurrent ankylosis then localized radiation therapy is suggested.[53]

Other Complications

Limited range of motion may be due to coronoid impingement on the zygomatic arch. This should be recognized at the preoperative planning stage and coronoidectomy may be considered at the same surgical event but otherwise it is not routinely performed. Temporalis tendinitis is painful inflammation of the fibrous insertion at the bony coronoid interface and may only be relieved by surgically stripping off the tendon from the coronoid process. Frey syndrome is a rare complication of TMJ surgery and leads to facial sweating and flushing but can be managed with botulinum toxin administration. Damage to the facial (VII) nerve can occur and the risk increases with repetitive same site surgeries but nerve stimulation perioperatively can reduce the risk. Allergy to the device components may not be apparent until its implantation, however skin testing can be used to confirm suspicions and where positive, removal of the components may become necessary. Loosening of device or screw components is uncommon, particularly where micro-locking screws help limit micro-motion and where there are well-adapted fossa and ramal components.

EXPERT COMMENTARY

This well-written chapter nicely and briefly covers the challenge of replacement of the TM joint, one of the most complex and challenging joints in the body. While great progress has been made in this area, further improvements need to occur in surgical implants, planning, and procedures to address the failed primary trauma repair.

Here, the authors cover the history, indications, and present the case for and against the various techniques and choices of materials. While complete texts have been written on this subject, this chapter serves to introduce the reader to the subject, and the reading and reference list will challenge the more inquisitive practitioner. My recommendation is to seek a regional expert with whom you could consult for these challenging cases, and prepare yourself to expect less than perfection in the result.

REFERENCES

1. Giannakopoulos HE, Quinn PD, Granquist E. Posttraumatic temporomandibular joint disorders. *Craniomaxillofac Trauma Reconstruction.* 2009;2:91–102.
2. Mercuri LG. *Temporomandibular Joint Total Joint Replacement – TMJ TJR.* Basle: Springer International Publishing; 2016:p92–p94.
3. Mercuri LG. The use of alloplastic prostheses for temporomandibular joint reconstruction. *J Oral Maxillofac Surg.* 2000;58(70):75.
4. Samman N, Cheung LK, Tideman H. Overgrowth of a costochondral graft in an adult male. *Int J Oral Maxillofac Surg.* 1995;24:333–335.
5. Ellis E 3rd, Schneiderman ED, Carlson DS. Growth of the mandible after replacement of the mandibular condyle: an experimental investigation in *Macaca mulatta. J Oral Maxillofac Surg.* 2002;60:1461–1470.
6. Obeid G, Guttenberg SA, Connole PW. Costochondral grafting in condylar replacement and mandibular reconstruction. *J Oral Maxillofac Surg.* 1988;48:177–182.
7. He D, Ellis E 3rd, Zhang Y. Etiology of temporomandibular joint ankylosis secondary to condylar fractures: the role of concomitant mandibular fractures. *J Oral Maxillofac Surg.* 2008;66:77–84.
8. Davis B. Late reconstruction of condylar neck and head fractures. *Oral Maxillofacial Surg Clin North Am.* 2013;25:661–681.
9. Mercuri LG. Temporomandibular joint reconstruction. In: Fonseca R, ed. *Oral and Maxillofacial Surgery.* Vol. 51. Philadelphia, PA: Elsevier; 2008:945–960.
10. MacIntosh RB. The use of autogenous tissue in temporomandibular joint reconstruction. *J Oral Maxillofac Surg.* 2000;58:63–69.
11. Sawhney CP. Bony ankylosis of the temporomandibular joint: follow-up of 70 patients with arthroplasty and acrylic spacer interposition. *Plast Reconstr Surg.* 1986;77:29–40.
12. Takahashi T, Ohtani M, Sano T, et al. Magnetic resonance evidence of joint effusion of the temporomandibular joint after fractures of the mandibular condyle: a preliminary report. *J Craniomandib Pract.* 2004;22:1.
13. Goss AN, Bosanquest AG. The arthroscopic appearance of acute temporomandibular joint trauma. *J Oral Maxillofac Surg.* 1990;48:780.
14. Wong PK, Quinn JM, Sims NA, et al. Interleukin-6 modulates production of T lymphocyte-derived cytokines in antigen-induced arthritis and drives inflammation induced osteoclastogenesis. *Arthritis Rheum.* 2006;54:158.
15. Segami N, Miyamaru M, Nishimura M, et al. Does joint effusion on T2 magnetic resonance images reflect synovitis? Part 2. Comparison of concentration levels of proinflammatory cytokines and total protein in synovial fluid of the temporomandibular joint with internal derangements and osteoarthrosis. *Oral Surg Oral Med Oral Pathol Oral Radiol Endod.* 2002;94:515.
16. Nogami S, Takahashi T, Ariyoshi W. Increased levels of interleukin-6 in synovial lavage fluid from patients with mandibular condyle fractures: correlation with magnetic resonance evidence of joint effusion. *J Oral Maxillofac Surg.* 2013;71:1050–1058.
17. Mercuri LG. Alloplastic temporomandibular joint reconstruction. *Oral Surg.* 1998;85:631–637.
18. Takatsuka S, Narinobou M, Nakagawa K, Yamamoto E. Histologic evaluation of articular cartilage grafts after discectomy in the rabbit craniomandibular joint. *J Oral Maxillofac Surg.* 1996;54:1216–1225.
19. Reitzik M. Cortex-to-cortex healing after mandibular osteotomy. *J Oral Maxillofac Surg.* 1983;41:658–663.
20. Lienau J, Schell H, Duda G, et al. Initial vascularization and tissue differentiation are influenced by fixation stability. *J Orthop Res.* 2005;23:639–645.
21. Henry CH, Wolford LM. Treatment outcomes for temporomandibular joint reconstruction after Proplast–Teflon implant failure. *J Oral Maxillofac Surg.* 1993;51:352.
22. Liedberg J, Panmekiate S, Petersson A, Rohlin M. Evidence-based evaluation of three imaging methods for the temporomandibular disc. *Dentomaxillofac Radiol.* 1996;25:234–241.
23. Costa ALF, Yasuda CL, Appenzeller S, et al. Comparison of conventional MRI and 3D reconstruction model for evaluation of temporomandibular joint. *Surg Radiol Anat.* 2008;30:663–667.
24. Lexer E. Joint transplantations and arthroplasty. *Surg Gynecol Obstet.* 1925;40:782–809.
25. Gillies HD. *Plastic Surgery of the Face.* London: Oxford University Press; 1920.
26. MacIntosh RB. The use of autogenous tissues for temporomandibular joint reconstruction. *J Oral Maxillofac Surg.* 2000;58:63–69.
27. Kaban LB, Bouchard C, Troulis MJ. A protocol for management of temporomandibular joint ankylosis in children. *J Oral Maxillofac Surg.* 2009;67:1966–1978.
28. Link JO, Hoffman DC, Laskin DM. Hyperplasia of a costochondral graft in an adult. *J Oral Maxillofac Surg.* 1993;51:1392–1394.
29. Ko EW, Huang CS, Chen YR. Temporomandibular joint reconstruction in children using costochondral grafts. *J Oral Maxillofac Surg.* 1999;57:789–798.
30. Saeed NR, Kent JN. A retrospective study of the costochondral graft in TMJ reconstruction. *Int J Oral Maxillofac Surg.* 2003;32:606–609.
31. Medra AM. Follow up of mandibular costochondral grafts after release of ankylosis of the temporomandibular joints. *Br J Oral Maxillofac Surg.* 2005;43:118.
32. Garcia RG, Gias LN, Campo FJR. Vascularized fibular flap for reconstruction of the condyle after mandibular ablation. *J Oral Maxillofac Surg.* 2008;66:1133–1137.
33. Guyot L, Richard O, Layoun W, et al. Long-term radiological findings following reconstruction of the condyle with fibular free flaps. *J Craniomaxillofac Surg.* 2004;32:98–102.
34. Nahabedian MY, Tufaro A, Manson PN. Improved mandibular function after hemimandibulectomy, condylar head preservation, and vascularized fibular reconstruction. *Ann Plast Surg.* 2001;46:506–510.
35. Saeed NR, Hensher R, McLeod NMH, et al. Reconstruction of the temporomandibular joint autogenous compared with alloplastic. *Br J Oral Maxillofac Surg.* 2002;40:296–299.
36. van Loon JP, de Bont GM, Boering G. Evaluation of temporomandibular joint prostheses: review of the literature from 1946–1994 and implications for future prosthesis designs. *J Oral Maxillofac Surg.* 1995;53:984–996.
37. Jameson SS, Baker PN, Mason J, et al. Independent predictors of failures up to 7.5 years after 35386 single-brand cementless total hip replacements: a retrospective cohort study using National Joint Registry data. *Bone Joint J.* 2013;95B:747–757.
38. Mercuri LG, Wolford LM, Sanders B, et al. Custom CAD/CAM total temporomandibular joint reconstruction system: preliminary multicenter report. *J Oral Maxillofac Surg.* 1995;53:106–115.
39. Mercuri LG, Edibam NR, Giobbie-Hurder A. Fourteen-year follow-up of a patient-fitted total temporomandibular joint reconstruction system. *J Oral Maxillofac Surg.* 2007;65:1140–1148.
40. Wolford LM, Pitta MC, Reiche-Fischel O, et al. TMJ Concepts/Techmedica custom-made TMJ total joint prosthesis: 5-year follow-up study. *Int J Oral Maxillofac Surg.* 2003;32:268–274.

41. Giannakopoulos HE, Sinn DP, Quinn PD. Biomet microfixation temporomandibular joint replacement system: a 3-year follow-up study of patients treated during 1995 to 2005. *J Oral Maxillofac Surg.* 2012;70:787–794, discussion 795–6.

42. Lobo Leandro LF, Ono HY, de Souza Loureiro CC, et al. A 10-year experience and follow-up of three hundred patients fitted with the Biomet/Lorenz microfixation TMJ replacement system. *Int J Oral Maxillofac Surg.* 2013;42:1007–1013.

43. Mercuri LG. *Temporomandibular Joint Total Joint Replacement – TMJ TJR.* Basle: Springer International Publishing; 2016. Ch. 8.

44. Mercuri LG, Psutka D. Perioperative, postoperative, and prophylactic use of antibiotics in alloplastic total temporomandibular joint replacement surgery: a survey and preliminary guidelines. *J Oral Maxillofac Surg.* 2011;69:2106–2111.

45. Speculand B. Current status of replacement of the temporomandibular joint in the United Kingdom. *Br J Oral Maxillofac Surg.* 2009;46:146.

46. Fitzgerald RH Jr, Nolan DR, Ilstrup DM. Deep wound sepsis following total hip arthroplasty. *J Bone Joint Surg.* 1977;59:847–855.

47. Wolford LM, Rodriguehaves DB, McPhillips A. Management of the infected temporomandibular joint total joint prosthesis. *J Oral Maxillofac Surg.* 2010;68:2810–2823.

48. Mercuri LG. Avoiding and managing temporomandibular joint total joint replacement surgical site infections. *J Oral Maxillofac Surg.* 2012;70:2280–2289.

49. Fortin PR, Clarke AE, Joseph L. Outcomes of total hip and knee replacement: preoperative functional status outcomes after surgery. *Arthritis Rheum.* 1999;42:1722–1728.

50. Lingard EA, Katz JN, Wright EA. Predicting outcome of total knee arthroplasty. *J Bone Joint Surg Am.* 2004;86:2179–2186.

51. Wolford LM, Mercuri LG, Schneiderman ED, et al. Twenty-year follow-up study on a patient-fitted temporomandibular joint prosthesis: the Techmedica/TMJ Concepts device. *J Oral Maxillofac Surg.* 2015;73(5):952–960.

52. Movahed R, Mercuri LG. Management of temporomandibular joint ankylosis. *Oral Maxillofacial Surg Clin North Am.* 2015;27:27–35.

53. Reid R, Cooke H. Postoperative ionizing radiation in the management of heterotopic bone formation in the temporomandibular joint. *J Oral Maxillofac Surg.* 1999;57:900–905.

Maxillofacial Prosthodontics

Ghassan G. Sinada, Majd Al Mardini, Marcelo Suzuki

BACKGROUND

The replacement of missing structures in the head and neck region has been a concern for many centuries, with the fabrication of maxillofacial prosthetic restorations being mentioned since the 16th century, with the first mention often credited to Ambroise Paré in 1541.[1–3] Although the concern was often the restoration of a pleasing appearance, addressing the functional disruption was also part of the treatment, with clinicians being able to achieve the desired outcome with varying degrees of success.

Maxillofacial prosthetics is often described as "the art and science of anatomic, functional, or cosmetic reconstruction by means of nonliving substitutes of those regions in the maxilla, mandible, and the face that are missing or defective because of surgical intervention, trauma, pathology, developmental or congenital malformation."[2]

Maxillofacial prosthetic rehabilitation is best understood when the treatment is put in context with the overall patient care. In order to achieve the desired outcome, head and neck surgeons, plastic surgeons, oral surgeons, and the maxillofacial prosthodontist should all be involved in the treatment plan process, so proper site preparation in anticipation of prosthetic reconstruction can be successful. The concept of multidisciplinary care is very evident in the management of patients who will require maxillofacial prosthetic rehabilitation, as this interaction will facilitate the fabrication of a prosthesis, which can restore the patient to near normal function and esthetics in many cases.

The general goals when dealing with maxillofacial patients should be to restore form, function, and esthetics.[1–4] Prosthodontic rehabilitation aims to create maintainable health for the total masticatory system. This means freedom from disease in all masticatory structures, a healthy maintainable periodontium, stable temporomandibular joints, stable occlusion, healthy maintainable teeth, comfortable function, and of course, optimum esthetics. Practicing without a clear and comprehensive understanding of these goals exacts a costly penalty in missed diagnosis, unpredictable treatment results, and lost productive time.[5]

Prosthetic reconstruction of the trauma patient can be difficult due to the deformity created and the loss of vital structures. Oftentimes the construction may not be accomplished without several revisions on the site. Initial treatment will always involve closing the wound and stabilizing the patient, so prosthetic reconstruction does not become a relevant aspect of treatment until several months after the initial incident.[6–8]

ORAL AND DENTAL ANATOMY EVALUATION

It is important for the medical personnel treating head and neck patients (otolaryngologists, plastic surgeons, and speech pathologists, among others) to understand the oral cavity and dental anatomy, so they can identify and accurately communicate findings with their dental colleagues, as teeth and anatomical landmarks of the jaws are usually used as reference for the prosthetic planning before and after the surgery. In general terms, the most commonly used scheme for identification of adult teeth involves the sequential numbering (from 1 to 32) starting from the right maxillary third molar (tooth number 1), and moving across to the contralateral third molar (tooth 16), starting again from the lower left third molar (tooth 17) across to the right mandibular third molar (tooth 32). All missing and impacted teeth should be counted in this system. Anatomical structures of importance for retention and support of prostheses include the tuberosity, alveolar ridge, the hard palate on the maxilla, the alveolar ridge, the retromolar pad, and buccal shelf on the mandible.

An essential principle in prosthodontics is the determination of the correct physiologic maxillo-to-mandibular position.[4] This relationship must always be determined before we can determine the correct alignment and occlusal position of a prosthesis. The maxilla is affixed to the skull and the mandible can be considered a moving entity. As such, the functional movements of the mandible constitute the most fundamental basis for ideal prosthesis design. Therefore, we must consider the envelope of function as it is not merely an academic exercise. The range and limits of mandibular movement are indirectly related to the limits imposed by the postsurgical anatomy. Surgery affects the maxillomandibular ligaments, bone, muscle, and the temporomandibular joints. How much or how little varies from person to person and is affected by the surgery.

It is also important for those involved in treatment to be able to recognize the oral pathology resulting from poor oral health status. For example, advanced periodontal disease, gross dental caries, and excessive plaque and calculus formation are indicators of poor oral hygiene. These findings should be noted when referring the patient to the clinician who will perform a thorough radiographic and dental examination. Commonly in trauma patients previous dental casts are not available, so this examination may include acquisition of impressions from dental and facial structures as needed. The casts fabricated from these impressions can be used as aids in the treatment planning and posttreatment rehabilitation. Furthermore, the identification of hopeless teeth (i.e., severely decayed, extensive fractures) that need to be extracted will be made as well as weighing the need for any restorative treatments. Assessment of available soft and hard tissue can also be done at this appointment and, if possible, further advance imaging is obtained to evaluate available bone for future placement of osseointegrated dental implants.

Preservation of tissue at the time of surgery should be carefully examined, as it may require further revisions of the surgical site, as the remaining tissue can create challenges during prosthetic reconstruction.[8,9] It is important for the surgeon and the prosthodontist to understand the limitations of each case to better prepare the site for future prosthetic reconstruction.[6,8,10]

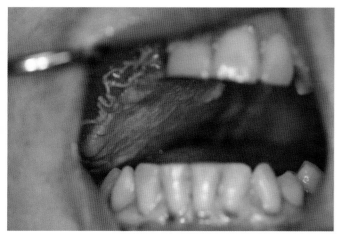

Fig. 3.11.1 Bulky free flap reconstruction, preventing the possibility of prosthetic reconstruction.

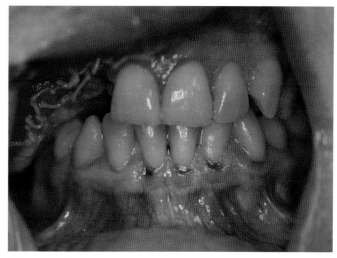

Fig. 3.11.2 Teeth opposing the reconstructed site contacting the free flap reconstruction. This can cause severe damage to the tissue and should be avoided.

Assaults, motor vehicle collisions, falls, and gunshot wounds are the major causes of fractures in the head and neck area. The resultant defect can significantly impact the patient functions, as the separation between the oral and nasal cavity can be compromised, causing air leakage during normal functions.[6,7]

Ideally, the defect created can be reconstructed with primary closure. This is the best outcome for the patient, as little to no disruption will occur. However, the defect created can be too big for primary closure to occur, and hard and soft tissue transfers to reconstruct the area are not possible due to concerns regarding morbidity of the donor site, cost of the procedure and hospitalization time, patient desire to avoid further surgery, or other health problems. In these situations, reconstruction with a prosthesis is indicated.[2]

During the initial fracture reductions and reconstruction, it is important to preserve as much as possible of the existing structures.[2,3,4,6,8] For instance, if the patient is edentulous, the hard palate is responsible for primary retention, support, and stability of a prosthesis. Without compromising the surgical outcome, surgeons should be encouraged to preserve as much of the hard palate and alveolar bone as possible. On a dentate patient, besides the preservation of bone, maintaining key teeth can dramatically improve prosthetic outcome, as the remaining dentition can be used for retention and stability.

As is often the case, a revision surgery may be required to further improve the reconstruction or address some common problems (i.e., excessive tissue scarring and contractures) to help the patient regain normal or close to normal function. During this revision procedure, if prosthetic reconstruction is going to be recommended, the consideration for lining the surgical site with keratinized tissue should be made, as a split-thickness skin graft placed during the surgical procedure – after a few weeks of maturation – can be easily maintained by the patient, in addition to being a stable area for the prosthesis. Also, during closure of the wound, the surgeon should remove any tissue tags or redundant tissue, as these structures can prevent proper prosthetic extension.[2-5]

If reconstruction using free tissue flaps is planned, an attempt should be made to keep the flap from being too bulky, as this extra tissue will require subsequent surgical revisions to allow proper space for the fabrication of a prosthesis (Figs. 3.11.1 and 3.11.2).

It is important also to emphasize that in an ideal situation, a team approach will be used from the beginning of treatment. This will result in the best outcome for patient rehabilitation.[2,3,4,6,7,8,11]

INTRAORAL PROSTHETIC REHABILITATION

The maxillofacial prosthetic rehabilitation is usually achieved in three different phases: surgical, interim, and definitive. This process usually is completed within a year, depending on the clinical situation and treatment needs.

The surgical phase occurs at the time of surgery; in the case of the maxilla, when a surgical obturator is placed to reestablish the separation between the oral and nasal cavities, while restoring proper palatal contour. This is a very important procedure, as the prosthesis will help maintain proper speech and swallowing function immediately after surgery, thus decreasing the need for a nasogastric tube, and speed recovery and discharge from the hospital. The surgical obturator will also serve to maintain proper lip and cheek support during the initial healing, and decrease the facial contracture that can happen due to scarring of the tissues. Finally, this prosthesis will serve to maintain a split-thickness skin graft in place, which is part of site preparation for prosthetic reconstruction. In the case of traumatic injury, this step is usually not possible as the fabrication of the surgical prosthesis cannot be accomplished prior to the surgery.

After initial healing has taken place (10–14 days), the surgical obturator is replaced with an interim obturator. While a surgical obturator may not have replaced any missing teeth as a result of the surgery, the interim obturator will most likely have teeth so the patient can slowly attempt to return to normal function. This prosthesis will be adjusted constantly as the surgical site heals, and the defect created will be changing in size and shape. The adjustments will require addition or removal of material accordingly, so optimal separation between oral and nasal cavity is maintained.

Once the healing of the surgical site has been completed, the fabrication of the definitive obturator begins. This prosthesis will further enhance esthetics and function.

In cases of mandibular involvement, the initial evaluation is very similar to that of the maxilla. However, it is important to emphasize that proper maintenance of the alignment of the remaining segments after the fracture reduction is a crucial step for subsequent prosthetic rehabilitation. If the alignment of the remaining mandible to the glenoid fossa and the temporomandibular joint is disrupted, damage to the surrounding areas will occur and the patient's normal mandibular motions will be affected, resulting in an improper occlusion. As a

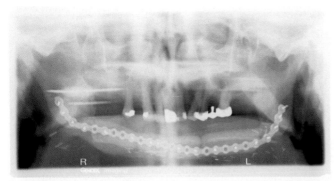

Fig. 3.11.3 Panoramic X-ray showing the fibula free flap reconstruction of the mandible.

consequence, the prosthetic reconstruction will be less than ideal, if not impossible.

To maintain proper alignment of the mandibular segments during mandibular surgery, the utilization of fixation plates and screws is a commonly available technique.[12] If no mandibular reconstruction is being planned due to the amount of tissue loss, the removal of the condyle and the remaining ramus on the affected side should be completed, to prevent the medial migration towards the maxilla, and decrease the chances of complications due to compromised function and prosthetic rehabilitation.[2–4]

Reconstructive surgery using free flaps and bone transplantation has greatly improved the surgical outcome for patients requiring a surgical procedure, which will affect the continuity of the mandible[12] (Fig. 3.11.3). Virtual surgical planning utilizing CT scans can also allow the members of the surgical and reconstructive team to rehearse the procedures to be done, and evaluate the outcome. This has become an invaluable tool, allowing for the fabrication of individualized reconstruction plates,[13] cutting guides for the harvesting of bone grafts,[14,15] and stents for the placement of osseointegrated dental implants.[15]

The placement of a split-thickness skin graft in conjunction with vestibuloplasty surgery will help reestablish a stable tissue foundation for the prosthesis.[2–4] These procedures, along with the utilization of osseointegrated implants, have made the fabrication of a stable mandibular prosthesis a predictable treatment modality.[15–20]

Prosthetic rehabilitation follows a similar pattern to that applied to the maxilla. A surgical prosthesis would usually be in place to help stabilize a split-thickness skin graft and to recreate the vestibule in preparation for the final prosthesis. The interim prosthesis will help reestablish the occlusal relationship and help the patient learn how to function and maintain the prosthesis. The final or definitive mandibular prosthesis will be fabricated once complete healing is achieved and the site is mature for reconstruction.

SOFT PALATE EVALUATION

When a defect involving the soft palate is present, the first decision needs to be a determination if surgical reconstruction is possible or not, as disruptions to the soft palate will cause severe problems with speech and swallow and as a consequence, severely impair the patient's overall quality of life.[21]

Soft palate reconstruction is often difficult, and although surgical techniques involving free tissue transfers have been developed and utilized to address these defects, rehabilitation with a prosthesis can deliver a successful and predictable result; although the results are not comparable to preoperative baseline measurements.[22,23]

When the soft palate is involved, a determination should be made whether the remaining soft palate will be useful in the prosthetic rehabilitation or not. Usually, the remaining soft palate is nonfunctional, and its removal will allow for easier access to the pharynx and the fabrication of the prosthesis. In short, the normal velopharyngeal closure occurs with the medial and anterior movement of the lateral and posterior pharyngeal walls contacting the posteriorly and superiorly lifting velum. Lateral soft palate defects can be easily restored with the addition of a pharyngeal extension to the prosthesis. Small mid-soft palate defects are generally harder to restore, especially when located close to the junction of the hard and soft palate. These patients will usually have problems with fluid leakage due to the mobility of the area during function.

A total soft palatectomy can facilitate the prosthetic rehabilitation, as it will create a static velar prosthesis. The appliance will be molded to the moving posterior and lateral pharyngeal walls at the anterior extent of their movement during speech and swallowing, creating an appropriate seal during these functions.

The decision to maintain or remove the soft palate should be discussed when further surgical revisions are being planned, as this can affect the success of the prosthetic outcome. Clinical experience and understanding of the prosthetic soft palate rehabilitation can better prepare the surgeon for making the final decision of whether to remove or maintain the remaining soft palate.

TONGUE EVALUATION

Lesions to the tongue are usually one of the most challenging problems both surgically and prosthetically. Loss of part or all of the tongue will disrupt proper swallowing, speech, and saliva control, in addition to the possible facial disfigurement caused by the injury. The majority of injuries are a result of falls, seizures, blunt force mechanisms, or an iatrogenic cause. Often, the injury created is minor and no treatment may be indicated, as the wound will heal on its own.[24]

An understanding of how normal speech is produced is important in the rehabilitation process, so the prosthetic treatment can be tailored to address the specific impairment the patient is experiencing.[25] In the case where the anterior portion of the tongue is lost, a significant interference with speech intelligibility will be noted. In such a scenario, a consultation with a speech pathologist is an extremely valuable tool for the successful rehabilitation of the patient.[2,3,26] In most cases the defect created is small and mobility of the tongue is not greatly affected. For such conditions the prosthesis of choice may be a palatal augmentation prosthesis.[2,3,27] This prosthesis will have the palatal portion recontoured to compensate for the lack of appropriate movement after the trauma. Further follow-ups with the speech pathologist will help determine the areas where the prosthesis will need to be further adjusted, to optimize the patient's speech and swallowing.

If the patient is missing the majority of the tongue bulk, a prosthesis replacing it will need to be individually evaluated in an attempt to determine its success,[26,27] but usually the prognosis is poor[28] due to the impairment to normal functions the loss of the tongue will create. In this scenario, the surgical reconstruction with a free flap, to add bulk to the floor of the mouth, can improve function by creating bulk in the oral cavity to decrease resonance,[29] and can also facilitate the prosthetic rehabilitation by decreasing the needed extent of the palatal augmentation prosthesis to contact the remaining tongue.

EXTRAORAL EVALUATION

Extraoral defects can involve severe tissue loss and deformity. Vehicular collisions (car, motorcycle, bicycle), assaults, and gunshot wounds are

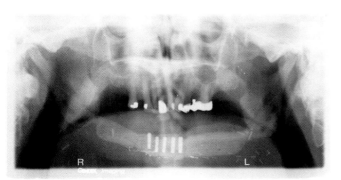

Fig. 3.11.4 Placement of mandibular implants and removal of reconstruction plate after healing. Removal of reconstruction plates can facilitate the placement of implants, since fixation screws are not interfering with osteotomies for implants.

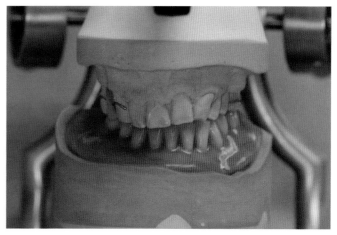

Fig. 3.11.5 Maxillary and mandibular casts mounted on semiadjustable articulator (Hanau Wide-Vue, Whip Mix Corp., Louisville, KY) and teeth arrangement of mandibular prosthesis.

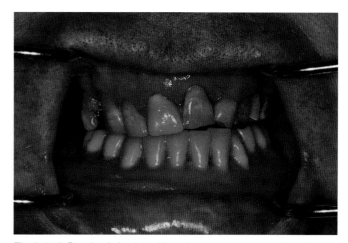

Fig. 3.11.6 Prosthesis in place. Note the accurate reproduction of teeth relationship.

the major causes of facial injuries. However, improvements in safety (use of seat belts, air-bags, and helmet wear) have dramatically reduced the numbers of facial trauma associated with vehicle injuries, with minor trauma as a result. Assaults usually produce facial fractures easily managed with "routine" maxillofacial reconstructive surgery.

Gunshot wounds produce more severe tissue loss and deformity. An entry and an exit wound will be created, with damage caused initially by the speed of the projectile, followed by bone fragments serving as secondary projectiles, causing further soft tissue damage on the exit wound. The type of firearm, location of the initial contact, and angle will further affect the defect created.

As noted earlier, the first concern should always be the stabilization of the patient and reduction of fractures when possible. Surgical revisions and reconstructions (prior to any prosthetic consideration) will be paramount to the successful rehabilitation of such patients, as well as proper psychological support.

Other possible causes of facial wounds are burns (electrical or acid), which often cause severe deformation with little to no tissue loss. These wounds may cause deformities that cannot be addressed with plastic surgery or prosthetics, and consideration should be given to a larger procedure (alloplastic transplantation) to restore the patient.

OSSEOINTEGRATED DENTAL IMPLANTS

The location of osseointegrated dental implants should be driven by the prosthetic needs of the treatment[30] (Fig. 3.11.4). This will ensure proper occlusion and function. Dental implants help in the retention of fixed,[30] removable[30] or extraoral prostheses.[31] The most common design of dental implants is the root-form design.[30,32] Implants can be placed in one or two stages. In general, the first stage is the placement of the implant in bone. Once placed, the site is closed and the implant is left covered and healing for 3 to 6 months for optimal osseous growth around the implant. This phenomenon is called osseointegration, which is defined as "intimate bone contact to the surface of an implantable biomaterial, detectable under optical microscope observation."[33] The second stage will have the implants uncovered and a healing cap or screw will be placed to allow for their use in the prosthetic phase of the treatment (Fig. 3.11.5).

Osseointegrated dental implants have been utilized routinely in dentistry for years, and their use for the rehabilitation of maxillofacial defects has become a common treatment choice to overcome the challenges in anatomy, and the lack of a stable tissue bed for prosthetic rehabilitation[15–18,34,35] (Fig. 3.11.6).

CONCLUSION

The common goal of the surgeon and prosthodontist should be to preserve and restore. The postsurgical condition of the mandible and the maxilla, the remaining musculature, and the oral mucosa is of major importance. These are the foundation tissues that must support every rehabilitative prosthodontic effort. Dental complications are directly proportional to the degree that these tissues are compromised by surgery. Surgical preparation for prosthodontic rehabilitation provides better results. A combined clinical evaluation should include:
1. Assessment of existing oral structures and their function.
2. Retaining or removing teeth.
3. Placement of osseointegrated implants.
4. Creating and maintaining intraocclusal space within the oral cavity.
5. Providing as much immobile tissues on load-bearing areas as possible.

In prosthodontic rehabilitation, surgical preparation and planning from the start of the case leads to more successful outcomes. The team should understand how surgery can impact the oral health of the patient. Whether to retain or remove teeth should be based on the defect in the area and what is best to restore that defect. The focus should be on the prosthodontic rehabilitation to achieve function, and that in turn guides the surgical plan.

The surgeon and prosthodontist should collaborate to preserve and restore tissues to a normal condition. The tissue must function in its anatomical place. However, if that tissue obstructs normal function, preserving it will impede the rehabilitation. In the latter case, better results may be achieved with a prosthesis. Surgical reconstruction alone may be the ideal choice for treatment, however, in most cases surgery is combined with prosthetic rehabilitation to achieve the best results possible.

EXPERT COMMENTARY

There are situations where reconstructive surgery is either not possible (globe, etc.) or not chosen by the patient, or where other comorbidities suggest the use of suitable prostheses. Therefore, every cancer surgeon of the head and neck, and every facial trauma surgeon should have good and frequent conversations with an excellent facial prosthetics expert about their patients' difficult problems, and it is the duty of the facial surgeon to consider and suggest that these opinions be obtained as suitable for their patients. Patients will then have the information to make more educated and complete decisions about their future care and options.

The patients will be grateful that this option has been explored, and frequently these options supplement and improve the results from standard surgical solutions. The patient's quality of life is frequently dramatically improved by these additions, and the patient is often grateful that long and complicated surgical options are not pursued. A long-term and good relationship with an excellent maxillofacial prosthodontist will be very beneficial to patients, and will reward the surgical practitioner with patients who are grateful that all options have been considered.

REFERENCES

1. Aramany MA. A history of prosthetic management of cleft palate: Paré to Suersen. *Cleft Palate J.* 1971;8:415–430.
2. Taylor TD, ed. *Clinical Maxillofacial Prosthetics.* Chicago, IL: Quintessence Publishing; 2000.
3. Beumer IIIJ, Marunick MT, Esposito SJ. *Maxillofacial Rehabilitation: Prosthodontic and Surgical Management of Cancer-Related, Acquired, and Congenital Defects of the Head and Neck.* 3rd ed. Chicago, IL: Quintessence Publishing.
4. Martin JW, Lemon JC, King GE. Oral and facial restoration with prosthetics. In: Knoll SS, ed. *Reconstructive Plastic Surgery for Cancer.* St. Louis, MO: 1996:130–138.
5. Dawson PE. *Functional Occlusion: From TMJ to Smile Design.* St. Louis, MO: Mosby Elsevier.
6. Kelly JF. Maxillofacial missile wounds: evaluation of long-term results of rehabilitation and reconstruction. *J Oral Surg.* 1973;31(6):438–447.
7. Wiens JP. Acquired maxillofacial defects from motor vehicle accidents: statistics and prosthodontic considerations. *J Prosthet Dent.* 1990;63(2):172–181.
8. King GE, Martin JW, Lemon JC, et al. Maxillofacial prosthetic rehabilitation combined with plastic and reconstructive surgery. *Compendium.* 1993;14(11):1390, 93–94, 96–99.
9. Robb GL, Marunick MT, Martin JW, et al. Midface reconstruction: surgical reconstruction versus prosthesis. *Head Neck.* 2001;23:48–58.
10. Sharma AB, Beumer J 3rd. Reconstruction of maxillary defects: the case for prosthetic rehabilitation. *J Oral Maxillofac Surg.* 2005;63(12):1770–1773.
11. Hickey AJ. Maxillofacial prosthetic rehabilitation following self-inflicted gunshot wounds to the head and neck. *J Prosthet Dent.* 1986;55–78.
12. Fonseca RJ, et al. *Oral and Maxillofacial Surgery.* Vol 3. Trauma. Philadelphia, PA: W.B. Saunders; 2000.
13. Kokosis G, Davidson EH, Pedreira R, et al. The use of computer-aided design and manufacturing in acute mandibular trauma reconstruction. *J Oral Maxillofac Surg.* 2018;76(5):1036–1043.
14. Ramella V, Franchi A, Bottosso S, et al. Triple-cut computer-aided design-computer-aided modeling: more oncologic safety added to precise mandibular modeling. *J Oral Maxillofac Surg.* 2017;75:1567.e1–1567.e6.
15. Tian T, Zhang T, Ma Q, et al. Digital workflow from visualized iliac bone grafting to implant restoration. *J Oral Maxillofac Surg.* 2017;75:1403.e1–1403.e10.
16. Bidra AS, Veeranki AN. Surgical and prosthodontic reconstruction of a gunshot injury of the mandible using dental implants and an acrylic resin fixed prosthesis: a clinical report. *J Prosthet Dent.* 2010;104:142–148.
17. August M, Bast B, Jackson M, Perrott D. Use of the fixed mandibular implant in oral cancer patients: a retrospective study. *J Oral Maxillofac Surg.* 1998;56(3):297–301.
18. Chiapasco M, Abati S, Ramundo G, et al. Behavior of implants in bone grafts or free flaps after tumor resection. *Clin Oral Implants Res.* 2000;11(1):66–75.
19. Goh BT, Lee S, Tideman H, Stoelinga PJW. Mandibular reconstruction in adults: a review. *Int J Oral Maxillofac Surg.* 2008;37:597–605.
20. Parel SM, Branemark PI, Jansson T. Osseointegration in maxillofacial prosthetics. Part I: Intraoral applications. *J Prosthet Dent.* 2004;55(4):490–494.
21. Seikaly H, Rieger J, Zalmanowitz J, et al. Functional soft palate reconstruction: a comprehensive surgical approach. *Head Neck.* 2008;30(12):1615–1623.
22. Bohle G, Rieger J, Huryn J, et al. Efficacy of speech aid prostheses for acquired defect of the soft palate and velopharyngeal inadequacy. Clinical assessments and cephalometric analysis: a memorial Sloan-Kettering Study. *Head Neck.* 2005;27:195–207.
23. Yoshida H, Michi K-I, Yamashita Y, Ohno K. A comparison of surgical and prosthetic treatment for speech disorders attributable to surgically acquired soft palate defects. *J Oral Maxillofac Surg.* 1993;51:361–363.
24. Bringhurst C, Herr RD, Aldous JA. Oral trauma in the emergency department. *Am J Emerg Med.* 1993;11(5):486–490.
25. McKinstry RE, Aramany MA, Beery QC, Sansone F. Speech considerations in prosthodontic rehabilitation of the glossectomy patient. *J Prosthet Dent.* 1985;53(3):384–387.
26. Lauciello FR, Vergo T, Schaaf NG, Zimmerman R. Prosthodontic and speech rehabilitation after partial and complete glossectomy. *J Prosthet Dent.* 1980;43(2):204–211.
27. Aramany MA, Downs JA, Beery QC, Aslan Y. Prosthodontic rehabilitation for glossectomy patient. *J Prosthet Dent.* 1982;48(1):78–81.
28. Taicher S, Bergen SF. Maxillary polydimethylsiloxane glossal prostheses. *J Prosthet Dent.* 1981;46(1):71–77.
29. Urken ML, Moscoso JF, Lawson W, et al. A systematic approach to functional reconstruction of the oral cavity following partial and total glossectomy. *Arch Otolaryngol Head Neck Surg.* 1994;120(6):589–601.
30. Misch CE. *Dental Implant Prosthetics.* 2nd ed. St. Louis, MO: Mosby Elsevier.
31. Parel SM, Branemark P-I, Tjellstrom A, Gion G. Osseointegration in maxillofacial prosthetics. Part II: Extraoral applications. *J Prosthet Dent.* 2003;55(5):600–606.
32. Misch CE. *Contemporary Implant Dentistry.* 3rd ed. St. Louis, MO: Mosby Elsevier; 2008.
33. Albrektsson T, Branemark P-I, Hansson HA, et al. Osseointegrated titanium implants. Requirements for ensuring a long-lasting, direct bone-to-implant anchorage in man. *Acta Orthop Scand.* 1981;52:155.
34. Huryn JM, Zlotolow IM, Piro JD, Lenchewski E. Osseointegrated implants in microvascular fibula free flap reconstructed mandibles. *J Prosthet Dent.* 1993;70:443–446.
35. Ch'ng S, Skoracki RJ, Sleber JC, et al. Osseointegrated implant-based dental rehabilitation in head and neck reconstruction patients. *Head Neck.* 2016;38(suppl 1):E321–E327.

Custom Craniofacial Implants

Jeffrey Lee, Chad Gordon, Michael J. Yaremchuk

BACKGROUND

Craniofacial injuries are ideally treated in the acute setting. In certain circumstances, it is appropriate for treatment to be delayed. Resuscitation and treatment of life-threatening injuries in multiple trauma victims may preclude facial trauma treatment. For example, the treatment for patients with intracranial hemorrhage involves removal of portions of the skull for surgical access. The resulting brain and dural injuries are addressed acutely, but the bony reduction is sometimes suboptimal or delayed, resulting in deformity. By necessity, resultant deformities are generally treated in a delayed fashion.

For delayed reconstructions, computer-aided design (CAD) and computer-aided manufacturing (CAM) implants can be a valuable adjunct. They can provide near anatomical replication of the cranial vault and facial skeleton. If one side of the face or vault is uninjured it can be "mirrored" to reconstruct the injured side. If that is not possible, the surgeon can design implants appropriate for the situation.

The use of alloplastic materials in the reconstruction of craniofacial deformities has both inherent advantages and limitations. The use of alloplasts avoids the morbidity of autogenous bone harvest. The use of CAD/CAM implants avoids intraoperative carpentry and therefore significantly reduces operative time. However, because alloplastic materials do not integrate into the bony skeleton, they are only used as non-load-bearing onlays except for the cranial vault, where they replace missing skull to restore contour and protect the brain.

CLINICAL PRESENTATION

Calvarial Deformity

These patients are typically ones who have undergone significant head trauma, often resulting in intracranial hemorrhage and emergent craniectomy. After an extended hospital course, they are often discharged to a rehabilitation facility and may regain some or most of their neurological function depending on their age. By the time they present for secondary reconstruction, they may have a noticeable depression at their craniectomy site. Some patients also undergo neurological deterioration that is related to the "Syndrome of the Trephined." This syndrome, also known as "sunken skin flap syndrome," is a poorly understood entity. It is characterized largely by neurological deficits after craniectomy and subsequent improvement after cranioplasty. Although the spectrum of deficits varies widely, most of the reported cases involve motor weakness, cognitive deficits, language deficits, or a combination of the three. In a recent literature review, the only consistent characteristic of those affected by the syndrome of the trephined was that greater than 90% exhibited a visibly sunken skin flap. Most patients have an improvement in their deficits within days after cranioplasty. Unfortunately, the pathophysiology is unknown. One of the leading theories is that the change in pressure seen by the brain without the structural support of the calvarium changes brain physiology, thereby causing neurological deficits.

Midface Deformity

These patients have typically undergone blunt facial trauma with subsequent facial fractures. Depending on the trauma burden, their facial fractures may or may not be treated operatively in the acute setting. For example, there may be a displaced zygoma fracture in a patient with concomitant head trauma and extremely labile vital signs which preclude operative repair. If the patient does not become stable within the first 4 weeks, repair may be deferred entirely. Alternatively, if a patient does have operative repair of facial fractures but the reduction is not perfect, they may still end up with facial asymmetries. In either case, patients present with facial deformities in a delayed fashion and have facial asymmetries such as brow malposition, lack of malar projection, enophthalmos, and/or lack of infraorbital rim definition.

Mandible Deformity

These patients have typically sustained a Le Fort pattern midface fracture as well as a mandible fracture. Operative treatment is aimed at restoring normal occlusion and involves open reduction, internal fixation, and sometimes maxillomandibular fixation. These are severe injury patterns and perfect bony reduction and facial symmetry are sometimes compromised in favor of achieving perfect occlusion. Depending on the location of the mandibular fractures, various parts of the mandible may be displaced to create a mandibular asymmetry, deformity, or bony step-offs that can be bothersome and warrant reconstruction.

RADIOLOGICAL EVALUATION

Dedicated CT scans of the face with thin cuts are the optimal imaging modality when evaluating a patient with posttraumatic deformity. These can be reformatted to create 3-dimensional reconstructions that can aid in creating molds for surgical planning or virtually designing custom implants.

CAD/CAM FACIAL IMPLANTS

Computerized tomographic (CT) scans are fundamental to CAD/CAM facial implant technology. Implementation of CAD/CAM implants is a multi-step process. It requires a CT scan with sufficient data to reconstruct an accurate 3D image. The resultant image can be used to design an implant virtually or to create a model of the 3D image on which an implant design is fashioned. Implants are subsequently manufactured using milling or 3D printing techniques.

This allows for millimeter precise assessment of the contour deficit: symmetry, height, width, projection, and its relationship to the entire facial skeleton. Applying knowledge of the normal skeletal relationship and aesthetic criteria, virtual surgery can be performed to design and to correct the posttraumatic deformities.

Implant Materials

Various materials are available for CAD/CAM implants. These include silicone rubber (Implantech, Ventura, CA), polyetheretherketone (PEEK, Johnson & Johnson), porous polyethylene (MEDPOR, Stryker Corporation, Kalamazoo, MI; OMNIPORE, Matrix Surgical, Atlanta, GA), and a porous composite material (HTR, Biomet, Jacksonville, FLA).

Each material has its advantages and disadvantages.

Silicone

Solid silicone or the silicone rubber used for facial implants is a vulcanized form of polysiloxane. Solid silicone has the following advantages: it can be sterilized by steam or irradiation, it can be carved with either a scissors or scalpel, and it can be stabilized with a screw or a suture. Because it is smooth, it can be removed quite easily. Disadvantages include the tendency to cause resorption of bone underlying it, particularly when used to augment the chin, the potential to migrate if not fixed, and the potential for its fibrous capsule to be visible when placed under a thin soft tissue cover.

Custom PEEK (Polyetheretherketone)

PEEK implants are extremely hard and inflexible. PEEK is most often used for cranial vault reconstruction where long incisions are possible allowing excellent exposure and access for implant placement. The more limited exposure for midface and mandible onlay reconstruction often requires PEEK implants to be segmented to allow implant placement. This makes reconstruction more tedious and time-consuming. Its rigidity precludes any imperfections in design to be accommodated by intraoperative manipulations of the implant.

Porous Polyethylene

Polyethylene is a simple carbon chain of ethylene monomer. The high density, porous variety – Medpor (Porex, Fairborn, GA) and Omnipore (Matrix Surgical, Atlanta, GA) – is used for facial implants because of its higher tensile strength. Its firm consistency resists material compression while still permitting some flexibility. It has an intramaterial porosity between 125 and 250 µm, which allows some fibrous ingrowth. The porosity of Medpor® and Omnipore has both advantages and disadvantages. The advantages of porous polyethylene include its tendency to allow soft tissue ingrowth, thereby lessening its tendency to migrate and to erode underlying bone. Its firm consistency allows it to be easily fixed with screws and contoured with a scalpel or power equipment without fragmenting. However, its porosity causes soft tissue to adhere to it, making placement more difficult and requiring a larger pocket to be made than with smoother implants. The soft tissue ingrowth also makes implant removal more difficult than with smooth surface implants. This material is the implant material of choice for the senior author [M.J.Y.].

HTR

HTR derives its name from the acronym for "hard tissue replacement" (Biomet, Jacksonville, FL). It is a porous composite of polymethylmethacrylate and polyhydroxyethyl methacrylate which allows some soft tissue ingrowth. A calcium hydroxide coating imparts a negative surface charge to encourage bony ingrowth and deter adhesion of bacteria to the implant. It is inflexible and relatively brittle, making implant placement through limited access and fixation difficult.

Indications

CAD/CAM implants have utility for calvarial, midface, and mandible reconstruction. CAD/CAM implants are most often used to reconstruct areas of skull loss. Defects may result from direct trauma, surgical decompression of intracranial pressure, or infection after craniotomy. Cranioplasty protects the brain from environmental trauma while restoring preinjury appearance facilitating integration into society. Cranioplasty often improves neurological function in those afflicted by the "Syndrome of the Trephined." CAD/CAM techniques using mirroring techniques of contralateral intact anatomy allow near anatomic preinjury contour. In addition to the aesthetic benefit, a preformed implant significantly decreases operative time.

Requisites for successful cranioplasty include avoiding implant contamination by communication with the frontal sinuses, ethmoid, or mastoid, elimination of dead space for fluid communication between the implant and the brain, appropriate fixation, and adequate soft tissue coverage. Fig. 3.12.1 shows a failed alloplastic cranial implant reconstruction resulting from frontal sinus communication and dead space between the implant and brain. Reconstruction required removal of the contaminated implant, isolation of the frontal sinus, obliteration of the dead space with a free tissue transfer, and tissue expander scalp reconstruction to assure adequate soft tissue coverage of the CAD/CAM porous polyethylene implant.

Significant dead space can also be treated by designing the implant to fill intracranial volume deficits. CAD/CAM cranial implants can be designed with ports allowing closed suction drains to be placed between the dura and implant thereby eliminating significant fluid collections.

It is not uncommon for prominent fixation hardware to erode through the scalp, as shown in Fig. 3.12.2.

This results in implant contamination and usually subsequent implant loss. Implants can be computer-designed to allow strategic lag screw fixation of the implant. The appropriate position and length of the screw is determined preoperatively by CT analysis and incorporated into the implant design (Omnipore, Matrix Surgical, Atlanta, GA). Video 3.12.1 demonstrates our lag screw technique.

CAD/CAM implants are particularly useful for reconstructing the complex curvature of the supraorbital rim (Fig. 3.12.3).

Midface

Midface injuries and their resultant deformity are most often the result of blunt trauma. Ideally, these facial injuries are treated in the acute phase. However, the severity of the overall trauma burden may obligate delayed treatment of non-life-threatening facial injuries resulting in deformation of facial anatomy. Clinical circumstances may limit the adequacy of acute treatment, also resulting in midface deformity. Secondary reconstruction of the midface can be extremely difficult to treat. Correction of midface asymmetry is improved by avoiding suboptimal exposure, and may require difficult osteotomies, creating gaps in bone after proper reduction requiring interpositional and onlay bone grafts (Fig. 3.12.4).

Two examples of untreated midface reconstructions with CAD/CAM implants are shown in Fig. 3.12.5. Access was obtained through intraoral and transconjunctival approaches.

Mandible

Compromised acute treatment or delayed treatment of mandible and maxillary fractures may result in malocclusion. Restoration of occlusion may require sagittal split or other osteotomies to create acceptable dental and condylar relations. The osteotomies may result in "bony step-off" deformities at the osteotomy sites and asymmetries in ramus height and angulation. CAD/CAM implants are invaluable in restoring

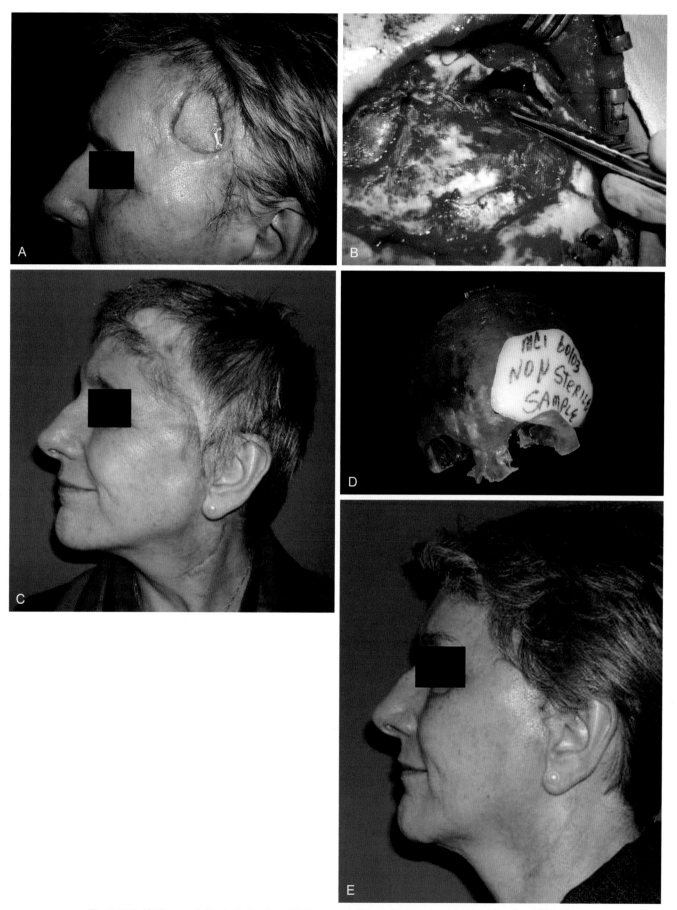

Fig. 3.12.1 (A) Exposed alloplastic implant. (B) Demonstration of deadspace underneath implant. (C) Patient after frontal sinus isolation and free flap coverage. (D) New implant design with the elimination of deadspace. (E) Patient after tissue expander reconstruction of the scalp.

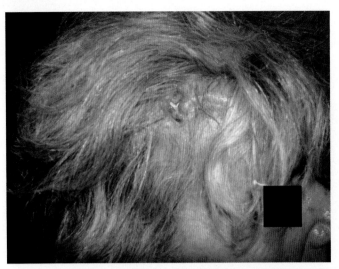

Fig. 3.12.2 Spontaneous exposure of prominent hardware.

mandible contour. The mandible is accessed through submental and posterior intraoral sulcus incisions (Fig. 3.12.6).

PREFERRED SURGICAL TECHNIQUES

Posttraumatic CAD/CAM implant reconstruction is technique-sensitive. The following tenets have reduced complications:

1. Meticulous preparation and draping of the operative field. Chlorhexidine mouthwashes are prescribed preoperatively to reduce intraoral contamination.
2. Meticulous hemostasis. Soft tissues are injected with epinephrine-containing solution prior to making incisions. Epinephrine-soaked neuropatties are routinely placed to minimize bleeding during the surgery.
3. Implants should not be placed under compromised tissue. For calvarial reconstruction this often requires preoperative tissue expansion or flap reconstruction. In the lower face, incisions should be remote from the implant. Implants are never placed near open wounds.
4. Obliterate dead space. Techniques used for cranial reconstruction have been discussed earlier in the text. All cranial and mandibular operative sites are treated with suction drains. Tissues damaged from blunt trauma or previous surgeries become less pliable and conformable thereby predisposing to dead space and hematoma collection.
5. Expose the area to be reconstructed widely to assure proper implant placement.
6. Immobilize the implant with rigid fixation.
7. Avoid prominent hardware.
8. Use perioperative antibiotics.

Evidence-Based Medicine

Unfortunately, there has not yet been one implant material that has been proven to be superior to others in the cranium, face, or mandible. For cranioplasty, there have been a variety of publications concluding that all the generally accepted alloplastic materials, including PEEK, titanium, porous polyethylene, and hydroxyapatite all have similar complication profiles and are similar to autologous bone grafting.[1–11] Regarding implant material in the face or mandible, there is less literature published when compared to cranioplasty. The existing literature concludes that silicone and porous polyethylene are safe and effective implant materials and have similar complication profiles. Currently,

there are no data to support the use of one alloplastic material over another so surgeon preference becomes the decision driver.[12–17]

POSTOPERATIVE COURSE

Postoperatively, patients remain on oral antibiotics for 1 week. If they have intraoral incisions, they use a chlorhexidine mouth rinse for 5 days. Sutures are left in for 7 days except for intraoral incisions which are closed with absorbable sutures.

Acute Complications

All alloplastic and autogenous materials are at risk for infection. Implant infections are usually as a result of inoculation at the time of surgery and usually present within 4–6 weeks. Signs and symptoms include fever, chills, leukocytosis, erythema around the surgical site, purulent drainage, or localized edema. Once diagnosed, the implant material should be removed entirely. On rare occasion, we have been able to salvage infected implants by acutely washing the wound and sterilizing or replacing the implant. Despite this, we do not advocate attempting implant salvage in the setting of infection and antibiotics will serve only to suppress an infection, and not eradicate it.

Long-Term Complications

Implant malposition or contour deformity after secondary reconstruction are possible. Depending on the type and location of the implant material, this can be as a result of implant malposition at the time of surgery, migration, or poor design of the implant itself. Fortunately, all these are potentially treatable with revision surgery. Custom implants typically have fewer problems with implant malposition. If the patient is unhappy with the contour of a custom implant, it is usually due to a design discrepancy, so it is important to discuss with the patient what kind of contour they desire in the preoperative visits.

Implant exposure is also a long-term risk for any implant. If there is good soft tissue coverage, it is rare for implants to become exposed. One exception is cranioplasty. Typically, neurosurgeons perform craniotomies with their scalp incision directly over their calvarial osteotomies. This unfortunately necessitates reconstructive surgeons placing the edges of the implant very close to or many times directly under the scalp incision. If there is any prominent hardware or "step-offs" in implant material, they can thin the scalp and ultimately erode, permitting exposure. This is because closure over the calvarium is usually tighter than in the face and therefore prominent hardware can cause pressure, thinning of soft tissue, possible necrosis, and soft tissue breakdown. It is for this reason that we use the radially based lag screw technique described previously to avoid any prominent hardware under the incision. We also make sure to "feather" the edges of the implant to eliminate step-offs, or shared edges in a non-custom implant with a contouring burr.

EXPERT COMMENTARY

There has been a longstanding controversy regarding autogenous versus alloplastic materials for secondary and primary reconstruction after facial/cranial injuries. Each option has its proponents, and experienced practitioners seem to have excellent possible results which are predicated upon logic and the desire for perfection improved by performance. Michael Yaremchuk and colleagues here present their masterful summary of the techniques they have perfected to use artificial materials with the best outcomes and minimal complications. The inquisitive reader is also referred to Yaremchuk's book [1] to further study the techniques which constitute the basis of good results with

Continued

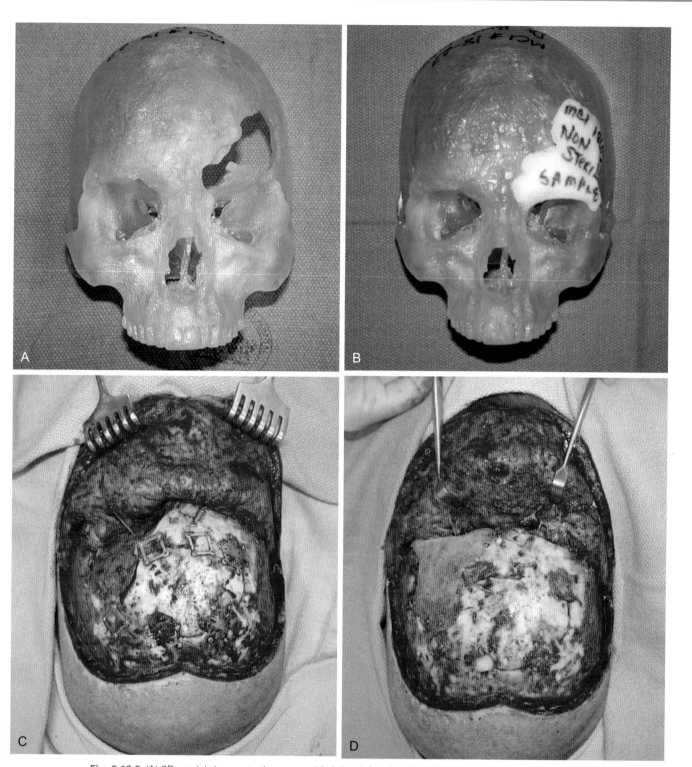

Fig. 3.12.3 (A) 3D model demonstrating supraorbital rim deformity. (B) CAD/CAM implants used for supraorbital rim deformity. (C) Intraoperative view of supraorbital rim deformity. (D) After implant placement.

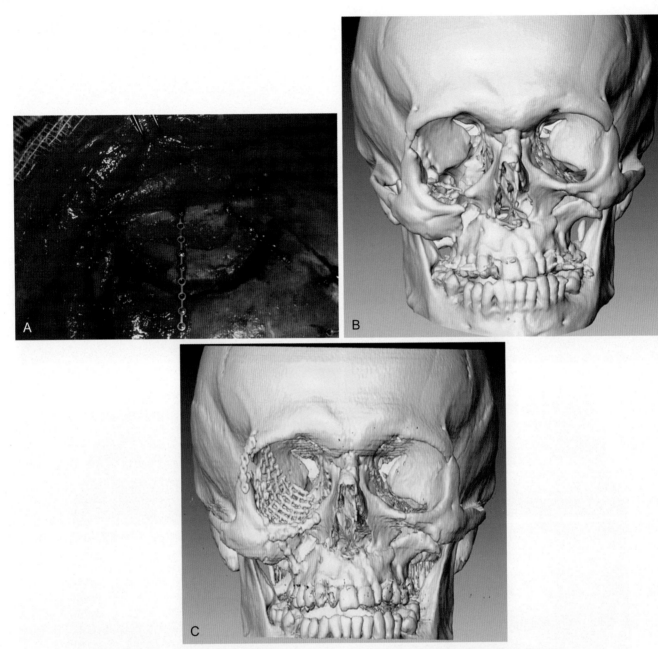

Fig. 3.12.4 (A) Patient with bone gaps after secondary reconstruction with osteotomies. (B) 3D reconstruction, patient 1 demonstrating bone gaps. (C) 3D reconstruction, patient 2 demonstrating bone gaps.

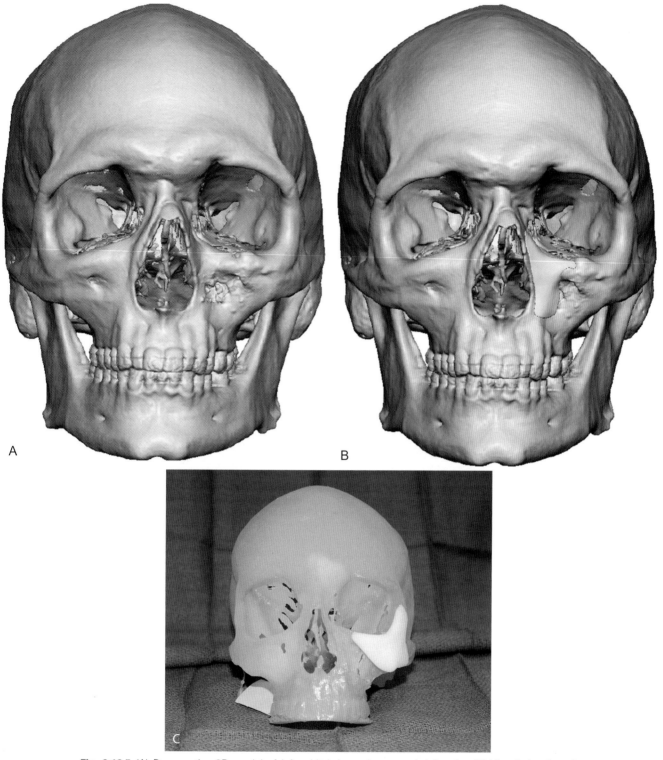

Fig. 3.12.5 (A) Preoperative 3D model of infraorbital rim and paranasal deformity. (B) Virtual planning of custom implant. (C) 3D model of patient with malar deformity and custom malar implant using CAD/CAM.

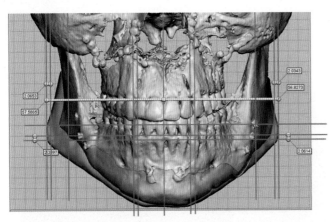

Fig. 3.12.6 Virtual design of mandible implants to correct asymmetries after sagittal split osteotomies.

REFERENCES

1. Honeybul S, Morrison DA, Ho KM, et al. A randomized controlled trial comparing autologous cranioplasty with custom-made titanium cranioplasty. *J Neurosurg*. 2016;1–10.

2. Sailer HF, Kolb E. Application of purified bone morphogenetic protein (BMP) preparations in cranio-maxillo-facial surgery. Reconstruction in craniofacial malformations and post-traumatic or operative defects of the skull with lyophilized cartilage and BMP. *J Craniomaxillofac Surg*. 1994;22(1):2–11.

3. Wallace RD, Salt C, Konofaos P. Comparison of autogenous and alloplastic cranioplasty materials following impact testing. *J Craniofac Surg*. 2015;26(5):1551–1557.

4. Zanaty M, Chalouhi N, Starke RM, et al. Complications following cranioplasty: incidence and predictors in 348 cases. *J Neurosurg*. 2015;123(1):182–188.

5. Zanotti B, Zingaretti N, Verlicchi A, et al. Cranioplasty: review of materials. *J Craniofac Surg*. 2016;27(8):2061–2072.

6. Kumar NG, Sreenivas M, Gowda S. Cranioplasty of large cranial defects with porous polyethylene implants. *J Craniofac Surg*. 2016;27(4): e333–e335.

7. Lindner D, Schlothofer-Schumann K, Kern B-C, et al. Cranioplasty using custom-made hydroxyapatite versus titanium: a randomized clinical trial. *J Neurosurg*. 2016;26:1–9.

8. Kung W-M, Lin F-H, Hsiao S-H, et al. New reconstructive technologies after decompressive craniectomy in traumatic brain injury: the role of three-dimensional titanium mesh. *J Neurotrauma*. 2012;29(11): 2030–2037.

9. Eufinger H, Wehmoller M, Machtens E, et al. Reconstruction of craniofacial bone defects with individual alloplastic implants based on CAD/CAM-manipulated CT-data. *J Craniomaxillofac Surg*. 1995;23(3): 175–181.

10. Chen TM, Wang HJ, Chen SL, Lin FH. Reconstruction of post-traumatic frontal-bone depression using hydroxyapatite cement. *Ann Plast Surg*. 2004;52(3):303–308.

11. Fiaschi P, Pavanello M, Imperato A, et al. Surgical results of cranioplasty with a polymethylmethacrylate customized cranial implant in pediatric patients: a single-center experience. *J Neurosurg Pediatr*. 2016;17(6): 705–710.

12. Chao JW, Lee JC, Chang MM, Kwan E. Alloplastic augmentation of the Asian face: a review of 215 patients. *Aesthet Surg J*. 2016;36(8):861–868.

13. Hammer B, Prein J. Correction of post-traumatic orbital deformities – operative techniques and review of 26 patients. *J Craniomaxillofac Surg*. 1995;23(2):81–90.

14. Tantawi D, Eberlin S, Calvert J. Midface implants. *Clin Plast Surg*. 2015;42(1):123–127.

15. Soares DJ, Silver WE. Midface skeletal enhancement. *Facial Plast Surg Clin North Am*. 2015;23(2):185–193.

16. Ridwan-Pramana A, Wolff J, Raziei A, et al. Porous polyethylene implants in facial reconstruction: outcome and complications. *J Craniomaxillofac Surg*. 2015;43(8):1330–1334.

17. Tepper OM, Sorice S, Hershman GN, et al. Use of virtual 3-dimensional surgery in post-traumatic craniomaxillofacial reconstruction. *J Oral Maxillofac Surg*. 2011;69(3):733–741.

Secondary Microvascular Reconstruction of the Traumatic Facial Injury

Isabel Robinson, J. Rodrigo Diaz-Siso, Eduardo Rodriguez

BACKGROUND

The preoperative planning and technical execution of craniofacial microsurgical reconstruction following traumatic injury is inherently complex. Patients may present with injury to any combination of tissue layers – including skin, vasculature, muscle, nerves, and bone – and reconstructive options span the entirety of the microsurgeon's armamentarium. These challenges are compounded in secondary reconstruction as prior reconstructive efforts may limit the surgical options available. Primary reconstruction often reduces the number of available recipient vessels and donor sites, while local tissue damaged by scarring and multiple operative attempts is more difficult to manipulate and more prone to complications, including necrosis and flap loss. An overly ambitious primary reconstruction may require an unplanned return to the operating room for secondary repair, which limits surgical options and reduces patient trust. However, when part of a pre-planned, multistaged surgical solution, secondary reconstruction can yield better functional and aesthetic outcomes than a single-stage operation.

Rodriguez et al. have previously described their approach to complex craniofacial reconstruction, which aims to optimize both functional and aesthetic outcomes.[1] In summary:

1. Aesthetic unit: the integrity of the aesthetic unit depends not only on soft tissue volume but also on adequate structural support.
2. Defect boundaries: when greater than 60% of an aesthetic unit is compromised, achieving an optimal result requires extending the defect boundaries to include the entire aesthetic unit so as to minimize scar burden and create unit homogeneity.
3. Tissue requirements: donor site selection must consider specific tissue deficiencies, including skin, mucosa, fat, muscle, and bone, as well as color match and volume requirements.
4. Bone and soft tissue support: deficient skeletal buttresses must be reconstructed with vascularized bone so as to provide adequate long-term support to the overlying soft tissues.
5. Soft tissue volume: the volume of soft tissue included in the reconstruction should be in slight excess of the base volume of the defect and should be vascularized so as to minimize resorption with the understanding that subsequent soft tissue contouring is preferable to additional tissue transfers.
6. Timing: early reconstruction minimizes morbidity by condensing the periods of healing from the initial injury and from the reconstruction into one event.
7. Secondary revisions: planned multistage reconstructions utilizing distant flaps for support and coverage followed by local flaps for color and contour improvement are preferable to unplanned secondary operations necessitated by complications or inadequate primary reconstruction.

All of these principles can help guide surgical decision-making when approaching the traumatic facial injury. However, the last two points – timing and secondary revisions – are particularly relevant to secondary microvascular reconstruction and will be discussed more extensively, along with the principle of tissue requirements.

SURGICAL ANATOMY

A wide variety of free flap options exist for the secondary reconstruction of traumatic defects of the face. The advantages and disadvantages of common donor sites are summarized briefly below.

Ulnar Artery Perforator Flap

First described by Lovie et al. in 1984,[2] the ulnar artery perforator flap provides thin, pliable tissue with a long pedicle, the ascending branch of the dorsal cutaneous branch of the ulnar artery. The donor site is less morbid than the neighboring radial forearm flap, and the skin of the ulnar forearm flap is less hirsute than its radial counterpart, making the former better suited for coverage of non-hair-bearing areas. The thinness of the flap precludes it from use in covering defects requiring bulky soft tissue or involving hardware, which can be exposed as the denervated flap thins over time.[3] Acceptance of the ulnar artery perforator flap by the microsurgical community has been sluggish owing to concerns over potential compromise to hand perfusion and innervation, despite long-term outcome analyses failing to demonstrate significant motor, sensory, or vascular impairment associated with ulnar forearm flap harvest.[4–6]

Anterolateral Thigh Flap

Since its introduction by Song et al. in 1984,[7] the anterolateral thigh flap (ALT) has become widely accepted as a workhorse flap for head and neck reconstruction. Its versatility in size and soft tissue components, reliable anatomy based off of the lateral circumflex femoral artery, and relative ease of harvest make the ALT a popular choice for the reconstruction of a wide range of head and neck defects. Disadvantages of the flap include its tendency – particularly in obese patient populations – to be especially bulky, its susceptibility to atrophy when muscle is included, and its potential to be hair-bearing.

Groin Flap

The groin flap, based off the superficial circumflex iliac artery, holds historical significance as the first successful free flap.[8] Advantages of the flap include its ability to be designed with muscle or as a perforator flap of variable depth and its easily concealed donor site with minimal morbidity. However, the utility of the groin flap is limited by its relatively short pedicle length and somewhat variable anatomic course.

Iliac Flap

First described by Acland in 1979,[9] the iliac flap provides substantial bone, muscle, soft tissue, and skin fed by the deep circumflex iliac artery (DCIA) and can be used for the reconstruction of extensive defects involving multiple tissue layers. The natural curvature of the iliac can approximate the angle of the mandible for jaw reconstruction, and the presence of vascularized bone provides the long-term bony support required for osseointegrated implants. Despite these advantages, its use as a vascularized bone flap has decreased with the advent of the free fibula flap owing to the iliac flap's higher donor site morbidity and shorter pedicle length. In cases where fibula-based reconstruction is not an option the iliac flap is a viable reconstructive modality for osseous or myo-osseous defects.

Free Fibula Flap

The free fibula flap (FFF), first described by Taylor for use in lower extremity salvage[10] and then by Hidalgo for mandibular reconstruction,[11] is one of the most commonly used vascularized osseous and osseocutaneous flaps. Its advantages include a substantial quantity of high-quality bone stock, its ability to include a wide range of tissues, and its flexibility in maneuvering those tissues without compromising blood supply. Disadvantages include variability in the pedicle length depending on the length of fibula being harvested and the potential for donor site morbidity including compromised ankle function, leg weakness, and great toe contracture.[12]

CLINICAL PRESENTATION

History

A meticulous assessment of the patient's injuries and surgical history is particularly critical when evaluating for secondary reconstruction, as prior reconstructive efforts are likely to limit the flap options available to the microsurgeon. The etiology of the injury must be ascertained and the patient's psychological state must be assessed. The patient's surgical history must be thoroughly reviewed and an inventory kept of available donor and recipient vessels. This practice is particularly critical when the patient is presenting from a different institution or when the secondary reconstruction is unplanned. If the secondary reconstruction is in response to an unforeseen complication of the primary reconstruction, the etiology of the primary failure must be ascertained so as to prevent a similar fate for the secondary reconstruction (as could be possible if the primary flap failed due to patient hypercoagulability).

Physical Examination

The goals for secondary craniofacial reconstruction depend on the patient's presentation and the extent of previous reconstructive efforts. Thorough, accurate physical examination is therefore critical in determining the reconstructive need. In performing the physical exam, it is helpful to follow an algorithmic approach in order to ensure complete evaluation and to resist the temptation to focus on the most immediately apparent defects. Step-wise evaluation moving from the superficial to deep tissue layers, with emphasis on the integrity of the facial coverage, lining, and support structures, can provide a straightforward system with which to approach patients.

Beginning superficially, observe the extent and location of the injury, taking note of the aesthetic unit(s) involved. Evaluate the quality of the skin, including areas of insufficient wound coverage, scarring, the positioning of hair-bearing skin, and texture or color mismatches between the local and free flap skin. Identify any contour deformities.

Assess the relevant muscular function, particularly the ability to smile and close the mouth for oral defects and the ability to close the eyes for periorbital defects. Evaluate specialized structures, including the oral and nasal mucosae, ocular conjunctivae, lacrimal apparatus, teeth, and tongue. Finally, examine the integrity of the underlying bone and cartilage, particularly the skeletal buttresses, which are critical for soft tissue support.[1,13] Bony structure evaluation is often greatly enhanced through the use of radiography.

RADIOLOGIC EVALUATION

CT scans with axial, coronal, and sagittal sections using both bone and soft tissue windows are the definitive imaging modality for craniofacial defects.[14–17] 3D CT scans[18–20] can more precisely evaluate spatial displacement and asymmetry in volume of bony structures. Computer-assisted digital cephalometric analysis systems can be used in soft tissue volume evaluation to quantify areas of excess, deficient, or asymmetrical soft tissue distribution.[21] Data from 3D imaging sources can be harnessed to create patient-specific implants and cutting guides, and virtual surgical planning using 3D scans from the patient can provide the surgeon with a more precise understanding of the patient's unique anatomy and defect prior to surgery.

SURGICAL INDICATIONS

Firm indications for secondary microsurgical craniofacial reconstruction are difficult to state given that craniofacial injuries encompass a broad range of anatomical, functional, and aesthetic defects. Indications depend on whether the secondary surgery is part of a planned, multi-stage reconstruction or the result of an unplanned complication such as flap loss. In considering the need for secondary microvascular reconstruction, it is critical to take into account the overarching treatment plan as well as the tissue layers involved.

For defects involving bony tissues, reconstruction is indicated when the skeletal buttresses are compromised. Skeletal buttresses are thick areas of bone that protect delicate facial structures by absorbing impact to the facial skeleton. They are also responsible for transferring the forces of mastication to the cranial base. The skeletal buttresses can be grouped into the vertical and horizontal buttresses. The vertical skeletal buttresses are stronger and include three paired buttresses – the naso-maxillary, zygomaticomaxillary, and pterygomaxillary – as well as one unpaired midline buttress, the frontoethmoid–vomerine buttress. The weaker horizontal skeletal buttresses include the frontal bandeau, inferior orbital rim, and lower transverse maxillary. Skeletal buttress integrity is critical for maintaining facial height, width, and projection, as well as allowing the placement of osseointegrated dental implants in the maxilla or mandible, and preventing periorbital complications.[22] In the lower two-thirds of the face, skeletal buttress integrity is critical for facilitating chewing, swallowing, oral competence, and speech. Microvascular mandibular reconstruction is indicated for mandibular defects greater than 5 cm, with flap selection dependent upon the location of the defect.[23] Hard tissue support must be established before any soft tissue reconstruction occurs or the surgeon risks the development of severe complications, including functional incompetence and extreme contour deformities. In cases in which the primary reconstruction simply "filled the hole and closed the wound" with soft tissues, without addressing the underlying structural deformity, secondary reconstruction may involve removal of the primary soft tissue flap and replacement with a composite flap involving bone. The decision to use vascularized or nonvascularized bone is complicated by the lack of high-level scientific evidence decisively demonstrating the superiority of one technique relative to the other.[24] Resorption rates of nonvascularized bone have been reported as high as 49.5% within 6 months,[25] although these rates are highly variable.[26,27] Several retrospective, single-institution studies have found that vascularized bone grafting yields higher bony union rates than its nonvascularized counterpart.[28,29] The unpredictability of nonvascularized bone graft resorption and union rates has prompted many surgeons to use vascularized bone graft for the reconstruction of extensive defects requiring hard tissues.

For extensive soft tissue defects without hard tissue involvement, or in cases in which the primary reconstruction restored skeletal buttress integrity, secondary reconstructive efforts can focus on returning an adequate amount of soft tissue to the affected area. In these cases, the quantity of soft tissue transferred should be in slight excess of the amount lost in the defect in order to account for expected tissue resorption. Keeping in mind that muscle, particularly when denervated, atrophies almost completely and substantially more than fat[3] and that nonvascularized tissue resorbs more extensively than vascularized tissue, vascularized fat is preferred for filling large soft tissue defects without a functional component.

Defects involving the oral or nasal mucosal linings must be repaired in order to guard against stenosis, contracture, and fistula. Muscle is preferred to skin for the reconstruction of lining surfaces due to its ability to mucosalize over time. Secondary reconstruction of mucosal surfaces is indicated in cases of insufficient or nonfunctional primary reconstruction, or as a second stage to replace skin from the primary reconstruction with mucosal tissue.

While many defects can be reconstructed with successful results, there are cases in which specialized structures, such as the eyelids or lips, prove particularly difficult to restore. These cases are often complicated by significant scarring and contracture from previous reconstructive efforts. Increasingly, vascularized composite allotransplantation of partial or full donor faces has been used to treat the most severe craniofacial defects. Traumatic injury currently accounts for the vast majority of defects warranting face transplantation, with mechanisms of injury including animal attacks, burns, and ballistic trauma.[30] A massive undertaking on the part of both the patient and the surgical team, face transplantation is reserved for the most extensive defects that severely impact a patient's function and quality of life despite conventional reconstructive efforts. When considering face transplantation, the benefits of recovering facial function and social reintegration must be weighed against the requirement for lifelong immunosuppression. Current face transplant efforts are limited by the difficulty of locating immunologically suitable donors. However, as immunosuppression modalities improve and donor pools are expanded, face transplantation may potentially grow into an accepted tool in the craniofacial surgeon's armamentarium for addressing the most complex facial defects.

SURGICAL TECHNIQUE

While specific surgical technique in secondary craniofacial reconstruction is largely a function of surgeon preference, there are several key principles that can help guide decision-making to optimize patient aesthetic and functional outcomes. Replacing lost tissues "in kind" as described by Gillies[31] is an age-old reconstructive principle that holds true in the setting of secondary microsurgical reconstruction, and involves identifying discrepancies between the tissues incriminated in the original defect and those used in the primary reconstruction, with emphasis on coverage, lining, and support. For example, a patient presenting with a full-thickness forehead defect involving both hard and soft tissue may have been primarily treated with a flap including only soft tissue. This "filling the hole" approach to primary reconstruction does not adequately

restore the underlying skeletal structure and thus requires secondary reconstruction with a flap involving hard tissue in order to restore normal contour and provide adequate soft tissue support. Replacing like with like is a guiding principle in secondary skin revision as well. Local advancement and transposition flaps are useful in covering de-epithelized free flaps with skin that more closely approximates the color and texture of the surrounding areas.

In deciding on the timing of a reconstruction, effort should always be made to begin the reconstructive process within the window of healing from the initial injury. This approach prevents the primary wound from healing extensively prior to reconstruction, thereby obviating the need to extend the borders of the defect by removing scar tissue when preparing the recipient site. Condensing the healing periods from the injury and reconstruction into one early phase significantly improves patient outcomes by reducing fibrosis and contracture.[32] Capitalizing on this opportunity for better results is only possible when the reconstructive stages are carefully planned shortly after the time of injury, such that primary wound closure and stabilization is followed by secondary reconstruction of the bony support and restoration of soft tissue deficits within the initial window of injury. Delaying decisive reconstruction risks the patient being lost to follow-up or developing severe complications including soft tissue collapse, stenosis, and fistula formation while awaiting secondary reconstruction.

Early restoration of critical bony and soft tissue elements can then be followed by planned secondary or tertiary revisionary procedures to improve soft tissue contour and color match. Intentionally oversized flaps can be debulked once soft tissue atrophy has occurred and distant flaps can be resurfaced with local skin advancement to reduce scar burden and improve the aesthetic result. Approaching the reconstruction as a multistage process rather than a single procedure reduces complications from overly ambitious surgeries and allows for better long-term outcomes. Unplanned salvage operations necessitated by severe complications damage patient trust and impair long-term aesthetic and functional results. By contrast, a clearly communicated and expertly executed reconstructive plan improves both the patient's long-term outcomes and psychological experience.

POSTOPERATIVE COURSE

While the postoperative course must be tailored to the individual needs of the patient, several aspects of postoperative care are universal. These include airway protection, diligent flap monitoring, perioperative antibiotics, deep venous thrombosis prophylaxis, and scar management. If a patient is judged likely to be unable to protect their airway following surgery, a tracheostomy may be established preoperatively when not preexisting from prior reconstruction. Patients requiring extensive oronasal reconstruction are particularly likely to require tracheostomy, while endotracheal intubation may suffice for patients with periorbital or scalp-based defects. While modalities like infrared spectroscopy[33] and implantable Doppler systems[34] exist to assist with flaps that are difficult to monitor, the effectiveness of these mechanisms is limited by their cost, the tendency for the probes to move, and the risk of false reassurance. As such, the gold standard in flap surveillance remains direct physical exam based on flap color, temperature, turgor, capillary refill, and the ability of flap puncture to induce hemorrhage. Clinical flap monitoring, as well as Doppler pencil probe monitoring of the anastomosis site, should occur every 30–60 minutes in the first 24 hours after surgery, then every hour on postoperative days 2 and 3 and every 6 hours for all subsequent days prior to discharge.

Care should be taken not to distort or compress either the donor or recipient site. For example, compression stockings should not be placed on a free fibula donor site. Prolonged sedation has not been shown to reduce flap complication rates and thus should be avoided to minimize the risk of intensive care unit-associated morbidities. Likewise, improved free flap outcomes have not been shown with the use of anticoagulants, antiplatelet therapy, or phosphodiesterase inhibitors.[35]

Nasogastric (NG) tube removal should be completed within 24 hours of the surgery and the patient's tolerance of oral secretions monitored. A liquid diet may be started within 48 hours if the patient is comfortably swallowing saliva, although the presence of sialorrhea should postpone any advances in diet. Facial structure physical rehabilitation should begin between postoperative days 7 and 10 with an emphasis on range of motion.

A minority of patients with complex oromandibular and oromaxillary defects require a gastrostomy tube placed preoperatively or may have presented with an existing gastrostomy tube from a prior surgery. In these cases the patient's preoperative and predicted postoperative functional level, nutritional status, and long-term surgical revision plan inform whether a gastrostomy tube is indicated.

COMPLICATIONS

Acute Complications

While complications related to flap failure are naturally at the forefront of the microsurgeon's mind, it is important to remain vigilant for potentially devastating complications that occur outside of the reconstructive zone. Airway collapse may be the most catastrophic acute complication following head and neck reconstruction. Edema can develop from fluid shifts following flap inset and compromise the endotracheal tube. This risk may be mitigated by preoperative tracheostomy. Carotid artery blow-out is a rare, major complication requiring emergent treatment. The surgeon performing secondary reconstruction ought to be particularly attendant to this risk, as both extensive surgery and wound breakdown predispose patients to developing carotid artery blow-out.[36]

Acute complications can occur in both the donor and recipient sites. Donor site complications are specific to the flap used and the tissues taken. The inability to close the donor site adequately predisposes the area to infection and wound dehiscence. Recipient site complications can include wound dehiscence, seroma, hematoma, infection, necrosis, venous congestion, vascular thrombosis, flap atrophy, and prosthesis exposure. Vascular integrity compromise can quickly develop into partial or total flap failure and thus diligent monitoring and prompt intervention, particularly in the first 48 hours following surgery, are critical for reducing rates of flap loss.

Long-Term Complications

Long-term complications can involve any or all tissue layers. One of the most common reconstructive complications is scarring. While difficult to avoid altogether, with careful flap design and revisionary procedures scars may often be hidden in the hairline, skin creases, or subunit borders to lessen their aesthetic burden. Failure to adequately restore the oral or nasal mucosa or the ocular conjunctiva can lead to fistula formation, contracture, or stenosis. The oral cavity is particularly vulnerable to infection and thus acutely dependent on its mucosa for disease prevention. Soft tissue is vulnerable to resorption and atrophy and so should be transferred in greater quantities than required by the defect in expectation of tissue loss. Tertiary debulking procedures can improve contour deformities resulting from excess soft tissue transfer once the threat of resorption has subsided. Denervated muscle flaps are more prone to atrophy than adipose flaps[3] and risk exposure of underlying hardware, so neurotized flaps should be considered during surgical planning.

CASE EXAMPLES

The following cases illustrate the principles discussed above regarding subunit-specific reconstruction and the benefits of planned second stage reconstructions compared to unplanned secondary salvages.

Case 1

A 34-year-old woman presented with enophthalmos and temporal hollowing following several failed attempts to reconstruct her orbit after sustaining a gunshot wound. She was treated with a fibula flap to repair her orbital floor and temporal fossa. The flap was composed of 5 cm of vascularized bone and a 10 cm × 7 cm skin island. The donor site was closed with a split-thickness skin graft. She had no complications and no secondary procedures. (See Fig. 3.13.1.)

Case 2

A 45-year-old woman sustained trauma to the right periorbit following a high-speed motor vehicle collision. She received an ulnar forearm free flap with a 4 cm × 3 cm skin paddle after several reconstructive efforts failed to correct her soft tissue defect. The donor site was closed with a full-thickness skin graft. She had no complications and subsequently underwent flap debulking, local tissue advancement, and a full-thickness skin graft to ameliorate skin color discrepancies. (See Fig. 3.13.2.)

Case 3

A 45-year-old woman initially underwent soft tissue only reconstruction following bilateral naso-orbito-ethmoid, maxillary, and mandibular fractures from a self-inflicted gunshot wound. She developed complete midface collapse due to insufficient skeletal buttress support and was subsequently reconstructed with a DCIA-based iliac crest flap with internal oblique muscle to restore her midface skeletal support. A calvarial bone graft and paramedian forehead flap were used for tertiary nasal reconstruction. (See Fig. 3.13.3.)

Case 4

A 56-year-old woman sustained a self-inflicted shotgun wound resulting in a 12 cm bilateral dentoalveolar mandibular defect that was primarily reconstructed with rigid fixation of the midface fractures and a reconstruction plate spanning the mandibular defect. She was referred to the senior author 7 weeks after the initial injury for definitive secondary mandibular reconstruction. A free fibula osteocutaneous flap was used to reconstruct her left mandible and cheek. The mandibular hardware was removed due to pain 10 months after the secondary reconstruction. Mandibular form and function was deemed to be excellent 19 months postoperatively. (See Fig. 3.13.4.)

Case 5

A 22-year-old man underwent a sternocleidomastoid rotational flap for primary reconstruction of a mandibular fossa defect following a gunshot wound. The primary reconstruction was unable to correct the defect of the right dentoalveolus and ramus and he developed impaired mandibular function 11 months later, at which point he presented to the senior author. Secondary reconstruction was undertaken with a DCIA-based free iliac osteocutaneous flap including a 7 cm × 2 cm bone segment and 10 cm × 2 cm skin paddle. The postoperative course was complicated by venous congestion that necessitated partial soft tissue debridement, although the bone and the majority of the soft tissue were not compromised. Mandibular function was restored at 5 weeks after the secondary surgery and prosthetic dental implants were ultimately placed. (See Fig. 3.13.5.)

Text continued on p. 481

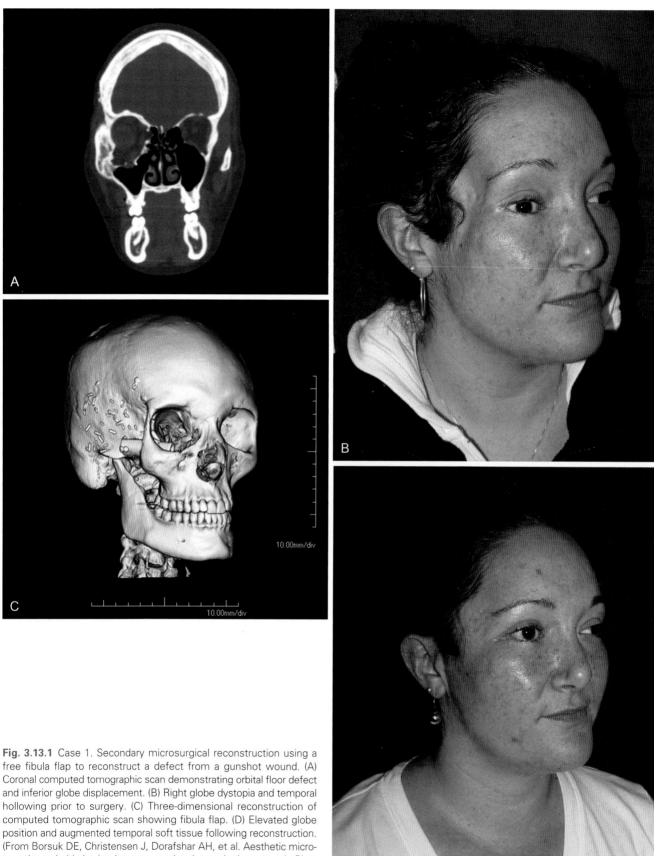

Fig. 3.13.1 Case 1. Secondary microsurgical reconstruction using a free fibula flap to reconstruct a defect from a gunshot wound. (A) Coronal computed tomographic scan demonstrating orbital floor defect and inferior globe displacement. (B) Right globe dystopia and temporal hollowing prior to surgery. (C) Three-dimensional reconstruction of computed tomographic scan showing fibula flap. (D) Elevated globe position and augmented temporal soft tissue following reconstruction. (From Borsuk DE, Christensen J, Dorafshar AH, et al. Aesthetic microvascular periorbital subunit reconstruction: beyond primary repair. Plast Reconstr Surg; 2013:131(2). 337–347.)

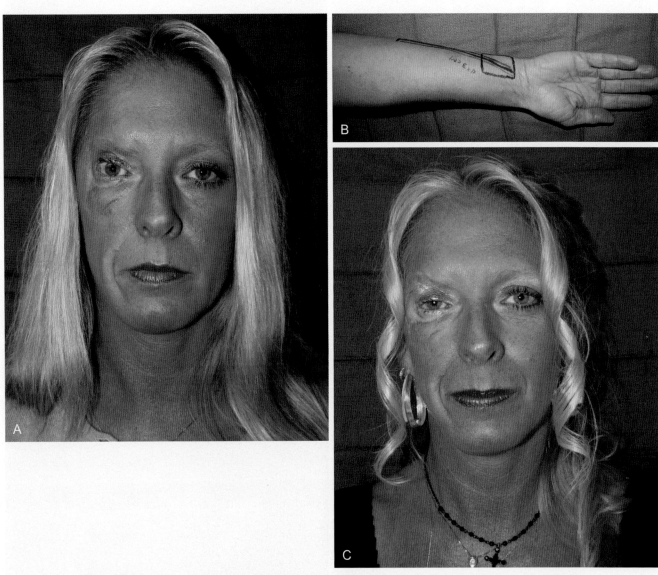

Fig. 3.13.2 Case 2. An ulnar flap was used to secondarily correct soft tissue deficiency in the periorbit resulting from a motor vehicle collision. (A) Outcome following initial procedure. (B) Flap outlined on the donor site. (C) The outcome following two revision procedures. (From Borsuk DE, Christensen J, Dorafshar AH, et al. Aesthetic microvascular periorbital subunit reconstruction: beyond primary repair. Plast Reconstr Surg; 2013:131(2). 337–347.)

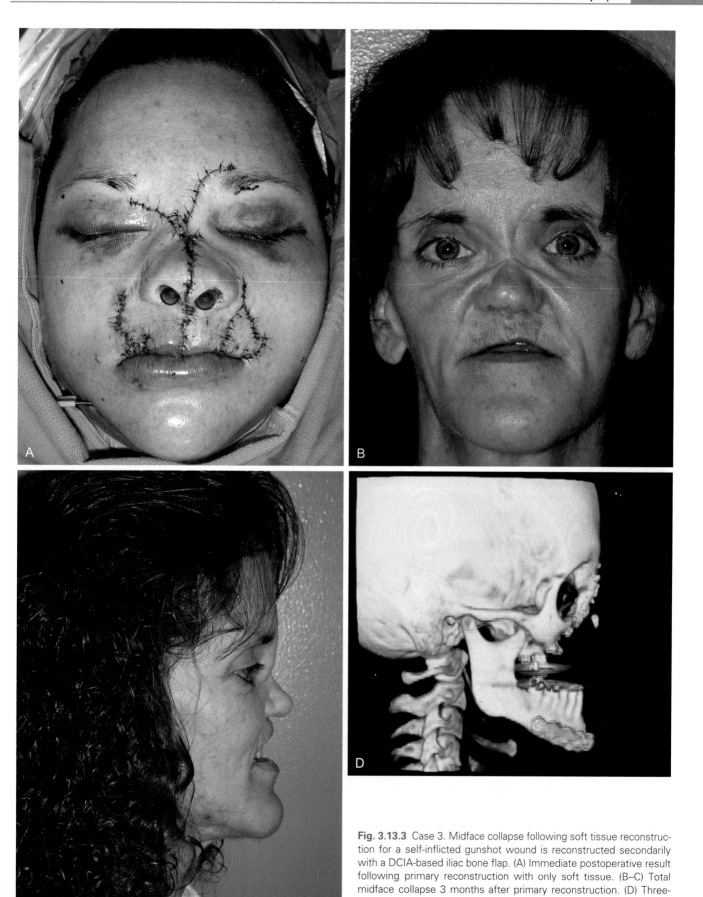

Fig. 3.13.3 Case 3. Midface collapse following soft tissue reconstruction for a self-inflicted gunshot wound is reconstructed secondarily with a DCIA-based iliac bone flap. (A) Immediate postoperative result following primary reconstruction with only soft tissue. (B–C) Total midface collapse 3 months after primary reconstruction. (D) Three-dimensional computed tomographic scan demonstrating the clinical diagnosis of total midface collapse. *Continued*

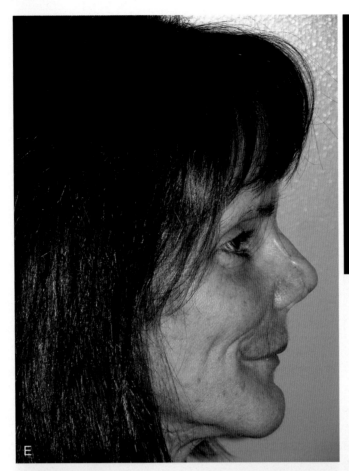

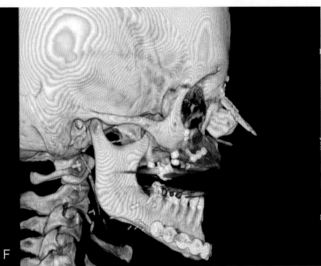

Fig. 3.13.3, cont'd (E) Clinical result 12 months following secondary reconstruction with a DCIA-based iliac bone flap to restore midface support. (F) Three-dimensional computed tomographic scan demonstrating result 12 months after secondary reconstruction. (From Rodriguez ED, Martin M, Bluebond-Langner R, et al. Microsurgical reconstruction of posttraumatic high-energy maxillary defects: establishing the effectiveness of early reconstruction. Plast Reconstr Surg. 2007;120(7):103s–117s.)

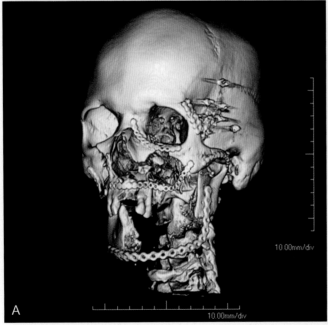

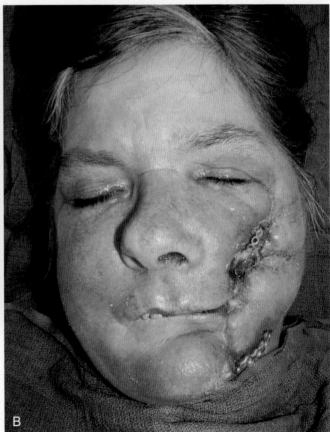

Fig. 3.13.4 Case 4. (A) Preoperative computed tomographic scan demonstrates a dentoalveolar mandibular defect. (B) Intraoperative photo depicting the mandibular and cheek defect.

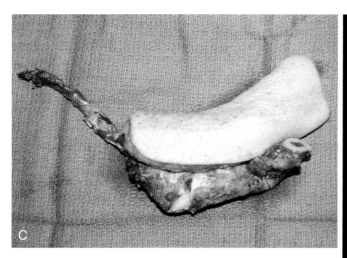

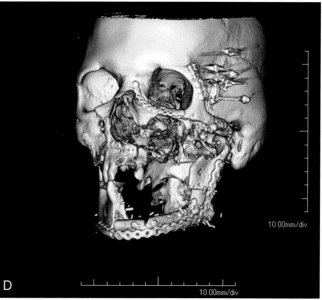

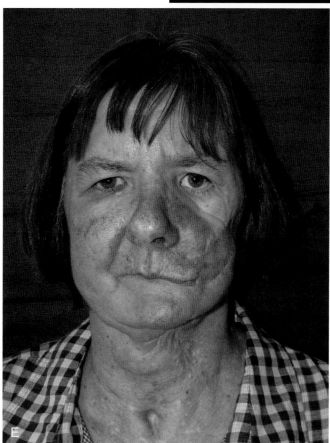

Fig. 3.13.4, cont'd (C) The fibula flap after osteotomy and rigid fixation to approximate the shape of the mandible. (D) Computed tomographic scan 1 year postoperatively demonstrating fibula free flap inset. (E) Clinical result 1 year postoperatively. (From Schultz BD, Sosin M, Mohan R, et al. Classification of mandible defects and algorithm for microvascular reconstruction. Plast Reconstr Surg. 2015;135(4)743e–754e.)

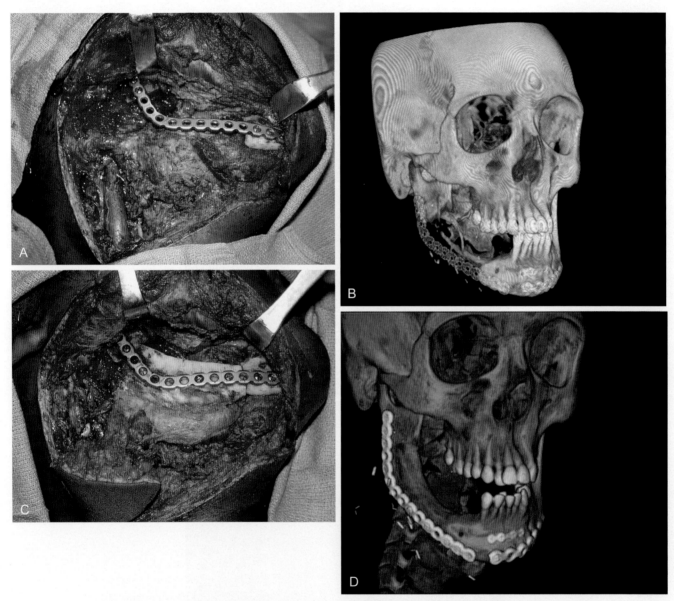

Fig. 3.13.5 Case 5. (A) Intraoperative demonstration of the right mandibular defect with the ipsilateral recipient vessels. (B) Preoperative computed tomographic scan demonstrating the right mandibular body and angle defect. (C) Iliac crest free flap inset. (D) Computed tomographic scan 1 year after secondary reconstruction demonstrating restoration of mandibular structure. (From Schultz BD, Sosin M, Mohan R, et al. Classification of mandible defects and algorithm for microvascular reconstruction. Plast Reconstr Surg. 2015;135(4)743e–754e.)

EXPERT COMMENTARY

Giles revolutionized secondary reconstructive plastic surgery in World War I with his innovative uses of pedicle flap reconstruction for defect fractures of the face. Dingman and Natvig [1], Converse [2], Rowe and Killey [3], and Irby [4] laid the foundation for modern open reduction of facial fractures in the 1970s–1990s, but the defect fracture needed the solution of microsurgery [4,5] and the principles of defect reconstruction of facial defects introduced in gunshot and shotgun wounds [5] which have become a fundamental part of facial reconstruction for cancer, congenital, and acquired facial defects and deformities [6–11]. The unusual background training of Rodriguez in four disciplines has allowed him to develop and perfect principles of facial reconstruction of traumatic and acquired facial defects [7], which have revolutionized the results available to patients unfortunate enough to have these previously unsolvable problems.

One would do well to thoroughly read and study the background papers of Rodriguez [7–12], who convinced the world of the validity of these concepts to gain further insight into the precise planning and organization required to successfully pursue this challenging and rewarding solution. Regrettably, many of the problems requiring these innovative solutions could have been solved by better/more timely management of the initial problem.

References

1. Dingman R, Natvig P. *Surgery of Facial Fractures*. Philadelphia, PA: W. Saunders; 1969:142–144.
2. Kazanjian VH, Converse JM. *Surgical Treatment of Facial Injuries*. 3rd ed. Baltimore, MD: Williams & Wilkins; 1974.
3. Rowe NL, Killey HC. *Fractures of the Facial Skeleton*. 2nd ed. London: E&S Livingstone; 1970:857–877.
4. Irby WB. *Facial Trauma and Concomitant Problems*. 2nd ed. St. Louis, MO: Mosby; 1979.
5. Gruss JS, Antonyshyn O, Phillips JH. Early definitive bone and soft-tissue reconstruction of major gunshot wounds of the face. *Plast Reconstr Surg*. 1991;878:436.
6. Clark N, Birely B, Manson PN, et al. High-energy ballistic and avulsive facial injuries: classification, patterns, and an algorithm for primary reconstruction. *Plast Reconstr Surg*. 1996;98:583–601.
7. Robertson B, Manson P. The importance of serial debridement and "a second look" procedures in high-energy ballistic and avulsive facial injuries. *Oper Tech Plast Reconstr Surg*. 1998;5(3):236–246.
8. Rodriguez E, Martin M, Bluebond-Langner R, et al. Microsurgical reconstruction of post-traumatic high-energy maxillary defects: establishing the effectiveness of early reconstruction. *Plast Reconstr Surg*. 2007;120(7):103S–117S.
9. Rodriguez E, Bluebond-Langner R, Park J, et al. Preservation of contour in periorbital and midfacial craniofacial microsurgery: reconstruction of the soft tissue elements and skeletal buttresses. *Plast Reconstr Surg*. 2008;121(5):1738–1747.
10. Rodriguez E, Bluebond-Langner R, Devgan L, et al. Correction of the recalcitrant post-traumatic periorbital soft tissue deformity: a novel microsurgical approach. *Plast Reconstr Surg*. 2008;121(6):1978–1981.
11. Sinno S, Rodriguez ER. Definitive management of persistent frontal sinus infections and mucocele with a vascularized free fibula flap. *Plast Reconstr Surg*. 2017;139:170.
12. Fisher N, Dorafshar A, Bojovic B, et al. The evolution of critical concepts in aesthetic craniofacial microsurgical reconstruction. *Plast Reconstr Surg*. 2012;130:389.

REFERENCES

1. Fisher M, Dorafshar A, Bojovic B, et al. The evolution of critical concepts in aesthetic craniofacial microsurgical reconstruction. *Plast Reconstr Surg*. 2012;130(2):389–398.
2. Lovie MJ, Duncan GM, Glasson DW. The ulnar artery forearm free flap. *Br J Plast Surg*. 1984;37(4):486–492.
3. Sosin M, Chaudhry A, De La Cruz C, et al. Lessons learned in scalp reconstruction and tailoring free tissue transfer in the elderly: a case series and literature review. *Craniomaxillofac Trauma Reconstr*. 2015;8(3):179–189.
4. Rodriguez ED, Mithani SK, Bluebond-Langner R, Manson PN. Hand evaluation following ulnar forearm perforator flap harvest: a prospective study. *Plast Reconstr Surg*. 2007;120(6):1598–1601.
5. Tan ST, James DW, Moaveni Z. Donor site morbidity of free ulnar forearm flap. *Head Neck*. 2012;34(10):1434–1439.
6. Sieg P, Dericioglu M, Hansmann C, et al. Long-term functional donor site morbidity after ulnar forearm flap harvest. *Head Neck*. 2012;34(9):1312–1316.
7. Song YG, Chen GZ, Song YL. The free thigh flap: a new free flap concept based on the septocutaneous artery. *Br J Plast Surg*. 1984;37(2):149–159.
8. McGregor IA, Jackson IT. The groin flap. *Br J Plast Surg*. 1972;25(1):3–16.
9. Acland RD. The free iliac flap: a lateral modification of the free groin flap. *Plast Reconstr Surg*. 1979;64(1):30–36.
10. Taylor GI, Miller GD, Ham FJ. The free vascularized bone graft: a clinical extension of microvascular techniques. *Plast Reconstr Surg*. 1975;55(5):533–544.
11. Hidalgo DA. Fibula free flap: a new method of mandible reconstruction. *Plast Reconstr Surg*. 1989;84(1):71–79.
12. Momoh AO, Yu P, Skoracki RJ, et al. A prospective cohort study of fibula free flap donor-site morbidity in 157 consecutive patients. *Plast Reconstr Surg*. 2011;128(3):714–720.
13. Muresan C, Hui-Chou HG, Dorafshar AH, et al. Forehead reconstruction with microvascular flaps: utility of aesthetic subunits. *J Reconstr Microsurg*. 2012;28(5):319–326.
14. Rowe LD, Brandt-Zawadzki M. Spatial analysis of midfacial fractures with multidirectional and computed tomography: clinicopathologic correlates in 44 cases. *Otolaryngol Head Neck Surg*. 1982;90(5):651–660.
15. Rowe LD, Miller E, Brandt-Zawadzki M. Computed tomography in maxillofacial trauma. *Laryngoscope*. 1981;91(5):745–757.
16. Gentry LR, Manor WF, Turski PA, Strother CM. High-resolution CT analysis of facial struts in trauma: 1. Normal anatomy. *AJR Am J Roentgenol*. 1983;140(3):523–532.
17. Gentry LR, Manor WF, Turski PA, Strother CM. High-resolution CT analysis of facial struts in trauma: 2. Osseous and soft-tissue complications. *AJR Am J Roentgenol*. 1983;140(3):533–541.
18. Zonneveld FW, Lobregt S, van der Meulen JC, Vaandrager JM. Three-dimensional imaging in craniofacial surgery. *World J Surg*. 1989;13(4):328–342.
19. Luka B, Brechtelsbauer D, Gellrich NC, Konig M. 2D and 3D CT reconstructions of the facial skeleton: an unnecessary option or a diagnostic pearl? *Int J Oral Maxillofac Surg*. 1995;24(1 Pt 2):76–83.
20. Kassel EE, Noyek AM, Cooper PW. CT in facial trauma. *J Otolaryngol*. 1983;12(1):2–15.
21. Chen SK, Chen YJ, Yao CC, Chang HF. Enhanced speed and precision of measurement in a computer-assisted digital cephalometric analysis system. *Angle Orthod*. 2004;74(4):501–507.
22. Bluebond-Langner R, Rodriguez ED. Application of skeletal buttress analogy in composite facial reconstruction. *Craniomaxillofac Trauma Reconstr*. 2009;2(1):19–25.
23. Schultz BD, Sosin M, Nam A, et al. Classification of mandible defects and algorithm for microvascular reconstruction. *Plast Reconstr Surg*. 2015;135(4):743e–754e.
24. Allsopp BJ, Hunter-Smith DJ, Rozen WM. Vascularized versus nonvascularized bone grafts: what is the evidence? *Clin Orthop Relat Res*. 2016;474(5):1319–1327.
25. Johansson B, Grepe A, Wannfors K, Hirsch JM. A clinical study of changes in the volume of bone grafts in the atrophic maxilla. *Dentomaxillofac Radiol*. 2001;30(3):157–161.
26. Mertens C, Decker C, Seeberger R, et al. Early bone resorption after vertical bone augmentation–a comparison of calvarial and iliac grafts. *Clin Oral Implants Res*. 2013;24(7):820–825.
27. Vermeeren JI, Wismeijer D, van Waas MA. One-step reconstruction of the severely resorbed mandible with onlay bone grafts and endosteal implants. A 5-year follow-up. *Int J Oral Maxillofac Surg*. 1996;25(2):112–115.
28. Pogrel MA, Podlesh S, Anthony JP, Alexander J. A comparison of vascularized and nonvascularized bone grafts for reconstruction of mandibular continuity defects. *J Oral Maxillofac Surg*. 1997;55(11):1200–1206.
29. Foster RD, Anthony JP, Sharma A, Pogrel MA. Vascularized bone flaps versus nonvascularized bone grafts for mandibular reconstruction: an

outcome analysis of primary bony union and endosseous implant success. *Head Neck.* 1999;21(1):66–71.

30. Sosin M, Rodriguez ED. The face transplantation update: 2016. *Plast Reconstr Surg.* 2016;137(6):1841–1850.

31. Gillies HD, Millard DR. *The Principles and Art of Plastic Surgery.* Boston, MA: Little; 1957.

32. Rodriguez ED, Martin M, Bluebond-Langner R, et al. Microsurgical reconstruction of posttraumatic high-energy maxillary defects: establishing the effectiveness of early reconstruction. *Plast Reconstr Surg.* 2007;120(7 suppl 2):103S–117S.

33. Cai ZG, Zhang J, Zhang JG, et al. Evaluation of near infrared spectroscopy in monitoring postoperative regional tissue oxygen saturation for fibular flaps. *J Plast Reconstr Aesthet Surg.* 2008;61(3):289–296.

34. Froemel D, Fitzsimons SJ, Frank J, et al. A review of thrombosis and antithrombotic therapy in microvascular surgery. *Eur Surg Res.* 2013;50(1):32–43.

35. Shen YF, Rodriguez ED, Wei FC, et al. Aesthetic and functional mandibular reconstruction with immediate dental implants in a free fibular flap and a low-profile reconstruction plate: five-year follow-up. *Ann Plast Surg.* 2015;74(4):442–446.

36. Khouri RK. Free flap surgery: the second decade. *Clin Plast Surg.* 1992;19(4):757–761.

Virtual Surgical Planning

Sashank Reddy, Alexandra Macmillan, Amir H. Dorafshar

BACKGROUND

Since its emergence in the late 1980s, computer-assisted surgery (CAS) has become an increasingly important adjunct to craniofacial reconstruction. The refinement of virtual surgical planning (VSP) coupled with the availability of 3-dimensional (3D) printing techniques has enabled easier and more predictable remodeling of the craniofacial skeleton. As these techniques continue to develop, they point to a future in which ever more elaborate craniofacial challenges can be tackled with more secure outcomes. In this chapter we discuss the utility of CAS techniques for primary and secondary trauma reconstruction and then consider the future of these approaches in craniofacial surgery.

The groundwork for contemporary CAS was established in the 1980s with the proliferation of CT scanning and the advent of computer-aided design and manufacturing (CAD/CAM) methods.[1,2] By enabling noninvasive, 3-dimensional visualization of the craniofacial skeleton, the former enabled much more accurate preoperative diagnosis and planning than was available from plain radiographs. Utilization of CAD/CAM in turn allowed that preoperative plan to be translated into adjuncts for surgery such as patient-specific cutting guides and implants. The integration of these techniques into a unified computer-assisted craniofacial surgery was first described by Toth et al. in 1988.[3] These authors generated patient-specific resin molds which were then used preoperatively to shape prosthetic implants and intraoperatively to guide bone shaping in a series of patients needing frontoorbital reconstruction. The subsequent revolution in digital image manipulation allowed this pioneering approach to be much more widely adopted.

CONTEMPORARY USES OF CAS

Currently CAS techniques are commonly used in elective craniofacial and orthognathic surgery as well as in craniofacial trauma reconstruction. The utility of these approaches has been widely chronicled in the literature.[4–9] Some of the broad categories of applications include VSP of osteotomies, segmental bone movements or reductions, virtual correction of occlusion, generation of customized cutting guides, and creation of patient-specific implants. These applications largely share a common workflow: (1) acquisition of high resolution CT images of the craniofacial skeleton; (2) conversion of these images to DICOM file format for use in digital image manipulation; (3) creation of 3D reconstructions of the craniofacial skeleton by a bioengineering company; (4) VSP teleconference between surgeons and biomedical engineers to discuss surgical plans; (5) creation of patient-specific implants, models, or cutting guides. Completion of this workflow can be accomplished in a week or less and has been shown to be cost-effective when considering its acceleration of operative times.[10] We next illustrate the use of CAS in primary and secondary trauma reconstruction.

PRIMARY RECONSTRUCTION

Utilization of CAS in primary craniofacial trauma reconstruction presents some challenges. The time required to complete CAS workflow may limit its utilization, though this process is becoming ever more expeditious. In general we advocate early treatment of facial fractures in order to achieve the most anatomic repairs and to minimize unfavorable scarring and soft tissue contraction.[11] However, in the severely injured trauma patient, where CAS techniques are most useful, there is often time between initial stabilization of injuries to other body systems and definitive repair of craniofacial injuries. Advantages of CAS in these situations include minimization of dissection and more accurate repairs through the use of pre-bent plates and cutting guides. These benefits are particularly valuable in severe craniofacial injuries in which multilevel trauma and comminution can disrupt normal anatomic relationships that guide repair. We present an example in which CAS proved valuable in reconstruction of the mandible.

We used CAS techniques to virtually reduce a severely comminuted mandible fracture following a blast injury (Fig. 3.14.1). The patient was involved in a chemical explosion at work and suffered injuries to his lower face including degloving of skin and soft tissues of the right cheek and open fractures of the right mandibular body and parasymphyseal region with significant comminution. After primary stabilization and placement of a tracheostomy at the regional burn center, the patient was transferred to our care for management of his facial injuries. The numerous fragments of mandibular bone – some of marginal viability – made accurate anatomical reduction challenging. Proper reduction and fixation was further complicated by the need to minimize additional soft tissue dissection for fear of compromising blood supply to the bone. For these reasons, we conducted a VSP planning session in which major fragments were brought into alignment virtually. Additionally, proper occlusion was established in this forum and used to guide design of a pre-bent reconstruction plate spanning the aligned fragments. This plate was milled and shipped to our center in 5 days. Intraoperatively, the patient's existing traumatic lacerations were extended and conservative debridement of clearly nonviable soft tissue and bone was performed. After simplification of smaller fracture fragments through a combination of bridle wiring and 1 mm superior border plates, the patient was placed in maxillomandibular fixation using Erich arch bars and elastics. These were secured to major fracture fragments with bone reduction forceps and digital manipulation. The custom plate was then readily adapted to the reduced mandible and secured using locking screws. The patient has gone on to heal with restoration of premorbid occlusion at his most recent 2-month follow-up.

SECONDARY RECONSTRUCTION

The improved preoperative diagnosis and planning afforded by VSP is particularly useful in complex secondary reconstructions. These cases are

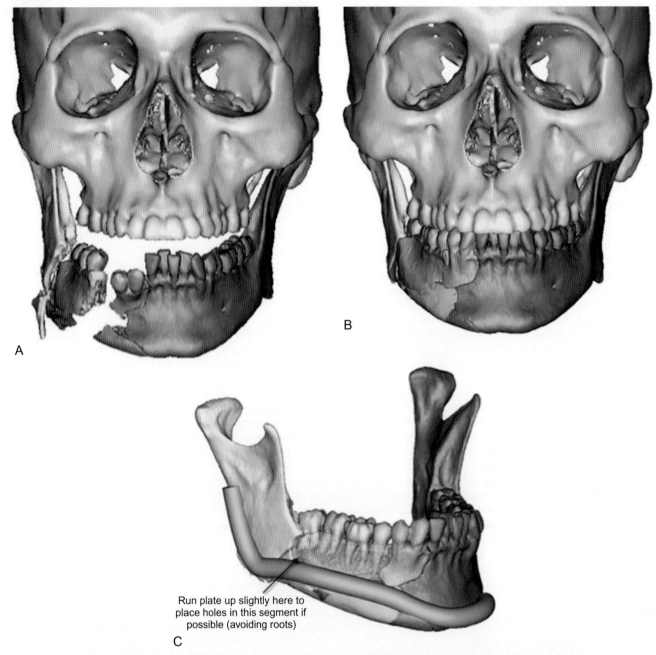

Run plate up slightly here to
place holes in this segment if
possible (avoiding roots)

Fig. 3.14.1 Computer-aided design and manufacturing (CAD/CAM) guided repair of complex mandibular fractures sustained in an industrial explosion. Simulated surgical plan illustrating (A) preoperative injury pattern, (B) virtual reduction and restoration of occlusion, and (C) planned placement of custom-milled plate with avoidance of tooth roots.

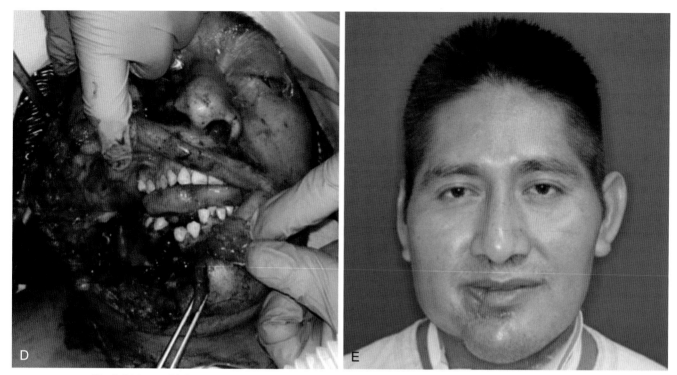

Fig. 3.14.1, cont'd Photographs showing (D) preoperative appearance with extensive soft tissue damage and comminution of mandible and (E) postoperative restoration. The virtual surgical plan and customized titanium plate enabled accurate anatomical alignment allowing for satisfactory postoperative occlusion and restoration of function.

challenging due to anatomic distortions and scarring caused by primary surgery, the requirement for debridement or corrective osteotomies, and the effacement of bony landmarks due to malunion or nonunion. In these cases the craniofacial surgeon must often remove what was suboptimal from the original surgery before crafting a *de novo* patient-specific solution. We describe some examples in which these principles are utilized to effect secondary repair of the mandible and orbit.

Mandible

We have used VSP to correct malunion of an edentulous mandible (Fig. 3.14.2). Accurate repair of mandible fractures in edentulous patients is challenging, as the lack of occlusal guidance makes accurate reduction difficult and poor bone stock complicates fracture healing.[12] In this example, the patient was a 69-year-old man who sustained bilateral body fractures after a fall 7 months prior to our repair. He originally underwent open reduction and internal fixation with miniplates, but this was complicated by plate failure. A revisional surgery was performed with hardware removal and reconstruction using a single load-bearing reconstruction bar spanning both fractures. This repair was complicated by malunion, however. Therefore, on presentation to our institution, the patient had an anterior open-bite with inability to masticate. As the patient was edentulous in both mandible and maxilla, VSP was instituted to place the mandible in a more functional position. Prefabricated cutting guides were generated to ensure accurate realignment of the malunited mandible and a pre-bent reconstruction plate was obtained to secure the osteotomized segments. Using these adjuncts repair was performed expeditiously. The patient achieved anatomic

union and was able to masticate with the aid of dentures at a 6-month follow-up.

Orbit

Fabrication of patient-specific implants is one of the more useful aspects of CAS in trauma reconstruction. We generated a custom orbital implant to precisely restore orbital volume in a patient with persistent enophthalmos following a motor vehicle accident. The 19-year-old man originally underwent repair of his right orbitozygomaticomaxillary complex fracture in Saudi Arabia. He presented to our clinic with enophthalmos of the right eye secondary to an inadequately repaired right orbital floor fracture, a poorly reduced and malpositioned right zygoma, and lower lid laxity. He underwent a staged repair with initial removal of periorbital and midfacial hardware through right eyebrow, transconjunctival, and intraoral vestibular incisions. Osteotomies at the zygomaticofrontal suture, orbital rim, zygomatic arch, and the zygomaticomaxillary buttress were performed and the fully mobilized zygoma was repositioned 5 mm superiorly and 2 mm medially (Fig. 3.14.3). Eight months later the patient returned with his zygoma in much better position and attention was turned to correcting the patient's enophthalmos and lid laxity. Through a right transconjunctival incision with lateral canthotomy, the orbital floor plate was freed from extensive scar and removed. A customized orbital implant was inserted to reconstruct the floor and medial wall and restore orbital volume. Prominent midfacial hardware was removed at the same time. A lateral canthopexy was performed prior to closure. The patient has healed well and is satisfied with his improved facial symmetry.

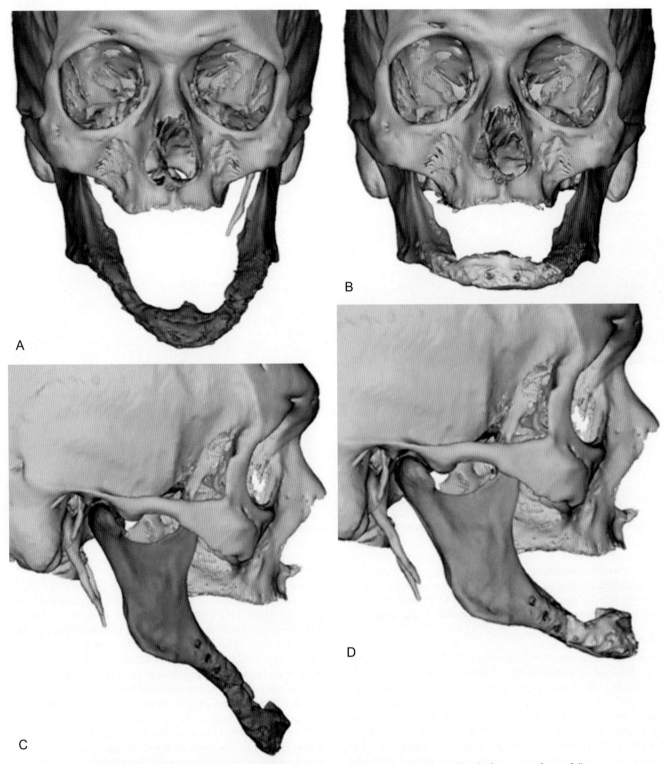

Fig. 3.14.2 A 69-year-old man with an edentulous mandible sustained bilateral body fractures after a fall. Failure of the original operation led to nonunion and malocclusion (A,C). Virtual surgical plan with repositioning of mandible is illustrated (B,D), along with pre- and postoperative photographs (E,F). He was able to masticate with the aid of dentures 6 months postoperatively.

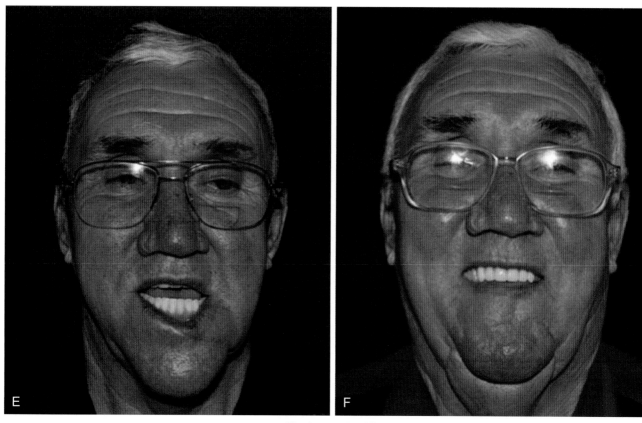

Fig. 3.14.2, cont'd

Free Tissue Transfer

Restoration of major bony and soft tissue losses in complex craniofacial trauma can necessitate free tissue transfer. When these injuries are treated secondarily, the reconstructive challenge is magnified by loss of normal anatomical relationships. Use of VSP is particularly helpful in these situations. Malunited bones can be osteotomized and realigned, abnormal tissues and implants removed, and new tissues docked into defects virtually. This expedites preoperative planning and allows for the fashioning of cutting guides that accelerate intraoperative execution. We provide an example in which these techniques were used to effect secondary reconstruction of the maxilla and orbit in a patient with significant ballistic injury.

The patient was a 19-year-old man who presented with severe secondary deformities following a gunshot wound to the face. He presented several months after his initial operative stabilization with maxillary malunion, enophthalmos, and malocclusion as well as a large oronasal fistula. The decision was made to proceed with debridement of necrotic maxilla, removal of hardware including his orbital implant, and reconstruction with free tissue transfer. A virtual planning session allowed simulation of maxillary resection and fibula placement and crafting of corresponding cutting guides. Through the use of these adjuncts, the patient's maxilla was resected leaving only the left posterior maxilla intact. This was mobilized via Le Fort I osteotomy and the free segment was placed in its premorbid position with proper occlusion using Ivy loops. After securing this segment to the zygoma with titanium plates, the right orbital rim and floor plates were removed and devitalized bone and soft tissue resected. Using prefabricated cutting guides a free myo-osteocutaneous fibula flap was harvested, segmented, and used to fill the large defect. Anastomosis was performed to the left facial vessels.

The segmented fibula was used to reconstruct the missing maxilla and medial orbital wall with additional free bone graft used to reconstruct the orbital floor (Fig. 3.14.4). The muscle and cutaneous portions of the flap were used to close the oronasal fistula and restore intraoral mucosal integrity. The patient has gone on to heal well from this extensive surgery, and following subsequent vestibuloplasty and soft tissue adjustments, is functioning well with good oral continence.

FUTURE OF CAS IN CRANIOFACIAL SURGERY

The examples above represent a small subset of the ways in which CAS currently expedites craniofacial reconstruction. The full flowering of these approaches, however, will require overcoming some of the existing impediments to their use, principally the time and cost associated with the CAS workflow. Recent trends such as the availability of low cost, in-office 3D printers, and the development of open source VSP software promise to bring the benefits of CAS to more patients. We next examine some of the more interesting applications of these technologies.

Rapid Prototyping

The emergence of low-cost consumer 3D printers coupled with CAD/CAM software is enabling more surgeons to use CAS. The situation is analogous to the development of desktop publishing in the 1980s, in which digital illustration and word processing on personal computers was coupled to consumer laser printers. Prior to this era, the inconvenience and expense of producing professionally printed materials meant that they were largely the province of businesses and were generated rarely. Desktop publishing enabled individuals to print high-quality documents with less time and expense, and this in turn led to more

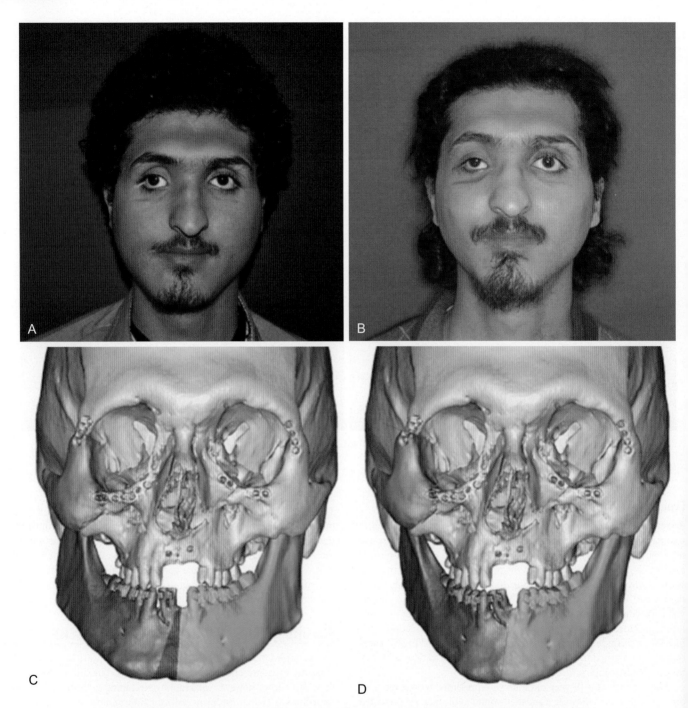

Fig. 3.14.3 A 19-year-old man with prior unsuccessful attempts to repair right orbitozygomaticomaxillary complex and mandibular fractures. Preoperative appearance (A) illustrates right enophthalmos secondary to an inadequately repaired right orbital floor fracture, a poorly reduced and malpositioned right zygoma, lower lid laxity, and widened intergonial width. After zygomatic and mandibular osteotomies and repositioning (C–D), placement of a customized orbital implant to reconstruct the floor and medial wall and restore orbital volume, he demonstrates improved facial symmetry (B). The surgical plan shows (C) preoperative appearance, and (D) result of intraoperative repositioning. The segment of the surgical plan in red illustrates a wedge of bone to be removed intraoperatively in order to reduce intergonial width (C).

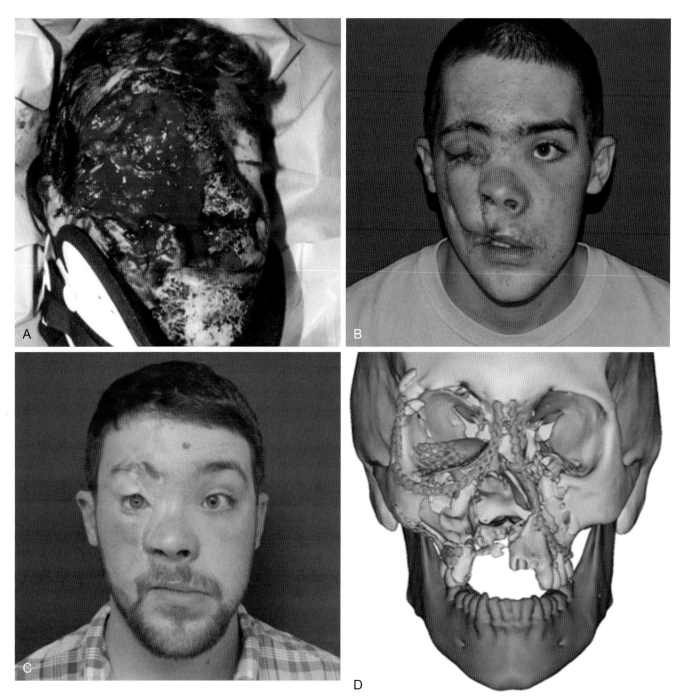

Fig. 3.14.4 A 19-year-old man with a maxillectomy defect following initial operative stabilization of fractures from a gunshot wound (GSW) required further reconstruction. Photographs demonstrate (A) extensive facial injuries secondary to the initial injury, (B) initial postoperative appearance following free fibular reconstruction using the VSP. The patient underwent further revisional surgeries to improve soft tissue contour (C), and is satisfied with the result. A planning session allowed visualization of (D and G) preoperative extent of injury, (E and H) simulation of maxillary osteotomies, and (F and I) reconstruction of the maxilla with placement of a free myo-osteocutaneous fibula flap. Simulation illustrating development of fibular cutting guides is demonstrated (J). *Continued*

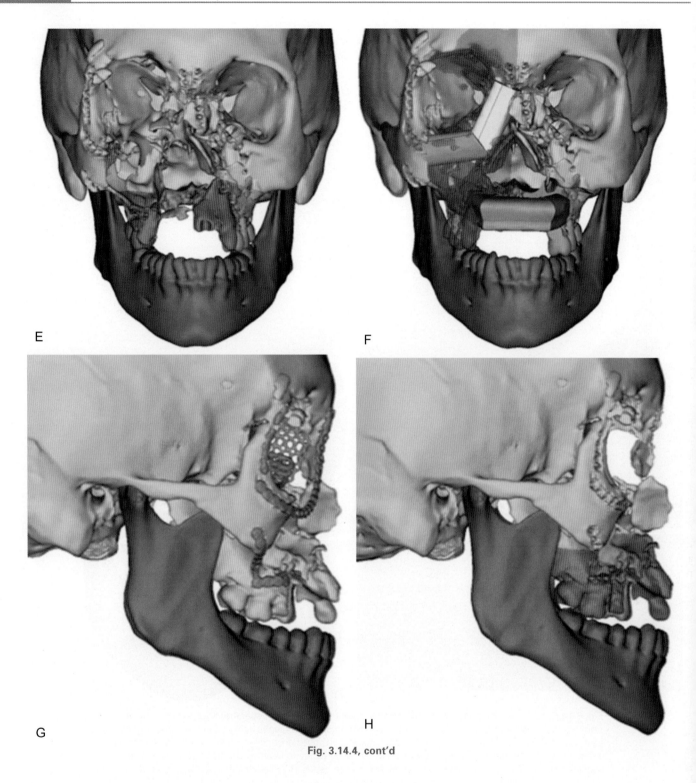

E

F

G

H

Fig. 3.14.4, cont'd

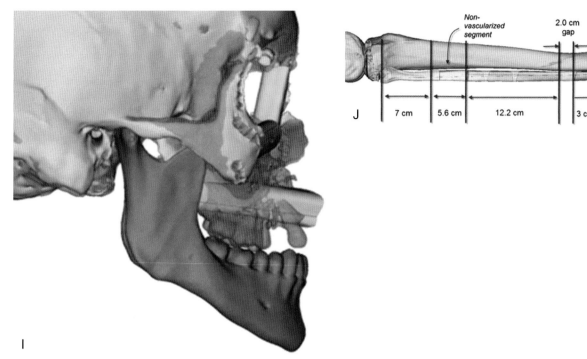

J   7 cm   5.6 cm   12.2 cm   3 cm   7 cm

Non-vascularized segment   2.0 cm gap

I

Fig. 3.14.4, cont'd

exploratory, provisional production of documents. We expect a similar proliferation of uses of CAS techniques as 3D printers and associated software become more available. Notably FDA requirements currently preclude implantation of titanium implants 3D printed in-house, thus requiring outsourcing at present to companies with FDA approval.

One example of "consumer" use of CAS technologies is provided by Dang et al., who used the approaches in reconstruction of the pre-maxilla.[13] The patient was an 18-year-old woman who was kicked by a horse resulting in fracture of the maxillary alveolus with loss of teeth numbers 11 and 12. The authors imported high-resolution CT images into an open source modeling program called 3D slicer (slicer.org). An STL file was generated and further refined using CAD/CAM software provided by Autodesk. The resulting digital file was used to generate a 3D physical model of the patient's defect using a MakerBot Replicator. The model, which was made of polylactic acid (PLA), was sterilized and used intraoperatively to plan and shape a bone graft harvested from mandibular symphysis. While the authors do not provide a cost estimate for their CAS workflow, the materials costs were less than US$2, the 3D printer they used can be obtained for a few thousand dollars, and the software was either open source or available through an academic license. The entire production took less than 14 hours.

Utilizing a similar workflow, Mendez and colleagues generated a 3D physical model of a patient's frontoorbital region illustrating a post-traumatic defect.[14] The model was sterilized and used intraoperatively to shape a split calvarial bone graft. Using the adjunct the reconstruction was performed expeditiously in 4 hours. The model itself was generated in 14 hours with a materials cost of $25. As these cases demonstrate, having a physical model of the defect enables a graft of the exact size to be obtained, limiting donor site morbidity and time of harvest. As costs drop further we expect more groups to utilize these approaches.

While CAS techniques have largely been used in reshaping the cra-niofacial skeleton, they are also useful in guiding soft tissue reconstruc-tion. Cho and colleagues recently described the use of 3D printing of a complex calvarial defect model.[15] This was subsequently used as a

template for liquid silicone application to generate a model of missing soft tissue envelope. The flexible, 3D model was then applied to guide the design of an anterolateral thigh flap for free tissue transfer. The resulting flap was precisely contoured to the patient's anatomy, limiting donor site morbidity and accelerating flap harvest. Future applications of CAS to soft tissue reconstruction can extrapolate from these approaches. For example, volumetric imaging systems like Dolphin may be used to generate models of missing soft tissue that can guide skin paddle design in fibular flap reconstruction or estimate tissue harvest for parascapular or anterolateral thigh flaps to restore missing craniofacial soft tissues. These approaches will enhance the ultimate appearance of craniofacial reconstructions.

One of the most exciting future applications of CAS in craniofacial surgery involves coupling custom implants with bioactive substances such as cells and growth factors. A number of experimental studies have demonstrated the utility of these approaches for regenerating craniofacial bone and soft tissues. Hung and colleagues, for example, used decellularized bone matrix combined with synthetic polycapro-lactone polymers to generate hybrid osteoinductive scaffolds.[16] These materials showed improved cell adhesion, and when used with adipocyte-derived stem cells (hASCs), were able to heal critical-sized calvarial defects in mice. The ready availability of hASCs in liposuction aspirates makes this type of cell-based approach more plausible for translational medicine than other stem cell strategies.

A major challenge to these approaches is securing regulatory approval for implantation of bioactive prosthetics, cells, and tissues. Yet as the successful use of 3D printed bladders in human clinical trials has dem-onstrated, these challenges are surmountable.[17] Furthermore, one of the major osteoinductive proteins, BMP2, has already been FDA approved for use in craniofacial surgery. We anticipate the combination of patient-specific implants, growth factors, and stem cells to yield reconstruc-tions with custom living tissue. All of this points to a future of more natural reconstruction for the most challenging craniofacial trauma patients.

EXPERT COMMENTARY

The roots of the current use of computer-assisted surgery, virtual surgery planning, and 3D printing extend to the 1980s, where the inventive use of computed tomography scans led to the planning of operations and their execution on the computer. It was not long before 3D printing would generate models helpful in surgery. We now can educate a generation of surgeons with virtual operations. Surgeons have been way behind other professionals, like engineers and airline pilots, in their use of virtual simulation, but our younger generation has vigorously embraced it, and the techniques indeed increase the organization, accuracy, and ease with which tough cases are handled. Two examples where the techniques have "shortened the learning curve" are the orbit and the occlusion. Both areas require some of the most demanding perfection in the face, and the use of these techniques of analysis and planning has produced many "experts" who would not have achieved that degree of expertise without those techniques of analysis and preparation. So read thoroughly, prepare your challenging cases, and enjoy the perfection achieved by these techniques of planning and analysis.

REFERENCES

1. Vannier MW, Marsh JL, Warren JO. Three dimensional CT reconstruction images for craniofacial surgical planning and evaluation. *Radiology.* 1984;150(1):179–184.
2. Arridge S, Moss JP, Linney AD, James DR. Three dimensional digitization of the face and skull. *J Maxillofac Surg.* 1985;13(3):136–143.
3. Toth BA, Ellis DS, Stewart WB. Computer-designed prostheses for orbitocranial reconstruction. *Plast Reconstr Surg.* 1988;81(3):315–324.
4. Fisher M, Medina M 3rd, Bojovic B, et al. Indications for computer-aided design and manufacturing in congenital craniofacial reconstruction. *Craniomaxillofac Trauma Reconstr.* 2016;9(3):235–241.
5. Hammoudeh JA, Howell LK, Boutros S, et al. Current status of surgical planning for orthognathic surgery: traditional methods versus 3D surgical planning. *Plast Reconstr Surg Glob Open.* 2015;3(2):e307.
6. Mahoney N, Grant MP, Susarla SM, Merbs S. Computer-assisted three-dimensional planning for orbital decompression. *Craniomaxillofac Trauma Reconstr.* 2015;8(3):211–217.
7. Rudman K, Hoekzema C, Rhee J. Computer-assisted innovations in craniofacial surgery. *Facial Plast Surg.* 2011;27(4):358–365.
8. Seruya M, Borsuk DE, Khalifian S, et al. Computer-aided design and manufacturing in craniosynostosis surgery. *J Craniofac Surg.* 2013;24(4):1100–1105.
9. Zhang W, Li B, Gui H, et al. Reconstruction of complex mandibular defect with computer-aided navigation and orthognathic surgery. *J Craniofac Surg.* 2013;24(3):e229–e233.
10. Seruya M, Fisher M, Rodriguez ED. Computer-assisted versus conventional free fibula flap technique for craniofacial reconstruction: an outcomes comparison. *Plast Reconstr Surg.* 2013;132(5):1219–1228.
11. Fisher M, Dorafshar A, Bojovic B, et al. The evolution of critical concepts in aesthetic craniofacial microsurgical reconstruction. *Plast Reconstr Surg.* 2012;130(2):389–398.
12. Broyles JM, Wallner C, Borsuk DE, Dorafshar AH. The role of computer-assisted design and modeling in an edentulous mandibular malunion reconstruction. *J Craniofac Surg.* 2013;24(5):1835–1838.
13. Dang P, Lafarge A, Depeyre A, et al. Virtual surgery planning and three-dimensional printing template to customize bone graft toward implant insertion. *J Craniofac Surg.* 2017;28(2):173–175.
14. Mendez BM, Chiodo MV, Patel PA. Customized "in-office" three-dimensional printing for virtual surgical planning in craniofacial surgery. *J Craniofac Surg.* 2015;26(5):1584–1586.
15. Cho MJ, Kane AA, Hallac RR, et al. Liquid latex molding: a novel application of 3D printing to facilitate flap design. *Cleft Palate Craniofac J.* 2016.
16. Hung BP, Naved BA, Nyberg EL, et al. Three-dimensional printing of bone extracellular matrix for craniofacial regeneration. *ACS Biomater Sci Eng.* 2016;2(10):1806–1816.
17. Atala A. Tissue engineering of human bladder. *Br Med Bull.* 2011;97:81–104.

Posttraumatic Facial Pain

A. Lee Dellon*

BACKGROUND

In order for a person to perceive facial pain, there must be a peripheral nerve pathway for neural impulses to travel from the site of injury into the central nervous system. The classic facial pain, "trigeminal neuralgia" or "tic douloureux" is *not* what this chapter is about, as that perceived pain originates within the central nervous system. Facial injury most often involves branches of the trigeminal nerve (TN) to the forehead (frontal branch, V_1), midface (maxillary branch, V_2), and mandible (mandibular branch, V_3) (Fig. 3.15.1).

There is no published epidemiologic study about the incidence or prevalence of posttraumatic facial pain. The most recently reported description of 21,000 craniofacial injuries in almost 10,000 patients did not include facial pain.[1] There have been observational studies related to the frontal bone (V_1) where 5 (13%) of 43 patients had chronic frontotemporal "headache pain."[2] These patients each had a fracture of the anterior table of the frontal sinus. In another observational study, related to zygoma fractures (V_2), 76% of 25 patients, at a mean of 6.3 months post-injury, were found to have abnormal cutaneous pressure thresholds in the distribution of the infraorbital nerve on the side with the fracture.[3] The difference between the 13% prevalence of facial pain, and the 76% prevalence of sensory abnormalities is due to the difference in the question asked and the method of investigation in the study of craniomaxillofacial trauma.

While the TN is a cranial nerve, once its branches leave the cranium, they become covered with Schwann cells, and therefore behave like a peripheral nerve in that they can regenerate. If they can regenerate, then they can form a painful neuroma. *This insight provides the basis of treatment of painful neuromas of the trigeminal nerve.* While injuries and painful sequelae of injured trigeminal nerves have been described classically,[4,5] and those descriptions remain valid, what remains unresolved is the surgical approaches to treat injuries to V_1, V_2, and V_3. An approach to the treatment of posttraumatic facial pain has been described in which the TN is considered as a peripheral nerve.[6,7]

As with every peripheral nerve injury, if the nerve provides sensibility to an area of critical importance, like the lip, then reconstruction is the appropriate surgical choice.[8–10] If the nerve does not provide critical sensibility to an area, like the forehead, then interruption of nerve function,[11] with appropriate treatment to the proximal end of the nerve, is the surgical choice.[12] The "appropriate treatment" for the proximal end of the injured TN will be discussed in detail later in this chapter (Box 3.15.1).

*Declaration of interest: Conssultant to Axogen, Inc., and royalties received on AcroVal.™

BOX 3.15.1 Clinical Pearl

- If a nerve provides critical sensibility to an area, like the lip, then reconstruction is the appropriate surgical choice.
- If a nerve does not provide critical sensibility to an area, like the forehead, then resection (interruption of function) of that nerve is the appropriate surgical choice.

For the purposes of this chapter on posttraumatic facial pain, the "face" will be defined as including skin that is innervated by branches of the cervical plexus, as these can be injured and the pain perceived as facial in origin (Fig. 3.15.1). Also for the purposes of this chapter, "headaches," including frontal, temporal, nasal, and occipital, will be included to provide a basis for approaching posttraumatic pain in a surgical manner distinct from the approach to the classic migraine, which is not posttraumatic in origin. Additionally, posttraumatic occipital injuries may give pain that radiates to the frontal region, and needs to be distinguished for diagnosis and appropriate treatment by doing nerve blocks (Figs. 3.15.2 and 3.15.3) or Botox® (onabotulinumtoxinA) injections.[13]

Aesthetic surgery of the face and neck can be considered as trauma, and, as such, this chapter will include facial pain that results secondary to cosmetic surgery, and the surgical approaches to correct this origin of posttraumatic facial pain.

Finally, this chapter will not include discussion of intrinsic temporomandibular joint (TMJ) disorders, although a peripheral nerve approach to denervation of the TMJ has been described[14,15]; nor will this chapter discuss other rare pain disorders, such as Eagle's syndrome[16] (orofacial pain related to the stylohyoid ligament), or persistent burning mouth syndrome.[17]

DIFFERENTIAL DIAGNOSIS OF POSTTRAUMATIC FACIAL PAIN

Posttraumatic facial pain must first be proven to be due to an injury to a peripheral nerve that is part of the craniofacial skeleton. This implies that *there has to be a history of trauma to the head and neck region*. A history of facial or cranial surgery is a history of trauma.

History

In obtaining the history from the patient, the most commonly overlooked source of posttraumatic facial pain is previous *neurosurgery procedures*, such as those for Chiari malformation (Fig. 3.15.4A), that require incisions at the base of the occiput, or those for brain tumor, such as acoustic neuroma,[18] which are in the postauricular, mastoid

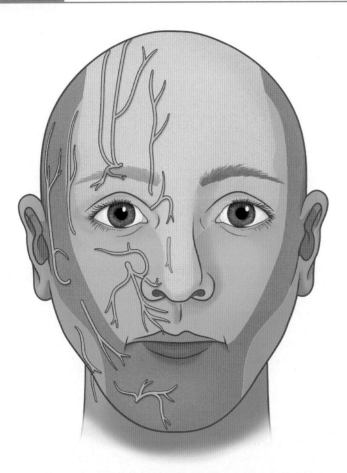

Fig. 3.15.1 Both the trigeminal nerve and the cervical plexus innervate the face. Trigeminal branches: V₁, frontal branch (*orange*), V₂, maxillary branch (*green*), V₃, mandibular branch (*pink*). Cervical branches (*blue*).

area. Other less common causes related to neurosurgery are cerebrospinal shunt placements, burr holes, and the anterior site of tong placements. The next most frequently missed history point is a previous *motor vehicle accident* with a whiplash injury, which can cause pain related to the anterior scalene becoming adherent to the cervical and brachial plexus,[19] or with an airbag inflation. Be sure to ask about childhood injuries to the craniofacial skeleton, such as a baseball (Fig. 3.15.4B) hitting the face, a fall from a bike, or other sports accidents, which must include heading a ball in soccer and concussion. Especially if the pain is related to V₂ or V₃, inquire about dental surgery, particularly dental implants (Fig. 3.15.4C). Finally, when asking about previous facial surgery, ask directly about cosmetic surgery such as facelift (Fig. 3.15.4D), cheek implants, or jaw surgery, such as chin implant or orthognathic surgery.

Nerve Blocks

Compression of the trigeminal ganglion or its nerve roots intracranially will cause facial pain that will *not* be relieved by a nerve block of the peripheral TN branches. It is now accepted that traditional trigeminal neuralgia is a vascular compression of the Gasserian ganglia roots by a branch of the inferior cerebellar artery, which is best treated by an intracranial vascular decompression, as originally described by Jannetta, in 1967.[20,21] Therefore, a nerve block, as depicted in Fig. 3.15.2, will document that pain is from an injury to a peripheral branch of the TN, and not from intracranial vascular compression if (1) the expected skin territory goes numb after the local anesthetic is injected, and if

(2) the pain is relieved. This holds true for nerve blocks to the cervical plexus (Fig. 3.15.2, and the occipital nerves (Fig. 3.15.3).

Imaging

While the computed tomography (CT) scans usually cannot demonstrate nerves directly, the injury to a bone adjacent to the known anatomical location of a nerve supports the diagnosis of posttraumatic facial pain due to that nerve. This is demonstrated in Fig. 3.15.5A where the left orbital floor is lower than it is on the right, and the infraorbital canal is deformed on the left. In Fig. 3.15.5B, the right infraorbital nerve is injured at the location of the fixation plate at the infraorbital rim. Another example is given in Fig. 3.15.6, where the right inferior alveolar nerve was injured twice; the first time with a screw designed to hold a bone graft prior to dental implant placement, and then a second time, when a metal clip was placed on the mental nerve at the mental foramen. The application of 3T MRI to the cranial nerves has brought a new dimension to being able to evaluate posttraumatic facial pain and is the best way to document vascular compression of the trigeminal ganglia and its roots.[22]

Neurosensory Documentation of Trigeminal Nerve Function

An injured sensory nerve will develop a pattern of function that relates to the degree of nerve compression and a pattern that can identify nerve regeneration. Normative data for the one-point static- and moving-touch, and two-point static- and moving-touch was reported in 2007 using the Pressure-Specified Sensory Device™.[23] The use of this device (previously marketed by Sensory Management Services, Inc., Baltimore, MD, now marketed as AcroVal™ Neurosensory and Motor Testing Systems by Axogen, Inc., Alachua, FL) has been reviewed extensively recently.[24] By measuring the cutaneous pressure threshold of appropriate target skin areas, a patient's subjective complaints can be documented, as related to complete loss of function, compression, or nerve regeneration for trigeminal nerve branches, as illustrated in Figs. 3.15.7–3.15.9.

Psychological Evaluation

While it is appreciated that living with chronic facial pain can cause depression, frustration, anxiety, household problems, loss of work, and narcotic addiction, it is not so commonly appreciated that either the injury itself of the interactions with the medical profession can cause posttraumatic stress disorder (PTSD).[25,26] At the time of the initial encounter with the patient, it is appropriate, indeed mandatory that medication either be prescribed for anxiety, depression, PTSD, or that referral to a psychiatrist be suggested so these medications can be prescribed. Most patients usually will have tried or already be on a neuropathic pain medication and a narcotic. It is critical that caring for this patient be done in conjunction with a pain management physician.

SURGICAL TREATMENT OF A PAINFUL NEUROMA (BOX 3.15.2)

Every divided peripheral nerve will sprout proximally and attempt to reconnect with its distal branches, guided by the gradient of new nerve growth factor produced by the distal Schwann cells. Nerve regeneration will proceed along the remaining distal basement membrane that survives after Wallerian degeneration. With the exception of the olfactory and optic nerves, which are extensions of the central nervous system, all other cranial nerves, will regenerate. Of course this applies to the cervical plexus (C₂, C₃, C₄, and C₅) and occipital nerves, which are the dorsal cutaneous branches of the occipital nerves C₁, C₂, and C₃.

When the nerve is first divided, there will be numbness in the distal skin target territory. Then, if the regenerating nerves connect to their

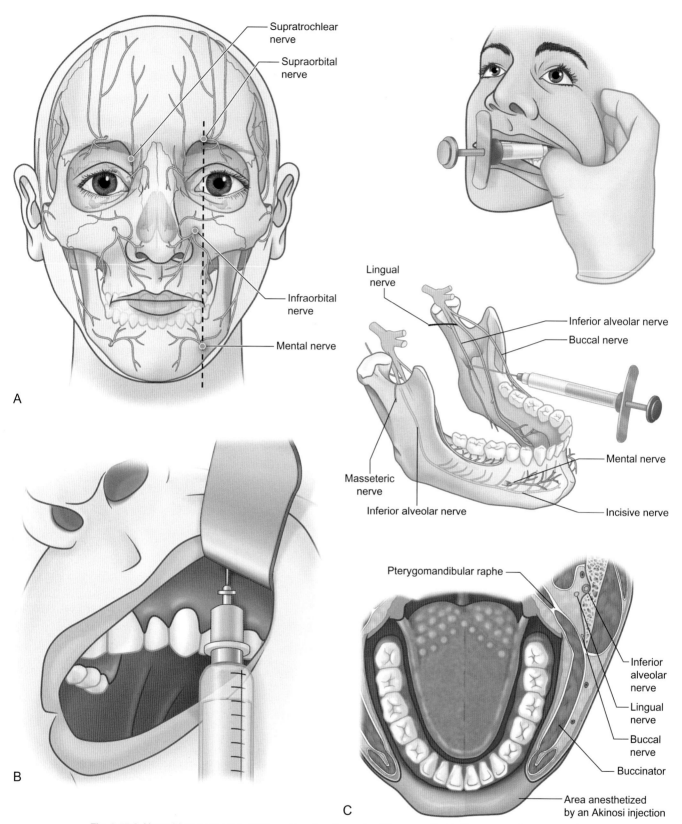

Fig. 3.15.2 Nerve blocks are essential in making the diagnosis of the nerve that is the source of posttraumatic facial pain. (A) Technique for blocking V_1, V_2, and V_3 through the skin. (B) Technique for blocking the anterior superior branch of V_2 which separates from the infraorbital nerve at or near the infraorbital foramen. (C) Technique for intraoral block of the inferior alveolar branch of V_3.

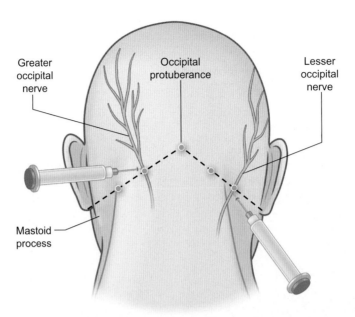

Fig. 3.15.3 Nerve block technique for the greater and lesser occipital nerves.

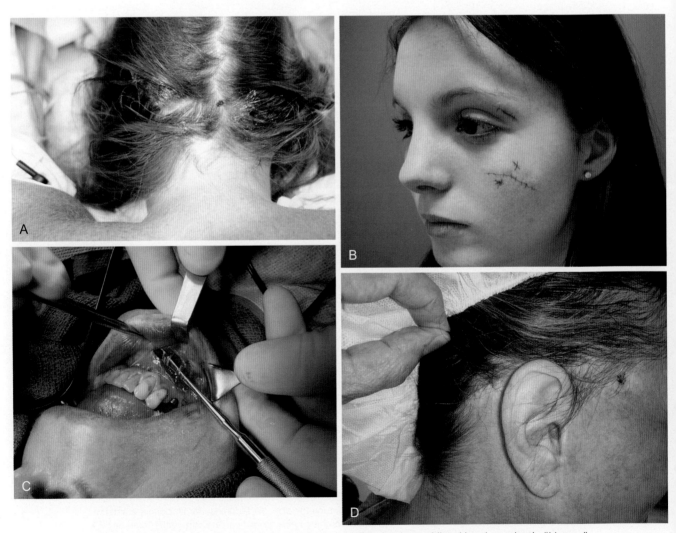

Fig. 3.15.4 Identification of posttraumatic facial pain can often be done while taking the patient's "history." (A) Scar from previous Chiari malformation surgery has injured occipital nerve branches. (B) Scars from being hit in the cheek with a baseball causing a zygoma fracture and eyebrow laceration have injured the zygomaticotemporal and zygomaticofacial branches of the frontal branch of the trigeminal nerve (V_1 and V_2). (C) Placement of dental implant has injured the terminal branch of the inferior alveolar nerve (V_3). (D) Facelift surgery has injured the greater auricular and lesser occipital branches of the cervical plexus.

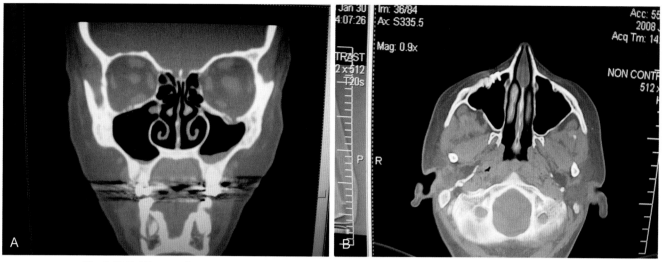

Fig. 3.15.5 CT scans document injury to the left (A) infraorbital nerve in the orbital floor, and right (B) infraorbital nerve next to a fixation plate at the infraorbital rim.

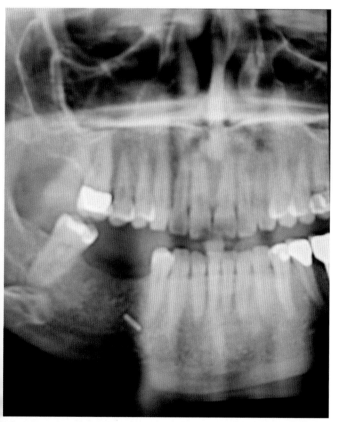

Fig. 3.15.6 Bone grafting was attempted to fill this right lower mandibular gap in order to facilitate a dental implant. The screw to hold the graft injured the inferior alveolar nerve. An attempt was made to treat the painful lip by placing a metal clip along the mental nerve at the mental foramen, further aggravating the nerve injury.

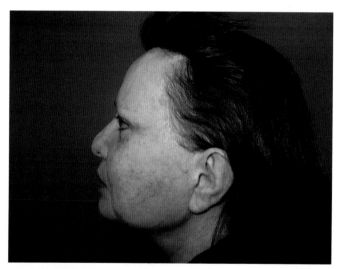

Fig. 3.15.7 This woman has had her second brow lift using an anterior hairline approach, and developed severe forehead pain and frontal headaches. Neurosensory testing demonstrated complete absence of static two-point discrimination on the right (red bars absent) and almost complete loss of sensibility on the left (blue bars), in the skin territories of the supraorbital and zygomaticotemporal nerves. The indicated treatment for this woman is to resect the damaged supraorbital and zygomaticotemporal nerves.

BOX 3.15.2   Clinical Pearl

- Treatment of a painful neuroma requires neuroma resection, as the neuroma is the source of the painful neural impulses.
- To prevent recurrent neuroma formation, the proximal end of the nerve must be placed into a "quiet" place, away from tension, traction, and touch.
- While muscle targets are available for cervical plexus and occipital nerves, muscle targets are *not* available for trigeminal nerve branches.
- *Unique operative solutions are required for each trigeminal nerve branch that has a painful neuroma*

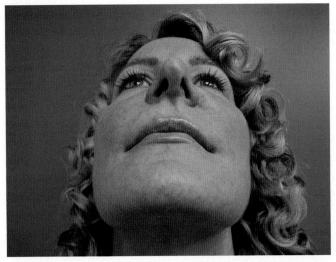

Fig. 3.15.8 This woman had bilateral upper lip and paranasal pain bilaterally after a rhinoplasty. Neurosensory testing of the cheek and upper lip bilaterally demonstrated preserved static two-point discrimination, although it required greater than normal pressure to be perceived and the static two-point discrimination threshold was abnormal. This is consistent with mild chronic compression, equal bilaterally, and observation with percutaneous massage of steroid into the nasal bone osteotomy sites was advised.

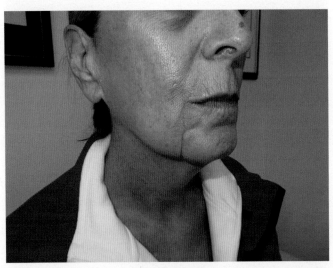

Fig. 3.15.9 This woman is 5 months following a dog bite to the lower right lip, with partial crush to the right upper jaw as well. Her neurosensory testing demonstrates a nerve regeneration pattern on the right for each of the three skin territories tested. She was advised that her pain should continue to improve with time, which it did.

distal targets, there will be the perception of buzzing and tingling as a normal consequence of regeneration. These are paresthesias. These perceptions may be perceived as uncomfortable or even painful, and then are termed dysesthesia. If during the course of regeneration the sprouts become entrapped in the healing process of the injury, a neuroma will form, which is just multiple small axon sprouts becoming embedded in scar. Not all neuromas are painful, in which case there is an area of numbness and no pain. If a localized area of pain exists at the site of an injury, with a distal decrease in sensibility, then a neuroma has formed.

While more than 200 papers have been published about techniques to prevent neuroma formation, the only approach that has proven

---

> ### BOX 3.15.3 **Clinical Pearl**
> - The surgical treatment for a chronic nerve compression is neurolysis.
> - If pain persists post-neurolysis, then nerve resection may be appropriate.

successful over a long period of time, and for peripheral nerves of the upper and lower extremity, is to place the proximal end of the nerve into a muscle sufficiently large and with little excursion.[27–30]

If a skin target is of critical sensibility, such as the lip, then the approach to the painful neuroma of the inferior alveolar nerve is to interrupt the pain pathway proximal to the injured nerve, and reconstruct the nerve, relieving pain and attempting to restore function.

For each of the specific nerve environments to be discussed in the rest of this chapter, this approach will be presented individually, but, in general, branches of the cervical plexus will be implanted into the sternocleidomastoid muscle, the occipital nerves will be implanted into the neck muscles deep to the trapezius (splenius capitus, and semispinalis capitus). There are no sufficiently large muscles on the facial skeleton into which a nerve can be implanted. In the hand, when no muscles sufficiently large are available, a digital nerve can be implanted into a medullary cavity of bone. There are no medullary bone cavities sufficient to do this in the facial skeleton. The approach to the TN branches is unique, and the author's current approach will be presented in the sections to follow.

FRONTAL BRANCH OF THE TRIGEMINAL NERVE (V₁)

Supraorbital, Supratrochlear and Infratrochlear Nerves

The anatomy of these nerves is well described classically.

With a blunt injury to the forehead, these nerves may be contused, subsequently swell, and then become adherent to the surrounding corrugator muscles and superior orbital ridge/trochlea. This creates a *chronic nerve compression*, which will differ in its symptoms and approach from that for a painful neuroma. With compression, the forehead skin will have decreased, but not absent, sensation; the sensation present will still be normal, not dysesthetic, and there will be a mild Tinel sign or tenderness over the nerves at the superior orbital ridge. A nerve block will relieve the pain as a diagnostic test, Botox injection into the corrugator muscles may give sufficient relief for several months at a time, and neuropathic pain medication may be of value. *The symptoms may be identical to the frontal headaches of migraine, but differ in the history of trauma. Frontal migraine patients do not have a history of trauma.* With a diagnosis of compression, the surgical approach should be a neurolysis, attempting to preserve function while relieving pain (Fig. 3.15.10 and Box 3.15.3). The patient should be counselled that the decompressed nerve may result, for about 3 months, in dysesthesias as neural regeneration occurs, although most commonly relief is experienced quickly. The patient should be counselled that if the symptoms persist 6 months or more after neurolysis, then it is appropriate to resect the injured nerves. This neurolysis differs from that typically described for the frontal migraine patient in that an upper eyelid incision, instead of an "endoscopic browlift" approach,[31] is used, thereby permitting a neurolysis into the orbit including a division of the band across the supraorbital notch.

With a sharp or open injury to the forehead, these nerves will be directly damaged. They may or may not have been repaired primarily. The diagnosis of this form of chronic pain is a neuroma of the supraorbital and/or supratrochlear nerve. A resection of these neuromas and treatment by end-to-end coaptation by means of a neural conduit has been described.[32] A series of six patients was reported. Preoperative

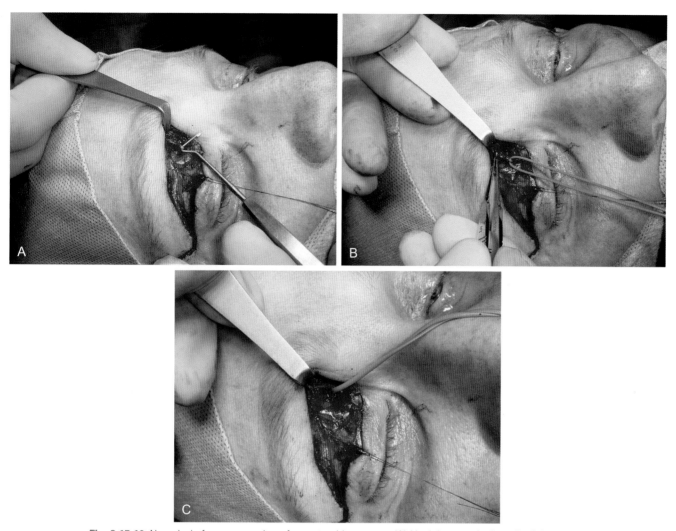

Fig. 3.15.10 Neurolysis for compression of supratrochlear nerve. (A) Hook is around a branch of the nerve. (B) Microscissors used to excise portions of corrugator muscle. (C) Completion of neurolysis.

mean pain (VAS) was 9.2 and postoperative mean pain was 1.5 ($p =$ .03). Mean follow-up was 14 months. No surgical complications were reported.

With or without a repair, if forehead and anterior scalp pain persist despite scar massage, neuropathic pain medication, and steroid injection, then *a surgical approach to the painful neuroma* is appropriate. This is illustrated in Fig. 3.15.11. After protecting the globe, and injecting the local anesthetic, an upper eyelid incision is made, taken deep to the orbicularis muscle, and then the dissection is directed along the orbital septum to the superior orbital rim. The branches of the supraorbital nerve are identified within the orbit, blocked with 1% lidocaine with epinephrine, dissected about 1.5–2 cm into the orbit, cauterized with a bipolar coagulator set at low level, and then sharply divided with a microscissors, allowing the proximal end to retract into the orbit and above the orbital fat. The supratrochlear nerve is treated in a similar manner, taking care not to injure the superior oblique muscle as it courses around the trochlea. My personal experience with the first 5 patients having this approach has been reported.[12] The mean preoperative pain (VAS) was 9 and the mean postoperative pain level was 0.6 ($p <$.001). The mean follow-up was 19.6 months, range 12–34 months. There were no surgical complications (Table 3.15.1). This experience has been confirmed since then with two more patients.

Anterior Ethmoidal Nerve

This is a branch of the frontal nerve, the external nasal nerve, that exits the medial wall of the orbit with the anterior ethmoidal artery, then proceeds within the mucous membrane of the lateral wall of the nose to exit distally between the nasal bone and the upper lateral cartilage to innervate the lateral nasal skin. The first report of injury to this nerve was in 1991, and 6 patients were reported to be helped by removal of this nerve endonasally.[33] The anterior ethmoidal nerve was mentioned in the differential diagnosis of nasal pain subsequently, but none of their four reported cases included an injured anterior ethmoidal nerve.[34] In my experience, this nerve can be injured during tumor surgery, cosmetic surgery, with blunt trauma, and during endonasal surgery. It can be resected directly through an upper eyelid incision, dissecting along the medial orbital wall until the nerve and vessel are identified. It is then blocked with 1% lidocaine with epinephrine, cauterized with a bipolar coagulator set at low level, and then sharply divided with a microscissors, allowing the distal end to retract into the ethmoids medial to the globe (Fig. 3.15.12). It may be necessary to resect also the infratrochlear nerve to relieve pain in the medial orbital/glabellar region.

Zygomaticotemporal Nerve

This is a branch of the frontal nerve that traverses a small foramen in the superior lateral orbital wall to enter the infratemporal fossa where

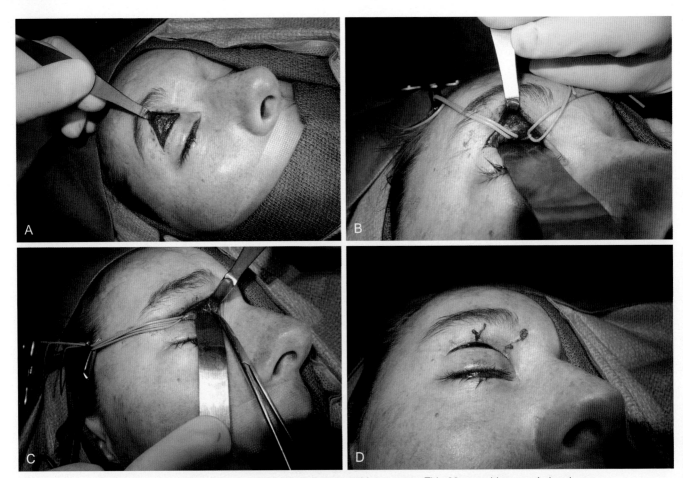

Fig. 3.15.11 Resection of the supraorbital and supratrochlear nerves. This 33-year-old woman's head was injured in a motor vehicle collision. The nerves were repaired primarily at the time of soft tissue closure 5 years previously. Her frontal headaches and pain have not been controlled with maximum medical treatment, and her pain is relieved with nerve blocks. She has had 2 years of Botox treatments. (A) The forehead and glabellar scars are evident. The dissection proceeds deep to the orbicularis oculi to the superior orbital ridge. (B) Within the orbit, two branches of the supraorbital nerves are encircled with vessel loops. (C) The supratrochlear nerve is identified. (D) Resected portions of the nerves are seen. The proximal ends are left within the orbit overlying the orbital fat.

TABLE 3.15.1 Outcomes From Resecting Supraorbital and Supratrochlear Neuromas, Leaving Proximal End Within Orbit

Name	Age (yr)	Initial Injury	Time From T^0 to OR (months)	Operation Done	Follow-Up (mth)	Result (E,G,F,P)
1	19	Fall, bike	120	R SOx R STx	34	E
2	18	Fall, bench	148	R SOx R STx	18	G
3	56	Tether ball	84	R SOx R STx R ZTx	20	E
4	51	WC tire Rim & fracture	60	R SOx R STx R ZTx	24	E
5	67	2nd brow	36	L SOx L STx	12	E

T^0 = initial injury; OR = operation; T^0 to OR = duration of symptoms prior to neuroma resection; R = right side; L = left side; SOx = resection supraorbital nerve; STx = resection supratrochlear nerve; WC = worker's compensation claim patient; E = excellent; G = good; F = fair; P = poor.

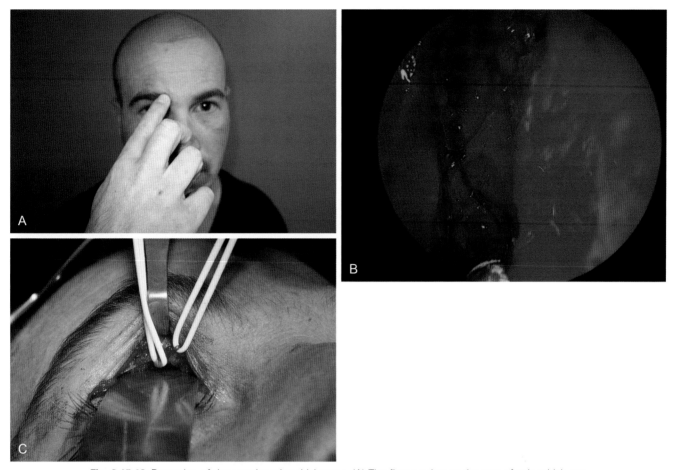

Fig. 3.15.12 Resection of the anterior ethmoidal nerve. (A) The finger points to the area of pain which can be triggered by pressing deeply into the medial orbit. The patient perceives numbness over the distal lateral side of the nose. He had a previous nasal injury in an altercation. (B) Endonasal view after endoscopic resection of the anterior ethmoidal nerve, at which time a metal clip was placed on the vessel/nerve, leading to his persistent pain. (C) A medial orbital approach identified the anterior ethmoidal nerve, which was divided and the proximal end allowed to remain within the orbit.

it pierces the temporalis fascia to innervate an area of skin that partially overlaps the auriculotemporal nerve territory.

The distinction of doing a neurolysis of the zygomaticotemporal (ZT) nerve versus a resection has been emphasized recently, with an approach using an anterior hairline incision. Among the 19 patients reported, equally good results were obtained with neurolysis as in those with resection of the nerve.[35] An intraoperative decision was made based upon the appearance of the ZT nerve as to whether to preserve it, or resect it and implant the proximal end into the temporalis muscle.

Other surgical approaches to the ZT nerve include a direct incision in the skin, appropriate for an older individual, or an approach through the lateral orbit (Fig. 3.15.13).

Zygomaticofacial Nerve

This nerve leaves from the floor of the lateral orbit, through a short tunnel, and exits directly over the zygoma. It can be directly injured with blunt trauma, without a zygoma fracture, the difference being pain directly in this spot, without measurable sensory loss, and without numbness in the infraorbital nerve distribution. This nerve can be injured during placement of a cheek implant. My preferred approach is through the upper buccal sulcus, directly to the foramen, and simply avulsing this nerve branch leaving its proximal end within the foramen. If an existing scar is present, it can be opened to reach this nerve. If

the pain recurs, the nerve can be resected within the orbit using a lower eyelid or transconjunctival approach.

Infraorbital Branch of the Trigeminal Nerve (V$_2$)

The anatomy of the infraorbital nerve (ION) has been well described with the exception of its anterior superior alveolar nerve (ASAN). The location of the ASAN has been defined recently, which permits a separate anatomical approach to its resection, permitting preservation of sensation to the lateral nose, cheek, and upper lip.[36]

There are no published outcome studies of the surgical approach to treat the ION.

The typical injury to the ION occurs from an orbital floor or zygoma fracture (Fig. 3.15.5). The pain distribution is the classic skin distribution of the ION, but may not include the anterior maxillary teeth, depending upon where the ASAN branches from the ION. For compression of this nerve due to blunt trauma, which may include a subperiosteal face lift, a surgical approach through the orbital floor can be used (Fig. 3.15.14) or a surgical approach under the upper lip can be used to approach the ION (Fig. 3.15.15).

For a true neuroma of the ION, a resection must be done, and the location into which to place the proximal end remains undefined. The choice is to (1) resect the neuroma and leave the proximal end within the floor of the orbit, after perhaps opening the roof of the tunnel, or

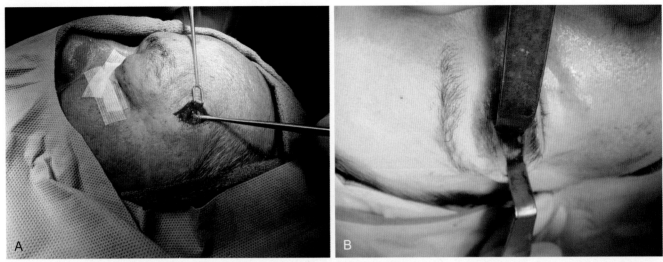

Fig. 3.15.13 Zygomaticotemporal nerve surgical approaches. (A) Left side of elderly man employs a direct approach with the incision positioned into a smile line. The divided nerve can be implanted into the subjacent temporalis muscle. (B) Right side, with retractor gently displacing the globe medially to give access to the zygomaticotemporal nerve entering the foramen, at which location it can be divided.

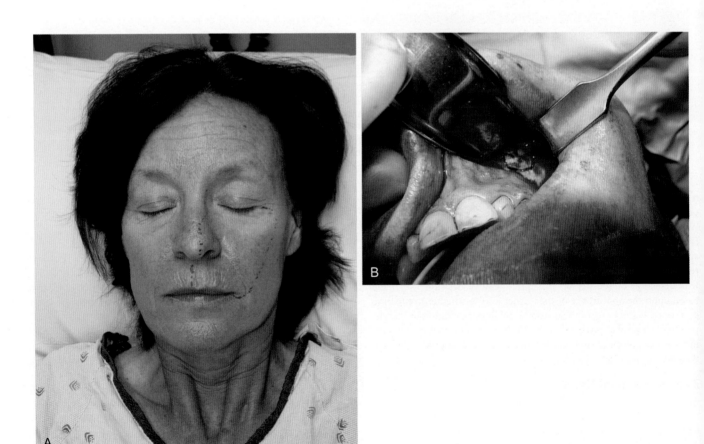

Fig. 3.15.14 The infraorbital nerve: neurolysis. This can be approached through an incision under the upper lip. (A) The typical outline of paresthesias and pain in a woman who had a zygoma fracture. (B) Surgical approach, beneath the upper lip, with infraorbital nerve entrapped in the healed fracture site. Bone to be removed is outlined to complete the neurolysis. (Courtesy Christopher Williams, MD, Denver, Colorado.)

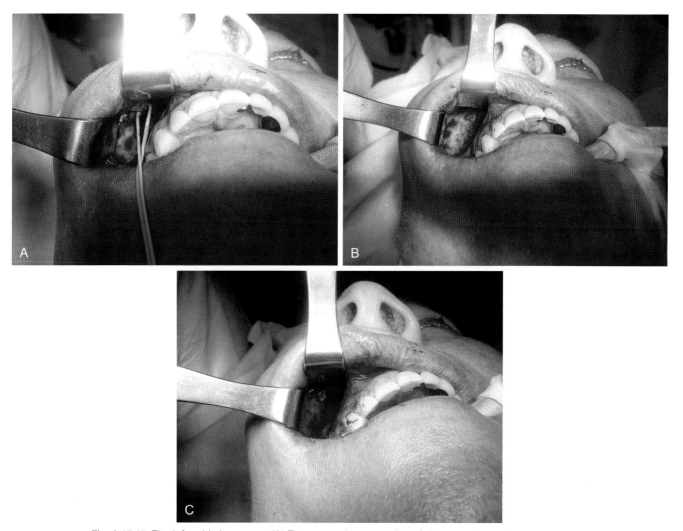

Fig. 3.15.15 The infraorbital neuroma. (A) The approach to resection of the nerve shown here is below the upper lip. (B) The proximal end of the infraorbital nerve has been resected to a level within bone. (C) The exit of the canal in this patient was then "plugged" with AlloDerm™ (Life Cell, Inc.).

(2) resect the nerve through an approach through the superior buccal sulcus, leaving the proximal end to lie within the short bone canal (Fig. 3.15.15), or (3) resect the nerve through a Caudwell–Luc or endoscopic approach through the maxillary sinus, leaving the proximal end of the ION to remain "free" within the maxillary sinus, as has been reported for the treatment of a painful ASAN branch of the ION.[37]

In our one experience with pain related to the incisors, with normal sensation to the nose, cheek, and upper lip, the ASAN is found injured on the CT scan. Local anesthetic block relieves the pain. The surgical approach is illustrated in Fig. 3.15.16, where the ASAN was identified with an endoscope, thin bone removed, and the injured nerve divided adjacent to the ION, leaving the proximal end to lie within the maxillary sinus. This patient remains free of the pain he had for 11 years,[37] now with an 18-month follow-up.

Inferior Alveolar Branch of the Trigeminal Nerve (V₃)

The anatomy of the inferior alveolar nerve (IAN) is well described classically.

As discussed above, the patient presenting with a painful lip and decreased sensation after injury to the IAN can be treated by interruption of nerve function and implantation of the proximal end of the nerve into the medial pterygoid. However, because of the critical sensory

contribution of the IAN, interruption of function and then reconstruction of the IAN is the method of choice.

There has been one systematic review of reconstruction of the IAN.[38] Twenty-seven papers were found suitable for final analysis. Treatment depended on injury type, injury timing, neurosensory disturbances and intraoperative findings. Best functional recovery occurred after direct coaptation if nerve gaps were <10 mm; larger gaps required nerve grafting using either the sural or greater auricular as the donor nerve. Timing of microneurosurgical repair after injury remains debated, with most authors recommending surgery when neurosensory deficit shows no improvement 90 days after diagnosis. Nerve transection diagnosed intraoperatively was recommended to be repaired primarily at the time of injury. There was no consensus regarding optimal methods and timing for repair.

IAN reconstruction has been demonstrated before using either autograft,[8] nerve conduit (Fig. 3.15.17),[9] a transfer of the suprascapular nerve to the mental nerve,[10] or now, a nerve allograft.[39] A series of 7 patients has been reported recently in which nerve gaps of 5–7 cm were reconstructed with an Avance Allograft (Axogen, Inc., Alachua, FL). The nerve gaps resulted from tumor resection. Mean follow-up time was 17.7 months (range, 10–27.5 months). Mean VAS score reported was 3.7 (range, 0–7). Superficial pain and touch was recovered in 86%

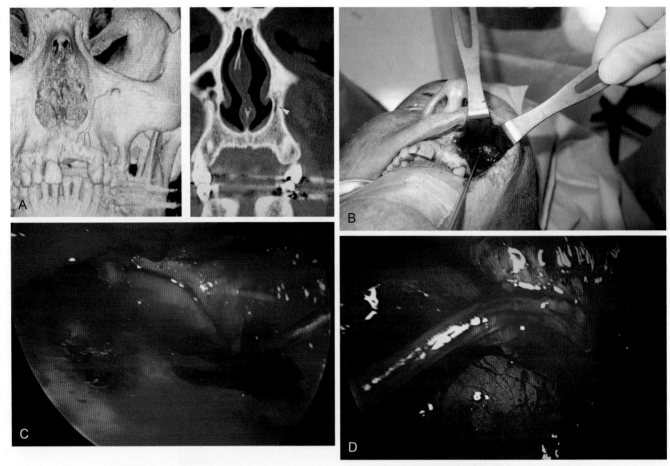

Fig. 3.15.16 The anterior superior alveolar branch (ASAN) of the infraorbital nerve (ION) can be injured during dental extraction or blunt cheek trauma. (A) Illustration of the ASAN path distinct from the ION and the CT scan showing injury to the left canalis sinuosus. (B) Note the sites of incisor teeth extraction, with surgical approach to the maxillary sinus. (C) A hook demonstrates the ASAN going from its infraorbital nerve origin on the right into the maxilla on the left. (D) Proximal end of ASAN will remain in the maxillary sinus.

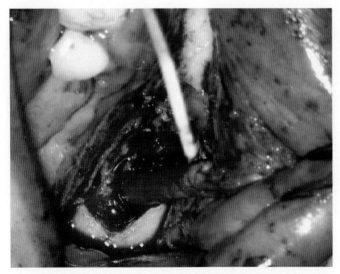

Fig. 3.15.17 The mental nerve can be reconstructed to provide lip sensation if the distal end of the inferior alveolar nerve is accessible at the mental foramen. Here a nerve conduit has been used for the reconstruction. (Courtesy Christopher Williams, MD, Denver, Colorado.)

of patients, and 14% had good tactile localization. An example of this type of reconstruction is given in Fig. 3.15.18 for a person whose pain was related to a screw being placed into the IAN during attempted dental implant reconstruction.

CERVICAL PLEXUS INJURY AND FACIAL PAIN

There are no comprehensive reports of facial pain due to injury to the cervical plexus, and yet the cervical plexus is often involved in trauma from cosmetic surgery, head and neck cancer surgery (Fig. 3.15.19), and blunt trauma. The classic anatomy of the cervical plexus is well described.

The most commonly injured sensory nerve during facelift procedures is the greater auricular nerve, with an incidence of 1.6% identified in a survey of aesthetic surgeons from the year 2000.[40] That survey was sent to 3800 members of the American Society for Plastic and Reconstructive Surgery and received 570 replies. In a more recent series, whose goal was to compare subcutaneous with or without SMAS plication to sub-SMAS plication surgical techniques, in a total group of 229 rhytidectomy patients, the incidence of injury to the greater auricular nerve was 5%–6% with all patients having sensory recovery by 6 months.[41] This group of patients overall averaged a 25% rate of complications.

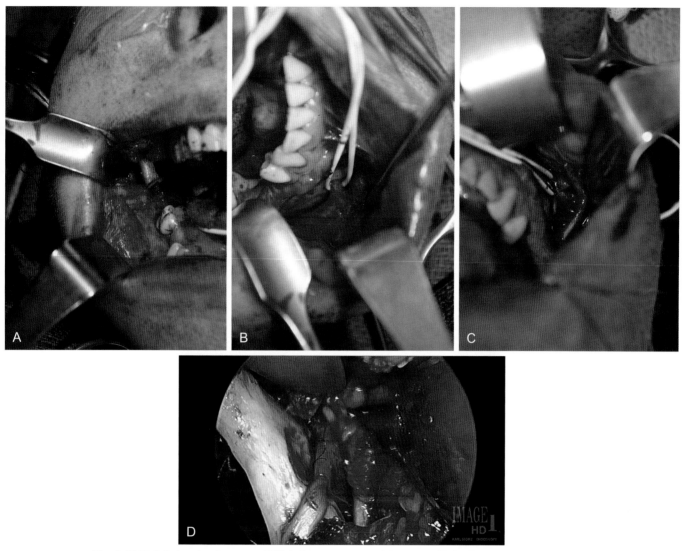

Fig. 3.15.18 Inferior alveolar nerve (IAN) being reconstructed from mandibular foramen to mental nerve, using a 7 cm Avance allograft (Axogen, Inc., Alachua, FL) that is "coupled" to the proximal end of the IAN with a nerve conduit or "connector." (A) View from front of oral cavity that demonstrates the teeth missing at site of IAN injury, with white vessel loop over the proximal IAN identified at site where the mandibular ramus is seen posteriorly. The nerve graft will be placed under the mucosa visible at site of tooth extraction. (B) The white vessel loop identifies the mental nerve. (C) The Avance allograft is seen, having been passed along the reconstruction pathway, and it lies next to the mental nerve prior to coaptation. (D) The proximal nerve connection in which an "connector" from Axogen is used to "couple" the Avance allograft to the proximal end of the IAN, just inferior to the lingula.

In contrast to that high percentage of complications is a series of 742 patients in which no sensory nerve injuries were reported.[42]

There is no published report of the success of treating neuromas of the cervical plexus. In my experience, the approach used to treat any other neuroma has been very successful, such that if the patient receives relief of pain after a block of the cervical plexus at the point of pain along the border of the sternocleidomastoid muscle (SCM), the success from resecting this branch and implanting it into the posterior border of the SCM is 90% good to excellent relief of pain.[43] In our series of 12 patients with cervical plexus injury, there were injuries to the supra-scapular branch in 6 patients, injuries to the lesser occipital branch in 4 patients, injuries to the greater auricular branch in 4 patients and injuries to the transverse cervical branch in 3 patients. Eight patients had an injury to just one branch, 2 patients had an injury to two branches, and 2 patients had an injury to three branches. Three facelift patients had bilateral symmetrical cervical plexus nerve injuries.[44]

For **the greater auricular branch**, an incision is made at the site of the painful Tinel sign, usually about one-third of the length of the SCM down from the mastoid. The nerve is identified in the scar tissue and is traced proximally into healthy tissue. Before cutting this nerve, intra-operative electrical stimulation is done to avoid injury to the spinal accessory nerve. The spinal accessory nerve also exits from beneath the SCM, going into the posterior cervical triangle. Then the greater auricular nerve is blocked with the local anesthetic, cauterized with the bipolar coagulator, the distal neuroma resected and the proximal end implanted deeply into the posterior border and deep side of the SCM. This sequence

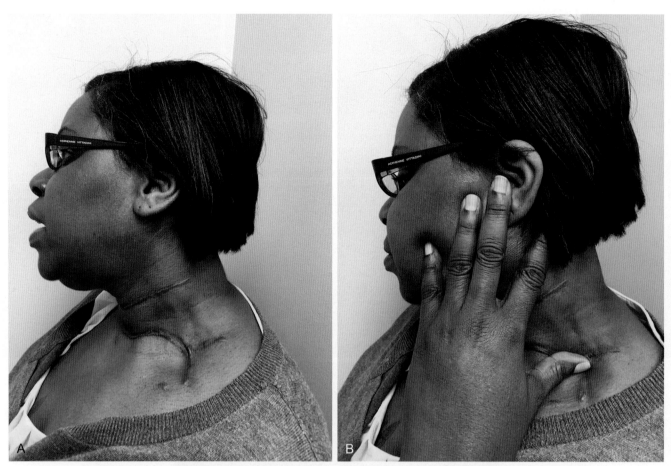

Fig. 3.15.19 Cervical plexus injury following modified radical neck for thyroid cancer. (A) Scars used for the surgical approach. (B) Area of pain demonstrated by spread of patient's fingers showing all branches of the cervical plexus except the lesser occipital nerve.

is illustrated in Fig. 3.15.20. The patient is typically numb prior to surgery but must be advised that they will be possibly more numb after surgery.

The **transverse cervical branch** anatomy is least understood. It has been a cause of failure in the author's first two patients, as the incision was too high, and the nerve found was probably not this branch. Injury to the transverse cervical branch comes most often from stretch/traction during the platysma or SMAS plication.[44] A symptom the author now attributes to this injury is neck tightness and trouble swallowing. The cervical plexus block can demonstrate relief. Release of the platysma where it is attached to the mastoid may be necessary. There will be numbness in the neck and about the mandible. During surgery the incision must be made further down on the SCM, about half way down. Intraoperative electrical stimulation is critical to avoid injury to the marginal mandibular branch of the facial nerve. As with the greater auricular nerve, once the transverse cervical branch has been found, it is blocked, cauterized, and implanted into the underside of the SCM (Fig. 3.15.21).

The **entire cervical plexus** can become injured and be perceived as facial pain and frontal headaches in relation to blunt trauma to the face and neck. It was observed that patients having a decompression of the brachial plexus remarked that besides their hand and shoulder symptoms being relieved, they also had relief of the facial pain, TMJ pain, and temporal or frontal headache relief. In a retrospective study, 75% of patients with these complaints at the time they presented for

brachial plexus problems had relief following anterior scalenectomy.[45] An example is given in Fig. 3.15.22. The explanation for this is that in some people the anterior scalene originates from more proximal transverse processes of the cervical vertebra than normal, and in this position the anterior scalene can compress the cervical plexus.

The **supraclavicular branch** is not covered in this chapter as it does not cause facial pain.

The **lesser occipital branch** will be covered in the next section, related to occipital pain.

OCCIPITAL NERVES AND FACIAL PAIN

The occipital nerves innervate the posterior scalp and not the face. However, it is common for injuries to the occipital nerves to cause sufficient pain that this pain seems to radiate into the frontal region to cause frontal headaches, and pain "behind the eye." It is also meaningful to discuss trauma to these nerves and the implications for treating these nerve injuries in contrast to classic, nontraumatic migraine headaches, according to the paradigm presented in this chapter related to neurolysis versus nerve resection.

It is beyond the scope of this chapter to discuss migraine headaches, but the distinction is to be made that the person with migraine headaches does not have a history of trauma. Conversely, the person who has had head trauma and has headaches is often lumped under the category of "migraines," but actually has posttraumatic injury of the

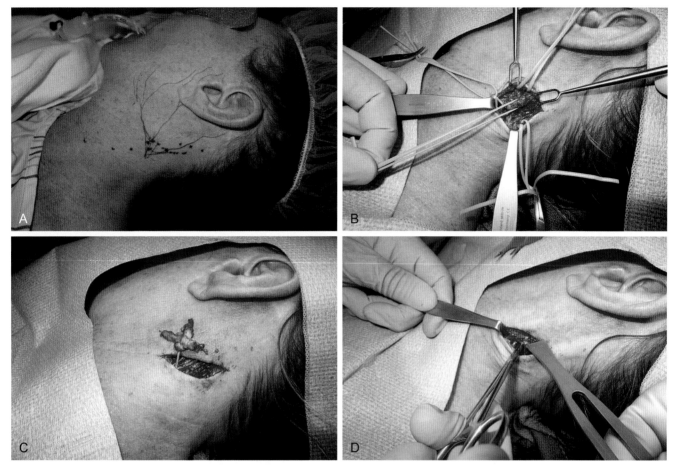

Fig. 3.15.20 Greater auricular branch of cervical plexus injured during facelift. (A) Area of pain is outlined. (B) The greater auricular nerve is identified going into the scar. (C) The neuroma attached to the nerve. (D) After neuroma resection, the proximal end of the nerve is implanted into the underside of the sternocleido-mastoid muscle.

occipital nerves. In the author's view this distinction makes a critical difference in determining the most appropriate first choice for surgical treatment, and it makes a critical difference in assessing outcomes of those surgical treatments (Box 3.15.4).

Bahmon Guyuron, MD, deserves the credit for listening to his patient's observations that following endoscopic brow lift they had relief of frontal headaches. A PubMed Review, as of September 28, 2016, lists 53 references for the search "Guyuron, Migraine." He applied his prior knowledge of nerves of the head and neck to the problem of "headache." However, he extrapolated from frontal headaches to occipital headaches, where the cosmetic approach to brow lifting does not really transpose. To his credit, there are now 5-year outcomes of his approach[46] and a randomized controlled study.[47] His observations and findings have enabled help to many sufferers.

In this chapter, an attempt is made to apply peripheral nerve approaches to "headache" pain. Careful reading of much of the "migraine" surgery literature demonstrates that surgeons employ both neurolysis and resection of nerves in the same anatomic area. Here we ask, "Is this the most appropriate approach?" and if not, how do we proceed into the future to gain better understanding of the pathophysiology of pain related to "headache." I have suggested that the neuropathophysiology of migraine results from a combination of referred pain and double crush along the TN's frontal branches, for example with compression of the supraorbital nerve being interpreted as pain from the meningeal

branch of the frontal nerve along that same nerve.[48] Most often this occurs in a person with central sensitization.[48]

A recent systematic review of "peripheral nerve interventional treatments for chronic headaches" selected 26 studies from an initial 250 search results.[49] Of these, 14 articles studied nerve decompression, 9 studied peripheral nerve stimulation, and 3 studied radiofrequency ablation (RFA). When study populations and results were pooled, a total of 1253 patients had undergone nerve decompression with an 86% success rate, 184 patients were treated by nerve stimulation with a 68% success rate, and 131 patients were treated by RFA with a 55% success rate. When compared to one another, these success rates were all statistically significantly different. Neither nerve decompression nor

> ### BOX 3.15.4   Clinical Pearl
>
> Unfortunately, "*occipital neuralgia*" is the term applied to the symptoms resulting from neural impulses from the three occipital nerves, whether the origin of those signals is from a nontraumatic or a traumatic origin. Unknowingly, failure to distinguish between these two etiologies leads to confusion as to whether the initial surgical approach should be a neurolysis or a resection of the involved nerves, and failing to make this distinction in outcome studies results in confounded data that cannot be interpreted appropriately.

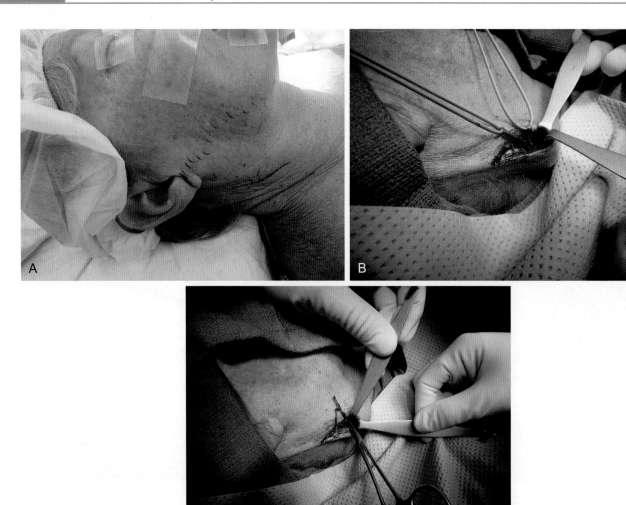

Fig. 3.15.21 Transverse cervical branch of the cervical plexus injured during facelift. (A) Area of pain is outlined. (B) Two branches of the transverse cervical nerve are identified. Note incision is lower than the one for the greater auricular nerve approach. (C) The nerve is implanted into the sternocleidomastoid muscle.

RFA reported complications requiring a return to the operating room, whereas implantable nerve stimulators had a 31.5% rate of such complications. Minor complication rates were similar among all three procedures. *This review did not distinguish between patients who had head trauma, and those that did not. It did not distinguish differences in outcome related to neurolysis or nerve resection.* In a subsequent publication,[50] these same authors recommended nerve resection for patients whose first operation "failed," but did not discuss whether those failed patients originally had posttraumatic occipital nerve injuries as the source of their pain.

Three different occipital nerves must be considered in the pain mechanism: going from lateral to medial, these are the lesser occipital nerve (LON), the greater occipital nerve (GON), and the third occipital nerve (TON). There is no accepted standard incision to be used (Fig. 3.15.23 and Box 3.15.5), but each of these nerves should be treated the same in each patient that has surgery for occipital headaches, whether that be a neurolysis for traditional migraine, or resection for posttraumatic occipital pain.

Neurolysis of the occipital nerves should be reserved for the first approach to occipital migraine surgery and this is illustrated in Fig. 3.15.24, with

BOX 3.15.5   Clinical Pearl

While there is no standard incision used to approach the three occipital nerves, each of these nerves should be treated the same in each patient that has surgery for occipital headaches, whether this be neurolysis for traditional migraine or resection for posttraumatic occipital pain.

the neurolysis continued proximally until there are no more fibrotic bands about the occipital nerves.

The **lesser occipital nerve** can be approached through a cervical incision if a more distal incision has already been used, or if the trauma occurred near the mastoid or from facial cosmetic surgery (Fig. 3.15.25), in which case the proximal end of the nerve should be implanted into the SCM. If this same patient has trigger points over the GON and TON, then a second transverse incision can be made and the proximal end of those nerves implanted into the muscle layer deep to the trapezius.

The **greater occipital nerve** can be injured anywhere along its axis, with deeper locations being the problem in whiplash-type injuries, and

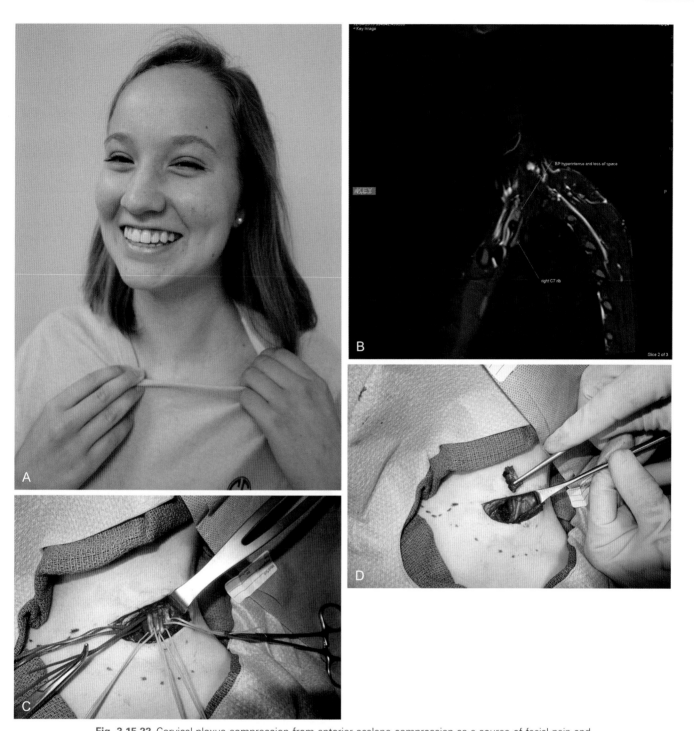

Fig. 3.15.22 Cervical plexus compression from anterior scalene compression as a source of facial pain and headache. (A) High school student who was injured while "heading" a soccer ball giving kinetic energy or stretch/traction to the anterior scalene muscles. (A) View of her smiling 3 weeks after resecting the anterior scalene muscle, showing 4 cm scar in her neck. (B) She was born with a cervical rib, seen here on the 3T MRI, which causes brachial plexus compression as well as causing pressure on the cervical plexus at the origins of the scalene muscles from the transverse processes of cervical vertebra. (C) Intraoperative view after anterior scalenectomy showing from lateral (in blue vessel loops) to medial (in red vessel loop), anterior and posterior divisions of upper trunk, middle trunk, lower trunk, and subclavian artery. (D) Removal of the cervical rib.

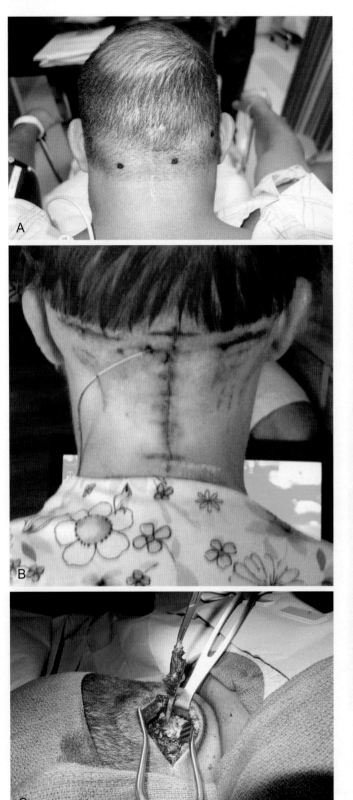

Fig. 3.15.23 Variety of incisions used for occipital nerve exposure. (A) A midline. (B) A midline plus bilateral transverse. (C) Transverse incision here shown with a neuroma of the greater occipital nerve. The hair can be shaved, or not shaved.

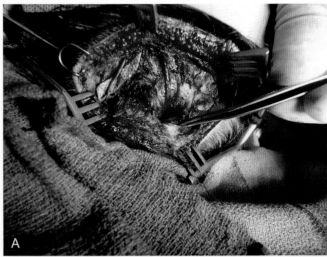

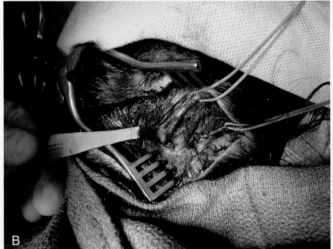

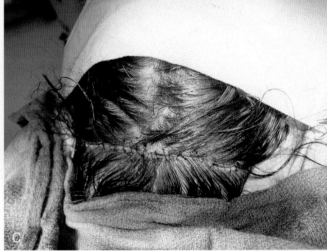

Fig. 3.15.24 Neurolysis of the greater (GON) and lesser (LON) occipital nerves in a patient with occipital migraine. (A) Left side, the GON and LON are seen after completion of the neurolysis. An indentation in the LON is noted and the GON is inflamed. (B) The dissection on the right side. (C) A single long transverse incision was used.

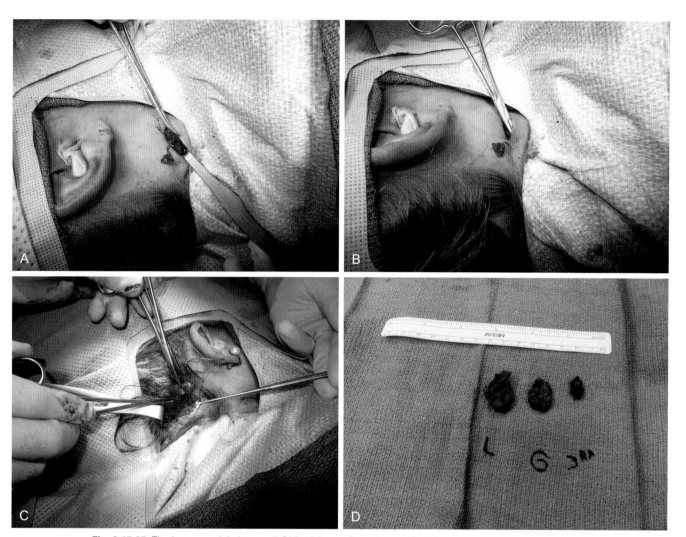

Fig. 3.15.25 The lesser occipital nerve (LON) originates from the cervical plexus as its most superior branch. Therefore, depending upon the mechanism of injury or previous surgery, a neck incision, instead of an occipital incision, may be chosen. (A) The location of the incision to approach the LON is noted in the upper neck with the LON identified. (B) The LON excised with the proximal end being implanted into the sterno-cleidomastoid muscle. (C) A transverse incision used to identify the neuromas of the greater occipital nerve (GON) and the 3rd occipital nerve (TON). (D) The three excised neuromas, LON, GON, and TON, after implanting the GON and TON into the splenius capitus muscle.

superficial locations being involved after previous neurolysis attempts, or "failed" previous "occipital neuralgia" surgery (Figs. 3.15.23C and 3.15.25). The GON must be dissected to within the splenius capitus muscle, and the proximal end implanted there, well away from the incision.

The **third occipital nerve** is the most medial. There can be anatomical variation in which the GON is small and the TON is large, and where the TON crosses towards the GON. This nerve must be dissected proximally and implanted into the splenius capitus muscle, too (Fig. 3.15.25).

EXPERT COMMENTARY

Most facial injury textbooks do not have a chapter on facial pain, and yet our study [1] of long-term follow-up of facial injury patients would indicate that it is a significant persistent post-injury symptom. "If you don't ask, you won't know."

Dr. Dellon's lifetime study of nerves and his interest in posttraumatic facial pain is summarized in this chapter, providing real definitive diagnostic and therapeutic options for this common but underappreciated posttraumatic sequela. Injections, neurolysis, division/implantation, and repair with and without neural

tubes provide us with real and definitive ideas, diagnosis and help for these patients.

Reference

1. Girotto J, MacKenzie E, Fowler C, et al. Long term physical impairment and functional outcomes following complex facial fractures. *Plast Reconstr Surg.* 2001;108: 312–328.

REFERENCES

1. Gassner R, Tuli T, Hächl O, et al. Cranio-maxillofacial trauma: a 10 year review of 9,543 cases with 21,067 injuries. *J Craniomaxillofac Surg.* 2003;31(1):51–61.
2. Sivori LA 2nd, de Leeuw R, Morgan I, Cunningham LL Jr. Complications of frontal sinus fractures with emphasis on chronic craniofacial pain and its treatment: a review of 43 cases. *J Oral Maxillofac Surg.* 2010;68(9):2041–2046.
3. Fogaça WC, Fereirra MC, Dellon AL. Infraorbital nerve injury associated with zygoma fractures: documentation with neurosensory testing. *Plast Reconstr Surg.* 2004;113(3):834–848.
4. Sweet WH. Controlled thermocoagulation of trigeminal ganglion and rootlets for differential destruction of pain fibers: facial pain other than trigeminal neuralgia. *Clin Neurosurg.* 1976;23:96–102.
5. Vijayan N, Watson C. Site of injury headache. *Headache.* 1989;29(8):502–506.
6. Williams CG, Dellon AL, Rosson GD. Management of chronic facial pain. *Craniomaxillofac Trauma Reconstr.* 2009;2(2):67–76.
7. Rosson GD, Rodriguez ED, George P, Dellon AL. Surgical algorithm for treatment of post-traumatic trigeminal nerve pain. *Microsurgery.* 2010;30(8):614–621.
8. Crawley WA, Dellon AL. Inferior alveolar nerve reconstruction with a polyglycolic acid bioabsorbable nerve conduit. *Plast Reconstr Surg.* 1992;90(2):300–302.
9. Evans GR, Crawley W, Dellon AL. Inferior alveolar nerve grafting: an approach without inter-maxillary fixation. *Ann Plast Surg.* 1994;33(2):221–224.
10. Mucci SJ, Dellon AL. Restoration of lower-lip sensation: neurotization of the mental nerve with the supraclavicular nerve. *J Reconstr Microsurg.* 1997;13(3):151–155.
11. Dellon AL. Interruption of nerve function. In: Marsh J, ed. *Current Therapy in Plastic and Reconstructive Surgery.* New York: BC Decker, Inc.; 1989:174–183.
12. Dellon AL. Treatment strategy for supraorbital and supratrochlear neuroma. *J Trauma Treatment.* 2014;3:213.
13. Janis JE, Barker JC, Javadi C, et al. A review of current evidence in surgical treatment of migraine headaches. *Plast Reconstr Surg.* 2014;134(4 suppl 2):131S–141S.
14. Davidson JA, Metzinger SE, Tufaro AP, Dellon AL. Clinical implications of the innervation of the temporomandibular joint. *J Craniofac Surg.* 2003;14(2):235–239.
15. Dellon L, Maloney CT Jr. Denervation of the painful temporomandibular joint. *J Craniofac Surg.* 2006;17(5):828–832.
16. Ata-Ali J, Ata-Ali F, Melo M, et al. Eagle syndrome compared with stylohyoid syndrome: complete ossification of the stylohyoid ligament and joint. *Br J Oral Maxillofac Surg.* pii: S0266-4356. 2016;(16):30173–30175.
17. Sotorra-Figuerola D, Sánchez-Torres A, Valmaseda-Castellón E, Gay-Escoda C. Continuous neuropathic orofacial pain: a retrospective study of 23 cases. *J Clin Exp Dent.* 2016;8(2):e153–e159.
18. Ducic I, Felder JM 3rd, Endara M. Postoperative headache following acoustic neuroma resection: occipital nerve injuries are associated with a treatable occipital neuralgia. *Headache.* 2012;52(7):1136–1145.
19. Zhang Z, Dellon AL. Facial pain and headache associated with brachial plexus compression in the thoracic inlet. *Microsurgery.* 2008;28(5):347–350.
20. Jannetta PJ. Arterial compression of the trigeminal nerve at the pons in patients with trigeminal neuralgia. *J Neurosurg.* 1967;26(1):Suppl:159–162.
21. Barker FG 2nd, Jannetta PJ, Bissonette DJ, et al. The long-term outcome of microvascular decompression for trigeminal neuralgia. *N Engl J Med.* 1996;334(17):1077–1083.
22. Seeburg DP, Northcutt B, Aygun N, Blitz AM. The role of imaging for trigeminal neuralgia: a segmental approach to high-resolution MRI. *Neurosurg Clin N Am.* 2016;27(3):315–326.
23. Dellon AL, Andonian E, DeJesus RA. Measuring sensibility of the trigeminal nerve. *Plast Reconstr Surg.* 2007;120(6):1546–1550.
24. Karagoz H, Ozturk S, Siemionow M. Comparison of neurosensory assessment methods in plastic surgery. *Ann Plast Surg.* 2016;77(2):206–212.
25. Sherman JJ, Carlson CR, Wilson JF, et al. Post-traumatic stress disorder among patients with orofacial pain. *J Orofac Pain.* 2005;19(4):309–317.
26. Glynn SM, Shetty V, Elliot-Brown K, et al. Chronic posttraumatic stress disorder after facial injury:1-year prospective cohort study. *J Trauma.* 2007;62:410–418.
27. Dellon AL, Mackinnon SE, Pestronk A. Implantation of sensory nerve into muscle: preliminary clinical and experimental observations on neuroma formation. *Ann Plast Surg.* 1984;12:30–40.
28. Meyer RA, Raja SN, Campbell JN, et al. Neural activity originating from a neuroma in the baboon. *Brain Res.* 1985;325:255–260.
29. Dellon AL, Mackinnon SE. Treatment of the painful neuroma by neuroma resection and muscle implantation. *Plast Reconstr Surg.* 1986;77:427–436.
30. Dellon AL, Aszmann OC. Treatment of dorsal foot neuromas by translocation of nerves into anterolateral compartment. *Foot Ankle.* 1998;19:300–303.
31. Guyuron B, Tucker T, Davis J. Surgical treatment of migraine headaches. *Plast Reconstr Surg.* 2002;109(7):2183–2189.
32. Ducic I, Larson EE. Posttraumatic headache: surgical management of supraorbital neuralgia. *Plast Reconstr Surg.* 2008;121(6):1943–1948.
33. Golding-Wood DG, Brookes GB. Treatment of post-traumatic external nasal neuralgia. *Rhinology.* 1991;29(4):315–320.
34. Rozen T. Treatment of post-traumatic external nasal neuralgia. *Headache.* 2009;49(8):1223–1228.
35. Peled ZM. A novel surgical approach to chronic temporal headaches. *Plast Reconstr Surg.* 2016;137(5):1597–1600.
36. Olenczak JB, Hui-Chou HG, Aguila DJ 3rd, et al. Posttraumatic midface pain: clinical significance of the anterior superior alveolar nerve and canalis sinuosus. *Ann Plast Surg.* 2015;75(5):543–547.
37. Dorafshar A, Dellon AL, Wan E, et al. Injured anterior superior alveolar nerve endoscopically resected within maxillary sinus. *Craniomaxillofac Trauma Reconstr.* 2017;10(3):208–211.
38. Kushnerev E, Yates JM. Evidence-based outcomes following inferior alveolar and lingual nerve injury and repair: a systematic review. *J Oral Rehabil.* 2015;42(10):786–802.
39. Salomon D, Miloro M, Kolokythas A. Outcomes of immediate allograft reconstruction of long-span defects of the inferior alveolar nerve. *J Oral Maxillofac Surg.* 2016;74(12):2507–2514.
40. Matarasso A, Elkwood A, Rankin M, Elkowitz M. National plastic surgery survey: face lift techniques and complications. *Plast Reconstr Surg.* 2000;106(5):1185–1195.
41. Rammos CK, Mohan AT, Maricevich MA, et al. Is the SMAS flap facelift safe? A comparison of complications between the sub-SMAS approach versus the subcutaneous approach with or without SMAS plication in aesthetic rhytidectomy at an academic institution. *Aesthetic Plast Surg.* 2015;39(6):870–876.
42. Rawlani V, Mustoe TA. The staged face lift: addressing the biomechanical limitations of the primary rhytidectomy. *Plast Reconstr Surg.* 2012;130(6):1305–1314.
43. Mustoe TA, Rawlani V, Zimmerman H. Modified deep plane rhytidectomy with a lateral approach to the neck: an alternative to submental incision and dissection. *Plast Reconstr Surg.* 2011;127(1):357–370.
44. Brown D, Dellon AL. Cervical plexus injuries. *Plast Reconstr Surg.* 2018;141:1021–1025.
45. Zhang Z, Dellon AL. Facial pain and headache associated with brachial plexus compression in the thoracic inlet. *Microsurgery.* 2008;28:347–350.

46. Guyuron B, Kriegler JS, Davis J, Amini SB. Comprehensive surgical treatment of migraine headaches. *Plast Reconstr Surg*. 2005;115(1):1–9.
47. Guyuron B, Reed D, Kriegler J, et al. Placebo-controlled surgical trial of the treatment of migraine headaches. *Plast Reconstr Surg*. 2009;124(2):461–468.
48. Dellon AL. Migraine and peripheral nerves. In: *Pain Solutions*. 3rd ed. Lightning Press. 2013:399–401.
49. Ducic I, Felder JM 3rd, Fantus SA. A systematic review of peripheral nerve interventional treatments for chronic headaches. *Ann Plast Surg*. 2014;72(4):439–445.
50. Ducic I, Felder JM 3rd, Khan N, et al. Greater occipital nerve excision for occipital neuralgia refractory to nerve decompression. *Ann Plast Surg*. 2014;72(2):184–187.

Secondary Nerve Reconstruction

Robin Yang, Anthony P. Tufaro

BACKGROUND

Injury to the peripheral nerve branches of the craniofacial region can arise from a variety of surgical procedures. Common elective procedures such as dentoalveolar surgery, dental implant placement, endodontic treatment, orthognathic surgery, and facial esthetic surgery can result in injury to branches of the trigeminal nerve.[1] Often overlooked in the evaluation of traumatic injury to the craniofacial skeleton or the surrounding soft tissue, is injury to the peripheral branches of the trigeminal nerve. Nerve injuries in facial trauma can be the result of direct injury to the area, traction or avulsion during repair, or aberrant scar/bone formation. Injuries can often lead to frustration and anger on the part of the patient, possibly leading to litigation.[2]

By definition, if postoperative pain persists for greater than 6 months, the diagnosis of chronic facial pain is made.[3] Most patients with postoperative pain can be managed nonoperatively, however those patients who qualify for surgical treatment should be managed in an algorithmic manner. In a retrospective review by Susarla et al., patient satisfaction following trigeminal nerve repair was strongly correlated with improvement in neurosensory examination.[4] Practitioners operating on the craniofacial skeleton should be familiar with the diagnosis and treatment of acute and chronic postoperative pain and relay the appropriate goals and expectations from both nonsurgical and surgical limbs. Persistent postoperative pain in the trauma setting may be multifactorial, particularly in the patient with a history of complex craniofacial injuries. Any attempt to treat the pain must be preceded by a thorough evaluation of the possible causative agents of the patient's problems. Malunion, nonunion, malocclusion, internal derangement of the TMJ and functional shortening of traumatized musculature can all lead to ongoing postoperative pain. The identification of a nerve injury as the causative factor may require the use of diagnostic nerve blocks, imaging and detailed examination, combined with a knowledge of the basic physiology of peripheral nerve injuries.

TRIGEMINAL ANATOMY

Due to the high volume of dentoalveolar surgery in the mandible, the inferior alveolar and lingual branches of the third trigeminal nerve are the most commonly injured. However, the incidence of injury to other branches of the trigeminal nerve in trauma patients is probably underreported. Manson et al. reported that a third of their patients with isolated traumatic Le Fort fractures complained of chronic facial pain. In addition, most of these patients showed some improvement after surgical intervention.[5,6] Unfortunately, the true incidence and evaluation of chronic facial pain in the trauma patient is often difficult to study due to the fact that many of these patients are lost to follow-up.

The most common sensory nerves encountered in craniofacial trauma are the supraorbital/supratrochlear, infraorbital, zygomaticofacial, inferior alveolar, and the lingual nerves.

The three branches of the trigeminal nerve, ophthalmic, maxillary, and mandibular nerves, exit the skull through separate foramina: superior orbital fissure, foramen rotundum, and foramen ovale respectively (Fig. 3.16.1). The largest branch of the ophthalmic nerve is the frontal branch. This branch will divide within the orbit to give the terminal branches of the supraorbital and supratrochlear nerves. These nerves give sensation to the upper eyelid as well as the central or lateral forehead. Classically, these nerves can be released from their bony foramina or notch to gain release of the forehead soft tissue to facilitate access to the upper facial skeleton via a coronal approach (Fig. 3.16.2).

The maxillary division carries sensory information from the lower eyelid, cheek, upper lip, upper teeth, and associated mucosa. The zygomatic nerve gives its terminal branch as the zygomaticofacial nerve that supplies sensation to the lateral cheek and portions of the forehead. The terminal branch of the maxillary nerve exits the facial skeleton as the infraorbital nerve. This nerve is encountered regularly in midface injuries as well as orbital floor fractures (Fig. 3.16.3). The mandibular division is the largest branch of the trigeminal nerve. Before the mandibular nerve enters the medial mandible at the lingula, it will bifurcate and the lingual branch will course within the soft tissue of the floor of the mouth, where it will be in intimate association with the submandibular duct. The terminal branch of the mandibular nerve will enter the medial mandible within the inferior alveolar canal and exit at the mental foramen to give sensation to the mandibular dentition, mucosa, and lower lip. Both of these nerves can be encountered in mandibular fractures as well as soft tissue injuries to the submandibular region (Fig. 3.16.4).

PERIPHERAL NERVE INJURY AND HISTOPATHOLOGY

Peripheral nerve injuries were historically first classified by Sir Herbert Seddon in 1943. This was based on gross and histological changes rather than the actual mechanism of injury. He initially described three types of nerve injuries.

Neurapraxia is a discrete area of local conduction block along the course of the nerve.[7,8] The nerve is in continuity and there is no Wallerian degeneration. Recovery is generally expected within 12 weeks. There will be no Tinel sign at the site of the lesion. This injury is associated with localized pressure such as a tourniquet or a retractor. Axonotmesis indicates direct axonal damage, and finally neurotmesis would involve transection of the peripheral nerve. Wallerian degeneration occurs in both axonotmesis as well as neurotmesis. The degeneration

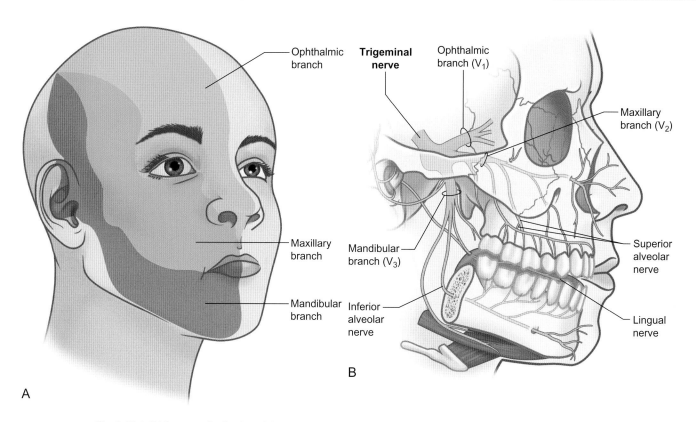

Fig. 3.16.1 (A) Sensory distribution of the trigeminal nerve. (B) Anatomical distribution of the terminal branches of the trigeminal nerve.

TABLE 3.16.1	**Classification of Nerve Injury**		
Seddon	**Sunderland**	**Injury**	**Prognosis**
Neuropraxia	Degree I	Conduction interruption	Excellent recovery
Axonotmesis	Degree II	Axonal rupture without loss of basal lamina tubes	Excellent recovery
Neurotmesis	Degree III	Some scar, rupture of axons and basal lamina tubes	Incomplete recovery
	Degree IV	Complete scar and block of conduction	No recovery
	Degree V	Complete transection	No recovery

occurs distal to the site of injury with recovery in axonotmesis but not in neurotmesis. Sunderland expanded on the initial work of Seddon and emphasized five degrees of nerve injury. First- (neuropraxia) and second- (axonotmesis) degree injuries can recover spontaneously, whereas fourth- and fifth-degree nerve injuries are not expected to recover spontaneously (Table 3.16.1).

Nerve injuries can also be grouped via their mechanism of injury. The clinical scenario of nerve injury can help manage expectations of spontaneous recovery and can also provide the practitioner a systematic algorithm for managing nerve injuries.[9]

CLINICAL PRESENTATION

History and Physical Exam

Each patient evaluated for neurosensory complaints undergoes a careful history. The history should be focused on their chief complaint (i.e., numbness, allodynia, paresthesia, and effect on daily activities). The history should also include any details on trauma, operative intervention, and progression of affected area. An initial Likert scale for pain assessment is also utilized for a baseline assessment. The physical exam is still the gold standard and most reliable method for evaluating a

neurological defect. Sensation or the lack of sensation can be examined using any standard techniques. The senior author prefers the use of the "ten test." The quick and easy ten test sensory exam uses the patient's subjective perception to moving light touch in order to elicit differences in sensation between the affected side and the control side (Fig. 3.16.5). The examiner lightly touches the normal side of the face and the affected side simultaneously, and the patient is asked how sensation in the affected area compares to the normal area on a scale of 1 to 10. The evaluation of sensory deficits can also be reproducibly evaluated by using 2-point discrimination and comparing the result to known standards. On the motor side of the nervous system drop out of motor axons is exhibited by weakness in the affected muscles. Drop out or loss of axons on the sensory side of the nervous system is exhibited by an increase in the 2-point discrimination. Physical examination should be correlated with the history of trauma or surgical intervention. Often the neurological problem can easily be determined.

Radiological imaging studies, such as fine-cut CT scans and/or magnetic resonance neurography, can be used to determine if a specific nerve branch is involved in a fracture that would require surgery on the cranial vault or maxillofacial skeleton (Fig. 3.16.6). Once the specific branch or branches of the trigeminal nerve were identified, a nerve

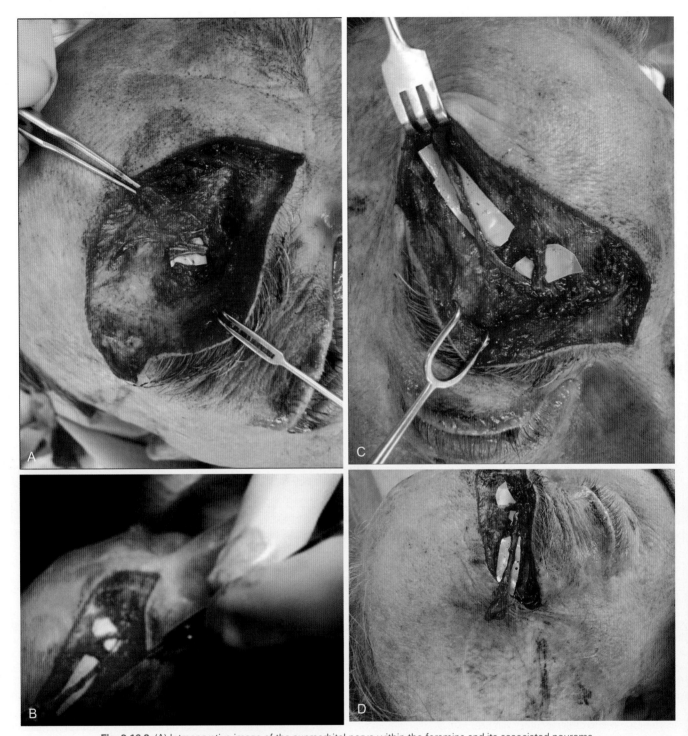

Fig. 3.16.2 (A) Intraoperative image of the supraorbital nerve within the foramina and its associated neuroma. (B) Identification of lateral branch leading to a neuroma. (C) Lateral branch terminating in a neuroma. Seen directly under the laterally placed retractor. (D) Neuroma clearly seen at the end of the proximal nerve stump. (Courtesy Dr. Anthony P. Tufaro.)

block with 1% xylocaine and 0.5% bupivacaine without epinephrine is used. If pain relief was seen, then the patient can decide if that sensory distribution of nerve loss would be acceptable. It is necessary to identify a target nerve with diagnostic blocks before any surgery can be planned. If no specific target nerve can be identified, blocked, and the patient rendered pain free, the diagnostic checklist must be reviewed.

Surgical Indications

Indications for surgery are primarily dependent on the patient's chief complaint, medical history, and also timing of injury. When there is a high index of suspicion that a specific nerve transection is encountered, there is no reason to wait for exploration and repair of the nerve. Nerve

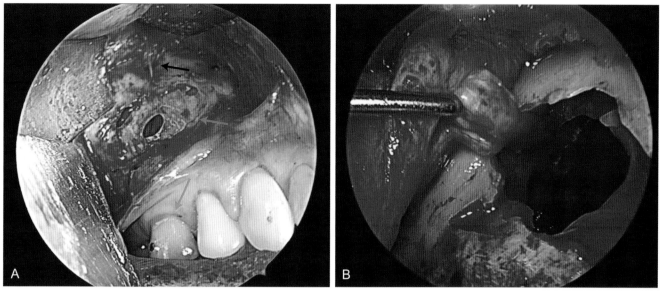

Fig. 3.16.3 (A) Intraoperative photograph of the terminal branch of the maxillary division (V₂). *Black arrow* points to the compression of the nerve as it leaves the foramen within the anterior wall of the maxilla. A portion of the anterior wall of the maxilla is removed and the maxillary sinus membrane (*blue arrow*) is visible. The location of the nerve is usually above the roots of the maxillary first molar (*green arrow*). (B) Surgical decompression of the nerve by removing the compressive bone surrounding the nerve. (Courtesy Dr. Amir Dorafshar and Dr. Lee Dellon.)

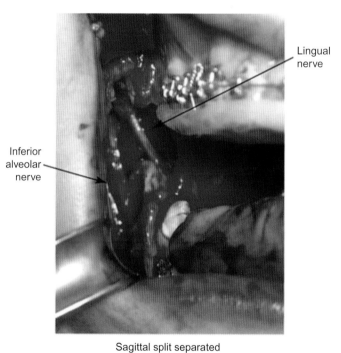

Fig. 3.16.4 Intraoperative photo of the mandibular nerve in a bilateral sagittal split osteotomy. (Courtesy Dr. Anthony P. Tufaro.)

repair in the acute setting can generally be repaired primarily, whereas those repaired after the first week may need secondary repair with possible grafting or extensive mobilization of the nerve ends. The delayed repair allows for the development of dense fibrous scar between the nerve ends and further distance between the transected ends. However, often in the craniofacial region, traumatic neurological injuries present in a delayed fashion.[10]

Surgical Algorithms

The author prefers to use the algorithm in Fig. 3.16.7 when presented with a neurological injury from maxillofacial trauma. As a rule, a patient who presents with a neurosensory deficit with a facial injury that was repaired, or considered nonoperative, can be observed for sensory recovery up to 12 weeks. Once improvement ceases, there is not an expectation of further recovery. Depending on the level of the sensory deficit, the patient's subjective assessment of his/her status, and any associated functional impairment, a treatment plan can be presented. Appropriate intraoperative management of facial fractures should include the management of the soft tissue and the terminal branches of the trigeminal distribution. If repair or the fracture itself results in nerve injury, these injuries should be addressed at that time. If the operator is unable to perform neurological microsurgery, then appropriate documentation of the nerve injuries should be performed, and the patient should be referred for specialty care. If possible, the injured nerve or nerve ends can be tagged with a Prolene suture to facilitate its identification at the secondary repair.

There should be special consideration in patients who present with neurosensory deficits of the inferior alveolar or lingual nerves after sagittal split osteotomies or mandibular third molar extractions. The algorithm in Fig. 3.16.8 is useful for the evaluation and planning of patients who present with V₃ neurosensory deficits. During third molar extraction, occasionally due to the anatomy of the dental roots, iatrogenic inferior alveolar nerve injury can be visualized. If there is visualization of an injured nerve, immediate referral to a nerve microsurgeon should be initiated. These patients should be monitored for improvement or development of pain. If neurosensory deficit after 12 weeks does not show any improvement, the patient should be given the option for surgical repair (details of surgical technique described later).

During the sagittal split osteotomy, if an inferior alveolar nerve injury is observed, the nerve should be repaired at that time. If the operator is unable to repair the injury, the two ends of the nerve should be placed in close proximity within their bony canal. Subacute (within

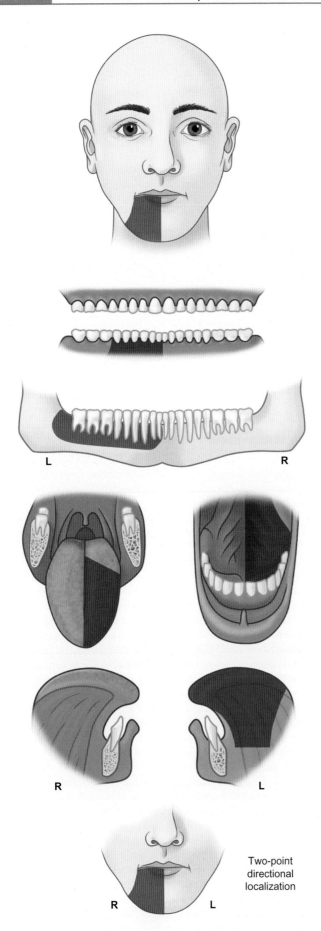

Two-point
directional
localization

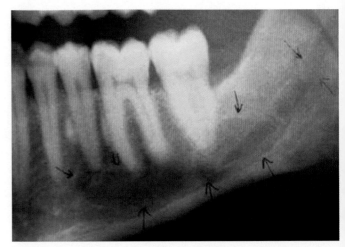

Fig. 3.16.5 Clinical document used to note sensory defects. The clinician can fill in the areas with a neurosensory defect. (From Bagheri, SC, Meyer RA. Management of trigeminal nerve injuries. In: Current therapy in oral and maxillofacial surgery. Philadelphia, PA: Saunders; 2012, Fig. 29.4.)

Fig. 3.16.6 Section of a preoperative dental panoramic X-ray (panorex). Surgical extraction of a wisdom tooth resulted in iatrogenic damage to the inferior alveolar nerve. The arrows point to the discontinuity of the nerve as well as increased radiolucencies most likely representing abnormal neuroma formation. (Courtesy of Dr. Anthony P. Tufaro.)

2 months) exploration and nerve repair should be avoided as the area of injury is under high inflammatory condition which will make repair and visualization very difficult.

SURGICAL TECHNIQUES

Approaches to the Infraorbital Nerve

The infraorbital nerve is often encountered in midface fractures. Nerve injury can occur during the initial traumatic event or often an avulsive injury can occur from a retraction-type mechanism. Approaches to the infraorbital nerve exploration can be performed with an intraoral buccal–vestibular incision between the central incisor and the maxillary first molar (Fig. 3.16.3). Subperiosteal dissection will often reveal the nerve exiting its foramen of the maxilla. Often these patients complain of pain. Simple division of the nerve has been shown to provide relief from pain.[10] The proximal end of the nerve can be implanted into muscle or soft tissue to attempt to form another neuroma.[11]

Approaches for the Lingual Nerve

Injuries to the lingual nerve can usually be accessed via an intra-oral incision. This is especially true if the injury results from a third molar extraction (Fig. 3.16.4). A gingival crestal flap along the buccal aspects of the mandibular posterior teeth along with a posterior–lateral release along the retromolar fossa is combined with a similar lingual crestal incision and flap. Careful dissection and elevation of a full mucoperiosteal flap along the lingual periosteum will reveal the entirety of the lingual nerve. The lingual nerve is appropriately treated based on the intraoperative findings.

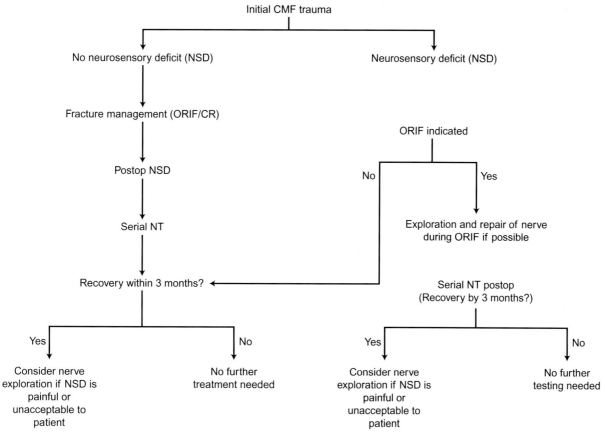

Fig. 3.16.7 Algorithm for neurological deficit from maxillofacial trauma. CR, closed reduction; NT, neuro testing.

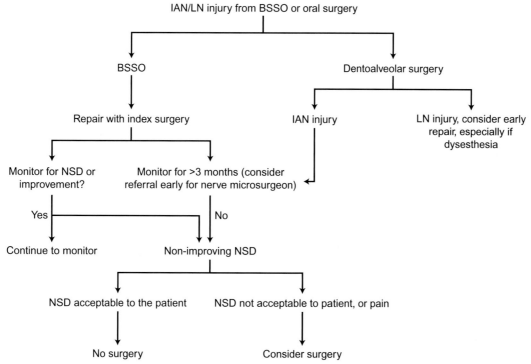

Fig. 3.16.8 Algorithm for inferior alveolar nerve (IAN) or lingual nerve (LN) injury. BSSO, bilateral sagittal split osteotomy; NSD, neurosensory deficit.

Approaches for the Inferior Alveolar Nerve

Injuries to the IAN (inferior alveolar nerve) within the mandibular canal due to iatrogenic causes (third molar extraction or sagittal osteotomies) can be accessed via an intraoral or an extraoral incision.[12,13] The authors prefer an extraoral incision well positioned in a submandibular neck crease (Fig. 3.16.9).[14] A subplatysmal flap is elevated to the inferior border of the mandible with care to avoid the marginal mandibular branch of the facial nerve. The masseter muscle is elevated to expose the body of the mandible. Injecting 1 mL of methylene blue deep into the mucobuccal fold along the area of intraoral injury prior to making the neck incision can help guide the extent of the osteotomies. Buccal cortical osteotomies are performed and elevated off of the mandible to expose the inferior alveolar canal and its contents (Fig. 3.16.10). Mobilization and repair of the affected portion of the nerve is then performed (Fig. 3.16.11). Often the lateral cortical bone is not replaced to avoid compression of the repaired nerve. The incision is closed in a layered fashion with approximation of the pterygomasseteric sling and platysma.

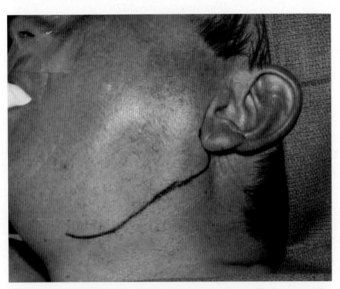

Fig. 3.16.9 Markings used prior to extraoral approach for access to the infraorbital nerve. (Courtesy Dr. Anthony P. Tufaro.)

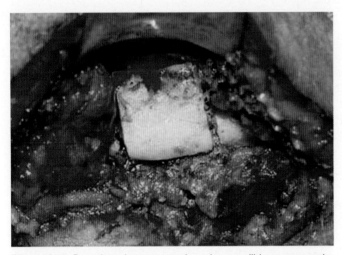

Fig. 3.16.10 Buccal corticotomy used on the mandible to access the contents of the infraorbital canal within the cortex of the mandible. (Courtesy Dr. Anthony P. Tufaro.)

Nerve Repair Technique/Timing

There is no consensus literature regarding the timing or method of IAN reconstruction. In contrast, upper extremity nerve repair/management is well studied and documented. The RANGER Study registry initiated in 2007 concluded that nerve allografts offer an effective method of reconstruction for peripheral nerve gaps in the upper extremity when compared to traditional autografts.[15] An additional large prospective trial, performed by Weber et al., did not show any significant differences in outcome between patients undergoing autologous nerve grafting/end-to-end repair of peripheral nerves or patients undergoing repair with a polyglycolic acid conduit.[16]

Primary repair is often the main goal and can result in the best outcome.[17] As a general guideline, primary tension-free repair should be attempted. Often this is not possible for the IAN due to the bony canal it is housed in. If a nerve gap is encountered the use of an autologous nerve (usually sural nerve or greater auricular nerve) has been the traditional method of reconstruction. Another option is the use of decellularized human nerve grafts. Lastly, a nerve conduit or cuff can be used without end-to-end repair of the nerve itself. The tube or cuff can help guide the growing axons to reach the adjacent nerve stump (Fig. 3.16.11B).

In regard to the inferior alveolar and the lingual nerves, a large retrospective study performed by Bagheri et al. did not find any significant differences in the type of surgical repair of the nerve. Two factors – age above 50 as well as time from injury to repair (over a year) – were associated with significantly less recovery of sensory function.[18,19] The authors' own series of IAN repair using a polyglycolic acid nerve conduit showed comparable results of sensory recovery (60%) and pain relief (100%) in addition to being cost-effective, reducing operative time, and eliminating donor site morbidity.[14] It is important to advise the patient that pain relief is often a more reliable outcome of the surgery and full sensory recovery is not a realistic expectation.

FOLLOW-UP

Postoperative Care

Most patients in the postoperative period can complain of increased paresthesia and occasional electrical shocks. Often these shocks can extend beyond the area of injury. If needed these shocks can be managed with neuromodulating medications such as gabapentin, or nortriptyline. If the patient has a history of chronic pain, a consultation to a pain specialist may be indicated to allow appropriate management of narcotics and other services. Neurosensory recovery should be monitored and documented appropriately. Physical therapy and neurosensory rehabilitation should be initiated early in the healing process to assist in sensory re-education.

EXPERT COMMENTARY

A number of years ago, nerve injuries of the face were identified on physical examinations, but treatment was not pursued. Today, nerve injuries of the motor (facial) and sensory (trigeminal) branches of the face are identified, quantified, and selected for treatment with surgical decompression or repair, or observation as decided by anatomy, the skill and interest of the surgeon, and the patient.

Therefore precise diagnoses and treatment plans are developed according to the history and physical findings and a plan for treatment or observation is developed, and perhaps confirmed with peripheral nerve consultants. This chapter outlines those steps permitting us to more effectively manage the overall patient and their injuries with new and up-to-date advice available.

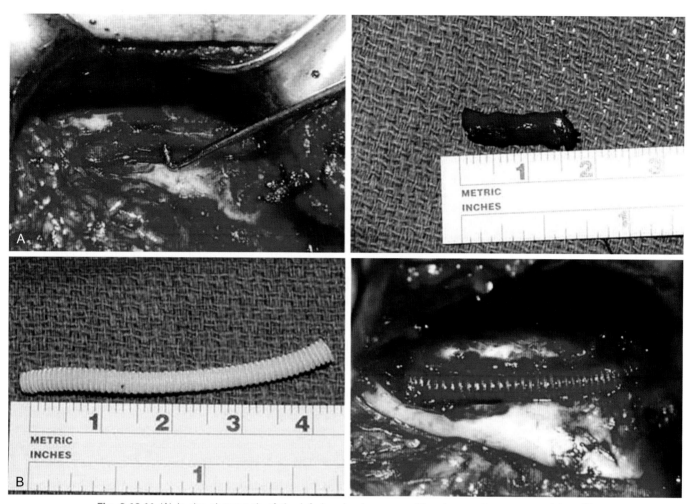

Fig. 3.16.11 (A) In-situ photograph of the inferior alveolar nerve with subsequent neuroma excision. (B) Reconstruction of the inferior alveolar nerve with a polyglycolic nerve tube. (Courtesy Dr. Anthony P. Tufaro.)

REFERENCES

1. Ziccardi V, Steinberg M. Timing of trigeminal nerve microsurgery: a review of the literature. *J Oral Maxillofac Surg.* 2007;65:1341–1345.
2. Chaushu G, Taicher S, Halamish-Shani T, Givol N. Medicolegal aspects of altered sensation following implant placement in the mandible. *Int J Oral Maxillofac Implants.* 2002;17:413–415.
3. Pinsky JJ, Crue BL. Intensive group psychotherapy. In: Wall PD, Melzack R, eds. *Textbook of Pain*. Edinburgh: Churchill Livingstone; 1984:823.
4. Susarla S, Kaban L, Donoff RB, et al. Does early repair of lingual nerve injuries improve functional sensory recovery? *J Oral Maxillofac Surg.* 2007;65:1070–1076.
5. Gregg JM. Studies of traumatic neuralgias in the maxillofacial region: surgical pathology and neural mechanisms. *J Oral Maxillofac Surg.* 1990;48:228–237, Discussion 238–239.
6. Girotto JA, MacKenzie E, Fowler C, et al. Long-term physical impairment and functional outcomes after complex facial fractures. *Plast Reconstr Surg.* 2001;108:312–327.
7. Seddon HJ. Three types of nerve injury. *Brain.* 1943;66:237–288.
8. Seddon HJ, Medawar PB, Smith H. Rate of regeneration of peripheral nerves in the man. *J Physiol.* 1943;102:191–215.
9. Mackinnon SE. New directions in peripheral nerve surgery. *Ann Plast Surg.* 1989;22:257–273.
10. Rosson G, Rodriguez E, George P, Dellon A. Surgical algorithm for treatment of post-traumatic trigeminal nerve pain. *Microsurgery.* 2010;30(8):614–621.
11. Dellon AL, Andonian E, DeJesus RA. Measuring sensibility of the trigeminal nerve. *Plast Reconstr Surg.* 2007;120:1546–1550.
12. Hwang K, Lee WJ, Song YB, et al. Vulnerability of the inferior alveolar nerve and mental nerve during genioplasty: an anatomic study. *J Craniofac Surg.* 2005;16:10–14.
13. Hillerup S. Iatrogenic injury to the inferior alveolar nerve: etiology, signs and symptoms, and observations on recovery. *Int J Oral Maxillofac Surg.* 2008;37:704–709.
14. Mundinger G, Prucz RB, Rozen S, Tufaro A. Reconstruction of the inferior alveolar nerve with bioabsorbable polyglycolic acid nerve conduits. *Plast Reconstr Surg.* 2012;129(1):110–117.
15. Cho MS, Rinker BD, Weber RV, et al. Functional outcome following nerve repair in the upper extremity using processed nerve allograft. *J Hand Surg Am.* 2012;37(11):2340–2349.
16. Weber RA, Breidenbach WC, Brown RE, et al. A randomized prospective study of polyglycolic acid conduits for digital nerve reconstruction in humans. *Plast Reconstr Surg.* 2000;106:1036–1045.
17. Dodson TB, Kaban LB. Recommendations for management of trigeminal nerve defects based on a critical appraisal of the literature. *J Oral Maxillofac Surg.* 1997;55:1380–1386.
18. Bagheri SC, Meyer RA, Sung C, et al. A retrospective review of microsurgical repair of 186 inferior alveolar nerve injuries. *J Oral Maxillofac Surg.* 2010;68:243–253.
19. Bagheri SC, Meyer RA, Khan HA, et al. A retrospective review of microsurgical repair of 222 lingual nerve injuries. *J Oral Maxillofac Surg.* 2010;68:715–723.

Facial Transplantation

Joseph Lopez, Eduardo D. Rodriguez, Amir H. Dorafshar

BACKGROUND

Facial Transplantation Experience

The first facial transplantation was completed in France in 2005. Since that time, over 37 facial transplantations have been performed around the world. Of these cases, at least 28 have been the result of facial trauma.[1,2] In fact, most of these cases have been performed secondary to ballistic injuries (n = 15), burn injuries (n = 8), or animal attacks (n = 3). As the number of new vascularized composite allotransplantation (VCA) centers continues to expand across the globe, face transplantation has emerged as a viable treatment modality for the management of severely disfigured patients following facial trauma.

The early success of facial transplantation for severe facial disfigurements has addressed the difficulties often associated with complex facial trauma reconstruction. Facial trauma is associated with significant bony and soft tissue loss. In the case of ballistic injuries, extensive bony and soft tissue damage results from the kinetic injury dissipated by the impact of the bullet. Moreover, significant damage can occur due to the trajectory of the bullet.[3,4] Unfortunately, the complexity of trauma-related injuries to the face makes the reconstructive effort difficult and often inadequate with conventional surgical techniques. Classically, reconstructive surgeons managed these injuries via multiple stages, often utilizing free tissue transfer reconstruction and other plastic surgery techniques. With immunosuppressive regimens now capable of achieving long-term allograft acceptance and current conventional reconstructive methods unable to achieve optimal facial aesthetic results, facial transplantation is now considered by some as a viable first-line treatment option in the patient with a central avulsive facial injury pattern.

SURGICAL INDICATIONS

Indications

Patient selection is the most important factor to consider before facial allotransplantation. The experience of the senior authors has revealed that proper evaluation and selection is the most important determinant of outcomes after facial allotransplantation. A multidisciplinary approach must be taken to not only assess the surgical indications for facial allotransplantation but also the psychological and social factors that may impact outcomes.[5] These psychological and social factors are critical since postoperative rehabilitation, therapy, and correctional surgery are necessary postoperatively for optimal aesthetic and functional results.

Given that facial allotransplantation is still in its infancy, surgical indications for facial allotransplantation have yet to be fully established. Although this is a topic of great controversy, most reconstructive surgeons agree that patients with severe central avulsive facial trauma, with functional limitations (i.e., oral competence) not amenable to reconstruction using classical reconstructive techniques, should be considered as potential candidates for facial allotransplantation. Patients with central avulsive facial trauma meet this criterion, since they typically present with naso-orbital-ethmoid fractures, eyelid and nasal defects, anterior maxilla, palate, and mandible fractures, and defects of the upper/lower lips and tongue. This typical injury pattern, considered by some as "unreconstructable," is completely addressed with facial allotransplantation in a single procedure. Traumatic burn injuries that result in extensive soft tissue loss of the lips and eyelids are also considered potential indications for facial allotransplantation (Fig. 3.17.1).

Although absolute indications are still controversial, most reconstructive surgeons agree on the establishment of strict exclusion criteria.[6] These criteria are established to reduce the risks associated with transplantation (Box 3.17.1). For example, most agree that patients under the age of 18 should be excluded due to the difficulties of informed consent in this population. Additionally, patients over the age of 65 are generally excluded due to the known higher malignancy risk associated with immunosuppression therapy, although these are relative contraindications and not absolute.

Relative Indications

As the facial transplantation experience grows, improvements in immunoregulatory regimens may potentially increase the indications for facial allotransplantation to smaller defects. Currently, autologous reconstruction options for the oral commissure, nose, and periorbital complex are limited. The current standard of care for oral commissure reconstruction is hallmarked by oral incompetence. Furthermore, current techniques give the oral commissure an unnatural appearance, particularly when attempting to recreate the dry and wet mucosa. Similarly, few nasal reconstructive surgeons can achieve both satisfactory function and appearance for total nasal defects. Additionally, it is rare for large eyelid defects to result in functional protection and lubrication of the globe with a normal appearance. Given these shortcomings along with the success of transplanting these facial units as part of larger facial transplants, it is reasonable to predict superior outcomes transplanting these units in isolation compared to autologous reconstruction. With the risks of current lifelong immunosuppressive regimens, the benefits of such small facial unit transplantations need to be considered carefully in the context of the individual patient. Facial unit transplantation may be more conceivable at this stage in the setting of concurrent solid organ or other VCA from the same donor, as it would not significantly increase the potential morbidity of the procedure. Conversely, unit transplantation results in less morbidity if rejection requires explantation, and may allow for investigational immunotherapy trials with less risk posed in the event of rejection.

CLASSIFICATION

A classification system that accurately describes facial defects is necessary to: (A) document facial deformities; (B) develop treatment

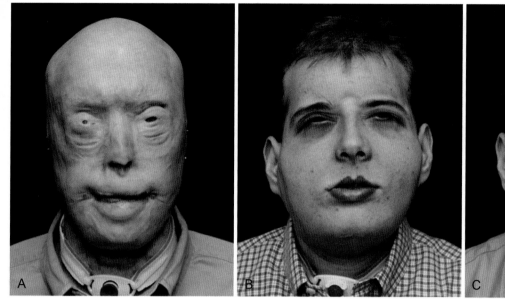
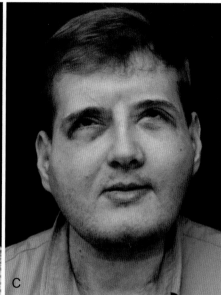

Preoperative: **August 2014**   Postoperative: **November 11, 2015**   Postoperative: **August 3, 2016**

Fig. 3.17.1 Facial transplantation of entire face and scalp soft tissue envelope. (A) Preoperative view; (B) early postoperative view; (C) approximately 1 year postoperatively. (Copyright Dr. Eduardo Rodriguez.)

BOX 3.17.1 Criteria to Consider When Selecting Candidates for Facial Allotransplantation

Age	Patients over 18 years and under 65 years
Vision	Although some centers believe that eyesight is important for functional recovery, many others do not believe blindness to be an absolute contraindication
Psychosocial assessment	Motivation for transplantation, social support system/family structure, emotional and cognitive preparedness, body image adaptation, history of medication compliance/substance abuse need to be evaluated

TABLE 3.17.1 Soft Tissue Classification System for Facial Allotransplantation

Type	Functional Subunit	Anatomic Defects
0	Oral subunit	Upper lip, lower lip, and oral commissures
1	Oral–nasal subunit	Septum, nasal cartilage, and nasal soft tissues, with or without defects in type 0
2	Oral–nasal–orbital subunit	Lower eyelids and malar soft tissues, with or without defects in type 1
3	Full facial subunit	Palpebral and frontal regions, can include all soft tissues of the face

TABLE 3.17.2 Bone Classification System for Facial Allotransplantation

Type	Defect
M	Presence of mandibular defect
A	Maxillary alveolus (Le Fort I segment)
B	Nasal bones, maxilla, zygoma, vomer, ethmoid, inferomedial orbital bones, and defects in type 1 (Le Fort III segment)
C	Frontal bone, supraorbital rims, and defects in type 2 (Monobloc advancement segments)

algorithms; and (C) develop indications for facial allotransplantation. The senior authors devised a working classification of facial allotransplants based on soft tissue functional–aesthetic subunits and the Le Fort classification for the craniofacial skeleton (Fig. 3.17.2).[7] Soft tissue defects were categorized into four zones (Table 3.17.1) and bony defects were classified into four types (Table 3.17.2). Based on this proposed classification, the senior authors believe that a predictable and modifiable treatment algorithm can be developed for the planning of facial allotransplantation. Although the application of this classification system is still in its infancy, we expect that future studies will examine its potential for advancing the field of facial allotransplantation.

SURGICAL TECHNIQUES

Donor Procedure

Donor procurement has been extensively described by the senior authors in previous publications.[8] In short, full facial allotransplantation is executed by sequential soft tissue and bony dissection. Before division of the pedicles, stereolithographic modeling can be used to tailor donor bony segments. This also allows for the pre-bending of plates before the beginning of ischemia time. After division of the pedicles, the allograft

is taken to the back table where it is flushed with University of Wisconsin solution and then placed on ice.

Recipient Procedure

The recipient is brought to the adjacent donor operating room and the recipient dissection is started almost concurrently with the donor harvest procedure. This often requires a second team to minimize fatigue and optimize efficiency. Since most recipients have had multiple previous

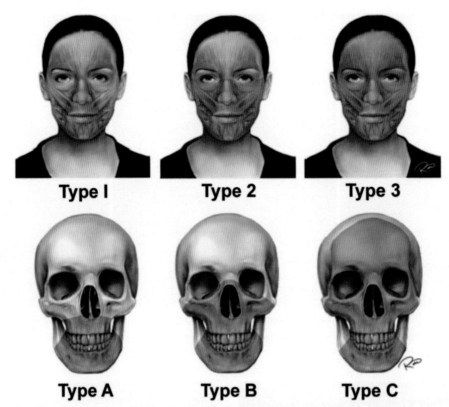

Fig. 3.17.2 Diagram of the classification system for facial transplantation illustrates the extent of each soft tissue (above, shaded red) and bony defect (below, shaded green). (From Mohan R, Borsuk DE, Dorafshar AH, et al. Aesthetic and functional facial transplantation: a classification system and treatment algorithm. Plast Reconstr Surg 2014; 133(2): 386–397.)

operations and extensive scarring from trauma, preparation of the recipient may take a long time (the first face transplant performed by the senior author required a recipient dissection time of 17 hours). Cutting guides and stereolithographic models can be utilized to optimize surgical efficiency (Fig. 3.17.3).[9]

Skeletal Fixation and Microvascular Anastomoses

The midface and mandibular segments are fixated using titanium miniplates. This is followed by insetting of bilateral donor external carotid arteries, which are anastomosed to the recipient vessels, typically the external carotid, facial, or internal maxillary arteries. The donor internal jugular veins can be anastomosed to the recipient internal jugular veins bilaterally, if available. Total ischemia time should be kept to a minimum to minimize the detrimental effects of ischemia–reperfusion injury.

Nerve Coaptation

Nerve regeneration is critical for optimization of functional facial allografts, however, recipient motor nerve anatomy often dictates the options for neurorrhapy and, ultimately, functional results. The initial trauma, scarring, and previous reconstructive procedures can often result in limited or damaged nerves. When possible, terminal nerve coaptation is preferable to main trunk repair to decrease the length required for nerve regeneration. Motor nerve branches to the orbit, upper lip, commissure, and lower lip should be prioritized for nerve coaptation to optimize functional results. Optimal neurorrhaphy can provide improvements in speech and swallowing. Improvement in voluntary and involuntary blink are possible, with the potential to improve the patient's ability to protect their globes and preserve vision.[10] Lastly, donor sensory nerves (supraorbital, infraorbital, inferior alveolar nerves)

are dissected as well while recipient sensory nerves are also isolated for coaptation.

Salivary Glands

Management of the salivary glands in facial transplantation has varied, without thorough reporting in the literature.[11] Transplanting the entire parotid gland reduces operative time in an otherwise lengthy procedure, but can result in excessive bulk and risk of salivary leak. Removing the entire gland without nerve dissection reduces concern for salivary leak and facial bulk, but may require nerve grafts. Finally, excision of the superficial lobe alone allows for maintenance of the entire facial nerve as needed, while reducing bulk, but significantly adds to operative time and can still risk salivary leak. All options present risks and benefits and must be thoroughly discussed and planned prior to performing facial allotransplantation.

POSTOPERATIVE COURSE

Immunosuppressive Regimen

Immunosuppression regimens following facial allotransplantation mirror those utilized in solid organ transplantation. All facial allotransplantation patients undergo induction therapy in the operating room, most commonly composed of antithymocyte globulin or alemtuzumab. Induction is then followed by triple drug maintenance therapy composed of mycophenolate (MMF), tacrolimus (FK506), and steroids.[12,13] Mycophenolate mofetil (MMF) has been used in all facial transplant recipients at a therapeutic range of 40–50 ng/mL. Tacrolimus is the mainstay of treatment and it is maintained at therapeutic blood levels of 10–15 ng/mL. Steroid boluses are typically started at very high doses

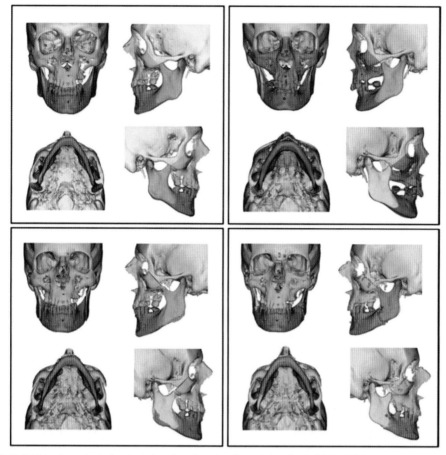

Fig. 3.17.3 Virtual surgical planning showing the planning of the donor (above, left) and recipient (above, right) osteotomies with simulated donor–recipient hybrid (below, left) and true postoperative (below, right). (From Brown EN, Dorafshar AH, Bojovic B, et al. Total face, double jaw, and tongue transplant simulation: a cadaveric study using computer-assisted techniques. Plast Reconstr Surg 2012;130(4): 815–823.)

on postoperative day 0 but are weaned over the next few weeks with the goal of removing steroids from the immunosuppressive regimen altogether or converting to a low-dose maintenance dose. Using the above foundation of induction therapy followed by triple drug maintenance therapy, with the goal of weaning steroid and calcineurin inhibitors, facial allografts can be maintained successfully.

Cellular Immunoregulation

Several of the facial allotransplants to date have had a vascularized bone marrow component included in the allograft. Additionally, three facial transplantation patients have had additional donor bone marrow cell infusions. One of these patients has even been found to exhibit signs of microchimerism in peripheral blood samples.[14] The experience with upper extremity transplantation at the University of Pittsburgh and the Johns Hopkins Hospital has been that upper extremity allografts can be maintained with tacrolimus therapy alone following cellular infusion of donor bone marrow cells (i.e., the Pittsburgh Protocol). Several laboratories in the United States and around the world are currently studying similar cellular augmentation strategies combined with novel targeted immunoregulatory therapy with the goal of reducing immunosuppression regimens and achieving allograft tolerance.

Monitoring of Rejection

All facial allografts have exhibited signs of acute rejection usually within the first several weeks and all within the first year of transplantation.

Therefore, monitoring of rejection is critical for graft maintenance. Previous studies have demonstrated that the skin is the most antigenic component of a VCA graft.[15] This provides VCA an advantage over solid organ transplantation since the skin allows for direct visualization of the immunological status of the allograft. Rejection of VCA allografts typically presents with erythema, edema, desquamation, and, ultimately, tissue necrosis. Confirmation of rejection must be performed by obtaining a skin biopsy. This biopsy is then utilized for histopathological diagnosis. Rejection is graded using the Banff 2007 Working Classification of Skin-Containing Composite Tissue Allograft Pathology (Table 3.17.3).[16]

More recently, several groups have advocated for the use of sentinel flaps, which can be used to monitor rejection at sites distant from the facial allograft. In an effort to avoid trauma to the facial allograft (for obvious aesthetic reasons and due to limited tissue availability), sentinel flaps have been used to monitor rejection episodes in previous series.[17] Sentinel flaps are small free alloflaps taken from the donor and transplanted to sites on the recipient. Previous experience with the use of sentinel flaps has shown that there exists a strong correlation in rejection grades between the facial allograft and sentinel flaps. Noninvasive monitoring of rejection is an ongoing area of study by several laboratories. Most of these research endeavors have focused on the use of high resolution ultrasound and photography to detect rejection.[18] It is the goal that some of these innovations may be used in the near future.

ACUTE COMPLICATIONS

Acute Rejection

All face transplantation recipients have experienced some form of acute rejection (Fig. 3.17.4). Acute rejection episodes are typically easily managed with steroids and maintenance therapy modifications (e.g. increased MMF or FK506 trough levels), however steroid-resistant rejection episodes may occur and these may require further interventions such as plasmapheresis or immunosuppression medication changes (e.g. transition from tacrolimus to sirolimus). The use of other immuno-modulating agents such as monoclonal antibodies is currently an area of study in VCA laboratories.

Infections

Infection control is extremely important in the setting of immunosuppression. In fact, infections can be life-threatening if severe. Immunosuppressed patients are both susceptible to bacterial and viral infections. Early postoperative bacterial infections seem to be common after facial and hand transplantation. Therefore, appropriate bacterial prophylaxis is imperative. For example, all facial transplant recipients should be placed on trimethoprim-sulfamethoxazole (400 mg/day for 6 months) for prevention of *Pneumocystis carinii*. Furthermore, viral prophylaxis for cytomegalovirus (CMV) infection is needed. Experience with upper extremity transplantation suggests that CMV infection may be more common in VCA than in solid organ transplantation.[19] The senior

TABLE 3.17.3	2007 Banff VCA Working Classification for Skin Allograft Rejection	
Grade	**Inflammatory Infiltrate**	**Involvement of Epithelium**
0 (no rejection)	None/rare	None
I (mild rejection)	Mild perivascular	None
II (moderate rejection)	Moderate to severe perivascular	Mild (limited to spongiosis or lymphocytic exocytosis)
III (severe rejection)	Dense	Apoptosis, dyskeratosis, and/or keratinolysis
IV (acute necrotizing rejection)	Frank necrosis of the epidermis or its structures	–

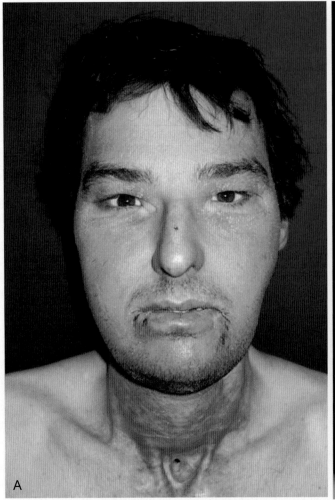
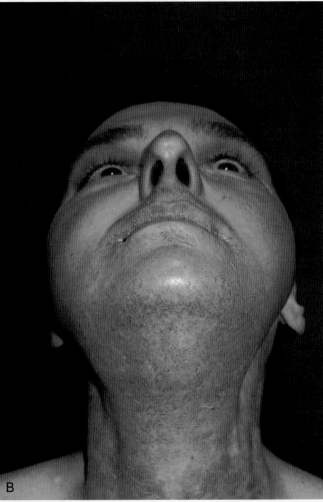

Fig. 3.17.4 Postoperative views showing facial allograft acute rejection. (Copyright Dr. Eduardo Rodriguez.)

authors recommend that all facial transplant recipients should be placed on valganciclovir (900 mg/day for 6 months) as prophylaxis.

LONG-TERM COMPLICATIONS

Revision Surgery

As with any reconstruction, secondary procedures are necessary to fully optimize reconstructive outcomes. The ultimate goal of facial allotransplantation is to restore facial function in the setting of an aesthetically balanced face. Due to the transfer of a large en-bloc segment from an individual with size discrepancies, the immediate posttransplantation result is often suboptimal. Furthermore, postoperative edema ensues immediately after surgery, causing contour irregularities that make the immediate postoperative result aesthetically unpleasing. Once facial edema resolves and scars have matured, the true outcome can be assessed. This typically occurs several months after facial allotransplantation and a careful exam is necessary at that time to fully evaluate the final aesthetic result. First, dental and skeletal relationships need to be evaluated to assess for malocclusion. Malocclusion can develop after facial allotransplantation due to initial allograft size discrepancies, poor preoperative planning, unstable skeletal movement/rotation, or over-manipulation of the temporomandibular joint position intraoperatively. Correction of postoperative malocclusion that has failed conservative management should be managed surgically to achieve optimal facial function. Most, if not all, facial allografts are based on anterior circulation, and traditional Le Fort I osteotomy may put the maxilla at risk for devascularization. Therefore, re-fracturing along the lines of maxillary/zygomatic osteosynthesis or mandibular osteotomy may be better choices in this setting. Maxillary advancement with Le Fort III osteotomy along the original lines of osteosynthesis was performed safely and successfully by one of the senior authors (E.D.R.) in the setting of class III malocclusion. Secondly, careful attention to facial suspensory ligaments must be performed to prevent significant soft tissue descent. Disruption of suspensory ligaments during transplantation can result in significant tissue descent over time and appropriate anchoring must be performed to prevent this risk either during transplantation or during subsequent secondary procedures. Lastly, careful attention to the distribution of soft tissue bulk along facial aesthetic subunits must be performed to optimize normal facial contours. Scar revisions, soft tissue re-suspension, debulking, and dental implants have all been safely performed as revisionary procedures by the senior authors, with no complications.[20]

Secondary procedures after facial allotransplantation are not benign. Although it is important to fully optimize both the functional and aesthetic result after transplantation, the desire to achieve optimal results must be weighed against the increased risk of revisionary surgery in an immunocompromised patient with poor wound healing and the propensity to contract infections. Furthermore, careful surgical planning is necessary with even the most minor of secondary procedures. Since the facial allograft is dependent on its vascular pedicles, incisions and secondary osteotomies must be carefully planned to reduce the risk of devascularization of the facial allograft.

Chronic Rejection

Chronic rejection has been extensively studied in solid organ transplantation and is defined as a low-grade injury to the vascular endothelium leading to irreversible allograft damage.[21] This "low-grade injury" results in what is defined as obliterative arteriopathy, and results from a chronic inflammatory response at the perivascular level of the allograft arteries. Per the latest reports, only a handful of facial transplant recipients have developed clinicopathological findings suggestive of chronic rejection.[22] Morelon et al. were the first to report clinically documented evidence of

chronic rejection in a face transplant recipient.[23] This case demonstrated that chronic rejection can proceed at the skin through the development of scleroderma-like features rather than graft vasculopathy. Unfortunately, this patient went on to develop partial loss of the facial allograft several years later.[24] Experimental evidence has shown that VCA allografts can indeed undergo classic perivascular chronic rejection features. Unadkat et al., utilizing a rat hindlimb transplant model, found that repeated episodes of acute rejection can cause perivascular changes consistent with chronic rejection.[25] Similarly, Mundinger et al., using a nonhuman primate facial allotransplantation model, found that numerous acute rejection events can lead to histological changes consistent with chronic rejection.[26] Although the molecular and cellular mechanisms behind the process of chronic rejection have not been fully elucidated, future basic science studies will explore this complex process more thoroughly. Additionally, prolonged survival of face allotransplantation recipients will inevitably provide more clinical evidence regarding the unknown risk factors associated with the development of chronic rejection in VCA.

EXPERT COMMENTARY

This is the first book on facial injuries to include a chapter on facial transplantation, by two members of the team that did the most extensive transplant to date at that time at the University of Maryland in 2012, and the team that popularized the principle of skeletal + soft tissue transplantation, a principle which, in retrospect, seems axiomatic, but which was proved by this remarkable case. In terms of how much to transplant, it stands to reason that the bone has to "fit" the soft tissue, and how can this occur with the mismatched parts from different individuals or with partial (only the soft tissue) transfers?

The long-term risks and success of these heroic transplantations are still to be chronicled, and it would be wise to realize that the previously unwanted patient – the self-inflicted shotgun wound to the face – has now become the most desired transplant candidate. Too often these patients are also the victims of the medical and surgical care provided, where late and inadequate treatment fix forever the results of deformity and make transplantation the only reasonable salvage. Today, transplantation attractiveness to surgeons causes little comprehensive treatment to be given to these patients, and a rapid progression to transplantation is accepted, perhaps compromising their long term health from immunosuppression. I have found almost all of these patients to be quite stable after the event *if* their reconstruction is reasonable, in contrast to some of the literature, the exception being those with advanced cancer or terminal neurological illness who will again repeat (understandably) the suicide process.

That being said, those suffering the loss of the central midface, the soft tissue and the lips and/or extensive third-degree burns, seem reasonable candidates for this heroic operation, and certainly the talented teams organized by Rodriguez et al. have achieved dramatic results in this pioneering surgery, and we are in awe of their expertise and inspiring progress.

I personally look forward to the next chapter of this work, which is partial facial transplantation in those with more limited but functionally significant and unfixable central defects.

REFERENCES

1. Khalifian S, Brazio PS, Mohan R, et al. Facial transplantation: the first 9 years. *Lancet.* 2014;384(9960):2153–2163.
2. Sosin M, Rodriguez ED. The face transplantation update: 2016. *Plast Reconstr Surg.* 2016;137(6):1841–1850.
3. Christensen J, Sawatari Y, Peleg M. High-energy traumatic maxillofacial injury. *J Craniofac Surg.* 2015;26(5):1487–1491.
4. Meningaud JP, Hivelin M, Benjoar MD, et al. The procurement of allotransplants for ballistic trauma: a preclinical study and a report of two clinical cases. *Plast Reconstr Surg.* 2011;127(5):1892–1900.

5. Siemionow MZ, Zor F, Gordon CR. Face, upper extremity, and concomitant transplantation: potential concerns and challenges ahead. *Plast Reconstr Surg.* 2010;126(1):308–315.

6. Wo L, Bueno E, Pomahac B. Facial transplantation: worth the risks? A look at evolution of indications over the last decade. *Curr Opin Organ Transplant.* 2015;20(6):615–620.

7. Mohan R, Borsuk DE, Dorafshar AH, et al. Aesthetic and functional facial transplantation: a classification system and treatment algorithm. *Plast Reconstr Surg.* 2014;133(2):386–397.

8. Dorafshar AH, Bojovic B, Christy MR, et al. Total face, double jaw, and tongue transplantation: an evolutionary concept. *Plast Reconstr Surg.* 2013;131(2):241–251.

9. Dorafshar AH, Brazio PS, Mundinger GS, et al. Found in space: computer-assisted orthognathic alignment of a total face allograft in six degrees of freedom. *J Oral Maxillofac Surg.* 2014;72(9):1788–1800.

10. Sosin M, Mundinger GS, Dorafshar AH, et al. Eyelid transplantation: lessons from a total face transplant and the importance of blink. *Plast Reconstr Surg.* 2015;135(1):167e–175e.

11. Frautschi R, Rampazzo A, Bernard S, et al. Management of the salivary glands and facial nerve in face transplantation. *Plast Reconstr Surg.* 2016;137(6):1887–1897.

12. Kueckelhaus M, Fischer S, Seyda M, et al. Vascularized composite allotransplantation: current standards and novel approaches to prevent acute rejection and chronic allograft deterioration. *Transpl Int.* 2016;29(6):655–662.

13. Schneeberger S, Khalifian S, Brandacher G. Immunosuppression and monitoring of rejection in hand transplantation. *Tech Hand Up Extrem Surg.* 2013;17(4):208–214.

14. Schultz BD, Woodall JD, Brazio PS, et al. Early microchimerism after face transplantation detected by quantitative real-time polymerase chain reaction of insertion/deletion polymorphisms. *Transplantation.* 2015;99(7):e44–e45.

15. Lee WP, Yaremchuk MJ, Pan YC, et al. Relative antigenicity of components of a vascularized limb allograft. *Plast Reconstr Surg.* 1991;87(3):401–411.

16. Cendales LC, Kanitakis J, Schneeberger S, et al. The Banff 2007 working classification of skin-containing composite tissue allograft pathology. *Am J Transplant.* 2008;8(7):1396–1400.

17. Kueckelhaus M, Fischer S, Lian CG, et al. Utility of sentinel flaps in assessing facial allograft rejection. *Plast Reconstr Surg.* 2015;135(1):250–258.

18. Kueckelhaus M, Imanzadeh A, Fischer S, et al. Noninvasive monitoring of immune rejection in face transplant recipients. *Plast Reconstr Surg.* 2015;136(5):1082–1089.

19. Avery RK. Update on infections in composite tissue allotransplantation. *Curr Opin Organ Transplant.* 2013;18(6):659–664.

20. Mohan R, Fisher M, Dorafshar A, et al. Principles of face transplant revision: beyond primary repair. *Plast Reconstr Surg.* 2014;134(6):1295–1304.

21. Yates PJ, Nicholson ML. The aetiology and pathogenesis of chronic allograft nephropathy. *Transpl Immunol.* 2006;16(3–4):148–157.

22. Kanitakis J, Petruzzo P, Badet L, et al. Chronic rejection in human vascularized composite allotransplantation (hand and face recipients): an update. *Transplantation.* 2016;100(10):2053–2061.

23. Petruzzo P, Kanitakis J, Testelin S, et al. Clinicopathological findings of chronic rejection in a face grafted patient. *Transplantation.* 2015;99(12):2644–2650.

24. Morelon E, Petruzzo P, Kanitakis J, et al. Face transplantation: partial graft loss of the first case 10 years later. *Am J Transplant.* 2017;17(7):1935–1940.

25. Unadkat JV, Schneeberger S, Horibe EH, et al. Composite tissue vasculopathy and degeneration following multiple episodes of acute rejection in reconstructive transplantation. *Am J Transplant.* 2010;10(2):251–261.

26. Mundinger GS, Munivenkatappa R, Drachenberg CB, et al. Histopathology of chronic rejection in a nonhuman primate model of vascularized composite allotransplantation. *Transplantation.* 2013;95(10):1204–1210.

Page numbers followed by "*f*" indicate figures, "*t*" indicate tables, and "*b*" indicate boxes.